Nutrition:
An Integrated Approach

Nutrition:
An Integrated Approach
Approach
Second Edition

RUTH L. PIKE
The Pennsylvania State University

MYRTLE L. BROWN
National Academy of Sciences-
National Research Council.

John Wiley & Sons, Inc. New York • London • Sydney • Toronto

Library of Congress Cataloging in Publication Data:

Pike, Ruth L
Nutrition, an integrated approach.

Bibliography: p.
Includes index.
1. Nutrition.   I. Brown, Myrtle Laurestine,
1926-   joint author.   II. Title.
DNLM: 1. Nutrition.   QU145 P636n

QP141.P53 1975   612′.3   75-1488
ISBN 0-471-68977-7

preface

What started out to be a revision has become almost a completely rewritten book. In addition to bringing the subject matter in this rapidly changing field up to date, we have reorganized it and presented it in a more logical fashion.

The book is now divided into five parts. Part I, "The Nutrients," is essentially the same as it was in the previous edition but it has been expanded. Part II, "Physiological Aspects of Nutrition," includes a new chapter on digestion and an enlarged section on absorption. Another new chapter is devoted to exchange and transport as well as mechanisms of homeostatic control. Since the nutrients must go through the intestinal mucosa and be transported to the cells to participate in metabolism, it seemed logical to place this material before the section on the cell. Part III, "The Cell," presents the basic biochemical cytology that is important to the nutritionist. As in the first edition, the nutrients are brought to the organelles within the cell, the locus of physiological and biochemical action. Where possible, basic reactions in cellular metabolism are discussed in terms of the complex multicellular organism. Each of these chapters has been rewritten and expanded. Two new chapters have been added: an introductory one on the methods used in studying cellular structure and mechanisms, and a chapter of the Golgi apparatus. Part IV, "Specialized Cells," is a new section that replaces the single chapter in the previous edition. The cells discussed are the ones that we think are of special interest to the nutritionist. Parts III and IV may contain more detail than some nutritionists believe is essential; others, however, will agree that the nutritionist must understand cell structure to understand how the nutrients participate as part of the dynamic complex of the cell. Part V, "The Complex Organism," includes a new chapter presenting the fundamental concepts underlying growth and development. Two chapters in the previous edition have been omitted. "Nutrients in Foods" was primarily a discussion of methodology; this material now has been incorporated into other parts of the book. Instead of the chapter on "Interrelationships of Nutrients," we have shown the interrelationships throughout the book because, indeed, they are interrelated in metabolism.

Our purpose is the same: to integrate the contributions of related scientific disciplines with the study of nutrition; to foster a questioning attitude; and to emphasize the depth and limitations of present knowledge.

We thank Dr. Helen G. Oldham for counsel and help in the preparation of the manuscript; Dr. Marian E. Swendseid for carefully reading the manuscript and making suggestions; and Dr. Lawrence M. Marshall for critically reading portions of the material.

Again we are indebted to Dr. Harald Schraer, who prepared many of the electron micrographs for our use.

If there are errors in the text, we assume full responsibility for them.

Ruth L. Pike
Myrtle L. Brown

contents

part one   The Nutrients   1

1.   Historical Perspective   3
2.   Carbohydrates, Lipids, Proteins, Nucleotides,
     and Nucleic Acids   18
3.   Water-Soluble Vitamins   80
4.   Fat-Soluble and Other Vitamins   140
5.   Minerals and Water   180

part two   Physiological Aspects of Nutrition   211

6.   Digestion and Absorption   213
7.   Nutrient Exchange and Homeostatic Control   302

part three The Cell   335

8.   Orientation to Cellular Nutrition   336
9.   The Plasma Membrane   351
10. The Nucleus   391
11. The Cytoplasmic Matrix and Endoplasmic
     Reticulum   423
12. The Golgi Apparatus   471
13. The Mitochondria   490
14. The Lysosomes and Microbodies   532

part four   Specialized Cells   565

     15.   Hepatocytes   569
     16.   Erythrocytes   594
     17.   Bone Cells   616
     18.   Muscle Cells   646
     19.   Nerve Cells   667
     20.   Adipose Cells   708

part five   The Complex Organism   727

     21.   Cellular Growth   729
     22.   Body Composition   757
     23.   Determination of Nutrient Needs: Energy,
          Protein, Minerals   814
     24.   Determination of Nutrient Needs: Vitamins   874
     25.   Dietary Standards   895
     26.   Nutrition Surveys   933

Bibliography   957

Index   1057

Nutrition:
An Integrated Approach

part one

the nutrients

Chapter 1   Historical Perspective
Chapter 2   Carbohydrates, Lipids, Proteins, Nucleotides, and
             Nucleic Acids
Chapter 3   Water-Soluble Vitamins
Chapter 4   Fat-Soluble and Other Vitamins
Chapter 5   Minerals and Water

The material in the following four chapters should be familiar to the student, but since it is fundamental to the integrated study that follows and since memories sometimes falter, it is included either for surreptitious reading or careful study, whatever the need may be.

Nutrition is the science that interprets the relationship of food to the functioning of the living organism. It includes the intake of food, liberation of energy, elimination of wastes, and all the syntheses that are essential for maintenance, growth, and reproduction. These fundamental activities are characteristic of all living organisms from the simplest to the most complex plants and animals.

1

Nutrition is a relatively new science that evolved from chemistry and physiology just as biophysics has more recently evolved from biology and physics. Recognition of nutrition as an independent field of study came only after the beginning of this century following a developmental period that stemmed from the experiments of Antoine Lavoisier almost 200 years earlier. Lavoisier's work formed the basis for the studies on respiratory exchange and calorimetry, the beginnings of scientific nutrition. Almost 100 years elapsed before carbohydrates, fats, and proteins were identified as the sources of energy for the animal body. By the end of the nineteenth century the significance of protein as a source of nitrogen and the necessity for certain minerals in the diet were established. During the early part of this century conclusive evidence was obtained indicating that proteins varied in their ability to support growth and maintenance. Furthermore it was established that purified diets containing only the major foodstuffs (including suitable protein sources) and minerals were inadequate to maintain life. It was therefore obvious that natural foods carried other substances yet to be identified.

Investigations with laboratory animals led to the crude separation of fat-soluble and water-soluble fractions from foods that contained the essential factors, but it was not until the 1930s that the majority of the vitamins were identified, isolated from foods, and synthesized in the laboratory. The development of methods for synthesizing the vitamins was a crucial step in the future of nutritional research. It then became possible to develop a completely synthetic diet that could support the life of laboratory animals, and research could be directed toward elucidating the functional roles of individual nutrients.

However crude the early work appears from the vantage point of current methodology and instrumentation, much of it was sophisticated, elegant in design, and carefully executed; this work provided the basic information that is the core of the science of nutrition.

chapter 1
historical perspective

1. Ancient and Medieval Ideas
2. The Phlogiston Theory of Combustion
3. Studies on Respiration: Development of Calorimetry
4. Later Calorimetric Studies
5. Studies on the Physiology of Digestion
6. Nutrition in Early Twentieth-Century America
7. Recognition of Mineral Requirements
8. Development of the Vitamin Theory
9. Significance of Protein Source: Identification of the Essential Amino Acids
10. Conclusion

"What little we know, what little power we possess, we owe to the accumulated endeavors of our ancestors. Mere gratefulness would already oblige us to study the history of the endeavors, our most precious heirlooms. But we are not to remain idle spectators. It is not enough to appreciate and admire what our ancestors did, we must take up their best traditions, and that implies expert knowledge and craftsmanship, science and practice."

George Sarton, *The History of Science and the New Humanism*, 1956

ANCIENT AND MEDIEVAL IDEAS

Before the eighteenth century little of a truly scientific nature was accomplished in the development of nutrition or, in fact, of any science. The ancient Greek philosophers apparently were interested in science, but logical reasoning, rather than experimentation, was the Greek way.

Hippocrates (460-364 B.C.) wrote the following passage that is accurate in essence although somewhat imprecise in detail.

"Growing bodies have the most innate heat; they therefore require the most food, for otherwise their bodies are wasted. In old persons, the heat is feeble and therefore they require little fuel as it were to the flame, for it would be extinguished by much..."

For nearly 1500 years after Hippocrates' time, little was accomplished in the development of science. The alchemists of the Middle Ages were devoted to the task of transforming common metals into gold, and medical knowledge had advanced little beyond the knowledge possessed by the ancient civilizations. It was not until the sixteenth century that the intellectual climate again became conducive to scientific development; interest revived in the relation of man to his environment and particularly to the air surrounding him. It was in the seventeenth century that van Helmont (1577-1644), a Belgian nobleman, discovered the lethal effect of carbon dioxide. In the same period, Sanctorious (1561-1636) published the results of experiments on himself clearly indicating that a major pathway of excretion from the human body was the "insensible perspiration," a loss of body weight not accountable by measurements of urine and feces and thus presumed to be expelled into the surrounding air. The sketch of Sanctorius sitting in his chair-scale has escaped few students of nutrition.

THE PHLOGISTON THEORY OF COMBUSTION

A major contribution to scientific thought at the beginning of the eighteenth century, unfortunately, was a misconception, the phlogiston theory of combustion that was promoted by Stahl (1660-1734), a German chemist. Although the theory was accepted by a majority of scientists of the period, it was based apparently on no more than a lively flight of imagination. Stahl maintained that all combustible materials contained phlogiston, which passed from them into the atmosphere when the substances were burned. The phlogiston theory, along with the generally held misconception that air was an elemental substance, profoundly influenced scientific thinking and interpretation of new discoveries for almost a century. Consequently, Black (1728-1799) termed carbon dioxide "fixed air"; Cavendish (1731-1810) called hydrogen "inflammable air" and believed it to be phlogiston. Rutherford's (1749-1810) "residual air" was what we now know as nitrogen. Two independent discoverers of oxygen, Priestley (1733-1804) and Scheele (1742-1786), used the terms "dephlogisticated air" and "fire air."

It was in a scientific climate dominated by misconception that Lavoisier began his experiments on combustion that led to studies on animal respiration and paved the way for the development of modern calorimetry.

STUDIES OF RESPIRATION: DEVELOPMENT OF CALORIMETRY

The truly great scientist not only observes phenomena (which any-one can do) but has the genius to interpret his findings and the strength to bear the consequences of possible failure. As Szent-Györgyi (1957) stated:

"There is but one safe way to avoid mistakes; to do nothing, or, at least, to avoid doing something new...The unknown lends an insecure foothold and venturing out into it, one can hope for no more than that the possible failure will be a honorable one."

Antoine Lavoisier (1743-1794) was one of the first to repudiate Stahl's theory of phlogiston.[1] By repeating experiments previously performed by some of his contemporaries of the late eighteenth century, for example, heating mercury oxide with carbon, Lavoisier

---

[1]As the result of a long series of experiments, Lavoisier established the law of the conservation of mass, a concept later refined by Einstein. For this reason Lavoisier is known as the father of modern chemistry as well as the father of nutrition.

concluded that "fixed air" (carbon dioxide) was formed by the combination of carbon and "air eminently respirable" (oxygen). In his *Reflections upon Phlogiston* he stated, "All the phenomena of combustion and calcination are much more readily explained without phlogiston than with phlogiston." (See Lusk, 1928).

Thus without the impediment of the phlogiston theory, Lavoisier went on to apply his theory of combustion to the problem of the origin of animal heat. Experimenting with guinea pigs and later with his assistant, Seguin, as subjects, Lavoisier measured body heat loss, oxygen consumed, and carbon dioxide expired and concluded that respiration is a combustion process similar to what happens when substances are burned outside the body. Furthermore, he was able to show that heat production in the animal body is directly related to oxygen consumption.

"Respiration is only a slow combustion of carbon and hydrogen which is entirely similar to that which obtains in a lamp or lighted candle and from this point of view, animals which respire are truly combustible bodies which burn and consume themselves. In respiration as in combustion it is the air which furnishes the heat—if animals do not repair constantly the losses of respiration, the lamp soon lacks oil, and the animal dies, as a lamp goes out when it lacks food." (See Lusk, 1928).

Measurements taken in the fasting and resting state, as initially performed by Lavoisier, represent essentially the basal metabolism. In another series of experiments in which Seguin was the subject, Lavoisier showed that oxygen consumption and therefore heat production was increased above the basal state by a decrease in environmental temperature, ingestion of food, and by physical exercise. The following table indicates the relative increases in oxygen consumption under the conditions of his experiment.

There were some technical inaccuracies in Lavoisier's work and in his interpretation of the data. His figures for oxygen consumption were too high, and he erroneously believed that carbon dioxide and water were formed in the lungs. However, in spite of these errors, refinements in instrumentation and in scientific thought have added little to the general concepts derived from his experiments. The increase in oxygen consumption following ingestion of food was later described by Rubner (1854-1932) as the *specific dynamic*

Condition	Environmental Temperature	Liters Oxygen Absorbed per Hour
Without food	26	24
Without food	12	27
With food		38
Work (9.195 foot pounds— without food)		65
Work (9.195 foot pounds— with food)		91

From G. Lusk, *The Elements of the Science of Nutrition.* 4th ed., W. B. Saunders Co., 1928, p. 19.

effect of food (Rubner, 1902). The effects of temperature and exercise on oxygen consumption and body heat production have been confirmed repeatedly and are basic tenets of modern calorimetry.

Lavoisier, however, did not recognize the nature of the foodstuffs and believed that elemental carbon and hydrogen were oxidized in the body. Francois Magendie (1783-1855), an early nineteenth century physiologist, was the first to distinguish between the different kinds of foodstuffs (carbohydrate, fat, and protein). Even so, this information was not applied to studies of respiratory exchange for many years. Regnault (1810-1878), however, showed that the ratio of carbon dioxide to oxygen consumed varied with kind of food (Regnault and Reiset, 1849). This ratio is now called the *respiratory quotient* (RQ).

LATER CALORIMETRIC STUDIES

Liebig (1803-1873), of the nineteenth century German school, apparently recognized that proteins, carbohydrates, and fats were oxidized in the body, and he then calculated energy values for some foodstuffs. He proposed that since only proteins contain nitrogen, the nitrogen of the urine must arise from protein in the body (Liebig, 1842). He erroneously believed that muscular work caused the metabolism of protein and that oxygen caused the destruction of carbohydrate and fat.

The first report of a balance-type experiment is credited to

Boussingault (1802-1887), a Frenchman and contemporary of Liebig. He measured carbon, hydrogen, oxygen, nitrogen, and salts of a cow's food and excreta. During the same period in Germany, Bidder (1810-1894) and Schmidt (1822-1894) performed a similar experiment but also related their balance data to the animal's respiratory exchange, a closer approximation to modern calorimetric method (Bidder and Schmidt, 1852). In their writings, they described a *typical minimum* of necessary metabolism which is apparent in experiments when no food is given. This typical minimum is now referred to as the *resting metabolism*.

Voit (1831-1908) was a particularly gifted student of Leibig and was distinguished not only by his own work but also by that of his students: Rubner (1854-1932), Atwater (1844-1907), Lusk (1866-1932), and many others. In the late nineteenth century the laboratory at Munich was the center for calorimetric studies; researchers from many countries went there to learn the most advanced techniques. From a series of calorimetric and balance experiments, Voit was able to disprove two theories proposed by his former professor, Liebig. He demonstrated first that protein metabolism is *not* affected by muscular work and second that oxygen consumption is not the cause of metabolism but, instead, that oxygen consumption is the result of cellular metabolism (Voit, 1881). Voit said, in what appears to be advanced thinking for his day:

"The life of the body is the sum of the action of all the thousands of minute workshops. A combination with oxygen is not first necessary, but there is a breaking up into various constituents which, under certain circumstances may remain unoxidized...What the eye of the layman regards as rest is in reality an interminable movement to and from of the finest cellular particles, the most complicated of all processes."

Obviously Voit suspected that even the apparently inert constituents of body tissues existed in a dynamic state (proved many years later by Schoenheimer, 1942) and, furthermore, that the balance experiments that scientists then performed were but a first step in unraveling the mysteries of cellular metabolism.

Rubner was one of Voit's most outstanding students. While still an assistant in Voit's laboratory, he determined caloric values of urine and feces under varying conditions of dietary intake; these figures formed the basis for later calorimetric work. Rubner proved conclusively that for the resting animal, heat production is equivalent to heat elimination, thus confirming that the law of conservation of energy (proposed in 1845 by Mayer (1814-1878) and in 1847 by Helmholz (1821-1894) and implied in Lavoisier's experiments) was applicable to the living organism as well as to inanimate matter. Furthermore, Rubner related heat production in the basal state to surface area, which also had been implied by experiments conducted previously by Regnault in France. The caloric values for different kinds of foodstuffs were determined by Rubner, and average values were calculated for carbohydrates, proteins, and fats. Rubner's computed caloric values are very nearly the same as those now used in dietary calculations.

STUDIES ON THE PHYSIOLOGY OF DIGESTION

At the same time that chemists were delving into the composition of foods and the mysteries of metabolism, physiologists were attempting to elucidate the mechanisms involved in digestion, the means by which food becomes available to the body for oxidation.

Some of the first experimental work on the digestive process was done by Reaumur in 1752. When he administered perforated metallic tubes containing food to birds that normally regurgitate indigestible residues remaining at the completion of digestion, he found that the regurgitated tubes were empty. This was obvious proof that something had occurred in the stomach other than grinding or crushing. A fascinating review of his and other early experiments is presented by Rose (1959) in an essay introducing a facsimile reprint of a dissertation presented to the University of Pennsylvania by John R. Young (1782-1804) entitled *An Experimental Inquiry into the Principles of Nutrition and the Digestive Process* (Young, 1803).

In the following century and a half, the physiological and biochemical aspects of the digestive process were studied and fairly well clarified through the work of many investigators and the dedication of several subjects with fistulas. First came the published work of Beaumont (1785-1853) in 1833 reporting observations on his patient, Alexis St. Martin, who had the misfortune of receiving a gunshot wound that, after healing, left him with an opening, or fistula, directly into the stomach. Beaumont not only treated but immortalized his patient by using him as the subject for a series of studies on digestive processes. By introducing specific foods into the stomach through the fistula (always with a string attached), Beaumont was able to ascertain the relative rates of digestion for different kinds of foodstuffs. He also described gastric juice and identified the acid as hydrochloric. He noted the movements of the stomach and was probably the first to report the effects of the emotions on gastric motility and secretion. This work suggested to Claude Bernard (1813-1878) the use of artificial fistulas in laboratory animals for the study of gastrointestinal function.

At the beginning of this century, W. B. Cannon (1871-1945) at Harvard University did much definitive work on motility and secretion of the gastrointestinal tract and trained a generation of physiologists. Through happenstance, other investigators and subjects with fistulas teamed together: Fred, at the University of Chicago, served as laboratory worker and experimental subject for Carlson, Luckhardt, and their associates who did much to advance the work started by Cannon; and Tom, at Cornell University Medical School, who had a long association with Wolf and Wolff as helper and subject in the laboratory and was the true subject of their now-classic volume, *Human Gastric Function* (1947) and its sequel, *The Stomach* (Wolf, 1965).

NUTRITION IN EARLY TWENTIETH CENTURY AMERICA

Up until the late nineteenth century most of the outstanding laboratories for physiological research were in the great European universities. Americans who wished to work with the leaders in these areas were obliged to go to the centers abroad to further their studies. Atwater (1844-1907) was among the first to make an outstanding contribution to the development of nutritional science in this country. After spending a year in Voit's laboratory he returned in 1888 to become chief of the newly organized Office of Experiment Stations of the U.S. Department of Agriculture. With the physicist, Rosa, he was responsible for the construction of the first calorimeter, which could be used for studying the energy exchange of man. Atwater and Bryant (1899), also of the Department of Agriculture, published a compilation of the composition of a large number of foods and forerunner of the classic tables of food composition now known as *Handbook 8* (Watt and Merrill, 1963).

Lusk, who also studied with Voit and Rubner at Munich, upon returning to this country began work on intermediary metabolism and on the specific dynamic effect of foods. He built a small calorimeter at the Cornell Medical College for use with small animals and babies and was instrumental in promoting the construction of a calorimeter at Bellevue Hospital in New York. Lusk's book, *The Science of Nutrition,* which went through four editions between 1906 and 1928, is a classic work and should be familiar to every serious student of nutrition.

A second large calorimeter was built in this country by Armsby (1853-1921) at The Pennsylvania State University. It was originally used for the study of energy exchange of large farm animals. Later this calorimeter was used for studies with human subjects (Swift et al., 1957). The calorimeter still remains in perfect working condition, and the building housing it has become the Armsby Museum (Fig. 1.1).

At the beginning of the twentieth century considerable work had been done on energy exchange and on the nature of the major foodstuffs. The proximate composition (carbohydrate, fat, protein, fiber, water, and ash) and the energy value of a large number of foods was known. Nutritional science was coming of age, however, as evidenced by the *Laws of Nutrition,* summarized by C. F. Langworthy (1864-1932), an associate of Atwater in the U. S. Department of Agriculture (Langworthy, 1897-1898).

Laws of Nutrition

1. All nitrogen is supplied by food, that is, none from atmosphere.

2. All nitrogen is excreted in urine and feces, none as gaseous nitrogen.

3. The animal adjusts itself to its nitrogen intake and comes into N-balance, in which state the intake and output are equal.

4. A certain amount of food material, that is, protein, fat, and carbohydrate, is required for maintenance. Mineral is also

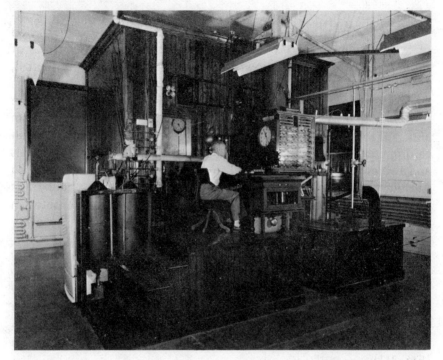

Fig. 1.1 The Armsby respiration calorimeter at The Pennsylvania State University. Seated at the controls is Dr. Raymond W. Swift.

essential, but very little is known regarding the kind and amount necessary.

5. A more abundant ration is required for muscular work, fattening, and milk production.

6. Food supplied in excess of all needs is stored, in part at least, as reserve material, principally as fat and glycogen.

7. The body comes into nitrogen equilibrium at different levels of protein intake.

8. Body fat may be formed from food fat (precipitated as such), or from carbohydrate, and doubtless from protein also.

9. As furnishers of energy the different nutrients may replace each other in approximately the following ratios: protein: fat: carbohydrates as 1: 2.5: 1. That is, having the requisite amount of nitrogen for repair or some vital process not understood, or both, it is, theoretically and within certain limits, unimportant which nutrient supplies the necessary energy.

10. The nutrients of the food combine within the body with oxygen of the air and undergo combustion, thus liberating energy for the body.

No argument can be raised against Langworthy's laws. Fundamentally, they are as valid today as when he stated them. The vitamins remained to be discovered and it was within the next 10 years that these essential food factors also were recognized.

RECOGNITION OF MINERAL REQUIREMENTS

Knowledge of mineral needs grew as data accumulated on the composition of body tissues and fluids. The mineral structure of bone and teeth was recognized by early workers although the element calcium was not discovered until 1808. In the latter part of the nineteenth century, however, the necessity for small amounts of calcium for blood coagulation had been demonstrated by the addition of calcium precipitants, such as oxalate and citrate, to blood.

The iron content of blood and various tissues was known well before the beginning of this century. Boussingault (1802-1887), for example, published data on the iron content of animals and believed iron to be an essential nutrient. Liebig suggested that oxygen was carried in blood by iron in the corpuscles. From Grecian times iron compounds had been used therapeutically, but the significance of the element in the treatment of anemia was not discovered until about 1840. Even with this knowledge available, however, the necessity of iron as a dietary constituent appears generally to have been ignored.

Liebig was aware of the differences in the distribution of sodium and potassium in the animal, and Boussingault had observed the deleterious effects of salt-free diets on animals. It was the observation that dogs deprived of sodium chloride died earlier than animals given no food, however, that lead to the conclusion that certain mineral constituents of animal tissues are essential to life and consequently must be necessary in the diet (Forster, 1873).

The significance of electrolyte concentrations in body fluids received most attention from the work of Ringer (1835-1910). Ringer (1895) found that solutions containing a combination of the chlorides of sodium, potassium, and calcium were satisfactory in maintaining the functional integrity of isolated animal tissues. Individually any one of these compounds was detrimental to isolated muscle activity, but the antagonistic effect could be removed by addition of the other salts (Locke, 1895). Early in this century Loeb (1859-1924) continued the work on salt antagonism and observed the effect of various concentrations of salts on living tissues. No combination tested was more favorable than the equivalent of the concentrations found in blood. Thus it was firmly established that the presence of certain salts in living tissues was not the result of incidental contamination, but that mineral elements were, indeed, nutrients essential to animal functioning and therefore they must be supplied in the diet.

The general belief at the beginning of the twentieth century was that sodium chloride, calcium, phosphorus, and probably iron were the minerals significant in animal nutrition. Little attention was given to other elements known to be present in tissues in relatively small amounts. The importance of the trace elements in animal nutrition was accepted more readily following the discovery of other essential micronutrients: the vitamins.

DEVELOPMENT OF THE VITAMIN THEORY

Recognition of the existence of organic compounds present in minute amounts in foods came less than 15 years after the beginning of this century. Dietary deficiency diseases, however, had been known for many years. Lind's (1716-1794) famous *Treatise on Scurvy* (Lind, 1753) was published just 10 years after the birth of Lavoisier. A syndrome described as beriberi, which could be prevented by dietary means, was reported to occur among Japanese sailors (Takaki, 1887). Three years later in the Dutch East Indies Eijkman (1858-1930) produced beriberi in birds (see Janson, 1956). Holst (1860-1931), working in Sweden, produced scurvy in guinea pigs and was able to cure the disease by feeding fresh fruits and cabbage (Holst and Frölich, 1907). Except for the realization that the diseases were of dietary origin, however, none of these investigators was aware that specific nutrients were involved in their etiology.

Near the end of the nineteenth century chemical methodology had progressed considerably so that relatively purified foodstuffs could be isolated from foods. Purified foodstuffs provided the tool needed for studying the physiological effects of various combinations of the nutrients then believed to be essential and thus for determining the function of individual foodstuffs in biological systems. Animal feeding experiments, however, produced unexpected results.

One of the first recorded studies was that of Lunin (1853-1937), who found that mice fed a purified diet simulating milk died within one month, but others fed fluid milk survived and were healthy for twice as long (Lunin, 1880). Purified diets supplemented with small doses of whey were found to be as effective as milk in experiments conducted by Pekelharing (1848-1922). He concluded that the active substance was not one of the major foodstuffs and, moreover, stated,

"If this substance is absent, the organism loses its power properly to assimilate the well-known principal parts of food, the appetite is lost and with apparent abundance the animals die of want." (See van Leersum, 1926.)

Frederick G. Hopkins (1861-1947) in England performed similar experiments with purified diets and independently reached a similar conclusion. However, Hopkins also clearly recognized the relationship between the *accessory food factors* (vitamins) and the dietary deficiency syndromes that had been observed for centuries (Hopkins, 1912). The theory that certain disease syndromes were the result of a dietary lack of specific substances present in foods was proposed also by Casimir Funk (1884-1967) in his classical paper, "The Etiology of the Deficiency Diseases" (Funk, 1912), which reviews much of the early history of beriberi and scurvy. Funk's outstanding contribution was to propose a name for the unknown accessory food factors. He chose *vitamines*, inspired by the knowledge that the factors were essential for life (vita) and that the antiberiberi factor that he was attempting to isolate was an amine. Vitamine thus was a misnomer and was modified to *vitamin* at the suggestion of Sir Jack Drummond (1891-1952) who proposed at the same time the alphabetical nomenclature for the vitamins (Drummond, 1920). Acceptance of the vitamin theory was not immediate in all circles of thought (new ideas rarely are!), but with the discovery of vitamin A by McCollum (1879-1967), the vitamin era in nutrition investigations was securely launched (McCollum and Davis, 1913).

Details of the discovery, isolation, and synthesis of each of the vitamins are too voluminous to record at this point and will be discussed in the chapter on the vitamins. The furor created by the discovery of the minute factors in food reached a peak between 1930 and 1940. The literature of this period is crowded with new discoveries, wrong turns, and rediscoveries. In the excitement attending the discovery of the vitamins, many nutritionists tended toward overenthusiasm rather than the restraint more typical of new ideas. This overenthusiasm probably helped to encourage the development of the multimillion dollar vitamin business now supported by our population with money that could best be spent at the local food market.

SIGNIFICANCE OF PROTEIN SOURCE: IDENTIFICATION OF THE ESSENTIAL AMINO ACIDS

At about the same time that the existence of minute quantities of accessory food factors was emerging, evidence also began to accumulate suggesting that dietary proteins varied widely in their ability to support growth and life in laboratory animals. The essential nature of protein as a source of nitrogen had been suggested by the work of Magendie (1816) and later was confirmed by Mulder (1802-1880), who coined the term protein from the Greek word *proteus,* which roughly may be translated as "first." It was clearly recognized then that protein was necessary for life in a more fundamental way than could be attributed to either carbohydrate or fat. Liebig also recognized the nitrogen-containing components of food as necessary for tissue building and suggested that urinary nitrogen could serve as a measure of protein destruction in the body (Liebig, 1842). Later, Voit established the principle of nitrogen equilibrium (Bischoff and Voit, 1860). This method remains as the most widely used criterion for evaluating protein metabolism and requirements.

By 1900, 16 different amino acids had been isolated from hydrolysates of various biological materials (see McCollum, 1957), but the nature of protein composition was poorly understood. Mulder (1839; 1848) had proposed that only one protein was present in any one food although the proteins differed among different foods; this view was accepted by Liebig. It was not until the beginning of this century that T. B. Osborne (1859-1929) in work begun in the 1890s with R. H. Chittenden (1856-1943) at Yale was able to demonstrate conclusively that foods (and thus other biological materials) contained not one, but a mixture of several different proteins (see Osborne, 1924). The availability of the isolated proteins enabled Osborne in the classic animal feeding experiments performed with L. B. Mendel (1872-1935), also at Yale, to demonstrate differences in the capability of individual proteins to promote growth and to maintain life (Osborne and Mendel, 1911). This work, along with the studies of Hopkins on the essential nature of tryptophan, provided the framework for the basic understanding of proteins and amino acids in nutrition (Willcock and Hopkins, 1906-1907). This work was carried further by W. C. Rose (born 1887), a former student of Mendel at Yale, and culminated in the identification and isolation of the final essential amino acid, threonine. For the first time it was demonstrated by Rose and his associates at the University of Illinois that rats could be reared to maximum growth on mixtures of purified amino acids (McCoy et al., 1935-1936). The isolation of the essential amino acids made possible the later studies on amino acid requirements of experimental animals and humans and provided the fundamental information necessary for exploring the intermediary metabolism of proteins.

CONCLUSIONS

It was the intention of this chapter to reveal the general development of nutrition as a field of scientific study. Much of significance has, of necessity, been omitted as, for example, the discovery of the essential fatty acids (Burr and Burr, 1929). These and other historical developments will be discussed in later chapters, but much still remains for the interested student to search out for himself.

chapter 2

carbohydrates, lipids, proteins, nucleotides, and nucleic acids

1. **Carbohydrates**
   a. Monosaccharides; Monosaccharide Derivatives
   b. Oligosaccharides
   c. Polysaccharides
   d. Mucopolysaccharides
2. **Lipids**
   a. Fatty Acids
   b. Prostaglandins
   c. Acyl Glycerols
   d. Phospholipids
   e. Sphingolipids
   f. Steroids and Sterols
   g. Fat Consumption Patterns and Ischemic Heart Disease

3. **Proteins**
   a. Amino Acids; Functions of Amino Acids
   b. Protein Structure; Spatial Arrangement of the Protein Molecule
   c. Protein Classification
   d. Protein and Amino Acid Deficiency
4. **Complexes of Carbohydrates, Proteins, and Lipids**
   a. Glycoproteins
   b. Glycolipids
   c. Lipoproteins
5. **Nucleotides and Nucleic Acids**
   a. Nucleotides: ATP and cAMP
   b. Nucleic Acids: DNA and RNA

"I, too, dislike it: there are things that are important beyond all
  this fiddle.
Reading it however with a perfect contempt for it, one discovers in
it after all, a place for the genuine.
  Hands that can grasp, eyes
  that can dilate, hair that can rise
    if it must, these things are important not because a
high-sounding interpretation can be put upon them but because
    they are
  useful..."

Marianne Moore, *Poetry*

CARBOHYDRATES

Carbohydrates are defined as polyhydroxy aldehydes and ketones and their derivatives and vary from simple three-carbon sugars to complex polymers. Most carbohydrates conform to the general formula $(CH_2O)_n$, but the classification of carbohydrates includes compounds that are not true hydrates as the name implies. For example, deoxyribose contains 5 carbon atoms, 10 hydrogens, but only 4 oxygens rather than 5 as is customary for a pentose. Moreover, some compounds that are properly classified as carbohydrates in terms of chemical properties contain nitrogen or sulfur in addition to carbon, hydrogen, and oxygen.

Carbohydrates are classified into three main groups: monosaccharides, or simple sugars; oligosaccharides, of which the most prevalent in nature are the disaccharides; and polysaccharides, the most complex of the carbohydrates. Many of the compounds to be discussed in this chapter are of biological importance. Only three, however, are significant as dietary sources of carbohydrate. Starch is by far the most important source of carbohydrate in the human diet amounting to approximately 50 percent of total carbohydrate in the American diet, but often as much as 75 percent of total carbohydrate in some of the developing countries. Sucrose ranks next in importance comprising about 25 percent of total carbohydrate intake. In the last 70 years the intake of complex carbohydrate in the diet of Americans has decreased, and the intake of sucrose has markedly increased (Friend, 1967). Lactose or milk sugar comprises approximately 10 percent of the total carbohydrate intake in the United States but, of course, is of little significance in nonmilk-drinking populations. For a comprehensive listing of the carbohydrates present in a large variety of foods see Hardinge et al. (1965).

Biologically the carbohydrates are a significant source of energy for cellular metabolism, but they also serve functional and structural roles in the animal body.

Monosaccharides

Monosaccharides are, as the name implies, the simplest of the carbohydrates. This classification includes a series of aldehydes (aldoses) and ketones (ketoses) grouped according to the number of carbon atoms in the chain: trioses, tetroses, pentoses, hexoses, and heptoses (Table 2.1). These sugars may be more definitively described according to structure and number of carbon atoms as aldotrioses, ketotrioses, and so on.

Table 2.1 MONOSACCHARIDES

Classification	Aldoses	Ketoses
Trioses ($C_3H_6O_3$)	Glyceraldehyde	Dihydroxyacetone
Tetroses ($C_4H_8O_4$)	Erythrose	Erythrulose
	Threose	
Pentoses ($C_5H_{10}O_5$)	Xylose	Xylulose
	Ribose	Ribulose
	Arabinose	
Hexoses ($C_6H_{12}O_6$)	Glucose (dextrose)	Fructose (levulose)
	Galactose	
	Mannose	Sorbose
Heptoses ($C_7H_{14}O_7$)		Sedoheptulose

With the possible exception of the hexoses, monosaccharides are of little dietary significance. Both glucose and fructose have long been known to occur in free form in certain fruits and in honey.

Recently small amounts of mannose have also been detected in a few fruits (see Herman, 1971). However, it appears at present that only the pentoses and hexoses play fundamental roles in cellular metabolism although trioses, tetroses, and sedoheptulose are important intermediates in the metabolism of carbohydrate in animal cells. Indeed, the simple triose, glyceraldehyde, is potentially the building block of all cell carbohydrates as will be seen in the later discussion of carbohydrate metabolism (Chapter 13).

Pentoses.

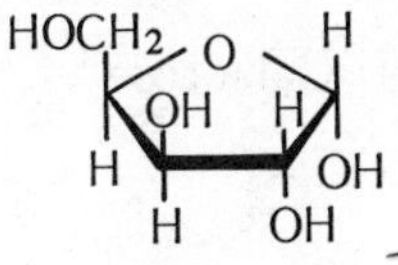

D-Xylose

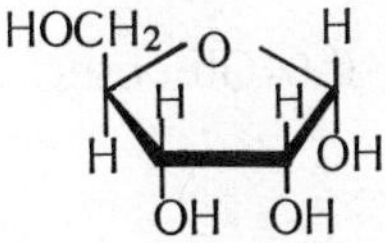

D-Ribose

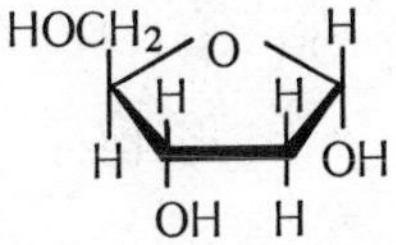

2-Deoxy-D-ribose

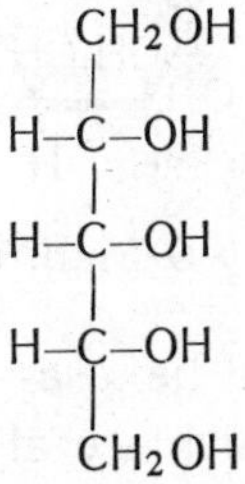

$$CH_2OH$$
$$H-C-OH$$
$$H-C-OH$$
$$H-C-OH$$
$$CH_2OH$$

Ribitol

Pentose sugars are readily synthesized in the cell. Ribose is the most important of the pentoses in biological systems and can be converted to deoxyribose and ribitol, neither of which can be classified strictly as a carbohydrate. Deoxyribose has two hydrogen atoms attached to carbon atom 2, instead of one hydrogen atom and one hydroxyl group. Both ribose and deoxyribose are constituents of a nucleic acid that bears their name: ribonucleic acid (RNA) and deoxyribonucleic acid (DNA). Ribose also is a constituent of many other nucleotides including the adenosine phosphates (ATP, ADP, AMP) and the nicotinamide adenine dinucleotides (NAD, NADP). Deoxyribose is encountered less frequently as a nucleotide constituent.

Ribitol, a reduction product of ribose, is a component of the vitamin, riboflavin, and therefore, like ribose and deoxyribose, performs a functional role in cell metabolism.

Hexoses.

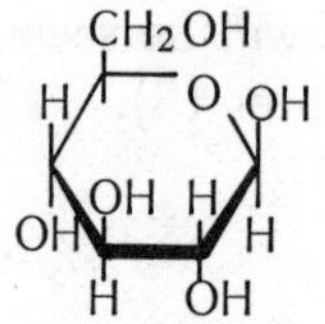

β-D-Glucose

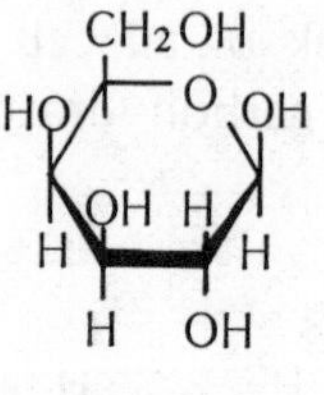

β-D-Galactose

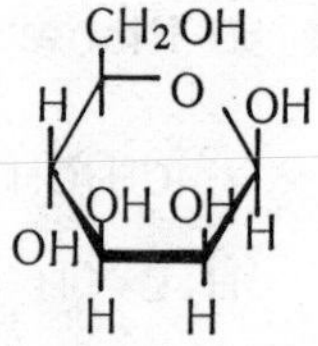

β-D-Mannose

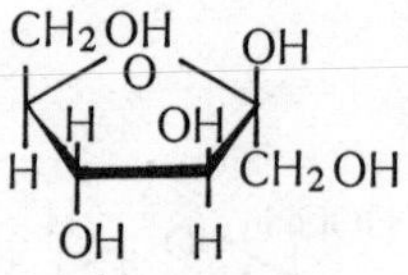

β-D-Fructose

The principal hexoses are glucose, galactose, mannose, and fructose. The first three are aldohexoses; fructose is a ketohexose. Glucose is the central compound in the catabolism and synthesis of carbohydrates and is the form in which carbohydrate is supplied to the cell from body fluids. Glucose concentration in the blood is closely regulated (see Chapter 15). Its presence in blood apparently was first detected in 1844 by Schmidt (collaborator with Bidder on metabolic studies; see Chapter 1). The sugar is a metabolic substrate for all cells, but cells of nerve tissue and lens of the eye are normally entirely dependent on glucose as a source of energy. However in starvation or other conditions of excessive lipolysis, brain tissue switches to ketone bodies as the primary source of energy (see Chapter 15). Fructose and galactose are converted to the storage carbohydrate, glycogen, in the liver and thus may give rise to glucose and contribute to the cell energy supply.

The hexoses and their derivatives also are constituents of a large number of complex substances that are synthesized by the cell as structural components and secretions. These substances generally consist of combinations with proteins or lipids and hence are known as glycoproteins, mucopolysaccharides, or glycolipids. Mannose, for example, is of little significance as a direct energy source for the cell, but it is an important constituent of both glycoproteins and glycolipids. Two six-carbon deoxy sugars, L-rhamnose (6-deoxy-L-mannose) and L-fucose (6-deoxy-L-galactose) also are components of the glycoproteins of cell membranes.

Monosaccharide Derivatives

Like all monosaccharides, the metabolically active forms of the hexoses are the phosphorylated derivatives. For example, it is glucose-6-phosphate, shown below, and not the free sugar that holds the central position in the metabolism of carbohydrate. All of the phosphorylated sugars involved in carbohydrate degradation and and synthesis exist as fleeting intermediaries and thus are active metabolites that do not accumulate within the cell to any great extent. Indeed, the bulk of carbohydrates within the cell exist in the form of the complex polysaccharides.

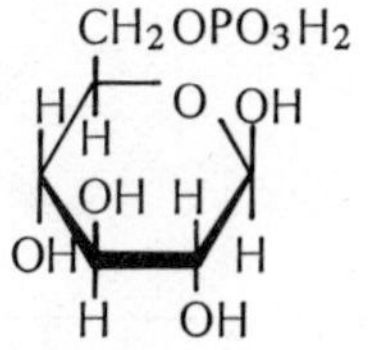

$$CH_2OPO_3H_2$$

β-D-Glucose-6-phosphate

Certain of the other commonly occurring sugar derivatives are shown in Table 2.2; for simplicity, derivatives of glucose are used to illustrate structural characteristics. Of these compounds, the amino and acetyl amino sugars are significant components of the complex structural carbohydrates.

Oligosaccharides

Of the oligosaccharides the most common are the disaccharides: sucrose, lactose, and maltose. The general class of oligosaccharides, however, includes sugars containing any number from 2 to as many as 10 monosaccharide units joined together through the hydroxyl groups of each sugar with the loss of one molecule of water. This

Table 2.2 MONOSACCHARIDE DERIVATIVES

Derivative	Characteristic Grouping	Structure
Amino sugars	Hydroxyl group is replaced by an amino group.	β-D-Glucosamine
Acetyl amino sugars	Acetyl group is attached to the nitrogen of an amino sugar.	N-Acetyl-β-D-glucosamine
Uronic acids	Primary alcohol group is oxidized to a carboxyl group.	β-D-Glucuronic acid
Glyconic acids	Aldehyde group is oxidized to a carboxyl group.	D-Gluconic acid (glyconic acid)
Sugar alcohols	Aldehyde or ketone group is reduced to an alcohol group.	D-Glucitol (sorbitol)

type of bonding, or glycosidic linkage, is common to the disaccharides and other more complex carbohydrates. Most generally, it is the 1,4- or 1,6-linkage, the hydroxyl group on C-1 of one molecule in a glycosidic bond to the hydroxyl on C-4 or C-6 of another monosaccharide unit.

Sucrose, the most widely distributed of the disaccharides, on hydrolysis yields glucose and fructose. Lactose is found only in milk and is composed of glucose and galactose. Maltose contains two molecules of glucose and is formed by the partial hydrolysis of starch; it is of little dietary significance except perhaps for the habitual beer drinker.

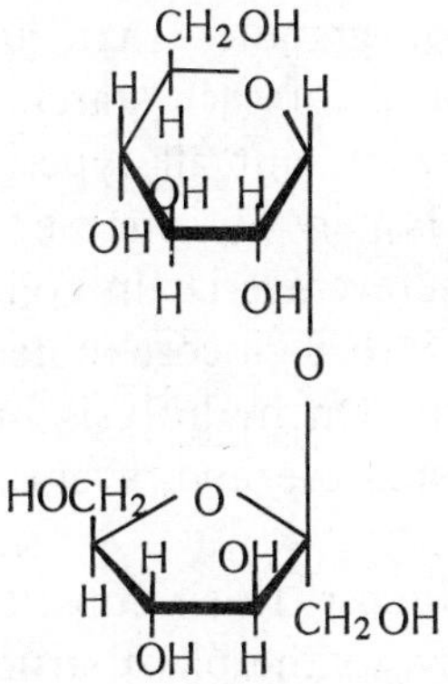

Sucrose

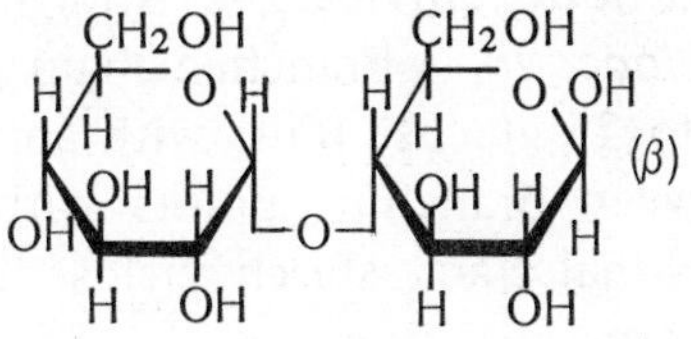

Maltose

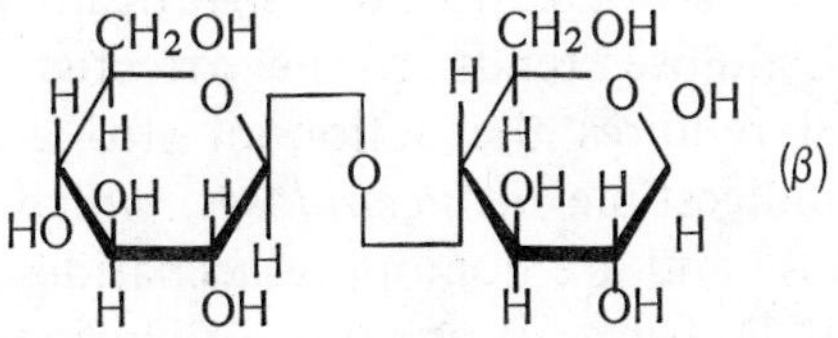

Lactose

The disaccharides are unimportant in the metabolism of the animal cell and contribute to body function solely through their products of digestion, the monosaccharides. Sucrose, if injected into the blood stream of an animal, for example, cannot be metabolized and is rapidly excreted intact. Synthesis of lactose is a highly specialized function both in terms of site (cells of the mammary glands) and period of the life cycle (lactation).

Polysaccharides

Polysaccharides are complex polymers containing only one mono-saccharide, *homopolysaccharides,* or several different monosaccha-rides or monosaccharide derivatives, *heteropolysaccharides.* Many polysaccharides exist in the plant and animal kingdoms. However, only a few of these are known to be significant in mammalian nutrition, either as dietary constituents or as animal cell metabolites.

The most common digestible polysaccharide in plants is *starch,* a polymer of glucose. Starch is present primarily in the cells of grains, fruits, and tubers in the form of granules that, under microscopic examination, appear to be typical for each starch. The composition of starches also differs somewhat, but all types con-tain both *amylose,* a straight chain polymer of glucose, and *amylopectin,* a branched-chain polymer. The average chain contains 20 to 25 glucose units with approximately 5 to 8 glucose molecules between branching points within the chain. On hydrolysis in the intestinal tract, starch yields dextrins and maltose and, eventually, glucose.

Cellulose is a straight chain polymer of glucose. It is a constituent of the cell walls of plants and gives rigidity to the plant structure much as the skeleton supports the animal body. It is not attacked by digestive enzymes of the human, and although it provides bulk to the diet it does not contribute significantly to the nutrition of body cells. Cellulose tends to be affected little by usual acid hydrolysis and requires the action of strong mineral acids. Plants also contain indigestible *hemicelluloses,* which are unrelated chemi-cally to cellulose and are homopolysaccharides containing D-xylose. Pectin, present in fruits, is an indigestible heteropolymer and con-tains arabinose, galactose, and galacturonic acid.

Some partially digestible polysaccharides also occur in foods and together comprise roughly 2 percent of the total carbohydrate intake. Inulin, galactogens, mannosans, and pentosans are homo-polymers of fructose, galactose, mannose, and pentoses, respectively. Raffinose, a heteropolymer, contains glucose, fructose, and galac-tose.

Glycogen is the only homopolysaccharide of importance in animal metabolism. Its presence in liver was first detected in 1856 by Claude Bernard, who recognized the relationship between the glycogen of liver and the sugar present in the blood. Subsequently Voit proved that the common monosaccharides give rise to liver glycogen. Although the total quantity of glycogen in the animal body is low, considerably less than one-tenth percent of the total body weight, its role is primarily that of a storage carbohydrate, similar to the role of starch in plant cells. It occurs predominantly in the liver where it is important in the homeostatic mechanism regulating glucose level of the blood. In skeletal muscle, glycogen serves as a source of energy for muscle contraction.

Glycogen is a branched-chain polymer of 6000 to 30,000 glucose units. It is similar to amylopectin in structure but is more highly branched. The average chain length is only 10 to 14 glucose units with 3 to 4 glucose units between branching points. The size of the molecule varies with its source and with the metabolic state of the animal. Muscle glycogen is estimated to have a molecular weight of about 10^6 whereas the liver glycogen molecule is much larger, approximately 5×10^6. Both molecules, however, constantly change in size as glucose molecules are added or removed.

Glycogen is of no importance as a dietary source of carbohydrate. When animals are slaughtered, the small amount of glycogen in the body is quickly degraded and has practically disappeared by the time the meat reaches the consumer's table.

Mucopolysaccharides

The mucopolysaccharides (sometimes called acidic glycoaminoglycans) are heteropolysaccharides and occur in combination with protein in both body secretions and structures. Many mucopolysaccharides tend to be highly viscous and are responsible for the viscosity of body mucous secretions. They are generally components of the extracellular, amorphous ground substance that surrounds the collagen and elastin fibers and the cells of connective tissue and may be involved in the induction of calcification, control of metabolites, ions, and water, and the healing of wounds. Mucopolysaccharides, along with glycoproteins and glycolipids, also form the cell coat that is present in most animal cells. The cell coat is visible by electron microscopy but is not a well-defined structure as is the cell wall of plant cells. For this reason the cell coat permits more intimate interaction between the cells and between the cell and its environment.

Mucopolysaccharides contain amino sugars, either D-glucosamine or D-galactosamine together with uronic acids, either D-glucuronic acid or L-iduronic acid; in addition they may contain acetyl or sulfate groups. Two compounds that are generally included in the mucopolysaccharide classification do not follow the usual pattern of composition. Keratan sulfate, which is found in connective tissues, contains D-galactose instead of a uronic acid component. Heparin is similar in composition and is synthesized and stored in the mast cells of connective tissue.

Hyaluronic acid is a typical mucopolysaccharide. It is a component of the ground substance of intercellular material; the human umbilical cord and cattle synovial and vitreous fluids are the most common sources of hyaluronic acid, but it is widely distributed and is found in most connective tissues. Its name is derived from hyaloid (vitreous) and uronic acid. Hyaluronic acid is composed of equimolar proportions of D-glucuronic acid and acetyl glucosamine occupying alternating positions in the molecule. The structure is shown below.

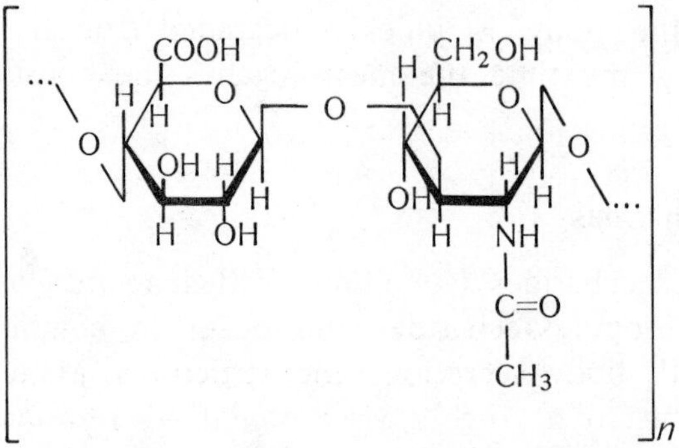

Repeating unit of
hyaluronic acid

The molecular weight varies depending on the source with reported values ranging from a few hundred thousand to well over a million. Large polymers of hyaluronic acid form a mesh that enables it to bind a large amount of water. In loose connective tissue such binding of tissue fluid forms a jellylike matrix filling the space between capillaries and cells. The large amount of fluid that is held by the polymers permits diffusion of solutes between capillaries and cells. In the synovial cavity, the viscosity of the synovial fluid assists in the lubrication of joints.

Chondroitin and *chondroitin sulfates* are polysaccharides containing D-glucuronic acid and acetyl galactosamine. Their general structure is similar, but they differ in the content and location of sulfate ester groups in the molecule. Chondroitin contains only a small number of sulfate ester groups, whereas both chondroitin 4- and chondroitin 6-sulfates (previously known as chondroitin sulfates A and C) contain one sulfate group for each disaccharide grouping. Their structures are shown below.

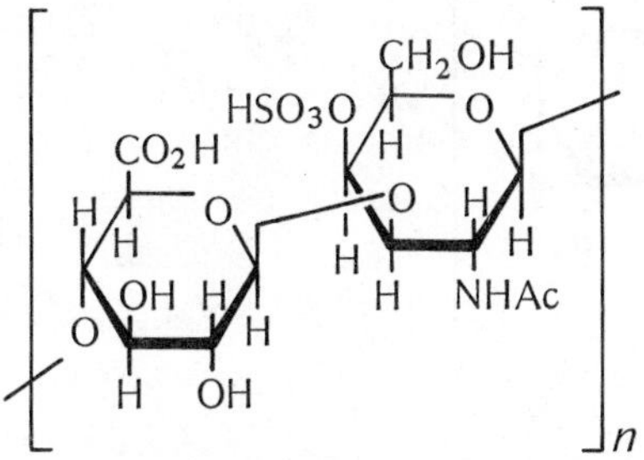

Chondroitin 4-sulfate 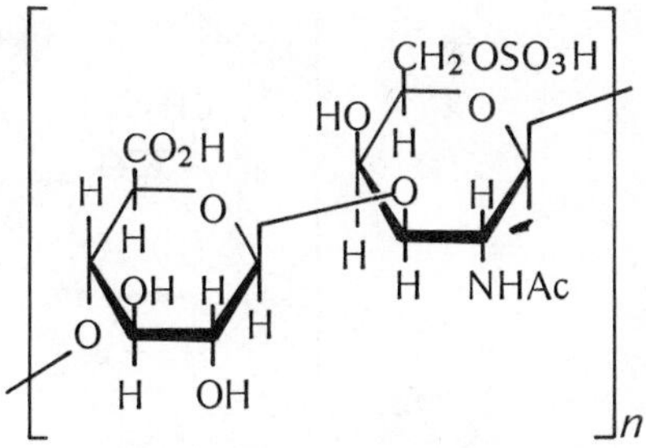   Chondroitin 6-sulfate

Chondroitin sulfates have a high viscosity and a capability for binding water and, in connective tissue, apparently play a role similar to that of hyaluronic acid. In addition, these compounds are distinguished by the ion-binding capacity of the sulfate groups. Chondroitin is a component of the cell coat (see Chapter 9), and chondroitin 4-sulfate is the principal organic component of the ground substance of cartilage and bone (see Chapter 17).

Dermatan sulfate (formerly chondroitin sulfate B or β-heparin) contains largely L-iduronic acid in place of D-glucuronic acid; iduronic acid is a derivative of the obscure hexose, idose. It has been suggested, however, that dermatan sulfate is a hybrid molecule containing both iduronic acid and glucuronic acid (Fransson, 1970). Dermatan sulfate generally occurs in tissues that are rich in collagen (Meyer et al., 1956). Its biological role appears to be different from the chondroitin sulfates, and it is present mainly in the skin.

Keratan sulfate (keratosulfate) is composed of D-galactose, N-acetyl-D-glucosamine and sulfate groups in a molar ratio of 1:1:1. Certain sources also have been found to contain a 6-deoxy-hexose (which is presumed to be L-fucose), sialic acid, and amino acids (Jeanloz, 1970). The function of keratan sulfate is not known. Apparently it is related to the blood group substances; it is degraded by enzymes that also degrade blood group substances, but not by hyaluronidases and chondrosulfatases. In addition, after removal of the sulfate groups, the desulfated keratan sulfate strongly cross-reacts with antibodies that also cross-react with blood group substance A (Hirano et al., 1961). The basic structure of keratan sulfate is shown below.

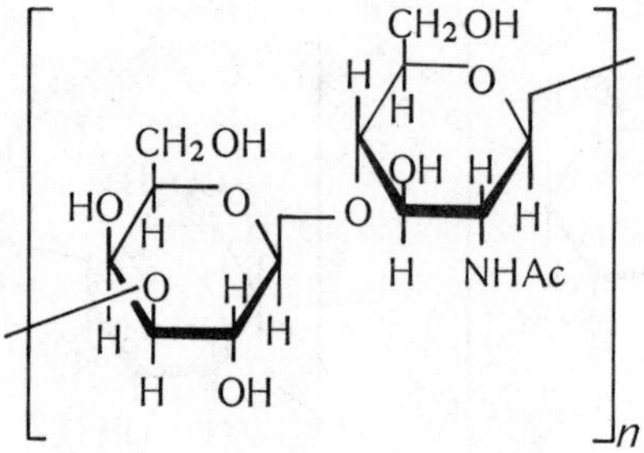

Keratan sulfate

Heparin (or α-heparin), the naturally occurring anticoagulant in blood and other tissues contains glucosamine, glucuronic acid, and varying proportions of sulfate and acetyl groups. Its structure is not entirely clear. It is produced by mast cells of the connective tissue and is stored as granules within the cells. The heparin content of tissues correlates with the number of mast cells present. These cells are particularly numerous in the loose connective tissue along the path of small blood vessels. Heparin is secreted into the intercellular substance and functions there to prevent the fibrinogen that escapes from capillaries from forming fibrin clots. It also functions in the formation or activation of lipoprotein lipase, which clears chylomicrons from the plasma (see Chapter 20). There is an insufficient amount of heparin in the bloodstream to perform these functions, but the mast cells along the capillaries supply additional amounts.

For detailed information concerning the structure and function of the mucopolysaccharides, see Balazs (1970) and Jeanloz (1970).

LIPIDS

Lipids include all substances that are extractable from biological materials with the usual fat solvents (ether, chloroform, benzene, carbon tetrachloride, acetone, etc.). Certain lipids are an energy source for the cell, others are structural compounds (particularly important are the lipid constituents of cell and organelle membranes), and still others function as hormones. This diversity of function recalls the not-too-remote past when lipids were considered to be inert constituents of adipose cells. The work of Schoenheimer (1942) established the concept of the dynamic state of lipid metabolism and led to a new appreciation of adipose tissue as an active participant in the metabolic scheme.

Of the many compounds classified as lipids, only a fraction is significant in the diet, or in the structure and function of the animal cell. The following classification is limited to lipids of importance in animal nutrition and excludes the fat-soluble vitamins that, although properly classified as lipids, will be discussed in a separate section on the vitamins, following the classic practice of nutritionists. Glycolipids and lipoproteins also will be discussed in a later section.

A. Simple Lipids
   1. Fatty acids
   2. Neutral fats (mono-, di-, and triacyl glycerols)
   3. Waxes (esters of fatty acids with higher alcohols)
     a. Sterol esters (i.e., cholesterol esters with fatty acids)
     b. Nonsterol esters (i.e., vitamin A esters, etc.)
B. Compound Lipids
   1. Phospholipids
     a. Phosphatidic acids, lecithins, cephalins, etc.
     b. Plasmalogens
     c. Sphingomyelins
   2. Glycolipids (carbohydrate-containing)
   3. Lipoproteins (lipids in combination with protein)
C. Derived lipids, alcohols (including sterols and hydrocarbons)

Fatty Acids

The fatty acids, the simplest of the lipids, are defined as monocarboxylic acids that tend to be more soluble in organic solvents than in water. The molecule consists of a polar carboxyl group that is soluble in water and a nonpolar hydrocarbon chain that is insoluble in water but soluble in the common organic solvents. The solubility of fatty acids in water therefore is fairly high for those of low chain length but decreases markedly as chain length increases.

The names and structures of some common fatty acids are shown in Tables 2.3 and 2.4. Note that for the unsaturated fatty acids (Table 2.4) two different systems for abbreviated formulas are given, one based on the position of double bonds from the carboxyl carbon, the other on the position of the first double bond from the terminal methyl group of the fatty acid molecule.

Table 2.3   SOME NATURALLY OCCURRING SATURATED FATTY ACIDS

Common Name	Chemical Name	Formula[a]
Butyric	n-Butanoic	$CH_3CH_2CH_2COOH$
Caproic	n-Hexanoic	$CH_3(CH_2)_4COOH$
Caprylic	n-Octanoic	$CH_3(CH_2)_6COOH$
Capric	n-Decanoic	$CH_3(CH_2)_8COOH$
Lauric	n-Dodecanoic	$CH_3(CH_2)_{10}COOH$
Myristic	n-Tetradecanoic	$CH_3(CH_2)_{12}COOH$
Palmitic	n-Hexadecanoic	$CH_3(CH_2)_{14}COOH$
Stearic	n-Octadecanoic	$CH_3(CH_2)_{16}COOH$
Arachidic	n-Eicosanoic	$CH_3(CH_2)_{18}COOH$
Behenic	n-Docosanoic	$CH_3(CH_2)_{20}COOH$
Lignoceric	n-Tetracosanoic	$CH_3(CH_2)_{22}COOH$

[a]Abbreviated formulas indicate the number of carbon atoms, followed by a colon and O denoting no. double bonds in the molecule; thus butyric acid may be written as 4:0 or $C_{4:0}$.

Most naturally occurring fatty acids are straight-chain saturated or unsaturated acids containing an even number of carbon atoms. Those in animal products generally contain 16 to 26 carbon atoms. Palmitic acid and stearic acid are by far the most commonly occurring and widely distributed of the saturated fatty acids whereas oleic acid and linoleic acid are the most prevalent of the unsaturated. These four fatty acids account for over 90 percent of the fatty

Table 2.4 SOME NATURALLY OCCURRING UNSATURATED FATTY ACIDS

Common Name	Chemical Name	Formula	Abbreviated Formulas	
			Carboxyl Series[a]	Omega Series[b]
Monoenoic				
Palmitoleic	*cis*-9-Hexadecenoic	$CH_3(CH_2)_5CH=CH(CH_2)_7COOH$	9-16:1	(9-)16:1ω7
Oleic	*cis*-9-Octadecenoic	$CH_3(CH_2)_7CH=CH(CH_2)_7COOH$	9-18:1	(9-)18:1ω9
Dienoic				
Linoleic	*cis, cis*-9,12-Octadecadienoic	$CH_3(CH_2)_3(CH_2CH=CH)_2(CH_2)_7COOH$	9,12-18:2	(9,12-)18:2ω6
Trienoic				
Linolenic	All-*cis*-9,12,15-Octadecatrienoic	$CH_3(CH_2CH=CH)_3(CH_2)_7COOH$	9,12,15-18:3	(9,12,15)18:3ω3
Tetraenoic				
Arachidonic	All-*cis*-5,8,11,14-Eicosatetraenoic	$CH_3(CH_2)_3(CH_2CH=CH)_4(CH_2)_3COOH$	5,8,11,14-20:4	(5,8,11,14-)20:4ω6

[a]Using palmitoleic acid as an example, 9 = position of double bond from the carboxyl carbon; 16 = length of carbon chain; 1 = number of double bonds in the molecule. It may also be written $\Delta^9 C_{16:1}$.

[b]Also using palmitoleic acid as an example, 9, 16, and 1 are the same as above; ω7 denotes the position of the double bond from the terminal (or omega) methyl carbon. It may also be written as simply 16:1ω7.

33

acids in the average American diet. Fatty acids of shorter chain length are for the most part minor constituents of plant and animal fats. However, butyric acid and myristic acid occur in milk fat in large amounts, and about 60 percent of the fatty acid in coconut oil consists of lauric acid and fatty acids of shorter chain length.

Odd-numbered and branched-chain fatty acids occur in some cells (Kingsbury et al., 1961). Certain fish and bacteria contain fairly high amounts of odd-numbered fatty acids; the occurrence of these compounds in some common sources is shown in Table 2.5.

Table 2.5 OCCURRENCE OF ODD-NUMBERED FATTY ACIDS

Source	Percent Odd of Total Fatty Acids
Olive oil	<0.4
Chicken fat	0.4 - 1.5
Lard	0.8
Menhaden	2.4, 3.0
Mullet	19.1, 20.4
Tuna	4.2
Rat liver	2.9, 0.5
Human (depot fat)	1.1
Human (erythrocytes)	0.8
Euglena gracilis	33.4
Ochromonas danica	<1

Adapted from H. Schlenk, *Fed. Proc., 31:* 1431 (1972).

The polyunsaturated acids—linolenic, linoleic, and arachidonic—have often been designated the *essential fatty acids* (EFA). Of these three, linoleic acid is most abundant in human diets. Essential fatty acid activity, however, is shared by other unsaturated acids having the 9,12 double bond (counting from the carboxyl group) of the C_{18} acids or the 11, 14 bond of the C_{20} acids. Some new synthetic odd-numbered fatty acids also have been shown to possess EFA activity (Schlenk, 1972). The essentiality of linoleic acid in the diet of the rat was first demonstrated by Burr and Burr (1929) who found that the acid would prevent or cure a characteristic dermatitis observed in rats fed a fat-free diet. Other effects of EFA deficiency in the rat are shown in Table 2.6. Later Wiese et al. (1958) demonstrated a requirement for linoleic acid in human infants. The dietary requirement for the human adult, however, appears to be negligible since tissue stores of essential fatty acids in the adult apparently are high.

Table 2.6 MAJOR EFFECTS OF EFA DEFICIENCY IN THE RAT

1. Skin symptoms	Dermatosis; increased water permeability; drop in sebum secretion; epithelial hyperplasia.
2. Weight	Decrease.
3. Circulation	Heart enlargement; decreased capillary resistance; increased permeability.
4. Kidney	Enlargement; intertubular hemorrhage.
5. Lung	Cholesterol accumulation.
6. Endocrine glands	(a) *Adrenals.* Weight decreased in females and increased in males.
	(b) *Thyroid.* Reduced weight.
7. Reproduction	(a) *Females.* Irregular estrus and impaired reproduction and lactation.
	(b) *Males.* Degeneration of seminiferous tubules.
8. Metabolism	(a) Changes in fatty acid composition of most organs.
	(b) Increase in cholesterol levels in liver, adrenals, and skin.
	(c) Decrease in plasma cholesterol.
	(d) Changes in swelling of heart and liver mitochondria and uncoupling of oxidative phosphorylation.
	(e) Increased triglyceride synthesis and release by the liver.

From M. I. Gurr and A. T. James, *Lipid Biochemistry: An Introduction*, Cornell University Press, Ithaca, 1971, p. 56.

The animal cell is capable of forming certain unsaturated fatty acids. Linoleate, linolenate, oleate, and palmitoleate are all precursors for the biosynthesis of individual "families" of polyunsaturated fatty acids (Table 2.7). The omega nomenclature described by Guarnieri and Johnson (1970) is particularly useful when considering the interconversions of unsaturated fatty acids because any new double bonds must be introduced between the carboxyl group and the first double bond of the fatty acid molecule. Therefore, in this type of conversion, the terminal double bond remains fixed. Thus, linoleate ($18:2\omega6$) may be converted to arachidonate ($20:4\omega6$), but little or no conversion of other acids to linoleate occurs. In contrast, plant cells are able to introduce a second double bond

Table 2.7 PATHWAYS FOR BIOSYNTHESIS OF POLYUNSATURATED FATTY ACIDS

Linoleic   ω6 family   18:2 — 18:3 → 20:3 → 20:4 → 22:4 → 22:5
                              ↗ 20:2

Linolenic   ω3 family   18:3 → 18:4 → 20:4 → 20:5 → 22:5 → 22:6

Oleic   ω9 family   18:0 → 18:1 → 18:2 → 20:2 → 20:3

Palmitoleic ω7 family   16:0 → 16:1 — 18:1 — 18:2 → 18:3 → 20:3 → 20:4
                              ↗ 16:2   ↗ 20:2

Adapted from H. W. Sprecher, Fed. Proc., 31:1451 (1972).

between carbon atoms 12 and 13 of oleic acid to form linoleic acid.

Because of the double bonds in the molecule, unsaturated fatty acids may exist as isomers. This type of isomerism is known as *cis-trans* isomerism and involves changes in the geometrical configuration of the molecule. *Cis* isomerism results in a doubling back of the molecule in a horseshoe-like configuration whereas *trans* isomerism has the effect of extending the molecule. As an illustration, the *cis* and *trans* forms of the C_{18} monounsaturated acid are shown below.

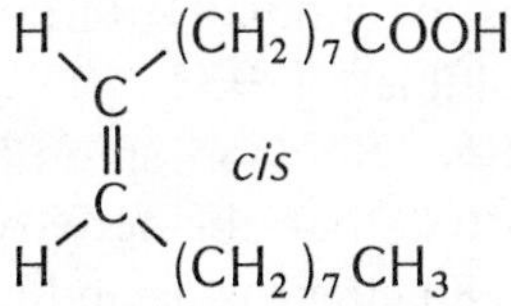

Oleic acid 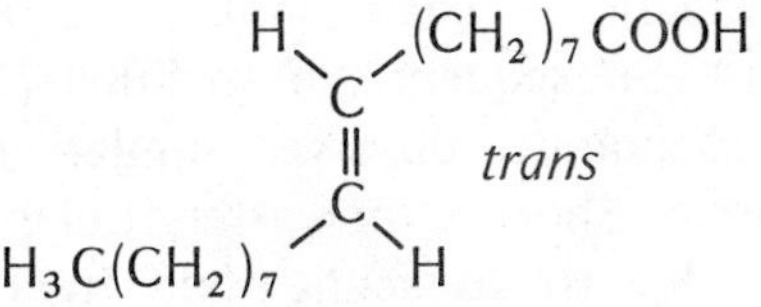   Elaidic acid

In either case, however, the hydrocarbon chain of a fatty acid does not exist as a long straight chain but, instead, in a zigzag conformation. When a *cis* double bond is present the molecule becomes bent, and the bending is more drastic as the number of double bonds increases as shown below. The zigzagging along with the bending of the molecule makes for a bulky structure instead of the tidy straight chain suggested by the formula. The molecular configuration of the fatty acids play an important role in both the structure and function of membranes (see Chapter 9).

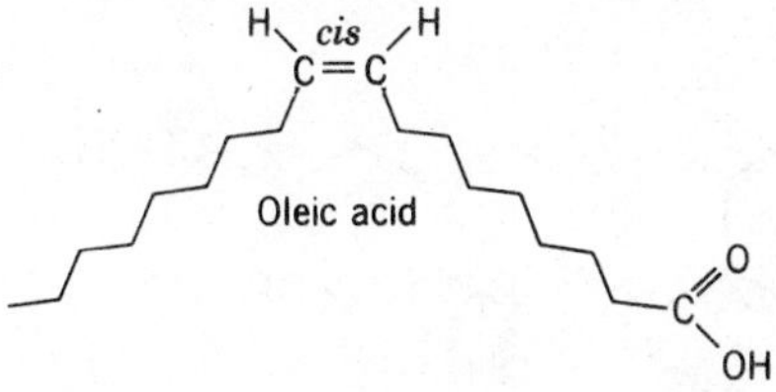

Oleic acid (one *cis* bond) 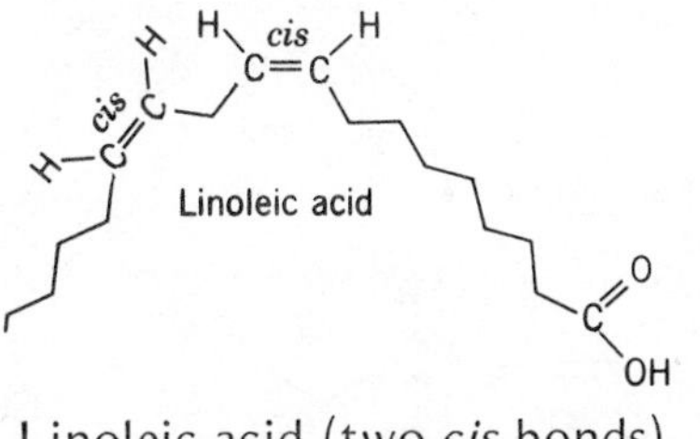   Linoleic acid (two *cis* bonds)

Most naturally occurring fatty acids are largely of the *cis* configuration although conversion to the *trans* form results from heating or hydrogenation. However, *trans* fatty acids also exist in natural fats and oils. In cow's milk, for example, *trans* unsaturated fatty acids comprise about 8 percent of total fat and about 20 percent of total unsaturated fatty acids (Woodrow and de Man, 1968).

Protaglandins

Essential fatty acids are precursors of a ubiquitious family of lipids—the prostaglandins. These compounds have hormone-like activity and are among the most potent biological substances known. The first indication of the existence of this new family of compounds came when Kurzrok and Lieb (1930) reported that human seminal fluid produced both relaxation and strong contractions when applied to isolated strips of human uterine tissue. Subsequently both Euler (1934) and Goldblatt (1933, 1935) independently observed similar effects of seminal fluid on smooth muscle. Shortly thereafter, Euler (1935) reported that the activity was due to an acidic lipid fraction that he named prostaglandin. More than 25 years passed, however, before the structure was determined by Bergström et al. (1962) using a variety of techniques including mass spectrometry, X-ray crystallography, and nuclear magnetic resonance. Two years later the essential fatty acids were found to be precursors (Bergström et al., 1964; Van Dorp, 1964).

Work on the prostaglandins then mushroomed. As of the end of 1972, 14 different compounds have been identified, each having 20 carbon atoms and the same basic molecule of prostanoic acid. The carbon chains are bonded in the middle by a five-member ring. On the basis of the structural arrangement of double bonds, hydroxyl and ketone groups, the acids have been divided into four

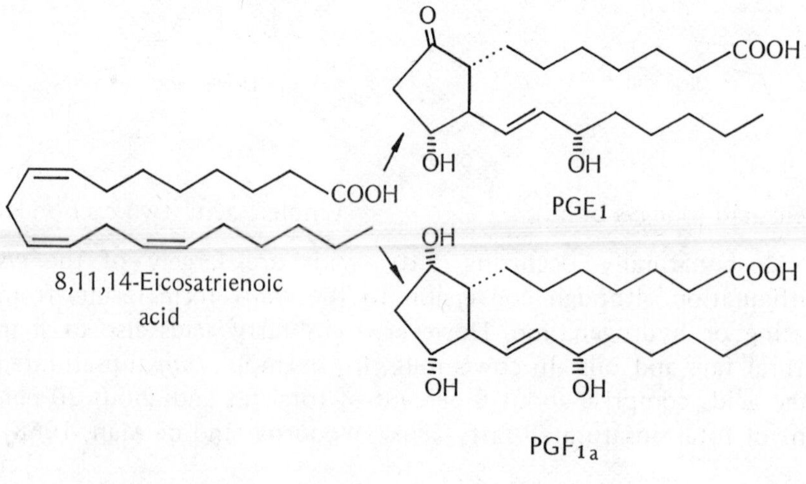

8,11,14-Eicosatrienoic acid

PGE_1

PGF_{1a}

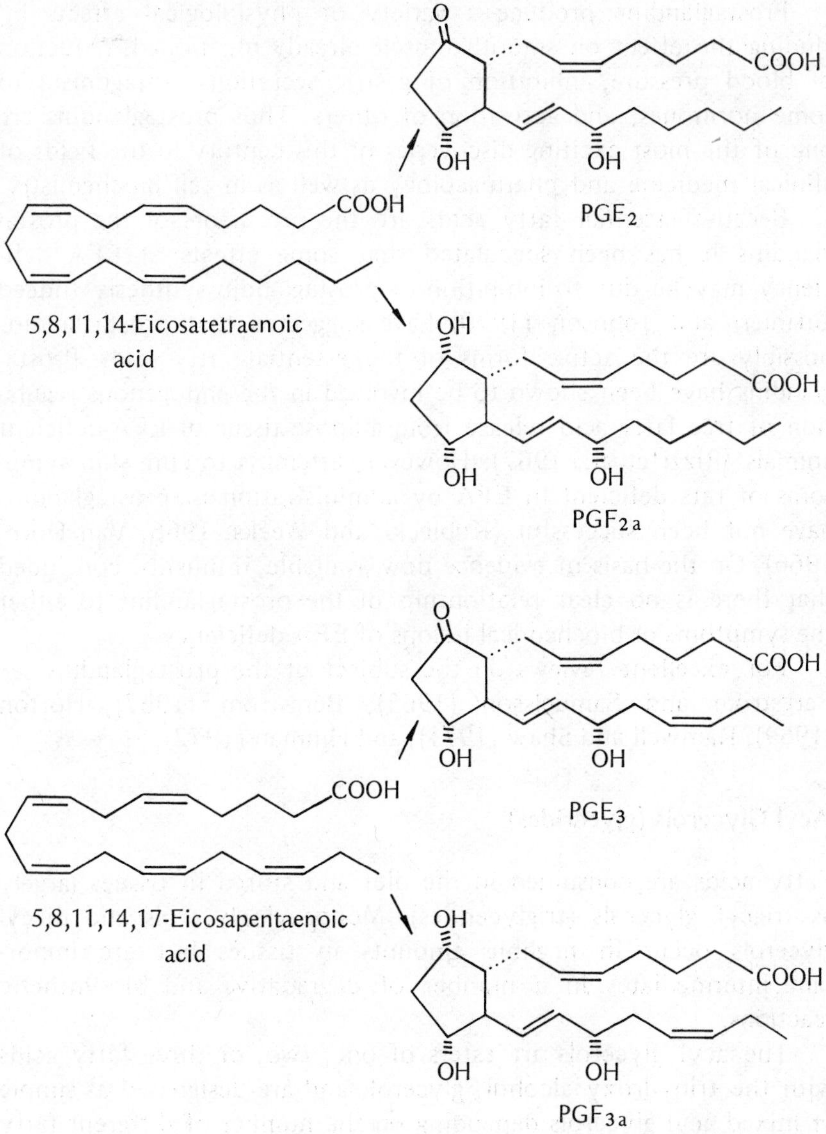

5,8,11,14-Eicosatetraenoic
acid

PGE₂

PGF₂ₐ

PGE₃

5,8,11,14,17-Eicosapentaenoic
acid

PGF₃ₐ

categories: A, B, E, and F. Six primary prostaglandins of the E and F categories occur in most cells and arise from eicosatri-, tetra- and pentaenoic acids as shown above. These are converted to the eight secondary natural prostaglandins that have been identified. It is not unlikely that yet other of these compounds will subsequently be discovered.

Prostaglandins produce a variety of physiological effects including the effect on smooth muscle already mentioned, reduction of blood pressure, inhibition of gastric secretions, antagonism to some hormones, and activation of others. Thus prostaglandins are one of the most exciting discoveries of this century in the fields of clinical medicine and pharmacology as well as in cell biochemistry.

Because essential fatty acids are the precursors of the prostaglandins it has been speculated that some effects of EFA deficiency may be due to inhibition of prostaglandin synthesis. Indeed Guanieri and Johnson (1970) have suggested that prostaglandins possibly are the active forms of the essential fatty acids. Prostaglandins have been shown to be involved in the endogenous regulation of free fatty acid release from adipose tissue of EFA-deficient animals (Bizzi et al., 1967). However, attempts to cure skin symptoms of rats deficient in EFA by administration of prostaglandins have not been successful (Kupiecki and Weeks, 1966; Van Dorp, 1966). On the basis of evidence now available, it must be concluded that there is no clear relationship of the prostaglandins to either the symptoms or biochemical lesions of EFA deficiency.

For excellent reviews on the subject of the prostaglandins see Bergström and Samuelsson (1965), Bergström (1967), Horton (1969), Ramwell and Shaw (1971), and Hinman (1972).

Acyl Glycerols (glycerides)

Fatty acids are consumed in the diet and stored in tissues largely as triacyl glycerols (triglycerides). Monoacyl glycerols and diacyl glycerols occur in neglible amounts in tissues but are important intermediates in a number of degradative and biosynthetic reactions.

The acyl glycerols are esters of one, two, or three fatty acids with the trihydroxy alcohol, glycerol, and are designated as simple or mixed acyl glycerols depending on the number of different fatty acids present in the molecule. (The location of the fatty acids in the molecule is shown by the system designated below.) Tristearin, for example, indicates a simple triacyl glycerol containing only stearic acid in the molecule, whereas 1-oleo-2-stearo-3-palmitin is a triglyceride containing oleic, stearic, and palmitic acids. As mentioned before, these acids along with linoleic acid are the most widely distributed of the fatty acids. Generally, triacyl glycerols in biological systems contain different fatty acyl groups.

$$1 \text{ or } \alpha \ CH_2\,OH$$
$$2 \quad \beta \ CHOH$$
$$3 \quad \alpha' \ CH_2\,OH$$

Glycerol

$$CH_2-O-\overset{\overset{\displaystyle O}{\|}}{C}-R$$
$$CHOH$$
$$CH_2\,OH$$

Monoacyl glycerol
(monoglyceride)

$$CH_2-O-\overset{\overset{\displaystyle O}{\|}}{C}-R$$
$$CH-O-\overset{\overset{\displaystyle O}{\|}}{C}-R$$
$$CH_2\,OH$$

Diacyl glycerol
(diglyceride)

$$CH_2-O-\overset{\overset{\displaystyle O}{\|}}{C}-R$$
$$CH-O-\overset{\overset{\displaystyle O}{\|}}{C}-R$$
$$CH_2-O-\overset{\overset{\displaystyle O}{\|}}{C}-R$$

Triacyl glycerol
(triglyceride)

Triacyl glycerols are classed as fats or oils depending on the state of the acyl glycerol at room temperature, which depends on the fatty acid composition. In general, acyl glycerols containing a high proportion of short chain (less than eight carbon atoms) or unsaturated acids have a low melting point and are liquid (oils) at room temperature. The longer chain saturated fatty acids produce a fat of higher melting point that is solid at room temperature.

Triacyl glycerols are a form of stored energy in animal tissues (adipose cells) and are commonly referred to as neutral fat. The capacity to store fat in the animal body unfortunately appears to be unlimited. Fatty acids are released from adipose cells in free form. These are designated both as FFA, free fatty acid and NEFA nonesterified fatty acids. Once released from neutral fat the FFA are transported in the blood bound to serum albumin (Goodman, 1957).

Although triacyl glycerols containing exclusively fatty acids with chain length of 6 to 12 carbon atoms are rare or nonexistent in nature, such compounds, called medium chain triglycerides or MCT, have been synthesized. The synthetic MCT contain approximately 75 percent caprylic acid (C_8), 22-23 percent capric (C_{10}), 1 percent each of caproic (C_6) and lauric (C_{12}), and traces of other fatty acids such as palmitic, stearic, and linoleic (Greenberger and Skillman, 1969). These compounds are liquid at room temperature due to the low melting points of the shorter chain fatty acids.

Because of the shorter hydrocarbon chain the MCT are also more soluble in water than the naturally occurring triacyl glycerols containing the long chain fatty acids. They are readily absorbed from the gastrointestinal tract and do not require bile salts for absorption. For these reasons the MCT appear to have therapeutic value in the treatment of a number of diseases including tropical and nontropical sprue, pancreatic insufficiency, and other conditions affecting intestinal absorption.

Phospholipids

$$
\begin{array}{l}
CH_2-O-C \overset{\displaystyle O}{\parallel} R_1 \\
\quad\quad\quad\quad O \\
CH-O-C \overset{\displaystyle \parallel}{} R_2 \\
\quad\quad\quad OH \\
CH_2-O-P=O \\
\quad\quad\quad OH
\end{array}
$$

Phosphatidic acid

Phosphatidic acids are compounds consisting of glycerol, two fatty acids, and a phosphate group and, as the structure suggests, they easily give rise to triacyl glycerols or to phospholipids. Because they are active intermediates in the biosynthesis of other lipid compounds, the phosphatidic acids do not accumulate in tissues in significant amounts.

Phospholipids differ chiefly in the specific compound attached to the phosphate group of the phosphatidic acid core. The fatty acids present in the molecule are usually saturated in the a-position (palmitic or stearic) and unsaturated in the β-position (oleic or linolenic). The phospholipid structures are shown in Table 2.8.

Phospholipids have the useful property of attracting both water-soluble and fat-soluble substances due to the hydrophilic (water-attracting) phosphoryl grouping and the hydrophobic (water-repelling) fatty acids in the molecule. In combination with protein, they are constituents of cell membranes and membranes of subcellular particles where they serve as a liaison between fat-soluble and water-

Table 2.8 GLYCEROL PHOSPHOLIPIDS

Name	Characteristic Group	Structure
Phosphatidyl cholines (lecithins)	Choline	$$\begin{array}{l} CH_2OCOR^1 \\ \mid \\ R^2COOCH \\ \mid \quad\quad\quad O \\ \mid \quad\quad\quad \| \\ CH_2-O-P-OCH_2CH_2\overset{+}{N}(CH_3)_3 \\ \quad\quad\quad\;\; \mid \\ \quad\quad\quad\;\; O^- \end{array}$$
Phosphatidyl ethanolamines (cephalins)	Ethanolamine (aminoethanol)	$$\begin{array}{l} CH_2OCOR^1 \\ \mid \\ R^2COOCH \\ \mid \quad\quad\quad O \\ \mid \quad\quad\quad \| \\ CH_2-O-P-OCH_2CH_2\overset{+}{N}H_3 \\ \quad\quad\quad\;\; \mid \\ \quad\quad\quad\;\; O^- \end{array}$$
Phosphatidyl serines (cephalinlike compounds)	Serine	$$\begin{array}{l} CH_2OCOR^1 \\ \mid \\ R^2COOCH \\ \mid \quad\quad\quad O \quad\quad\quad\quad \overset{+}{N}H_3 \\ \mid \quad\quad\quad \| \quad\quad\quad\quad\; \mid \\ CH_2-O-P-OCH_2CH_2 \\ \quad\quad\quad\;\; \mid \quad\quad\quad\quad\quad COO^- \\ \quad\quad\quad\;\; OH \end{array}$$

(continued)

Table 2.8 (continued)

Name	Characteristic Group	Structure
Phosphatidyl inositols (inositides or lipositols)	*Myo*-inositol	
Plasmalogens	Ethanolamine One fatty acid replaced by a long-chain unsaturated ether	

Structure 1 (Phosphatidyl inositols):

$$CH_2OCOR^1$$
$$R^2COOCH \quad\quad O$$
$$CH_2-O-\overset{\displaystyle O}{\underset{\displaystyle OH}{P}}-O-\text{(inositol ring: OH, OH, OH, OH, OH)}$$

Structure 2 (Plasmalogens):

$$\alpha CH_2OCH=CHR^1$$
$$R^2COOCH\beta \quad\quad O$$
$$CH_2-O-\overset{\displaystyle O}{\underset{\displaystyle O^-}{P}}-OCH_2CH_2\overset{+}{N}H_3$$

44

soluble materials that must penetrate the membrane and interact once they have gained entry. In this structural role, phospholipids are not generally available as an energy source. Even a starved animal will retain the phospholipid necessary to maintain the integrity of cells.

Sphingolipids

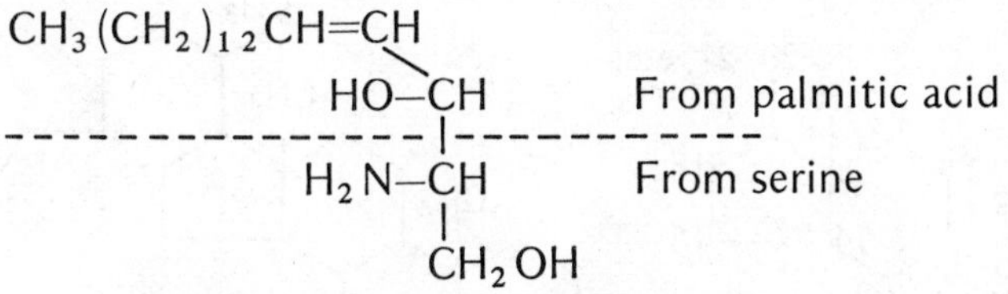

$$CH_3(CH_2)_{12}CH{=}CH$$
$$HO{-}CH \qquad \text{From palmitic acid}$$
$$H_2N{-}CH \qquad \text{From serine}$$
$$CH_2OH$$

4-Sphingenine (sphingosine)

Sphingolipids are classed as phospholipids but, in place of the glycerol characteristic of the glycerophospholipids, they contain 4-sphingenine (sphingosine), an 18-carbon monounsaturated alcohol derived from palmitic acid and the amino acid serine. Carbon atoms 1-3 form the glycerol-type part of the molecule; the structure differs from glycerol principally in that an amino group (from serine) is attached to the second carbon.

Sphingomyelins. Sphingomyelins occur in large amounts in the myelin sheath of nerve tissue and derive their name from this structure. The sphingomyelins contain phosphorylcholine attached to the terminal carbon atom of sphingosine and a fatty acid attached in amide linkage to the nitrogen of carbon 2.

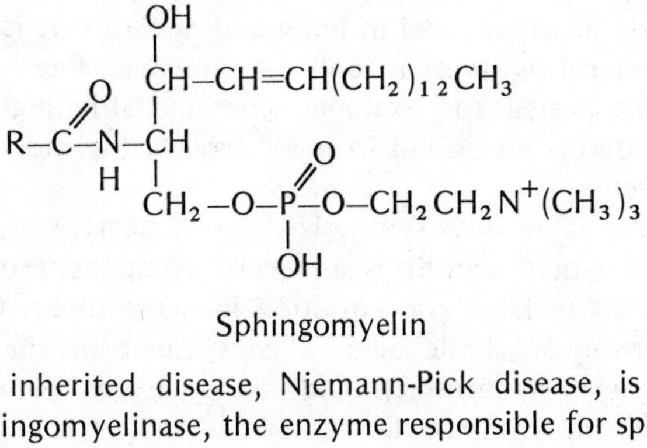

$$OH$$
$$\underset{H}{\overset{O}{\underset{\|}{R{-}C{-}N}}}{-}\overset{\overset{\displaystyle CH{-}CH{=}CH(CH_2)_{12}CH_3}{|}}{CH}$$
$$CH_2{-}O{-}\overset{\overset{\displaystyle O}{\|}}{P}{-}O{-}CH_2CH_2N^+(CH_3)_3$$
$$OH$$

Sphingomyelin

A rare inherited disease, Niemann-Pick disease, is due to the lack of sphingomyelinase, the enzyme responsible for sphingomyelin cleavage. The disease is characterized by deposition of sphingomyelin in almost every organ and tissue of the body and is usually fatal before the third year of life.

Steroids and Sterols

Cyclopentanoperhydrophenanthrene nucleus   Cholesterol

Steroid compounds are derivatives of a ring structure with the formidable name of the cyclopentanoperhydrophenanthrene nucleus. Certain steroids are characterized by a free hydroxyl group and thus behave chemically like alcohols. These alcohol-like steroids do not contain carbonyl or carboxy groups common to other steroids and are generally referred to as *sterols.* The most common sterol in animal tissues is cholesterol, which occurs in the free form or combined in ester formation with fatty acids. The proportion of free cholesterol to cholesterol esters varies considerably among different tissues. Sterol esters predominate in plasma and adrenals whereas nearly all cholesterol in brain and nerve tissue is in the free form. Cholesterol is present only in animals. Egg yolk, dairy products, and meats, for example, contain fairly high amounts. Many other sterols are found in plant tissues, the most important being β-sitosterol.

Cholesterol is readily synthesized from acetate in all animal tissues (see Chapter 15). It is a normal component of all body cells and occurs in large concentration in nerve tissue. Cholesterol is the precursor of cholic acid, a constituent of the bile acids (taurocholic and glycocholic), and its 7-dehydro derivative is a precursor of the vitamin D of animal tissues, cholecalciferol.

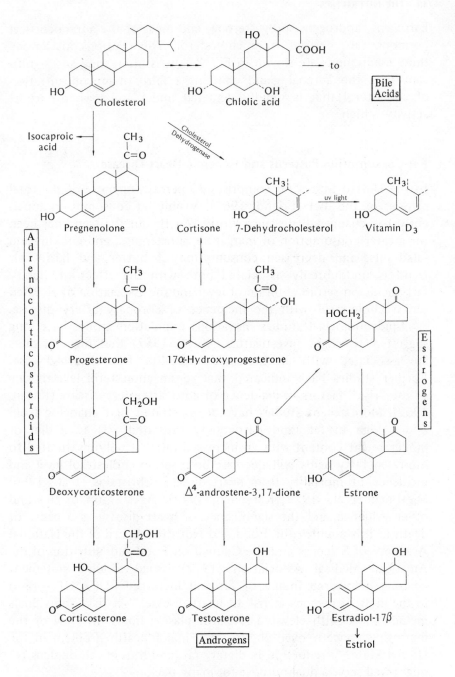

Fig. 2.1 Metabolic relationships among the steroids.

47

Estrogens, androgens, progesterone, and most of the adrenocortical hormones are derived from cholesterol. The relationships among these compounds are shown in Fig. 2.1. It is interesting and significant that the adrenal gland contains a fairly high concentration of cholesterol that is rapidly depleted under stress when cortical activity is high.

Fat Consumption Patterns and Ischemic Heart Disease

In the United States fat comprises 40 percent or more of the total calories of the diet (Friend, 1967). Visible fat consumption apparently has changed little since World War II, but the trend has been for greater consumption of margarine, shortenings, and cooking and salad oils, and decreased consumption of butter and lard. This trend is undoubtedly associated both with the effect of dietary fatty acids on serum cholesterol level and the association of elevated serum cholesterol with the incidence of coronary artery disease.

Epidemiological studies of various population groups have long suggested to some investigators (Keys, 1957) that high fat diets are associated with an increased mortality from heart disease. Further studies have indicated that serum cholesterol level is one of the "risk" factors in incidence of coronary artery disease (Kagan, 1962). More recent studies have demonstrated that changing from a diet high in fat (and particularly saturated fat) to a diet of moderate fat content with an increased ratio of polyunsaturated to saturated fatty acids will decrease both serum cholesterol level and incidence of mortality from heart disease (Christakis et al., 1966; Miettinen et al., 1972; Karvonen, 1972). As a result of this and other evidence and the significance of heart disease as a cause of death in this country the Food and Nutrition Board of the National Academy of Sciences and the Council on Food and Nutrition of the American Medical Association (1972) issued a joint statement advising a lowered intake of fat and increased PUFA:UFA ratio in the diets of persons at risk of heart disease. "At risk" individuals include those with elevated levels of plasma lipids. In view of the increasing concern over obesity as a major health problem in the United States, a reduction in dietary fat (and thus in caloric density) might well serve a dual purpose for many persons.

PROTEINS

Nearly half of the dry weight of a typical animal cell is protein. Structural components of the cell, antibodies, and many of the hormones are proteins, but as much as 90 percent of cellular proteins are the enzymes upon which fundamental cellular function depends. There may be as many as 1000 different enzymes in a single cell.

The protein molecule is a polymer of amino acids joined in peptide linkages. Although the molecular weight is usually high, there is a vast range in both structure and complexity of protein molecules. Hemoglobin, for example, has a molecular weight of about 64,500; myosin, a muscle protein, is estimated to have a molecular weight of about 468,000 (Klotz and Darnall, 1969). It is not uncommon for peptide structures of fairly low molecular weight (less than 10,000 and containing less than 100 amino acids) to be designated polypeptides rather than proteins. On the average, about 20 different amino acids occur in most proteins. The amino acids present, their position in the molecule, and the spatial arrangement of the molecule all determine the properties and characteristics of the protein. In turn the function of a protein depends, in large measure, on its structure (see Hess and Rupley, 1971).

Amino Acids

The amino acids are the fundamental units of protein structure. All amino acids contain at least one amino group ($-NH_2$) in the alpha position and one carboxyl, and all (except glycine) contain an asymmetric carbon atom. For this reason, they may exist as isomers. Most naturally occurring amino acids are of the L-configuration, although D-amino acids are not uncommon in some microorganisms. The presence of a D-amino acid oxidase in mammalian tissues, however, suggests that the D-forms may play some yet unrecognized role in mammalian protein metabolism.

The common amino acids and their formulas are shown in Table 2.9 and are grouped in the classical method according to

Table 2.9 AMINO ACIDS

Monoamino monocarboxylic

Glycine

$$H-CH-COOH$$
$$\quad\ \ |$$
$$\quad\ NH_2$$

Alanine

$$CH_3CH-COOH$$
$$\qquad\ |$$
$$\qquad NH_2$$

[a]Valine

$$CH_3$$
$$\quad\ \ \diagdown$$
$$\qquad CH-CH-COOH$$
$$\quad\ \diagup \qquad\ |$$
$$CH_3 \qquad\ NH_2$$

[a]Leucine

$$CH_3$$
$$\quad\ \ \diagdown$$
$$\qquad CH-CH_2-CH-COOH$$
$$\quad\ \diagup \qquad\qquad\ |$$
$$CH_3 \qquad\qquad\ NH_2$$

[a]Isoleucine

$$CH_3-CH_2-CH-CH-COOH$$
$$\qquad\qquad\ |\quad\ |$$
$$\qquad\qquad CH_3\ NH_2$$

Hydroxyl-containing

Serine

$$HO-CH_2-CH-COOH$$
$$\qquad\qquad\ |$$
$$\qquad\qquad NH_2$$

[a]Threonine

$$CH_3-CH-CH-COOH$$
$$\qquad\ |\quad\ |$$
$$\qquad OH\ NH_2$$

Sulfur-containing

Cystine (and cysteine)

$$S-CH_2-CH-COOH \qquad HS-CH_2-CH-COOH$$
$$|\qquad\qquad |\qquad\qquad\qquad\qquad\quad |$$
$$|\qquad\qquad NH_2\qquad\qquad\qquad\qquad NH_2$$
$$S-CH_2-CH-COOH$$
$$\qquad\qquad |$$
$$\qquad\qquad NH_2$$

[a]Methionine

$$CH_3-S-CH_2-CH_2-CH-COOH$$
$$\qquad\qquad\qquad\qquad\ |$$
$$\qquad\qquad\qquad\qquad NH_2$$

Aromatic

Tyrosine

$$HO-\langle\bigcirc\rangle-CH_2-CH-COOH$$
$$\qquad\qquad\qquad\qquad |$$
$$\qquad\qquad\qquad\quad NH_2$$

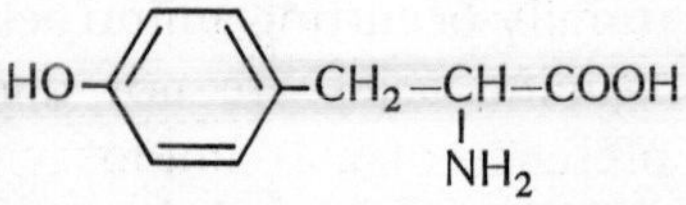

[a]Phenylalanine

$$\langle\bigcirc\rangle-CH_2-CH-COOH$$
$$\qquad\qquad\qquad |$$
$$\qquad\qquad\ NH_2$$

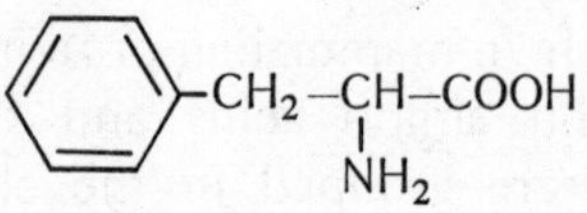

Table 2.9 (continued)

Heterocyclic
  Proline

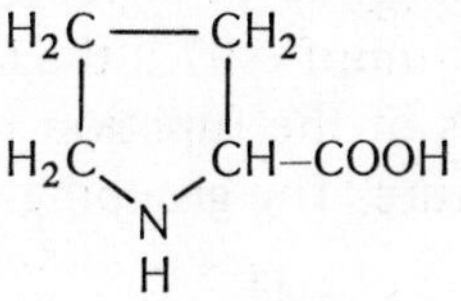

$$H_2C - CH_2$$
$$H_2C \diagdown \quad CH-COOH$$
$$N$$
$$H$$

Hydroxyproline

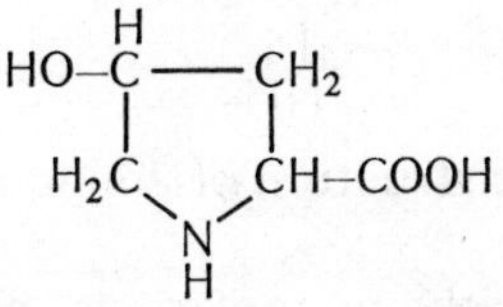

$$HO-\overset{H}{\underset{|}{C}} - CH_2$$
$$H_2C \diagdown \quad CH-COOH$$
$$N$$
$$H$$

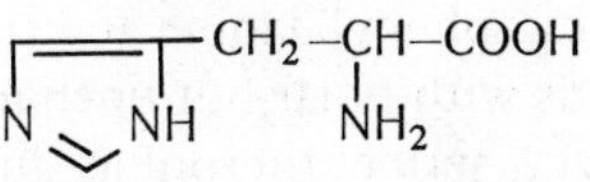

[b]Histidine

$$\overset{}{\boxed{}} - CH_2 - \underset{\underset{NH_2}{|}}{CH} - COOH$$
$$N \diagdown \; NH$$

[a]Tryptophan

$$CH_2 - \underset{\underset{NH_2}{|}}{CH} - COOH$$

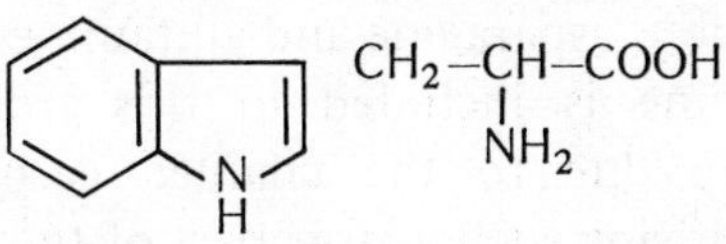

Diamino monocarboxylic (basic)
  Arginine

$$\overset{NH}{\underset{\|}{}}$$
$$H_2N - C - NH - CH_2 - CH_2 - CH_2 - \underset{\underset{NH_2}{|}}{CH} - COOH$$

[a]Lysine

$$H_2N - CH_2 - CH_2 - CH_2 - CH_2 - \underset{\underset{NH_2}{|}}{CH} - COOH$$

Monoamino dicarboxylic (acidic)
  Glutamic acid

$$HOOC - CH_2 - CH_2 - \underset{\underset{NH_2}{|}}{CH} - COOH$$

  Aspartic acid

$$HOOC - CH_2 - \underset{\underset{NH_2}{|}}{CH} - COOH$$

[a]Essential to the adult human.
[b]Essential to infants; may be essential to adults (Kopple and Swendseid, 1973).

their chemical nature. Amino acids also may be grouped according to the polarity of the R group attached to the alpha carbon atom. According to Conn and Stumpf (1972) the latter classification may be more significant in terms of the function that different amino acids perform in protein structure. The grouping is listed below:

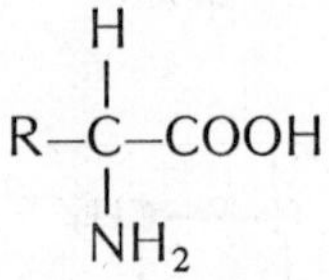

$$
\begin{array}{c}
H \\
| \\
R-C-COOH \\
| \\
NH_2
\end{array}
$$

Basic structure of amino acids

1. Amino acids with nonpolar or hydrophobic R groups:
   Aliphatic: alanine, valine, leucine, isoleucine, methionine.
   Aromatic: phenylalanine and tryptophan.
2. Amino acids with polar but uncharged R groups:
   Hydroxyl: serine, theronine, and tyrosine.
   Sulfhydryl: cysteine.
   Amide: asparagine and glutamine.
   (Glycine is included in this group because of its polar nature due to the charged carboxyl and amino groups comprising such a large part of the molecule.)
3. Amino acids with positively charged R groups:
   Amino: lysine
   Guanidine: arginine.
   Imidazole: histindine.
4. Amino acids with negatively charged R groups:
   Carboxyl: aspartic acid and glutamic acid.

Two diamino acids—ornithine and citrulline—probably do not

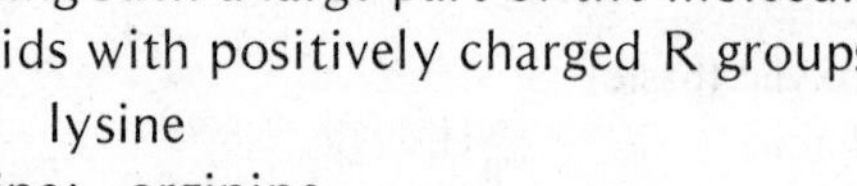

$$
NH_2-CH_2-CH_2-CH_2\underset{\underset{NH_2}{|}}{CH}-COOH
$$

Ornithine

$$
NH_2\overset{\overset{O}{\diagup\!\!\!\diagup}}{C}-NH-CH_2-CH_2-CH_2\underset{\underset{NH_2}{|}}{CH}-COOH
$$

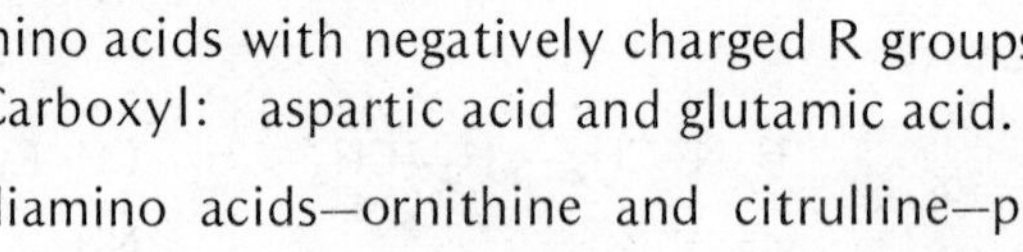

Citrulline

occur as constituents of protein molecules, but they are important intermediates in the formation of urea and thus contribute to the synthesis of arginine (see Chapter 15).

Functions of Protein and Individual Amino Acids. It would be impossible to discuss in detail the specific functions of all of the amino acids in the limited space that can be devoted to this subject. Certain reactions, however, will be mentioned briefly. It should not be assumed that these reactions are necessarily the most important of the many metabolic reactions in which the amino acids take part. Instead, they are merely examples intended to refresh memories and to stimulate further study.

Traditionally amino acids have been described as *ketogenic* and *glucogenic,* that is, they tend to give rise to acetoacetate or to carbohydrate intermediates. In light of the present knowledge of interrelated metabolic pathways, these terms are obsolete. Nonetheless, it is perhaps useful to remember that phenylalanine, tyrosine, leucine, and isoleucine are degraded in part to acetoacetate whereas other amino acids are degraded chiefly to pyruvate, oxaloacetate, α-ketoglutarate, succinate, and fumarate.

The dietary requirements of certain of the amino acids are influenced by the intake of other nutrients. For example, phenylalanine is converted to tyrosine in the animal cell. The dietary requirement for phenylalanine, therefore, is a function of the total aromatic amino acid content of the diet. Similarly, methionine may function metabolically as a precursor of other sulfur-containing amino acids so that both the dietary methionine and cystine determine the requirement for methionine. The relationship between tryptophan and nicotinic acid is another important example. Tryptophan may be metabolized to form nicotinic acid and, in so doing, contributes to the total amount of the vitamin available for cellular metabolism (see Chapter 3).

Many of the amino acids are precursors of other significant compounds required in metabolic processes. For example, tyrosine and, therefore, phenylalanine give rise to the hormones thyroxine and epinephrine. Glutamic acid, cysteine, and glycine are components of a tripeptide glutathione, which functions in cellular oxidation-reduction reactions. Sulfur-containing amino acids give rise to taurine, a bile acid component. Tryptophan may be metabolized to form serotonin (5-hydroxytryptamine), a tissue hormone that is found predominantly in serum, blood platelets, gastro-intestinal mucosa, and nerve tissue. Methionine provides methyl groups for synthesis of choline, creatine, and methylation of nicotinamide to its major excretion product N'-methylnicotinamide. Glycine contributes to the porphyrin ring of hemoglobin and, along with serine, provides part of the structure of the purines and pyrimidines of the nucleic acids. Two hydroxylated amino acids—hydroxyproline and hydroxylysine—are important constituents of collagen; approximately 12 percent of the total amino acid content of collagen is hydroxyproline.

This brief sketch should stimulate a thorough review of other equally important reactions in which amino acids are involved.

Protein Structure

The basic structure common to all proteins is the *peptide linkage,* which is formed by condensation of the carboxyl group of one amino acid with the amino group of another. In this way chains are created; these chains range from the smallest peptide units such as glutathione, which contains only 3 amino acids, to complex polymers of 1000 or more.

The sequence in which amino acids are arranged in the peptide chain is known as the *primary structure* of the molecule (Fig. 2.2). The proper sequence of amino acids tends to be a critical factor in protein function. In some heritable diseases, such as sickle cell anemia, the defect is due to the genetic substitution of only one amino acid for another in the hemoglobin molecule (see Chapter 16). Differences in the sequence of three amino acids in insulin from different species, however, do not affect the activity of the hormone, apparently because this three amino acid sequence is not an active site of the molecule (see Fig. 2.3).

Biological activity of a protein, however, depends not only on the sequence of the amino acids but also on the spatial arrangement of the long peptide chain. Although the peptide bond is the primary and also the strongest linkage in the protein polymer, other types of bonding occur. These additional linkages or *secondary bonds* are partly responsible for the arrangement of the molecule (see Fig. 2.2).

A very important linkage in the protein molecule is the hydrogen bond, a weak attachment between the hydrogen atom of an amino group and the oxygen of a carboxyl group (Fig. 2.4). A peptide

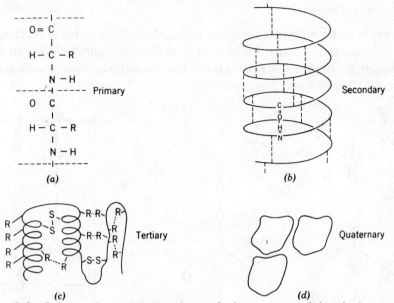

Fig. 2.2 Schematic representation of the structural levels in proteins. Amino acid chains are denoted by R, noncovalent interactions by · · ·. (From E. D. P. EdRoberts et al., *Cell Biology*, 5th ed., W. B. Saunders Co., Philadelphia, 1970, p. 53.)

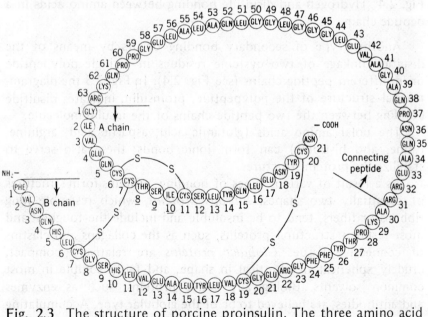

Fig. 2.3 The structure of porcine proinsulin. The three amino acid sequence (8, 9, 10) shows species difference: *cow:* Thr, Ser, Ile; *horse:* Thr, Gly, Ile; *sheep:* Ala, Gly, Val; *human:* Thr, Ser, Ile. [From R. E. Chance et al., *Science,* 161: 165 (1968).

chain may be held in a coiled or helical form by a series of hydrogen bonds that, although individually weak, are cumulatively strong enough to stabilize the structure. The uncharged polar amino acids are the sites of hydrogen bonding.

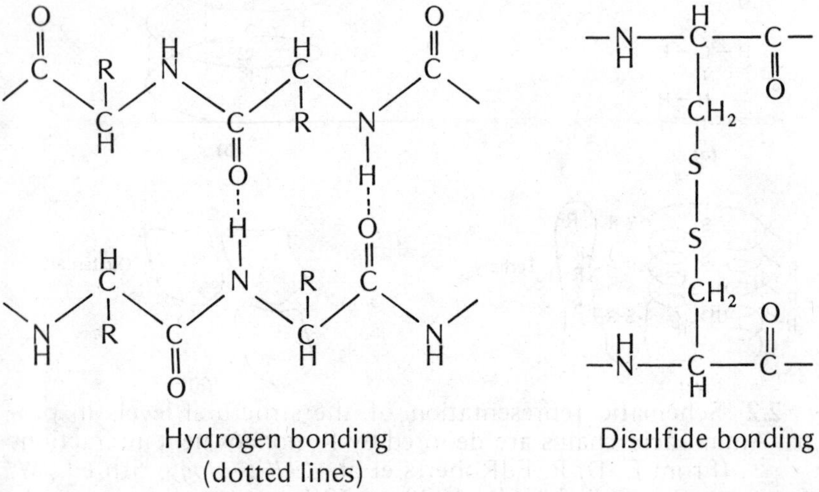

Hydrogen bonding
(dotted lines)

Disulfide bonding

Fig. 2.4 Hydrogen and disulfide bonding between amino acids in a peptide chain.

Another type of secondary bonding occurs by means of the disulfide linkage of two cysteine residues in a single polypeptide or in different peptide chains (see Fig. 2.4). In Fig. 2.3 the diagrammatical structure of the polypeptide, proinsulin, indicates disulfide bonding between the two peptide chains of the insulin molecule.

The polar amino acids (glutamic acid, aspartic acid, arginine, lysine, and histidine) can form ionic bonds; these also serve to stabilize the protein structures.

As a result of various types of bonding, proteins form structures of essentially two shapes. *Fibrous proteins*, which resemble long ribbons or fibers, tend to be insoluble and include the toughest and most resilient structural proteins, such as the collagens and elastins of connective tissue. *Globular proteins* are relatively compact, crudely spherical or elliptical in shape, and fairly soluble in most common solvents. Biologically active proteins, such as enzymes and antibodies, are believed to be of the globular type. Accumulating evidence indicates that the protein molecule tends to expose chiefly its polar groups to the aqueous environment of biological systems whereas nonpolar groups tend to be positioned internally.

In fibrous protein, hydrogen bonding predominates. Some fibers are essentially linear peptide chains bound together by hydrogen bonds that form a structure aptly described by Pauling as the *pleated sheet*. Most naturally occurring fibrous proteins, however, are probably arranged as α-helix chains coiled around each other to form a superhelix (Fig. 2.5). Both a right-handed α-helix and a triple helix are known to exist. Collagen is an example of a triple-stranded helix.

Globular proteins are formed into compact structures by the folding of one or more peptide chains due to secondary bonds between amino acids located at some distance from each other in the chain sequence. Some three-dimensional models have been determined, for example, for myoglobin (Kendrew, 1961). Both straight peptide chains and α-helix segments are present in this molecular structure. The secondary bonding appears to be chiefly by hydrogen and disulfide linkages.

The *tertiary structure* of a protein refers to the rigid compact structure of proteins produced by coiling and folding of the molecule (see Fig. 2.2). This structure is due to the various reactions

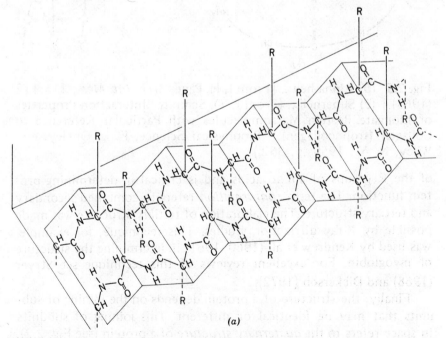

(a)

Fig. 2.5 (a) Pleated sheet structure of β-protein chains. (See the description in the text.) (From P. Karlson, 1963.)

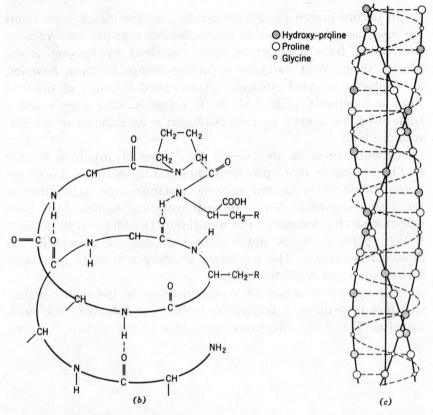

Hydroxy-proline
Proline
Glycine

Fig. 2.5 (*b*) Alpha-helix. [From I. H. Page, *Arch. Int. Med.*, 111:112 (1963).] (*c*) Superhelix. (From F. O. Schmitt "Interaction Properties of Elongate Protein Macromolecules with Particular Reference to Collagen (tropocollagen)," Biophysical Science, F. L. Oncley, ed., Wiley, N. Y., 1959, p. 352.)

of the R groups of amino acids and is critical in determining protein function. The term *conformation* refers to combined secondary and tertiary structure. The elaboration of tertiary structure was made possible by X-ray diffraction studies. This technique, for example, was used by Kendrew et al. (1960, 1961) indetermining the structure of myoglobin. For excellent reviews of this technique see Stryer (1968) and Dickerson (1972).

Finally, the structure of a protein depends on the joining of subunits that may be identical or different. This joining of subunits in space refers to the *quaternary structure* of a protein (see Fig. 2.2). Insulin, for example, contains two subunits, each of which is inactive alone as is its precursor, proinsulin (see Fig. 2.3). The antibody molecule functions as a trimer, and the plasma protein that binds both retinol and thyroxine for transport appears to be a tetramer (see Chapter 7). The number of subunits varies greatly among proteins from as few as two (which is commonly found) to as many as 2130 as in the complex protein, tobacco mosaic virus (Klotz and Darnall, 1969). For further details on quaternary structure of proteins see Klotz et al. (1970).

Protein Classification

Early systems devised for classification of proteins were based on solubility and chemical properties but such properties, determined on isolated proteins under laboratory conditions, are of only limited value when applied to living systems. The two broad structural groupings of proteins, fibrous and globular, while grossly related to biochemical function, are but a first step in the development of a classification of biological significance. As more data on protein structure become available it should be possible to establish a more precise system of classification with the ultimate aim of correlating structural characteristics with biochemical function (see Hess and Ruply, 1971).

Present information on structure and solubility may nevertheless be coordinated to provide a useful although likely an artificial and ill-defined system (Table 2.10). The problem of classification is further complicated by the realization that protein is usually present in the cell in combination with nonprotein substances, such as lipids, nucleic acids, carbohydrates, and various metals; these

Table 2.10 PROTEIN CLASSIFICATION

Protein	Characteristics	Example or Occurrence
Globular		
Albumins	Soluble in water, dilute salt solutions, dilute acids, and bases.	Lactalbumin Serum albumin
Globulins	Soluble in salt solutions, insoluble in water.	Serum globulin Myosin
Histones[a]	Basic proteins. Very soluble in most common solvents, fairly small molecules.	Nucleoprotein

Table 2.10 (Continued)

Protein	Characteristics	Example or Occurrence
Fibrous (scleroproteins)		
Collagens	Resistant to digestive enzymes; insoluble, converted to digestible proteins and gelatins on boiling; contain large amount of hydroxyproline; lack sulfur-containing amino acids.	Skin, tendons, bones
Elastins	Partially resistant to digestive enzymes; contain little hydroxyproline.	Arteries, tendons, elastic tissues
Keratins	Highly insoluble and resistant to digestive enzymes; high cystine content.	Skin, hair, nails
Proteids		
Nucleoproteins	Salts of basic protein or polypeptide and nucleic acids.	Chromosomes Nucleoli
Mucoproteins and	Protein or small polypeptide containing mucopolysaccharide; hexosamine content over 4%.	Glycoid of serum alpha globulin; submaxillary and gastric mucoids
Glycoproteins	Protein or small polypeptide containing mucopolysaccharide; hexosamine less than 4%.	Serum alpha, beta, and gamma globulins
Lipoproteins and	Complexes of protein and lipids having solubility properties of proteins.	Cell and organelle membranes
Proteolipids	Complexes of protein and lipids having solubility properties of lipids.	Myelin
Chromoproteins	Compounds consisting of proteins and a nonprotein pigment.	Flavoproteins Hemoglobin Cytochromes
Metalloproteins	Metals attached to protein; metals not part of a nonprotein prosthetic group.	Ferritin, Hemosiderin, Transferrin, Carbonic anhydrase
Phosphoproteins	Phosphoric acid joined in ester linkage to protein.	Casein of milk

[a]Protamines are polypeptides having similar solubility properties and containing as much as 70-80% of arginine.

conjugated proteins or *proteids* perform specific functions that neither constituent could properly perform alone. For example, neither the lipid nor protein moiety of a lipoprotein provides the requisite selectivity of a cell membrane; neither could riboflavin nor its associated protein individually perform the enzymatic function of a flavin nucleotide. In other words, neither protein nor any other cell constituents are apt to occur and function as single entities.

Protein and Amino Acid Deficiency

Uncomplicated protein or amino acid deficiency probably never occurs in man. The disease syndrome of kwashiorkor first described by Williams (1933) is believed to be due to protein deficiency, but it occurs to varying degrees in conjunction with calorie deficiency. For this reason the term protein-calorie malnutrition is preferred to the more limiting terms, kwashiorkor or marasmus (Behar et al., 1959) although the latter have not yet been discarded.

The disease syndrome is variable since the degree of both calorie and protein malnutrition, as well as other nutrients, will influence the biochemical and clinical changes (see Scrimshaw and Behar, 1959; McCance and Widdowson, 1968). In uncomplicated protein deficiency, for example, protein catabolism should be minimal; when total energy is the limiting factor, however, protein catabolism must increase to cover energy needs (see Chapter 23). Severe marasmus, or chronic starvation, is characterized by growth retardation, loss of body fat, and muscle wasting. When total caloric intake has been adequate or nearly adequate, as is possible when starchy low-protein foods are dietary staples, the symptoms are more toward changes associated with protein deficiency: pellagra-type dermatitis, fatty liver, changes in texture and pigmentation of hair, gastrointestinal disturbances, and diarrhea with resulting loss of electrolytes. The lesion appears to be the result of a deficiency of amino acids for protein synthesis and, indeed, most of the symptoms can be attributed to reduced synthesis. Analyses of liver biopsy samples suggest that approximately one-third of liver protein may be lost (Waterlow and Weisz, 1956). Enzyme changes are highly variable and depend both on the degree of deficiency and the tissue examined (Waterlow, 1959). Some differences and similarities in response to predominately protein deficiency (kwashiorkor) and calorie deficiency (marasmus) are shown in Table 2.11. The student is also referred to the excellent review by Waterlow and Alleyne (1971).

Table 2.11 COMPARISON OF CLINICAL AND BIOCHEMICAL LESIONS IN KWASHIORKOR AND MARASMUS

Lesion	Kwashiorkor	Marasmus
Cell division	Slightly below normal	Decreased
Basal O_2 consumption	Insignificant reduction	Decreased
Protein synthesis	Decreased	Equilibrium between growth rate and protein synthesis
Plasma proteins	Decreased	Normal or slightly low
Fatty liver	Present	Absent
Anemia	Moderate	Moderate
Blood glucose	Decreased	Decreased
Ratio of essential/ nonessential amino acids in serum	Decreased ratio	Normal ratio
Ratio of glycine, serine, and glutamic acid/branched-chain amino acids in serum	Increased ratio	Normal ratio
Hydroxyproline excretion	Decreased	Decreased
Serum FFA	Increased	Increased
Serum cholesterol, triglycerides, and phospholipids	Low	More normal

COMPLEXES OF CARBOHYDRATES, PROTEINS, AND LIPIDS

As mentioned earlier in this chapter, few nutrients occur or function alone in biological systems. The combinations are innumerable and many such unions will be discussed in later chapters. The following section is devoted to some of the more well-defined and identifiable complexes of carbohydrates, proteins and lipids. These include the glycoproteins, the glycolipids, and the lipoproteins.

Glycoproteins

Glycoproteins may be defined as biopolymers having amino acids and sugar residues linked covalently to each other (Montgomery,

1970). They differ from the mucopolysaccharide protein structures in that they contain considerably less carbohydrate. (The mucopolysaccharides, however, may be considered a type of glycoprotein.) The carbohydrate chains of glycoproteins are short, consisting of perhaps eight to ten saccharide units. D-galactose, N-acetyl-D-galactosamine, D-glucose, N-acetyl-D-glucosamine, D-mannose, L-fucose, and sialic acid (n-acetylneuraminic acid) comprise the bulk of the carbohydrate moiety. (Glucose, surprisingly, is relatively rare compared to the other sugars.) Of these compounds only sialic acid has not been discussed previously. The structure of this compound is shown below.

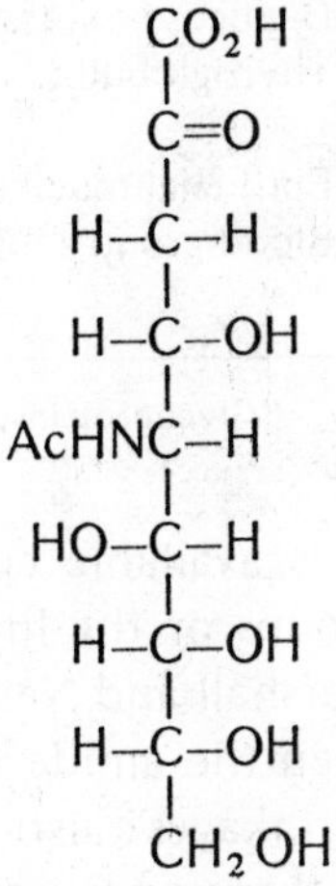

$$
\begin{array}{c}
CO_2H \\
| \\
C=O \\
| \\
H-C-H \\
| \\
H-C-OH \\
| \\
AcHNC-H \\
| \\
HO-C-H \\
| \\
H-C-OH \\
| \\
H-C-OH \\
| \\
CH_2OH
\end{array}
$$

Sialic acid (N-acetylneuraminic acid)

The amino acids and carbohydrates comprising the glycoprotein molecule are organized in two general ways. One type has a protein core, frequently of molecular weight less than 100,000, to which are attached a few oligosaccharide residues. The other type has a much higher molecular weight and is mainly carbohydrate in content and is organized as hundreds of small oligosaccharide residues covalently linked to a peptide core. The classification of some glycoproteins according to carbohydrate content is shown in Table 2.12, and the composition of some glycoproteins is shown in Table 2.13.

Table 2.12 CLASSIFICATION OF GLYCOPROTEINS ACCORD-
ING TO CARBOHYDRATE CONTENT

Classification	Example	Molecular Weight $\times 10^3$
Glycoproteins having one carbohydrate group in each protein group	Ovalbumin	44.5
	Soybean hemagglutinin	110
	Ceruloplasmin	143
	Transferrin	92
Glycoproteins having a few carbohydrate groups in each protein unit	Ovomucoid	28
	Fibrinogen	330
	Fetuin	46
	D-glucose oxidase	186
	Thyroglobulin	600
Glycoproteins having many carbohydrate groups in each protein unit	Epithelial mucins	1000
	Blood-group substance A	416

Adapted from R. Montgomery, "Glycoproteins," The Carbohydrates, Vol. IIB, Acad. Press, N. Y., 1970, pp. 627-709.

Very little information is available concerning the exact structure of the carbohydrate groups or the linkages of the carbohydrate
and peptide residues (see Marshall and Neuberger, 1970). A common
linkage appears to be between the amide nitrogen of asparagine and
N-acetyl-D-1-glucosamine. Linkages also may exist between the
hydroxyl group of serine or threonine and N-acetyl-D-galactosamine.
Another linkage common only to collagen unites the hydroxyl group
of hydroxylysine and D-galactose.

The class of glycoproteins includes a large number of biologically
active substances such as enzymes, hormones, and immunoglobulins
as well as structural components of blood vessels and skin. The
proteins in milk and egg white contain carbohydrates as do most
of the serum proteins. Examples of functions and types of glycoproteins are shown in Table 2.14.

Of particular interest are the glycoproteins associated with the
plasma membrane of the cells that coat the membrane surface
(see Chapter 9). These glycoproteins are likely involved in ion
transport and intercellular communication.

For a recent review of the glycoproteins see Sharon (1974).

Table 2.13 COMPOSITION OF SOME GLYCOPROTEINS. DATA ARE EXPRESSED AS MOLES OF COMPONENT PER MOLE OF GLYCOPROTEIN

	2	3	4	5	6	7
1	Human Parotid	"Principal Gastric	Human		Mouse H-2	Human Spleen
Glycoprotein	Glycoprotein	Glycoprotein"	Gastroferrin	α-Ovomucin	Antigen	HL-A
Aspartic acid	14.5	52	16	163	41	43
Threonine	0.9	580	76	124	31	20
Serine	11.4	296	40	134	28	23
Glutamic acid	45.9	87	19	189	54	67
Proline	73.8	418	49	90	29	23
Glycine	45.1	120	22	112	30	17
Alanine	1.2	210	25	80	30	43
Valine	1.3	58	16	100	23	18
½-Cystine		Trace	11	144	11	16
Methionine	0	0	3	13	9	5
Isoleucine	0.6	41	8	76	16	4
Leucine	1.4	81	13	106	36	43
Tyrosine	0	17	4	56	22	11
Phenylalanine	0	41	6	72	15	20
Lysine	11.0	29	11	91	18	33
Histidine	2.0	52	9	34	13	11
Arginine	10.8	52	9	45	21	16
Tryptophan				22		

(continued)

Table 2.13 (continued)

1 Glycoprotein	2 Human Parotid Glycoprotein	3 "Principal Gastric Glycoprotein"	4 Human Gastroferrin	5 α-Ovomucin	6 Mouse H-2 Antigen	7 Human Spleen HL-A
Glucose	+	0	0	0		4.4
Mannose		0	0	54		4.9
Galactose	+	3596	461	21		5.9
Fucose	8.9	2376	250	0		2.0
Sialic acid	2.2	133	30	7	2	0.4
Glucosamine	27.3	2726	+	63		6.1
Galactosamine		928	+	6		1.0
Total neutral sugar	22.6	5972	711	75	~17	17.2
Total hexosamine	27.3	3654	407	69	~13	7.1
Acetyl			~400			
Sulfate		1218	40	15		
10^3 x molecular weight	34.5	2040	263	210	55	45

From R. D. Marshall, "Glycoproteins," Ann. Rev. Biochem., 41: 693 (1972).

Table 2.14 DISTRIBUTION AND FUNCTION OF SOME GLYCO-
PROTEINS

Presumed Function	Name
Structural	Bacterial cell wall
	Collagen
	Mucopolysaccharides
Food reserve	κ-Casein
	Endosperm glycoproteins
	Ovalbumin, ovomucoid
	Pollen allergens
Enzyme	Bromelin
	Fungal glucoamylase
	Prothrombin
	Ribonuclease B
	Taka-amylase A
Transport	Ceruloplasmin
	Thyroglobulin
	Transferrin
Hormone	Erythropoietin
	Interstitial cell-stimulating hormone
	Thyroglobulin
Plasma and body fluids	Fetuin
	Fibrinogen
	α, β, and γ-Glycoproteins
	Plasminogen
"Protective"	Blood-group substances
	Epithelial mucins
	Fibrin
	γ-Globulins

From R. Montgomery, "Glycoproteins," The Carbohydrates, Vol. IIB, Acad. Press, N. Y., 1970, pp. 627-709.

Glycolipids

Glycolipids may be defined as compounds that have the solubility properties of a lipid and contain one or more molecules of a sugar. They are often associated with protein in biological systems. The classification of glycolipids is difficult and confusing as different terms are often used by different workers. For the purpose of this discussion we will follow the nomenclature developed by the IUPAC-IUB Commission on Biochemical Nomenclature (1967). Further we will be concerned only with those glycolipids of animal origin.

Many animal glycolipids are derivatives of a class of compounds known as *ceramides*. These compounds are formed from 4-sphingenine (sphingosine) in which the hydrogen of the amino group attached to carbon 2 is replaced by a long chain acyl group. The fatty acids vary depending upon the tissue source, but they usually contain 16 to 24 carbons and are generally saturated. Fatty acids from some tissue ceramides may contain hydroxyl groups at the carbon-2 position or they may contain an odd number of carbon atoms (see McKibbon, 1970). The sugars present in glycolipids are D-glucose, D-galactose, D-galactose-3-sulfate, L-fucose, 2-acylamido-2-deoxy-D-galactose, 2-acylamido-2-deoxy-D-glucose, and sialic acid. The carbohydrate components contain from one to seven monosaccharides linked in straight or branched chains and glycosidically linked to the primary alcohol group (C-1) of the sphingenine base.

The relationship of these principal glycolipids—the cerebrosides, sulfatides, and gangliosides—to the ceramides and the sphingenine molecule is shown in Table 2.15.

Cerebrosides (and sulfatides) are present in a large amount in the white matter of brain. The myelin cerebrosides are 1-*O*-β-D-galactopyranosylceramides. The fatty acids of brain cerebrosides generally contain 18 to 24 carbons; they may be even or odd numbered and often contain carbon-2 hydroxyl groups (Kishimoto and Radin, 1966). Cerebrosides are also found in other tissues including blood serum, erythrocytes, liver, spleen, and kidney, but the amounts present are usually considerably less than that found in brain myelin.

Gangliosides also are present in high amounts in brain tissue and in lesser amounts in other tissues. In many animal species 79 to 96 percent of the fatty acid in brain gangliosides is stearic acid (Trams et al., 1962).

A number of heritable diseases are due to enzyme deficiencies that result in the abnormal accumulation of glycolipids in various tissues. These include ganglioside accumulation in Tay-Sachs disease and neurovisceral gangliosidosis and cerebroside accumulation in

Table 2.15 RELATIONSHIP OF 4-SPHINGENINE TO CERA-MIDES AND GLYCOLIPIDS

$$
\begin{array}{ccccc}
 & \overset{\displaystyle RNH}{|} & \overset{\displaystyle OH}{|} & \overset{\displaystyle H}{|} & \\
R^1OCH_2-C & \!\!\!\!-\!\!\!\!- C & \!\!\!\!-\!\!\!\!- C & \!\!=\!\! C-C_{13}H_{27} \\
 & \underset{\displaystyle H}{|} & \underset{\displaystyle H}{|} & \underset{\displaystyle H}{|} &
\end{array}
$$

	R	R^1
4-Sphingenine	H	H
Ceramide	Long chain fatty acyl group	H
Cerebrosides[a] (1-O-monoglycosyl ceramide)	Long chain fatty acyl group	Glycosyl group
Sulfatides	Long chain fatty acyl group	Glycosyl sulfate (usually galactose sulfated at C-3)
Gangliosides	Long chain fatty acyl group	Oligosaccharide chain containing one or more sialic acid

[a] 1-O-diglycosylceramides ("cytosides") contain a lactosyl group at R^1.
1-O-oligoglyceramides contain an oligosaccharide chain at R^1.

Gaucher's disease, Fabry's disease, and metachromatic leucodystrophy. These diseases are usually fatal in early childhood. Victims of Fabry's disease, however, often survive well into adulthood.

The function of the glycolipids as components of the plasma membrane will be discussed in Chapter 9. For more detailed information concerning these compounds see Carter et al. (1965), McKibbin (1970), and Gurr and James (1971).

Lipoproteins

Lipids and proteins are associated in a wide variety of complexes that are significant in both the structure and function of cells. The exact nature of the lipid-protein bond is not well defined. Indeed much remains to be learned about these complex entities. Lipo-

Table 2.16 CLASSIFICATION AND COMPOSITION OF HUMAN SERUM LIPOPROTEINS

Class	Density Range[a] (g/ml)	S_f^b	Approximate Molecular Weight (in millions)	Composition (%)[b]			
				Protein	Triglyceride	Phospho-lipid	Others
Chylomicrons	0.95	400	10^3-10^4	2	83	7	8
VLDL	0.95-1.006	20-400	5-100	9	50	18	22
LDL	1.006-1.063	0-20	2-3	21	11	22	46
HDL	1.063-1.21	0-6	0.25	50	8	22	20

[a]Schumaker and Adams (1969).
[b]Gurr and James (1970).

proteins appear to be of two types. Those which exist as relatively discrete and identifiable macromolecules are called *soluble types*. Those that are aggregates of the complex membrane structure are called *membrane types or structural lipoproteins*. The latter type are those that are most difficult to characterize precisely.

Most soluble lipoproteins circulate in the blood plasma. Some are involved in blood clotting (see Barton, 1969 and Chapter 4 for further discussion of blood clotting factors). The combination of lipid and protein is advantageous because it makes possible the transport of a host of water-insoluble lipid compounds. The mechanism that permits lipid solubility is not well understood. It has been suggested that protein and more polar lipids form most of the lipoprotein surface whereas the less polar lipids, chiefly cholesterol esters and triacyl glycerols, form an inner core. Some experimental evidence supports this concept (see Scanu and Wisdom, 1972).

The ratio of lipid to protein in the serum lipoproteins varies widely and these variations affect their density. For this reason the serum lipoproteins may be separated and classified according to their density. Separations are accomplished by flotation in an ultracentrifuge with the rate of flotation expressed as an S_f value. Table 2.16 shows a classification and approximate composition of the major human serum lipoproteins that includes the chylomicrons, the very low density lipoproteins (VLDL), low density lipoproteins (LDL), and the high density lipoproteins (HDL). These fractions range in protein content from the lowest density chylomicrons containing 2 percent protein to the HDL containing 50 percent protein.

For a more detailed discussion of the lipoproteins see Tria and Scanu (1969) and Scanu and Wisdom (1972).

The structural lipoproteins that form an integral part of cell and organelle membranes will be discussed in Chapter 9.

NUCLEOTIDES AND NUCLEIC ACIDS

Nucleotides consist of three parts: a nonprotein heterocyclic nitrogen base, ribose (or deoxyribose), and a phosphate group (or groups). In most cases the base is a purine or pyrimidine, but one important nucleotide contains niacinamide. The latter will be discussed in Chapter 3. The structures of the purines and pyrimidines are shown in Fig. 2.6.

The nitrogen base is attached to carbon 1 of the pentose sugar that in turn is attached to the phosphate group at carbon 5. The basic structure of the nucleotides is shown below.

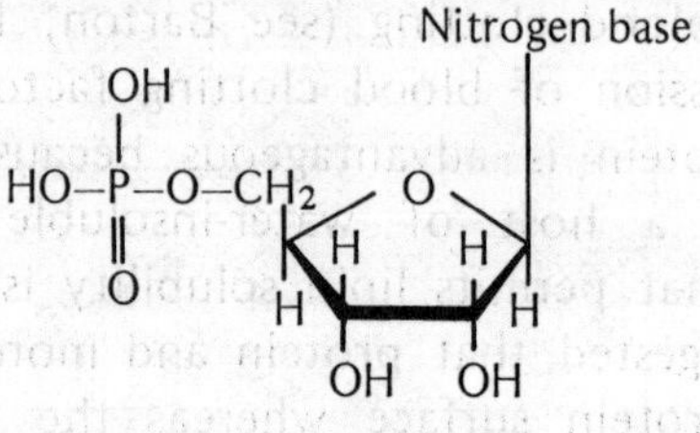

Nitrogen base

$$HO-\underset{\underset{O}{\overset{\parallel}{\underset{}{}}}{\overset{OH}{\underset{}{\overset{|}{P}}}}-O-CH_2$$

A ribose nucleotide

Nucleotides without the phosphate group are called nucleosides. Both take their names from the nitrogen base present in the formula. The purines and pyrimidines and their corresponding nucleosides and nucleotides are shown in Table 2.17.

Table 2.17 THE MAJOR PURINES AND PYRIMIDINES AND THEIR CORRESPONDING NUCLEOSIDES AND NUCLEOTIDES

Nitrogen Base	Nucleoside	Nucleotide
Purines		
Adenine (6-amino purine)	Adenosine	Adenosine monophosphate (AMP) or adenylic acid
Guanine (2-amino-6-oxypurine)	Guanosine	Guanosine monophosphate (GMP) or guanylic acid
Hypoxanthine (6-oxypurine)	Inosine	Inosine monophosphate (IMP) or inosinic acid
Pyrimidines		
Uracil (2,6-dioxypyrimidine)	Uridine	Uridine monophosphate (UMP) or uridylic acid
Cytosine (2-oxy-6-amino pyrimidine)	Cytidine	Cytidine monophosphate (CMP) or cytidylic acid
Thymine (5-methyl uracil)	Thymidine	Thymidine monophosphate (TMP) or thymidylic acid

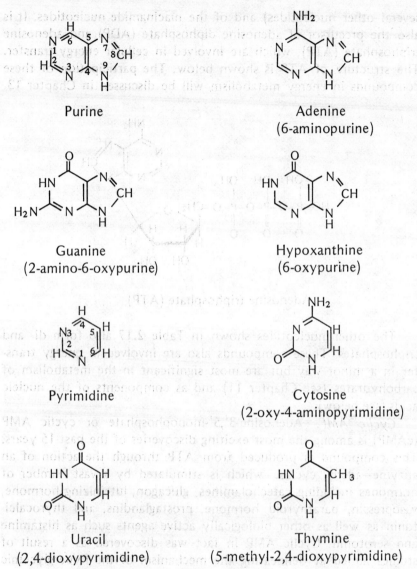

Fig. 2.6 Structure of the purines and pyrimidines.

The nucleotides are important in cellular metabolism. Nucleosides, as such, rarely are involved in metabolic reactions and are significant chiefly as components of the nucleotides.

Adenosine-5'-monophosphate (AMP) is one of the most important of the nucleotides. It is a part of the nucleic acids (as are several other nucleotides) and of the niacinamide nucleotides. It is also the precursor of adenosine diphosphate (ADP) and adenosine triphosphate (ATP), which are involved in cellular energy transfer. The structure of ATP is shown below. The participation of these compounds in energy metabolism will be discussed in Chapter 13.

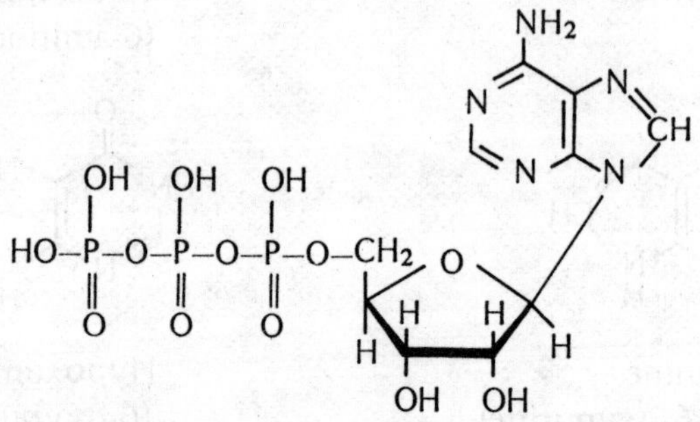

Adenosine triphosphate (ATP)

The other nucleotides shown in Table 2.17 also form di- and triphosphates. These compounds also are involved in energy transfer in a minor way but are most significant in the metabolism of carbohydrates (see Chapter 11) and as components of the nucleic acids (see below).

Cyclic AMP. Adenosine-3′,5′-monophosphate or cyclic AMP (cAMP) is among the most exciting discoveries of the past 15 years. This compound is produced from ATP through the action of an enzyme—adenyl cyclase—which is stimulated by a vast number of hormones including catecholamines, glucagon, luteinizing hormone, vasopressin, parathyroid hormone, prostaglandins, and thyrocalcitonin as well as other biologically active agents such as histamine and serotonin. Cyclic AMP in fact was discovered as a result of studies aimed at delineating the mechanism of the hyperglycemic action of epinephrine and glucagon (see Robison et al., 1971). The structure of cAMP is shown below.

Cyclic AMP has been described by Sutherland (see Robison et al., 1968) as a *second messenger* indicating that cAMP mediates the effects of hormones and other active agents. The number and variety of agents stimulating cAMP synthesis would suggest that

Adenosine-3',5'-monophosphate (cAMP)

the reactions influenced by this cyclic nucleotide are extremely varied. Indeed cAMP plays a regulatory role in cellular metabolism and controls the rate of a number of cellular reactions as varied as the synthesis and activity of proteins, glycogenolysis, lipolysis, steroidogenesis, and active transport. This ubiquitious compound will be discussed further in Parts III and IV. For excellent reviews on this subject see Robison et al. (1971), Hardman et al. (1971), and Jost and Rickenberg (1971).

Nucleic Acids

Nucleic acids are polynucleotides formed by the joining together of many mononucleotides. Two types of nucleic acids exist: deoxyribonucleic acid (DNA) and ribonucleic acid (RNA). They are distinguished by differences in the pentose in the molecule and by the structure of one of the four nucleotide bases present in the molecule.

DNA. DNA is made up of four nucleotides: AMP, TMP, CMP, and GMP that contain, respectively, the bases adenine, thymine, cytosine, and guanine. Deoxyribose is the pentose component. These four nucleotides are linked together in long polymeric chains, the 3-hydroxyl of the pentose joined to the phosphate of the adjacent nucleotide (Fig. 2.6). The pairing of the two strands always occurs by the sharing of three hydrogen bonds by cytosine and guanine and the sharing of two hydrogen bonds by adenine and thymine (Fig. 2.7). The pairing of bases and the double helical structure of the molecule discovered and described by Watson and Crick (1953) is characteristic of all DNA from the simplest

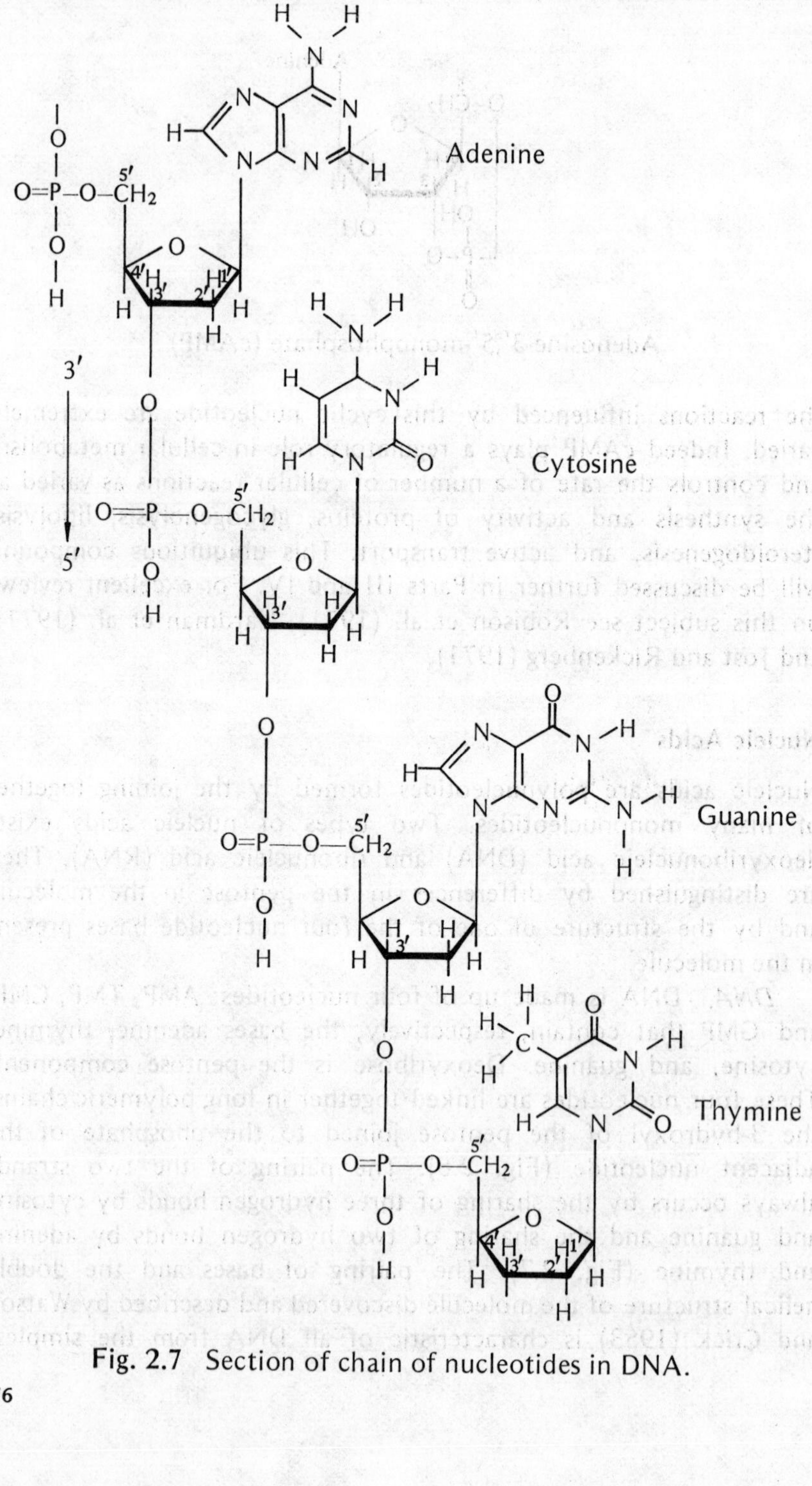

Fig. 2.7 Section of chain of nucleotides in DNA.

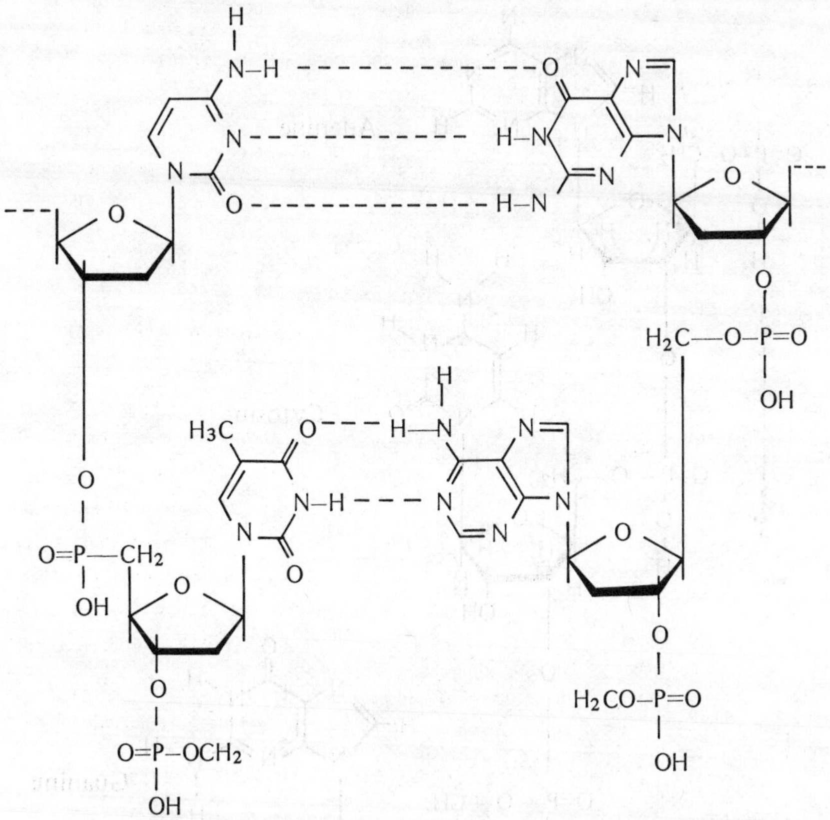

Fig. 2.8 Section of helix showing details of base-pairing.

one-celled organism to the most specialized cell of the largest mammals. The differences in the DNA, and therefore the differences in the genes and characteristics of species, are due to the order of the nucleotides in the strand and to the length of the strand which can vary from several thousand angstroms (Å) to several millimeters (1 mm = 10^7 Å). The sequence of the nucleotides in the strand provides the code for genetic information (see Chapter 10).

The established sequence of the nucleotides in one DNA strand will always determine the sequence in the paired strand. This provides the means whereby DNA can replicate itself and, barring error, transmit the exact code to a daughter cell. Replication takes place under the influence of the enzyme DNA polymerase. Kornberg (1960) purified DNA polymerase from *Escherichia coli* and found

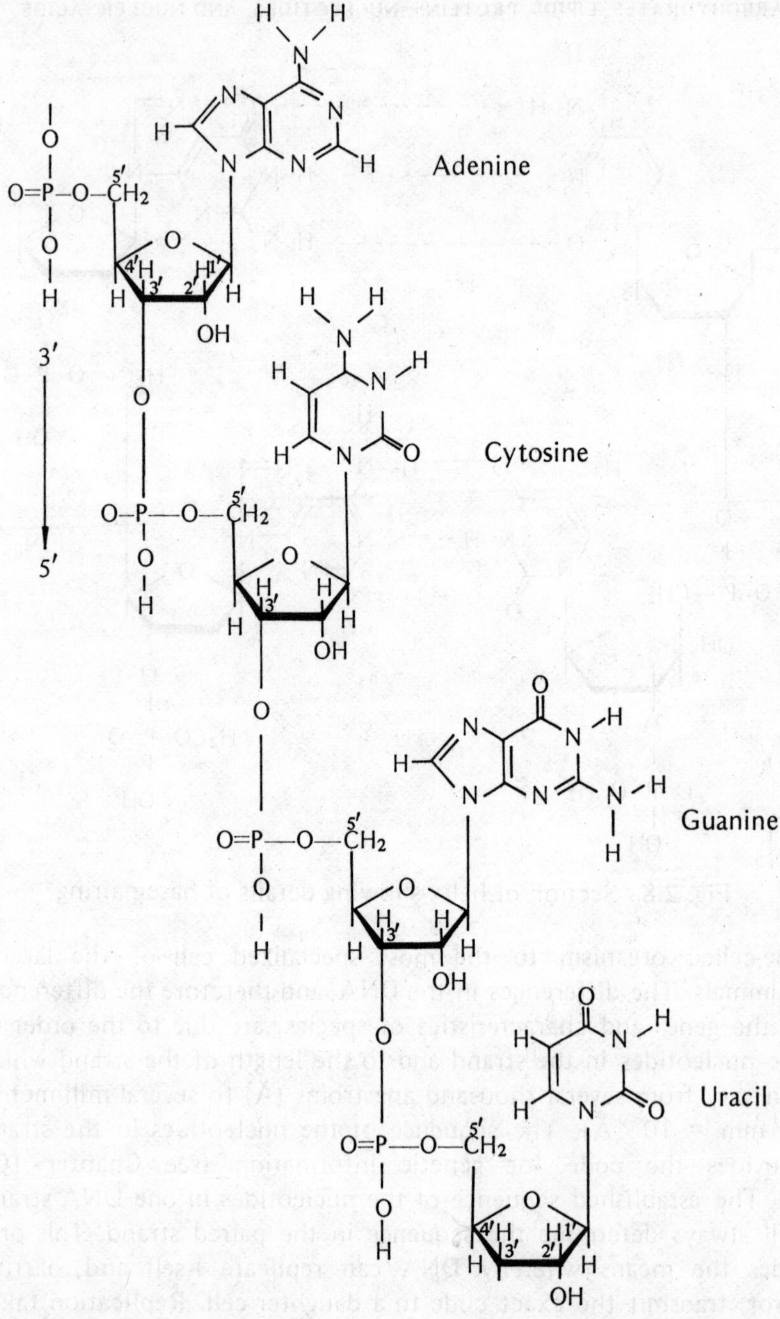

Fig. 2.9 Section of nucleotide chain of RNA showing substitution of ribose for deoxyribose and uracil for thymine.

that with the enzyme, a strand of DNA as a template, and a supply of nucleotides the synthesis of DNA could proceed *in vitro*. The enzyme produced long chains of nucleotides by base-pairing to produce a macromolecule with most of the properties associated with DNA isolated from nature.

RNA. The chemical constituents of RNA differ from those in DNA in two respects: the pentose is ribose instead of deoxyribose, and uracil is substituted for thymine, making the base content cytosine, guanine, adenine, and uracil (Fig. 2.9). When DNA acts as the template for the synthesis of a DNA strand, thymine will pair with adenine; however, when DNA is the template for RNA synthesis, uracil links with adenine. The regulation and separation of the two kinds of DNA template activity is undoubtedly under the control of specific mechanisms since they must and do occur at different times.

The structure of mRNA differs from DNA in that it is a single-strand polymer containing only hundreds of subunits, whereas DNA is a double helical structure with many thousands of subunits. Another type of RNA, transfer or soluble RNA (tRNA), is a single-strand polymer with about 70 subunits, but ribosomal RNA (rRNA) is a globular structure. These forms of RNA collaborate in the transfer and assembly of specific amino acids for protein synthesis and will be discussed in Chapter 11.

chapter 3

water-soluble vitamins

Water-Soluble Vitamins: Chemistry, Biochemical Function

a. Thiamin
b. Riboflavin
c. Niacin
d. Vitamin B$_6$
e. Pantothenic Acid

f. Folacin
g. Vitamin B$_{12}$
h. Biotin
i. Ascorbic Acid

The goal of vitamin research is to establish (1) the abnormalities that result when a vitamin is absent from the diet and therefore from cellular metabolism; (2) the metabolic functions that depend on the presence of the vitamin; and (3) a reconciliation between the two. The last goal is the most difficult to attain and, by far, the area in which least is known. In historical perspective and investigational procedure, knowledge of the deficiency disease syndromes must come first. For the modern nutritionist, however, it is clearly more important to think in terms of what vitamins *do* rather than the diseases they prevent.

Vitamins are chemically unrelated organic substances that are grouped together because each is essential in the diet in minute amounts and is required for specific metabolic reactions within the cell. Traditionally they are classified according to their solubility in water or fat and fat solvents and, from a physiological standpoint, this property determines the patterns of transport, excretion, and storage within the animal body. Several of the vitamins, while conveniently considered as a single substance, actually are a group of structurally related compounds that tend to behave alike physiologically. In general, however, physiological function tends to be limited to one active form to which the related forms are converted.

Whether a substance must be supplied intact to the cell or can be synthesized by the cell depends on the assortment of enzymes peculiar to the cell species. A substance, therefore, may be a vitamin for one species but not for another. The difference lies in whether the substance is required in the diet or whether it can be synthesized by the animal. The number of substances supplied by cellular synthesis tends to vary inversely with the complexity of the organism and appears to reflect an evolutionary adaptation as more complex organisms evolved from a simple one cell origin. Thus man is dependent on his environment for some nutrients that microorganisms and other lower forms of life can synthesize for themselves.

All of the vitamins of the B-complex are known to function as coenzymes. Coenzyme functions, however, have not yet been defined for the fat-soluble vitamins or for ascorbic acid. There seems to be little doubt, however, that all vitamins, like the hormones, play fundamental catalytic roles in specific metabolic reactions although some vitamins (e.g., ascorbic acid and vitamin E) also function in a more general fashion. It is conceivable that the apparent general function may be a secondary effect elicited by a single specific, yet unknown, biochemical action at a variety of sites.

A *coenzyme* may be defined as a small molecule loosely bound to an enzyme protein, or apoenzyme, and easily separated from the protein moiety by dialysis. A *prosthetic* group refers to a molecule that is firmly bound to the enzyme protein and that, on dialysis, remains bound to the enzyme protein. The distinction between the two is of little functional significance and, most often, the two terms are used interchangeably. Both serve as cofactors in enzymatic reactions and contain one of the active sites of the enzyme complex to which the substrate is attached. For most enzyme systems, the active site is a part of the vitamin structure.

Certain compounds similar in structure to the vitamin molecule (or to the portion of the molecule containing the active site) can replace the vitamin by attaching themselves to the enzyme. These substances are called *antimetabolites* or *metabolic antagonists*. They block the normal action of the coenzyme and, in effect, result in a cellular deficiency of the vitamin. Certain other antimetabolites exhibit antivitamin activity because they are capable of blocking biosynthesis of the coenzyme molecule; such compounds may or may not resemble the vitamin in structure. In either case, a condition similar to true vitamin deficiency is produced. Antimetabolites are useful in producing experimental vitamin deficiencies, especially those deficiencies that develop slowly from dietary restriction alone. Antimetabolites are also useful adjuncts in delineating the bio-chemical pathways in which the vitamin is involved and in relating metabolic disturbances to symptoms of deficiency. (For discussions of antimetabolites see Woolley, 1944, 1963; and Somogyi, 1966.)

Significantly, the vitamins were discovered not by their presence in the diet but because of their absence. A lack of most of the vitamins known to be required by the human results in typical clinical syndromes or symptoms that can be cured by adding the necessary vitamin to the diet. This negative approach to the function of the vitamins is a useful tool in research. The investigator obtains some clues to the metabolic role of nutrients when he observes the functional failures that result when the nutrient is absent from the diet.

Carefully controlled studies with many species of animals thus have helped to elucidate the role of vitamins in man since most monogastric mammals tend to metabolize most vitamins similarly. Even microorganisms, however, have contributed to knowledge of human nutrition and are useful as test organisms for nutrient analyses. The microbiological assay and the rat and chick bioassays all take advantage of the requirement of these species for specific nutrients since growth response due to an unknown amount of vitamin in food may be measured directly against response to a known amount of pure vitamin.

The clinical course of deficiency, however, may vary widely among species; symptoms observed in a rat, for example, often are quite different from those observed in chicks or in man. Biochemical lesions tend to be more similar.

To establish that vitamin deficiency results in growth failure or dermatitis or any other symptom establishes a nutrient as essential in the diet and defines the deficiency syndrome so that it can be recognized when it occurs naturally (Table 3.1). It does not, however, establish the function of the nutrient. Only by careful

Table 3.1 VITAMIN DEFICIENCY SYMPTOMS IN MAN

Vitamin	Symptoms
Thiamin	Beriberi: chiefly nervous and cardiovascular systems affected; mental confusion, muscular weakness, loss of ankle and knee jerks, painful calf muscles, peripheral paralysis, edema (wet beriberi), muscle wasting (dry beriberi), enlarged heart. Infantile beriberi: cyanosis, dyspnea, tachycardia, aphonia (soundless crying), eventual cardiac failure.
Riboflavin	Ariboflavinosis: cheilosis, angular stomatitis (fissures at the corners of the mouth), nasolabial dermatitis, photophobia, corneal vascularization (not specific).
Nicotinic Acid	Pellagra: bilateral dermatitis particularly in areas exposed to sunlight, glossitis, diarrhea, irritability, mental confusion, eventually delirium or psychotic symptoms.
Pyridoxine	Convulsions in infants. Experimental deficiency in man: seborrheic dermatitis, glossitis, angular stomatitis, abnormal EEG.
Pteroylglutamic acid (folic acid)	Glossitis, gastrointestinal disturbances, diarrhea, megaloblastic anemia.
Vitamin B_{12}	Pernicious anemia, generally due to genetic lack of intrinsic factor. Dietary deficiency occasionally seen in strict vegetarians.
Ascorbic acid	Scurvy: red, swollen, bleeding gums, perifolliculosis, poor wound healing, subcutaneous hemorrhage, swelling of joints.
Vitamin A	Night blindness (nyctalopia), hyperkeratinization of epithelial tissues, xerophthalmia.

and often tedious probing to determine the specific metabolic reactions affected by nutrient deficiency have the basic functions of many of the vitamins been delineated. If we think of cellular metabolism as a series of reactions that eventually lead to the complete oxidation of foodstuffs, or the synthesis of a phospholipid or of an enzyme protein, it is not difficult to visualize the havoc that could result if any *one* reaction in the chain is blocked. The experimental nutritionist plays the role of detective who follows a long list of clues before he finally establishes the motive and the culprit of a committed crime. The path is often long and arduous.

Thiamin

The disease beriberi had been known for several centuries before its dietary origin was recognized. Beriberi is characterized by extensive damage to the nervous and cardiovascular systems and may be accompanied by severe muscle wasting (dry beriberi) or edema (wet beriberi). In the late nineteenth century, Takaki, a surgeon in the Japanese navy, demonstrated that addition of meat and whole grains to the customary naval ration resulted in a marked decrease in the incidence of what was then known as "shipboard beriberi," Some 15 years after Takaki's finding, Eijkmann made his famous observations of a beriberi-type syndrome (characterized by a peculiar head retraction obviously of neurological origin) in birds maintained on a diet of highly polished rice. He was able to cure the disease with rice bran. The proper interpretation of Eijkmann's work, however, was left to Grijns, another Dutch physician, who theorized that the disease was due to the lack of a dietary constituent in polished rice that was present in the whole grain. It was not until 1926 that the vitamin was isolated by another group in the Dutch East Indies, Jansen and Donath. Ten years later Williams and Cline (1936) won the race to develop a successful method for synthesis of thiamin; this discovery led to large-scale commercial production of the vitamin.

Prior to the commercial synthesis of the vitamin, research on thiamin had been limited to a few laboratories. The yield of thiamin isolated from rice bran, for example, was in the order of 5 grams of the vitamin for every ton of bran. Availability of the synthetic vitamin permitted rapid treatment of patients known to be suffering from beriberi; only a few milligrams of the vitamin are necessary to promote dramatic improvement. The early history of thiamin and the drive to eradicate beriberi as a serious threat to the public health has been recorded by Williams (1961).

Chemistry. Thiamin is a relatively simple chemical compound composed of a pyrimidine and a thiazole ring; it is available commercially both in the hydrochloride and the mononitrate forms. Thiamin hydrochloride is a white crystalline solid and is stable when in dry form. It is highly soluble in water and fairly soluble in 95 percent alcohol and absolute ethyl alcohol. In acid solution the

Thiamin

vitamin is quite stable at temperatures up to 120°C. In alkaline solution the vitamin decomposes rapidly; decomposition is hastened by heat. Thiamin mononitrate is also a white crystalline substance. It is quite soluble in water and is more stable to heat than the hydrochloride. For this reason, thiamin mononitrate often is preferred for fortification of cereal products that have to be cooked.

When treated with potassium ferricyanide in alkaline solution, thiamin is converted to a fluorescent compound called thiochrome. This reaction is the basis for the most commonly used chemical determination for the vitamin (see *Association of Official Agricultural Chemists,* 1960; Association of Vitamin Chemists, 1966). Thiamin also reacts with diazotized para-aminoacetophenone to form a red-colored complex that can be measured spectrophotometrically. Various microbiological techniques also have been described (Baker and Sobotka, 1962; Baker et al., 1964; Baker and Frank, 1968). These methods are both sensitive and relatively simple in operation. Other more recent methods include reaction of thiamin with lithium picrolonate and with bromothymol blue, spectrophotofluorometric assay, paper chromatography, thin layer chromatography, electrophoresis, and polarography (see McCormick and Wright, 1970).

Biochemical Function. As early as 1911 the decarboxylation of pyruvic acid by yeast cells was known to depend on an enzyme—carboxylase. This reaction was shown to require Mg^{2+}. Twenty-five years later Peters (1936) reported that thiamin was necessary for carbohydrate metabolism in pigeons and that pyruvate accumulated in tissues of thiamin-deficient birds. This discovery marked the first time that the action of a vitamin had been defined in terms of intermediary metabolism (see Thompson, 1971). In the following year the coenzyme of the carboxylase enzyme was isolated from yeast by Lohmann and Schuster (1937) and shown to be thiamin pyrophosphate (TPP). The coenzyme was originally called co-carboxylase and later was known as diphosphothiamin.

Thiamin pyrophosphate (TPP)

Phosphorylation of free thiamin to the coenzyme requires ATP. The active site of the coenzyme at which combination with substrate takes place is carbon 2 of the thiazole ring, indicated in the formula for TPP by an asterisk. The carboxylase system is a mixture of thiamin, Mg^{2+} or Mn^{2+}, and the apoenzyme protein. Both a mono- and triphosphate of thiamin are known to be present in peripheral nerves and blood of rats (Rindi et al., 1968). Their presence in nerve tissue led to the suggestion that the mono- and triphosphates perform a useful function in nerve cells (Muralt, 1962). Apparently thiamin triphosphate can also function as a coenzyme for carboxylase and is more stable than TPP (see Pollak, 1969).

TPP functions in several critical metabolic reactions in mammalian cells.

1. Oxidative decarboxylation of a-keto acids to carboxylic acids.
   a. Pyruvic acid $\longrightarrow$ acetyl CoA
   b. a-Ketoglutarate $\longrightarrow$ succinyl CoA
2. Transketolase reaction of pentose phosphate shunt: transfer of an a-keto group from xylulose-5-phosphate to ribose-5-phosphate to form sedoheptulose-7-phosphate and glyceraldehyde-3-phosphate.

Thiamin is also known to be involved in the conversion of glyoxylate to carbon dioxide and formate. As a result, methyl glyoxal accumulates in thiamin-deficient rats (Liang, 1963).

Each of these reactions involves a cleavage of the carbon-carbon bond adjacent to an a-keto group and formation of an aldehyde or carboxyl group. Either Mg^{2+} or Mn^{2+} is required for enzymatic activity; apparently these ions are involved in binding TPP to the enzyme. A more detailed discussion of reactions involving TPP is given in Chapters 11 and 13; also see Sauberlich (1967); Krampitz (1969); and Ullrich et al. (1970).

Although the clinical syndrome of thiamin deficiency (see Table 3.1) and biochemical function of the vitamin are well defined, very little is known of how disturbances in metabolic function caused by thiamin deficiency lead to the pathology so characteristic of the disease. One of the first symptoms of thiamin deficiency in experimental animals, for example, is anorexia and subsequent loss of weight. Bai et al. (1971) reported that a decrease in transketolase activity of intestinal mucosa correlated more closely with the development of anorexia than did decrease in pyruvate dehydrogenase activity. This evidence, however, as the authors point out, does not establish that anorexia is the result of decreased mucosal transketolase activity. Instead, transketolase activity is known to be affected early in thiamin deficiency (Brin, 1962) and may well simply coincide with the development of anorexia.

Handler (1958) suggested possible mechanisms for the neurological damage associated with thiamin deficiency. One is that the deficiency results in the inability of nerve cells to obtain sufficient energy supply or essential metabolites due to a reduction in glucose oxidation. Another suggestion is that the buildup of toxic substances such as pyruvic acid or methyl glyoxal (pyruvic aldehyde) may cause certain symptoms. According to Handler the latter alternative seems most likely. Admittedly lack of energy per se would not seem to be entirely responsible for the syndrome peculiar to beriberi since deficiencies of other vitamins that do not result in beriberi also are known to interfere with the ultimate formation of ATP. Furthermore, it is known that brain transketolase is retained even as thiamine deficiency progresses to its terminal conclusion and that pyruvate dehydrogenase activity in brain falls long after its activity in heart, liver, and kidney have fallen sufficiently to result in a reduction in ATP formation (Dreyfus, 1969).

It is possible that thiamin exerts a specific effect in nerve tissue since it has been shown that stimulation of nerve fibers results in release of free thiamin and thiamin monophosphate. This finding is consistent with the occurrence of thiamin monophosphate in nerve tissue. However, neurological symptoms observed in rats are not correlated with accumulation of pyruvate in the blood (as suggested by Handler, 1958) and although glycogen has been shown to accumulate in glial cells in thiamin deficiency (Collins and Converse, 1970), there is no clear indication that the known blocks in carbohydrate metabolism are fundamental to the neurological disturbances in thiamin deficiency. It has been suggested that neurological changes are due to a specific failure in oligodendroglial cells by an as yet unknown mechanism but one that may be independent of thiamin coenzyme function (Cooper and Pincus, 1967; Dreyfus, 1969).

Similarly, although biochemical defects in heart tissue of thiamin-deficient rats have been studied extensively (Gubler, 1969; McCandless et al., 1970), the mechanism by which thiamin deficiency results in bradycardia and ultimately in heart failure are not resolved. Clearly, the problem of relating deficiency symptoms to biochemical lesions is a perplexing one; this problem exists not only for thiamin deficiency, however, but for other vitamin and mineral deficiencies as well.

Thiamin Metabolites. A large number of thiamin metabolites have been identified in mammalian urine. Several years ago Ziporin (1965) demonstrated that both pyrimidine and thiazole were excreted in the urine. Excretion of these two compounds remained at high levels even after thiamin excretion ceased on a thiamin-deficient diet. Thiamin, thus, is degraded by cleavage of the molecule to produce the pyrimidine and thiazole moieties. It is further degraded by splitting the thiazole ring so that carbon-2 is released as carbon dioxide (Balaghi and Pearson, 1966). Studies utilizing thiamin labeled with ^{14}C in both the pyrimidine and thiazole rings indicated at least 22 breakdown products from ^{14}C-labeled pyrimidine (Neal and Pearson, 1964) and 29 different products from ^{14}C-labeled thiazole (Balaghi and Pearson, 1966). A refined procedure for isolation of thiamin metabolites from urine has been described by Neal (1970) and with this procedure several additional degradation products have been identified.

Thiamin Antagonists. Although several thiamin antagonists are known (see Cerecedo, 1955; Rogers, 1970), the two most commonly used in experimental studies are oxythiamine and pyrithiamine. Oxythiamine is formed by substitution of an hydroxyl group for the amino group of the pyrimidine moiety of the thiamin molecule. Pyrithiamine results from the substitution of a pyridine ring for the thiazole ring of thiamin. It appears that, in general, thiamin activity is impaired when the number 2 position of the pyridine ring is changed. However, both the 2-ethyl and 2-propyl compounds possess thiamin activity to some degree.

Both oxythiamine and pyrithiamine possess potent antithiamin activity, but the mechanism by which they oppose thiamin function differs. Oxythiamine is readily converted to the pyrophosphate and competes with thiamin for its place in the TPP-enzyme systems. It markedly depresses appetite, growth, and weight gain and produces bradycardia, heart enlargement, and an increase in blood pyruvate. However, it does not produce neurological symptoms. Pyrithiamine exerts its antithiamin activity chiefly through its effect on thiamin kinase, the enzyme involved in formation of TPP. Thus pyrithiamine is not converted to the pyrophosphate but rather prevents conversion of thiamin to TPP. It has a specific and marked effect on the central nervous system and quickly produces the neurological symptoms of thiamin deficiency. Treatment with pyrithiamine results in loss of thiamin from tissues, bradycardia, and heart enlargement but does not produce an increase in blood pyruvate. In addition its effect on weight gain is considerably less than that of oxythiamine. The comparative physiological and biochemical effects of these two thiamin antagonists have been detailed by Steyn-Parvé (1967) and Gubler (1968).

Amprolium, the 2-*n*-propyl pyrimidine analog of thiamin, is used in the treatment of coccidiosis in chickens. When fed at high levels, this compound has antithiamin activity and has been used experimentally to some extent (see Brin, 1964; Rindi et al., 1966).

Substances with antithiamin activity also occur naturally in some foods. Originally the antithiamin factor was referred to as thiaminase and was presumed to be an enzyme that splits the thiamin molecule thus rendering the vitamin inactive. Thiaminase was discovered as the result of an outbreak of a paralyzing disease in silver foxes raised on a farm owned by one J. S. Chastek. The disease, called

"Chastek paralysis," was traced to raw fish fed to the animals and was later characterized by Green et al. (1942) as a thiamin deficiency. Heating or cooking destroyed antithiamin activity. Thiaminase has been found to occur in both fresh- and salt-water fish, and more recently in various plant sources.

In addition to the thermolabile thiaminase, a heat-stable substance with antithiamin activity also has been identified. This factor is a large molecule containing amino acids but does not appear to be a true protein and therefore is not likely an enzyme (see Gontzea and Sutzescu, 1968).

Riboflavin

In the early days of vitamin research it was believed that the antiberiberi factor represented a single vitamin. After thiamin was isolated, however, it became clear that at least two factors were involved, a heat-labile fraction that was the true antiberiberi vitamin and a heat-stable fraction essential for growth (Emmett and Luros, 1920). The latter fraction for some time was thought to be only one substance and was named vitamin B_2 in Great Britain and vitamin G in the United States. Subsequently the heat-stable fraction was shown to be not one vitamin but a mixture of several vitamins (later identified as riboflavin, vitamin B_6, niacin, and pantothenic acid). The orange-yellow color of riboflavin and its natural fluorescence in solution undoubtedly aided in its discovery since its presence in extracts from foods and other biological materials could be confirmed with the naked eye.

The vitamin was first isolated from egg white and called "oloflavin" (see György, 1954). Compounds later isolated by other

Riboflavin

groups from milk and liver were designated "lactoflavin" and "hepatoflavin." The name riboflavin was adopted only after the compound was shown to contain the sugar alcohol, ribitol, in the molecule. The name was changed to riboflavine, and then back to riboflavin (IUPAC, 1966).

Riboflavin was synthesized independently by Kuhn et al. (1935) and Karrer et al. (1935).

Chemistry. The chemical name for riboflavin is 6,7-dimethyl-9 (D-1'-ribityl) isoalloxazine. It is an orange-yellow crystalline substance that is very slightly soluble in water or acid solution. In neutral or acid media it is stable to heat. It is highly soluble in alkaline solution but is not stable to heat under alkaline conditions. In solution at any pH riboflavin is unstable to both visible and ultraviolet light. Hence special precautions must be taken when riboflavin is analyzed in the laboratory to avoid exposure of solutions to light. Analyses usually are carried out in a darkened room; as further precaution dark red glassware, which filters out the blue portion of the spectrum, should be used. The natural yellow-green fluorescence characteristic of riboflavin in solution is the basis for the fluorometric assay for the vitamin (see AOAC, 1960; Koziol, 1970). Riboflavin and its derivatives also may be determined by spectrophotometric and polarographic methods (see McCormick and Wright, 1971a) as well as microbiologically (Snell and Strong, 1939; Baker and Frank, 1968).

The vitamin is easily reduced to a colorless compound, leucoriboflavin, by hydrogen in the presence of a catalyst and sodium hydrosulfite or other reducing agents. In the analysis of riboflavin by the fluorometric technique, fluorescence has been measured before and after reduction of riboflavin by sodium hydrosulfite in order to correct for fluorescence produced by interfering substances. The reversible reduction takes place by a shifting of bonds in the isoalloxazine ring as shown below. The ease with which riboflavin can be reversibly reduced and oxidized is the basis for its function in cellular respiration.

Biochemical Function. Riboflavin is a constituent of two coenzymes: flavin mononucleotide (FMN) and flavin adenine dinucleotide (FAD). For the most part the vitamin is present in mammalian tissues as these two compounds. The identification of the flavin coenzymes dates back to the early 1930s when Warburg and Christian (1932) isolated a fluorescent oxidative enzyme from

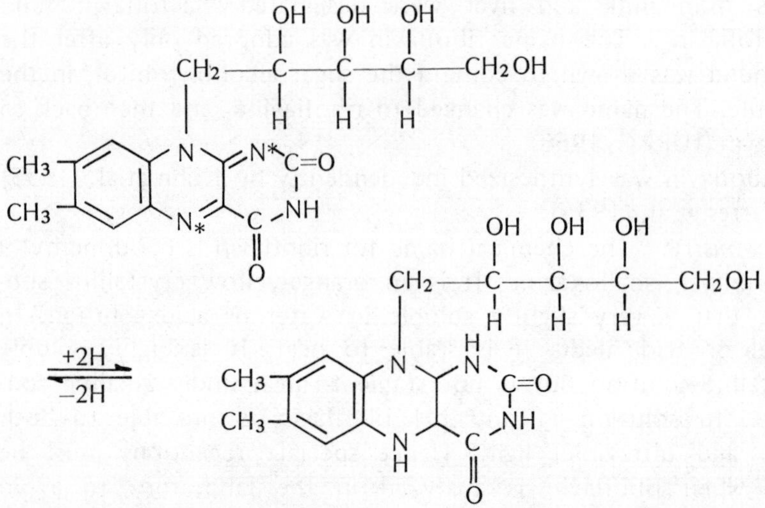

$$
\begin{array}{ccccc}
& OH & OH & OH & \\
& | & | & | & \\
CH_2 - C - C - C - CH_2OH & & & \\
& | & | & | & \\
& H & H & H &
\end{array}
$$

(Oxidized riboflavin isoalloxazine ring structure with CH$_3$, CH$_3$ groups, N, N*, C=O, NH, C, O)

$$\overset{+2H}{\underset{-2H}{\rightleftharpoons}}$$

(Reduced form with ribityl side chain: OH OH OH, CH$_2$—C—C—C—CH$_2$OH, H H H; ring with CH$_3$, CH$_3$, N, H, N, C=O, NH, NH, H, C, O)

yeast and were able to separate the enzyme into a protein and a yellow-pigmented component. Two years later, Theorell (1934) showed that the active component of the yellow enzyme was flavin phosphate. FAD was identified from a group of enzymes known as diaphorases, and its structure was determined by cleavage to riboflavin-5'-phosphate and adenosine-5'-phosphate (Abraham, 1939). The formulas for the two coenzymes are shown below.

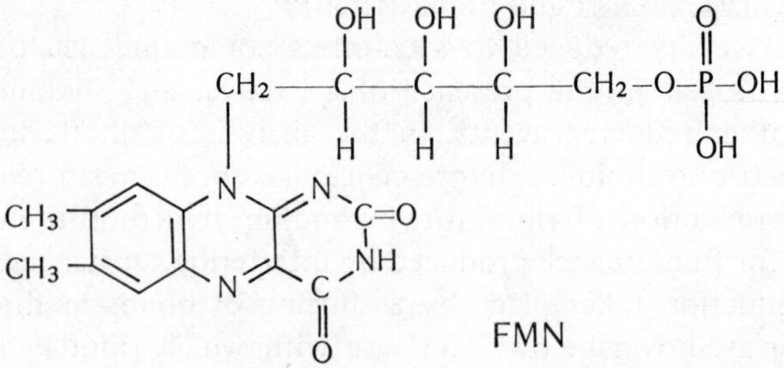

$$
\begin{array}{ccccc}
& OH & OH & OH & O \\
& | & | & | & || \\
CH_2 - C - C - C - CH_2-O-P-OH & & & \\
& | & | & | & | \\
& H & H & H & OH
\end{array}
$$

(FMN isoalloxazine ring structure with CH$_3$, CH$_3$, N, N, C=O, NH, C, O)

FMN

The riboflavin coenzymes function in a large number of enzyme systems and serve as carriers in the electron transport system leading to the formation of the high energy compound ATP (see Chapter 13). Essentially these coenzymes function in dehydrogenations in the course of which the coenzyme is reduced. In turn, the flavin enzymes become substrates for reactions involving other electron

FAD

acceptors resulting in the regeneration of the oxidized form of the coenzyme.

FMN is a part of the L-amino acid oxidase which participates in enzyme systems that oxidize L-a-amino acids and L-a-hydroxy acids to a-keto acids. FAD is a part of many enzyme systems including succinic dehydrogenase, xanthine oxidase, glycine oxidase, lipoyl dehydrogenase, NAD^+-cytochrome c reductase, and D-amino acid oxidase. Flavin enzymes also are involved in the specific dehydrogenation of adjacent carbon atoms resulting in the introduction of double bonds into certain molecules such as butyryl CoA and other acyl CoA compounds in the metabolism of fatty acids. Some of the flavoproteins contain a metal as, for example, xanthine oxidase that contains molybdenum and cytochrome c reductase that contains iron. For details of flavoprotein-catalyzed reactions see Wellner (1967) and Neims and Hellerman (1970).

A specific role for thyroid hormone in the biosynthesis of FMN and FAD has been proposed by Rivlin (1970). His hypothesis is based on the observation that flavoprotein enzymes are decreased in activity in hypothyroidism and increased in hyperthyroidism. Rivlin suggests that the thyroid hormone acts on the activity of the enzyme flavokinase, which catalyzes the conversion of riboflavin to FMN and, therefore, a lack of the hormone produces a cellular deficiency of riboflavin. This interesting speculation may have important significance in the understanding of the symptoms of hypothyroidism as well as of riboflavin metabolism.

The young growing rat is readily depleted of riboflavin when fed a diet lacking the vitamin; growth ceases and death ensues. It is interesting and puzzling, however, that a lack of this vitamin has not been shown to result in a discrete or lethal deficiency syndrome in the human. Clearly, the rat is more susceptible to a lack of dietary riboflavin than the human. One might theorize that in the human alternative pathways exist for performing the vital functions normally mediated through the flavoproteins, but it seems more likely that the human is not readily depleted of the vitamin. The fact that riboflavin is tightly bound to the enzyme protein, that is, it is technically a prosthetic group, may import a stability that the more loosely bound coenzyme vitamins do not have. Since riboflavin is associated with protein in metabolic systems and, therefore, in foods, it seems possible also that a riboflavin deficiency that is severe enough to result in debilitation or death does not occur except in conjunction with protein deficiency. In such a case the symptoms might merge into a variable syndrome such as the one observed in kwashiorkor and might well be obscured by the devastating effects of protein deficiency. Such speculation is interesting, but it is only speculation.

Riboflavin Metabolites. Apparently little degradation of riboflavin occurs in mammalian tissues. Following injection of $2\text{-}^{14}C\text{-}$riboflavin to rats, the vitamin is excreted rapidly in the urine (Yagi et al., 1966; Yang and McCormick, 1967). Only a trace of the radioactive riboflavin is converted to radioactive carbon dioxide (Yang and McCormick, ibid). In studies with humans given oral doses of riboflavin, however, West and Owen (1969) report the occurrence in the urine of at least three fluorescent compounds that were identified as degradative products of the vitamin: hydroxyethylflavin, formylmethylflavin, and an unknown compound designated as "Compound A." The amount of the compounds excreted represented considerably less than one percent of the dose of riboflavin fed to the subjects. Hydroxyethylflavin and formylmethylflavin were shown to be identical to riboflavin breakdown products that were isolated from the rumen and cecum of goats, and it was presumed that these metabolites originated from bacterial action in the intestinal tract and were absorbed as such.

Further breakdown of formylmethylflavin apparently occurs in animal tissues. This compound has been shown to be reduced by liver and kidney homogenates from goats, sheep, and cattle to hydroxymethylflavin (West and Owen, 1973). The enzyme responsible for the conversion has been found in tissues from other species including the rat, chicken, mouse, rabbit, and guinea pig (ibid).

Thus, there is yet no clear evidence of tissue breakdown of riboflavin. The continuous need for a dietary source of riboflavin appears, therefore, to be the result of a continuous loss of the vitamin via the urine rather than to any extensive tissue degradation.

Riboflavin Antagonists. Among the riboflavin antagonists galactoflavin (Emerson et al., 1945) in which the ribitol moiety is replaced by galactose is used most extensively in experimental studies. In man treatment with galactoflavin results in the usual effects on the mouth and skin (see Table 3.1). In addition a normochromic and normocytic anemia has been described (Lane and Alfrey, 1970). The anemia is accompanied by decreased incorporation of radioactive iron (^{50}Fe) into erythrocytes and bone marrow red cell hypoplasia (see Chapter 16). This condition is cured by riboflavin and is assumed to be a manifestation of riboflavin deficiency in man. A similar syndrome has been observed in baboons fed a riboflavin-deficient diet (Foy and Kondi, 1968).

Diethylriboflavin, another riboflavin antagonist, has been shown to possess a potent antivitamin effect in rats (see Lambooy, 1955). This compound has been found to be useful in studies designed to elucidate the mechanism of action of the flavoprotein enzymes. Other riboflavin antagonists also have been described (Lambooy, ibid). Some of these compounds have been shown to retard malignant tumor growth in experimental animals (see Rivlin, 1970a).

A substance antagonistic to riboflavin has been found to occur naturally in a limited number of foods, as for example the ackee nut that is consumed in Jamaica (Fox and Miller, 1960).

Niacin (nicotinic acid and nicotinamide)

Pellagra apparently has been known for several centuries and has long been associated with dietaries in which corn is a major staple food. The disease was endemic in the southern United States during the early part of the twentieth century and reached such proportions in institutions in the south that in 1914 a U.S. Public Health team headed by Dr. Joseph Goldberger was sent to the area to determine the cause and possible treatment of the disease. At that time it was generally believed that pellagra was caused either by an infectious agent or a toxic substance present in corn.

Goldberger's work on pellagra represents one of the most fascinating chapters in the history of nutrition. He observed that the disease occurred among institution inmates but not among staff who lived in the same environment but who invariably had a better diet including more animal protein food. Through carefully conducted studies he was able to produce pellagra in a group of prisoner volunteers by feeding them a diet similar to that consumed by persons who developed the disease (Goldberger and Wheeler, 1915). He was able to show also that the disease was not infectious since it could not be induced by exposure of healthy, well-fed volunteers to secretions or excreta from pellagrous patients (Goldberger, 1916). Finally, Goldberger and Wheeler (1928) produced black tongue in dogs, a disease comparable to human pellagra, by feeding a diet then known to produce pellagra in humans.

It was not until the middle 1930s that the pellagra-preventive factor in food was identified. Interestingly enough, nicotinic acid had been known for some time. It had even been isolated by Funk in the early part of this century when he was searching for an antiberiberi factor but was discarded when it was ineffective against beriberi! However, the discovery of nicotinamide as a component of coenzyme II (now NADP) by Warburg and Christian (1935) suggested that the substance was of metabolic importance. When Elvehjem et al. (1938) were able to cure black tongue in dogs with nicotinamide isolated from liver, the vitamin was firmly established as the pellagra-preventive factor. Subsequent treatment of pellagrous humans with the compound added final confirmatory evidence (Spies et al., 1938).

The history of pellagra and the discovery of niacin as the protective dietary component in the prevention of the disease have been reviewed by Sydenstricker (1958).

Chemistry. Niacin is the official name for the vitamin and includes both nicotinic acid and nicotinamide. Nicotinic acid is pyridine-3-carboxylic acid, a white crystalline solid that is easily converted to the physiologically active compound, nicotinamide. Both are soluble in water and in alcohol, but nicotinamide has a much higher solubility than nicotinic acid. Both are stable in the dry state and in solution at temperatures not exceeding 120°C.

$$\text{Nicotinic acid (with —COOH group)} \qquad \text{Nicotinamide (with —CONH}_2 \text{ group)}$$

Nicotinic acid   Nicotinamide

Chemical determination of the vitamin depends on the reaction of the pyridine with cyanogen bromide to form a yellow color (see György, 1950). Microbiological methods, however, appear to be more accurate (Snell and Wright, 1941; Baker and Frank, 1968). Other methods including fluorometry and gas chromatography have been described (see McCormick and Wright, 1970a).

Biochemical Function. Niacin functions metabolically as a component of the coenzymes nicotinamide adenine dinucleotide (NAD) and nicotinamide adenine dinucleotide phosphate (NADP). These coenzymes are not nucleotides in a strict chemical sense because they contain the sugar alcohol, ribitol, rather than ribose. The coenzymes were previously known as coenzymes I and II and then DPN and TPN. Like the flavin coenzymes the nicotinamide nucleotides function in the transfer of hydrogens (or electrons). In the reduced state they are designated NADH and NADPH. Hydrogens are attached at the number 4 carbon of the pyridine ring, indicated by asterisk in the formulas for the coenzymes.

The influence of these coenzymes is so widespread in cellular metabolic processes that a lack of the vitamin results in major damage to cellular respiration. Enzyme systems in which NAD participates include alcohol dehydrogenase, glycerolphosphate dehydrogenase, lactic dehydrogenase, and glyceraldehyde-3-phosphate dehydrogenase to name only a few. Either NAD or NADP participates in reactions involving isocitric dehydrogenase and glutamic dehydrogenase; NADP is specifically involved with malic enzyme and glucose-6-phosphate dehydrogenase.

Reduced NAD (NADH) usually donates its hydrogens to FAD and thus to the cell respiratory chain responsible for energy release (see Chapter 13). NADPH gives up its hydrogens most often to cellular biosynthetic processes. For example, the synthesis of fatty

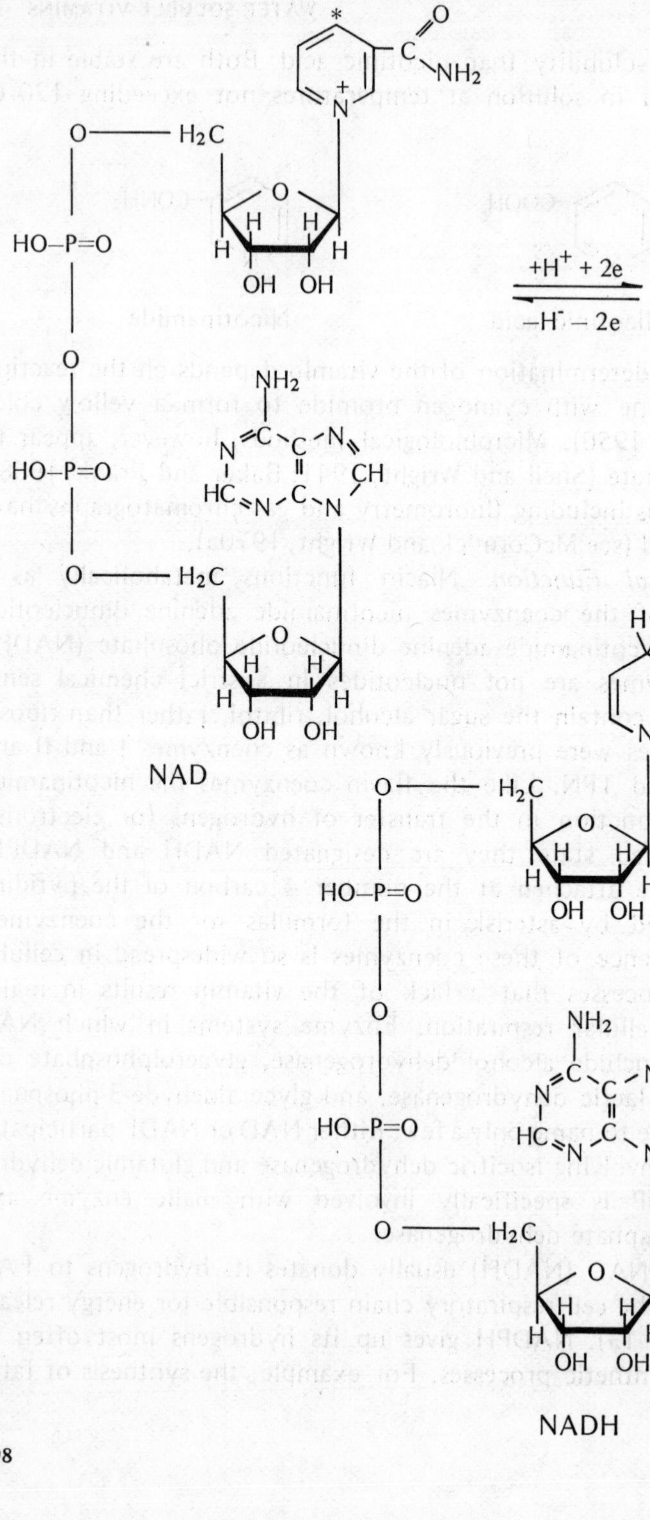

$$\dfrac{+H^+ + 2e}{-H^- - 2e}$$

NAD

NADH

NADP

acids specifically requires NADPH. For detailed discussion of reactions involving niacin coenzymes, see Chaykin (1967), Sund (1968), and Slater et al. (1970).

Niacin is synthesized by mammalian cells from the amino acid tryptophan (Krehl et al., 1945a, 1945b). Numerous studies with microorganisms and animal tissues helped to elucidate the pathway by which tryptophan is converted to the vitamin. The final step in the synthesis of niacin eluded investigators for many years but eventually was shown to involve the conversion of the key intermediate quinolinic acid to nicotinic acid mononucleotide (Nishizuka and Hayaishi, 1963) and thus to NAD (Fig. 3.1, pages 100-103). Nicotinic acid mononucleotide also is an intermediate in the conversion of nicotinic acid to NAD.

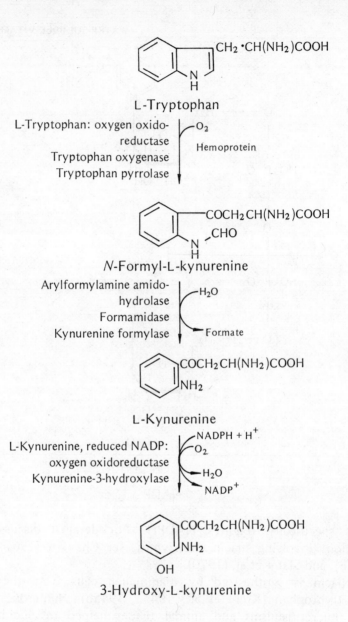

Fig. 3.1 Conversion of tryptophan to NAD. Adapted from S. Daglev and D. E. Nicholson, An Introduction to Metabolic Pathways, Wiley, N. Y., 1970, pp. 238-239.

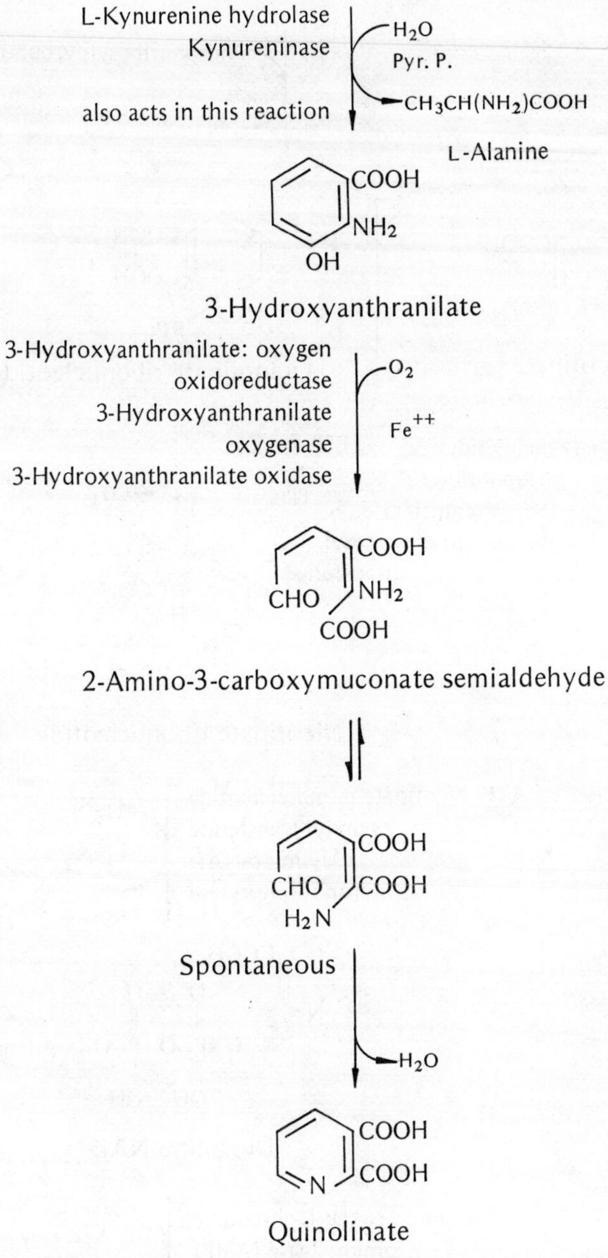

L-Kynurenine hydrolase
Kynureninase
also acts in this reaction
H2O
Pyr. P.
CH3CH(NH2)COOH
L-Alanine
COOH
NH2
OH
3-Hydroxyanthranilate
3-Hydroxyanthranilate: oxygen oxidoreductase
3-Hydroxyanthranilate oxygenase
3-Hydroxyanthranilate oxidase
O2
Fe++
COOH
CHO
NH2
COOH
2-Amino-3-carboxymuconate semialdehyde
COOH
CHO
COOH
H2N
Spontaneous
H2O
COOH
COOH
N
Quinolinate

Fig. 3.1 (continued)

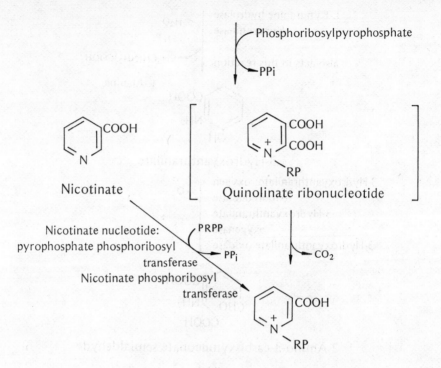

Nicotinate

Quinolinate ribonucleotide

Nicotinate nucleotide: pyrophosphate phosphoribosyl transferase

Nicotinate phosphoribosyl transferase

Nicotinate ribonucleotide

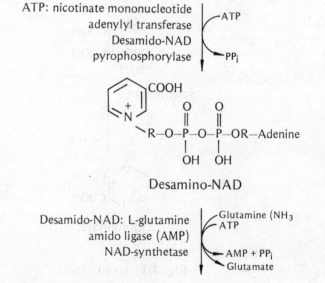

ATP: nicotinate mononucleotide adenylyl transferase

Desamido-NAD pyrophosphorylase

Desamino-NAD

Desamido-NAD: L-glutamine amido ligase (AMP)

NAD-synthetase

Fig. 3.1 (continued)

R represents the ribosyl group and RP ribosyl phosphate

Fig. 3.1 (continued)

Confirmation of nicotinic acid synthesis from tryptophan sup-ported early observations on the efficacy of animal protein in the prevention and cure of pellagra. Experiments with humans indicate that approximately 60 mg of tryptophan are equivalent to 1 mg of nicotinic acid (Horwitt et al., 1956a; Goldsmith et al., 1961). The total amount of available niacin in the diet thus may be expressed in terms of milligram equivalents (mg equiv), which includes both preformed niacin and niacin synthesized from tryptophan (see Chapter 25). Since food tables list niacin values in milligrams a rough calculation of available niacin may be made on the assump-tion that tryptophan comprises approximately 1 percent of dietary protein. The resulting figure added to preformed niacin yields total niacin in mg equiv.

The turnover of nicotinamide nucleotides in the mammalian body is very high (see Dietrich, 1971). However, under normal conditions the vitamin appears to be utilized efficiently. Metabolism of the nicotinamide nucleotides appears to be regulated both at the cellular (Gholson, 1966) and systemic levels (Deitrich et al., 1968) by an intricate series of enzyme activations and inhibitions involving the synthesis and degradation of the niacin coenzymes.

Thus as shown in Fig. 3.2 tryptophan and nicotinic acid are converted to NAD in the liver. Catabolism of NAD releases nicotinamide that, along with absorbed vitamin, is converted to NAD in other tissues where the cycle is repeated. Some nicotinamide is believed to be excreted into the gastrointestinal tract where it may be converted by intestinal bacteria to nicotinic acid. At least some of the nicotinic acid so formed may be absorbed and returned to the general circulation. Nicotamide also is converted in the liver to N^1-methyl nicotinamide, a major niacin metabolite that is excreted in the urine.

Niacin Metabolites. As mentioned above, in man and other monogastric animals nicotinamide is methylated before it is excreted.

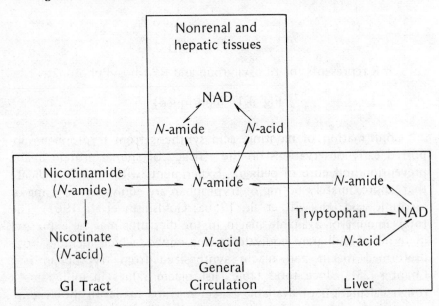

Fig. 3.2 Systemic pyridine nucleotide cycle. [From L. S. Dietrich, *Amer. J. Clin. Nutr.*, 24:802 (1970).]

N^1-methylnicotinamide and the 2- and 6-pyridones of N^1-methyl-nicotinamide are excreted in the urine. Other known metabolites of niacin are nicotinuric acid, nicotinamide-N-oxide, N^1-methyl-2-pyridone-5-carboxamide, and N^1-methyl-4-pyridone-3-carboxamide, and the more recently identified 6-hydroxynicotinamide and 6-hydroxynicotinic acid (Lee et al., 1969). Many of these compounds were identified in urine following injection of ^{14}C-labeled nicotin-amide or nicotinic acid. The compounds that were excreted have been shown to vary both with the form of the vitamin administered and the size of the injected dose.

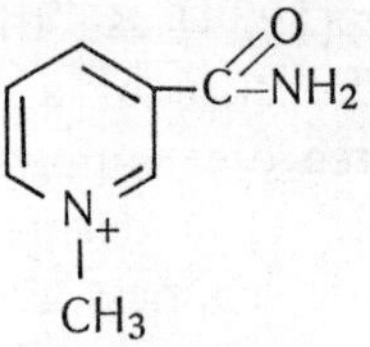

N'-methyl
nicotinamide

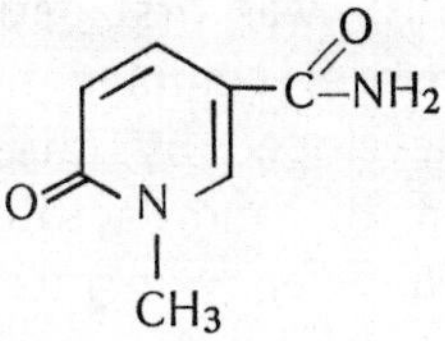

6-pyridone of
N'-methyl nicotinamide

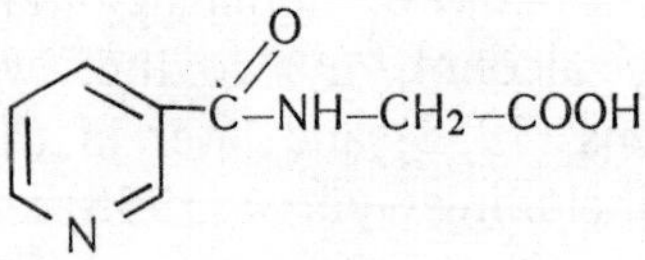

Nicotinuric acid

Niacin Antagonists. One of the first niacin antagonists to be discovered was 3-acetyl pyridine (Woolley, 1945), and this compound and 6-aminonicotinamide have received the most attention (Kodicek, 1966). Other niacin antagonists include pyridine-3-sulphonamide, 7-aminonicotinamide, and 4-acetyl pyridine.

The effect of predominantly maize diets in producing pellagra has been attributed to binding of niacin with a complex substance resistant to enzymes. This substance has been called *niacinogen*. The low incidence of pellagra in Mexico where maize is treated with lime led to the belief that lime treatment freed niacin and thus made the vitamin available for metabolism. Experiments designed to prove this hypothesis, however, failed to show any positive effect of lime treatment (Goldsmith et al., 1952). It now appears that maize contains an unidentified antiniacin substance that, in effect, increases the requirement for niacin since feeding maize to rats who do not require a dietary source of the vitamin causes disorders that can be alleviated by adding either niacin or tryptophan to the diet (see Gontzea and Sutzescu, 1968). The existence of such a substance has not yet been proved, and at this point the antiniacin action of maize still lies in the realm of speculation.

Vitamin B$_6$ (pyridoxine, pyridoxal and pyridoxamine)

The term vitamin B$_6$ is the official name for the 2-methyl pyridine derivatives having the biological activity of pyridoxine and includes the aldehyde, pyridoxal, and pyridoxamine.

Vitamin B$_6$ was first defined by György (1934) as "that part of the vitamin B complex responsible for the cure of a specific dermatitis developed by rats on a vitamin-free diet supplemented with vitamin B$_1$ and lactoflavin (riboflavin)." The dermatitis of vitamin B$_6$ deficiency in rats is a characteristic scaliness about the paws and mouth; these areas eventually become denuded as the scales slough off. Hence the vitamin was first identified as the rat antidermatitis factor. Alopecia (loss of hair) also is a commonly observed symptom of vitamin B$_6$ deficiency in rats.

The vitamin B$_6$ alcohol, pyridoxine, was isolated first by Kerestezy and Stevens (1938) and later in the same year by four independent groups including György (1938) and Lepkovsky (1938). Synthesis of the vitamin was accomplished in the following year by Harris and Folkers (1939). It was not until 1945, however, that the multiple nature of the vitamin was recognized and the other compounds of the complex identified as pyridoxal and pyridoxamine (Snell, 1945). Pyridoxine predominates in plant products, but pyridoxamine and pyridoxal are the principal forms of the vitamin in animal tissues (Rabinowitz and Snell, 1948).

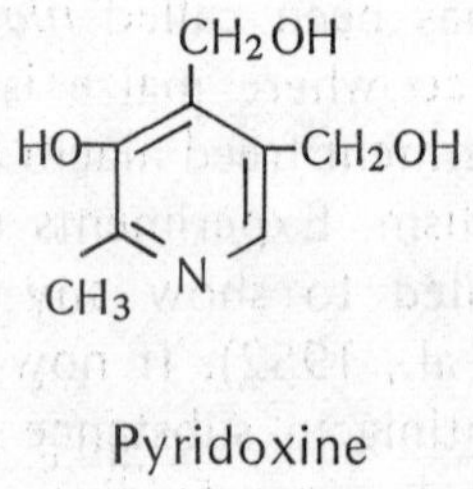

Pyridoxine

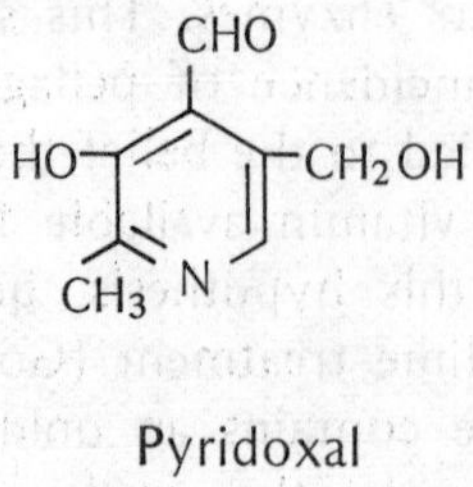

Pyridoxal

$$CH_2NH_2$$

HO—⬡—CH_2OH

CH_3 N

Pyridoxamine

Chemistry. Pyridoxine is readily soluble in water and slightly soluble in alcohol and acetone. It is stable to heat in acid solution and somewhat less stable in alkaline medium. It is quite unstable to visible and ultraviolet light in neutral and alkaline solution and therefore must be protected during laboratory analysis. In acid solution very little of the vitamin is destroyed by light.

The microbiological method of assay has long been a preferred method for determination of the vitamin, but it is complicated by differences in growth response of suitable microorganisms to the three forms of the vitamin. A satisfactory modification has been the separation of the three compounds on a chromatographic column and the assay of each by microbiological assay using *Saccharomyces carlsbergensis* as test organism (Toepfer and Lehmann, 1961; Brin, 1970). The three forms of vitamin B_6 also can be determined fluorometrically (see Toepfer and Polansky, 1964).

Chemical assay methods also have been developed. One involves the conversion of the three vitamin B_6 compounds to pyridoxic acid. Another involves the conversion of pyridoxine and pyridoxamine to pyridoxal and reaction of the aldehyde with cyanide to cyanhydrin. These methods among others have been reviewed by Storvick and Peters (1964).

Other more recent methods include assay by nuclear magnetic resonance spectroscopy, mass spectrometry and gas chromatography (see McCormick and Wright, 1970), and thin-layer chromatography and electrophoresis (Ahrens and Korytnyk, 1969).

Biochemical Function. The active form of vitamin B_6 is the coenzyme pyridoxal phosphate (PLP) identified by Umbreit and Gunsalus (1945). The coenzyme also has been referred to as codecarboxylase or cotransaminase. All three forms of the vitamin are converted to the active coenzyme or to their respective phosphates. Phosphorylation requires ATP.

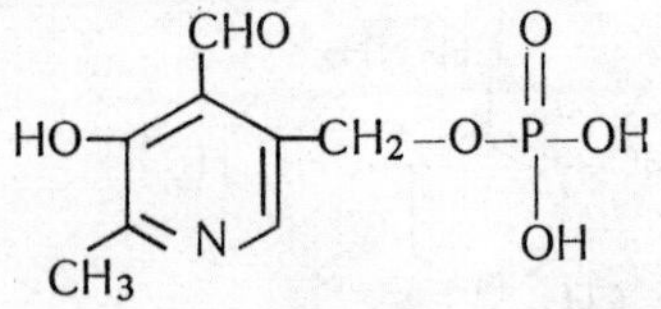

Pyridoxal phosphate

It has been generally presumed that the pathway for conversion of pyridoxine to PLP is by formation of pyridoxine phosphate and subsequent oxidation to PLP as demonstrated by Wada et al. (1959) in rat liver homogenates. In red cells, however, the pathway involves conversion of pyridoxine to pyridoxal phosphate and then to pyridoxal, which is gradually released into the plasma (Anderson et al., 1971). In mouse carcass, injected ^{14}C-pyridoxine is present primarily as pyridoxine and pyridoxal (McCoy and Columbini, 1972) indicating that the chief initial pathway in carcass is by way of oxidation of pyridoxine to pyridoxal. The major portion of vitamin B_6 in the animal body is present in muscle tissue.

PLP functions in nearly all reactions involved in the metabolism of amino acids including transamination, desulfhydration, decarboxylation, amine oxidation, and deamination. The general reactions are shown below.

1. Transamination

$$R_1CHNH_2COOH + R_2COCOOH \rightleftharpoons R_1COCOOH + R_2CHNH_2COOH$$

2. Desulfhydration

$$RCHSCHNH_2COOH + H_2O \longrightarrow RCH_2COCOOH + H_2S + NH_3$$

3. Decarboxylation

$$RCHNH_2COOH \longrightarrow RCH_2NH_2 + CO_2$$

4. Amine oxidation

$$RCH_2NH_2 + H_2O + O_2 \longrightarrow RCHO + NH_3 + H_2O_2$$

5. Deamination (dehydration)

$$RCHOHCHNH_2COOH \longrightarrow RCH_2COCOOH + NH_3$$

In addition PLP is required for many specific reactions of individual amino acids and is a coenzyme for phosphorylase (Cori and Illingworth, 1957).

Evidence suggests that the coenzyme is bound loosely to the ϵ-amino group of lysine of the apoenzyme molecule forming a Schiff's base. This reaction appears to occur in all enzymatic conversions requiring PLP. The formyl group of PLP appears to be the major site for coenzyme binding, but the phosphate group, 2-methyl group, 3-hydroxy group, and the heterocyclic N atom all are involved in coenzyme-apoenzyme interaction (Hayaishi and Shizuta, 1970). In fact, every side chain of the PLP molecule likely plays a role in apoenzyme binding, but the importance of the group involved varies from one enzyme system to another (see Fasella, 1967).

Not unexpectedly vitamin B_6 deficiency results in profound effects upon protein and amino acid metabolism. Since PLP is required for the action of the kynureninase enzyme involved in the metabolism of tryptophan (see Fig. 3.1), nicotinic acid formation may be reduced as a consequence of the deficiency. In addition, tryptophan metabolism is diverted from its normal course which results in the formation of xanthurenic acid, an abnormal metabolite of the amino acid. The excretion of xanthurenic acid following a test dose of tryptophan thus can be used as a means of detecting vitamin B_6 deficiency.

Vitamin B_6 also has been implicated in metabolic systems in which the mechanism of action is not clear. For example, it has been suggested that the vitamin is essential to the metabolism of unsaturated fatty acids, specifically in the conversion of linoleic acid to arachidonic acid (Witten and Holman, 1952). It has been suggested, however, that an effect of the vitamin on fatty acid metabolism is probably indirect (Mueller, 1964), and still other studies suggest no relationship between vitamin B_6 and essential fatty acid metabolism (Williams and Schier, 1961; Johnston et al., 1961). More recently Sato (1970) has presented evidence supporting a role of the vitamin in the conversion of γ-linolenate to arachidonate. The mechanism of action, however, has not been elucidated and, indeed, the specificity of PLP in this role remains controversial.

A number of genetic diseases involving vitamin B_6-dependent enzyme systems have been reported (see Mudd, 1971; György, 1971; Brown, 1972). Some of the reported diseases and the enzymes

Table 3.2   VITAMIN B_6 GENETIC DISEASES

Abnormal Condition	Biochemical Defect
Infant convulsive seizures	Decreased synthesis of γ-amino butyric acid due to reduced activity of glutamic decarboxylase.
Vitamin B_6-responsive anemia (microcytic, hypochromic)	Decreased formation of δ-aminolevulinic acid from glycine and succinyl CoA in heme synthesis.
Cystathionuria	Decreased interconversion of homoserine and cystathionine due to reduced activity of cystathionase.
Xanthurenic aciduria	Decreased conversion of kynurenine to anthranilic acid due to reduced activity of kynureninase.
Homocystinuria	Decreased conversion of homocysteine to cystathionine due to reduced activity of cystathionine synthetase.

and reactions affected are shown in Table 3.2. The basic defect in many of these diseases appears to be a decrease in binding of PLP to the apoenzyme. Although some of these defects respond to massive doses of the vitamin, other hereditary disorders of amino acid metabolism, many of which are associated with mental deficiency, are not responsive to vitamin B_6 therapy (see Berry, 1969).

Vitamin B_6 Metabolites.   A major metabolite of vitamin B_6 is 4-pyridoxic acid. Following injection of pyridoxine about 50 percent of the dose is excreted in the urine as pyridoxic acid. This compound can be measured fluorometrically (Reddy et al., 1958). Following oral dosage with the vitamin approximately 20 to 40 percent has been recovered in the urine as pyridoxic acid (Johansson et al., 1966; Tillotson et al., 1968).

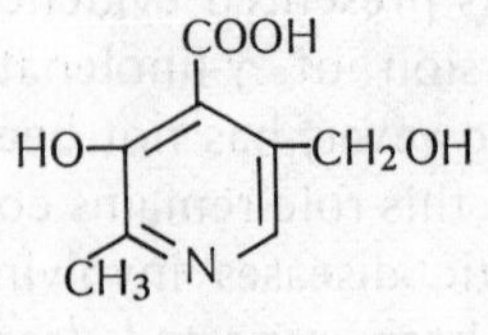

$$
\begin{array}{c}
\text{COOH} \\
\text{HO}\!-\!\overset{\displaystyle|}{\underset{\displaystyle CH_3}{\bigcirc}}\!-\!CH_2OH \\
N
\end{array}
$$

Pyridoxic acid

Pyridoxic acid is similar in structure to the vitamin but is inactive metabolically. An intermediary metabolite in the formation of pyridoxic acid has been identified in rat tissues as 4-pyridoxic acid 5'-phosphate (Contractor and Shane, 1970). Apparently pyridoxal phosphate is oxidized to pyridoxic acid phosphate, which is hydrolyzed to pyridoxic acid and excreted.

Other metabolites of vitamin B_6 have been found in urine. Those that have been identified include pyridoxal, pyridoxamine, PLP, pyridoxamine phosphate, and traces of pyridoxine. At least nine other unidentified compounds are excreted following a radioactive dose of vitamin B_6 (Tillotson et al., 1968).

Vitamin B_6 Antagonists. Of the many known vitamin B_6 antagonists (see Umbreit, 1955; Sauberlich, 1968; Hullar, 1969), 4-deoxypyridoxine has been utilized most frequently in experimental studies. The first studies of vitamin B_6 deficiency in man were made with the use of deoxypyridoxine (Mueller and Vilter, 1950).

4-Deoxypyridoxine   Isoniazid

Deoxypyridoxine apparently can be phosphorylated and thus competes with PLP for binding to the apoenzyme.

Isoniazid, a drug used in the treatment of tuberculosis, also is a potent antimetabolite of the vitamin B_6 group (Biehl and Vilter, 1954). This compound as well as other hydrazines form hydrazones with pyridoxal that inhibit pyridoxal kinase activity thus preventing formation of the coenzyme. Cycloserine, another antituberculosis drug, leads to an increased excretion of pyridoxine in the urine and, like isoniazid, produces neurological symptoms similar to those seen in vitamin B_6 deficiency (Cohen, 1969). Deoxypyridoxine does not produce the neurological symptoms.

Other vitamin B_6 antagonists include 4-methoxypyridoxine and toxopyrimidine, which have ring structures similar to the vitamin, and other structurally unrelated compounds such as penicillamine and semicarbazide.

Certain drugs such as amphetamine, chlorpromazine, reserpine, and birth control pills affect either the concentration of the vitamin in various tissues or enzymes involved in vitamin B_6 metabolism. The effect of birth control pills on vitamin B_6 requirement has received considerable attention. Much of the work has been reviewed by Mason et al. (1969), Brown et al. (1969), György (1971), and Brown (1972). Tryptophan metabolism is markedly affected in women taking the pill. This results in increased excretion of tryptophan metabolites and other biochemical manifestations of abnormal vitamin B_6 metabolism. Biochemical evidence of vitamin B_6 deficiency also has been observed in normal pregnancy (Wachstein, 1964). Brown et al. (1969) suggest that estrogen is responsible for the effect on tryptophan metabolism.

McCoy and Colombini (1972) have presented evidence that marijuana affects vitamin B_6 interconversions in brain. Mice were given the red oil of marijuana and sacrificed 30 minutes after administration of ^{14}C-pyridoxine. The percent of radioactivity retained in PLP and pyridoxal was decreased in brain while pyridoxine phosphate and pyridoxamine phosphate increased. The mechanism of action of marijuana on brain vitamin B_6 metabolism is not known.

Pantothenic Acid

Pantothenic acid was isolated and synthesized long before its metabolic role was identified. The vitamin was purified from liver and yeast along with pyridoxine, and the two vitamins were separated by adsorption chromatography. Pyridoxine was adsorbed on a column of Fuller's earth and subsequently eluted; pantothenic acid was not adsorbed and was recovered in the filtrate leaving the column. For this reason, pantothenic acid was designated the *filtrate factor* and pyridoxine, the *eluate factor.*

At about the same time several groups of investigators were searching for the identification of the vitamin known to be necessary for growth of lactic acid bacteria, prevention of dermatitis in chicks, and prevention of graying in black rats. Pantothenic acid was isolated by R. J. Williams and his associates (1938) and was synthesized by Stiller et al. (1940). Later tests with the purified vitamin proved it to be the factor required by bacteria, chicks, and rats for preventing the dissimilar deficiency symptoms.

Pantothenic acid attracted only mild interest for more than 10 years after it was recognized as a vitamin. The first breakthrough came with the identification of coenzyme A as the active factor required for metabolic acetylation processes (Lipmann and Kaplan, 1946); this discovery earned a Nobel Prize for Dr. Lipmann. The identification of pantothenic acid as a constituent of CoA was accomplished by a group in the same laboratory (DeVries et al., 1950). With this discovery the metabolic importance of pantothenic acid was clearly recognized.

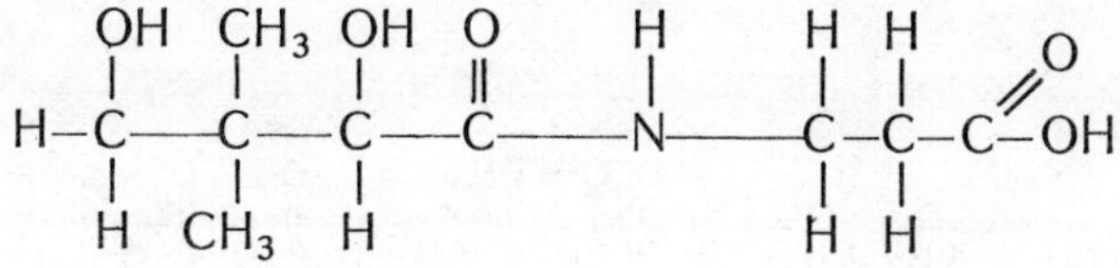

$$\underset{\displaystyle \underset{\text{Pantoic acid}}{\underbrace{}}}{\overset{\displaystyle \overset{OH\ \ CH_3\ \ OH\ \ O}{|\ \ \ \ |\ \ \ \ |\ \ \ \ \|}}{H-C-C-C-C}}-\underset{\displaystyle \underset{\text{β-Alanine}}{\underbrace{}}}{\overset{\displaystyle \overset{H\ \ \ \ H\ H}{|\ \ \ \ |\ |}}{N-C-C-C}}\overset{O}{\diagup}OH$$

Pantothenic acid

Chemistry.   The pantothenic acid molecule is a condensation product of β-alanine and a hydroxyl- and methyl-substituted butyric acid, pantoic acid. It is an unstable, pale yellow oil. Commercially it is available as the stable white crystalline calcium or sodium salt. The salt is soluble in water and glacial acetic acid. In neutral to slightly acid medium, pH 5-7, it is relatively stable at high temperatures.

Pantothenic acid may be assayed colorimetrically following reaction with 1,2-naphthaquinone-4-sulphonate or ninhydrin (Crokaert, 1949). Microbiological methods, however, are the most reliable methods for determination of the vitamin in biological materials (see AOAC, 1960). *Lactobacillus casei* (Pennington et al., 1940), *D. arabinosus* (Skeggs and Wright, 1944), and *Tetrahymena pyriformis* and *L. plantarum* (Baker and Frank, 1968) are among the organisms that have been used successfully. A major problem in the analysis is to free the vitamin from the coenzyme molecule. An intestinal phosphatase and a CoA-splitting enzyme from pigeon liver (Neilands and Strong, 1948) and diastase (Baker and Frank, 1968) are reported to yield good results.

Biochemical Function.   Unlike most vitamin coenzymes, pantothenic acid does not comprise the functional unit of coenzyme A (CoASH). The CoASH molecule contains β-mercapto ethylamine, adenine, ribose, and phosphoric acid in addition to the vitamin. Pantotheine, the β-mercaptoethylamine derivative of pantothenic acid, is the functional unit of CoASH. The sulhydryl group of β-mercaptoethylamine is the site at which acyl groups are linked for transport by the coenzyme. The discovery of the thioester linkage was reported by Lynen and Reichert in 1952. Since then CoASH has been demonstrated to be by far the most important acyl transfer coenzyme in biological systems.

Coenzyme A

The ability of CoASH to form thioesters with carboxylic acids is responsible for the vital role of the coenzyme in numerous metabolic processes. A key reaction is the formation of acetyl CoASH, *active acetate*, which condenses with oxaloacetate to form citrate and thus introduces two-carbon fragments into the tricarboxylic acid cycle, the common pathway of nutrient oxidation in the cell. In this critical function the vitamin influences the metabolism of carbohydrate, lipid, and protein (see Chapter 13). The coenzyme is necessary for fatty acid oxidation and synthesis, and for synthesis of cholesterol and phospholipid. These and other reactions involving CoASH will be discussed in subsequent sections.

Thioester   Acetyl CoASH

Pantothenic Acid Metabolites. Metabolic products of pantothenic acid have not been studied extensively. Although degradation products of the vitamin have not been identified it has been shown that pantolactone probably is not a metabolite of pantothenic acid in man (Sarett, 1945) as in some other species. Pantothenic acid administered orally or by injection is rapidly excreted in the urine (Silber and Unna, 1942). Larger amounts of the vitamin were excreted following oral dosage than after subcutaneous injection.

Pantothenic Acid Antagonists. A large number of pantothenic acid antagonists have been described (see Bird et al., 1955; Copping, 1966). The activity of some of these compounds, however, may vary among species. For example, pantothenol, a simple alcohol derivative of the vitamin, is a powerful antagonist for many bacteria but is utilized as readily as the vitamin by higher animals, including man.

The most important of the pantothenic acid antimetabolites in studies with experimental animals and man is ω-methyl pantothenic acid, a compound produced by substitution of a methyl group for the hydrogen in the pantoyl part of the molecule. This antagonist was used in the first studies of pantothenic acid deficiency in man (Bean and Hodges, 1954). Symptoms were observed in little more than a month in subjects given a diet deficient in pantothenic acid and administered the antagonist.

Other more recently reported pantothenic acid antagonists include homopantothenic acid (Nishizawa and Matsuzaki, 1969) and N'-substituted pantothenamides (Clifton et al., 1970).

Folacin (folic acid)

Many different species played significant roles in the identification of folacin as a vitamin. In the early 1930s Dr. Lucy Wills in India observed a megaloblastic anemia in pregnant women whose diets consisted primarily of white rice and bread. Since the anemia could be produced in monkeys maintained on a similar monotonous diet and also responded to supplements of yeast, it was apparent that the anemia was of nutritional origin (Wills, 1933). The unidentified factor was known as the Wills factor. Various other nutritional factors protective in other species were later shown to be identical with the original Wills factor: vitamin M, a factor protective against cytopenia in monkeys; factor U, a growth factor for chicks; vitamin B_c, protective against anemia in chicks; *L. casei* factor, necessary for growth of *Lactobacillus casei;* citrovorum factor, necessary for growth of *Leuconostoc citrovorum* (now *Pediococcus cervisiae).*

The name folic acid was proposed by Mitchell et al. (1941) for a compound isolated from spinach and shown to be necessary for growth of *Streptococcus faecalis R.* Eventually the structure and synthesis of pteroylglutamic acid were determined by Angier et al. (1946) and Pfiffner et al. (1946). A few years later it was clear that all the factors were forms of the vitamin now known as folacin, a collective term that comprises folic acid (monopteroyl-glutamic acid) and its derivatives.

Pteridine nucleus   *p*-Aminobenzoic acid   Glutamic acid

Pteroic acid

Folic acid (monopteroylglutamic acid)

Chemistry. Folic acid consists of a pteridine nucleus, *p*-amino-benzoic acid, and glutamic acid, hence the name monopteroyl-glutamic acid. The portion of the molecule containing pteridine and *p*-aminobenzoic acid is designated pteroic acid. At one time both *p*-aminobenzoic acid and pteroylglutamic acid were considered to be vitamins, but it is now apparent that the species requirement is for one or the other of the two. Pteroylglutamic acid (PGA) is the vitamin for most mammals, whereas *p*-aminobenzoic acid is essential to certain bacteria that are able to synthesize the larger molecule.

The compound is a dull yellow substance very slightly soluble in water. Its sodium salt is considerably more soluble. When in dilute acid solution pteroylglutamic acid is stable at temperatures below 100°C; stability to heat increases as pH increases. Solutions of both the acid and its salts are unstable to light.

Other biologically active forms of folic acid have been isolated from liver and yeast. These compounds contain three or more glutamic acid molecules. The tri- and heptaglutamyl peptides are most prevalent.

The microbiological procedure is preferred for the determination of folacin in biological materials. Because of the many different forms of the vitamin, major problems are encountered due to variance in response and to the small amounts and instability of many naturally occurring folates (see Baugh and Krumdieck, 1971). *Streptococcus faecalis, L. casei* and *Pediococcus cervisiae* have been used for assay. Of these *L. casei* appears to be most satisfactory for detection of folate nutritional status in man and animals (Baker et al., 1958; Cooperman, 1970). However, there is no one method at present that will measure *all* folic acid active compounds.

Enzymatic methods, radioisotope assay, and column chromatography have more recently been used for the determination of folic acid activity (see McCormick and Wright, 1971a). Chemical methods have been described, but these methods are generally unsuitable for the complexities of biological materials and are limited to assay of pharmaceutical preparations.

Biochemical Function. The active form of the vitamin is tetrahydrofolic acid (THFA). Folic acid is reduced to dihydrofolic acid by an enzyme, folic acid reductase. Dihydrofolic acid, in turn, is reduced to the active THFA. Both reductions require NADPH. The possible mechanisms of action have been discussed by Zakrzewski (1969).

Tetrahydrofolic acid (THFA)

Just as coenzyme A is a carrier for acyl groups, THFA is carrier for single carbon groups: formyl, formaldehyde, and methanol. One-carbon donors include formylglutamate, purines, serine, glycine, and histidine. Several coenzyme forms are involved in folate metabolism: N^{10}-formyl THFA, N^5-formyl THFA, $N^{5,10}$-methenyl THFA, $N^{5,10}$-methylene THFA, and N^5-formimino THFA. The interconversions of these compounds and some of the reactions in which they participate are shown in Fig. 3.3.

The formation of N^{10}-formyl THFA is a key reaction in the metabolism of folacin. This compound is generated from N^5-formyl THFA (folinic acid, citrovorum factor) or by addition of a formate group (donated by glycine) to THFA.

N^{10}-Formyl
tetrahydrofolic acid

$N^{5,10}$-Methenyl
tetrahydrofolic acid

N^{10}-formyl THFA undergoes ring closure to form the unstable $N^{5,10}$-methenyl THFA that, in turn, is reduced by NADPH to form. $N^{5,10}$-methylene THFA. Both formiminoglutamate, a product of histidine catabolism, and formiminoglycine give rise to N^5-formimino THFA, which also may be converted to $N^{5,10}$-methenyl THFA.

The single-carbon units transferred by THFA and its derivatives are important in the biosynthesis of purines and pyrimidines, in amino acid interconversions, and in certain methylation reactions. Some specific reactions in which THFA participates are conversion of glycine to serine, methylation of ethanolamine to choline, methylation of homocysteine to methionine, methylation of nicotinamide to N^1-methylnicotinamide, methylation of a pyrimidine intermediate to thymine, and introduction of carbons 2 and 8 in the purine ring structures. Vitamin B_{12} is intimately involved in some of these reactions. There is evidence that, in these instances, a methyl group is transferred from N^5-methyl THFA to form methyl-B_{12}.

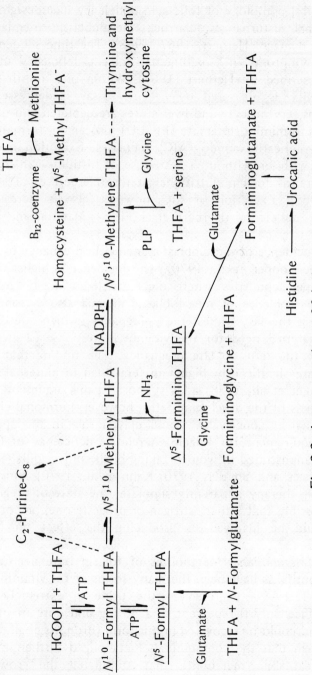

Fig. 3.3 Interconversions of folacin coenzymes.

119

The clinical pathology of folic acid deficiency includes glossitis, gastrointestinal disturbances, diarrhea, megaloblastic anemia, and neurological damage (Herbert, 1967, 1968). The time sequence of developing symptoms in experimental folacin deficiency in man has been described by Herbert (1967). Within one month serum folacin activity as measured by *L. casei* assay is depressed. By three months, erythrocyte and liver stores are depleted and urinary excretion of formiminoglutamate (FIGLU), urocanate, formate, and aminoimidazole carboxamide (AIC) increases. Excretion of these compounds with or without a test dose of histidine can be used as a measure of folacin nutritional status (Herbert et al., 1964; Herbert, 1968). Excretion of AIC, however, also is increased in vitamin B_{12} deficiency (Herbert et al., 1964; Marston and Allen, 1970).

A high incidence of megaloblastic anemia in pregnancy has been reported (see Cooper et al., 1970). The incidence is highest in the underdeveloped countries where diets are likely to be poor in quality. The incidence of megaloblastic anemia also is somewhat higher during the last trimester of pregnancy, which suggests an increased maternal need for the vitamin in response to increased demands by the fetus in late pregnancy. The finding that levels of folacin are significantly higher in fetal than in maternal blood at term (Baker et al., 1958) adds support to this argument. Aside from the needs of the developing fetus, however, hormonal changes during pregnancy conceivably could play a role in the apparent increased requirement for folacin. A relative deficiency of folacin has been demonstrated in women taking birth control pills (Streiff, 1970; Necheles and Snyder, 1970; Kahn et al., 1970). Since oral contraceptive therapy apparently simulates the state of pregnancy, it seems possible that either estrogen or progesterone, or both hormones, could be involved in producing the effect on folacin metabolism.

Folacin Metabolites. Metabolites of folacin have been as difficult to identify as have been the many forms of the vitamin itself. N^5-formyl THFA is excreted in the urine in extremely small amounts. Since only 0.1 percent of a 50 mg oral dose of pteroylglutamic acid could be recovered in this form (Broquist et al., 1951), it would seem that the compound is metabolized further in tissue cells. A heat-labile metabolite that stimulated the growth of *L. citrovorum* also has been identified in urine (Silverman et al.,

1956). Presumably this factor is N^{10}-formyl THFA. Other compounds isolated from human urine include xanthopterin (Koschara, 1936), isoxanthopterin (Blair, 1958), and biopterin (Patterson et al., 1956). It seems likely that they are true end products of folacin metabolism.

Folacin Antagonists. A large array of folacin antagonists have been identified (Burchenal, 1955; Robinson, 1966). Burchenal (ibid) has grouped the compounds with antifolacin activity into five classes: (1) the 9-methyl or 10-methyl glutamic acid derivatives that inhibit the growth of certain bacteria and animals; (2) the 4-amino pteroylglutamic acids (aminopterin) and its derivatives, many of which are active as cancer chemotherapeutic agents; (3) the 2,4-diamino pteridines that are active against bacteria only; (4) the diamino-dichlorophenyl pyrimidines that are active against both bacteria and animals and tend to be more effective and also more toxic than the 4-amino pteroylglutamic acids as cancer chemotherapeutic agents; and (5) the dihydrotriazines that are noncompetitive inhibitors of folacin for *S. faecalis* and *L. citrovorum.*

Of these five classes, the 4-amino derivatives of pteroylglutamic acid have been studied most extensively both in the induction of experimental folacin deficiency and as cancer chemotherapeutic agents. Aminopterin is the preferred antimetabolite for nutritional studies. It is partly competitive in action but certain cells, such as chick embryo osteoblasts and fibroblasts, and mouse liver can inactivate the antimetabolite; normal bone marrow or normal lymphoblastic and lymphocytes cannot (Jacobson and Cathie, 1960).

Beginning with the discovery by Farber et al. (1948) that aminopterin produced temporary remission in leukemia in children, several related compounds have been developed as cancer chemotherapeutic agents. Of these compounds amethopterin (Metrotrexate, MTX) has shown most promise against tumor growth. The selectivity of the antimetabolite in inhibiting tumor growth seems to depend on the vulnerability of rapidly proliferating tumor cells to folacin antagonists (see Hryniuk and Bertino, 1971). Both aminopterin and MTX inhibit dehydrofolate reductase activity by binding to the enzyme and thus preventing the formation of THFA. This site of action, however, does not seem to be primarily responsible for their anticancer effect (Wilmanns, 1971). Furthermore, it has been shown that resistance to the antagonists can develop through induction of additional dihydrofolate reductase and through a compensatory increase in thymidine kinase activity which permits tumor cell growth to continue. For these reasons, control and timing of dosage of the antagonist are critical determinants in the effectiveness of treatment.

Although a large amount of administered antagonist is recovered in the urine, contrary to earlier supposition, folate antagonists are metabolized to some degree by the animal body (Johns and Valerino, 1971). Tissue distribution of folate antagonists also has been extensively studied (Oliverio and Zaharko, 1971); these data provide valuable insight into the relative efficiency of antagonists in limiting tumor growth in various tissues.

Vitamin B_{12} (cyanocobalamin)

The search for vitamin B_{12} began with the discovery by Minot and Murphy (1926) of the efficacy of liver in the treatment of pernicious anemia, a disease characterized by a severe megaloblastic anemia and, if untreated, eventual extensive neurological damage. Much of the work leading to the isolation of the active principle in liver has been reviewed by SubbaRow et al. (1948). Crystalline B_{12} was isolated independently by two groups, Rickes et al. (1948) in this country and Smith and Parker (1948) in England and was shown to be active in the treatment of pernicious anemia (West, 1948). The substance was also shown to be identical with the *animal protein factor,* a growth factor present only in animal products, which had been known for some time and rightly believed to be an unidentified vitamin.

Chemistry. The vitamin B_{12} molecule is the most complex of the vitamins. Elucidation of the structure of the vitamin was accomplished seven years after its isolation and resulted from a brilliant series of x-ray crystallographic analyses by Hodgkin and associates (1955; 1957). The vitamin is distinguished by the presence of cobalt in the molecule, which is responsible for its dark red color.

The cobalt is bordered by a corrin ring that consists of four nitrogen-containing five-membered rings joined through three methylene bridges. The corrin ring is similar to the porphyrin ring of chlorophyll. (The term *corrinoids* applies to all compounds containing the corrin nucleus and though chemically related to the vitamin they are not synonymous with vitamin B_{12}.)

Vitamin B_{12}

Cyanocobalamin, the commercially available form of the vitamin, contains a cyanide group attached to the central cobalt (see formula). Apparently cyanide is present due to contamination from reagents used in isolation of the vitamin and little, if any, of the cyanide form occurs naturally (see Stadtman, 1971). However, other forms of the vitamin in which cyanide is replaced by another group occur in nature. For example, *hydroxycobalamin* (vitamin B_{12a}, vitamin B_{12b}) contains a hydroxyl group in place of cyanide; this compound has been isolated from liver extracts. Certain bacteria have been found to contain a *nitritocobalamin* (vitamin B_{12c}), a compound in which cyanide is replaced by nitrogen. In other cases, the dimethylbenzimidazole moiety is replaced by other nitrogenous bases. In pseudovitamin B_{12}, adenine is the nitrogenous base. Cobalamins containing 2-methyl adenine and guanine also occur in nature.

A major breakthrough in the chemistry of vitamin B_{12} came with the recent synthesis of the vitamin 25 years after its isolation (see Maugh, 1973). This work represented a joint effort directed by R. B. Woodward of Harvard University in the United States (who won the Nobel Prize in 1965 for the synthesis of chlorophyll) and A. Eschenmoser of the Eidgenössische Technische Hochschule, Zurich, Switzerland. The enormity of the task can be appreciated when one considers that the project involved 99 scientists from 19 countries working over a period of 11 years! The final stages of the synthesis begin with a compound aptly designated B-corrnor-sterone by Woodward because it is the "cornerstone" of the plan for completion of the cyanocobalamin molecule (Woodward, 1971).

Aside from the obvious contribution to scientific achievement, the synthesis of vitamin B_{12} may well have profound effects on commercial production of the vitamin. Vitamin B_{12} has been produced by bacterial fermentation processes and also can be recovered as a by-product of streptomycin and aureomycin antibiotic fermentations (Wuest and Perlman, 1968). What effect the chemical synthesis will have on industrial production remains to be seen.

Crystalline vitamin B_{12} is fairly soluble in water, ethyl alcohol, other lower alcohols, aliphatic acids, and phenols and is relatively stable in solution at pH values between 4 and 7. It decomposes rapidly at pH 2 or pH 9. Solutions of the vitamin are moderately sensitive to light. However, it is stable in the hydrated form and in triturates with sodium chloride and certain sugars. A mannitol triturate is a commonly available commercial preparation.

Both spectrophotometric and chemical methods of assay are suitable for determination of vitamin B_{12} in pharmaceutical preparations or in substances relatively free of interfering substances (see Rosenthal, 1968). However, for complex biological materials the microbiological assay is the preferred method of analysis. *Lactobacillus lactis* Dorner (LLD) has been used as a test organism for determining antipernicious anemia activity of liver extracts. Bioassays run with this organism aided in identifying the crystallized vitamin as the antipernicious anemia factor (Shorb, 1948). This organism is more erratic in response, however, than *L. leichmanii* (see AOAC, 1960 and U. S. Pharmacopeia, 1960). Methods using *Ochromonas malhamensis* and *Euglena gracilis*, z strain, are described in detail by Baker and Frank (1968) and are equally suitable for urine, blood, and animal tissues. Nuclear magnetic resonance and electron paramagnetic resonance spectroscopy appear to show promise as tools in the simultaneous identification of the various forms of the vitamin and its coenzymes (Hill et al., 1971).

Biochemical Function. The coenzyme form of vitamin B_{12} was discovered by Barker and his coworkers (1958) in the course of studying the conversion of glutamic acid to β-methylaspartate in an obscure anaerobic bacterium, *Clostridium Tetanomorphum.* They found that a derivative of pseudovitamin B_{12} was involved in the reaction. The same group later isolated a similar derivative containing 5,6-dimethylbenzimidazole from *C. tetanomorphum,* animal liver, and propionic acid bacteria (Weissbach et al., 1959). The structure of the coenzyme shown below was determined by Lenhert and Hodgkin (1961) using the x-ray crystallography technique, which had been instrumental in determining the structure of the vitamin.

The coenzyme contains a 5-deoxyadenine nucleoside in place of the cyanide (or hydroxyl) group of the vitamin molecule. The nucleoside is linked to the cobalt in the corrin ring through the 5-carbon of the deoxyribose moiety. This unusual binding of carbon linked covalently with cobalt had never before been demonstrated to occur naturally. It is now known that the chemical and biological reactivity of coenzyme B_{12} depends on the carbon-cobalt bond.

The coenzyme is easily degraded by visible light and although most of the vitamin apparently occurs naturally as the coenzyme, the extreme sensitivity of the coenzyme to light is probably responsible for what was once believed to be its elusive nature.

The coenzyme is known to participate in a number of enzymatic reactions in bacteria, but only two vitamin B_{12}-dependent enzyme systems, methylmalonyl CoA and methyl transferase (transmethylase), have been demonstrated in mammalian tissues (see Hogenkamp, 1968, Weissbach and Taylor, 1968, 1970; Stadtman, 1971).

Coenzyme B_{12}

Methylmalonyl CoA is the intermediary compound in the metabolism of propionate in mammalian tissues; the enzyme converts methylmalonyl CoA to succinyl CoA. The reaction is essentially a carbon-carbon bond cleavage (see below). In vitamin B_{12} deficiency excretion of methylmalonate in the urine is increased (Cox and White, 1962).

$$
\begin{array}{ll}
& \text{O} \\
& \parallel \\
\text{①} & \text{C–S–CoA} \\
& \mid \\
\text{②} & \text{CH–CH}_3 \\
& \mid \quad \text{③} \\
\text{④} & \text{COOH}
\end{array}
\qquad \rightleftharpoons \qquad
\begin{array}{ll}
& \text{O} \\
& \parallel \\
\text{①} & \text{C–S–CoA} \\
& \mid \\
\text{②} & \text{CH}_2 \\
& \mid \\
\text{③} & \text{CH}_2 \\
& \mid \\
\text{④} & \text{COOH}
\end{array}
$$

Methylmalonyl CoA   Succinyl CoA

The vitamin B_{12}-transmethylase is responsible for the methylation of homocysteine to form methionine and has been studied most extensively in *E. coli*. However, there is strong evidence that the enzyme is present also in mammalian liver (Loughlin et al., 1964; Dickerman et al., 1964) and possibly is quite similar to the system in *E. coli*. The reaction involves N^5-methyl THFA; the methyl group is transferred to homocysteine to form methionine and as a result, THFA is regenerated (see Figure 3.3).

The megaloblastic anemia and the changes in bone marrow associated with the pernicious anemia syndrome suggest that, like folacin, vitamin B_{12} is in some way essential for DNA synthesis which, in turn, is necessary for normal development of mature red blood cells (see Beck, 1968). However, neither the methylmalonyl CoA reaction nor methionine synthesis per se provide clear evidence of precisely how vitamin B_{12} is related either to folacin metabolism and one-carbon transfers or to DNA synthesis. In an attempt to clarify this, Herbert and Zalusky (1962) proposed that the function of vitamin B_{12} in DNA synthesis may be through its involvement in methionine synthesis and subsequent regeneration of THFA. If methionine synthesis is inhibited by vitamin B_{12} deficiency, then the ability to regenerate THFA from N^5-methyl THFA also would be inhibited (see Figure 3.3). Further, if the synthesis of methionine from homocysteine is the major pathway for regeneration of THFA, then a deficiency of vitamin B_{12} could result in an excess of N^5-methyl THFA (or "methylfolate block") and a consequent reduction in the methenyl and methylene derivatives responsible for purine synthesis. This theory was based on the observation that untreated pernicious anemia patients given a dose of folic acid showed a marked increase in N^5-methyl THFA in serum. Thus, if N^5-methyl THFA increased at the expense of THFA regeneration, this factor could account also for increased urinary excretion of FIGLU in vitamin B_{12} deficiency.

Weissbach and Taylor (1970), however, cite evidence apparently in conflict with the theory of N^5-methyl THFA build-up in serum. For example, studies with radioactive labeled folate administered to patients with pernicious anemia indicate that increased serum and urinary folate arise from mobilization of unlabeled folate from tissues (Chanarin and McLean, 1967) and that clearance of parentally administered N^5-methyl THFA from plasma is similar in patients with pernicious anemia and in normal controls. Furthermore, little change in serum N^5-methyl THFA was reported to occur in rats given a diet deficient in methionine and vitamin B_{12} than when supplements of either the amino acid or the vitamin were given (Vitale and Hegsted, 1969).

To complicate the picture further, a direct role of vitamin B_{12} in ribonucleotide synthesis in bone marrow also has been postulated (Beck, 1968). Although the evidence is inconclusive, enzymological studies suggest that bone marrow ribonucleotide reductase may be a B_{12}-dependent enzyme.

Thus, the mechanism of action of vitamin B_{12} in maintaining a normal blood picture remains obscure. However, the clinical symptoms and morphology of megaloblastic erythroid cells are well defined (see Beck, 1968; also see Chapter 16). Pernicious anemia (or vitamin B_{12} deficiency) is most often due to malabsorption of the vitamin that results from a hereditary lack of the factor required for vitamin B_{12} absorption (see Thedering, 1968; also see Chapter 6). However, since vitamin B_{12} occurs only in animal products, a dietary deficiency of the vitamin has been known to occur in complete vegetarians, that is, those persons who include no animal products in their diet.

Vitamin B_{12}, thus, is a vitamin in which cellular deficiency is the result, most often, not of a dietary lack but, instead, of the inability of the individual's absorptive mechanism to make the vitamin available for cellular metabolism.

Vitamin B_{12} Metabolites. Very little is known of the end products of vitamin B_{12} metabolism. Absorbed vitamin B_{12} that is not required immediately is stored in body tissues, particularly in the liver. Total body stores in the human have been estimated as 2-4 mg of which 30-60 percent is in the liver, 30 percent in muscle, skin, and bone, and smaller amounts in the lungs, kidneys, and spleen (Reisner, 1968). Surprisingly little vitamin B_{12} is stored in bone marrow. The vitamin is excreted in the urine, but when given in physiological amounts, a large amount is excreted in the bile (Reizenstein, 1959). In fact, more vitamin B_{12} is excreted daily in the bile than is contained in the entire blood volume. It is assumed that most of the B_{12} in bile is from hepatic stores. Fecal excretion, while higher than urinary excretion, is less than biliary loss. Thus some reabsorption of biliary vitamin B_{12} probably occurs.

Vitamin B_{12} Antagonists. Vitamin B_{12} analogs and antagonists have been reviewed by Friedrich (1966) and Moore and Folkers (1968). Although many derivatives of vitamin B_{12} possess vitamin activity, and many are antagonistic to bacterial growth and survival, relatively few compounds inhibit vitamin B_{12} activity in higher animals. The antagonists active in animals include a lactam of vitamin B_{12} prepared by Beiler et al. (1951) and several competitive inhibitors involving modification of one or more of the propion-amide sidechains of vitamin B_{12} (see Cuthbertson et al., 1956).

Biotin

Biotin was first described as the factor protective against egg-white injury. Rats fed large amounts of raw egg white developed an eczema-like dermatitis, paralysis of the hind legs, and a character-istic alopecia around the eyes, aptly termed *spectacle eye*. However, cooked egg white fed to rats was not toxic. A protective factor present in liver and yeast was designated vitamin H by György (1939), and the "factor protective against egg white injury" by Parsons et al. (1937). This factor was later designated biotin and was shown to be identical to *bios* or *Coenzyme R,* a growth factor for certain microorganisms that previously had been isolated from egg yolk as the crystalline methyl ester (Kögl and Tönnis, 1936). The synthesis of biotin was accomplished several years later by Harris et al. (1945).

The heat-labile biotin antagonist in raw egg white is avidin, a protein-carbohydrate compound that binds with biotin in the intes-tinal tract and thus inhibits biotin absorption.

Chemistry. Biotin is a relatively simple monocarboxylic acid. It is soluble in methanol, ethanol, acetone, and chloroform but is almost insoluble in water. Salts of the acid, however, are quite soluble. Biotin is destroyed by severe treatment with acids and alkalies but, in general, it tends to be more stable than most other vitamins to acid and alkali treatment.

$$
\begin{array}{c}
O \\
\parallel \\
C \\
{}_{2'} \\
HN^{3'} \quad {}^{1'}NH \\
| \qquad\qquad | \\
HC^{4'}_4 \!-\!\! {}^{5'}_3CH \\
| \qquad\qquad | \\
H_2C^5 \qquad {}^2C\!-\!(CH_2)_4COOH \\
\diagdown_S\diagup \quad H
\end{array}
$$

Biotin

A number of microorganisms have been tested for use in a biotin assay (see Baker and Frank, 1968), but because of a lack of specificity for the vitamin, few are suitable for determination of the vitamin in biological materials. Baker et al. (1962) found the flagellate, *Ochromonas danica,* to be both specific and sensitive as an assay organism for biotin. This organism has been used for biotin assay in blood, urine, and animal tissues. More recently a colorimetric reaction has been described that allows for separation of biotin and its analogs by paper or thin-layer chromatography (McCormick and Roth, 1970). Spectrophotometric techniques for determination of both biotin and avidin also have been developed (Green, 1970); these methods are somewhat less sensitive than the microbiological assay but are described as more convenient, more precise, and applicable over a wide range of pH and salt concentrations.

Biochemical Function. Biotin is known to function in two general types of carboxylation reactions. The first type is energy-dependent and involves the cleavage of ATP to ADP and inorganic phosphate (see below). Most biotin-requiring reactions in mammalian tissues appear to be of this type.

$$
\begin{array}{lll}
ATP + HCO_3^- & \qquad & ADP + Pi \\
 & \diagup\!\!\diagdown & \\
Biotin\text{-}protein & & {}^-O_3C\text{---}biotin\text{---}protein \\
 & \diagup\!\!\diagdown & \\
RCO_2^- & & RH
\end{array}
$$

The second type involves only an exchange of carboxyl groups; free CO_2 does not participate nor is ATP or any other energy source needed for the reaction.

Biotin appears to be very tightly bound to the enzyme protein through the ϵ-N-lysine moiety of the protein. The existence of ϵ-N-biotinyllysine (biocytin), was established by Lane and Lynen (1963) for propionyl carboxylase, a biotin-dependent enzyme. It appears that biotin is bound to this enzyme through an amide linkage between the ϵ-amino group of a lysine residue of the enzyme and the carboxyl group of the valeric acid side chain. Biocytin has been isolated as a hydrolysis product from other biotin-containing

$$
\underset{\text{Biocytin}}{\text{(biotin ring)}-(CH_2)_4-\overset{O}{\overset{\|}{C}}-\overset{H}{\overset{|}{N}}-(CH_2)_4-\overset{\overset{+}{N}H_3}{\underset{H}{\overset{|}{\underset{|}{C}}}}-CO_2^-}
$$

Biocytin

enzymes, and apparently this type of linkage is characteristic of all biotin-enzyme binding.

The biotin enzyme systems have been reviewed by Mistry and Dakshinamurti (1964) and Knappe (1970). Five biotin enzyme systems have been positively identified and are described below. The first four reactions are ATP-dependent; the fifth is a carboxyl transfer that does not require an energy source.

1. *Acetyl CoA carboxylase*

$$
\underset{\text{Acetyl CoA}}{CH_3COSCoA} + HCO_3^- + ATP \xrightarrow{Mg^{2+}} \underset{\text{Malonyl CoA}}{\overset{COO}{\overset{|}{C}H_2COSCoA}} + ADP + Pi
$$

This enzyme plays an essential role in the initial stage of the biosynthesis of fatty acids.

2. *β-Methyl crotonyl CoA carboxylase*

$$
\underset{\text{β-Methyl crotonyl CoA}}{\overset{CH_3}{\overset{|}{C}H_3C}=CHCOSCoA} + HCO_3^- + ATP \xrightarrow{Mg^{2+}} \underset{\text{β-Methyl glutaconyl CoA}}{\overset{CH_3}{\overset{|}{C}H_2\overset{|}{C}=CHCOSCoA}} + ADP + Pi
$$

This enzyme is involved in one step in the oxidative degradation of leucine to acetoacetate and acetyl CoA and catalyzes the conversion of the intermediary β-methyl crotonyl CoA to β-methyl glutaconyl CoA.

3. *Propionyl CoA carboxylase*

$$CH_3CH_2COSCoA + HCO_3^- + ATP \xrightarrow{Mg^{2+}} \underset{CH_3CHCOSCoA}{\overset{COO^-}{|}} + ADP + Pi$$

Propionyl CoA   Methylmalonyl CoA

Propionyl CoA arises from various pathways including degradation of isoleucine and the oxidation of odd-numbered fatty acids. Recently it has been shown by Travis et al. (1972) that linoleate is catabolized by way of propionyl CoA. Thus, the reaction is both biotin- and vitamin B_{12}-dependent (Dupont and Mathias, 1969). (Note that methylmalonyl CoA is an intermediary in the conversion of propionyl CoA to succinyl CoA.)

4. *Pyruvate carboxylase*

$$CH_3COCOOH + HCO_3^- + ATP \xrightarrow{CH_3COSCoA + Mg^{2+}} \underset{CH_2COCOOH}{\overset{COO^-}{|}} + ADP + Pi$$

Pyruvate   Oxalacetate

This enzyme appears to be dependent on the presence of acetyl CoA or propionyl CoA although acetyl CoA is not incorporated into the oxalacetate molecule.

5. *Methylmalonyl-oxalacetic transcarboxylase (methylmalonyl CoA pyruvate carboxyl transferase)*

$$\underset{CH_3CHCOSCoA}{\overset{COO^-}{|}} + CH_3COCOO^- \rightleftharpoons CH_3CH_2COSCoA + \underset{CH_2COCOO^-}{\overset{COO^-}{|}}$$

Methylmalonyl CoA   Pyruvate   Propionyl CoA   Oxalacetate

This enzyme differs from propionyl CoA carboxylase in that it involves a direct transfer of a carboxyl group, that is, it does not require CO_2 or energy to activate CO_2. Although this reaction has been demonstrated in mammalian tissues it may occur to a lesser extent than CO_2 fixation via propionyl CoA carboxylase.

Biotin also appears to be involved in the reaction leading to the formation of carbamyl phosphate, an important early step in the synthesis of pyrimidines, and in amino acid metabolism (Wellner et al., 1968). In fact, biotin profoundly affects the metabolism of carbohydrates, proteins, and lipids although the mechanism is far from clear and may, indeed, be only indirectly related to its known metabolic functions. Considerable attention has recently been directed to the relation of deficiency of the vitamin to hypercholesterolemia and hyperglycemia. Of special interest is the observation that in rats the relationship between biotin status and lipid metabolism appears to be related to other genetically transmitted metabolic phenomena (Marshall et al., 1972).

Biotin deficiency due to diet restriction is not known to occur in humans. The vitamin is widely distributed in foods. It also is synthesized in the gastrointestinal tract and some of this appears to be absorbed. A few cases of biotin deficiency due to excessive intake of raw eggs, however, have been reported (Scott, 1958; Baugh et al., 1968). Paradoxically, while egg white is the best known source of avidin, the biotin antagonist, egg yolk is a very rich source of the vitamin.

Biotin Metabolites. Very little breakdown of biotin apparently occurs in either rats or man (Fraenkel-Conrat and Fraenkel-Conrat, 1952; Wright et al., 1956). A high proportion of administered biotin is recovered intact in the urine. The rapid clearance of injected radioactive biotin in experiments with rats further suggests that the rat possesses a very low renal threshold for reabsorption of biotin (Lee et al., 1972). The same situation probably holds for the human as well. Biotin excretion in the human, like that of most water-soluble vitamins, is closely related to intake (Sydenstricker et al., 1942).

What degradation that does take place involves only the side chain of the vitamin. When ring-labeled ^{14}C-biotin is administered, little or no radioactive CO_2 is recovered in expired air (Dakshina-murti and Mistry, 1963; Lee et al., 1972). These data strongly suggest that the biotin ring remains intact.

In addition to the high amounts of intact biotin, however, small amounts of biotin metabolites have been recovered in the urine following administration of the radioactive vitamin. These include the *d*- and *l*-sulfoxides, bisnorbiotin (a compound with two carbons less in the side chain) and a neutral unidentified ketone (Lee et al., 1972). All of these compounds involve changes in the side chain of the vitamin. Incubation of radioactive biotin with liver tissue suggested that the sulfoxides are formed almost exclusively in the liver whereas bisnorbiotin appears to be formed in other organs as well.

In more recent studies (Lee et al., 1973), small amounts of biotin sulfone and tetranorbiotin (four carbons less in the side chain) also were recovered in urine. The excretion rate of the metabolites is exceedingly rapid, thus following the excretion pattern of the vitamin. Kidney clearance appears to be related to the degree of water solubility of the compounds excreted.

Biotin Antagonists. Avidin is the most important of the biotin antagonists in mammalian metabolism. As mentioned earlier, the antibiotin effect of this compound was responsible for the discovery of the vitamin. Avidin has been shown to be an oligomer with molecular weight of about 70,000 comprising four polypeptide chains and four binding sites for biotin (Green, 1968).

A number of other antagonists including desthiobiotin, desthioisobiotin, 4-imidazolidone-2-caproic acid, biotin sulfone, and ureylenecyclohexylvaleric acid are active against various bacteria and insects (Kodicek, 1966; Langer and György, 1968).

Ascorbic Acid

Historically the disease scurvy became widely recognized when man learned to build ships capable of long sea voyages, and it is probably true that on long-term explorations more deaths were caused by scurvy than any other single factor. The dietary prevention of scurvy was well documented by Lind in 1750. It is typical of the time span between discovery and application of knowledge that Lind's recommendation of providing fresh foods for sailors on long sea voyages was not introduced until some 30 years later when Captain Cook sailed to the Pacific and subsequently discovered the Hawaiian Islands.

The identification of ascorbic acid was aided by Holst and Frölich (1907) who accidentally produced scurvy in guinea pigs and thus provided a test animal for later studies. Of the mammals, only man, the monkey, and the guinea pig require the vitamin; other mammalian species possess the necessary enzyme to synthesize ascorbic acid.[1] The fruit bat, the pipistrelle and some birds of the Passeriformes order (Chaudhuri and Chatterjee, 1969; Chatterjee, 1970) as well as the channel and blue catfish (Wilson, 1973) have been shown to require the vitamin.

Ascorbic acid was isolated first by Szent-Györgyi (1928) from orange juice, cabbage juice, and adrenal cortex; he named the compound hexuronic acid in recognition of the six carbon atoms in the molecule and, at the time, was concerned chiefly with the reducing property of the acid. Four years later ascorbic acid was isolated again by Waugh and King (1932), who demonstrated its antiscorbutic activity in guinea pigs. The compound was subsequently shown to be identical with hexuronic acid by Svirbely and Szent-Györgyi (1932).

Chemistry. Ascorbic acid is a hexose derivative and is properly classified as a carbohydrate. It is a white crystalline substance, highly soluble in water, and also soluble in ethyl alcohol and glycerol. The vitamin is quite stable in the dry state but is easily oxidized when in solution. It is stable in acid solutions below pH 4.0 but the instability of ascorbic acid in solution increases markedly as the alkalinity of the solution increases. Ascorbic acid also is unstable in the presence of certain metals such as iron and copper.

Ascorbic acid   Dehydroascorbic acid   Diketogulonic acid

---

[1]Synthesis of ascorbic acid is by way of D-glucuronic acid →L-gluconic acid→L-gulonolactone→3-keto-L-gulonolactone→L-ascorbic acid. Species that require a dietary source of the vitamin lack the enzyme, L-gulonoxidase, which converts L-gulonolactone to 3-keto-L-gulonolactone.

Ascorbic acid (reduced ascorbic acid) is easily oxidized to form dehydroascorbic acid that is just as easily reduced back to the original form. The ease with which the two active forms of the vitamin are interconverted is probably related to at least some of the physiological properties of the vitamin. Further oxidation of dehydroascorbic acid results in formation of diketogulonic acid and loss of vitamin activity.

In mammalian tissues reduction of dehydroascorbic acid to reduced ascorbic acid appears to be aided by sulfhydryl compounds, for example, the tripeptide glutathione. In analytical procedures that measure only the reduced form of ascorbic acid, hydrogen sulfide may be passed through the solution for the same purpose.

The strong reducing property of ascorbic acid is the basis for an analytical procedure in which the dye 2,6-dichlorophenolindophenol is reduced by the vitamin; only the reduced form of the vitamin is measured by this method. Total ascorbic acid may be measured by reaction with 2,4-dinitrophenylhydrazine (Roe et al., 1948; Roe and Kuether, 1943). The latter method is probably the most widely used method today. Recently a new titrimetric method for the determination of ascorbic acid (Barakat et al., 1973) has been reported; the method is described as simple, rapid, and sensitive to as little as 25 μg. of the vitamin. Other methods for the determination of ascorbic acid have been reviewed by Roe (1961) and Olliver (1967).

Biochemical Function. The mechanism by which ascorbic acid acts in biological systems remains obscure; if a coenzyme form exists for the vitamin, it likely is a highly unstable molecule since it has eluded investigators for so long. Ascorbic acid is known to function as a reducing agent, but since in some cases other reducing agents perform equally well, the effect may be largely nonspecific for the vitamin.

Abnormalities of connective tissue observed in scurvy have long suggested that ascorbic acid is involved in the synthesis of collagen or mucopolysaccharides. There is now ample evidence to support a role of the vitamin in collagen biosynthesis as first suggested by the studies of Robertson and Hewett (1961). Stone and Meister (1962) and Peterkafsky and Udenfriend (1965) demonstrated that the vitamin is necessary for the hydroxylation of proline to form hydroxyproline, an unusual amino acid that occurs almost exclusively in collagen. In *in vitro* studies, Gottlieb et al. (1966) presented evidence of a collagenlike protein containing little hydroxyproline. This protein is formed in response to ascorbic acid deficiency or when hydroxylation is impaired by lack of oxygen and was believed to be responsible for the structural changes observed in scorbutic tissues. In *in vivo* experiments, however, Barnes (1969) reported that collagen synthesis is impaired in scorbutic animals but that there is not an accumulation of an unhydroxylated collagen precursor as was observed *in vitro*. These data suggested that proline (and lysine) are probably hydroxylated after incorporation into the polypeptide chain. According to this investigator, hydroxylation of proline apparently occurs to a very limited extent in scorbutic animals and a lack of the vitamin gives rise to partially hydroxylated peptides that do not accumulate in the body but rather are rapidly excreted.

Other hydroxylation reactions also have been reported to require the vitamin including the oxidation of tryptophan to 5-hydroxytryptophan (Cooper, 1961), the conversion of 3,4-dihydroxyphenylethylamine to norepinephrine (Levin et al., 1960) and hydroxylation of *p*-hydroxyphenylpyruvate to homogentisic acid in tyrosine metabolism (Sealock and Silbertsein, 1939). LaDu and Zannoni (1961) have suggested that in the latter reaction ascorbic acid acts not as a cofactor but instead, the vitamin appears to protect the enzyme, *p*-hydroxyphenylpyruvic acid oxidase, from inhibition by its substrate. Further, the protective action is necessary only when large amounts of tyrosine are being metabolized. Ascorbic acid does not seem to be necessary for tyrosine metabolism under normal dietary conditions.

Staudinger et al. (1961) reported that ascorbic acid participates between NADH and cytochrome b_5 in the electron transport chain (see Chapter 13) and suggested that this reaction is coupled with hydroxylation. In this case, dehydroascorbic acid would function as the electron acceptor as has been suggested in the hydroxylation of tryptophan (Cooper, 1961).

A role for ascorbic acid also has been demonstrated in the transfer of plasma iron to the liver and its incorporation into the iron storage compound, ferritin (Mazur, 1961). The reaction requires energy in the form of ATP. Ascorbic acid appears to be specific for this function and cannot be replaced by other reducing agents.

Ascorbic acid also is involved in the distribution of iron storage compounds (Lipschitz et al., 1971). In ascorbic acid-deficient guinea pigs, ferritin was reported to be decreased and hemosiderin increased in liver and spleen. When ascorbic acid was fed, the distribution of iron between these compounds returned to normal.

Thus, the participation of ascorbic acid in a number of metabolic reactions has been demonstrated and, for the most part, these reactions tend to relate to clinical symptoms of ascorbic acid deficiency. A role for the vitamin in the prevention of the common cold has been suggested when the vitamin is taken in massive doses (Pauling, 1970, 1971). Although there is some evidence that symptoms of a cold are somewhat lessened among persons taking large quantities of ascorbic acid (Anderson et al., 1972; Coulehan et al., 1974) any such effect likely should be classed as pharmacologic rather than physiologic. *In vitro* studies indicate that ascorbic acid is effective in the detoxication of histamine (Subramanian et al., 1973). Since histamine formation is known to be increased under many conditions of body stress (including the common cold) these workers suggest that any beneficial effect of ascorbic acid is due to its detoxication of excess histamine produced in response to stress.

Ascorbic Acid Metabolites. Very little is known of the end products of ascorbic acid metabolism. Apparently much of ingested ascorbic acid is excreted intact (Baker et al., 1971b). Various unidentified 6-carbon compounds are excreted following administration of labeled ascorbic acid but because of the labile nature of the vitamin, the identification of these compounds as true metabolites or as breakdown products in urine is difficult. Oxalate has been shown to be derived from ascorbic acid (Hellman and Burns, 1958; Baker et al., 1966) and more recently ascorbate-3-sulfate has been identified as an important metabolite of the vitamin (Baker et al., 1971a).

A small amount of ascorbic acid is excreted in expired air as CO_2, but only 2 percent of a radioactive dose of the vitamin has been accounted for in that form (Baker et al., 1971b). At least one source of CO_2 appears to be 2,3-diketo-L-gulonic acid that is formed by hydrolysis of dehydro-L-ascorbic acid. The enzyme involved is known to be aldonolactonase (see Kagawa and Shimazono, 1970). In turn, 2,3-diketo-L-gulonic acid is hydrolyzed to L-xylonic acid (or L-lyxonic acid) and CO_2.

In man catabolism of ascorbic acid appears to represent about 3 percent of the body pool per day. When subjects were depleted of the vitamin, a body pool of approximately 300 mg appeared to be associated with appearance of clinical symptoms of scurvy. The average pool of healthy male subjects was calculated to be 1500 mg. Once this level is reached, excretion of ascorbic acid in the urine markedly increases (Baker et al., 1971b).

Ascorbic Acid Antagonists. Only one antagonist of ascorbic acid, glucoascorbic acid, is known and it appears that this compound may have toxic as well as antimetabolite properties (Woolley and Krampitz, 1943). When fed to rats, mice, and guinea pigs, gluco-ascorbic acid induced growth failure and lesions similar but not identical to scurvy. Effects of the compound were alleviated by adding ascorbic acid to the diet of the guinea pig, which requires the vitamin, but not to rats or mice, which synthesize ascorbic acid (Woolley, 1944b). However, glucoascorbic acid was shown to inhibit oxidation of tyrosine by liver slices and addition of ascorbic acid removed the inhibition (Lan and Sealock, 1944) suggesting that glucoascorbic acid acts as an antimetabolite for at least some of the functions performed by the vitamin.

chapter 4
fat-soluble and other vitamins

1. **Fat-Soluble Vitamins: Chem-**
   istry, Biochemical Function
   a. Vitamin A
   b. Vitamin D
   c. Vitamin E
   d. Vitamin K

2. **Other Vitamins and Vitamin-**
   like Compounds
   a. Choline
   b. Inositol
   c. Lipoic Acid
   d. Ubiquinone

The fat-soluble vitamins appear to be more unlike the water-soluble vitamins in biological function than can be attributed to their solubility properties alone. Solubility, of course, affects the transport, distribution, storage, and excretion of the vitamins, but the concept of very fundamental differences in mode of action gradually is emerging. The search for a coenzyme function comparable to those of the B-vitamins is giving way to investigation of other mechanisms by which the fat-soluble vitamins exert their influence in biochemical systems.

Recent evidence suggests, for example, that vitamin D fulfills the functional requisites for classification as a hormone, that is, the active "vitamin" is elaborated by one organ but acts on other target organs. Although no such clearly defined mode of action has yet been attributed to the other fat-soluble vitamins, the separation of these substances from the water-soluble vitamins is far more than a question of solubility. They are, indeed, a class unto themselves.

Vitamin A (retinol, retinaldehyde, retinoic acid)

Vitamin A was the first of the accessory food factors to be identified as a component of specific foods. In 1913 McCollum and Davis reported that rats failed to grow on diets containing carbohydrate, protein, lard, and salts. Addition of an ether extract of butter or eggs promoted growth and established that the missing factor was a fat-soluble substance. A lack of the *fat-soluble growth factor* later was shown to result in necrosis of the cornea in rats. This condition was similar to an eye disease (xerophthalmia) seen in humans, then believed to be due to a lack of dietary fat. Mori (1922) clearly established that the disease was due to lack of a fat-soluble factor (vitamin A) but not to a lack of dietary fat per se.

By the middle 1920s the relationship between dark adaptation and vitamin A was established, but it was nearly 10 years later that Wald discovered that the pigment rhodopsin (visual purple), responsible for sight in dim light, contained vitamin A in combination with protein (Wald, 1933). Wald's subsequent elucidation of the reactions involved in bleaching and regeneration of rhodopsin still provides the only well-defined role of the vitamin in mammalian systems. For this contribution Wald was awarded the Nobel Prize for Medicine in 1967.

Early feeding experiments with rats indicated that vitamin A was associated with plants containing the yellow, orange, or red-colored carotene pigments. Moore (1930) demonstrated that the carotenes were related structurally to vitamin A and were converted *in vivo* to the vitamin.

Vitamin A was isolated in large amounts from fish liver oils by Karrer et al. (1931) and subsequently by several groups. It was not until the late 1940s, however, that synthetic vitamin A became available on the commercial market.

Vitamin A (all *trans*)

Chemistry. Vitamin A exists in animal products in several forms but occurs largely as the alcohol, retinol (Vitamin A_1). It is stored in the animal body in combination with fatty acids as retinyl esters; palmitic acid appears to be the preferred fatty acid. The vitamin molecule contains a β-ionone ring with an unsaturated side chain. The formula for retinol is shown above. A retinol isomer, dehydro-retinol (vitamin A_2) is found in liver oils from fresh water fish and some marine fish. This compound has an additional double bond between carbon atoms 3 and 4 in the ring and is about 40 percent as active as retinol (Shantz, 1948). The terms vitamin A_1 and vitamin A_2, however, are no longer used. All β-ionone derivatives other than the provitamin carotenoids are included under the descriptive term "vitamin A."

The alcohol is converted *in vivo* to an aldehyde, retinaldehyde (retinal), which has been isolated from the retina of the eye and is the form in which the vitamin functions in dark adaptation. Retinoic acid (vitamin A acid) is formed from retinol via retinalde-hyde in the animal body, but a reverse reaction does not occur. Synthetic retinoic acid, for example, will promote growth in animals, but it is not active in the visual process (Dowling and Wald, 1960) nor in the support of normal reproduction (Juneja et al., 1964).

Retinol is a nearly colorless oil and is soluble in all fat solvents. It is relatively stable to heat but is extremely unstable to oxidation and fairly unstable to light. The basis for the earliest chemical determinations for vitamin A is the Carr-Price reaction, in which the vitamin forms a blue color with antimony trichloride in chloroform (Carr and Price, 1926). Other methods include fluorometry (Hansen and Warwick, 1969) and thin-layer chromatography (Targan et al., 1965). Drujan (1971) has recently reviewed methods for determination of vitamin A.

Vitamin A activity in plants resides in the carotenoid pigments that are precursors to the vitamin in the animal body and, therefore, are designated the provitamins A. Conversion of the provitamins to the vitamin occurs in cells of the intestinal mucosa and, to some extent, in the liver and possibly in the kidney. Beta-carotene is the most widely distributed of the carotenoid pigments and is the most active in terms of vitamin A activity.

The β-ionone ring usually is essential for vitamin A activity. The β-carotene molecule is a double retinol structure (see formula) and theoretically should give rise to two molecules of retinol. Biologically, however, the activity of β-carotene is only about half that of retinol. The enzyme responsible for carotene cleavage to retinal has been referred to as β-15,15' dioxygenase (Olson and Hayaishi, 1965) and is known to split the two central carbon atoms of β-carotene in the presence of molecular oxygen to yield two molecules of retinal. Retinal so produced is converted to retinol by a nonspecific aldehyde reductase for which either NADH or NADPH can serve as cofactor (see Goodman, 1969; Olson and Lakshmanan, 1969). Some carotenoids may enter the lymphatic system intact and are converted to the vitamin in the liver or possibly in the kidney (see Chapter 6).

The disparity between the chemical structure and biological activity of carotene compounds is primarily the result of inefficiency of carotene absorption but also, in part, of the oxidation of some of the retinal formed from carotene cleavage to retinoic acid. The retinoic acid, in turn, is rapidly excreted from the animal body.

Many different carotenoids occur in nature. In addition to β-carotene, likely only α-carotene and cryptoxanthin are significant in human nutrition. The latter two carotenoids are about half as efficient as β-carotene in the ultimate yield of retinol. The biological activity of some carotenoids is shown in Table 4.1. With a few exceptions, the biologically active carotenoids contain an unsubstituted retinyl or a dehydroretinyl moiety. Carotenoids possessing no vitamin A activity are listed in Table 4.2.

Beta-carotene

The carotenoid pigments may be separated by column or thin-layer chromatography following extraction from tissues with a suitable solvent such as acetone or ethanol. The pigments are usually assayed by spectrophotometry (see AOAC, 1960) but also may be assayed by nuclear magnetic resonance, mass spectrophoto-

Table 4.1 ALL-TRANS CAROTENOIDS WITH VITAMIN A ACTIVITY

Compound	Moiety Structure[a]	Relative Biological Activity[b]
Retinol	—	200
3-Dehydroretinol	—	80
Hydrocarbons		
β-Carotene	(Retinyl:)₂	100
3-Dehydro-β-carotene	Retinyl:3-dehydroretinyl	75
α-Carotene	Retinyl:α-retinyl	53
γ-Carotene	Retinyl:geranyl-geranyl-4,8-diene	43
β-Zeacarotene	Retinyl:geranyl-geranyl-4-ene	40
Homo-β-carotene	Retinyl:retinylvinyl	20
Bis-3,3′-dehydro-β-carotene	(3-dehydroretinyl:)₂	38
Oxygenated derivatives		
Cryptoxanthin	Retinyl:3-hydroxyretinyl	57
Echinenone	Retinyl:4-ketoretinyl	44
5,6-Epoxy-β-carotene	Retinyl:5,6-epoxyretinyl	21
Torularhodin	Retinyl:geranyl-geranyl-4,8,12-tetraen-16-oic acid	<50
Apocarotenol derivatives		
β-Apo-14′-carotenol	Retinyl:ethanol	(7)
β-Apo-12′-carotenal	Retinyl:α-methylbutenal	(125)
Methyl β-apo-12′-carotenoate	Retinyl:methyl α-methylbutenoate	(200)
β-Apo-10′-carotenal	Retinyl:γ-methylhexadienal	(>100)
β-Apo-8′-carotenal	Retinyl:α,ε-dimethyloctatrienal	(40), 72

[a]Colon(:) indicates a double bond joining two moieties head to head.

[b]In reference to activity of β-carotene (=100).

Adapted from J. A. Olson and M. R. Lakshmanan, "Enzymatic Transformations of Vitamin A, with Particular Emphasis on Carotenoid Cleavage" in The Fat-Soluble Vitamins, H. F. DeLuca and J. W. Suttie, eds., University of Wisconsin Press, Madison, 1969.

Table 4.2 CAROTENOIDS WITHOUT VITAMIN A ACTIVITY

Compound	Moiety Structure[a]
Hydrocarbons	
Phytoene	(Geranyl-geranyl:)$_2$
Lycopene	(Geranyl-geranyl-4,8-diene:)$_2$
Decapopreno-β-carotene	(Retinylprenyl:)$_2$
retro-β-Carotene	(*retro*-anhydroretinyl:)$_2$
Oxygenated derivatives	
Zeaxanthin	(3-hydroxyretinyl:)$_2$
Isozeaxanthin	(4-hydroxyretinyl:)$_2$
Lutein	3-hydroxyretinyl:3-hydroxy-α-retinyl
5,6:5′,6′-Diepoxy-β-carotene	(5,6-epoxyretinyl:)$_2$
5,8:5′,8′-Diepoxy-β-carotene	(5,8-epoxyretinyl:)$_2$
Astacin	(3,4-diketoretinyl:)$_2$

[a]Colon(:) indicates a double bond joining two moieties head to head.

From J. A. Olson and M. R. Lakshmanan, "Enzymatic Transformations of Vitamin A, with Particular Emphasis on Carotenoid Cleavage" in The Fat-Soluble Vitamins, H. F. DeLuca and J. W. Suttie, eds., University of Wisconsin Press, Madison, 1969.

metry or radiochemical analysis (Britton and Goodman, 1971). If the goal of analysis is to determine vitamin A activity rather than carotene content per se, a bioassay method is preferred (see Harris, 1960; Ames, 1965).

Biochemical Function. A specific coenzyme function has not been demonstrated for vitamin A. Indeed there seems to be considerable opinion that vitamin A may be regarded as a hormone, albeit a hormone that must be supplied in the diet. A hormone has been defined by Wolf and De Luca (1970) as a substance secreted into the bloodstream that influences tissues and organs to differentiate and elaborate new cell types and new enzymes. If one disregards the fact that vitamin A (unlike the substances traditionally classified as hormones) cannot be synthesized by the animal body, then it would seem to comply with the Wolf-De Luca definition. These authors further suggest that because the vitamin is stored in the liver and secreted into the blood stream when needed, the liver thus behaves as an endocrine organ.

The physiological functions of vitamin A have been well defined for many years. The vitamin is necessary for growth, reproduction, the maintenance of epithelial tissues, and for normal vision. Of these functions, only the latter—the visual function—has been delineated in terms of biochemical action. The role of the vitamin in growth is least well understood. Its role in reproduction and epithelial tissues, although still an enigma, at least can be characterized by a series of events that are associated directly or indirectly with vitamin A.

In the visual function vitamin A is combined with a hexose and hexosamine-containing protein, opsin, to form the visual pigment rhodopsin. This pigment is present in the rod cells of retina of most, but not all, vertebrates. Functionally 11-*cis*-retinaldehyde is the active form of the vitamin moiety of rhodopsin and combines with opsin through an ε-amino group of a specific lysine residue of the protein and possibly through the sulfhydryl group of a cysteine residue (Heller, 1968). Other light-sensitive pigments also contain a form of vitamin A. Iodopsin, a pigment of the cone cells, contains retinaldehyde, but the opsin is different from that of rod cells; porphyropsin, found in rod cells of fresh-water fish, contains 3-dehydroretinaldehyde.

The reactions involved in the visual cycle were identified principally by Wald and his associates (see Wald, 1953). The pigment rhodopsin (visual purple) is bleached by light, resulting in liberation of protein and retinaldehyde in all *trans* form via a series of intermediary compounds (Matthews et al., 1964). In the dark, the pigment is regenerated; this process requires that retinaldehyde be isomerized back to the *cis* form. The series of reactions is shown in Fig. 4.1. Some of the vitamin is degraded in the overall process, and night blindness results when there is not sufficient vitamin present for regeneration of the rhodopsin molecule. The effect of light on degeneration of rhodopsin and the maintenance of rhodopsin content of the eye have been shown in rats to be highly dependent on the level of illumination to which the animals are exposed. Animals that were depleted of vitamin A and kept in the dark maintained rhodopsin content of the retina for five to six months while those kept in weak cyclic light lost rhodopsin continuously (Noell and Albrecht, 1971).

Both retinol and retinaldehyde will prevent night blindness, but retinoic acid is not effective in the visual process. As shown in Fig. 4.2, the alcohol and aldehyde forms of the vitamin are interconvertible. Retinoic acid is a normal metabolite of retinol and

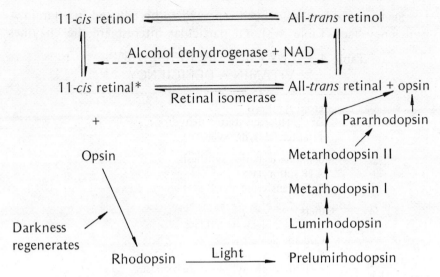

Fig. 4.1 Role of Vitamin A in the Visual Cycle. The asterisk (*) indicates the active form.

retinaldehyde, but it cannot be converted *in vivo* to either of these compounds. The acid, however, is fully active in promoting growth in experimental animals.

The role of the vitamin in the growth process is poorly understood. Vitamin A-deficient animals lack appetite and fail to grow. Loss of appetite has been attributed in part to loss of the sense of taste due to keratinization of taste buds and atrophy of accessory glandular tissue (Bernard and Halpern, 1968). Death appears to be due to infection. Bieri et al. (1969) found that conventional animals reared under standard laboratory conditions died within 54 days when fed a vitamin A-deficient diet whereas germ-free animals lived up to 272 days.

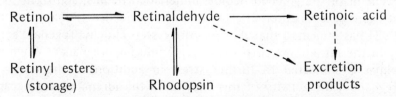

Fig. 4.2 Interrelationship between retinol, retinaldehyde, and retinoic acid.

Several enzymes have been reported to be reduced in vitamin A deficiency (see Table 4.3). Of particular interest are the enzymes

Table 4.3   ENZYMES DECREASED BY
VITAMIN A DEFICIENCY

Steroid synthesis
$\Delta^{5,3}\beta$-Hydroxysteroid dehydrogenase
11β-Steroid hydroxylase

Mucopolysaccharide synthesis
ATP sulfurylase
Sulfotransferase

Others
L-γ-Gulonolactone oxidase
Codeine demethylase
Squalene oxidocyclase
p-Hydroxyphenyl pyruvate oxidase
Oxidative phosphorylation

---

involved in steroid synthesis ($\Delta^{5,3}\beta$-hydroxysteroid dehydrogenase and 11β-steroid hydroxylase) and in mucopolysaccharide synthesis (ATP sulfurylase and sulfotransferase). The activity of these enzymes possibly could be linked with the function of vitamin A in reproduction in experimental animals and in the maintenance of epithelial tissues.

It would be tempting to conclude that the effect of vitamin A deficiency on reproduction, for example, is the result of a depression in activity of $\Delta^{5,3}\beta$-hydroxysteroid dehydrogenase. This enzyme catalyzes the conversion of $\Delta^{5,3}\beta$-hydroxysteroids to Δ^{4}-3-keto-steroids and, therefore, is involved in synthesis of steroid hormones (from cholesterol) in the adrenals, gonads, and placenta. One such reaction is the conversion of pregnenolone to progesterone, the precursor of the glucocorticoids, mineralocorticoids, androgens, and estrogens (see Chapter 2). Histochemical evidence (Pohanka et al., 1973) has indicated that $\Delta^{5,3}\beta$-hydroxysteroid dehydrogenase activity in the rat adrenal cortex is increased during pregnancy. When the animal is subjected to further stress in addition to the stress of pregnancy, the activity of this enzyme in the adrenal cortex became extremely intense. In vitamin A-deficient pregnant rats, however, pregnenolone prevented fetal resorption but progesterone was ineffective (Juneja et al., 1969). In addition Rogers and Bieri (1968) found that pair-fed rats and vitamin A-deficient rats showed similar activity for $\Delta^{5,3}\beta$-hydroxysteroid dehydrogenase.

The possibility that vitamin A is directly involved in synthesis of mucopolysaccharides has intrigued investigators for many years in view of the profound effects of vitamin A on epithelial tissues. Indeed the enzyme ATP sulfurylase (which activates sulfate) was reported some years ago to be depressed in the early stages of vitamin A deficiency. This finding has been both confirmed and contradicted by an almost equal number of subsequent studies. Experiments with pair-fed animals have led to the conclusion that inanition and stress, instead of a lack of vitamin A per se, are responsible for decreased activity of ATP sulfurylase (as well as $\Delta^{5,3}\beta$-hydroxysteroid dehydrogenase and L-gulono-γ-lactone oxidase) in vitamin A deficient animals (Rogers, 1969). Moreover, Olson (1969) has suggested that the effect of vitamin A deficiency on enzyme activity is greatly influenced by the nutritional state of the animal. Differences in diets used or previous nutritional state of the animal, therefore, could possibly account, in part, for discrepancies among laboratories. Thus, a possible coenzyme role for vitamin A in these enzyme systems remains questionable.

An alternative role for vitamin A in the maintenance of epithelial tissue integrity has been offered by DeLuca et al. (1972) who studied the effect of vitamin A deficiency on intestinal tissue. In most epithelial tissues, vitamin A deficiency is characterized by replacement of normal mucus-secreting cells by keratinized epithelia. Intestinal mucosa does not become hyperkeratinized but instead there is a significant reduction in the number of goblet cells. In addition, goblet cells were shown to contain a specific fucose-containing glycopeptide and the synthesis of this compound also is decreased in vitamin A deficiency. DeLuca and coworkers (1972) hypothesize that vitamin A, a short-chain polyprenol derivative, may function in mammals by forming retinyl-phosphate-sugar intermediates that act as donors of sugar to acceptor proteins in membrane structures. This hypothesis is based on an analogy between vitamin A function in higher animals and the known function of polyisoprenols in bacteria in the transfer of mono- or oligosaccharides into acceptor proteins to synthesize glycoproteins.

To add to the confusion concerning the mode of action of vitamin A, a role in protein synthesis and in electron transfer also has been postulated (see Wasserman and Corradino, 1971). In vitamin A-deficient rats, administration of the vitamin stimulated incorporation of labeled uridine into RNA of intestinal mucosa and liver (Zachman, 1967). Evidence for participation of vitamin A in electron transfer is indirect and is based on a chemical model using two nonbiological electron acceptors (Lucy and Lichti, 1969). The significance of the chemical model to the biochemical mode of action of the vitamin remains speculative. For reviews of vitamin A metabolism and function see Wolf and DeLuca (1970), Wasserman and Corradino (1971), and Underwood (1974).

Vitamin A Metabolites. For some time it has been thought that there is an active metabolite common to retinol and retinoic acid. This speculation was based primarily upon the knowledge that retinoic acid (as well as retinal and retinol) would support growth; yet the acid cannot be converted to the other forms of vitamin A and thus does not function in the visual process. Attempts to identify a common active form of the vitamin so far have been unsuccessful. Retinol metabolism appears to be highly regulated; thus it seems likely that the amount of a circulating active compound in the body is minute (Roberts and DeLuca, 1967; Emerick et al., 1967). Conversely, retinoic acid metabolism is extremely rapid (Zachman et al., 1966), and it is difficult to identify or to isolate a single active form from among its metabolic products.

End products of vitamin A are known to be excreted in urine and bile. Two specific compounds are identified as end products of vitamin A metabolism. A product of retinoic acid was isolated from rat tissues and shown to be 13-*cis*-retinoic acid (Zile et al., 1967). This compound also is present in ester form. Retinyl-β-glucuronide has been shown to be a major component of metabolites of retinoic acid in bile (Dunagin et al., 1965; 1966).

Roberts and DeLuca (1967) have studied the metabolism of vitamin A in the rat using radioactive retinol and retinoic acid labeled in the 15-C of the isoprenoid chain or 6,7-C position of the β-ionone ring and retinoic acid labeled in the 14-C position. These studies indicate that the side chain is oxidized to carbon dioxide whereas the β-ionone ring is excreted entirely through the urine and feces. The degradation of the isoprenoid side chain to CO_2 occurs mostly at the terminal 15-C and less at the 14-C. However, radioactivity in urine was largely from the 6,7-C of the ring. The recovery of radioactivity from ^{14}C-retinoic acid was nearly complete within 48 hours indicating that retinoic acid is not stored in the rat; this finding has been confirmed recently by Smith et al. (1973).

From these data Roberts and DeLuca (1967) suggested that at least three major pathways for the metabolism of vitamin A exist (Fig. 4.3). Pathway I assumes the excretion of an intact isoprenoid chain and is based on the percentage of the radioactivity accounted for from 15-^{14}C in urine and feces. Approximately 62-65 percent

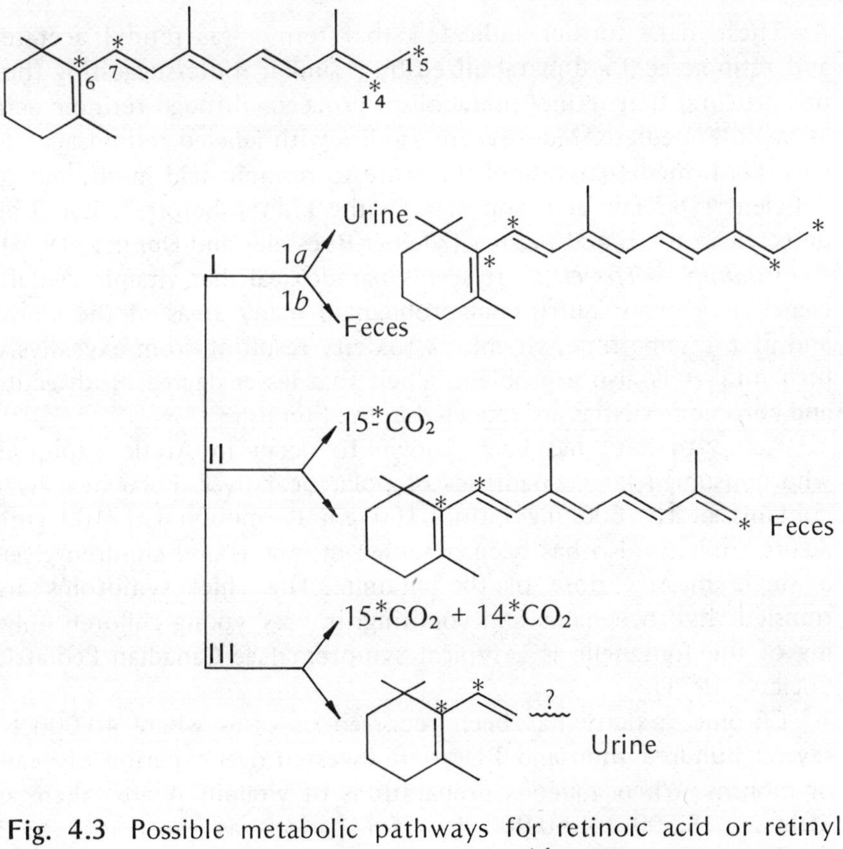

Fig. 4.3 Possible metabolic pathways for retinoic acid or retinyl acetate: * indicates the position of the ^{14}C label. The structures shown represent the portion of the retinoic acid or retinol molecule that would become incorporated into a product after metabolism by the suggested pathways. [From A. B. Roberts and H. F. DeLuca. *Biochem. J.*, 102:604 (1967).]

of labeled retinoic acid and 67-69 percent of retinyl acetate were accounted for by this pathway. Pathway II indicates the decarboxylation of 15-C with excretion of other labeled sites in the feces. Approximately 18-20 percent of retinoic acid and 9-12 percent of retinyl acetate were excreted via this route. Finally, pathway III considers the elimination of $^{14}CO_2$ from both 15-^{14}C and 14-^{14}C of the labeled compound and the appearance of the isoprenoid chain in the urine. The latter may include retinyl-β-glucuronic acid that, as mentioned previously, is found in bile of rats given retinoic acid.

These data further indicated that retinol (as retinyl acetate) and retinoic acid are metabolized by a similar route suggesting (but not proving) that retinol metabolism proceeds through retinoic acid as an intermediate. More recent studies with labeled retinyl acetate have confirmed that retinol gives rise to retinoic acid in vitamin A-deficient rats. The acid appeared in the kidney before it could be detected in the blood plasma (Kleiner-Boessaler and DeLuca, 1971).

Vitamin A Toxicity. It seems paradoxical that vitamin A deficiency is a major nutritional problem in many areas of the world and at the same time, vitamin A toxicity resulting from excessively high intakes is also a problem, albeit to a lesser degree. Both acute and chronic toxicities are reported in the literature.

Acute toxicity has been known to occur in Arctic explorers who consumed large quantities of polar bear liver. Polar bear liver contains nearly 600 mg retinol/100 gm (2 million I.U./100 gm). Acute toxicity also has been observed in infants and children given a single massive dose of the vitamin. The chief symptoms are transient hydrocephalus and vomiting. In very young children bulging of the fontanelle is a typical symptom (see Canadian Pediatric Society, 1971).

Chronic toxicity has been reported in cases where 40,000 to several hundred thousand I.U. were ingested over a period of years or months. When aqueous preparations of vitamin A are taken, as little as 18,500 to 60,000 I.U. for periods as short as 1 to 3 months may be toxic to children (Persson et al., 1965). Anorexia, loss of weight, nausea, vomiting, vague abdominal pain, and irritability are common symptoms. Drying and scaling of the lips and various types of skin rashes may occur without any other sign of toxicity. Loss of hair is not uncommon (Morrice et al., 1960). A characteristic symptom is pain and tenderness over the long bones, possibly with swelling of the joints. Other symptoms reported to occur include headache, pseudotumor cerebri, enlargement of the liver, spleen, and lymph glands, polydipsia, and polyuria (Dalderup, 1967; Meunter et al., 1971).

The clinical picture of vitamin A toxicity is variable, and one or two or many of the symptoms may be seen in any one case. It seems that many cases of minor chronic toxicity easily would not be detected. In clinically diagnosed cases, blood levels of vitamin A range from 250-6600 I.U./100 ml as compared with a normal range of 50-150 I.U. (Roe, 1966).

In experimental animals, excess vitamin A given during pregnancy resulted in congenital malformations in the young (Cohlan, 1953; Murakami and Kameyama, 1965). For further discussion of molecular effects of vitamin A excess see Chapter 14.

Vitamin A Antagonists. Several chemically unrelated compounds have been shown to be antagonistic to vitamin A. The nature of the antagonistic action is not known since the metabolic function of the vitamin itself is not understood. However, it appears that the antagonisms are quite different from those of the water-soluble vitamins which usually are associated with the coenzyme function of the vitamin.

Sodium benzoate (Meunier et al., 1949), monobromobenzene (Haley and Samuelsen, 1943), and citral (Leach and Lloyd, 1956) have been reported to produce toxic reactions in rats that could be counteracted by large doses of vitamin A. In the case of the first two compounds, it appears that the vitamin may act in some way as a detoxifying agent, and it seems possible that the mechanism is different for each of the toxic compounds. Citral, however, is somewhat similar in chemical structure to vitamin A and may be a more typical example of competitive antagonism at the molecular level.

A disease of cattle called *X* disease (bovine hyperkeratosis), which is caused by the contamination of feeds during processing with chlorinated naphthalenes, is similar to classic vitamin A deficiency. The disease may be alleviated by administration of vitamin A but is neither completely cured nor prevented by the vitamin (Copenhauer and Bell, 1954).

For further discussion of vitamin A antagonists see Green (1966).

Vitamin D (ergocalciferol, cholecalciferol)

It has been said facetiously that civilization changed vitamin D from a hormone into a vitamin. Certainly the ambiguous nature of this vitamin has been evident since Mellanby (1919) demonstrated the beneficial effect of cod liver oil and other foods in the prevention and cure of rickets, and in the same year Huldschinsky (1919) reported healing rickets in young children by exposure to sunlight or artificial ultraviolet light. In the middle 1920s Steenbock (1924) demonstrated that irradiation of foods also produced antirachitic activity. Later the phenomenon was shown to be due to activation of a sterol in foods. The Steenbock irradiation process was patented and royalties obtained helped to begin and continue to support the Wisconsin Alumni Research Foundation at the University of Wisconsin.

The factor responsible for prevention of rickets was named vitamin D and was clearly distinguished from the vitamin A also present in oils when it was discovered that antirachitic activity remained even after vitamin A activity had been destroyed by oxidation (McCollum et al., 1922). It was not until 1934, however, that it was demonstrated that the vitamin D synthesized in the animal body was chemically different from that derived from plant sources (Waddell, 1934).

Chemistry. Several forms of vitamin D exist; nearly all arise from the irradiation of sterols that are provitamins or precursors of the vitamin. The two most important forms of vitamin D in human nutrition are ergocalciperol and cholecalciferol. Ergosterol, which occurs in plants, is activated by sunlight to form ergocalciferol (vitamin D_2, calciferol). The form synthesized in animal epidermal cells is cholecalciferol (vitamin D_3) which is derived from 7-dehydrocholesterol. The formulas for these two forms of vitamin D are shown below.

Ergocalciferol differs from cholecalciferol only by a double bond at the 22,23 position and a methyl group at the 24 position. Both forms possess equal activity for man, the rat, and most mammalian species (Hess et al., 1925) with the exception of the newworld monkey (Hunt et al., 1967). However, ergocalciferol is only one-tenth as potent in curing rickets in chicks (Chen and Bosmann, 1964).

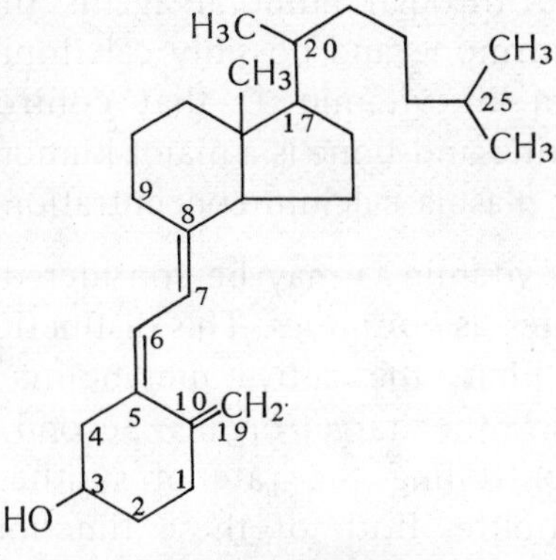

Vitamin D₃
Cholecalciferol

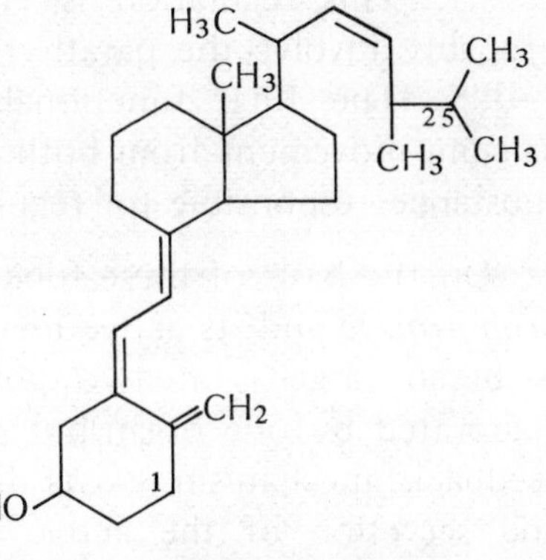

Vitamin D₂
Ergocalciferol

Although ultraviolet irradiation produces the vitamins from their sterol precursors, the active forms, ergocalciferol and cholecalciferol, are unstable to irradiation. Excessive irradiation will produce some toxic products. The vitamins D are not affected by oxidation or by temperatures below 140°C. In acid media the vitamins are relatively unstable, the instability increasing with increase in temperature. In alkaline solution vitamin D compounds are stable even at elevated temperatures.

Assay of the vitamin may be accomplished by chromatographic separation of the vitamin from interfering substances such as inactive sterols and vitamin A, and spectrophotometric determination of the nearly purified vitamin. Antimony trichloride-acetyl chloride reagent may be used for color development (see AOAC, 1960; U. S. Pharmacopeia, 1960). The more recent gas chromatographic method is suitable for separation of the various forms of the vitamin (Sheppard and Hubbard, 1971). Other methods of analysis including bioassay techniques have been described by DeLuca and Blunt (1971).

Biochemical Function. The biochemical function of vitamin D has been succinctly summarized by Omdahl and DeLuca (1973).

"1. Vitamin D must first be metabolically altered before it functions.

"2. Functional metabolites of vitamin D are generated in organs other than their sites of action.

"3. The rates of synthesis and secretion of these functional forms are feedback regulated.

"4. This regulation is effected through humoral agents that probably involve the parathyroid hormone and possibly calcitonin.

"5. The final functional form of vitamin D that controls calcium movement from both intestine and bone is a major humoral substance responsible for regulating plasma calcium concentration."

On the basis of these functions, vitamin D may be considered a *prohormone* and its active metabolites as *hormones*. This distinction is based largely on two points. First, the active metabolite is elaborated by one organ but acts on other target organs. Second, a feedback mechanism exists for controlling the rate of synthesis and secretion of the active metabolite. Both of these functions comply with the classic definition of a hormone, but not a vitamin, at least not in the same sense that we have come to think of the action of the water-soluble vitamins.

The overall effect of vitamin D is to bring about the mineralization of bone. In absence of the vitamin, rickets (or demineralization of bone) results. The mechanism by which vitamin D accomplishes mineralization lies in stimulating the absorption of calcium and phosphate from the intestinal lumen to the blood (Nicolaysen, 1937). Thus, plasma calcium and phosphorus levels are elevated so that these ions are present in good supply in the extracellular fluid surrounding the sites of calcification. The possibility that vitamin D functions in a more direct fashion in calcification of bone remains speculative. However, the vitamin is known to stimulate the mobilization of calcium from bone to blood.

The observation that a lag period of from 10-12 hours occurs after administration of vitamin D to rachitic animals before functioning of the calcium transport system or mobilization of calcium from bone led to the belief that some transformation of the vitamin was required before it became active *in vivo*. Following the preparation of a tritiated vitamin D, extensive work began in DeLuca's laboratory leading to the discovery of the active metabolite of the vitamin (see DeLuca, 1973; Omdahl and DeLuca, 1973; Wasserman and Corradino, 1973). It was reported that 25-hydroxycholecalciferol was the metabolically active form of vitamin D_3 (Blunt et al., 1969) and later 25-hydroxyergocalciferol as the active form of vitamin D_2 (Suda et al., 1969). The conversion of cholecalciferol to $25(OH)D_3$ was shown to occur in the liver under the influence of an enzyme calciferol-25-hydroxylase. This enzyme has recently been shown to be regulated by a feedback mechanism. Rats pretreated with labeled or unlabeled vitamin D_3 showed decreased levels of liver calciferol-25-hydroxylase activity and the degree and length of low activity depend upon the amount of vitamin administered (Bhattacharyya and DeLuca, 1973). The regulation of enzyme activity may be important both in protecting against vitamin D toxicity and in conserving vitamin D during periods when dietary intake and/or formation of vitamin D in skin are low.

Direct evidence suggesting that $25(OH)D_3$ was responsible for vitamin D action was obtained using perfused small intestine from vitamin D-deficient rats. Calcium transport was measured after addition of either 25 μg of $25(OH)D_3$ or 250 μg of vitamin D_3. The $25(OH)D_3$ induced a rise in calcium transport within two hours, whereas the vitamin D_3 had no effect (Olson and DeLuca, 1969). The two-hour delay in action suggested that perhaps $25(OH)D_3$ might have to be converted further. This anticipated next step was demonstrated almost simultaneously at the Cambridge laboratory (Lawson et al., 1971) and De Luca's laboratory at Wisconsin (Holick et al., 1971) in rats, and shortly thereafter confirmed in human subjects (Mawer et al., 1971). The active form of vitamin D was isolated and identified on the basis of mass spectrometry and specific chemical reactions as $1,25-(OH)_2 D_3$. The kidney was shown to be the site at which $1,25-(OH)_2 D_3$ is synthesized (Fraser and Kodicek, 1970). This metabolite was shown to act much more rapidly than $25(OH)D_3$ in both the calcium transport system and the bone calcium mobilization system. Further, $1,25-(OH)_2 D_3$ is about 10 times more potent than the $25(OH)D_3$ compound in the prevention and cure of rickets (Tanaka et al., 1973). The pattern of distribution of radioactive vitamin D_3 is closely correlated with the presumed sites of vitamin D_3 metabolism and possible sites of action. Following injection of ^{14}C-labeled vitamin D_3 into mice there was a high accumulation of radioactivity in the liver at short survival times (1 and 8 hours). At longer survival times there was a high and well localized uptake in the kidneys while concentration in liver became considerably lower (Dencker and Tjalve, 1973).

The synthesis of $1,25-(OH)_2 D_3$ is under feedback regulation by calcium availability. This finding helps to explain the well-known ability of man and experimental animals to adapt to low levels of dietary calcium by increasing calcium absorption. Indeed,

Boyle et al. (1971) demonstrated that rats fed low-calcium diets synthesize large amounts of $1,25\text{-}(OH)_2D_3$ whereas when calcium intake is increased the synthesis of $1,25\text{-}(OH)_2D_3$ is reduced. These data are in accord with the more recent finding of a feedback mechanism regulating the activity of calciferol-25-hydroxylase activity as mentioned previously. Furthermore, when $1,25\text{-}(OH)_2D_3$ synthesis is depressed, another metabolite identified as $24,25\text{-}(OH)_2D_3$ is formed (Holick et al., 1972). This compound is very active in intestinal calcium transport but has only slight activity in mobilization of calcium from bone.

More recently a third metabolite of vitamin D_3 has been identified. It is $1,24,25\text{-}(OH)_3D_3$ which is generated from $25(OH)D_3$ (Holick et al., 1973). This compound is preferentially more active in inducing calcium transport in the intestine than in mobilizing calcium from bone. It is about 60 percent as effective as vitamin D_3 in curing rickets.

Evidence suggests that parathyroid hormone stimulates synthesis of $1,25\text{-}(OH)_2D_3$ (Garabedian et al., 1972; Fraser and Kodicek, 1973). The feedback mechanism is shown in Fig. 4.4. When serum calcium falls below the norm of 10 mg per 100 ml the parathyroid glands are stimulated to secrete parathyroid hormone, which stimulates synthesis of $1,25\text{-}(OH)_2D_3$ in kidney. This compound then stimulates calcium intestinal absorption and mobilization from bone. When serum calcium returns to normal, the parathyroid secretion is cut off, and the feedback loop is completed (see Omdahl and DeLuca, 1973). The role of the parathyroid hormone in calcium metabolism in bone will be discussed in Chapter 17.

Vitamin D appears to be rather widely distributed in lipid-rich tissues in the animal body. Recent studies with ^{14}C-labeled vitamin D_3 suggest that adipose tissue and skeletal muscle are the major storage sites of unaltered cholecalciferol in the rat and in the human (Mawer and Schaefer, 1969; Holman et al., 1970; Rosenstreich et al., 1971; Mawer et al., 1971). The liver, although prominent in vitamin D metabolism, is not an important site for prolonged storage of the vitamin.

Vitamin D Metabolites. In addition to $25(OH)D_3$, $1,25\text{-}(OH)_2D_3$ and $24,25(OH)_2D_3$, a $25,26(OH)_2D_3$ derivative also has been isolated (Suda et al., 1970). The latter compound is active in calcium intestinal transport but has little activity in the laying down

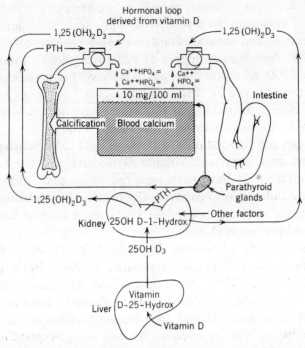

Hormonal loop
derived from vitamin D

Fig. 4.4 Schematic designation of hormonal control loop for vitamin D metabolism and function. A drop below set point for serum calcium of 10 mg per 100 ml prompts a proportional secretion of parathyroid hormone that acts to increase bone resorption and thus elevates serum calcium. Parathyroid hormone also directs metabolism of 25-OH-D$_3$ to 1,25-(OH)$_2$D$_3$ in the kidney, where "hormone" 1,25-(OH)$_2$D$_3$ acts both on bone and on intestine to mobilize calcium from bone and intestinal contents. As serum calcium increases toward its set point, parathyroid hormone secretion is proportionately decreased. [From J. L. Omdahl and H. F. DeLuca, *Physiol. Rev.*, 53: 327 (1973).]

or mobilization of calcium from bone. Because other sterols are known to be hydroxylated in this manner prior to cleavage and elimination from the body, it has been suggested that this reaction may be a final step in the degradation of vitamin D$_3$

Other unidentified inactive compounds formed from vitamin D$_3$ also have been detected (Ponchon and DeLuca, 1969).

Vitamin D Toxicity. Vitamin D toxicity in humans is more likely to occur in infants and young children, but toxic symptoms have been reported in adults as well. In mild toxicity, hypercalcemia is the chief symptom. In severe toxicity, typical facies, supravalvular aortic stenosis, and mental retardation have been reported (Anning et al., 1948; American Academy of Pediatrics, 1963). Intakes in the range of 2000 to 3000 I.U. per day have been associated with hypercalcemia. However, lower intakes also have been implicated (Taussig, 1966) and individual hypersensitivity to the vitamin may be a causal factor in such cases (Fraser et al., 1966).

Although the population at risk is believed to be relatively small, the dangers associated with vitamin D toxicity and the rather low levels of intake that have been reported to be toxic prompted the American Academy of Pediatrics Committee on Nutrition (1965) to recommend extreme caution in supplementation of foods other than milk with vitamin D.

Excessive levels of vitamin D_2 (150,000 I.U. daily for 10-14 days) were found to stimulate oxidation of tissue lipids (Spirchev and Blazheievich, 1969). Antioxidants and especially tocopherols reduced peroxidation and deposition of calcium in aorta and kidney. The effect of vitamin D and the opposing effect of tocopherols and antioxidants was believed to be due to corresponding effects on mitochondrial and lysosomal membranes (see Chapter 9). This finding may prove to be significant in explaining the mechanism of vitamin D toxicity.

Other attempts have been made to counteract the effects of excess vitamin D in experimental animals. Calcitonin, which inhibits bone resorption and resulting hypercalcemia, was shown to be partially effective in rats with vitamin D toxicity (Mittelman et al., 1967; Frankel and Yasamura, 1971). However, chondroitin A, which inhibits calcification, did not prevent deposition of calcium in blood vessels, kidney and other soft tissues (Robbins et al., 1969).

Vitamin D Antagonists. No antagonists of vitamin D are known at present.

Vitamin E

Vitamin E has been known as the antisterility vitamin since its discovery in 1922 by Evans and Bishop as the fat-soluble factor that prevented resorption of fetuses in female rats and testicular degeneration in males. The early history of the vitamin has been reviewed by Evans (1963) including the work of Karrer,

Fernholz, the Emersons, and others in the isolation and synthesis of the tocopherol compounds. The name tocopherol was derived from the Greek *tokos* (childbirth) and *phero* (to bear), but the influence of the tocopherols is vastly greater than the original designation implies.

Chemistry. Two distinct classes of compounds comprise the vitamin E group. They are all derivatives of chroman-6-ol. The first series—the tocopherols—derive from tocol, which contains a 16-carbon saturated isoprenoid side chain. The second series, the tocotrienols, contain a triply unsaturated side chain. Within each series the compounds differ only in the number and position of methyl groups in the ring structure. The ring structure of the corresponding tocotrienol is similar to the tocopherols designated α, β, γ, δ (see Table 4.4). Alpha tocopherol is the most widely distributed in nature and is the most active biologically of the compounds. The formula is shown below.

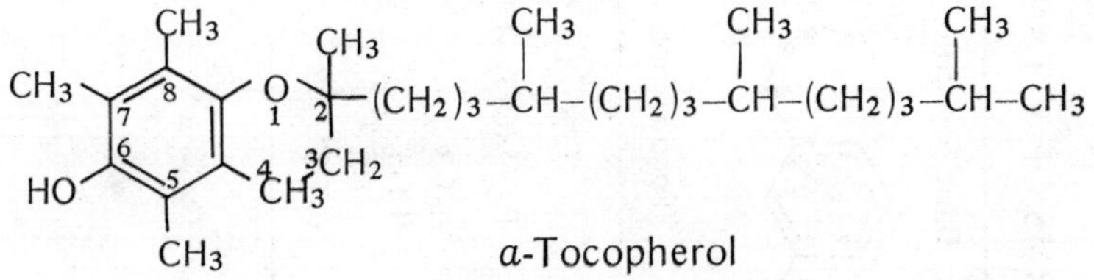

α-Tocopherol
(5,7,8-trimethyltocol)

Vitamin E is found mostly in plants and is present in highest concentration in many of the seed oils such as soybean, cottonseed, corn, sunflower, and wheat germ oil. Olive, coconut, and peanut oils are low in the vitamin. Animal tissues also contain little vitamin E; that present is mostly α-tocopherol.

The vitamin is a potent antioxidant and functions, at least in part, in protecting other nutrients, such as vitamin A and poly-unsaturated fatty acids, from destructive oxidation. The tocopherols are themselves easily oxidized, and this property presents problems in analyses for the vitamin particularly in its isolation. The early chemical assay for tocopherol is based on the Emmerie and Engel reaction, the reaction of tocopherols with ferric chloride to yield ferrous chloride which, in turn, reacts with α-α'-dipyridyl to yield a red-colored complex (see Quaiffe and Harris, 1948). This method has almost completely given way to gas-liquid chromatography as the preferred method of assay (see Kofler et al., 1962;

Table 4.4 NATURALLY OCCURRING FORMS OF VITAMIN E

	CH₃ Substitution

Basic Structure

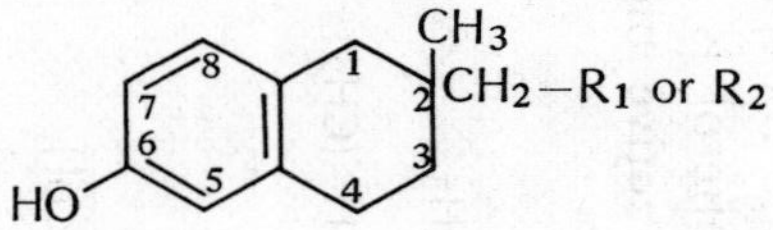

$$CH_2-R_1 \text{ or } R_2$$

Tocotrienols

$$R_2 = (CH_2-CH=C-CH_2)_3H$$ with CH_3

	CH₃ Substitution
α-T-3	5,7,8-Trimethyl
β-T-3	5,8-Dimethyl
γ-T-3	7,8-Dimethyl
δ-T-3	8-Methyl

Tocols

$$R_1 = (CH_2-CH_2-CH-CH_2)_3H$$ with CH_3

| α-T |
| β-T |
| γ-T |
| δ-T |

Sheppard et al., 1971; Ames, 1972). The determination of individual tocols and tocotrienols by partial purification using thin-layer chromatography and subsequent identification as their trimethylsilyl ethers using gas-liquid chromatography has been reported (Slover et al., 1968). Chemical assay, however, provides little indication of biological activity. The classic bioassay procedure measures the amount of tocopherol that will prevent fetal resorption in female rats or testicular degeneration in male rats on a tocopherol-free diet. A more recent bioassay procedure measures the amount of tocopherol that will prevent hemolysis of erythrocytes from tocopherol-deficient rats when erythrocytes are incubated with dialuric acid or dilute hydrogen peroxide (Rose and György, 1952; Century and Horwitt, 1965). This method, in effect, measures the extent of lipid peroxidation in erythrocyte membranes. A new method for determination of lipid peroxidation involving ethane evolution recently has been described (Riley et al., 1974).

   Biochemical Function.   A coenzyme function for vitamin E has not been demonstrated and in spite of a tremendous amount of research the role of the vitamin in biological systems is still controversial. At least three schools of thought currently exist regarding the biochemical function of vitamin E. One maintains that the vitamin functions primarily as an antioxidant and that symptoms of vitamin E deficiency are secondary to *in vivo* damage to sensitive cell structures produced by intermediates of lipid peroxidation. That is, in the absence of the vitamin, free radicals arise, and these may interact at critical enzyme sites and structural membranes (Tappel, 1962; 1970). Another view of the vitamin suggests that deficiency symptoms cannot be explained by lipid peroxidation and that a more specific (although presently unknown) role exists (Boguth, 1967; Green and Bunyan, 1969). A third viewpoint embraces the two, that is, vitamin E functions as an antioxidant in preventing certain symptoms of deficiency but, in other cases, it functions in a more specific manner (Scott, 1970).

   In support of the latter theory, Wasserman and Taylor (1972) have classified vitamin E deficiency diseases into two categories: those that respond to an antioxidant as well as to the vitamin and those that respond to the vitamin but are not affected by antioxidants. The antioxidant-responsive symptoms include encephalomalacia, *in vitro* erythrocyte hemolysis, formation of ceroid pigments, and reproductive failure in some species (Table 4.5).

Table 4.5 THE VITAMIN E DEFICIENCY DISEASES

Disease	Experimental Animal	Tissue Affected	Severity Dependent Upon Dietary PUFA	Prevented by			
				Vitamin E	Selenium	Synthetic Antioxidants	Sulfur Amino Acids
REPRODUCTIVE FAILURE							
Embryonic degeneration							
Type A	Female rat, hen, turkey	Vascular system of embryo	Yes	Yes	No	Yes	No
Type B	Cow, ewe	Vascular system of embryo	No	No[a]	Yes[b]	No	No
Sterility	Male rat, guinea pig, hamster, dog, cock	Male gonads	No	Yes	No	No	No
LIVER, BLOOD, BRAIN, CAPILLARIES, ETC.							
Liver Necrosis	Rat, pig	Liver	No	Yes	Yes	No	No
Erythrocyte Hemolysis	Rat, chick, man (premature infant)	Erythrocytes	Yes	Yes	No	Yes	Yes

Condition	Species	Tissue affected					
Plasma Protein Loss	Chick, Turkey	Serum albumen	No	Yes	Yes	No	No
Anemia	Monkey	Bone marrow	No	Yes	No	Yes	No
Encephalomalacia	Chick	Cerebellum	Yes	Yes	No	Yes	No
Exudative Diathesis	Chick, turkey	Vascular system	No	Yes	Yes	No	No
Kidney Degeneration	Rat, monkey, mink	Kidney tubular epithelium	Yes	Yes	Yes	No	No
Depigmentation	Rat	Incisors	Yes	Yes	No	Yes	No
Steatitis (yellow fat disease)	Mink, pig, chick	Adipose tissue	Yes	Yes	No	Yes	No
NUTRITIONAL MYOPATHIES							
Nutritional muscular dystrophy Type A	Rabbit, guinea pig, monkey, duck, mouse, mink	Skeletal muscle	No	Yes	No	No?	No
Type B	White muscle disease of lamb, calf, kid	Skeletal and heart muscles	No	No[a]	Yes[b]	No	No
Type C	Turkey	Gizzard, heart	No	No[a]	Yes	No	No
Type D	Chicken	Skeletal muscle	No[c]	Yes	No	No	Yes

From M. L. Scott, The Fat Soluble Vitamins, H. F. DeLuca and J. W. Suttie, eds., The Univ. of Wisconsin Press, Madison, 1969, p. 357.

[a] Not effective in diets severely deficient in selenium.
[b] When added to diets containing low levels of vitamin E.
[c] A low level (0.5%) of linoleic acid is necessary to produce dystrophy; higher levels did not increase vitamin E required for prevention.

The symptoms which respond to vitamin E but do not respond to antioxidants include muscular dystrophy in most species, testicular degeneration in the rat, and anemia in monkeys. Thus, it seems likely that vitamin E functions in living systems both as an antioxidant *and* in some possibly more specific but as yet unknown role.

The delineation of tocopherol function is complicated by variations in response of different species to the vitamin and by the relation of vitamin E to other dietary factors. Some symptoms of deficiency are accentuated by dietary polyunsaturated acids; other symptoms may be prevented by nonspecific antioxidants, by selenium, or by sulfur-containing amino acids.

The relationship between dietary PUFA and vitamin E is well documented in experimental animals (Dam, 1962) and man (Horwitt, 1962). The requirement for vitamin E is increased as the PUFA content of the diet is increased and, consequently, the severity of symptoms due to a lack of vitamin E in the diet is increased by the level of dietary PUFA.

Most (but not all) of the symptoms of vitamin E deficiency can be prevented by a nonspecific antioxidant (Table 4.5). Encephalomalacia and exudative diathesis in chicks are typical examples of this phenomenon. The clinical signs of encephalomalacia are ataxia, spasms, or paralysis. Exudative diathesis is characterized by accumulation of fluid in subcutaneous tissues, muscles, or connective tissues and is caused by exuding of plasma from the capillaries. These symptoms were first described by Pappenheimer and Goettsch (1931) and do not occur in chicks given a fat-free vitamin E-deficient diet. Furthermore, ceroid pigmentation, a yellow-brown coloration of adipose tissue, liver, and other tissues that is highly characteristic of vitamin E deficiency, is known to be dependent upon the *in vivo* autoxidation of polyunsaturated acids (Dam and Granados, 1945). On the other hand, fetal resorption has been shown to be prevented in rats on a vitamin E-low diet by the antioxidant diphenyl-β-phenylenediamine (Draper et al., 1964) but not by ethoxyquin, which is active against encephalomalacia. However, ceroid pigments have been observed in uterus and fallopian tubes of vitamin E-deficient rats (Raychaudhuri and Desai, 1971). This finding suggested that lipid peroxidation resulting in tissue damage could be responsible for the irreversible loss of fertility.

Similarly, Nogichi et al. (1973) have shown that both vitamin E and selenium will prevent exudative diathesis in chickens on a diet low in selenium and vitamin E. Selenium appears to act by destroying peroxides that form within the capillary cell; vitamin E may act within the cell lipid membrane where it neutralizes free radicals, thus preventing a chain-reaction autoxidation of the capillary membrane lipids.

To add to the confusion, muscular dystrophy in some species responds to vitamin E only whereas in the chick cystine or methionine are also effective. In the turkey selenium is the only known preventive agent (Table 4.5).

Anemia in the monkey, however, appears to be the result of a specific vitamin E effect on hematopoiesis in bone marrow rather than red cell destruction by membrane peroxidation (Fitch, 1968). It could be postulated, therefore, that the vitamin E-responsive anemia observed in children with protein-calorie malnutrition derives from the same defect as that which occurs in monkeys on a vitamin E-deficient diet (Majaj et al., 1963; Majaj, 1966). Indeed, Murty et al. (1970) and Caasi et al. (1973) have presented evidence of a direct effect of vitamin E on heme biosynthesis. Vitamin E deficiency in the rat was shown to lead to decreased activity of bone marrow δ-aminolevulinic acid synthetase and hepatic δ-aminolevulinic acid dehydratase. Studies on the incorporation of glycine-2^{14}C and δ-aminolevulinic acid into bone marrow heme indicated that in bone marrow the defect was at the level of the first enzyme whereas in liver the defect appears to be primarily at the second. The failure to maintain heme synthesis in vitamin E-deficient rats was reflected partially by lowered levels of the heme protein enzymes catalase and tryptophan oxygenase, and of microsomal cytochrome P-450 and microsomal cytochrome b_5. The activity of nonheme enzymes was not affected by vitamin E deficiency, which suggests that the effect of the vitamin on heme synthesis is due to a specific, although as yet unknown, role of the vitamin.

Tappel (1970) has proposed a theory by which antioxidants, selenium, and the sulfur-containing amino acids all fit into the damage to protein and enzymes produced by lipid peroxidation. Free radical intermediates of lipid peroxidation react with proteins and enzymes such that cross-linking of the molecular structure results in loss of solubility and destruction of amino acids comprising these structures. Methionine, cystine, histidine, and lysine are among the most labile of the amino acids (Roubal and Tappel,

1966) and the sulfhydryl enzymes are most susceptible to inactivation (Chio and Tappel, 1969). Malonaldehyde produced by peroxidizing lipids may be the active compound responsible for the intra- and intermolecular cross-linking of the enzyme structure that results in loss of activity. According to Tappel (1970) vitamin E functions as an inhibitor of lipid peroxidation. Sulfhydryl compounds react in small amounts as free radical scavengers and as peroxide decomposers. Selenoamino acids react similarly but also protect the enzyme structure apparently by binding reversibly to enzyme sulfhydryl groups. Whether this hypothesis can explain the role of vitamin E in heme synthesis remains to be seen.

Vitamin E Metabolites. Very little is known of the metabolic fate of vitamin E. The formation of a dimer and a trimer in rat and pig liver has been reported as the result of a-tocopherol oxidation (Csallany and Draper, 1963; Draper et al., 1967). Neither compound evidenced vitamin E activity, but they are believed to be formed in animal tissues since oral administration of the synthetic dimer indicated extremely poor absorption from the intestinal lumen. It does not seem likely, therefore, that these compounds are formed in the gut.

Two minor metabolites of vitamin E have been identified. Alpha-tocopherol-p-quinone was identified in rat liver and adipose tissue (Csallany et al., 1962; Weber and Wiss, 1963). This compound has little or no biological activity. Alpha tocopheronic acid was isolated from urine (Simon et al., 1956) after administration of massive doses of vitamin E. This compound is believed to be formed via a-tocopherol quinone that is itself a minor metabolite of the vitamin which is excreted partially through the feces.

Vitamin E Antagonists. No true metabolic antagonists of vitamin E are as yet known.

Vitamin E Toxicity. Available evidence suggests that vitamin E has a low level of toxicity in the human (Hillman, 1957) and, in general, there has been little concern over the likelihood of overdosing. Hypervitaminosis E, however, has recently been demonstrated in chicks given 2200 I.U. vitamin E/kg of diet (March et al., 1973). Depression in growth, bone calcification, hematocrit levels, and in respiration of skeletal muscle mitochondria was observed as well as increased prothrombin times. The effects on bone calcification and prothrombin time suggested that requirements for vitamin D and vitamin K were increased by hypervitaminosis E.

Large doses of vitamin E have been proposed by various individuals and groups for the treatment of heart disease, infertility, muscular dystrophy as well as numerous other ailments. There is no present convincing evidence, however, in favor of giving vitamin E supplements for any of these disorders (Committee on Nutritional Misinformation, 1973; Olson, 1973). In view of the recent evidence of hypervitaminosis E in chicks, the possibility of adverse effects occurring in man as a result of overzealous supplementation with vitamin E should be reevaluated.

Vitamin K

Vitamin K was identified in 1935 by Dam as a factor present in green leaves which prevented a hemorrhagic syndrome observed in chicks maintained on a low fat diet. The new fat-soluble vitamin was designated vitamin K for the Danish word, *koagulation.* The purified compound was isolated from alfalfa by Dam and associates in 1939 (see Dam, 1948).

Chemistry. Vitamin K exists in nature in two series of compounds: the phylloquinone (K_1) series and the menaquinone (K_2) series. A third series is related to the synthetic compound, menadione (2-methyl-1,4-naphthoquinone or vitamin K_3), a ring compound which is the basic structure of the naturally occurring vitamins and is about twice as active biologically as vitamins K_1 and K_2 under most conditions.

Menadione

The naturally occurring vitamins are 2-methyl-1,4-naphthoquinones substituted in the 3-position by isoprenoid chains. Vitamin K_1 contains a monounsaturated side chain with 20 C atoms (2-methyl-3-phytyl-) and occurs in green plants. The K_2 compounds contain a polyunsaturated side chain with 30-45 C atoms comprised of 6-9 isoprenoid units (2-methyl-3-difarnesyl-). These compounds are synthesized in many microorganisms including bacteria of the intestinal tract of a large number of species. Phthiocol

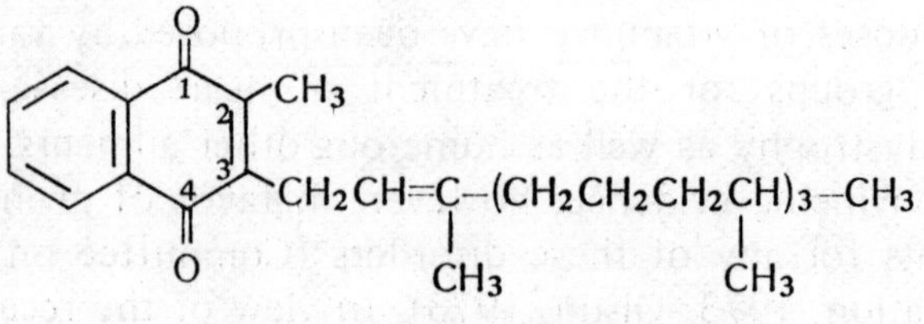

Vitamin K_1 (phylloquinone)

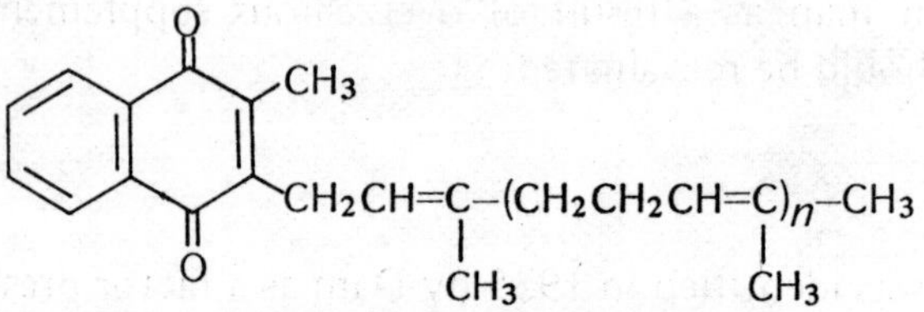

Vitamin K_2 (menaquinone)

(2-methyl-3-hydroxy-1,4-naphthoquinone), a pigment first isolated from bacteria, also has vitamin K activity.

All of the naphthoquinones are soluble in fat solvents; the synthetic compound is soluble in boiling water.

One of the first methods for the assay of vitamin K was a color reaction with sodium ethylate (Dam-Karrer reaction), which forms an unstable violet-blue color that quickly changes to red. Spectrophotometric measurement can be made when the color changes to a stable reddish brown. Other methods of analysis include ultraviolet spectroscopy, polarography, thin-layer chromatography and gas chromatography (see Sommer and Kofler, 1966; Sheppard, 1971). A crucial part of any assay for the vitamin is its separation from interfering substances such as other quinones, chlorophyll, and carotenoid pigments.

Biological activity may be determined by a chick bioassay in which blood clotting time or whole blood prothrombin level is the criterion for measuring vitamin K activity. The relative potency of the various forms of vitamin K has been reviewed in detail by Griminger (1966).

Biochemical Function. The active form of vitamin K and its specific role in mammals are not known. The vitamin is known, however, to be essential for the synthesis of prothrombin and of other factors involved in blood clotting.

Early work by Dam et al. (1936) and Quick (1957) indicated that prothrombin was lacking in hemorrhagic disease of chicks and that the disease was of dietary origin. The deficiency was later shown to be due to a lack of vitamin K (Brinkhous, 1940). For many years it was thought that vitamin K exerted its influence on blood clotting only through its effect on prothrombin synthesis in liver (see Ferguson, 1946). However, during the 1950s, three other factors involved in the complex series of events leading to blood coagulation were shown to be vitamin K-dependent: Factor IX, Factor VII, and Factor X (see Table 4.6).

Table 4.6 SCHEME OF BLOOD COAGULATION

Phase 1. Generation of thromboplastin
Platelet phosphatides
+ Factor VIII (antihemophilic globulin, AHG)
+ *Factor IX* (plasma thromboplastin component, PTC)   } Plasma thromboplastin
+ Factor XI (plasma thromboplastin antecedent, PTA)
+ Factor XII (Hageman factor)

Phase 2. Activation of thromboplastin
Plasma thromboplastin
+ Factor V (labile factor)
+ *Factor VII* (stable factor)   } Activated thromboplastin
+ *Factor X* (Stuart-Prower factor)
+ Ionic calcium (factor IV)

Phase 3. Conversion of prothrombin
Activated thromboplastin
+ *Prothrombin* (factor II)   } Thrombin

Phase 4. Conversion of fibrinogen
Thrombin
+ Fibrinogen (factor I)   } Fibrin
+ Factor XIII (fibrin stabilizing factor)

From C. A. Owen, Jr.,"Vitamin K X. Deficiency Effects in Animals and Human Beings" in The Vitamins, Vol. III, W. H. Sebrell, Jr. and R. S. Harris, eds., Acad. Press, N. Y., 1971, p. 472.

The first factor to be discovered was called stable factor (Owen and Bollman, 1948) later shown to be two factors, Factor VII (Koller et al., 1951) and the Stuart-Prower factor or Factor X (Hougie et al., 1957). Factor IX was first identified as plasma thromboplastin component (PTC) factor in this country (Aggeler et al., 1952; Schulman and Smith, 1952) and Christmas factor in England (Biggs et al., (1952).

How vitamin K functions in the synthesis of blood coagulation factors remains speculative. Studies with actinomycin D suggested to Olson (1964) that vitamin K was involved in the control of DNA-directed mRNA synthesis. Subsequent investigations by Olson and other laboratories, however, indicated that vitamin K acts beyond the DNA level and possibly at the ribosomal level or in the transformation of a precursor protein to a final product. As an alternative hypothesis, Olson (1970) has proposed that the vitamin acts to regulate the biosynthesis of prothrombin and other vitamin K-dependent clotting proteins by binding with a hypothetical regulatory protein which has a recognition site for the prothrombin mRNA. Other reports gave evidence that the vitamin K-dependent clotting factors are present in the liver as a completed polypeptide chain. Studies by Shah and Suttie (1971) with cycloheximide, an antibiotic that inhibits protein synthesis, suggested that vitamin K acts to convert a protein of short biological half-life to prothrombin. Johnson et al. (1971) suggest that vitamin K functions by attaching the carbohydrate moiety to the completed polypeptide chain of the glycoprotein, prothrombin. Pereira and Couri (1971) also propose that vitamin K acts prior to or at the point of attachment of glucosamine to a precursor polypeptide chain to form thrombin. This hypothesis seems to be favored by a number of investigators (see Wasserman and Taylor, 1972).

A more recent finding adds indirect evidence to support this hypothesis. Johnson et al. (1972) have isolated a protein from plasma, "protein X," which is significantly increased in blood of vitamin K-deficient rats or warfarin (a vitamin K antagonist)-treated rats. As the level of protein X increased, the level of prothrombin decreased. In rats given vitamin K the reverse relationship between prothrombin and protein X was observed. These workers suggest that protein X may be the polypeptide chain awaiting attachment of the carbohydrate moiety to form prothrombin. Characterization of protein X may well bring the elucidation of vitamin K action closer.

Vitamin K Metabolites. Little is known of the breakdown products of vitamin K. An unidentified water-soluble factor with vitamin K-activity was isolated from pig liver (Lev and Milford, 1966) and from urine of rats (Wiss and Gloor, 1966). An inactive compound identified as a lactone formed from menaquinone or phylloquinone was reported by Gloor et al. (1966).

Labeled menadione is converted to menaquinone-4 in the rat and apparently biological activity depends on this conversion (Taggart and Matschiner, 1969). Similarly, menaquinone-4 appears in the liver of vitamin K-deficient rats following a single injection of vitamin K (Matschiner and Taggart, 1968). At least four significant inactive metabolites are secreted into the bile of rats, the most important being the glucuronide of 2-methyl-1,4-naphthoquinone, which apparently is formed in extraheptaic tissues (Losito et al., 1967).

The principal forms of the vitamin found in human liver are phylloquinone and menaquinone-7. However, various other menaquinone compounds are also present including menaquinone-9, -9(H_2), -9(H_4), -10, -10(H_2), -10(H_4), and -11 (Duello and Matschiner, 1972).

Shearer and Barkhan (1973) have reported on the excretion of vitamin K metabolites in urine of man following oral and intravenous administration of radioactive phylloquinone. At least three different glucuronide conjugates were detected. Treatment with dilute acid produced a neutral metabolite resembling phylloquinone-γ-lactone suggesting that the lactone originally identified by Wiss and Gloor (1966) may be an artifact resulting from the methods for isolating the metabolite. The biological activity of the compounds identified by Shearer and Barkhan (1973) was not established.

Vitamin K Antagonists. A number of vitamin K antagonists are known. The hemorrhagic effect of a substance present in spoiled sweet clover was isolated and identified by Campbell and Link (1941) as dicoumarol. This compound is one of a large number of 3-substituted 4-hydroxy coumarin compounds with anti-vitamin K activity. It is assumed that coumarin antagonists compete directly with vitamin K at the site where vitamin K exerts its biological activity. Warfarin, the rodenticide, and Tromexan, which is used clinically in the treatment of thromboembolisms, are dicoumaral derivatives. The anticoagulant effect of these compounds is reversed by phylloquinone or menaquinones but not by menadione.

A number of 1,3-indanedione derivatives also possess anti-vitamin K activity (see Arora and Mathur, 1963) and more recently 2-chloro-3-phytyl-1,4-naphthoquinone was shown to be a competitive antagonist of vitamin K (Lowenthal and MacFarlane, 1967). For a detailed discussion of vitamin K antagonists, see Green (1966).

Choline

$$\underset{\underset{\underset{CH_3}{|}}{HO-N}}{\overset{\overset{CH_2CH_2OH}{|}}{}}\overset{CH_3}{\underset{CH_3}{\diagdown}}$$

Choline

Choline is a trimethylated hydroxide compound and occurs in biological tissues in the free form and as a component of lecithin, acetylcholine, and certain of the plasmalogens and sphingomyelins. Choline is important as a source of labile methyl groups and is also synthesized by methylation of dimethylaminoethanol, the needed methyl group being supplied by methionine (Fig. 4.5).

A choline deficiency has never been demonstrated in man, and it is not known if a dietary supply is required in addition to that formed by biosynthesis. Because choline is widely distributed in plant and animal tissues, however, it seems unlikely that a deficiency

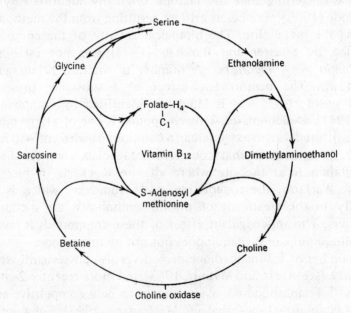

Fig. 4.5 Labile methyl metabolism.

would occur except under the most severe circumstances. Choline is known to be required by a number of animal species including the rat, the chick, the pig, and the dog. For this reason it is classified as a vitamin.

The two most significant results of choline deficiency in rats are fatty liver (Best and Huntsman, 1932) and hemorrhagic degeneration of kidneys (Griffith and Wade, 1939). In rats fed a choline-deficient diet, these conditions can be prevented by other methyl donors, betaine and methionine, or by folic acid and vitamin B_{12}. The coenzymes of the latter two nutrients catalyze reactions leading to *de novo* synthesis of methyl groups that can be transferred to homocysteine to form methionine (Fig. 4.5). Perosis or slipped tendon disease is the chief sign of choline deficiency in poultry. This disease responds to treatment with choline, but not to betaine, methionine, folic acid, or vitamin B_{12} (Table 4.7).

Table 4.7   EFFECT OF CHOLINE AND OTHER DIETARY FAC-
TORS ON SYMPTOMS PRODUCED BY CHOLINE
DEFICIENCY

Symptom	Choline	Methionine	Betaine	Folic acid + Vit. B_{12}
Fatty liver (rats)	+	+	+	+
Hemorrhagic kidneys (rats)	+	+	+	±
Prevention of perosis (chicks and turkeys)	+	—	—	—

Adapted from T. H. Jukes, Fed. Proc., 30:156 (1971).

There are three important pathways for choline metabolism in the animal body: (1) formation of phospholipids via phosphoryl-choline; (2) oxidation to betaine, a source of labile methyl groups; and (3) formation of acetylcholine, a neurotransmitter.

One of the earliest effects of choline deficiency in the rat is an interference with the secretion of triglycerides in the form of low-density lipoproteins from liver into the plasma. This defect seems to be the major cause for development of fatty liver in choline deficiency (Mookerjea, 1971).

The hemorrhagic kidney disease in choline-deficient weanling rats has been hypothesized to be due to two factors. First, decreased acetylcholine concentration in the kidney results in increased production of renal vasopressin and necrosis of the proximal convoluted tubules. Secondly, choline deficiency has been shown to result in a deficiency of the factor V involved in blood clotting. The latter could account for massive hemorrhages observed in kidneys of depleted animals. Working alone, neither factor likely could account for the hemorrhagic disease, but concomitantly, these two factors could cause the hemorrhagic degeneration observed in choline-deficient weanling rats (Wells, 1971).

Perosis in poultry appears to be independent of the labile methyl function of choline in that it is not alleviated by the usual methyl donors. It is possibly due to a defect in phospholipid synthesis and thus to effects on cell membrane function (Griffith and Nyc, 1971).

It has been tempting to speculate that choline deficiency could be involved in the fatty liver induced by protein-calorie malnutrition. Obviously, a deficiency of protein would indicate a deficiency of methionine and, thus, the possibility of a deficiency of labile methyl groups. At least one study has shown a positive effect of choline administration in treatment of fatty liver of protein-calorie malnutrition (Meneghello and Neimeyer, 1950). These results, however, have not been confirmed.

Myo-inositol

Myo-inositol

Inositols are cyclic alcohols (cyclohexanehexols) that, because of the presence of several hydroxyl groups and the configuration of the molecule, are related chemically to the sugars. Like the sugars, myo-inositol is a white crystalline substance and has a sweet taste. Several isomers of inositol exist in nature. Myo-inositol occurs in animal tissues as a constituent of phospholipids. In plants it is usually found as phytic acid, the hexaphosphate ester of inositol. It is present mostly in seeds and whole grains. Large amounts of phytic acid in the diet may interfere with the absorption of calcium and iron (see Chapter 5). Paradoxically, a beneficial effect of phosphates primarily in the form of phytates of whole grain cereals has been demonstrated in the prevention of dental caries (McClure, 1964).

In rats, myo-inositol deficiency results in an alopecia which presents a specific bilateral pattern (Woolley, 1941), one characteristic of which is the "spectacled eye" condition similar to biotin deficiency. In fact, it has been shown that myo-inositol alleviates to a large extent the spectacled eye produced by biotin deficiency (Lindley and Cunha, 1946). It has been postulated that the effect of myo-inositol is through stimulation of intestinal or tissue synthesis of biotin.

There is no evidence that myo-inositol is required in the diet of man. However, it is widely distributed in the body of man and has been demonstrated to exert a lipotropic action in patients with fatty infiltration of the liver (Milhorat, 1971).

Myo-inositol is thought to have three metabolic pathways in the animal body: (1) oxidation to CO_2, (2) synthesis of phospholipids, and (3) use in gluconeogenesis (Alam, 1971). Myo-inositol gives rise to glucose through glucuronic acid in the following sequence:

D-Glucuronic acid ⟶ L-Gulonic acid
↓
D-Xylulose ← Xylitol ← 3-Oxogulonic acid
↓
Pentose phosphate shunt
↓
Glucose

It is through this reaction that myo-inositol may be used in gluconeogenesis or oxidized to CO_2. The role of myo-inositol as a component of phospholipids appears to account both for its wide distribution in the animal body and for its apparent lipotropic action.

Lipoic Acid

$$CH_2 \diagup \overset{CH_2}{\diagdown} CH-(CH_2)_4COOH$$
$$S——S$$

Oxidized lipoic acid

$$CH_2 \diagup \overset{CH_2}{\diagdown} CH-(CH_2)_4COOH$$
$$\underset{SH}{|} \qquad \underset{SH}{|}$$

Reduced lipoic acid

Lipoic acid was discovered as a growth factor for certain micro-organisms (see Gunsalus, 1953). It likely is not a vitamin for mammals since it appears to be synthesized in adequate amounts in the mammalian cell. It is a coenzyme for a number of enzyme systems, the most significant of which are the pyruvate dehydrogenase complex and the α-ketoglutarate dehydrogenase complex (see Schmidt et al., 1969).

Lipoic acid exists in the oxidized (disulfide) and the reduced (sulfhydryl) form. In the pyruvate and α-ketoglutarate dehydrogenase systems, lipoic acid works along with thiamin in the transfer of acyl groups that, in effect, are generated by lipoic acid. The latter compound reacts with an acylol-thiamin complex to form a larger complex that rearranges to yield a free thiamin residue and an acyl-lipoic acid complex. (In the course of the reaction the acylol moiety is oxidized to an acyl group and the oxidized lipoic acid is reduced.) Finally, the acyl group is transferred to coenzyme A and the reduced lipoic acid is oxidized by an FAD-enzyme to yield the oxidized lipoic acid (see Chapter 13).

In enzyme binding, lipoic acid seems to be bound to the lysine residues of the enzyme protein. Hydrolysis of lipoic acid-protein complexes yields ϵ-N-lipoyl-L-lysine, a compound that is similar to biocytin (ϵ-N-biotinyl-L-lysine).

Lipoic acid, thus, is of vital importance in cellular oxidative processes. It is, however, of little significance as a dietary component in mammals.

Ubiquinone

Ubiquinone$_{10}$

Ubiquinone (coenzyme Q) is a collective name for a group of lipid-like compounds consisting of a substituted benzoquinone ring with a long isoprenoid side chain. Several forms of the compound exist in nature varying only in the number of isoprenoid units in the chain. Ubiquinone$_{10}$ is the form that is commonly found in mammalian respiratory systems. Ubiquinones with six to nine isoprenoid units are found in lower organisms. A chemically similar compound, plastoquinone, is found in plant tissues and apparently is functionally analagous to the ubiquinones in animal tissues.

Ubiquinone is synthesized in animal tissues and for this reason it is not a true vitamin. It functions in cellular electron transport, acting between the flavin coenzymes and the cytochromes (see Chapter 13). Like all quinones, ubiquinone is easily reduced to the hydroquinone.

Ubiquinone has been reported to improve reproductive performance of rats on a vitamin E-deficient diet (Scholler et al., 1968; Jones et al., 1971). The physical performance of genetically dystrophic mice also has been reported to be improved by administration of hexahydrocoenzyme Q_4, which can substitute for ubiquinone$_{10}$ (Scholler et al., 1968). Ubiquinone has also been shown to be of value in treatment of anemia of severe human malnutrition (Majaj and Folkers, 1968), and a deficiency of ubiquinone has been suspected in some cases of human heart disease (Littaru et al., 1971). As diverse as these conditions appear to be, it seems that the major contribution of ubiquinone may be in improving oxidative metabolism in the affected organs. The possibility of the use of ubiquinone in clinical medicine, therefore, appears to be a fertile field for further investigation.

chapter 5
minerals and water

1. Calcium
2. Phosphorus
3. Magnesium
4. Sodium
5. Chloride
6. Potassium
7. Sulfur
8. Iron

9. Other Trace Elements
   a. Copper
   b. Iodine
   c. Manganese
   d. Molybdenum
   e. Fluoride
   f. Selenium
   g. Zinc
   h. Chromium
   i. Nickel, Silicon, Tin, and Vanadium
10. Water

"...Fish, amphibian, and reptile, warm-blooded bird and mammal—each of us carries in our veins a salty stream in which the elements sodium, potassium and calcium are combined in almost the same proportions as in sea water. This is our inheritance from the day, untold millions of years ago, when a remote ancestor, having progressed from the one-celled to the many-celled stage, first developed a circulatory system in which the fluid was merely the water of the sea. In the same way, our lime-hardened skeletons are a heritage from the calcium-rich ocean of Cambrian time. Even the protoplasm that streams within each cell of our bodies has the

chemical structure impressed upon living matter when the first
simple creatures were brought forth in the ancient sea....''

Rachel Carson, *The Sea Around Us*

The bulk of the total mineral content of the animal body is
represented by the skeletal minerals. Lesser amounts of minerals
are constituents of essential molecules such as thyroxine and hemoglobin, or exist as free ions, or more frequently are loosely bound
to proteins and other substances in the body tissues. Activation of
cellular enzyme systems, the critical pH of body fluids necessary
for the control of metabolic reactions, and the osmotic balance
between the cell and its environment all largely depend on the
mineral elements present in the cellular medium.

The minerals that are known to be essential, and that are present
in fairly large quantities, are calcium, phosphorus, potassium,
sodium, chloride, magnesium, and sulfur. The principal minerals
present in micro quantities are iron, copper, cobalt, manganese, zinc,
iodine, and molybdenum. Accumulating evidence indicates that selenium, fluoride, and chromium are essential elements for most species
and that nickel, silicon, tin, and vanadium are essential for some
animals and likely also for man.

Essential elements characteristically tend to concentrate in body
tissues in a fairly consistent fashion; absorption from the gut and
excretion through the kidney, bile, or other intestinal secretions
are precisely regulated by body homeostatic mechanisms. However,
the homeostatic mechanism can be overloaded when excessive
amounts gain entrance to the body through food, water, or air.
A number of minerals that in minute amounts are essential to body
functioning are toxic when accumulated in large amounts. Iron,
zinc, and manganese as well as some of the newly detected essential
trace minerals are in this category.

In order to analyze minerals that are present in biological
materials the elements must be freed from the organic complexes

to which they are bound. Removal of organic substances is accomplished by ashing. Dry ashing involves heating the dried material to high temperatures in a muffle furnace; wet ashing is accomplished by digesting with strong acids. When minerals are present in fairly large amounts, methods of assay are usually quite precise. A number of reasonably simple colorimetric methods have been used for years (see Sandell, 1959; AOAC, 1960). Trace minerals, however, present more difficult analytical problems most of which are being met by newer methods such as emission spectrography, absorption spectrometry, neutron activation, gas-liquid chromatography, and spark-source mass spectrometry (see Mertz, 1971; Livingston and Wacker, 1971; Laitinen, 1972).

CALCIUM

The human body contains about 22 gm Ca/kg fat-free body weight, about 99 percent of which is concentrated in the hard structures of bones and teeth. The precise composition and structure of bone salt are not known; it is generally assumed to resemble a hydroxyapatite similar to $Ca_{10}(PO_4)_6(OH)_2$ (see Bronner, 1964). Other minerals such as magnesium, sodium, and strontium in combination with phosphates and carbonates or citrates are adsorbed on the surface of bone crystals or trapped in the lattice-like network characteristic of bone (see Chapter 17). Some minerals such as strontium likely are not essential to bone structure but are probably incidental though harmless contaminants. In other cases, such as lead poisoning, the accumulation of the contaminant in bone could be lethal.

In an equally fundamental role, a small amount of calcium is essential in fluids bathing the cell; an even smaller amount occurs in the intracellular fluid. The level of calcium circulating in blood remains remarkably constant at about 10 mg/100 ml and normally varies within no more than 10 percent. Slightly less than half of the calcium in blood and other fluids exists as the free ion; about the same amount is bound to protein, mainly albumin and globulins, and very small quantities are complexed with organic acids such as citrate or inorganic acids such as sulfate or phosphate.

In addition to its structural role as component of bones and teeth, ionic calcium of body fluids is essential for a variety of processes. A major role of calcium appears to be in the regulation of ion transport across cell membranes; other influences of the ion may be a direct result of this basic function.

The level of circulating calcium is independent of dietary intake. Regulation of serum calcium is achieved by the balanced effect of parathormone, which increases serum calcium partly through stimulation of bone resorption and calcitonin, which decreases serum calcium and inhibits bone resorption (see Chapter 17). Abnormalities leading to hyper- or hypocalcemia are relatively rare. An increase in serum calcium leads to respiratory or cardiac failure; a decrease results in tetany.

Calcium in body fluids exerts a profound effect upon neuro-muscular irritability. A role of calcium in muscle contraction was suggested as early as 1882 by Ringer, who showed that the contraction of excised heart muscle depended on the concentration of calcium in solutions bathing the muscle. (Muscle contraction and the effect of calcium will be discussed in detail in Chapter 18).

The role of calcium in blood clotting has been mentioned in connection with vitamin K. Apparently extremely minute quantities of calcium are required for prothrombin activation since blood clotting proceeds normally even in the presence of hypocalcemic tetany. Calcium also is involved in maintaining the integrity of the intercellular cement substance. Calcium is necessary for the activation of certain enzymes including pancreatic lipase, plasma lipo-protein lipase, phospholipase A and phosphorylase kinase, and the release of neurotransmitters such as acetylcholine, serotonin, and norepinephrine (see Chapter 19).

The metabolism of calcium in relation to vitamin D has been discussed in Chapter 4 and will be discussed further in Chapter 17.

Calcium and ^{90}*Strontium.* The metabolism of strontium has been studied chiefly in relation to the radioactive compound ^{90}Sr, an atmospheric fallout contaminant. Strontium metabolism is simi-lar in most respects to calcium metabolism, although strontium is less well controlled homeostatically. The two minerals tend to be associated in foods and in deposition in the animal body; strontium, like calcium, tends to accumulate in bone.

The body absorbs and retains calcium in preference to stron-tium and this selective behavior has been termed *discrimination* by Comar et al. (1956). Metabolically, strontium is discriminated against in favor of calcium and as calcium intake increases, strontium absorption decreases. Conversely, normal renal clearance of strontium is about four times that of calcium (Nordin et al., 1967). The ability of the animal body to discriminate between the two elements is believed to protect against a large buildup of strontium in the body.

PHOSPHORUS

The human body contains roughly 12 gm P/kg fat-free tissue; of this amount, about 85 percent is contained in the inorganic phase of skeletal structures. The phosphorus content of plasma is about 3.5 mg/100 ml plasma; when red cell phosphorus is also included the total phosphorus content of blood ranges between 30-45 mg/100 ml blood.

Organic phosphates are a part of the structure of all body cells and are intimately involved in cellular functions. Phosphorus is a constituent of the high energy compound ATP and thus is necessary for energy transductions essential for all cellular activity. The oxidation of carbohydrate leading to the formation of ATP also requires phosphorus since phosphorylation is an obligatory step in the metabolism of the monosaccharides. The active coenzyme form of certain of the B vitamins also function as the phosphorylated derivatives. Phospholipids are constituents of all cellular membranes and are active determinants of cellular permeability. DNA and RNA, the genetically significant compounds responsible for cell reproduction and therefore for growth and all protein syntheses, are phosphorylated compounds. Indeed, all nucleotides contain phosphorus.

A dietary deficiency of phosphorus is not likely to occur in the human. Because of its metabolic significance in both animal and plant tissue the mineral is widely distributed in foodstuffs. A phosphorus depletion syndrome, however, has been observed in grazing animals subsisting on grasses and hay that are high in calcium but low in phosphorus. The syndrome is characterized by anorexia, weakness, stiff joints, and fragile bones.

The ratio of dietary calcium to phosphorus is critical to the rat deprived of vitamin D and, in fact, rickets can be produced in the rat only by wide variations in the dietary ratio of the two minerals. However, Malm (1953) and Spencer (1965) found no adverse effect on either mineral absorption or retention when the ratio of the two minerals was varied in the diets of human subjects. The intake of phosphorus is almost always higher than that of calcium in human diets. In rats, supplementation of a cariogenic diet with inorganic phosphate has been shown to reduce the incidence of dental caries (McClure, 1958). There are suggestions that phosphates may play a similar protective role in man. For example, the incidence of dental caries appears to be lower in the southern states than in the north of the United States. The use of large amounts of self-rising flour containing considerable amounts of inorganic phosphates has been cited as a contributing factor (see Shaw and Sweeney, 1973).

The significance of the calcium to phosphorus ratio in the diet, however, is far from clear. Krishnarao and Draper (1972) report that high intakes of phosphorus in adult rats and mice increase bone resorption and that this effect can be prevented in older animals if the phosphorus content of the diet is lowered during middle age. Krook et al. (1972) suggest that periodontal disease resulting from resorption of alveolar bone is the first manifestation of osteoporosis and that these conditions are caused by a lack of calcium and/or an excess of phosphorus in the diet. Further studies are needed to clarify the role of phosphorus (and calcium) in dental health and in the etiology of osteoporosis. The answer may lie not in the actual amount of either nutrient in the diet per se but, instead, in the ratio of the two minerals.

MAGNESIUM

Of the total body magnesium, about 0.5 gm/kg fat-free tissue, roughly 60 percent is located in bone. The function of magnesium in hard tissues is not known; one-third of it is in combination with phosphate, and the remainder appears to be adsorbed loosely on the surface of the mineral structure. A small amount of magnesium is dissolved in the extracellular fluid and is easily exchanged with that adsorbed at the bone surface. Only 1-3 mg/100 ml is present in serum; of this about 35 percent is bound to protein or complexed with other substances and is not available for exchange.

Within the cells of soft tissues the concentration of magnesium is greater than any other mineral except potassium. Loss of magnesium from the body therefore is usually associated with tissue breakdown and cell destruction. Magnesium is required for cellular respiration, specifically in oxidative phosphorylation leading to formation of ATP. In fact, magnesium is necessary for all phosphate transferring systems and in certain tissues, such as heart, a major fraction of the Mg present is complexed with ATP, ADP, and AMP (Polimeni and Page, 1973). In some phosphate transfers, magnesium may be replaced by manganese as activator for enzyme activity. Calcium ions antagonize the activity of certain magnesium-activated enzymes including pyruvate phosphokinase, ATPase, and inorganic pyrophosphatase.

Magnesium is the activator for all enzymic reactions requiring TPP: oxidation of pyruvate, conversion of a-ketoglutarate to succinyl CoA, and the transketolase reaction of the pentose monophosphate shunt. Various reactions in the metabolism of lipid and protein also require magnesium: transfer of CoA to acetate and to cholic acid forming acetyl CoA and cholyl CoA, and synthesis of DNA and RNA. For a review of magnesium metabolism see Aikawa (1963) and Wacker and Parisi (1968).

Acute magnesium deficiency in the rat was first described by Kruse et al. (1932) and is characterized by neuromuscular hyperirritability and tetany. The syndrome is similar to the tetany that results from hypocalcemia. Chronic deficiency produces alopecia, skin lesions, and swollen gums. High calcium intakes tend to aggravate symptoms of magnesium deficiency and, as a result, magnesium requirement of experimental animals is raised in order to counteract the effect of calcium (Morris and O'Dell, 1963).

Shils (1964) has described experimental magnesium deficiency in two adult male volunteers. Personality changes, muscle tremor, lack of coordination, and gastrointestinal disturbances developed after three months on the deficient diet. In addition, serum calcium and potassium decreased as serum magnesium decreased and rose to normal when magnesium therapy was instituted. This finding confirms the suggestion of a metabolic relationship between calcium and magnesium and suggests that potassium also is involved.

Magnesium deficiency does not appear to be a problem in most human dietaries since the mineral element is widely distributed in foodstuffs. In a normal adequate diet about 30 percent of the total magnesium intake may come from green vegetables that contain the magnesium porphyrin, chlorophyll.

Magnesium deficiency, however, may occur in man as a result of prolonged episodes of vomiting or malabsorption as in severe diarrhea. Gastric juice contains a fair amount of magnesium and excessive vomiting could result in substantial losses of the mineral in addition to the loss resulting from the failure to retain ingested food. Certain drugs—ammonium chloride and mercurial diuretics—result in loss of magnesium through the urine (Martin et al., 1952). Magnesium deficiency has been reported in children with protein-calorie malnutrition due primarily to diarrhea which increases fecal loss of the mineral (Caddell, 1969). Recovery was more prompt when diets were supplemented with magnesium (ibid).

Hypomagnesemia is associated with chronic alcoholism and with the neuromuscular symptoms of alcoholic withdrawal (Mendelson et al., 1969). When pancreatitis is also present, magnesium replacement therapy becomes an important part of treatment because magnesium (and calcium) in blood may be decreased due presumably to deposition in areas of adipose tissue (Hersh and Siddiqui, 1973). Magnesium content of adipose tissue has been shown to be markedly increased in humans dying from acute pancreatitis and in animals in whom pancreatitis was induced experimentally.

It has been suggested recently that cellular loss of magnesium may be a primary biochemical mechanism in the etiology of various types of myocardial lesions (Seelig and Heggtveit, 1974). The high content of magnesium in hard water has been cited as a possible reason for the lower incidence of sudden death from heart disease in areas of hard water as compared to soft water areas.

SODIUM

The value of salt has been recognized for centuries. The common expressions "salt of the earth" and "worth his salt" and even the word "salary" all derive from the high value placed upon salt throughout history. The requirement for sodium is not well defined, but human dietaries generally contain more sodium than necessary. Tissue formation, as in growth, requires about 1.1-2.2 mg/kg of tissue gained; the requirement for maintenance should be considerably less. Intakes vary widely; about 10 gm NaCl/day appears to be usual for most Americans, whereas intakes of 30-40 gm/day are not uncommon in Oriental countries where soy sauces and sodium glutamate are favored as flavoring agents.

The human body contains about 1.8 gm Na/kg fat-free body weight, most of which is present in extracellular fluids. The content of serum normally is about 140 mEq/liter (300-355 mg/100 ml). Since sodium is the chief cation of the extracellular fluid, the control of body fluid osmolarity and therefore body fluid volume is largely dependent on sodium ions and the ratio of sodium to other ions.

Sodium is capable of permeating the cell membrane, and muscle contraction and nerve transmission involve a temporary exchange of extracellular sodium and intracellular potassium (see Chapters 18 and 19). The subsequent transfer of sodium out of the cell is by means of an active mechanism or *pump* (see Chapter 9). A very small amount of sodium occurs intracellularly.

In bone, sodium is bound for the most part on the surface of bone crystals. The amount present in bone is by no means small and accounts for 30 to 45 percent of total body sodium. This reservoir apparently is part of the active labile sodium pool in the body (see Chapter 17).

Sodium metabolism is regulated primarily by aldosterone, a hormone of the adrenal cortex that promotes the reabsorption of sodium from the kidney tubules. In the absence of this hormone, sodium excretion is increased and symptoms of deficiency ensue. Other adrenal mineralocorticoids, deoxycorticosterone and hydrocortisone, are involved in regulation of sodium excretion but are less potent in action.

Dietary deficiency of sodium probably never occurs in the human. The element is widely distributed in foodstuffs. Plant sources contain less than animal products and are therefore prominent on low sodium diets. Processed foods of all kinds tend to have a high sodium content since many sodium compounds are used in preserving, tenderizing, and flavoring.

Excessive losses of sodium may result from vomiting, diarrhea, or profuse sweating. Depletion is usually, although not always, associated with concurrent water loss and it is the balance of sodium and water losses that will determine whether serum sodium is increased, decreased, or remains normal. Rogers et al. (1963) have reported that men deprived of food in an arctic environment lose large amounts of sodium during the first days of starvation, but because this loss is accompanied by diuresis, serum sodium levels remain unchanged. Their results, therefore, point to an isotonic contraction of the extracellular fluid.

The results of sodium depletion are closely related to the state of water balance. If only sodium is lost and water is retained, serum sodium concentration eventually will decrease, as when water only is replaced following excessive sweating. As a result, water will migrate into the cells and symptoms of water intoxication develop: loss of appetite, weakness, mental apathy, and muscle twitching. If sodium loss is accompanied by water loss, symptoms of extracellular fluid depletion develop: low blood volume, high hematocrit, collapse of veins, low blood pressure, and muscle cramps.

Sodium balance is so well controlled by homeostatic mechanisms in normal individuals that little attention is usually given to sodium intake. However, evidence suggests that an increase in body mass and body water, such as occurs during pregnancy, increases sodium requirement up to ten times that for maintenance in the adult rat (Pike et al., 1966). When this increase in intake is not available the sodium conserving mechanisms operate to increase sodium reabsorption. The resulting stress during pregnancy in rats has been documented through electron microscopic and histochemical evidence as severe pathology in the adrenal gland (Šmiciklas et al., 1971a, 1971b) and by changes in the secretory capacity of the adrenal (Khokhar and Pike, 1973). These findings further support the suggestion that the common practice of restricting salt intake in pregnancy be critically evaluated (Committee on Maternal Nutrition, 1969). Pitkin et al. (1972) estimate that the pregnant woman requires 25 gm of sodium chloride per day, about 7 gm above usual intakes.

CHLORIDE

The chloride ion is the major anion of the extracellular fluid and occurs for the most part in combination with sodium, although small amounts may be bound loosely to protein and other substances. Less than 15 percent of the total body chloride is located intracellularly. Chloride in blood easily transfers between the blood fluid and erythrocytes in what is commonly known as the *chloride shift,* a primary homeostatic mechanism for the control of blood pH.

Although chloride is generally considered with sodium, with which it functions in maintenance of extracellular fluid pH and osmolarity, the chloride ion also functions as activator for amylases and obviously is essential for the formation of gastric hydrochloric acid. It is interesting that although chloride is generally transported across biological membranes by passive diffusion, in gastric and intestinal mucosa the chloride ion is actively transported (see Chapter 6).

The same factors that affect sodium loss from the body tend to affect chloride loss. Vomiting leads to high losses because of the hydrochloric acid content of gastric secretions. In normal individuals, dietary chloride intake is of little practical significance.

POTASSIUM

Potassium is the chief cation of the intracellular fluid and functions, as does sodium, as a major contributor to normal fluid pH and osmolarity. The human body contains about 2.6 gm K/kg fat-free body weight. Nerve and muscle cells are especially rich in potassium, but all cells, both plant and animal, tend to concentrate the mineral.

The ion is found in small amounts in extracellular fluid; serum level is 5 mEq/liter (14-22 mg/100 ml). Apparently potassium is capable of transferring across the cell membrane with somewhat greater ease than sodium. During muscle contraction and nerve transmission, potassium diffuses out of the cell as sodium enters and is transported back into the cell when sodium is extruded (see Chapters 18 and 19).

The potassium ion is necessary for carbohydrate and protein metabolism, but the mechanism by which it acts is not clear. Both glycogen formation and glucose degradation require potassium. Protein synthesis also requires potassium. The effect of the ion, however, appears to be on amino acid uptake by the cell rather than on the incorporation of amino acids into the protein molecule.

A deficiency of potassium is unlikely to occur as a result of dietary lack. Body potassium may be depleted, however, in conditions resulting in excessive excretion through the kidney: renal disease, hyperfunction of the adrenal cortex, diabetic acidosis, and treatment with mercurial diuretics. Losses through the gastro-intestinal tract may result from excessive vomiting or diarrhea.

The effect of potassium deficiency is primarily on the muscles and is characterized by muscular weakness that, in skeletal muscle, may result in paralysis. Diarrhea and intestinal distention are common manifestations of the effects of potassium deficiency on gastro-intestinal smooth muscle. Weakness of vascular and cardiac muscle leads to tachycardia and hypotension.

Potassium therapy is tricky, particularly if solutions are given by intravenous route. Too rapid infusion of potassium salts into the bloodstream may result in hyperkalemia, which is even more serious than hypokalemia. Muscle weakness and central nervous system changes result and, if unchecked, may lead to death.

SULFUR

The bulk of the sulfur present in the animal body is derived from the three sulfur-containing amino acids: methionine, cystine, and cysteine, which provide the sulfur needed for synthesis of other sulfur-containing compounds. Inorganic sulfates and sulfides are a small fraction of the total sulfur. Thiamin and biotin also contribute small amounts of sulfur to the total body supply.

The metabolic importance of some sulfur-containing compounds resides in the easy interconvertibility of disulfide and sulfhydryl groups in oxidation-reduction reactions. The reduction of cystine (disulfide) to cysteine (sulfhydryl) demonstrates the kind of reaction involved.[1]

$$
\begin{array}{ccccc}
\text{S} \relbar\joinrel\relbar\joinrel\relbar \text{S} & & & \text{SH} \\
| \qquad\qquad | & & & | \\
\text{H--C--H} \quad \text{H--C--H} & \xrightleftharpoons[-2H]{+2H} & \text{H--C--H} \\
| \qquad\qquad | & & & | \\
\text{H--C--NH}_2 \quad \text{H--C--NH}_2 & & & \text{H--C--NH}_2 \\
| \qquad\qquad | & & & | \\
\text{COOH} \qquad \text{COOH} & & & \text{COOH} \\
\end{array}
$$

Cystine   Cysteine

[1] The cystine content of hair and animal fur is roughly 15 percent; human hair contains somewhat more cystine than that of other species. The presence of disulfide or sulfhydryl bonds in the protein molecule forms the molecular basis for the permanent wave. Disulfide bonds are opened and reformed in a second position; hence the proper curl is held in place.

The activity of glutathione (γ-glutamyl-cysteinyl-glycine) in oxidation-reduction reactions depends upon the sulfhydryl group of cysteine in the molecule. Similarly, the sulfhydryl groups of CoASH and lipoic acid are the active sites of these molecules (see Chapter 3).

In addition to its role in oxidation-reduction reactions, sulfur is a component of other essential compounds and active metabolites. Taurine, the precursor to the bile acid taurocholic acid, is formed from cystine by way of cysteine. The mucopolysaccharides, specifically, the chondroitin sulfates and heparins, contain sulfated sugar derivatives; incorporation of sulfates into the sugar molecule appears to be influenced by vitamin A. Sulfates are also metabolically important in detoxication reactions and form esters with potentially toxic compounds. Prior to ester formation sulfates are activated by ATP, which gives rise to 3-phosphoadenosine 5′-phosphosulfate (PAPS); the reaction requires magnesium. This compound was originally designated active sulfate by Hilz and Lipmann (1955).

IRON

The human body contains about 75 mg Fe/kg fat-free body weight. Most of the body iron occurs as protein chelates in which heme compounds predominate. The heme molecule is comprised of ferrous or ferric iron in the center of a porphyrin ring. Hemoglobin contains four porphyrin units bound to the protein globin (see Chapter 16). Myoglobin, a similar type of compound present in skeletal and heart muscle, contains only one ferrous porphyrin group per molecule. Both hemoglobin and myoglobin enter into a reversible combination with oxygen; myoglobin has the greater affinity and this property enables it to serve as a cell reservoir of oxygen. About three-fourths of the total body iron is contained in these two compounds.

In addition to the large amount of iron in the erythrocytes iron is also present in serum in ferric form bound to a specific β-globulin, transferrin. Transferrin is a glycoprotein containing 5.9% carbohydrate and has a molecular weight of 81,000 (Katz, 1970). The concentration of transferrin is influenced by the availability of body stores of iron and by the rate of erythropoiesis (see Chapter 7). Serum iron ranges from 70-140 μg/100 ml, although approximately 360 μg or more could be bound to the protein present. The quantitative ability of transferrin to bind iron is designated *iron-binding capacity* of serum. Practically no ionic iron exists in the animal body.

Less than 0.3 percent of total body iron is present in the form of intracellular heme enzymes. Catalases and the cytochromes of the cellular electron transfer system function by virtue of the readily reversible reduction of ferric to ferrous iron. Certain other enzymes classed as metalloflavoproteins contain iron in a nonheme structure: succinic dehydrogenase, DPNH-cytochrome reductase, and xanthine oxidase. Aconitase, which catalyses the conversion of citric acid to isocitric acid in the tricarboxylic acid cycle, may require iron as a specific cofactor but apparently does not contain iron as a part of the molecule.

A large amount of iron, about 26 percent of total body content, is stored in cells of liver, spleen, and bone in the form of two compounds, ferritin and hemosiderin; lesser amounts are stored in other tissues. These compounds are iron-protein complexes containing ferric hydroxide and are closely related in structure. Ferritin is a polyhydroxy iron polymer with a molecular weight of about 150,000 surrounded by a protein coat of molecular weight 465,000. The specific protein to which iron is attached is known as apoferritin. The hemosiderin molecule apparently is more complex. When normal amounts of iron are stored, ferritin appears to predominate; when large stores accumulate, the storage form is chiefly hemosiderin. Apparently ferritin is a constituent of the hemosiderin structure, and grouping of ferritin molecules occurs as the compound accumulates. Ferritin has a high capacity for iron storage incorporating as much as 4500 atoms as the ferric oxide hydrate (Macara et al., 1972).

Virtually all metabolic processes involving iron are dependent upon the interconversion of ferrous and ferric iron (Frieden, 1973). As shown in Fig. 5.1, iron is present in the ferrous state in hemoglobin and in the ferric state in methemoglobin, transferrin, and ferritin. The oxidation of ferrous to ferric iron is catalyzed by a copper-containing enzyme, ceruloplasmin (ferroxidase-I), and a second enzyme identified as ferroxidase-II by Topham and Frieden (1970). (These enzymes are found in the human; other ferroxidases have been identified in other species.) Both enzymes contain copper, but ferroxidase-II contains less copper than ceruloplasmin and has a higher molecular weight.

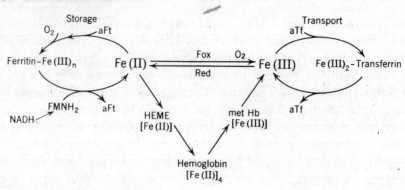

Fig. 5.1 The ferrous to ferric cycles in iron metabolism and their importance in the storage, transport, biosynthesis, and catabolism of iron. A key influence is exerted by the ferroxidases (Fox I, Fox II), copper enzymes which catalyze the oxidation of Fe(II) to Fe(III) and the ferrireductases. [Diagram modified from Frieden, 1973a].

The degradation of hemoglobin is discussed in detail in Chapter 16. It is enough to mention here that the pathway is through oxidation to methemoglobin, which contains ferric iron, and which is degraded to yield iron, globin, and protoporphyrin. Iron so released is reused for synthesis of hemoglobin or other iron-containing compounds. The globin portion gives rise to its component amino acids, and the protoporphyrin is degraded to form the bile pigments.

In simplest terms iron serves a primary role in the animal body as a mediator of oxidative processes. Heme compounds are the carriers of oxygen to tissue cells and the transporters of hydrogen to molecular oxygen as a part of the cellular electron transport system. In iron deficiency, the lowered capacity to provide oxygen is largely responsible for the fatigue and apathy characteristic of iron-deficiency anemia, and, for that matter, of all anemias.

Iron-deficiency anemia occurs almost exclusively in young children and women of child-bearing age. Because iron is conserved by the body, adult males rarely develop the anemia of iron-deficiency except following excessive blood loss (see Chapter 23). It should be made clear, however, that there are many types of anemias. Of the nutritional anemias, iron-deficiency anemia is by far the most common.

A role for iron has been demonstrated in the synthesis of collagen. Iron is required for the hydroxylation of both proline

Heme compds are carriers of:

1) O_2 to tissue cells

2) transporters of hydrogen to molecular O_2
   as a part of E.T.S.

Primary role is as a mediator of oxidative process.

Lowered capacity to provide O_2 is largely responsible
for the fatigue & apathy characteristics of
Fe-def. anemia

Fe - in synthesis of collagen.

" required for the hydroxylation of Pro & ~~Lys~~
+ Lys in protocollagen, a step wh. is required
before the molecule is extruded from the
cell into the extra-cellular matrix

and lysine in protocollagen, a step which is required before the molecule is extruded from the cell into the extracellular matrix. In *in vitro* studies in which connective tissue was incubated with a chelating agent, hydroxylation was inhibited and protocollagen remained within the cells. Evidence suggests that an iron-containing enzyme catalyzes the hydroxylation and that the iron is likely in the ferrous state (Prockop, 1971).

OTHER TRACE ELEMENTS

For many years the importance of trace elements in human dietaries was given little attention. The following statement from the first edition of this book was typical of the prevailing opinion.

"Trace elements are required in extremely small amounts in the diet and are so widely distributed in foodstuffs that even diets inadequate in other respects usually contain sufficient quantities of these nutrients."

With the development of improved methodology for the detection of trace elements and the resulting intensified research in this area, it is now clear that some human dietaries *are* marginally deficient in some trace elements and that functional impairments due to these deficiencies may be more prevalent than has been suspected.

Many of the difficulties of trace element research have been the result of the relative insensitivity of methods for detecting the minute amounts present in biological materials and to the inability to prevent contamination during feeding experiments. A further problem seems to lie in the traditional definition of an essential nutrient: a substance, necessary for life, whose absence from the diet will result in typical symptoms. It is now recognized that the definition is likely too rigid for defining the essentiality of a trace element because at present the demonstration of the complete absence of a trace element is still virtually impossible even with the most highly refined techniques available. Some investigators as, for example, Mertz (1970), have offered a more practical definition of essentiality: "An element is essential if its deficiency reproducibly results in impairment of function from optimal to suboptimal." This definition may well prove to be a more valid one for other nutrients as well (see Chapters 23 and 24).

Because of the small amounts of trace minerals present in the body, it is clear that they play primarily catalytic roles in cellular metabolism and therefore function in much the same way as vitamins. Some, such as cobalt and iodine, appear to function entirely as components of larger molecules whose metabolic role, however, also is fundamentally catalytic. The essential compounds or enzymes with which some of the more significant trace minerals are associated are shown in Table 5.1.

Deficiencies of several of the trace elements have been known to occur naturally in cattle and sheep allowed to graze on pastures in which the soil was grossly deficient in an essential mineral. Some pathological conditions observed in grazing animals, however, also may result from toxic effects of excessive amounts of certain elements in the soil. Experimental studies have for the most part been performed on animals, and these studies have provided useful clues to mineral function in man. A few rare disease conditions that occur in humans appear to result in or from abnormalities in trace mineral metabolism. Some of these diseases will be mentioned briefly in the section that follows.

Copper

The human body contains 1.5-2.5 mg Cu/kg fat-free body weight. The mineral is distributed in all body tissues, but liver, brain, heart, and kidney contain the highest amounts. In blood, copper appears to be about equally divided between plasma and erythrocytes; plasma contains about 110 μg/100 ml and erythrocytes, 115 μg/ 100 ml. About 90 percent of the plasma copper is present as the a_2-globulin copper complex, ceruloplasmin. Ceruloplasmin has a molecular weight of 151,000 and contains eight atoms of copper. In erythrocytes about 60 percent of copper is bound by another metalloprotein, erythrocuprein.

Copper deficiency has been produced in rats, swine, dogs, and other species and has been observed in domestic animals grazing on copper-deficient soil. Symptoms of copper deficiency include anemia, hypopigmentation, and changes in the texture of hair, abnormalities in bone structure, failure of myelination, and central nervous system defects. Hart et al. (1928) first reported that copper

Table 5.1   FUNCTIONS OF TRACE MINERALS

Mineral	Enzymes or Essential Compounds
Cobalt	Constituent of vitamin B_{12}
Copper	Tyrosinase, cytochrome oxidase, ceruloplasmin (ferroxidase-I), other ferroxidases
Iodine	Constituent of thyroxine
Manganese	Kinases, peptidases, arginase
Molybdenum	Xanthine oxidase, aldehyde oxidase
Selenium	Metabolism of tocopherol and sulfur amino acids Glutathione peroxidase
Zinc	Carbonic anhydrase, peptidases, dehydrogenases

is essential for the utilization of iron for hemoglobin formation in rats. Detailed studies were later carried out in swine by Cartwright and Wintrobe (1964) who observed defects in bone and central nervous system similar to those seen in domestic animals. A condition known as *swayback* is observed in young lambs born of mothers grazing on copper-deficient soil; this condition is associated with cerebral demyelinization. Sheep and cattle develop osteoporosis and spontaneous fractures. Merino sheep that normally have a crimpy wool grow relatively straight wool.

Many of these conditions can be associated with known biochemical functions of copper. Ceruloplasmin, for example, is necessary for oxidation of ferrous to ferric iron. Thus, lowered ceruloplasmin levels interfere with hemoglobin formation. Copper *Cu-Fe relation* also influences iron absorption and mobilization from liver and other tissue stores. Copper enzymes catalyze oxidation reactions. Enzymes involved in the oxidation of cytochrome *c* and mono- and diamines are copper-containing proteins. Certain other enzymes such as lecithinase and oxaloacetic decarboxylase are activated by copper. A copper-containing enzyme plays an important role in connective tissue metabolism (see Carnes, 1971), specifically in the oxidation of ε-amino groups of lysine side chains necessary for cross-linkage of the polypeptide chains of elastin and collagen. In copper deficiency there is an accumulation of soluble protein with decreased cross-linking. The activities of bone amine oxidase and cytochrome oxidase also are reduced. A decrease in the enzyme tyrosinase that is necessary for melanin formation is associated with hypopigmentation.

Low serum copper levels have been observed in conditions associated with protein loss from the body such as protein-calorie malnutrition and the nephrotic syndrome. Hypocupremia also occurs in patients with Wilson's disease and in infants maintained for long periods on milk only (Cordano et al., 1964). Hypercupremia is associated with many viral and microbial infections, leukemias, some anemias, myocardial infarction, cirrhosis, nephritis, and Hodgkin's disease (see Sandstead et al., 1970; McCall et al., 1971).

Iodine

As far as is known the role of iodine in the animal body is related solely to its function as a constituent of thyroxine and other related compounds synthesized by the thyroid gland. The adult body contains 10-20 mg iodine, of which 70-80 percent is concentrated in the thyroid gland. However, iodine is present in all tissues; next to thyroids, the ovaries, muscle, and blood have the highest amounts.

The element is absorbed as iodide that, in the thyroid gland, is quickly oxidized to iodine and bound to the tyrosine residues of thyroglobulin, a glycoprotein of relatively high molecular weight (670,000). Thyroglobulin contains 120 tyrosine molecules of which roughly two-thirds are available for iodine binding. In the thyroglobulin molecule, iodine is present primarily as 3-monoiodotyrosine; 3,5-diiodotyrosine; 3,5,3',5'-tetraiodothyronine (thyroxine, T_4) and 3,5,3'-triiodothyronine (T_3). These compounds are shown in Fig. 5.2. The active hormones are T_4 and T_3.

Proteolysis of thyroglobulin yields T_4 and T_3 to the bloodstream in a ratio of about four to one. T_4 is bound to a specific carrier protein (thyroxine-binding protein) that also transports retinol; only minute amounts of free T_4 are present in plasma. T_3 is very loosely bound to protein and, as a result, it passes from the blood to cells rapidly. T_3 thus accounts for 30-40 percent of total thyroid hormone activity by virtue of its easy availability.

The ratio between bound and free thyroxine may be a significant factor in the control of thyroid hormone distribution among

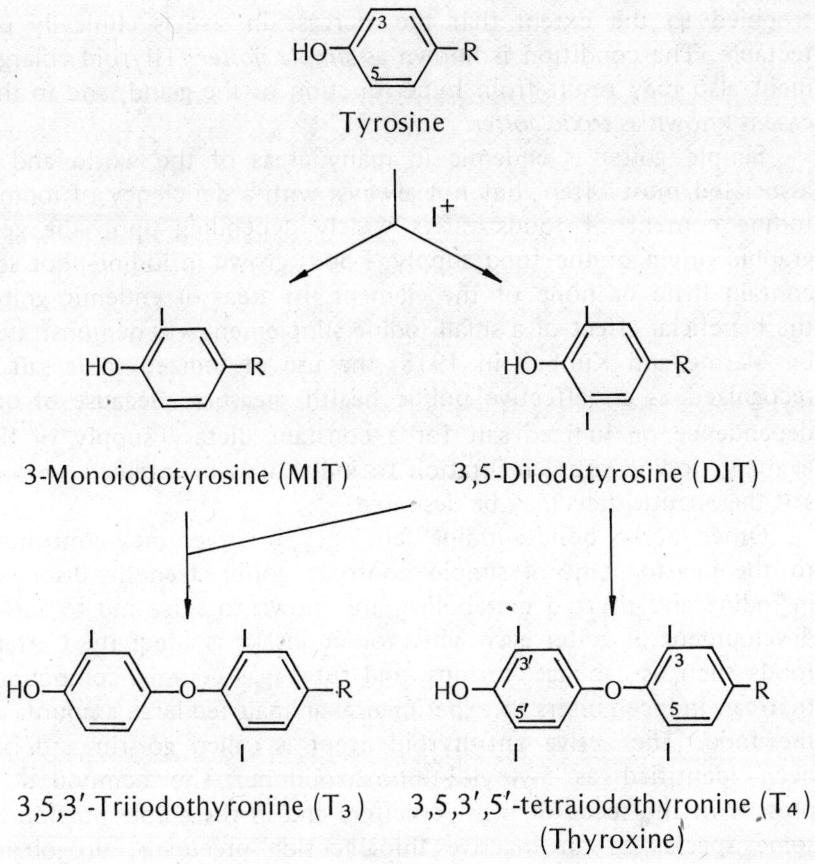

Fig. 5.2 Iodinated compounds.

body tissues. It has been suggested, though not proven, that the concentration of free hormone in blood and extracellular fluids determines the rate at which thyroxine is transferred to its metabolic target sites (Robbins and Rall, 1960).

The function of thyroxine and therefore of iodine is in the control of cellular energy transductions. Thyroid activity is under the influence of thyrotropin or thyroid-stimulating hormone (TSH) secreted by the anterior lobe of the pituitary, and it is essentially a feedback mechanism triggered by the level of circulating thyroid hormone. When blood hormone level is low, TSH stimulates the thyroid to increased production and release of iodinated compounds. As a result, thyroid cells increase in size. With continued stimulation (as when blood level remains low) the gland becomes hypertrophied to the extent that the increase in size is clinically detectable. The condition is known as *simple goiter*. Thyroid enlargement also may result from hyperfunction of the gland, and in this case is known as *toxic goiter*.

Simple goiter is endemic in many areas of the world and is associated most often, but not always, with a deficiency of iodine. Iodine content of foods varies widely depending upon the geographic origin of the food supply. Foods grown in iodine-poor soil contain little or none of the element. In areas of endemic goiter the beneficial effect of a small iodine supplement was demonstrated by Marine and Kimball in 1918; the use of iodized table salt is recognized as an effective public health measure. Because of our dependence on iodized salt for a constant dietary supply of the element, iodine supplementation to individuals maintained on low salt therapeutic diets may be desirable.

Other factors besides iodine deficiency, however, may contribute to the development of simple nontoxic goiter. Genetic disorders in iodine and thyroid metabolism are known to exist and to foster development of goiter even when iodine intake is adequate. Certain foods such as cabbage, turnips, and rutabagas contain compounds that can induce goiters in experimental animals fed large amounts of the food. The active antithyroid agent is called goitrin and has been identified as 5-vinyl-2-thiooxazolidone. The compound is present in the seeds of most crucifera and in the edible portion of some species as an inactive thioglycoside precursor, progoitrin, from which the active goitrin is formed by hydrolysis in the seed or in the gastrointestinal tract. It is doubtful that humans consume enough of any potentially goitrogenic food to seriously affect thyroid activity, but it is possible that goitrogenic foods may accentuate the effects of low iodine intake. The subject of goitrogens has been reviewed by Clements (1960), who cites a suspected incidence of goiter caused or intensified by consumption of milk from cows grazed on pastures of high goitrogenic content. No other similar incident apparently has been reported. The content of progoitrogenic compounds in 65 species of cruciferae was reported by Daxenbichler et al. (1964).

The thyroid hormones accelerate cellular reactions in nearly all cells of the body resulting in increased oxygen consumption and an increase in basal metabolic rate. The hormones have a profound effect upon growth. A part of the effect of the hormones is the result of an increase in enzyme activity; a large number of enzymes are reported to be affected by administration of thyroxine. Thyroid hormones also influence protein synthesis. In liver, thyroid hormones accelerate the rate of transfer of amino acids from tRNA to ribosomes. Specific effects of thyroid hormones on mitochondrial membrane will be discussed in Chapter 13.

Manganese

The adult human body contains about 20 mg manganese. The highest concentration is in bone where it is found in both inorganic salts and in the cells of the organic matrix. Pituitary, liver, pancreas, gastrointestinal tissue, and lactating mammary glands also contain relatively high concentrations. An interesting observation has been that the lactating mammary glands of the rabbit contain about 10 times as much manganese as the nonlactating tissue (Fore and Morton, 1952). The significance of this finding is uncertain.

Manganese deficiency has not been identified in the human, but deficiencies have been produced in rats, chicks, swine, and other species. Invariably skeletal development is affected, resulting in shortened and often deformed limbs. Disturbances in reproductive function, in the central nervous system, and in lipid metabolism also have been observed (Underwood, 1971). Loss of equilibrium, ataxia, and incoordination resulting from defects in the otic membrane have been observed in young rats born of manganese-deficient mothers (Hurley and Emerson, 1959).

A specific biochemical role for manganese was for many years difficult to define. In vitro manganese activates many enzyme systems but because other divalent ions, especially magnesium, are equally effective, a specific role for manganese does not seem likely. Pyruvate carboxylase, the biotin-dependent enzyme, was the first manganese-containing enzyme to be discovered (Scrutton et al., 1966). It contains four atoms of manganese per mole of protein. An effect of manganese deficiency upon pancreatic islet and beta cells and consequently upon glucose utilization has been demonstrated (Everson and Shrader, 1968), but the mechanism by which manganese acts is unclear. A specific role for manganese in the synthesis of mucopolysaccharides has been demonstrated (Leach and Muenster, 1962). This function has been studied primarily in chicks which develop a syndrome known as "slipped tendon" as a result of manganese deficiency. Cartilage from manganese-deficient chicks contains less hexuronic acid than from normal chicks. At least two enzyme systems appear to be the sites of manganese function: (1) the polymerase system which is responsible for polysaccharide chain elongation and (2) the galactosyltransferase system which incorporates galactose into the protein component of the molecule (Leach, 1971).

Manganese toxicity has been reported in miners of manganic oxide who acquire toxic levels of the mineral through inhalation of ore dust. The toxic syndrome appears to be similar to viral encephalitis and in severe cases is characterized by tremor, a peculiar mask-like facial expression, and incoordinated body movements. This syndrome has been reviewed in detail by Cotzias (1958).

Molybdenum

The molybdenum content of tissues of all animal species is very low. In adult man the liver contains about 3.2 ppm and kidney about 1.6 ppm. Molybdenum content of muscle, brain, lung, and spleen ranges from 0.14 to 0.20 ppm (see Underwood, 1971). Body content of molybdenum is increased markedly by unusually high intakes of the element. It is reduced, however, by high intakes of inorganic sulfate even in the presence of high levels of molybdenum.

Molybdenum is a component of xanthine oxidase and aldehyde oxidase. Both enzymes contain FAD as well as molybdenum and both function in electron transport. Xanthine oxidase catalyzes the oxidation of purines, pterins, and reduced pyridine nucleotides. In its reduced form, xanthine oxidase participates in the conversion of Fe^{3+}-ferritin to Fe^{2+}-ferritin. Molybdenum like copper, thus, is intimately involved in the metabolism of iron (see Seelig, 1972).

There is little concrete evidence establishing the quantitative requirement for molybdenum in the human or rat, although there is evidence of a quantitatively significant requirement in the chick (Reid et al., 1956). The species difference may be due to differences in nitrogen metabolism. The chick metabolizes all nitrogenous compounds to uric acid, and therefore likely has a greater requirement for xanthine oxidase (and molybdenum) than man and the rat, who normally degrade only purines and similar compounds to uric acid.

The effects of excess molybdenum in cattle, however, have been known for almost 25 years. The disease *teart* occurs in cattle maintained on pastures with high molybdenum content and is characterized by diarrhea and general wasting. Administration of copper or methionine has been shown to offset effects of experimental molybdenum toxicity (see Miller and Engel, 1960).

Fluoride

Fluoride is present in humans and other animals in highly variable amounts depending upon the diet and water supply. It is not known if fluoride is essential to life. However, fluoride has been shown to be essential for optimal growth of rats (Schwarz and Milne, 1972) and normal reproduction in mice (Messer et al., 1972). Hence it is assumed that fluoride is an essential nutrient.

The beneficial effect of fluoride in the prevention of dental caries is well documented. In areas where small amounts of fluoride (1-2.5 ppm) are present naturally in the water supply and in communities where fluoride (1 ppm) was added to the drinking water the incidence of dental caries is remarkably low. The epidemiological study conducted in Newburgh and Kingston, New York, as well as other similarly conducted studies, clearly demonstrated that 1 ppm fluoride added to drinking water in areas lacking fluoride reduced dental caries and was entirely compatible with health of the population (Ast et al., 1956).

High levels of fluoride occur naturally in drinking water in some areas. Bartlett, Texas, is one such area in the United States where fluoride content of the water supply is roughly 8 ppm. Consistently high intakes of fluoride result in strong but esthetically unattractive teeth that are covered with whitish to gray or black spots; the condition is known as *mottled enamel*. Fluorosis of bone, a condition clinically similar to arthritis, has been reported in populations living for many years in areas of high fluoride water content, at least 8 ppm, and results from an excessive accumulation of fluoride in bone. Nikiforuk and Grainger (1964) calculate, however, that an individual consuming daily 1-1½ liters of water containing 1 ppm fluoride could not possibly accumulate enough of the element to cause fluorosis even if this level of fluoride were taken in every day over a lifetime of 65 years.

The mechanism by which fluoride protects the integrity of tooth structure is not fully understood. It appears that fluoride is deposited in the tooth enamel and in bones as a part of the mineral salt structure. It would seem, then, that the effect of fluoride is localized at the tooth surface and that deposition of fluoride results in a chemical structure more resistant to acid-producing bacteria.

Violent public opposition of fluoridation in areas that would benefit from addition of small amounts of the mineral to the public water supply is clearly based on ignorance and unreasonable emotion. All scientific information supports fluoridation as a significant factor in the control of dental caries. Some evidence suggests that fluoride therapy is beneficial in the treatment and possible prevention of osteoporosis (Rich and Ensinck, 1961; Sognnaes, 1965; De Gubareff and Platt, 1969). Final proof of the value of fluoride in treatment of osteoporosis remains to be established.

For further discussion of fluoride see McClure (1970) and Gedalia and Zipkin (1973).

Selenium

Early reports of an unidentified factor capable of preventing and curing symptoms of vitamin E deficiency in rats and chicks referred to the compound as *factor 3*. The elusive factor was identified by Schwarz and Foltz (1957) as an inorganic selenium compound. Since that time a tremendous amount of research energy has gone into attempts to delineate the complex relationship between vitamin E and selenium. More recently attention has been given to selenium as an essential nutrient quite apart from its relationship to vitamin E metabolism.

Selenium is clearly implicated in the metabolism of tocopherol compounds but the mode of action is far from certain. Interrelationships between vitamin E and selenium are complicated by further interrelationships with sulfur-containing amino acids, antioxidants, and other nutrients. Selenium can replace tocopherol in the prevention of some vitamin E deficiency symptoms (liver necrosis in rats, exudative diathesis in chicks) but has no effect on other tocopherol deficiency syndromes (muscular dystrophy in chicks, encephalomalacia in chicks, fetal resorption in pregnant rats). Cystine or methionine, however, will prevent muscular dystrophy in chicks, and antioxidants will prevent encephalomalacia in chicks (Scott, 1962). Apparently only vitamin E will prevent the resorption syndrome in rats (see Chapter 4).

Selenium has been shown to be a required nutrient for several species. Chicks fed a selenium-deficient diet showed severe degeneration and fibrosis of the pancreas that could be prevented by adding a small amount of selenium to the basal ration (Thompson and Scott, 1970). Addition of selenium also improved growth. Rats fed a selenium-low diet grew and reproduced normally but the young receiving the same diet grew slowly, were virtually hairless, and failed to reproduce. Addition of selenium to the diet reversed these effects (McCoy et al., 1969).

Selenium has been demonstrated to participate in two enzyme systems in bacteria (see Stadtman, 1974) and one in mammalian tissues, glutathione peroxidase of rat erythrocytes (Rotruck et al., 1972; 1973). In chicks, glutathione peroxidase of plasma is high when the diet contains selenium but drops to a low level in selenium-deficient chicks (see Scott, 1973). The drop in glutathione peroxidase activity occurs just prior to the onset of exudative diathesis.

Selenium is believed to be essential in human nutrition. In children with protein-calorie malnutrition, supplementation with selenium improved weight gain and reticulocyte response (Schwarz, 1961; Hopkins and Majaj, 1967). Blood levels of selenium in children with protein-calorie malnutrition are lower than those of normal children and persist for several months following rehabilitation (Burk et al., 1967). No other cases of possible selenium deficiency have been demonstrated in the human.

In greater than trace amounts, selenium is toxic to animals. A syndrome called both "alkali disease" and "blind staggers" has been known since the middle of the nineteenth century, but it was not until the 1930s that the disease was recognized as the result of high concentration of selenium in soils. In experimental animals, selenium toxicity is more severe at low levels of dietary protein. Sulfate and some forms of arsenic appear to be effective in counteracting selenium toxicity (see Underwood, 1971). Some studies have suggested that, at high levels of intake, selenium is a carcinogen in rats; the evidence is inconclusive. In contrast, there are suggestions that trace amounts of selenium may be protective against human cancer (see Scott, 1973). This problem also needs further study.

Zinc

The adult human body contains about 2-3 gm zinc. Zinc is present in most tissues of the animal body. Extraordinarily high concentrations occur in choroid of the eye and in male reproductive organs. Liver, voluntary muscle, and bone contain considerably less but more than other tissues. Most of the zinc in blood is present in the erythrocytes; almost all of the zinc occurs associated with carbonic anhydrase.

Parakeratosis, a naturally occurring disease of pigs and cattle, has been shown to be due to zinc deficiency. High levels of calcium accentuate the development and the severity of the disease. This antagonistic action of calcium appears to be mediated primarily through a reduction in zinc absorption (Forbes, 1960).

In rats, zinc deficiency is characterized by growth failure, testicular atrophy, decreased size of the accessory sex glands, and dermatitis and keratinization of epithelial tissues. Delayed healing of experimental wounds has been observed in the zinc-deficient rat (Sandstead et al., 1970).

Zinc deficiency in humans was first described by Prasad et al. (1963) in areas of the Middle East where the diet consisted chiefly of cereals with little or no animal protein. The syndrome is similar to that seen in experimental animals: severe growth retardation resulting in dwarfism, hypogonadism, and low levels of zinc in plasma and red blood cells. Treatment with zinc resulted in improved growth and sexual development and a return of zinc blood levels to normal. More recently, hypogeusia (decreased taste acuity) has been shown to be a consequence of zinc deficiency (Henkin et al., 1971). Marginal zinc deficiency in a group of children in the United States has been reported (Hambidge et al., 1972). The symptoms were poor appetite, poor growth, hypogeusia, and low levels of zinc in the hair; all symptoms were improved by zinc therapy. The observation that wound healing in man can be accelerated by treatment with zinc sulfate (Pories et al., 1967) further suggests that marginal zinc deficiencies may not be uncommon.

Zinc is a component of a number of metalloenzymes including the pancreatic peptidases, carbonic anhydrase, alcohol dehydrogenase, and other dehydrogenases. The activities of certain other enzymes are increased by addition of zinc *in vitro*, but since other metal ions also are effective the action of zinc is largely nonspecific. Zinc is involved in protein synthesis. The ion is bound to RNA; in zinc deficiency synthesis of RNA, DNA, and protein is impaired (Wacker, 1962). A role for zinc in connective tissue metabolism seems very likely, but the mechanism by which it acts is not known (Westmoreland, 1971).

Zinc metabolism is affected by a variety of disease states: many infections, myocardial infarction, nephrosis, uremia, and post-alcoholic cirrhosis. In the latter condition, serum zinc levels are about 50 percent of normal. The syndrome has been described as a conditioned zinc deficiency (Vallee et al., 1957).

Chromium

The adult body contains little chromium, probably less than 6 mg. There is great variation depending upon geographic location. Concentrations are reported to decline with age (Mertz, 1969).

In studies with rats, Schwarz and Mertz (1959) showed that chromium is required for glucose metabolism and suggested that the element probably acts as a cofactor with insulin. Later, Schroeder (1966) demonstrated growth retardation and a syndrome similar to diabetes mellitus in chromium-deficient rats, thus establishing the essentiality of the element for this species.

The mode of action of trivalent chromium in glucose metabolism is not clear. It has been suggested that chromium may aid in the binding of insulin to cell membranes and in this way facilitate the action of insulin. Chromium therapy has been used in cases of diabetes in humans and in cases of impaired glucose tolerance in children with protein-calorie malnutrition. The results have been variable (see Sandstead et al., 1970). It is clear, however, that trivalent chromium is effective in some cases of impaired glucose tolerance and suggests that in these cases, a marginal chromium deficiency may exist (Hambidge, 1974).

Schroeder et al. (1962) have compiled extensive data on the distribution of chromium in both plant and animal tissues.

Nickel, Silicon, Tin, and Vanadium

Nickel, silicon, and vanadium have been shown to be essential for animals by a number of investigators (see Nielsen and Sandstead, 1974). At least one report indicates that tin is essential for growth of rats (Schwarz et al., 1970). The implications of these findings for human nutrition are not well defined at this time, but it seems very likely that these trace elements are also human nutrient requirements. Vanadium has long been considered of questionable significance in human nutrition, although approximately 20 mg are present in the human body (see Oser, 1965). Tin and nickel have generally been considered environmental contaminants with no function in mammalian metabolism. Until recently, silicon has been ignored (see Carlisle, 1974). Undoubtedly there is yet much to be learned of the significance of trace elements in metabolism and in human diets.

WATER

Water is by far the most critical of all nutrients. Animals will succumb to water deprivation sooner than to starvation. Water is an essential component of all cell structures and is the medium in which all the chemical reactions of cellular metabolism take place. Just as the life of the one-celled organism depends upon contact with its watery environment for sustenance, the cells of higher organisms are dependent upon the aqueous medium within and surrounding cell structures.

The water available to the animal body includes that present in liquids and solid food consumed, and water formed in the cells as a result of the oxidation of foodstuffs. This endogenous water is designated *metabolic water* or *water of oxidation*. Metabolic water amounts to roughly 15 percent of the daily total water available from an ordinary intake of food and drink. The water of oxidation has been computed for the major foodstuffs by Newburgh et al. (1930) and Peters et al. (1933). The figures vary slightly for carbohydrate and protein, as shown below.

Foodstuff (100 gm)	Water of Oxidation (gm)	
	Newburgh	Peters
Protein	41	40
Carbohydrate	60	56
Fat	107	107

The total amount of water available to the body thus may be calculated when the composition of the diet as well as the consumption of water and other beverages are known. Accurate determination of water balance, for example, must include the metabolic water. The data shown in Table 5.2 illustrate a typical water balance.

Table 5.2   DAILY WATER BALANCE

Water Intake	Grams	Water Output	Grams
Drinking water	400	Skin	500
Water in other beverages	580	Expired air	350
Preformed water in solid foods	720	Urine	1100
Metabolic water	320	Feces	150
Total	2020	Total	2100

From I. S. Kleiner and J. M. Orten, *Biochemistry*, 7th ed., C. V. Mosby Co., St. Louis, Mo., 1966, p. 650.

The animal body contains more water than any other compound. Approximately 70 percent of the fat-free body is water. Water is compatible with more substances than any other known solvent, and therefore it is an ideal medium for transporting nutrients to the cells and for the chemical reactions of cellular metabolism to take place. Its role, however, is more than that of a passive reaction medium; in hydrolytic and hydration reactions, water is an active participant in body metabolism.

The regulation of body temperature is dependent partially upon the high conductivity property of water to distribute heat evenly within the body and eventually to remove by vaporization the excess heat released by metabolic reactions within the cells. (As environmental temperature decreases, radiation and conduction are more important means of disposing of body heat.) Drastic changes in body temperature, moreover, are prevented by other properties of water: high specific heat and high latent heat of vaporization. In other words, more heat is required to change water from liquid to vapor or liquid to solid than almost any other substance. These properties alone establish water as a superior medium for metabolic activity. Sudden and violent changes in temperature obviously would disrupt the enzymatic machinery of the animal cell.

Excessive water loss from the body, as in profuse sweating, diarrhea, or prolonged episodes of vomiting, results in dehydration and in loss of electrolytes. The danger of replenishing the body water without concurrent repletion of electrolytes leads to water intoxication and has been discussed in the section on sodium. Body water distribution and compartments are discussed in Chapters 7 and 22.

part two
physiological aspects of nutrition

Chapter 6   Digestion and Absorption
Chapter 7   Nutrient Exchange and Homeostatic Control

The integration of biological mechanisms and the arbitrary divisions between branches of the biological sciences are well illustrated by the chapter title. Nutritionists refer to the physiological aspects of nutrition; physiologists to the nutritional aspects of physiology, and biochemists to the nutritional or physiological aspects of biochemistry. Each, however, is concerned with the biochemical activity in the physiological process of digestion through which nutrients are released and converted to forms capable of passing through a membrane. Understanding the details of the actual process of membrane transport calls for the talents of the biophysicist. The simpler the organism, the fewer the membranes or barriers to be crossed before entering cellular metabolism. In the complex organism, the first barrier is the intestinal mucosal membrane that is, in reality, the lumenal surface of each cell in the sheet of epithelium lining the tract. The accepted nutrients must then leave the cell, enter the extracellular fluid, the transport system and, eventually, leave the capillaries to enter the external environment, or the fluid, surrounding each of the individual cells throughout the body. It is at this point that the nutrients function and, depending upon perspective, come within the purview and, hence, the domain of the cell physiologist, geneticist, molecular biologist, biophysicist, biochemist, and nutritionist. Such convergence of

211

interest has led to the enormous acceleration of activity in this area of investigation in recent years. It is inevitable that progress toward an understanding of the common denominator should be the cooperative achievement of such a spectrum of scientific disciplines. The divisions of science, like the joinings and juxtapositions of a mosaic, are a means to an end and should not be permitted to detract from the unity of the image. If it is recognized that there is a broad spectrum of knowledge that sometimes can be examined only in segments, then we can proceed with what might otherwise have been considered a parochial view: the physiological aspects of nutrition.

chapter 6
digestion and absorption

1. Gastrointestinal Hormones
2. Digestion
   a. Carbohydrates
   b. Lipids
   c. Proteins
3. Absorption
   a. Mucosal Structure
   b. Mucosal Function
      1. Carbohydrate Absorption
      2. Amino Acid Absorption
      3. Lipid Absorption
      4. Cholesterol Absorption
      5. Nucleic Acid Absorption
      6. Water-Soluble Vitamin Absorption
         a. Ascorbic Acid
         b. Thiamin
         c. Riboflavin
         d. Pyridoxine
         e. Folacin
         f. Vitamin B_{12}
         g. Myoinositol
7. Fat-Soluble Vitamin Absorption
   a. Vitamin A
   b. Vitamin D
   c. Vitamin E
   d. Vitamin K
8. Water and Electrolyte Absorption
9. Mineral Absorption
   a. Calcium
   b. Iron
   c. Other Minerals
   c. Conclusion
4. Fecal Excretion
5. Epilogue

In order to discuss the activities of the gastrointestinal tract in the preparation of food for absorption into the body, one must assume that it is taken into the mouth, however eagerly or reluctantly. However, admission of food to the gastrointestinal tract, the obvious first step, does not assure admission to the body. Despite the activities of the tract in the breakdown of the complex foodstuffs, they are still "outside." Only after each of the individual nutrients breaches the barrier of the intestinal mucosa are they "in." Absorption, then, is the final and crucial hurdle. After that hurdle is passed, what were the foods become the nutrients en route to their site of action: the cells.

All cells depend on their external environment for their supply of nutrients. In a complex organism only those cells forming the mucosa of the gastrointestinal tract are in direct contact with the essential nutrients available in the external environment. It becomes obligatory, therefore, for these mucosal cells to take in all the nutrients essential not only for their own metabolism, but also for that of the whole organism. The mucosal cells are uniquely adapted to perform this primary function: transporting from the external environment (lumen of the tract) to the internal environment (extracellular fluid) the nutrients essential for all of the cells that comprise the total organism. As a corollary to this function, the cells also can exert control over the quantities of certain nutrients absorbed, such as iron, an excess of which leads to physiological embarrassment. Unfortunately, this capacity for exclusion does not extend to surplus energy-yielding nutrients that may also lead to embarrassment.

Disorders of nutrition may be due to failure at any step: inadequate intake, impaired digestion, or inefficient absorption. Despite seemingly adequate intake, psychomotor effects on motility of the gastrointestinal tract may so rush the passage of foods that breakdown and absorption cannot take place; genetic error may interfere with synthesis of enzymes or accessory factors essential to the digestive process; parasitic infestation, a fortuitous nutritional arrangement for the parasite, may prove rather less fortunate for the deprived host.

GASTROINTESTINAL HORMONES

Early studies on the motility and secretory activity of the gastro-intestinal tract indicated that control was not only by the autonomic nervous system but also by a series of gastrointestinal hormones whose release is stimulated when specific hormones reach particular loci in the tract. Hormones were originally identified by four primary actions (Table 6.1). In subsequent years three purified

Table 6.1 IDENTIFYING ACTIONS OF GASTROINTESTINAL HORMONES

Hormone	Action	Reference
Secretin	Stimulates secretion of HCO_3 and H_2O	Bayless and Starling, 1902
Gastrin	Stimulates gastric secretion of acid	Edkins, 1906
Cholecystokinin (CCK)	Contracts gallbladder	Ivy and Oldberg, 1928
Pancreozymin (PZ)	Stimulates pancreatic secretion of enzymes	Harper and Raper, 1943

gastrointestinal hormones (Table 6.2) were shown to participate in the four primary actions originally identified (Grossman, 1970). Other hormones with possible actions on gastrointestinal secretion have been suggested; for example, a glucagon-like substance in the intestinal wall and a gastric-inhibitory polypeptide that could be like enterogastrone (Andersson, 1973). Recent studies have implicated cAMP and the prostaglandins in key regulatory roles in gastrointestinal tract function (Levin, 1973; Wilson, 1972).

Table 6.2 PARTICIPATION OF THREE PURE GASTROINTES-
TINAL HORMONES IN FOUR PRIMARY FUNCTIONS

| Hormone | Gastric H$^+$ | Pancreatic | | Gallbladder Contraction |
		HCO$_3$	Enzymes	
Secretin	--	++	+	+ with CCK
Gastrin	++	+	++	+
Cholecystokinin-pancreozymin (CCK-PZ)	+ - with gastrin	+	++	++

From M. I. Grossman, 16th Nobel Symposium, Frontiers of Gastro-Intestinal Hormone Research 1970.
+ Stimulates.
++ Stimulates strongly.
- Inhibits.
--Inhibits strongly.

DIGESTION

Carbohydrates

Some polysaccharides such as the celluloses, hemicelluloses, and pectins are completely indigestible; but inulin, galactogens, mannosans, and raffinose that occur in certain fruits and vegetables are partially digested to monosaccharides.

The only polysaccharides in food that are digested to any degree by man are the starches that are glucose polymers. They must be broken down into monosaccharides, the molecules suitable for passage through the intestinal mucosal cells. This process of digestion could start in the mouth since a salivary amylase is secreted that can hydrolyze cooked starch to maltose *in vitro*; its efficacy *in vivo*, however, depends on the amount of time that the enzyme remains in contact with substrate. Generally, eating habits permit too short a time for enzyme-substrate interaction and activity is, therefore, insignificant. After the food reaches the stomach further amylase activity depends on the time it takes for the pH to be brought below the 6.6-6.8 range, which is optimum for amylase. Davenport (1971) suggests that up to 50 percent of the starch may be broken down depending on the rate of gastric mixing and emptying time.

No carbohydrate-digesting enzymes are secreted into the gastric juice. Theoretically there is a possibility of some acid hydrolysis of sucrose taking place in the stomach but it is probably negligible (Dahlqvist and Borgstrom, 1961). Therefore, no further digestion of carbohydrate takes place until the stomach contents, or *chyme*, enter the duodenum.

The major carbohydrate-digesting enzyme, α-amylase, is secreted with the pancreatic juice and is effective on raw as well as cooked starch. It hydrolyzes the α-1,4 glucosidic bonds. If the starches are unbranched, the end products are maltose and maltotriose; but if the starches are branched, there will be, in addition, a mixture of dextrins averaging six glucose residues per molecule containing the 1,6 linkages. A striking adaptation in pancreatic enzyme activity has been shown to occur with long-term alterations in the diet. In Desnuelle's laboratory (Marchis-Mouren et al., 1963) an eight- to tenfold increase in rate of amylase synthesis has been shown to occur in rats with a diet high in carbohydrate compared to a diet high in protein. At the same time, there was a two- to threefold decrease in the rate of synthesis of chymotrypsinogen, a protease precursor.

No further hydrolysis of carbohydrate takes place in the intestinal lumen since the disaccharidases (see Table 6.4) responsible for the final hydrolysis are located in the outer protein coat of the membrane of the intestinal mucosal cells (Miller and Crane, 1961a, 1961b; Eichholz and Crane, 1965; Overton et al., 1965). The development of disaccharidase activity within the villus cells as they migrate up toward the tip was demonstrated by Dahlqvist (1967) and the higher enzyme activity was observed in the region of the villi where the most active absorption of monosaccharides occurred.

Although the detection in the intestinal lumen of monosaccharides or the various enzymes responsible for the final stages of hydrolysis has been cited as evidence of lumenal digestion, this can be easily explained. Either the membrane-bound enzyme may be at the outermost edge of the intestinal coat permitting hydrolysis while the disaccharides are still in the lumen, or desquamation of mucosal cells from the tip of the villi contributes the membrane-bound enzymes to the lumenal contents. According to Ugolev (1965), hydrolysis on the external surface of the cell, or membrane digestion, is midway between digestion and absorption and ensures absorption at the final stages of hydrolysis. This is brought about by the intestinal enzymes present in or on the brush borders of the cells themselves. Thus, the digestion taking place in the lumen and in the membrane are interacting mechanisms that provide optimum conditions for absorption. Ugolev (1965) suggests a three-link system: hydrolysis in the lumen—membrane digestion—absorption. This relationship is depicted in Fig. 6.1. Membrane digestion takes place not only for the final hydrolysis of carbohydrates but also for the lipids and proteins to be discussed subsequently.

A disaccharidase deficiency would prevent the final hydrolysis of carbohydrate prior to its absorption and produce a condition of disaccharide intolerance (Dahlqvist, 1962). Accumulation of disaccharides in the lumen is associated with diarrhea, flatulence, nausea, and a sense of fullness—partly due to the osmotic activity of the disaccharides and partly due to bacterial fermentation. Any condition that produces damage to the mucosa by preventing the rapid proliferation of cells, such as occurs in protein-calorie malnutrition or celiac disease (Plotkin and Isselbacher, 1964), would be associated with enzyme deficiency. Inability to hydrolyze lactose has been reported and attributed to a defect in lactase synthesis (Holzel et al., 1959). Low levels of lactase activity and the consequent lactose intolerance have been observed in 30 percent of apparently healthy white adults (Friedland, 1965; Newcomer and McGill, 1966) and 80 percent of non-white subjects (Bayless and Rosensweig, 1966). Some attribute this to a genetic defect (Huang and Bayless, 1968), and others suggest that it is an acquired trait due to regression of enzyme activity in a postweaning diet that is low in lactose (Bolin et al., 1969). The rapid rise in lactase activity in the days prior to birth and the regression of lactase activity as part of the normal growth pattern has been observed in all mammals studied (Deren, 1968). The fall in lactase and an associated rise in sucrase and maltase activities accompanies the change in carbohydrate substrate presented to the tract: lactose in milk is the only sugar fed to mammalian neonates, and maltose, sucrose, and polysaccharides predominate in postweaning and adult diets.

Over the world more people are lactose-intolerant than tolerant. Since lactose tolerance was observed in 90 percent of the North European adults, and in 80 percent of the population of two

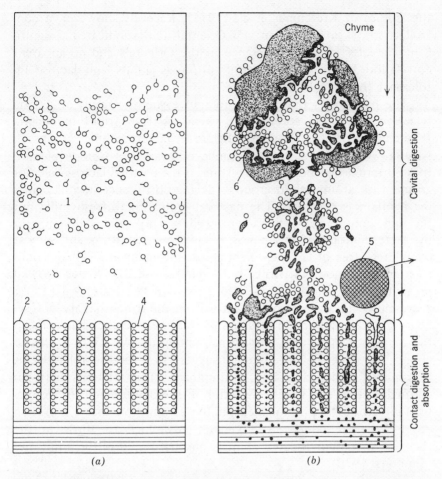

Fig. 6.1 Detailed diagram of relation between cavital and membrane digestion in the intestinal cavity in the presence (a) and absence (b) of foodstuff. (1) Enzymes in intestinal cavity (distributed chaotically); (2) microvilli; (3) enzymes on surface of microvilli (strictly orientated; (4) pores of brush border; (5) microbes not penetrating brush border; (6, 7) food substances at various stages of hydrolysis. [From A. M. Ugolev, *Physiol. Rev.,* 45:557 (1965).]

nomadic pastoral tribes in Africa, it was suggested that tolerance is the result either of the continued presence of milk in the adult diet or an evolutionary process of natural selection (Kretchmer, 1972). The thesis that continued ingestion of milk is responsible for continued lactase synthesis has some support in the studies of Kretchmer et al. (1971). Recently, however, a controlled study on Caucasian and Oriental adults indicated a significantly greater lactose intolerance in the Orientals and no apparent correlation between milk consumption as adults and lactose intolerance (Nandi and Parham, 1972).

The hypothesis that lactose tolerance was the result of genetic selection has been studied in several African tribes in Nigeria (Kretchmer, 1972). Two of the four largest ethnic groups in Nigeria were pastoral for thousands of years and lactose-tolerant. In an intermarried population of one of the pastoral lactose-tolerant groups with an intolerant group, a decided difference in milk drinking habits was observed. The pastoral group drank fresh milk, but the milk consumed by the town dwellers who were predominantly the lactose-intolerant group was in a fermented form and almost completely free of lactose. Even lactose-intolerant individuals could tolerate it without difficulty but their lactose intolerance showed up in tests. American blacks who arrived in this country 10 to 15 generations ago were predominantly from the tribes that are lactose-intolerant. The mixing in of genes for lactose tolerance has reduced the incidence of lactose intolerance among the American blacks to about 70 percent. The findings suggest that lactose tolerance is transmitted genetically and is dominant. The relations between cultural history and genetic selection in the development of lactose-tolerant groups is promulgated on the assumption that a mutation developed that conferred a genetic advantage to those in the societies that domesticated animals and used milk in the adult diet (Simoons, 1970).

The prevalence of lactose intolerance in older children and adults of some racial groups—in fact, the majority of the human species—brings into question the use of large scale supplementary feeding of whole or skim milk powder in many countries. This has prompted the publication of a report by the United Nations Protein Advisory Group (1972) alerting authorities about the problem and suggesting that gradual introduction of milk may be advisable.

In a lactose tolerance test 50 gm of lactose are administered, an amount equivalent to the lactose content of one quart of milk. Although a high incidence of lactose intolerance to a test dose was observed in Eskimo adults and children (Bell et al., 1973), all of the adults and children could consume one cup of milk without adverse effects. Stephenson and Latham (1974) have also shown that individuals with positive tests for lactose intolerance can consume nutritionally useful quantities of milk without developing symptoms of intolerance.

Sucrase deficiency has also been detected in children, as well as deficiencies in maltase and isomaltase (Semenza et al., 1965).

Lipids

The gastric digestion of dietary lipids is hampered by the action of acid and pepsin in the stomach which break up fat emulsions resulting in the formation of large globules of fat. This fat, like that in a gravy boat, floats on the surface and is last to enter the duodenum. Although a gastric lipase is secreted, it is not of major physiological importance. It is a tributyrase and responsible mainly for the hydrolysis of tributyrin to free fatty acids. The activity of this lipase decreases with increasing chain length of the fatty acids in the triacyl glycerols. This enzyme is virtually ineffective for releasing fatty acids with 10 carbons or more.

The presence of fat in the duodenum elicits the release of the postulated hormone, enterogastrone, which is purported to decrease gastric secretion and motility thereby slowing gastric emptying time. Whether the inhibitory mechanism is due to a distinct and separate hormone or a combination of other effects is still a moot question (Andersson, 1967). Nevertheless, the rate at which fat enters the duodenum is regulated and appears to be correlated with the capacity of the lipolytic enzymes from the pancreas to handle entering fat.

In the duodenum, the major source of lipolytic enzymes is the pancreatic juice. Several pancreatic hydrolases have been identified. A glycerol ester hydrolase, which hydrolyzes insoluble esters of glycerol, and a cholesterol esterase, which hydrolyzes esters of cholesterol, are both dependent on bile salts for their action. The bile salts along with fatty acids and glycerol have a detergent action on fat and aid in the emulsification of triacyl glycerols. Since pancreatic lipase acts on the interface of triacyl glycerol emulsions, it follows that there is increased activity with increased surface area. Bile salts also promote the downward shift in lumen contents to a pH of 6.0, which is the optimum for pancreatic lipase activity. The pancreatic lipases have a specificity for the 1 and 3 positions of the triacyl glycerol molecule. If short chain fatty acids are in the 2 position, these may be hydrolyzed to a considerable degree. However, since short and medium chain fatty acids isomerize at a high rate, it is possible that isomerization to the 1 position might account for the hydrolysis (Benzonana et al., 1964). The major end products following triacyl glycerol lipolysis by pancreatic lipase, therefore, are the 1-, 3-fatty acids and the remaining 2-monoacyl glycerols. Furthermore, bile salts along with monoacyl glycerol and fatty acids play a fundamental role in the formation of aggregates called *micelles* (Johnston, 1968). Under normal conditions, conjugated bile salts in the intestinal lumen are above the concentration critical for micellar formation. As a result, monoacyl glycerols liberated from triacyl glycerols are immediately trapped by the bile salts to form micelles which then dissolve free fatty acids. Cholesterol and fat-soluble vitamins are also dissolved in the micelles (Davenport, 1971). According to Hofmann and Borgström (1962), mixed micelles of fatty acids, cholesterol, and monoacyl glycerols with bile salts acting as detergents are brought into contact with the microvilli of the intestinal mucosa. The role of the micelle in lipid and in fat-soluble vitamin absorption will be discussed in a later section.

The enzymes located in the intestinal mucosal cells and concerned with lipid digestion are a lipase (Holt and Miller, 1962) and lecithinase (Winkler et al., 1967). The appearance of these enzymes in the lumen is due to the sloughing off of cells.

Abnormalities of lipid digestion can occur as the result of interference with enzyme synthesis, which may be due to a genetic defect, or to interference with enzyme secretion associated with pancreatic disease. In either case, undigested lipid remaining in the lumen will result in a condition known as *steatorrhea* in which the stools are fatty, bulky, and very light in color. Lipid in the stools would, of course, carry with it lipid-soluble substances. As a result, the disorder that develops is due not only to deficiency of lipid as an energy source but also to the deficit of essential linoleic acid and fat-soluble vitamins. Cases of congenital pancreatic lipase deficiency have been described (Sheldon, 1964).

The detergent action of bile salts may not always be to an individual's advantage. Many patients with gastric ulcers have been found to have bile salts in the stomach that apparently were carried there by regurgitation of intestinal contents during digestion. The detergent action of the bile is believed to break the gastric mucosal barrier making it vulnerable to self-digestion, or ulceration (Davenport, 1972).

Proteins

The distention of the stomach as well as the chemical stimulation produced by the presence of food liberates the hormone gastrin (see Table 6.2) from the gastric mucosa. Gastrin then stimulates the parietal cells of the mucosa to secrete hydrochloric acid. The hydrochloric acid plays a dual role in protein digestion: it promotes the swelling of protein and it activates pepsinogens (protease precursors) secreted by the zymogenic cells of the mucosa. The activation process is autocatalytic, that is, after the initial conversion of pepsinogen to pepsin, the pepsin itself can activate additional pepsinogen. From three to seven pepsins have been identified depending on the method of separation. The physiological significance of the various pepsinogens and pepsins that have been identified is not clear (see Davenport, 1971). Pepsins hydrolyze the peptide bonds between the aromatic amino acids, phenylalanine or tyrosine, and a second amino acid to give polypeptides of varying lengths.

Additional protein-digesting enzymes present in the gastric secretion are a gelatinase that liquifies gelatin, and rennin that, in the presence of calcium ions, changes casein to a coagulated form, paracasein, and thereby slows the passage of milk through the stomach. Rennin is present in the stomach of the calf but whether or not it is present in the stomach of the human infant is questioned.

The mechanisms by which the stomach protects itself from both the strong acid and the proteolytic enzymes has been the subject of both speculation and sound research. The known physical and chemical mechanisms by which the stomach maintains its mucosal barrier are interestingly discussed by Davenport (1972).

The efficiency of peptic digestion of protein can vary enormously from person to person, and the protein entering the duodenum from the stomach is a mixture of intact protein, large polypeptides, and not more than 15 percent as amino acids.

The action of the gastric proteolytic enzymes is halted when the acid contents of the stomach reach the duodenum and the pH is increased from approximately 2.0 to about 6.5. However, acid chyme entering the duodenum elicits the secretion of the hormone secretin which stimulates the secretion of an aqueous, enzyme-poor pancreatic juice. The products of protein digestion entering the duodenum stimulate the secretion of another hormone, cholecysto-kinin-pancreozymin (CCK-PZ), which affects the enzyme content but not the volume of pancreatic juice. A recently identified peptide separated from CCK-PZ and named chymodenin (Adelson and Rothman, 1974) elicits the specific increase in secretion of chymo-trypsinogen. This suggests that there may be other analogous pep-tides that are enzyme-specific which selectively regulate the secretion of a particular enzyme in the pancreatic juice.

The zymogens, or inactive proteolytic enzymes, in the pan-creatic juice are trypsinogen, chymotrypsinogen, and procarboxy-peptidase. Activation is triggered by the conversion of the trypsino-gen to trypsin by the enzyme enterokinase secreted by the intestinal mucosa. After this initial activation, trypsin becomes the activator of the rest of the pancreatic enzymes, all of which are secreted in precursor form. Small quantities of trypsin can also act autocata-lytically activating more trypsinogen. Activation, in each case, is cleavage of a peptide bond adjacent to an arginine or a lysine residue near the beginning of the chain of the zymogen (Neurath, 1964). It appears that a further change is required in the activation of procarboxypeptidase.

The pancreatic proteolytic enzymes are classified as the endo-peptidases, trypsin and chymotrypsin; and the exopeptidases, amino-peptidase and carboxypeptidase. These enzymes can perform their proteolytic functions whether or not peptic digestion has taken place. The endopeptidases cleave peptide bonds in the inner portion of the molecule. Trypsin's action takes place at a bond where a dibasic amino acid contributes the carboxyl group, whereas chymo-trypsin hydrolyzes the bond where an aromatic amino acid con-tributes the carboxyl group. The products of endopeptidase action are small polypeptides and amino acids. Additional amino acids are liberated by the action of the exopeptidases that cleave the end peptide linkage with a free amino group, the aminopeptidases, or the linkage with the free carboxyl group, the carboxypeptidases. The aminopeptidases usually require Mn^{2+} or Mg^{2+} as cofactors and the carboxypeptidases contain a metal, usually Zn^{2+} or Cu^{2+} firmly bound to the active site (Neurath, 1964). Removal of the metal leads to a loss of enzyme activity.

The final cleavage of the small peptides to amino acids is accomplished by the aminopeptidases and dipeptidases secreted by the intestinal glands. This occurs not in the lumen of the tract but in the mucosal cell membranes. The reported appearance of intestinal proteolytic enzymes in the contents of the small intestine is acknowledged to be due to the sloughed off mucosal cells since carefully prepared cell-free juice is free of intestinal digestive enzymes (see Davenport, 1971). For detailed discussion of protein digestion see Wiseman (1974).

The coordinated timing and action of hormonal secretion and neuromuscular and secretory activity with the presence of substrate results in the orderly and sequential digestive process that has been presented. A summary of the gastrointestinal hormones released by the mucosal membranes when specific substances reach particular loci in the tract is presented in Table 6.3. Table 6.4 summarizes the source and action of the various digestive enzymes and accessory factors.

Table 6.3 SOME ACTIONS OF GASTROINTESTINAL HORMONES

	Gastrin	CCK-PZ	Secretin	Glucagon
H_2O-electrolyte secretion				
Stomach	+	+	–	–
Pancreas	+	+	+	–
Liver	+	+	+	+
H_2O-electrolyte absorption				
Ileum	–	–	–	
Gallbladder	0	0	–	
Enzyme secretion				
Stomach	+	+	+	0
Pancreas	+	+	+	–
Endocrine secretion				
Secretin	+			
Gastrin			–	
Insulin	+	+	+	+
Glucagon	0	+	0	

From M. I. Grossman, 16th Nobel Symposium, Frontiers of Gastro-Intestinal Hormone Research, 1970.

+ Stimulates.
– Inhibits.
0 No effect.

Table 6.4 SOURCE AND ACTION OF DIGESTIVE ENZYMES

Source of Secretion	Stimulus	Enzyme or Secretory Product	Action
Mouth			
Salivary glands (3 pair)	Psychic, Mechanical, Chemical	Salivary amylase	Glycogen, Starch, Dextrin → branched oligosaccharides, some maltose. Action of minor importance
Stomach			
Gastric glands (35,000,000)	Reflex, Gastrin	HCl	Pepsinogen → pepsin; Fe^{3+} → Fe^{2+}; Swelling of proteins; Antibacterial effect
		Mucin	Acid-combining power; Protective to mucosa
		Intrinsic factor	Essential for absorption of vitamin B_{12}
		Pepsins	Hydrolyze peptide bonds between aromatic and dicarboxylic acids → large polypeptides and amino acids
		Gelatinase	Liquifies gelatin
		Tributyrase	Tributyrin → free fatty acids
		Rennin (?)	Casein → paracasein (? in infants)

Pancreas
Exocrine secretion

Secretion	Enzyme	Action
Secretin		
Cholecystokinin-pancreozymin		
	Trypsinogen	Activated by enterokinase and by trypsin
	Chymotrypsinogen	Activated by trypsin
	Procarboxypeptidase	Activated by trypsin
	Endopeptidases	
	Trypsin	Protein and polypeptides → small polypeptides
	Chymotrypsin	Protein and polypeptides → small polypeptides
	Exopeptidases	
	Carboxypeptidase A	Polypeptides with free carboxyl group → lower peptides and aromatic amino acids
	Carboxypeptidase B	Polypeptides with free carboxyl group → lower peptides and dibasic amino acids
	Elastase	Hydrolyzes fibrous proteins
	Collagenase	Hydrolyzes collagen
	Ribonuclease	Ribonucleic acid → nucleotides
	Deoxyribonuclease	Deoxyribonucleic acid → nucleotides
	α-Amylase	Starch → dextrins and maltose
	Lipase (requires bile salts)	Fats → monoacyl glycerols, fatty acids, glycerol
	Phospholipase A	Lecithin → lysolecithin (= removal of one fatty acid)
	Retinyl ester hydrolase	Hydrolyzes retinyl esters
	Cholesterol esterase (requires bile salts)	Free cholesterol → esters of cholesterol with fatty acids

(continued)

Table 6.4 (continued)

Source of Secretion	Stimulus	Enzyme or Secretory Product	Action
Small intestine Most enzymes located in microvilli of mucosal cells	Enterocrinin	Aminopeptidases	Polypeptides with free amino group $\longrightarrow$ lower peptides and free amino acids
		Dipeptidases	Dipeptides $\longrightarrow$ amino acids
		Nucleotidase	Nucleotides $\longrightarrow$ nucleosides and H_3PO_4
		Nucleosidase	Nucleosides $\longrightarrow$ purines, pyrimidines, and pentose
		Alkaline phosphatase	Organic phosphates $\longrightarrow$ free phosphates
		Monoglyceride lipase	Monoglycerides $\longrightarrow$ fatty acids and glycerol
		Lecithinase	Lecithin $\longrightarrow$ fatty acids, glycerol, phosphoric acid, and choline
		Disaccharidases	
		Sucrase	Sucrose $\longrightarrow$ glucose and fructose
		Maltase	Maltose $\longrightarrow$ glucose
		Lactase	Lactose $\longrightarrow$ glucose and galactose
Gallbladder Liver	Cholecystokinin Hepatocrinin	Bile	Emulsifies fat Stabilizes emulsions Neutralizes acid chyme Accelerates action of pancreatic lipase Path for pigment and cholesterol excretion

Although digestion has been discussed solely in terms of the gastrointestinal tract and its secretions, a variety of other neural and hormonal influences are intimately concerned with the efficiency of operation of the tract in the digestive process. Some of these relationships are shown in Fig. 6.2.

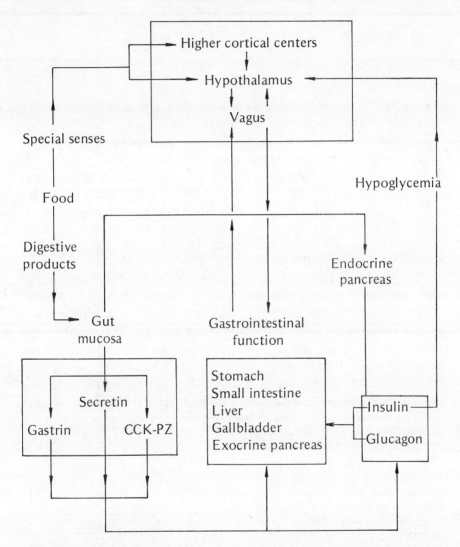

Fig. 6.2 Neural-hormonal relationships in digestion. [From V. L. W. Go and W. H. J. Summerskill, *Amer. J. Clin. Nutr.*, 24:160 (1971).]

The amino acids released in the mucosa, like the mono-saccharides, fatty acids, and glycerol, can now make the final transition from being constituents in food to nutrients and metabolites in the body. They are now ready for the final hurdle through the mucosal cell, the intricate process of absorption.

ABSORPTION

Mucosal Structure

The small intestine is approximately 380 cm long but with an epithelial lining that presents a surface area many times this linear measurement. The entire lining has its surface extended by villi, fingerlike protuberances extending into the lumen, each of which is 0.5-1.5 mm long. There are 20-40 villi per mm^2, giving a total estimated surface of approximately 300 m^2 (Blankenhorn et al., 1955) or about 3000 square feet! This enormous surface area is further increased by the brush borders, revealed by the electron microscope to be microvilli, which extend from the entire free surface of the villi epithelial cells (Fig. 6.3).

In man and other mammals, the microvilli of the absorptive cells average 1 μ in length and 0.1 μ in width (Palay and Karlin, 1959a) becoming increasingly longer along the villi, attaining greatest length and number toward the tip. There may be 2000-4000 microvilli on the free surface of each intestinal cell and in one mm^2 of intestine, the estimates range from 50,000-200,000 (Ugolev, 1965) to 200,000,000 (DeRobertis et al., 1970), increasing the effective absorptive surface of the intestine approximately thirtyfold.

The microvilli appear to be excrescences of the plasma membrane of the villus epithelial cell and the narrow spaces between them ap-

Fig. 6.3 The brush border or microvilli of two adjacent intestinal villi showing the surface coat which is a product of the cells whose surface it covers. Among the probable functions of this coating is the role as barrier to large particles while permitting substances in solution, emulsified lipid and colloidal particles to pass freely. It is resistant to a wide variety of proteolytic and mucolytic agents. Intestinal epithelium of cat. Magnification 51,000. (Courtesy of Dr. Susumu Ito.)

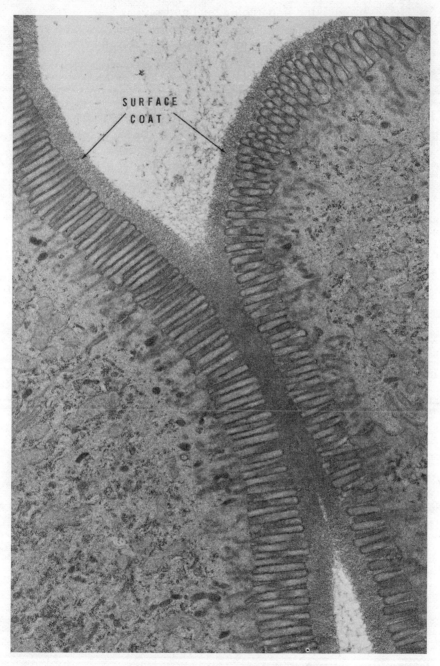

SURFACE
COAT

pear to act as sieves or pores for molecules being absorbed or, as will be discussed later, undergoing final hydrolysis.

At the base of the villi, and with epithelium continuous with the villus epithelium, are the crypts of Lieberkühn. These are simple tubes 0.3-0.5 mm deep. Each villus has three of them, and they comprise the proliferative area, the area of mitotic activity, where the epithelial cells of the intestinal mucosa are formed. Cells formed in the crypts migrate up the length of the villus and are extruded from the tip into the intestinal lumen when their short (1 to 3 day) life span is completed (Leblond and Messier, 1958). The average height of a column of cells in the crypt is 30 cells and each of these columns produces one new cell every three hours. However, each villus loses one cell per hour from its tip; consequently cellular production from three crypts is needed to maintain each villus. The extrusion of these cells into the intestine of man is estimated to be at a rate of 20-50 million cells per minute and amounts to 250 gm of cells each day (Davenport, 1971). The cells therefore increase in age as they approach the tip of the villus. With increasing age comes increased efficiency, the absorptive capacity being greater in the oldest cells (Padykula, 1962). The villus cell clearly exemplifies the manner in which morphological differentiation and development are correlated with the development of specific functional capabilities (Rubin, 1971). The undifferentiated crypt cell acquires numerous enzymes, receptors, and carriers to become the highly selective and biochemically sophisticated mature cell. It functions impressively but reaches its nadir and oblivion in short order.

The extremely rapid rate of renewal of mucosal cells has been demonstrated by following the incorporation of tritiated thymidine into newly synthesized DNA by autoradiography techniques. Lipkin (1965) has shown that most of the epithelial lining of the human tract is replaced in 3 to 6 days. The mean rate of cell proliferation was calculated as 1 to 2 cells/100 cells/hour. A similar technique used earlier in rats and mice indicated that replacement of the epithelial lining occurred within 2 to 3 days (Hooper, 1956). The very brief life span of the intestinal epithelial cell (compared to 120 days for the erythrocyte and far slower rates for connective tissue and muscle cells) makes it very clear why the intestinal mucosa is an early target when there is interference with cell division as in vitamin B_{12} deficiency.

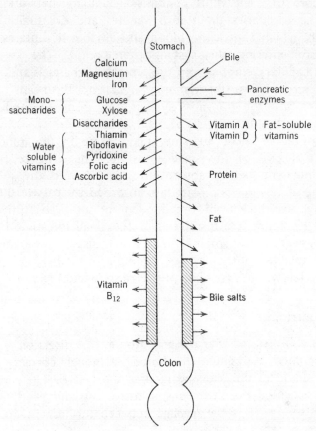

Fig. 6.4 Known sites of absorption in the small intestine. (From C. C. Booth, *Handbook of Physiology*, Section 6, Vol. III C. F. Code, ed., American Physiological Society, Washington, D. C., 1968, p. 1524.)

A reduction in the number of microvilli has been observed in various malabsorption syndromes (Ugolev, 1965). Stanfield et al. (1965) have reported that in infants with kwashiorkor there are gross changes in the appearance of the villi: flattening, broadening, and atrophy, drastically decreasing the membrane surface. They also observed associated disaccharidase deficiency. It appears reasonable to suggest that the severe protein deficiency of kwashiorkor prevents the rapid cellular proliferation of the mucosa, which normally offsets the desquamation of cells from the villus tip, and that this in time leads to the atrophy observed.

The core of each villus contains a capillary network and a lacteal. The capillaries drain into venules and eventually to the portal vein, which carries the blood and all that it contains to the liver before entering the systemic circulation. The lacteal or lymphatic capillary empties into the lymphatic channels and, via the left thoracic duct, into the systemic circulation. By means of these two entries into the transport system, the absorbed products of digestion reach the distant cells of the organism.

Absorption of most nutrients takes place in the duodenum, the proximal end of the small intestine. The distance traveled by each nutrient before absorption is related to the rate and mechanism of absorption. Materials absorbed by passive diffusion are usually absorbed from the duodenum; some absorption also occurs in the ileum, the distal end of the small intestine. It is the ileum, however, that contains the active transport mechanism for absorbing specific nutrients, for example, vitamin B_{12} (Booth, 1968). The known sites for absorption are shown in Fig. 6.4.

Mucosal Function

Often it is glibly stated that the end products of digestion leave the intestinal lumen and enter the blood. Although correct, such a statement discloses the end and ignores the means. The end result is fact and accepted, but the means is illusive, intriguing and, in many ways, mystifying. It is the passage between the lumens, intestinal and vascular, where the excitement is.

It had been assumed until relatively recently that digestion in the intestinal lumen was carried to the stage of monosaccharides, amino acids, fatty acids, and glycerol, forms that could pass through hydrolytic digestive actions do not take place in the lumen of the small intestine but occur in the membrane itself. This would appear to be a clever means of ensuring that the products of the hydrolysis are efficiently shunted into the channels for which they were intended. For discussion of membrane digestion see Ugolev (1974).

The primary assignment and main function of the intestinal mucosal cell, thus, is absorption. The mucosal membrane is the first in the series of membranes interposed between the incoming nutrients and the cells to which they must be transported for metabolism. Once inside the mucosal cell, the nutrients must traverse the cell, leave through the serosal membrane, and ultimately enter the interstitial fluid. From this compartment the nutrients finally can pass through the wall of the vascular or lymphatic capillary and be transported to other loci for metabolism. The mucosal cell, therefore, must participate actively or passively in the transport of any substance from the lumen of the small intestine into the body. If this specialized membrane either fails to accept or rejects specific molecules, the effects will eventually become apparent in the metabolism of the total organism. For discussion of hereditary disorders of intestinal transport, see Milne (1974).

The mechanisms of membrane transport will be discussed in Chapter 9.

Carbohydrate Absorption. It has been known for over 60 years that the small intestine absorbs certain hexoses faster than others (Csaky, 1963). The first suggestion of selectivity of the intestinal membrane for simple sugars was made by Cori (1925). He found that sugars administered to rats by stomach tube disappeared from the intestine at strikingly different rates: galactose > glucose > fructose > mannose > xylose > arabinose. It was established that galactose and glucose were actively absorbed against a concentration gradient and that fructose, mannose, xylose, and arabinose did not enjoy active transport. The minimal structural requirements for active transport of sugar by the intestine suggested by Wilson and Landau (1960) and by Crane (1960) provided an explanation for the differences in rate. For active transport, the sugar must contain six carbons in the form of a D-pyranose ring with an intact —OH at the carbon-2 position (Fig. 6.5). It therefore became understandable, on the basis of the minimal structural requirements, why certain of the sugars were transported against a concentration gradient and others were not (Table 6.5).

Table 6.5 PARTIAL SPECIFICITY OF SUGAR ACTIVE TRANSPORT IN HAMSTER SMALL INTESTINE *IN VITRO*

Actively Transported	Not Actively Transported
Glucose	Fructose
Galactose	Mannose
3-O-Methylglucose	Xylose
1-Deoxyglucose	2-Deoxyglucose
6-Deoxyglucose	Sorbitol
6-Deoxy-D-galactose	6-Deoxy-L-galactose

From R. K. Crane, *Fed. Proc.*, 21:891 (1962).

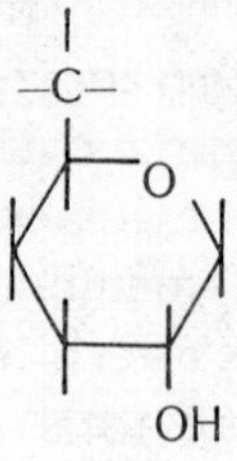

$$-\overset{|}{\underset{|}{C}}-$$

Six carbons
Intact —OH at carbon 2
D-pyranose ring

Fig. 6.5 Minimal structural requirements for active transport of sugar by intestine. [From R. K. Crane, *Physiol. Rev.,* 40:789 (1960); Wilson et al., *Fed. Proc.,* 19:870 (1960).]

Despite the inability of fructose to qualify structurally for active transport and its consequent slower rate of absorption than galactose and glucose, it does enjoy a faster rate of movement than mannose, xylose, and arabinose. It has been shown that this is due to the conversion of fructose to both lactic acid (Wilson and Wiseman, 1954) and to glucose (Hers and Kusaka, 1953) in the intestinal mucosal cell, each of which can then pass through the cell into the blood (Fig. 6.6). The absence of fructokinase and or glucose-6-phosphatase from intestinal mucosal cells accounts for species difference in the ability to convert fructose. Whereas both enzymes are present in guinea pig mucosa (Darlington and Quastel, 1953; Kiyasu and Chaikoff, 1957), preparations from neither rats

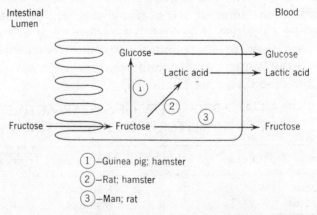

Fig. 6.6 Pathways of fructose in epithelial cell in small intestine. (From T. H. Wilson, *Intestinal Absorption,* W. B. Saunders Co., Phila. 1962, p. 94.)

nor humans have shown evidence of glucose-6-phosphatase (Ginsburg and Hers, 1960), and therefore these species are believed to be unable to convert fructose in the intestinal mucosal cell.

Although the exact mechanism of transport is not known, the current consensus is that there is a carrier on the lumenal border of the epithelial cell membrane to which the sugar becomes attached (White and Landau, 1965). Sugars that are actively transported inhibit each other; this suggests that there is a shared common carrier and pathway for these sugars (Jorgensen et al., 1961). In fact, Alvarado (1966) postulates a common polyfunctional carrier that has individual binding sites for sugars, neutral and basic amino acids, and for Na^+.

The story of the attempts to unravel the intricacies of sugar transport across the intestinal mucosa illustrates another instance where a forgotten discovery was rediscovered after a lapse of almost 60 years. Schultz and Curran (1968) point to the report of Reid (1902) as the first indication that the presence of Na^+ in the intestinal lumen enhanced the absorption of glucose. The importance of Na^+ in the small intestine for the active transport not only of sugars but also amino acids and other nonelectrolytes was then rediscovered and extensively studied (Csaky, 1961; Bihler and Crane, 1962; Riklis and Quastel, 1958; Schultz et al., 1966).

According to Crane (1965), the glucose associates with a carrier and with Na^+ in the microvilli and the complex travels to the inner side of the membrane where it dissociates, releasing glucose and Na^+ into the cytoplasm. The Na^+ is then actively transported out of the cell. The stored energy in ATP in the cell, trapped through the metabolism of glucose molecules previously brought in or by fatty acids (Crane and Mandelstam, 1960) illustrates a reciprocity; Na^+ helps to move glucose into the cell and the metabolic energy in ATP moves Na^+ out.

In the epithelial cell, Na^+ translocation can occur either through the serosal membrane or back through the brush border. A suggested mechanism is one in which the ion site on the carrier has one shape when Na^+ accompanies sugar across the membrane, and assumes another shape when the site accommodates K^+ going out (Fig. 6.7). The Na^+, however, must then be removed from the cell against a gradient. Another energy-requiring carrier system, the sodium pump (see Chapter 9) transports Na^+ across the membrane

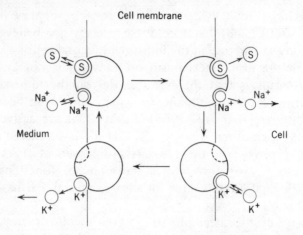

Fig. 6.7 Model of mobile carrier with two sites illustrating the influence of intracellular K+. (From R. K. Crane, *Handbook of Physiology,* Section 6, Vol. III, C. F. Code, ed., Amer. Physiological Society, Washington D. C., 1968, pp. 1335.)

in exchange for K+. The model proposed by Crane (1968) of the functional activities of the disaccharidases in the membrane and Na+ involvement in the mechanism of active sugar transport is shown in Fig. 6.8. For further details, see Crane (1974).

Na+ concentration also has an effect on the transport of many substances other than sugars: amino acids (Csaky, 1963; Christensen, 1962), uracil (Csaky, 1963), and bile salts (Playoust and Isselbacher, 1964), to name a few. In fact, Crane (1965) suggests that the Na+-dependent transport system appears to be ubiquitous, and it will be referred to again in subsequent sections.

Amino Acid Absorption. Of the total protein in the intestinal lumen, a relatively small part is derived from the ingested food; the major portion is derived from endogenous sources: digestive secretions and desquamated cells. The digestive secretions in man can contribute from 60 to 260 gm protein/24 hr as calculated by Nasset (1965). In addition, Nasset estimates that 90 gm protein/day are released into the lumen by desquamated cells. In a feeding experiment using labeled protein it was found that the endogenous protein diluted that obtained from food by approximately sevenfold (Nasset and Ju, 1961). However, all the protein that enters the lumen can be hydrolyzed and absorbed,

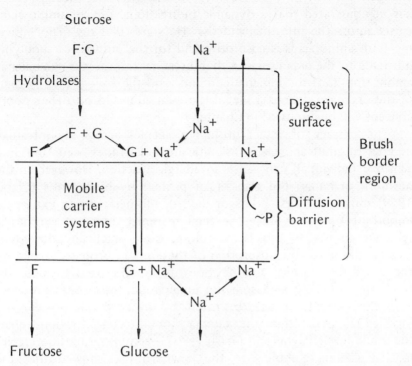

Fig. 6.8 Model of functional activities of the brush border membrane of intestinal epithelial cell. (Adapted from R. K. Crane, *Handbook of Physiology*, Section 6, Vol. III, American Physiological Society, Washington, D. C., 1968, p. 1338.)

thereby constituting a large and mobile protein reserve. Nasset suggests that the hydrolysis of the protein mixture in the lumen yields an amino acid pool with a relatively constant molar ratio regardless of the type and amount of protein ingested. Further, such a mechanism can prevent acute and large fluctuations in the amino acid mixture presented for absorption; but it can operate effectively only in the well-nourished organism that has readily available protein reserve in the glands and mucosa of the digestive system.

In addition to the contribution of the obvious sources of

endogenous protein to the lumen of the intestine, Jacobs (1965) has demonstrated that a dynamic bidirectional flux of amino acids exists across the intestinal mucosa. He states that the major movement of amino acids is absorptive and for the purpose of supplying nutrients to the organism, but that intestinal transport is in a balance among the diet, the lumenal contents, and the endogenous systems of the organism. Jacobs' concept is presented in Fig. 6.9. The "pool" concept will be discussed in Chapter 7.

The passage of intact protein molecules across the intestinal mucosa of adult animals is insignificant, but it does occur and, in a sensitive individual, can cause an allergic reaction. However, in the newborn mammal, the transfer of protein by pinocytosis (Clark, 1959) during the first hours or days of life performs an extremely important function. Since the fetal mammal does not synthesize its own antibodies and is, therefore, born practically devoid of gamma globulins, the absorption of these intact proteins carried by the colostrum allows the newborn to obtain passive immunity from the mother. For reasons not understood, the intestinal mucosa loses this capacity to absorb protein by the time milk proteins are ingested at which time the gamma globulin concentration equals the adult level. Payne and Marsh (1962), administering fluorescein-labeled gamma globulins to the newborn pig, showed that the intestinal cells absorbed the gamma globulin until they became so packed that the nuclei were pushed aside. When the cells apparently could take in no more, the gamma globulin passed into the lym-

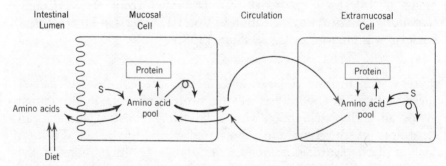

Fig. 6.9 Bidirectional flux of amino acids. Balance of amino acids from the dietary source to the amino acid pool. S represents synthetic reactions that feed amino acids to the pool. Looped arrow represents degradation to nonamino acid compounds from the pool. [Adapted from F. A. Jacobs, *Fed. Proc.*, 24:946 (1965).]

phatics. This capacity to absorb intact protein ceased when the microvilli of the epithelial cells were exposed to a yet to be identified protein contained in milk. The transfer of passive immunity by absorption of intact gamma globulin from colostrum apparently occurs in all mammals and is one of the strongest arguments for breast feeding in humans.

Amino acid absorption is rapid and active. It has been established by a long series of studies, reviewed by Wilson (1962), that active transport systems for the neutral amino acids, all of which share a common membrane carrier, depend on the following criteria: optical specificity (the D-stereoisomer does not appear to be transported actively); an intact carboxyl group; an a-amino group; an a-hydrogen; pyridoxal phosphate; and solubility of the side chain in the lipid-rich membrane of the mucosal cells. Wilson (1962) suggests that the solubility of the side chain in the lipid-rich membrane is decisive in permitting the carboxyl group, amino group, and a-hydrogen to gain access to the active site of the carrier.

This hypothesis has the support of Reiser and Christensen (1965) who found that among the neutral amino acids that inhibit valine absorption by rat intestine, those with very lipophilic side chains had a greater effect than did those amino acids that were poorly lipophilic. This may be related to the finding of Imami et al. (1970) that vitamin E is specifically concerned with the transport of valine across the membrane of the intestinal mucosal cells in the rat. A hypothetical interaction of a neutral amino acid and the membrane carrier is shown in Fig. 6.10.

The basic amino acids lysine, arginine, and ornithine share a carrier system with cystine. Wiseman (1956) has shown that the rate of transport for these amino acids is one-tenth to one-twentieth the rate for glycine and alanine. Information concerning the common carrier for these amino acids was revealed when it was shown that the genetic defect that led to cystinuria prevented the absorption from the intestine of lysine and ornithine as well as cystine (Milne et al., 1961). It was later shown that arginine absorption was also reduced in cystinurics (Asatoor et al., 1962). Apparently a similar carrier is present in both the kidneys and the intestines for these amino acids. The defect in the intestinal carrier is of doubtful clinical importance since absorption abnormalities become apparent only when large quantities of the affected amino acids are presented for absorption in a limited time. However, the defect in renal

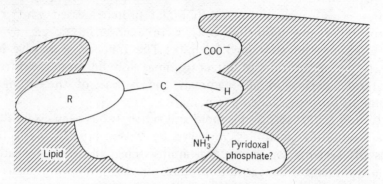

Fig. 6.10 Hypothetical interaction of neutral amino acid with the membrane carrier. Stereospecificity suggests that transport system interacts with at least three groups on the asymmetric carbon. (From T. H. Wilson, *Intestinal Absorption*, W. B. Saunders Co., Phila. , 1962, p. 123.)

absorption in cystinurics involving the same carrier protein is clinically important (Milne, 1968).

The betaine transport system appears to be shared by proline and hydroxyproline. Wilson (1962) suggests that this is probably the system normally utilized by these two amino acids since competition for the neutral amino acid transport system might lead to their exclusion.

The absorption of glutamic and aspartic acids is still not entirely clear. It had been suggested that these were not actively transported since relatively small amounts were recoverable in the portal blood after feeding. However, Neame and Wiseman (1957) have shown in dogs that introduction of glutamic acid into the lumen resulted in an increase in alanine in the blood rather than glutamic acid. Transamination during glutamic acid absorption has also been demonstrated for the cat and rabbit (Neame and Wiseman, 1958) and the rat (Peraino and Harper, 1962).

Christensen (1963) has discussed the effect of one amino acid on the transport of other amino acids sharing the same transport group. Levels of amino acids of particularly high transport affinity, such as phenylalanine or methionine, can inhibit others in the same transport group. However, in certain cases they may exert a positive influence on the uptake of others. Figure 6.11 illustrates the pumping of methionine into the cell against a concentration gradient

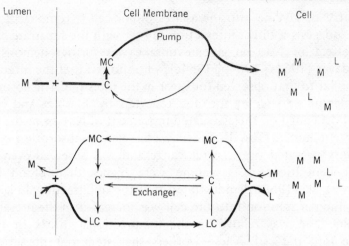

Fig. 6.11 Visualization of the way an amino acid entering by uphill transport may serve by exchange to drive uphill transport of an amino acid entering by a passive exchange diffusion. M = methionine entering by "uphill" system; L = leucine concentrated into cell by exchange for accumulated methionine molecules. [Adapted from H. N. Christensen, *Fed. Proc.*, 22:1110 (1963).]

and because of its affinity for a second transport system, it can cause an exchange and consequent accumulation in the cell of another amino acid, in this case, leucine.

Competition among the groups of amino acids for the shared transporting mechanism is a "first come, first served" basis. The relative absorption rates of the eight essential amino acids have been studied in man using a perfusion technique (Adibi and Gray, 1967). A consistent sequence was observed in the way the amino acids were absorbed from the mixture indicating a specific affinity of each amino acid for the transport mechanism as well as competition among them for the carrier. Supportive data based on *in vitro* work with rat intestine indicate that methionine, isoleucine, leucine, and valine have the greatest affinity for the carrier and were most rapidly bound; whereas threonine had the lowest affinity and was most slowly absorbed. From these data it is assumed that methionine and branched-chain amino acids, having highest affinity for carriers, would therefore have the greatest rates of absorption and would inhibit transport of the amino acids having lower affinities.

The dependence of amino acid transport upon Na^+, shown for the entry of glycine into the ascites tumor cell (Kromphardt et al., 1963), suggests a direct interaction of Na+ with the substrate carrier. This effect of Na+ on glycine uptake was further demonstrated by Vidaver (1964a, 1964b, 1964c), who showed that the interaction was similar to that observed for sugar in the intestine. The absorption of L-alanine *in vivo* in the dog reported by Fleshler and Nelson (1970) depended on the associated movement of Na+ from the blood to the gut lumen. The dependency of L-alanine absorption on Na+ transport operated over a wide range and was observed even when the concentrations of L-alanine were higher than blood levels. Curran et al. (1968) demonstrated that the unidirectional Na+ flux from mucosal solution into the cell was increased in the presence of L-alanine and was related to the unidirectional influx of the L-alanine into the cell. These workers suggested that the effect of L-alanine in stimulating Na+ transport was the result of an interaction at the mucosal border of the cell leading to an increased rate of Na+ entrance into the intestinal cell.

Pyridoxal appears to play a part in the uptake of amino acids by intestinal cells but the way in which it augments amino acid absorption is not known. Christensen (1962) suggests that perhaps pyridoxal decreases loss of amino acids from cells by altering membrane permeability.

For further details on amino acid absorption see Wiseman (1974).

Lipid Absorption. Lipid absorption has been a subject of controversy since 1856 when Claude Bernard observed that the lymphatics distal to the pancreatic duct became cloudy after a fat-containing meal. He suggested that pancreatic juices were involved and that absorption was by way of the lymphatic system. A brief history of some of the early investigations and speculations concerning fat absorption are well told by Johnston (1963; 1968) and are, therefore, only briefly reviewed here.

The mechanism by which fat reaches the lymphatics was debated with great fervor by two opposing schools. The adherents of the *particulate theory* held that triacyl glycerols were absorbed as fine emulsions and crossed the intestinal epithelial cells to enter the lymphatic ducts in the villi. The opposing school, adherents of the *lipolytic theory*, held that triacyl glycerols had to be completely hydrolyzed to fatty acids before they could be absorbed. The lipolytic theory gained more adherents, and it was generally accepted that hydrolysis was complete in the lumen. It was granted that emulsification was advantageous but not obligatory prior to hydrolysis. Following hydrolysis, it was hypothesized that the fatty acids and glycerol were taken into the mucosal cells and reconverted into fats which appeared as small globules. This theory remained popular well into the 1930s. At that time Verzar (see Verzar and McDougall, 1936), a strong proponent of the lipolytic theory, emphasized the importance of bile acids in the solubilization of the fatty acids and suggested that a-glycerolphosphate might be involved in the resynthesis of the triacyl glycerols.

The suggestion that some fat was partitioned into the portal circulation and other fat into the lymph and that bile salts, monoacyl glycerols, and fatty acids were involved in the emulsification of triacyl glycerols (Frazer, 1918) remained dormant for 25 years and then emerged in the 1960s with the work of Borgström (1962; 1963) and Hofman and Borgström (1962; 1963) establishing the importance of micelles in lipid absorption. It is now generally accepted that fatty acids and 2-monoacyl glycerols in the lumen, together with bile salts, are absorbed in micellar form. According to Johnston (1968), in the conversion of fats from an emulsion phase to a micellar phase, the diameter of the particles is reduced approximately 100 times and the surface area increased 10,000 times. In terms of volume, one emulsion particle can form approximately 1×10^6 micelles.

The mechanism by which micelles penetrate the membrane of the mucosal cell is not completely understood. Earlier it had been suggested that entry of lipid into the cell was by pinocytosis (Palay and Karlin, 1959; Ashworth et al., 1960). However, in a study combining biochemical and electron microscopic techniques, Ashworth and Johnston (1963) found that the pinocytotic inclusions in the intestinal epithelium were no greater in fed than in fasted rats and concluded that the quantitative role of pinocytosis in fat absorption remained indefinite. However, morphological investigations involving the electron microscope have yielded evidence that minute particles of lipid diffused into the cell (Sjöstrand, 1963; Cardell et al., 1965), and that there was little or no entry through pinocytosis (Phelps et al., 1964; Rubin, 1966; Porter, 1969). Biochemical and autoradiographic data support the hypothesis that the intestinal uptake of lipids in micellar form occurs by simple diffusion (Strauss, 1964; 1966; 1968), and that chemical synthesis of higher acyl glycerols within the cell was subsequent to diffusion of lipid into the cells, and independent of uptake (Strauss and Ito, 1965).

Recently Ockner et al. (1972) reported the presence of a binding protein for long chain fatty acids in jejunal mucosa and other mammalian tissues. The fatty acid binding protein (FABP) was offered as an explanation for the differences in intestinal absorption among fatty acids. Binding appeared to be related to length and saturation of the fatty acid chains. Unsaturated long chains were bound to a greater extent than medium chain fatty acids. These investigators also suggested that the observed difference in rate of esterification of fatty acids in the intestinal mucosal cell—unsaturated more rapid than saturated—might be due to different rates of translocation of the fatty acids from the membrane of the cell to the site of activation within the cell. The possibility also exists that FABP might regulate or modify the intracellular metabolism of fatty acids through its effect on translocation.

Whatever the means of entry into the cell, 2-monoacyl glycerols and fatty acids are esterified into triacyl glycerols by the enzymes in the cell (Isselbacher, 1965; Barrnett and Rostgaard, 1965). The major steps in triacyl glycerol formation, either through phosphatidic acid or the direct interaction of monoacyl glycerols with fatty acyl CoA to form di- and then triacyl glycerols, were investigated by Isselbacher (1965) who found all of the enzymes involved in the microsomal fraction of the cell (Fig. 6.12). Although both a hydrolytic and a synthetic pathway are depicted, it is suggested that the predominant one under physiologic conditions is the synthetic one.

The source of a-glycerophosphate that forms the glycerol backbone of the triacyl glycerol is a subject of controversy. It had been generally believed that the glycerol liberated in the lumen by the complete hydrolysis of triacyl glycerol could not be reused for triacyl glycerol synthesis. The investigators supporting this hypothesis suggested that the acyl glycerol glycerol came from glycolysis in the mucosal cell. These conclusions were based on labeling experiments and on the assumption that the intestine did not contain a glycerokinase (Buell and Reiser, 1959). However, Haessler and Isselbacher (1963) have demonstrated that glycerol is metabolized by intestinal mucosa and that it can serve as a precursor of glycerophosphate. In addition, it was shown by these workers and by Clark and Hubscher (1962) that a glycerokinase was present in the cytoplasm of the

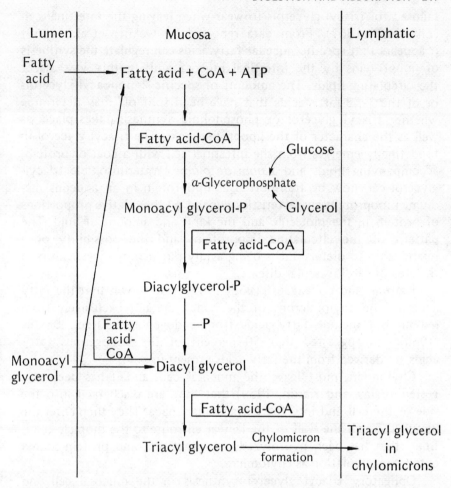

Fig. 6.12 Major biochemical reactions in transport of long chain fatty acids and monoacyl glycerols by intestinal mucosa. [From K. J. Isselbacher, *Fed. Proc.*, 24:16 (1965).]

intestinal mucosal cells and acted in the formation of glycerophosphate from glycerol and ATP. It remains to be determined which pathway is the major one.

The *chylomicron*, a low density lipoprotein, is the final product in the metamorphosis of lipid in the intestinal cell. In addition to the triacyl glycerols, it contains phospholipids, cholesterol and cholesterol esters, and a protein component. The protein of the chylomicron is synthesized in the cell and is the protein traveling coat tailored for triacyl glycerols to wear when leaving the intestinal cell (Zilversmit, 1967). From data reported by Ockner et al., (1969) it appears that specific micellar fatty acids can regulate the synthesis of lipoproteins by the intestinal mucosa and, in this way, affect the circulating lipids. The amounts of specific 2-monoacyl glycerols or of the 1-, 3-fatty acids that have been split off may determine whether triacyl glycerol or phospholipid synthesis takes place, as well as the character of the lipoprotein coat. The triacyl glycerol in food finally emerges from the intestinal cell with a coat of protein, accompanying lipids and a *nom de plume.* Water-insoluble triacyl-glycerol can now be transported as lipoprotein in an aqueous medium. Lipoprotein characteristics depend on the relative proportions of protein in the molecule and the kind and amount of lipid. The pattern of the circulating lipoproteins and the possibility of a relationship to dietary fat is being avidly pursued by investigators in the area of cardiovascular disease.

Karman and colleagues (1962; 1963) have shown that the fatty acids in the chylomicrons of the lymph are not exclusively from fed fat but include fatty acids from endogenous sources. Baxter (1966) has suggested that 50 percent of the endogenous fatty acids are derived from the fatty acids present in bile.

Chylomicra must leave the mucosal cell, and it has been suggested (Palay and Karlin, 1959) that they are discharged into the side of the cell and into the extracellular space. They then enter the lymph through the wall of the lacteal en route to the thoracic duct. Lipid that has been hydrolyzed, resynthesized, and protein-coated enters the circulation as chylomicra.

Obligatory triacyl glycerol synthesis in the mucosal cell and subsequent entry into the lymph occurs only for the long chain fatty acids and monoacyl glycerols. Those fatty acids with a chain length of 10 carbons or less are transported unesterified and leave the mucosa via the bloodstream. Triacyl glycerols containing fatty acids of medium chain length have been shown to enter the mucosal cell without prior hydrolysis and to be subjected to hydrolysis after entry by a lipase or esterase present in the microsomal fraction (Playoust and Isselbacher, 1964). These medium chain fatty acids then leave the cell and enter the blood for transport (Fig. 6.13).

The major portion of ingested phospholipid undergoes complete hydrolysis in the lumen to fatty acids, glycerol, phosphate, and

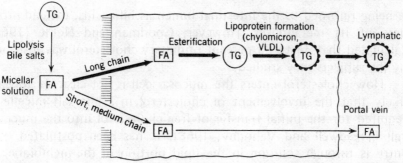

Fig. 6.13 A scheme showing the major steps in lipid uptake by the mucosal cell, its metabolism, and its exit into the lymph as chylomicra or short-chain fatty acids. (Adapted from K. J. Isselbacher and R. M. Glickman, *Transport Across the Intestine*, W. L. Burland and P. D. Samuel, eds., Churchill Livingstone, Edinburgh, 1972, p. 245.)

other compounds. Absorption presumably parallels that of the breakdown products from ingested triacyl glycerols.

The fate of circulating lipid may range from the evanescent provider of energy, to the invisible component of cell substance, to the far-too-visible package of adipose tissue stored for future contingencies that all too often fail to materialize.

Cholesterol Absorption. Cholesterol in the lumen of the intestine is derived from both endogenous and exogenous sources. Most of the endogenous cholesterol, which comprises about one-half of the total, is derived from bile. Cholesterol esters comprise about 15 percent of the cholesterol in the lumen. They cannot be absorbed intact but must be hydrolyzed before the cholesterol moiety can be transferred through the mucosa (Hyun et al., 1964). The esters, therefore, will remain in the lumen for either eventual hydrolysis and absorption, or will continue on to the large intestine and be excreted.

The presence of fatty acids, particularly oleic acid, stimulates the absorption of cholesterol (Treadwell et al., 1962). These authors have also shown that absorption is stimulated by pancreatic juice which increases the level of cholesterol esterase in the mucosa, thereby promoting micellar formation and entrance into the cell, and by bile which influences the level of esterifying activity and chylomicron formation in the cell. Cholesterol absorption is particularly difficult to study because at the same time that it is being absorbed it is being returned to the intestinal lumen as bile acids, the end products of its metabolism. However, Goodman and Noble (1968) calculated that 34 to 63 percent of dietary cholesterol was absorbed by the subjects they studied.

How cholesterol enters the mucosal cell is not clear. It appears likely that the involvement of cholesterol in a bile salt micelle is required for the initial transfer of free cholesterol into the mucosal cell (Treadwell and Vahouny, 1968). It has been postulated that entry is through solution in the lipid portion of the membrane. It has also been suggested that the cholesterol in micellar form in the lumen is transferred to a mucoprotein carrier on the cell surface (Green, 1963).

It had been believed that plant sterols were not absorbed and that they, in fact, blocked the absorption of cholesterol (Blomstrand and Ahrens, 1958). This block in absorption was attributed to competition for a carrier and the ingestion of plant sterols was recommended in order to reduce the quantity of cholesterol absorbed. However, it has been shown that the phytosterols that occur in plants can be absorbed by the same mechanism and influenced by the same factors as cholesterol but that the quantity absorbed is considerably less (Swell et al., 1959a; 1959b). From a study on humans, Grundy et al. (1969) concluded that with large dosee of plant sterols absorption of both endogenous and exogenous cholesterol was impaired, and this was reflected in increased fecal excretion. Whether the decreased absorption was due to competitive inhibition of absorption, esterification, or micelle formation was not clear. However, when reabsorption was diminished by feeding plant sterols, cholesterol synthesis increased.

The location and physical state of the cholesterol after entrance into the mucosal cells are uncertain (Treadwell and Vahouny, 1968). Once in the cell, exogenous cholesterol mixes with endogenous free cholesterol. Movement through the cell is slow. It has been suggested that cholesterol may enter the triacyl glycerol droplets in the cell and leave with the triacyl glycerols to enter the lymph (Wilson, 1962). The major portion of cholesterol in the lymph is esterified with fatty acids which are apparently drawn from pools of fatty acids derived from both exogenous and endogenous sources. The absorption of cholesterol is, therefore, intimately related to and possibly dependent upon the concurrent absorption of fats. Fig. 6.14 illustrates the degree of synchronization required to bring

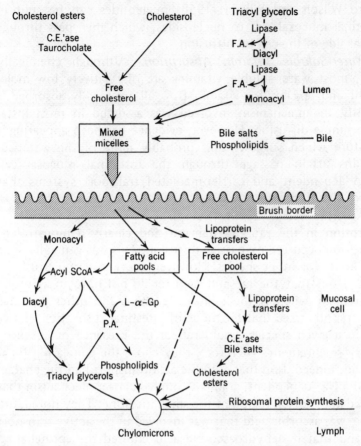

Fig. 6.14 Mechanism of cholesterol absorption. C.E.'ase, cholesterol esterase; F.A., fatty acids; Diacyl, diacyl glycerols, Monoacyl, monoacyl glycerols; L-a-GP, L-a-glycerophosphate; P.A., phosphatidic acid. (From C. R. Treadwell and G. V. Vahouny, *Handbook of Physiology*, Section 6, Vol. III, American Physiological Society, Washington, D. C., 1968, p. 1432.)

lipids including cholesterol and cholesterol esters from the lumen of the intestinal tract to the point of incorporation into chylomicrons which leave the cell for transit to the lymph.

For comprehensive accounts of lipid absorption, see Treadwell and Vahouny (1968); Brindley (1974); Borgström (1974).

Nucleic Acid Absorption. Nucleic acids are almost completely absorbed from the small intestine after being split to the free base or only partially fragmented to nucleotides or nucleosides. According to Wilson and Wilson (1958) nucleotides can be split in the intestinal mucosal cell to nucleosides, which then pass through the serosal side of the cell by diffusion.

Water-Soluble Vitamin Absorption. Although chemically diverse, most water-soluble vitamins are of relatively low molecular weight and, except for vitamin B_{12}, all are readily absorbed. Until recently the mechanism involved was assumed in most instances, to be simple diffusion. However, evidence has been appearing in the literature which suggests that probably more of the water-soluble vitamins attain passage through the intestinal mucosal cell via energy-dependent and carrier-mediated transport systems than by passive diffusion.

Ascorbic Acid. Spencer et al. (1963) studied ascorbic acid absorption in the rat and hamster and clearly demonstrated that absorption occurred by passive diffusion. This was generally accepted as a model for other species. However, Stevenson and Brush (1969) pointed out that the rat and hamster do not have an ascorbic acid requirement whereas the guinea pig, man, and other primates do. They hypothesized that the mode of intestinal absorption of ascorbic acid in a given species would reflect the presence or absence of a dietary requirement. Therefore, they chose the guinea pig for study and did, indeed, find that ascorbic acid transport had the characteristics of a Na^+-dependent, gradient-coupled carrier mechanism that was located in the distal region of the small intestine. They noted, further, that it was ascorbic acid that was involved in the active transport system and that if dehydroascorbic acid entered the epithelial cell its absorption rate was very low. Since they were unable to demonstrate a similar active transport system in the rat, they suggested that a species-specific transport mechanism for ascorbic acid is related to a species-specific nutrient requirement. In a study involving intubation of humans, Nicholson and Chornock (1942) found that ascorbic acid was taken up very rapidly and efficiently by the jejunum. They estimated the absorptive capacity of the small intestine to be as much as 20-40 gm day that is, of course, greatly in excess of the NRC Recommended Allowance. This divergence in suggested intake and absorptive capacity is interesting to note and perhaps to investigate in light of the arguments presented by those espousing greatly increased ascorbic acid intakes.

Thiamin. The absorption of this vitamin is rapid and largely from the proximal small intestine. Since the absorptive capacity for thiamin in man is very restricted, amounting to only a few milligrams per dose, it was attributed to a special mechanism (Morrison and Campbell, 1960). Studies on everted sacs of rat intestine provided no evidence of concentration against a gradient, nor was the movement of thiamin affected by the addition of either substrates or inhibitors (Turner and Hughes, 1962). It was concluded, therefore, that absorption was by passive diffusion and that the rate was sufficient to account for daily uptake of the vitamin from the diet. However, *in vivo* data from chicks using intestinal loops and a thiamin antagonist suggested that thiamin uptake may be an active process superimposed on some passive absorption (Polin et al., 1963). Later studies on everted sacs in rats did demonstrate a net transport of thiamin against a concentration gradient with the serosal concentration increasing up to 2.1 times the initial concentration (Ventura and Rindi, 1965). Both metabolic inhibitors and reductions in incubation temperatures depressed serosal accumulation of thiamin, supporting the conclusion that an active transport mechanism was operating. Pyrithiamin was shown to inhibit uphill transport of thiamin whereas oxythiamin did not. Since pyrithiamin but not oxythiamin is a potent inhibitor of thiamin phosphorylase from rat intestine, it was concluded that phosphorylation is the basic mechanism of intestinal uphill transport of thiamin (Ventura and Rindi, 1965).

Alcoholic patients frequently exhibit a marked reduction in thiamin absorption (Leevy and Baker, 1968). In a study on normal human volunteers and alcoholic patients, Thomson et al. (1970) found thiamin absorption after a 20 mg dose to malnourished alcoholics was one-third that of normal volunteers. With nutritional improvement, thiamin absorption returned to normal in the alcoholics. Since these investigators observed that an increase in thiamin intake above 10 mg did not significantly increase its level in the blood or urine, they concluded that intestinal transport of thiamin invokes a rate-limiting process. The maximum absorption of thiamin in normal man after a single dose was approximately 8.3 mg (Thomson and Leevy, 1972). Although the exact relationship between phosphorylation of thiamin and its intestinal transport was not established, it was assumed that thiamin primarily utilized that mechanism for absorption (Rindi et al., 1966). However, it is not the phosphorylation step that is the rate-limiting one since thiamin propyl disulfide, which is also phosphorylated, is not rate-limited (Thomson et al., 1971). The phosphorylation step, therefore, is not the one that is vulnerable to malnutrition or other conditions such as alcoholism. Thomson and Leevy (1972) suggest that the decrease in thiamin absorption in alcoholic patients and in those with intestinal resections is due to a decrease in the number of receptor sites available. The time lapse observed for the restoration of normal thiamin absorption after thiamin administration to malnourished alcoholic patients probably is associated with regeneration of mucosal cells with adequate receptor sites.

Riboflavin. According to Spencer and Zamchek (1961) riboflavin absorption occurs through passive diffusion in the proximal part of the small intestine. This study was carried out using the everted sac technique in the rat and hamster. In studies of riboflavin and riboflavin-5′-phosphate (flavin monophosphate, FMN) absorption, it was found that absorption took place only in the proximal small intestine and that the site could be saturated (Levy and Jusko, 1966; Jusko and Levy, 1970). Extensive evidence has been presented that FMN is rapidly and almost completely dephosphorylated to free riboflavin in the small intestine (Jusko and Levy, 1957). A specialized transport process involves subsequent rephosphorylation of riboflavin to FMN in the intestinal wall (Jusko and Levy, 1967). An apparent conflict exists when it is suggested that riboflavin absorption is carried out by simple diffusion (Spencer and Zamchek, 1961) and requires phosphorylation (Jusko and Levy, 1967), since phosphorylation of riboflavin to FMN requires ATP. One wonders whether the specialized transport process may, indeed, be an energy-requiring or active transport mechanism.

In a study on humans ranging in age from 0.25 to 40 years, Jusko et al. (1970) observed increased absorption with increased age when FMN was administered orally. The authors suggested that retention of the vitamin at intestinal absorption sites was responsible but indicated that secretions, motility, and length of the intestine might also be involved in the increase in riboflavin absorption with age. Although the dephosphorylation rate was ruled out since phosphatase decreases rather than increases with age, no mention was made of the possibility that retention of the vitamin might be due to the increased number of absorption sites or, perhaps, to an increased rephosphorylation rate with age. Further work is needed to clarify the mechanism.

Pyridoxine. The absorption of pyridoxine was investigated by Booth and Brain (1962) using tritium-labeled pyridoxine hydrochloride. Absorption was remarkably rapid in the rat and occurred primarily in the jejunum although some absorption also took place in the ileum. The criteria for passive diffusion were that absorption of the oral dose was in the proximal part of the intestine and that the site of absorption was independent of the dose given. It was concluded, therefore, that pyridoxine absorption occurred by passive diffusion. In a study on humans using tritiated pyridoxine (Brian and Booth, 1964), absorption was maximal between 60 and 90 minutes. There was no effect on the amount of pyridoxine absorbed in conditions that contributed to malabsorption such as steatorrhea or resection of major sections of the small intestine. Again, it was concluded that passive diffusion accounted for pyridoxine absorption. The ability of pyridoxine to alter membrane permeability had been suggested by Christensen (1962) as a factor promoting the active absorption of amino acids from the small intestine. Whether the entry of pyridoxine accompanies the active transfer of amino acids as part of an interdependent or reciprocal arrangement has not been suggested but should not be overlooked. If this should be the case, then considerably more work will be necessary before the mechanism of pyridoxine absorption is clarified.

Folacin. The absorption of this vitamin has been attributed to passive transport by some (Turner and Hughes, 1962) but to active transport by others (Herbert and Shapiro, 1962; Cohen et al., 1964). Most naturally occurring folates found in food are in the form of polyglutamates. Only monoglutamates are detected in the serum. It was concluded, therefore, that the polyglutamates must be deconjugated before absorption takes place (Rosenberg et al., 1969; Bernstein et al., 1970; Butterworth et al., 1969). Whether the enzymatic deconjugation of the polyglutamates takes place in the lumen or within the mucosal membrane has not been established but the proximal portion of the small intestine is the primary site for absorption (Hepner et al., 1969) and it occurs more distal than pyridoxine (Booth, 1968). In a series of studies on dogs, employing folic acid conjugates with side chains of varying lengths, it was shown that the intestinal mucosa was capable of absorbing the diglutamate as well as the monoglutamate (Baugh et al., 1971), and that the rate of absorption was inversely proportional to the length of the γ-glutamyl side chain. However, Butterworth et al. (1969), using labeled synthetic folates administered orally to human subjects, found that only the monoglutamate was absorbed.

Baugh et al. (1971) clarified another point of controversy when they demonstrated that folic acid was absorbed unaltered from the intestine. The intestine had been believed to be the site of methylation (Chanarin and Perry, 1969) but work with humans confirmed that methylation took place in the liver (Melikian et al., 1971).

Folate deficiency has been observed in women taking oral contraceptives (Shojania et al., 1968). In a clinical study Strieff (1970) found that absorption of polyglutamates was decreased by 50 percent when oral contraceptives were used. Similar findings were reported by Necheles and Snyder (1970). Strieff (1970) concluded, therefore, that interference by oral contraceptives probably occurred at the step of enzymatic deconjugation. Since the average American diet contains sufficient folate, even if absorption is reduced by 50 percent, Strieff did not think that folic acid deficiency was likely to develop. However, the chance of folate deficiency developing when the folate intake is low should not be overlooked. Another interesting relationship between oral contraceptive agents and folates was presented by Bovina (1971) who found in rats that estrogen administration facilitated conversion of folate to the coenzyme form. If this also occurs in humans, it could mean that enhanced utilization of folates could offset reduced absorption by women taking oral contraceptives. It is apparent that further work is essential in order to obtain a clearer understanding of the mechanism of folic acid absorption. For comprehensive reviews of folic acid absorption in man, see Gerson and Cohen (1972); Matthews (1974).

Vitamin B_{12}. The absorption of vitamin B_{12} is unique and, despite extensive study, some of its aspects remain obscure. Vitamin B_{12} is the largest and most complex of the B vitamins and for the absorption of microgram quantities of this large molecule the presence of a still larger molecule, gastric intrinsic factor (IF) is required.

The chemistry of IF has been studied intensively and a highly purified form has been prepared that is active at a dose as small as 50 μg, one-millionth the dose of 30 years ago. All preparations contain both peptide and carbohydrate moieties, with a ratio of protein to carbohydrate of 3:2 (Highly et al.,1967), and with a molecular weight of approximately 50,000 (Grasbeck et al., 1966). The polysaccharide moiety contains up to 5 percent fucose and 10 percent hexosamine and hexoses. Neuraminic acid is also present. The chemical characteristics of IF are closely related to those of the mucopolysaccharides forming the cell coat (see Chapter 9), and this is interesting in light of the function of IF in absorption. The specific affinity of IF-B_{12} for the absorption site has suggested that the binding forces are similar to those concerned in antigen-antibody reactions (Hughes-Jones, 1963). Many excellent review articles on both the historical and current concepts concerning IF are available (Ellenbogen and Highley, 1963; Herbert and Castle, 1964; Castle, 1968; Glass, 1974).

Certain facts about IF and its relationship to vitamin B_{12} are known. It is generally acknowledged that IF is secreted by the cells in the fundic region of the stomach. In the rat and mouse the cells that appear to be responsible for the secretion of IF are the chief or pepsinogen-secreting cells, whereas in human preparations the secretory activity appears to be confined to the parietal or acid-secreting cells (Hoedemaker et al., 1964). The IF secreted into the stomach binds with vitamin B_{12}, part of which is released from food by cooking and part of which enters bound to animal protein and then is released in the acid medium of the stomach by gastric protease (Abels and Schilling, 1964). The binding capacity of IF for vitamin B_{12} is its unique biological property and is related to the absorption of the vitamin. The nature of the bond or bonds between the two molecules, or the bonding sites, remains unknown (see Castle, 1968). It has been suggested that possibly one mole of IF binds two moles of vitamin B_{12} (Gräsbeck et al., 1965) or that IF is a dimer. Once binding has taken place, advantages accrue to each molecule: the thermolability of IF and its sensitivity to proteolytic enzymes is abolished; and vitamin B_{12} is navigated to the most distal sections of the small intestine and zeroed in on target site for adsorption.

Recently the pancreas has been implicated in the protection and maintenance of the IF-B_{12} complex in a form available for absorption. Toskes et al. (1971) found that vitamin B_{12} malabsorption which accompanied pancreatic insufficiency was corrected by administration of pancreatic extract. In a subsequent study employing partially depancreatized rats as an animal model (Toskes and

Deren, 1972), vitamin B_{12} absorption was found to be defective but could be corrected by the administration of pancreatic extract. The authors postulate that the pancreatic extract either protects the complex or blocks an inhibitor of complex formation.

The site for passage through the mucosa has been determined in man, monkey, rat, dog, and other animals. The absorption of vitamin B_{12} by the ileal cells has been established (Booth and Mollin, 1959), and it has been further shown by transplant experiments that the absorptive capacity is due to specific characteristics of these cells rather than to their distal location in the tract (Drapenas et al., 1963). Histochemical staining of the ileal cells has shown high concentrations of certain enzymes on the mucosal surface (Wilson, 1962). The specific receptor sites postulated by Abels et al. (1959) and Herbert (1958) were shown to be on the microvilli or brush border of the ileal mucosal cells (Donaldson et al., 1967; Rothenberg, 1968; MacKenzie et al., 1968).

The attachment of IF-B_{12} complex to the ileal cell surface does not appear to be an energy-requiring process since it occurs almost immediately and is not affected by oxygen or temperature (Donaldson et al., 1967). It would seem, therefore, that the process is one of physical adsorption. The receptor site for the complex, like IF itself, probably is a glycoprotein or a mucopolysaccharide. This is consistent with both the location of the site on the microvillus surface and with the character of the attachment that probably takes place (MacKenzie and Donaldson, 1969). Studies on both everted sacs and ileal homogenates (Herbert, 1959; Herbert et al., 1964) have demonstrated that divalent cations are required and that, in the presence of Ca^{2+}, the IF-B_{12} complex can attach to the receptor sites on the surface of the ileal mucosal membrane (Fig. 6.15). It appears that the IF molecule has different binding sites for vitamin B_{12} and Ca^{2+} since the initial complexing of IF and B_{12} does not require Ca^{2+} but the attachment of the complex to the receptor does (Castle, 1968). Since a proper fit into the receptor site appears to require the prior complexing of IF with vitamin B_{12}, an insufficient quantity of IF leads to inadequate vitamin B_{12} absorption. However, if excessive quantities of IF are present in the lumen some IF molecules may attach to receptor sites without the vitamin, thereby blocking receptor sites for the IF-B_{12} complex.

How the vitamin B_{12} molecule progresses from the receptor site through the cell and into the circulation is not known. The

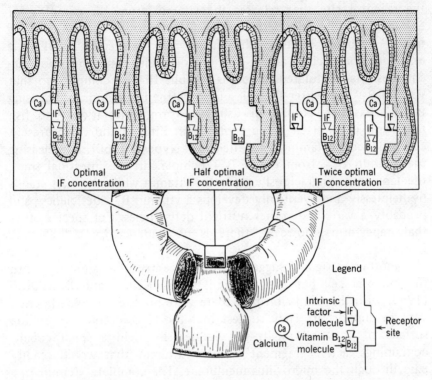

Fig. 6.15 Mechanism of vitamin B_{12} absorption and intrinsic factor action. [From V. Herbert et al., *Medicine*, 43:679 (1964).]

location of receptor sites on the microvilli has suggested to some that the mode of entrance of vitamin B_{12} into the cell is by pinocytosis, especially if entry occurs as the large IF-B_{12} complex (Abels et al., 1959; Wilson, 1963). This, however, is purely speculative since there is no experimental evidence to support it.

If pinocytosis were the means of entry, the need for Ca^{2+} would be clearer since calcium ions are required in other systems for pinocytosis to take place (Brandt and Freeman, 1967). Adsorption of the complex to the cell surface in the presence of Ca^{2+} would presumably initiate the pinocytosis (MacKenzie and Donaldson, 1969). Another suggestion (Gräsbeck, 1967) is that the receptor site in the mucosa is part of a carrier that becomes complete and operative when the IF-B_{12} complex is attached to it. The complex in that way is transported through the membrane and into the cell.

If the vitamin B_{12} is absorbed alone, there must be a system at the receptor site that releases the vitamin from the complex for entrance into the cell. Herbert et al. (1964) suggest that a "releasing factor" probably exists. Such a factor may be specific for IF or it may be nonspecific acting on mucoproteins and mucopolysaccharides. Its postulated action is to split IF-B_{12} complex so that vitamin B_{12} can enter the cell and leave the IF behind. A "releasing factor" has been found in fish tapeworm. Infestation with fish tapeworm is reported to be common in Finland and when present can produce a vitamin B_{12} deficiency (Nyberg, 1960). By releasing the vitamin B_{12} from the IF-B_{12} complex in the intestinal tract, the tapeworm ungraciously grabs the vitamin while the host stands by helplessly and eventually develops a vitamin B_{12} deficiency, and probably a variety of other nutrient deficiencies. For species other than tapeworms, however, there is no evidence for a "releasing factor."

Another intriguing suggestion for the entry of vitamin B_{12} into the mucosal cell has been offered by MacKenzie and Donaldson (1969) with the admission that there were no relevant experimental data to support it. They suggest that the IF-B_{12} complex on the surface of the cell might be digested to yield a small cobalt-containing "active fragment" of the vitamin that would readily pass through the microvillus membrane. The complete vitamin B_{12} molecule would then be resynthesized within the cell from the absorbed precursor in a manner analagous to the hydrolysis and re-synthesis of triacyl glycerols during lipid absorption.

Whatever the mechanism, there are just two choices: either the entire IF-B_{12} complex enters the cell, or the complex is split and vitamin B_{12} enters alone. If the complex enters the cell, there are again two choices: either the complex is split in the cell and vitamin B_{12} leaves alone, or the entire IF-B_{12} complex passes into the circulation. A molecule as large as IF-B_{12} would surely have to leave the cell via the lymphatics, but 95 percent of absorbed vitamin B_{12} has been shown to leave the mucosa via the portal vein and no IF has been found there (Boass and Wilson, 1964). It must be assumed, therefore, that IF is left behind, either at the mucosal barrier or in the cell. Regardless of whether the vitamin B_{12} is liberated before or after the complex enters the cell, once within the cell the vitamin combines with cell protein and is transported slowly across the cell for passage into both the blood and lymph. The vitamin B_{12}-binding protein in plasma, transcorrin, is an a_1-globulin, and it is in this form that the vitamin is transported, perhaps in a manner analagous to the transport of iron as transferrin (Herbert et al., 1964).

It is apparent that many questions remain to be answered about the complex mechanism of vitamin B_{12} absorption. The unique gastric secretion responsible for delivering minute quantities of the vitamin to the absorption site has certain characteristics that invite speculation about the mechanism. IF chemically resembles the "fuzz" or cell coat that is mucopolysaccharide or mucopolypeptide material synthesized within the cell and extruded to its surface (see Chapter 12). Particular carbohydrate groups in the cell coat function in recognition and adhesion, in selective passage through the membrane and in provision of specific receptor sites. If the information carried by some proteins is enhanced by the addition of particular carbohydrate chains that confer different types of specificity, Whaley et al. (1972) suggest that such carbohydrate-containing materials on the surface of the cell would have particular informational characteristics that are capable of influencing a wide range of cellular activities. This concept, carried one step further, suggests the possibility of a "detachable" or "shuttle" form of cell coat synthesized and extruded by cells in the gastric mucosa. This cell coat recognizes and adheres to the surface of the ingested vitamin B_{12} molecule and the IF-B_{12} complex detaches from the rest of the cell coat. The complex travels to the ileum where it recognizes specific receptor sites in the coat of the ileal cells, perhaps as an antibody recognizes an antigen, and adhesion takes place. Selective passage through the membrane follows. Simplistic? Perhaps. But often, and probably unavoidably, attempts to unravel a mechanism produce unnecessary and tangential complexities. The classic simplicity and elegance of many physiological phenomona become apparent only much later in time when conjecture yields to fact. The hypothesis we propose is entertaining, but we recall that the late A. J. Carlson of the University of Chicago warned his students that it was all right to entertain an hypothesis as long as the hypothesis doesn't entertain you.

For additional insight into the mechanism of vitamin B_{12} absorption, see Matthews (1974).

Myo-inositol. The absorption of myo-inositol from segments of hamster small intestine fulfills all the current criteria of active absorption: accumulation against a concentration gradient, energy-dependence, Na+-dependence, and phlorizin sensitivity (Caspary and Crane, 1970). Phlorizin, a potent inhibitor of sugar entry into the cell (Lotspeich and Wheeler, 1952), acts at a superficial level in the mucosa (Parsons et al., 1958). It was shown to be a strictly competitive inhibitor for the sugar substrates (Alvarado and Crane, 1962) and was also shown to interact competitively with the myo-inositol binding site (Caspary and Crane, 1970). However, the affinity for the myo-inositol site was 10- to 100-fold less than it was for the common sugar-binding site. The pathway for myo-inositol to cross into the mucosal cell was not the same as D-glucose but there was an interaction between the two at the level of translocation.

Whether the water-soluble vitamins or vitamin-like substances not discussed are absorbed by mechanisms other than simple diffusion is a moot question. Convincing evidence, as yet, is not available.

Fat-Soluble Vitamin Absorption. The fat-soluble vitamins are usually associated with the other lipids in the diet. Their absorption is assumed to depend on those conditions that favor lipid absorption, including the presence of bile. Only recently have some of the mechanisms of absorption become clear and, as is usually the case, the unraveling of the mechanisms illumined some links between the fat-soluble vitamins and other nutrients. Relationships which had been the subjects of conjecture can now be explained on a more rational basis.

Vitamin A. The absorption of vitamin A has been studied extensively in rats and chicks as well as in humans. Although some species differences have been shown, the similarities among species are striking. Absorption of both the provitamin, β-carotene, and preformed vitamin A occur primarily from the duodenum and the jejunum.

Cleavage of β-carotene to form vitamin A occurs mainly in the intestinal mucosa during absorption although some cleavage can occur in the liver in those species that can absorb some intact carotenoids. At either location, β-carotene is cleaved in a two-step process to form two molecules of retinal. The reaction depends on molecular oxygen reacting with the two central carbon atoms of β-carotene (Goodman and Huang, 1965). The enzyme involved is

β-carotene-15-15[1] dioxygenase, the carotene cleavage enzyme (Olson and Hayaishi, 1965). In addition, a detergent-lipid mixture is necessary for the *in vitro* reaction (Goodman et al., 1967) suggesting that a bile-lipid combination is probably active under physiological conditions. Cleavage in the intestine is followed by the reduction of retinal to retinol in the mucosal wall. The enzyme involved in the rat is an aldehyde reductase that requires either NADH or NADPH and resembles the alcohol dehydrogenase enzymes isolated from many tissues (Fidge and Goodman, 1968). The retinol is then esterified to retinyl ester. The retinyl esters so formed from β-carotene are indistinguishable from those derived from preformed vitamin A (Goodman, 1969a), and travel in the lymph with them (see below). Although the rat cannot, man can absorb a small amount of dietary β-carotene unchanged (Goodman et al., 1966), and this also leaves the mucosal cell via the lymph.

See Olson and Lakshmanan (1970) for a review of the mechanisms of carotenoid cleavage.

Retinyl esters are the principal form in which vitamin A is present in food. The hydrolysis of retinyl esters is a prerequisite for absorption and retinol is released through the action of pancreatic hydrolase (Mahadevan et al., 1963a; 1963b). Bile is essential for both the activation of the enzyme and the incorporation of the released retinol and remaining unhydrolyzed retinyl esters into micellar solution. The retinol and its esters are picked up from the micelle by the microvilli of the mucosal cell. The retinol passes directly into the cell but those retinyl esters that escape enzymatic hydrolysis in the lumen are met by a retinyl ester hydrolase oriented on the outer surface of the microvilli (David et al., 1966). The retinol so formed can then pass into the mucosal cell. Once inside the cell, reesterification takes place, preferentially with palmitic acid (Mahadevan and Ganguly, 1961), although some retinyl stearate, oleate, and linoleate are also formed (Goodman et al., 1966). The retinyl esters leave the mucosal cell as chylomicrons in the lymph. The fatty acid composition of chylomicra and of lymphatic triacyl glycerols and cholesterol esters usually reflect the composition of ingested fat. Retinyl esters, however, are unique in that both in man and in the rat they are predominantly palmitates regardless of the type of dietary fat consumed (Goodman et al., 1966; Mahadevan et al., 1963a).

Retinal fed to rats appears in the tissues and blood, and as retinol and its esters in the mucosal cell (Deshmukh et al., 1965). *In vitro* studies with everted sacs from rat intestine incubated with retinal demonstrated the formation of large amounts of retinol, retinyl esters, and retinoic acid (Deshmukh et al., 1967). Since the alcohol and acid can diffuse out of the cell readily, Ganguly (1969) speculated that ester formation was either a trapping mechanism of a means to protect retinol from the retinol dehydrogenase in the mucosa.

Retinoic acid was not found in animal tissues after feeding and it was assumed, therefore, that it was not absorbed. This obviously was not the case since it was shown to promote growth in animals on a vitamin A-deficient diet (Arens and van Dorp, 1946) although it did not prevent blindness (Dowling and Wald, 1960). Further study revealed that retinoic acid could be detected in the blood of man (Jurkowitz, 1962) and chicks (Krishnamurthy et al., 1963). It was then found to be absorbed by rats via the portal blood but rapidly removed from tissues (Deshmukh et al., 1964). When Fidge et al. (1968) fed labeled retinol or retinal, the label was recovered in the lymph associated with retinol and its esters; but in the bile a significant portion was associated with retinoic acid. These data clearly indicated that retinoic acid could be absorbed and, furthermore, that fed retinol and retinal could be oxidized in the mucosa to retinoic acid. The oxidation of retinol to retinoic acid however is not reversible.

The chylomicra containing retinyl esters, and any β-carotene that was absorbed intact, enter the systemic blood via the thoracic duct. The retinoic acid as such, or as the glucuronide, enters the portal blood directly. In the absence of bile, retinal or its ester may also enter the portal system. All meet once again in the liver, which is equipped with a battery of enzymes capable of performing all the transformations performed by the intestinal mucosal cell. Retinol is released from the retinyl esters to be reesterified (Lawrence et al., 1966) and packaged for storage as liver lipoprotein (Krishnamurthy, 1958). As in the intestine, the hepatic retinol is esterified primarily with palmitic acid. Liver stores of these retinyl esters are available for hydrolysis to retinol, which is the form in which vitamin A is transported through the plasma to the cells.

The transport of the retinol is in conjunction with and dependent on a specific protein—retinol-binding protein (RBP)—and plasma prealbumin, both of which are believed to be synthesized in the liver.

RBP has recently been purified (Kanai et al., 1968). It has the characteristic electrophoretic mobility of an a_1-globulin and a molecular weight of approximately 21,000. The usual concentration in the plasma is about 3-4 mg/100 ml (Goodman, 1969b). In the plasma it is associated with another larger protein with the mobility of prealbumin. One molecule of RBP is complexed with one molecule of the larger protein, and cooperatively they transport one molecule of retinol. The RBP interacts with retinol, a lipid-protein interaction, and with prealbumin, a protein-protein interaction (Goodman, 1970). Goodman (1969) suggests that this arrangement with the prealbumin may serve to stabilize and protect the retinol-RBP and, because of the size of the resulting molecule, prevent loss of the retinol-RBP through glomerular filtration.

An interesting observation on the prealbumin that binds with RBP is that it is the same one that binds with thyroxine (Purdy et al., 1965; Oppenheimer et al., 1965). The binding sites are different and the presence of RBP does not affect the capacity or affinity of the prealbumin for thyroxine, nor does the presence of thyroxine affect the affinity of the prealbumin for RBP. A model for the retinol transport system in human plasma first suggested by Goodman (1970) to be a dimer with binding sites for both RBP and thyroxine, has since been revised. Morgan et al. (1971) present data that strongly suggest that the human prealbumin exists as a tetramer with subunits that are very similar and probably identical in primary structure. The manner in which the four subunits of prealbumin associate to form a molecule with one binding site for thyroxine and one for RBP has not been determined. The nature of the binding sites will undoubtedly become clearer when the three dimensional structure of the prealbumin is determined.

A summary of the related steps in vitamin A absorption from ingestion to transport in the systemic blood as retinol bound to RBP and prealbumin is shown in Fig. 6.16. For reviews of vitamin A absorption see Ganguly (1969), Olson (1969a; 1969b), and Olson and Lakshmanan (1970).

A relationship between vitamin A status and the regulation of RBP release from the liver has been demonstrated in the rat (Muto et al., 1972). With the development of a vitamin A deficiency, serum vitamin A values decreased gradually to extremely low levels as did

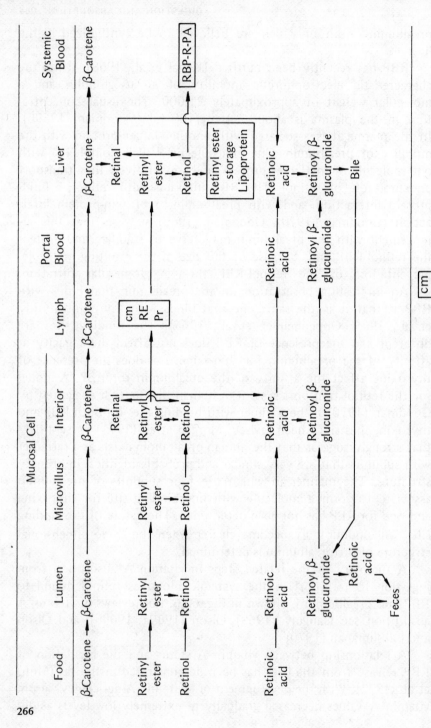

Fig. 6.16 Summary of steps in vitamin A absorption in man. $\boxed{\begin{array}{c}\text{cm}\\\text{RE}\\\text{Pr}\end{array}}$ = chylomicron containing retinyl ester

RBP. However, there was a time lag of about three days for the RBP levels. After three to four weeks of deficiency most of the circulating RBP was present without attached retinol. When vitamin A was fed orally to deficient rats a very rapid increase in serum RBP level occurred within five hours, indicating that a pool of previously formed RBP was present in the liver and was released into the serum when vitamin A became available. The suggestion was offered that vitamin A deficiency primarily interferes in some way with the secretion of RBP from the liver rather than with its synthesis.

The absorption of both the carotenoids and preformed vitamin A is promoted by the presence of bile salts in the intestinal lumen. The detergent properties of the bile acids contribute to the emulsification of lipids in the intestinal lumen and, in addition, to the activation of pancreatic hydrolases for digestion of complex lipid materials. A detergent-lipid mixture has been implicated in the activity of the carotene cleavage enzyme (Goodman et al., 1967), and bile salts are probably involved in the *in vivo* reaction. Bile salts also play a role in the formation of the micelles that participate in bringing retinol and its esters to the microvillus surface for transport into the mucosal cell.

It is the unique molecular structure of bile salts that enables them to behave in aqueous solutions as amphipathic molecules forming mixed micelles. Since solubilization into micelles facilitates the absorption of polar lipids and is a prerequisite step in the absorption of nonpolar lipids, the role of bile salts was studied in relation to the solubilization of polar retinol and of nonpolar β-carotene. The presence of polar lipids in complex micelles is known to enhance the solubilization of nonpolar solutes and El-Gorab and Underwood (1973) have presented *in vitro* data indicating the solubility of retinol to be approximately 7 to 9 times greater than that of β-carotene. They suggested that the two molecules are solubilized independently in different regions of the complex lipid-bile salt micelles and that this might be related to the size of the micelle formed. In a subsequent study, El-Gorab (1974) suggested that the polar retinol expands the size of the micelle by aggregating at the periphery and thereby increasing the inner volume of the complex. This increase in inner volume enables the nonpolar β-carotene to enter the center of the micelle and be carried to the membrane-binding sites for uptake (Fig. 6.17). Bile salts, therefore, are involved

Nonpolar molecule (β-carotene)
Polar molecule (vitamin A)

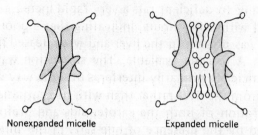

Nonexpanded micelle   Expanded micelle

Fig. 6.17 Expansion of the inner volume of a micelle by the aggregation of polar retinol at the periphery and of nonpolar β-carotene in the center. (By permission from M. El-Gorab.)

indirectly in vitamin A absorption through their role in lipid digestion and are more directly involved in vitamin A and carotene absorption through their participation in the formation of mixed micelles.

Low intakes of dietary fat have been associated with inefficient absorption of the carotenoids. This assumes great importance when the major portion of the vitamin A in the diet is in the form of the provitamin. In a vegetarian population in Central Africa, Roels et al. (1958) found that the carotene absorbed by children depended on the amount of fat that was consumed and not upon the amount of carotene in the diet. The addition of small amounts of fat to the diet improved the absorption of carotene, increased serum vitamin A levels, and was associated with a reduction of the symptoms of vitamin A deficiency. Furthermore, disturbances in fat absorption, such as occurs in celiac disease, interferes not only with the absorption of carotene but also of vitamin A (Breeze and McCoord, 1939). However, the effect on vitamin A is much less than on carotene. The incidence of night blindness was reduced in a study group not with the addition of carotene alone, but when both fat and carotene were added to the diet (Roels et al., 1963).

Another factor affecting vitamin A absorption is the state of vitamin E nutriture. Vitamin A absorption is markedly impaired in vitamin E-deficient rats. When an oral supplement of D-a-tocopherol was fed to vitamin E-deficient rats, absorption of orally fed vitamin

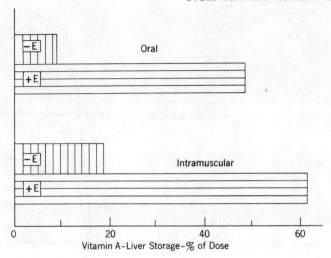

Fig. 6.18 Effects of vitamin E and vitamin A utilization in vitamin E-deficient rats. [From S. R. Ames, *Amer. J. Clin. Nutr.*, 22:934, (1969).]

A increased approximately sixfold (Ames, 1969). An intramuscular injection of an emulsified form of vitamin A evoked no response in vitamin E-deficient rats, but with the simultaneous injection of vitamin E the response was marked (Fig. 6.18). Thus, the effect produced by vitamin E is not solely in the lumen of the intestinal tract. The mechanism involved is not clear but may be related to the action of vitamin E in preventing peroxidative destruction of certain labile substances such as vitamin A, both in the lumen and in the tissues.

A relationship between dietary protein deficiency and low plasma vitamin A values was reported for children with kwashiorkor (Trowell et al., 1954; Arroyave et al., 1959; Gopalan et al., 1960). Since the dietary sources of vitamin A were probably not different in children with and without kwashiorkor in the same population group, interference with utilization of vitamin A was postulated and studied (Arroyave et al., 1959). Plasma levels of vitamin A were determined in children with kwashiorkor after a test dose of vitamin A palmitate was administered by stomach tube. Skim milk therapy was then instituted for five days and was followed by a repetition of the test dose procedure. The results are shown in Fig. 6.19. It was not apparent from these data whether the difference

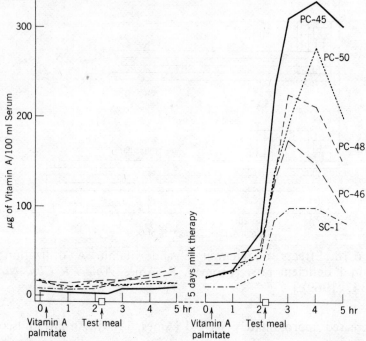

Fig. 6.19 Response to oral vitamin A palmitate in children with kwashiorkor before and after 5 days of therapy. Children were given 75,000 μg of vitamin A as palmitate orally followed by a glass of either skimmed milk or cornstarch gruel 2 hr later. Blood samples for vitamin A analysis were taken at the intervals indicated and the entire test repeated after 5 days of intensive therapy based on the administration of adequate quantities of half-skimmed milk. [From G. Arroyave et al., *Amer. J. Clin. Nutr.,* 7: 185, (1959).]

in test response following skim milk feeding was due to intestinal function or to plasma transport. In a subsequent study (Arroyave et al., 1961), plasma vitamin A levels in children with kwashiorkor were markedly increased during the first 10 days of treatment even when no vitamin A was administered in the diet. That this was due to mobilization of liver stores for transport following protein therapy was corroborated by corresponding decreases in liver vitamin A in biopsy samples. However, the synthesis of protein for the transport of vitamin A turned out to be only half of the answer.

The other half of the answer appeared to be the synthesis of enzymes involved in the preparation of vitamin A esters for absorption from the intestinal lumen. Periera et al. (1967) concluded that interference with the absorption of naturally occurring vitamin A was probably at the level of hydrolysis and re-esterification. They found that vitamin A, when fed as a water dispersion of vitamin A palmitate to children with kwashiorkor, reached the plasma whereas vitamin A fed in oil did not. Absorption of vitamin A palmitate was slower in protein-deficient chicks, and the amount left in the intestinal tract was always higher. This was observed only when vitamin A was given as the ester and did not occur when retinol was fed. When absorption was bypassed by intravenous injection of vitamin A given as the palmitate, acetate, or alcohol, protein restriction had little effect on the rate of vitamin A disappearance from the blood or on liver storage. These data support the conclusion that the block occurs at the stage of hydrolysis in the intestinal lumen. Enzymes secreted by the pancreas are reduced in protein malnutrition (Scrimshaw et al., 1956) and a reduction in retinyl esterase may well be a rational explanation of the decreased vitamin A absorption accompanying protein deficiency.

Lest supposedly rational thinking based on too little accumulated data be accepted too readily, questions have been raised again as to whether the low levels of vitamin A in the livers of malnourished children are due to low protein or to low vitamin A intakes (Zaklama et al., 1972). Because liver vitamin A stores are generally accepted as the indicator of vitamin A nutrition (Smith and Malthus, 1962; Underwood et al., 1970), the effects of protein deficiency and of low vitamin A intake were evaluated in terms of liver vitamin A in rats. Low protein did not materially influence the level of liver vitamin A on either low or high oral retinyl palmitate supplements. The authors caution, as all reporters of animal data should, that interpretation of the results obtained in rats cannot be extrapolated to humans. They suggest that other—as yet unknown—factors may be involved in the apparent relationship between protein deficiency and vitamin A status in children with protein-calorie malnutrition.

Vitamin D. The mechanism of vitamin D absorption from the intestinal lumen is still not clear. Avioli (1970) refers to the "vitamin D information gap," which has resulted from recently accelerated vitamin D research in animals and the knowledge of vitamin D activity in man. Indeed, there is question as to whether it should even be called a vitamin; many believe its mode of action allies it more closely to the hormones. However, if vitamin D is present in or added to food, it becomes available as a nutrient, whether vitamin or hormone, only if it can penetrate the intestinal mucosa. *That* this occurs is not disputed, but *how* is still fairly vague and generalized. Only since the middle of the 1960s have specific data been forthcoming.

One of the first steps in attempting to ascertain how vitamin D was absorbed was to establish where in the intestinal tract absorption occurred. Establishing the location awaited methods and instruments capable of detecting very small quantities of vitamin D in tissues and fluids. Not until radioactive forms of the vitamin were available could serious work begin. Studies employing labeled vitamin D_3 fed to rats indicated that the primary site of absorption was the ileum (Norman and DeLuca, 1963; Callow et al., 1966). This was disputed by Schachter et al. (1964) who reported that the greatest capacity for absorbing vitamin D was in the midsection of the jejunum although absorption was also observed in most of the proximal three-fourths of the small intestine. Kodicek (1960) fed labeled vitamin D_2 to infants and found that 13 to 23 percent appeared in the feces within three days. It was assumed that the rest was absorbed. A later report on human adults (Thompson et al., 1965) indicated that vitamin D could be absorbed efficiently even if only a small remnant of the jejunum remained after intestinal resection. Whether the jejunum was indeed the primary site of vitamin D absorption, or whether adaptation had occurred and absorption took place there because that section was all that remained, was not apparent.

Observations of conditions that led to defective absorption of vitamin D established the importance of bile salts. In obstructive jaundice bile was prevented from entering the small intestine, and after intestinal resection bile salts could not be reabsorbed and recycled. In both conditions defective vitamin D absorption was reported (Schachter et al., 1964). Conditions that led to fecal excretion of fat such as celiac disease (Thompson et al., 1966a) were also accompanied by malabsorption of tritiated vitamin D_3 as was partial gastrectomy even in the absence of steatorrhea (Thompson et al., 1966b).

By cannulating the thoracic duct and following the absorption of tritiated vitamin D_3 in man, Blomstrand and Forsgren (1967) demonstrated clearly that bile salts were essential for vitamin D absorption. Further, they established that the pathway for absorption in man was through the lymph just as had been reported previously for rats (Schachter et al., 1964). From these data certain preliminary conclusions could be drawn: vitamin D probably is absorbed at the level of the jejunum; it is dependent upon the presence of bile; and it is carried in the chylomicra of the lymph.

Some studies reported that the vitamin D in the lymph of rats was in the form of esters that were identified as being primarily stearate, palmitate, oleate, and linoleate (Fraser and Kodicek, 1968a). These esters could be detected at the time vitamin D was being absorbed, suggesting that the intestine was the site of esterification (Fraser and Kodicek, 1968b). This conclusion, however, had to be modified when esters were also recovered in plasma, liver, and kidney but not in the intestine, after intravenous infusions of vitamin D. Other sites obviously were involved in esterification. In vitro studies were undertaken in an attempt to clarify not only the site but also the mechanism of esterification if indeed it did occur. When pancreatic juice and bile salts were present, vitamin D was esterified with oleic acid. It appeared that the enzyme involved was more closely related to the cholesterol-esterifying than to the retinol-esterifying enzyme (Fraser and Kodicek, 1968c). The presence of a cholesterol-esterifying enzyme in plasma and the esterification of vitamin D in vitro by plasma from rats (Glomset, 1962) suggested that the plasma was a site of vitamin D esterification. However, no definite conclusions could be reached concerning vitamin D esterification in conjunction with absorption, nor could it be decided if it was an obligatory step. It is clear that if the effectiveness of vitamin D administration depended on our understanding of how it gets through the intestinal mucosa, rickets would still be rampant.

There is no doubt that the vitamin D that appears in the intestinal lumen as part of a bile salt-lipid micelle is transported by some means into and through the mucosal cell. What, if anything, happens between its entrance into the mucosal cell and its exit through the lymph in the chylomicron fraction is not clear. It appears that the major transport form in the blood is the hydroxylated form, 25-hydroxycholecalciferol (25-$(OH)D_3$), which according to a report of Rikkers and DeLuca (1967) is complexed with an α_2-globulin.

The second hydroxylation to the active 1,25-dihydroxycholecalciferol $(1,25\text{-}(OH)_2D_3)$ occurs in the kidney (Fraser and Kodicek, 1971; Norman et al., 1971). Some of this form may also appear in transport since it travels to its site of activity in the small intestine for calcium absorption (Haussler et al., 1971; Omdahl et al., 1971) and to bone for calcium mobilization (Holick et al., 1972).

Vitamin E. The absorption of this vitamin is understood only in the most general terms. The superior biological activity of a-tocopherol over the other naturally occurring forms has been attributed in part to its more efficient intestinal absorption (Draper and Csallany, 1970). It is assumed that certain aspects of molecular structure may facilitate absorption but what these aspects are is not known (Bieri, 1970). Like other fat-soluble vitamins, vitamin E absorption from the intestinal lumen depends on the presence of both pancreatic secretions and bile (Greaves and Schmidt, 1937; Gallo-Torres, 1970b; MacMahon and Thompson, 1970). In man, conditions of pancreatic insufficiency or biliary obstruction have been associated with malabsorption of vitamin E (MacMahon and Neale, 1970; Binder et al., 1965) and, in fact, malabsorption of vitamin E is more marked than that of dietary triacyl glycerols (MacMahon and Neale, 1970). Pancreatic juice may supply a specific enzyme for the hydrolysis of vitamin E esters in the lumen and thereby account in part for malabsorption associated with pancreatic insufficiency (Gallo-Torres, 1970a). The essentiality of bile for vitamin E absorption is due to its role in formation of mixed micelles (MacMahon and Neale, 1970) which is more important in the absorption of nonpolar lipids such as a-tocopherol than for the absorption of polar lipids such as long chain fatty acids (MacMahon and Thompson, 1970).

The vitamin E that enters the mucosa apparently is not esterified and leaves unchanged via the lymph (Johnson and Pover, 1962). The lymphatic route has been clearly demonstrated by thoracic duct cannulation studies in rats (Gallo-Torres, 1970a; MacMahon and Thompson, 1970) and in humans (Forsgren, 1969). The vitamin E appears mainly in the chylomicra associated with β-lipoproteins. However, under abnormal conditions such as the absence of bile, a significant uptake of vitamin E can occur via the portal route (MacMahon et al., 1971). Losowsky et al. (1972) suggest that a previously demonstrated need for bile in the absorption of a-

tocopherol may be secondary to its effect on the absorption of fat and, in fact, demonstrated that better absorption of fat occurred when long chain triacyl glycerols were replaced by medium chain triacyl glycerols. In each case the major pathway of a-tocopherol absorption paralleled the fat absorption.

Although investigators have been searching long and hard for an enzymatically active metabolite of vitamin E in animal tissues, thus far none has been found and the existence of such a form is beginning to be doubted (Draper and Csallany 1969; 1970; Bieri, 1970). One can only conclude that a-tocopherol in the diet is absorbed through the intestinal mucosal cell and normally is transported via the lymph to the liver and many other tissues where it can be stored. Whether the storage form is different from the form in which it enters and leaves the liver is not known, nor has a specific carrier protein for its transport in the plasma been identified. A dynamic equilibrium exists between the vitamin E in the plasma lipoprotein and that in the erythrocytes (Kayden and Bjornson, 1972). These are all problems awaiting a solution.

Vitamin K. The vitamin K in the intestinal lumen is derived from two sources: that present in ingested food and that synthesized by the flora in the tract. Both sources are available for absorption. There is only general information concerning the passage of vitamin K from the intestinal lumen into the mucosal cell. Those factors that promote the absorption of fat, such as the presence of bile, are also important for the absorption of vitamin K; those conditions that lead to fat malabsorption will interfere with vitamin K absorption. In addition, because one source of intestinal vitamin K is that synthesized by intestinal flora, any condition that interferes with intestinal synthesis such as oral administration of antibiotics, will affect vitamin K availability and absorption.

There is no consensus, to our knowledge, on whether or not changes occur to the vitamin K in the mucosal cell. The assumption is that it leaves the cell in the form in which it entered and travels by way of the lymph, probably in the chylomicron fraction. However, there is no direct evidence to support this.

The vitamin K in the liver, at least in beef and horse liver, is that which is absorbed from the gut, and none appears to be in a form that is endogenous in origin (see Matschiner, 1970). Evidence from other species (Hamilton and Dalton, 1968) indicates that perhaps a form derived from metabolism is the form in the liver.

Very little is known about the mechanism of absorption and distribution of vitamin K in man. The importance of such information in relation to hypoprothrombinemia in newborn and young infants, as well as in adults, is evident. Only within the last several years has a labeled form of vitamin K become available that could be used in concentrations present in animal tissue. One hopes that some of the gaps in our knowledge concerning vitamin K absorption and transport will soon be filled.

Water and Electrolyte Absorption. The water and electrolytes in the lumen of the intestine represent both dietary intake and the endogenous water and electrolytes secreted into the lumen in the gastric juice, bile, and pancreatic and intestinal juices. Whereas the quantity of ingested water may amount to 1 to 2 liters per day, the *endogenous secretion* may amount to 7 to 8 liters. Since the feces normally hold only about 100 ml of water, the remainder passes back through the mucosal wall and into the body. Bland (1963) refers to this as "gastrointestinal circulation." At any one time, the amounts of fluid and electrolytes in the lumen are the consequence of the simultaneous fluxes from the lumen to the blood and from the blood to the lumen. Absorption, as defined by Berger (1960), is the net decrease in the amount of electrolyte or water in the lumen resulting from a flux out of the lumen that is greater than the flux into the lumen. Studies by Curran and Solomon (1958) suggest that water and salt transfer through the intestinal mucosa partially depends on the active metabolism of the mucosal cells. However, the mechanisms of transport have yet to be clarified to ascertain whether water movement follows the active transport of solutes or whether the primary movement is that of the solvent, water. The dependence of water transfer on temperature, oxygen, and glucose and its restraint by metabolic inhibitors suggests that the transfer is energy-requiring. Nevertheless, there is no strong evidence that water transport is an active process and, according to Schultz and Curran (1968), there is little need to suggest it since the results of all experimental work can be explained on the basis of simple physical forces that result from active solute transport. Surely, on a purely quantitative basis, it would seem that the energy requirement would be for the solute rather than for the very large volume of water and, indeed, this has been shown for the chloride ion

(Curran and Solomon, 1957). There is no evidence that water is transported in the absence of solute transport or an osmotic pressure difference. The role of the sodium ion in the active transport of glucose and amino acids across the intestinal mucosa has been discussed. In both instances, the transport of sodium and water across the mucosa is stimulated. For a detailed presentation see Schultz and Curran (1968); Fordtran and Ingelfinger (1968); Edmonds (1974).

Mineral Absorption. In general, the absorption of the divalent ions is slower than the rate of entrance for the monovalent ions. Calcium, for example, is abosrbed 50 times more slowly than sodium, yet its rate far exceeds that for iron, zinc, and manganese (Wilson, 1962). Limitations on the rate and the magnitude of absorption of specific ions appear to be related to the organism's inadequacy in handling its excretions or in coping with a surplus. The absorption of calcium and iron, two minerals long known to be essential and apt to be in short supply, has been subjected to considerable study.

Calcium, mangesium, and iron may form insoluble phytates with the phosphorylated myo-inositol present in whole grains and in some nuts and beans. The extent to which insoluble complex formation interferes with absorption, however, is not well defined. In the case of calcium, it appears certain that although high phytate intake initially inhibits calcium absorption, adaptation soon occurs (Irving, 1957).

The tempo of the research, especially in the area of calcium absorption, has become greatly accelerated as knowledge of vitamin D activity has unfolded. Many gaps in our knowledge still exist, but they are becoming smaller.

Calcium. The presence of relatively large amounts of calcium in the feces led to the early suggestion that this was the pathway of calcium excretion. However, the calcium in the lumen of the small intestine is a combination of dietary calcium and the endogenous calcium secreted into the gut as a constituent of the digestive juices (Bronner and Harris, 1956). Since the quantity of endogenous calcium is difficult to ascertain, studies reported calcium absorption as the difference between intake and fecal excretion. On this basis, Leichsenring et al. (1951) reported absorption of approximately 15 percent in college women. Reports on calcium absorption (intake minus fecal excretion) in infants and young animals showed that up to 80 percent of lumenal calcium is absorbed (Liu et al., 1940; Benjamin, 1943). When ^{45}Ca became available, studies were initiated to clarify some of the mechanisms of calcium absorption. Schachter and Rosen (1959), using everted gut sacs, observed that calcium passed through the mucosal membrane against a concentration gradient, indicating active transport. This suggestion was reinforced by the observation that transport was depressed by inhibitors of oxidative metabolism. In subsequent studies it was observed that absorption of calcium was greater from the duodenum and jejunum than from the more distal segments of the small intestine (Schachter et al., 1960). There was evidence also that the active transport system adjusted to meet the calcium needs of the organism and, therefore, could account for the greater efficiency that accompanied either decreased intake or increased need.

The effect of decreased intake became apparent when Kimberg et al. (1961) observed that net transport of calcium was approximately twice as great in duodenal segments from rats on a low compared to a high calcium diet. Cramer (1963) suggested that the decreased efficiency of absorption noted on the higher intakes might be due to saturation of the carrier system. The adjustment to the increased need during pregnancy had been observed in a study using everted sacs from rats. Sacs from rats in the third week of pregnancy transferred more calcium than did sacs from nonpregnant rats (Schachter et al., 1960). The effect of age was also an observed adaptation to increased need. Increased efficiency of calcium absorption during the stages when bone growth was most active indicated that young animals had a greater capacity to absorb this ion than adults. Active transport in old nongrowing rats was minimal (Schachter et al., 1960). Similarly, Cannigia and coworkers (1964) found little difference in the time it took for radioactive calcium to appear and to reach its maximum level in venous blood in nongrowing human subjects ranging from 29 to 70 years of age.

The association of calcium with lactose in milk and the observed beneficial effects of lactose on calcium absorption provide grist for the teleological mill. By design or not, the two are associated and their simultaneous presence in the intestinal lumen was shown to improve the absorption of ^{45}Ca (Lengemann et al., 1959). Suggestions were that this was due to the effect of lactose on intestinal flora and the consequent lowering of the pH or on calcium per se that maintained it in a form available for transport. Perhaps one could even suggest that lactose provided a split-and-serve package of metabolizable hexose for use at the membrane surface.

The observed adaptations all seemed geared toward adjusting supply to demand; they indicate gross effects but yield no information on the mechanisms involved.

The relationship of vitamin D to calcium metabolism and bone formation has long been known, but specific actions of the vitamin that could explain the effects on calcium absorption are just being revealed. Greenberg (1945) showed that the presence of vitamin D increased the absorption of radiocalcium from the intestine of the rachitic rat. Harris et al. (1965), using ^{47}Ca, studied the response of rachitic children to vitamin D administration and presented evidence to support the conclusion that a direct action of vitamin D on the intestinal mucosa leads to improved absorption of both dietary and digestive juice calcium. That the effect of vitamin D on calcium absorption was not due to the simultaneous presence of the two nutrients in the gut became evident when a lag in response following vitamin D administration was reported (Williams et al., 1961). This lag effect suggested to some investigators that the action of vitamin D was not directly on the mucosal membrane, but that its role was a more fundamental one. It became evident that an understanding of what happened during the lag period was essential if the action of vitamin D on calcium absorption was to be understood.

The lag between the administration of vitamin D and the response it evoked, that is, absorption of calcium, suggested that protein synthesis might be required for membrane transport but early evidence was conflicting (Zull et al., 1965; Norman, 1965). A protein formed in chick mucosa after vitamin D$_3$ was administered to a rachitic chick was identified by Wasserman and Taylor (1966) and designated *calcium-binding protein* (CaBP). CaBP was subsequently found in mucosal homogenates from rats (Schachter et al., 1967) and from other species (Wasserman and Taylor, 1970). The fact that this protein was not found in the mucosa of rachitic chicks but appeared after vitamin D treatment suggested that it was induced by vitamin D (Wasserman and Taylor, 1966). Ebel et al. (1969) reported the appearance of CaBP in intestinal homogenates at the same time that an increase in calcium absorption due to vitamin D was observed. Considerable evidence accumulated that strongly indicated that CaBP played an important role in calcium absorption (Wasserman and Taylor, 1968; Taylor and Wasserman, 1969). Its capacity to bind calcium and to form a complex with it suggested that CaBP was related to the movement of calcium through the intestinal mucosa. This suggestion was strongly re-inforced by the localization of CaBP in the microvilli of the intestinal absorptive cells (Taylor and Wasserman, 1970). It was also found in the goblet cells and Wasserman (1970) suggested that these cells might be a site either of synthesis or concentration.

If the lag period between the administration of vitamin D and the absorption of calcium involves the synthesis of a protein, how is vitamin D involved in stimulating the protein synthesis? After the physiologically active form of vitamin D_3 was identified as $1,25\text{-}(OH)_2 D_3$ (Fraser and Kodicek, 1971; Gray et al., 1971), the next step was to identify the receptor site for its action in initiating calcium transport from the intestine. It now appears that the active metabolite of vitamin D_3 becomes localized in the nucleus of the mucosal cell (DeLuca, 1969b). How it functions in the mucosal cell is not yet clear. The first step appears to be one of initiating the transcription of a specific DNA into mRNA. DeLuca (1971) has shown that intravenous administration of $25\text{-}(OH)D_3$ induced RNA synthesis within 15 to 30 minutes. Presumably the first step was a second hydroxylation to yield $1,25\text{-}(OH)_2 D_3$, which then initiated the transcription of a specific DNA. Whether the protein synthesized by the mRNA is an enzyme that is responsible for the formation of CaBP from a preexisting protein in the cell or whether it leads to the de novo synthesis of CaBP can only be conjectured at this time. That it probably is related to some aspect of CaBP synthesis is evident since synthesis of both RNA and protein have been shown to occur in intestinal mucosa as an effect of vitamin D administra-tion to vitamin D-deficient chicks (Norman et al., 1969). These investigators have hypothesized that vitamin D functions, as do other steroids, in activating the biochemical expression of genetic information and eliciting a physiological response. A schematic representation of vitamin D action in the mucosal cell according to Haussler (1974) is presented in Fig. 6.20. (For further discussion of protein synthesis, see Chapter 11.)

Schachter et al. (1961) proposed that calcium transport was a two-step process: uptake at the mucosal surface that is rate-limited but evidently not energy-coupled, and exit at the serosal surface against a concentration gradient. They concluded, on

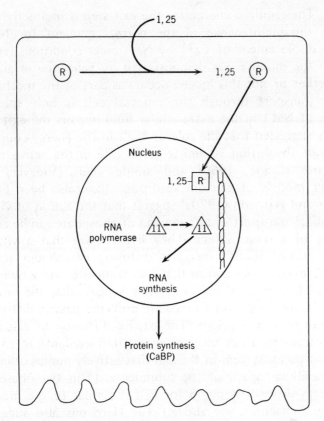

Fig. 6.20 Schematic representation of the initial events of the action of $1a,25\text{-}(OH)_2D_3$ on the intestinal mucosa cell. $1a,25\text{-}(OH)_2\text{-}D_3$ hormone, 1,25; cytosol receptor protein, R ; chromatin associated receptor, R ; DNA-dependent RNA polymerase II, II ; calcium binding protein, CaBP. [From: M. R. Haussler, *Nutr. Rev.* 32: 257 (1974).]

the basis of *in vitro* work, that the exit phase was energy-coupled and was dependent upon a metabolizable hexose and NaCl in the medium (Schachter et al., 1966; 1969). On the basis of these findings Schachter proposed a working model of the *calcium cation pump* (Schachter, 1970). He speculated that calcium binds to a protein whose synthesis is dependent upon vitamin D. This step is rate-limited by the availability of unbound CaBP. The calcium-protein complex traverses the cell and enters the membrane on the side away from the mucosal surface. When the calcium is exposed to the NaCl of the interstitial fluid, it is displaced from the protein by Na^+. The required energy for the exit step is indirectly available through the maintenance of the normal gradient for Na^+. The *in vitro* displacement of Ca^{2+} by Na^+ under conditions resembling those in the mucosa was demonstrated by Schachter et al. (1967), but whether or not this indeed occurs as part of the mechanism of calcium transport through the mucosal cell is only speculation. Absence of NaCl in the extracellular fluid impairs the exit process, and it is suggested that the role of NaCl in the energy-coupled step in calcium absorption is similar to its role in the active transport of glucose (Crane, 1960) and amino acids (Vidaver, 1964c).

Other models of calcium absorption have also been proposed. Harrison and Harrison (1970a) suggest that the action of vitamin D on intestinal transport of calcium and of phosphate can be explained in terms of a single effect. They hypothesize that a vitamin D-induced protein (CaBP) increases diffusion of calcium across the intestinal mucosal cell and in that way stimulates the active mucosal to serosal transport of calcium. They suggest that the vitamin D-induced factor might act to mediate both the passive diffusion and active transport of calcium. The passive diffusion of calcium into the cells leads to a net increase of calcium available to an energy-dependent pump system in the cell that actively pumps calcium into the extracellular space of the submucosa. (This two-phase system with energy-dependent pump for exit is similar to the model proposed by Schachter, see above.) The Harrisons also suggest that the increase in the calcium concentration in the cell compartment increases the transport of inorganic phosphate by a calcium-stimulated phosphate transport system.

Still another working hypothesis of vitamin D action in calcium transport has been suggested (DeLuca, 1971). Vitamin D_3 hydroxylated in the liver to $25\text{-}(OH)D_3$ is further hydroxylated in the kidney to $1,25\text{-}(OH)_2D_3$, which acts on the nuclear DNA, probably by unmasking the gene that codes for the calcium transport protein. This causes the transcription of an mRNA that, in turn, is responsible for the protein that binds calcium. The calcium transport protein then moves to the brush border surface. DeLuca postulates that a calcium-dependent ATPase system at the surface releases ATP, which is used to enhance the rate at which calcium is transferred from the lumen of the intestine into the cell. The absorbed calcium, he suggests, is taken

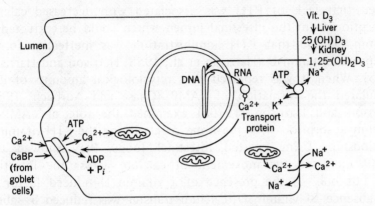

Fig. 6.21 Graphic representation of a working hypothesis of the mechanism of vitamin D action on intestinal mucosa. [Adapted from H. F. DeLuca, *Recent Progr. in Hormone Res.*, 27: 479 (1971).]

up by the mitochondria and subsequently released at the opposite side of the cell where a downhill sodium gradient introduces an additional push of calcium from inside the cell to the outside. The sodium-potassium gradient is maintained by the sodium-potassium ATPase system (Fig. 6.21).

Corradino (1973) has found that in chick intestine in organ culture the response to $1,25$-$(OH)_2 D_3$ was by far the most potent inducer of synthesis of CaBP. It acted more rapidly than vitamin D_3 to stimulate ^{45}Ca uptake. However, vitamin D_3 was also effective despite its lower potency.

Which of the working models described or perhaps yet to be formulated will eventually turn out to be closest to the answer, we cannot guess. It is not unlikely that threads of several may eventually be woven into the final story. The data that have been obtained from the various laboratories involved in exploring the intricacies of calcium absorption are gradually falling into place. There are many unproven assumptions, and even what some might consider wild guesses, to be sure; but the pattern is emerging and the story of how calcium absorption depends on prior absorption and activation of vitamin D is becoming clearer.

Another aspect to be considered in the story of calcium absorption is the mechanism through which parathyroid hormone (PTH) exerts influence on the absorption of calcium from the intestinal lumen and the relationship of PTH to vitamin D. It had been observed that lack of PTH was associated with decreased calcium absorption from the intestinal lumen which could be corrected by vitamin D, and that PTH administration was ineffective in the absence of vitamin D (Harrison et al., 1958; Harrison and Harrison, 1965). When it was reported that physiological amounts of PTH stimulated the formation of cAMP (Chase and Aurbach, 1968), Harrison and Harrison (1970b) examined the role of cAMP in calcium absorption with the hope of clarifying the PTH-vitamin D relationship. Using everted intestinal loops, they showed that cAMP increased the movement of calcium across the intestinal wall but only in the presence of a vitamin D-induced factor. In the absence of vitamin D, calcium transfer was reduced by about 50 percent. Thus, the effects of cAMP were similar to those of PTH itself, and suggested that PTH acts through stimulation of cAMP production. From their data they concluded that the energy-independent downhill transfer of calcium across the mucosal wall was enhanced by cAMP only when vitamin D was adequate. This does not explain the mechanism of interaction of cAMP and vitamin D that is yet to be resolved. For reviews of the interrelationships among calcium, vitamin D, PTH, and calcitonin, see Melancon et al. (1970); DeLuca (1971); Harrison and Harrison (1974). For further discussion of these interrelationships in bone metabolism, see Chapter 17.

Iron. The presence of relatively large amounts of iron in the feces and very small quantities in the urine led to the early obvious suggestion that iron, like calcium, was excreted into the lumen of the gastrointestinal tract. However, McCance and Widdowson (1937) clearly demonstrated that iron that was injected directly into the blood in large doses was not excreted either by way of the urine or feces. This work was subsequently confirmed by many investigators and by the use of radioactive iron. It is now fairly well established that there is a unidirectional movement of iron across the intestinal mucosal cell with no satisfactory means of excretion either through the gut or urine.

Excess iron that does enter by injection or by disruption of the normal regulation of iron absorptive processes has no means of exit and, as a result, accumulates in storage primarily in the liver but also in the spleen, bone marrow, and other cells as ferritin, or hemosiderin. Normally the body mass of iron is maintained within relatively narrow limits and, with the demonstrated inability to

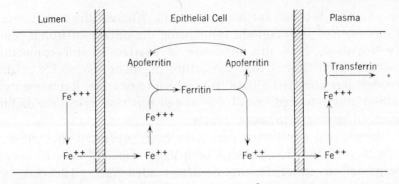

Fig. 6.22 "Mucosal Block" hypothesis. [From S. Granick, *Bull N. Y. Acad. Med.*, 30: 81 (1954).]

cope with excess by excretion, the only logical means of explaining what is termed "embarrassment of excess," a euphemism for toxicity, would be through control of entry. This, indeed, seems to be the case but the control mechanism remains unclear. Based on early suggestions that ferritin was involved in the control of iron absorption (Hahn et al., 1939; 1943) and that divalent iron was more readily absorbed than trivalent (Moore et al., 1944), the Mucosal Block Theory was proposed by Granick (1949; 1954). He postulated that the mechanism for regulation of iron absorption resided in the mucosal cells of the duodenum and upper jejunum. It was a function of the ferritin content of the cells and was an adjustable one in that it could range from almost complete restriction of entry to no restriction at all. The details which Granick proposed are shown in Fig. 6.22. He suggested that the change from ferric to ferrous iron occurred in the intestinal lumen prior to entry into the mucosal cell. Once inside the cell, the iron was oxidized and joined to the protein, apoferritin, which was synthesized in the cell, thereby forming ferritin. Passage through the serosal membrane in response to body need required the splitting of the iron from ferritin, its reduction and subsequent reoxidation upon entrance into the blood, where it attached to the specific iron-binding β_1-globulin, transferrin, or siderophilin as it is sometimes called. With iron release, the ferritin once again became apoferritin that could be degraded to amino acids. According to this scheme, apoferritin was continually being broken down and resynthesized. If iron was not needed to maintain the body mass of iron it remained in the mucosal cell as ferritin and, according to Granick, it was a high level of ferritin in the cells that blocked further absorption. Whereas the basic concept of mucosal cell iron content influencing the uptake of iron is generally accepted, how this influence is exerted is still conjecture, however sophisticated that conjecture might be. Granick's original proposal has provided a base from which to operate. Refinements of method and extended knowledge of cell function have provided the means of prying into some details.

Recent and conflicting data have been presented that show no difference in the iron content of isolated mucosal cells in normal compared to iron-deficient or iron-loaded rats (Balcerzak and Greenberger, 1968), guinea pigs (Pollack and Campana, 1970) or humans (Allgood and Brown, 1967). However, when Greenberger et al. (1969) found Fe^{2+} bound to brush borders of mucosal cells and found that the quantity could be depressed by prior iron loading and increased by prior iron depletion, they suggested that it was the iron in the brush border that was the regulator of transport. Bédard et al. (1971) also found that ^{55}Fe was quickly taken up by the brush border but that it then became localized within the cell mainly in areas rich in rough endoplasmic reticulum and free ribosomes.

Another approach using radioactive iron and a closed intestinal loop *in vivo* showed that, in the normal animal, tagged iron rapidly appeared in ferritin and this accounted for more than 90 percent of the radioactivity after one hour (Sheehan and Frenkel, 1972). Additional iron was present as unbound iron salts. With increased iron absorption induced by iron depletion, the major difference from the normal distribution pattern was the increase in proportion and quantity of free iron salts. These investigators concluded with the suggestion that iron absorption rates may be controlled in part by the rate of initial iron uptake by the mucosal cells and that a membrane transport mechanism exists which is mediated by the nonheme iron content of the mucosal cell or some portion thereof. They indicated that their suggestion is in accord with that of Conrad et al. (1964) that the mucosal cell iron was a factor in regulating uptake. This, of course, is in accord with Granick's prior proposal and that of Hahn et al. (1939; 1943) prior to that.

An extremely interesting report reviewing some of the work in Munro's laboratory (Munro and Drysdale, 1970) indicates that perhaps certain seemingly irreconcilable data are indeed compatible.

The distinctive aspect of ferritin is its capacity to bind iron and the amount that is bound ranges from none in the apoferritin to an amount one-quarter the weight of the protein (Harrison, 1964). The ferritin molecule is able to accumulate and release iron without disintegration (Mazur and Carleton, 1963). This information, newer methods available for isolating ferritin (Drysdale and Munro, 1965), and knowledge of the mechanisms regulating protein synthesis led Munro and his group to reinvestigate the role that iron plays in regulating the accumulation and turnover of ferritin protein in the cell. They showed unequivocally that iron administration led to *de novo* synthesis of apoferritin (Drysdale and Munro, 1966) and that iron was preferentially incorporated into newly synthesized apoferritin as compared with older ferritin molecules already partially filled with iron. They showed further that the newly synthesized ferritin molecules gave up their recently incorporated iron more readily than older iron-rich molecules (Drysdale and Munro, 1966). In other words, iron incorporated into newly formed partially filled ferritin was more labile, and iron in filled and older ferritin molecules was more inert. It followed, then, that large amounts of iron introduced into the cell would fill ferritin molecules more rapidly and provide more of the relatively inert variety of ferritin. This was first studied in the liver cell and then in the intestinal mucosal cell where the same mechanism of regulation was operative (Smith et al., 1968).

The investigations of Munro's group led them to believe that the synthesis of apoferritin induced by iron was a cytoplasmic one, and this fit in with the assumption that proteins synthesized for export are synthesized on membrane-attached ribosomes, whereas proteins retained within the cell are synthesized on polysomes free in the cytoplasm (Takagi and Ogata, 1968). Indeed, Hicks et al. (1969) showed that ferritin protein was formed by RNA located on free polysomes in the cell. Bédard et al. (1970) observed the majority of the absorbed radioactive iron in the rough endoplasmic reticulum and in the ribosome-containing areas of the cytoplasm in their studies of iron absorption in mouse duodenum. Fig. 6.23 presents the mechanism Munro and Drysdale (1970) proposed whereby available iron regulates both synthesis and breakdown of ferritin protein.

An interesting aspect of the work reported from Munro's

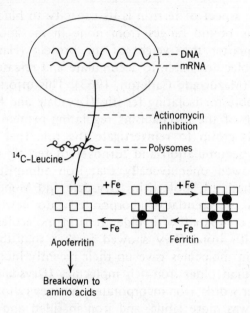

Fig. 6.23 Suggested mechanism by which the availability of iron regulates both the synthesis and degradation of ferritin protein. [From Munro and Drysdale, *Fed. Proc.*, 29: 1469 (1970).]

laboratory is the use of leucine-^{14}C to carry the label for the protein ferritin, in contrast to most other studies that used labeled iron. This may help to explain the apparently conflicting results obtained in investigations of iron absorption. One would expect that an iron label would indicate the total iron taken into the cell and not just the iron that is incorporated into ferritin. The distribution of the label among the iron components of the cell had been one of the points of controversy (Balcerzak and Greenberger, 1968; Greenberger et al., 1969; Bédard et al., 1971; Sheehan and Frenkel, 1972). Leucine can, of course, be incorporated into other cell proteins, and Drysdale and Munro (1966) demonstrated a steady and low level of incorporation of leucine into mixed liver protein after iron administration and a significant peak .into ferritin (Fig. 6.24). Because of the variable content of iron in the ferritin molecule, it would seem that the label appearing in the protein moiety should more accurately signal the ferritin synthesis induced by iron. The work reported from Munro's laboratory does not resolve

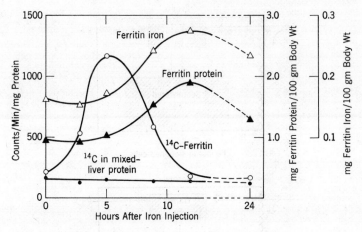

Fig. 6.24 Uptake of leucine-^{14}C into liver ferritin and into mixed liver proteins after a 2-hr pulse dose of leucine-^{14}C given to rats at various times after injection of iron. Each rat received 400 μg of iron/100 gm of body wt, followed at 1, 3, 7, 10, and 22 hours by 5 μCi of leucine-^{14}C/100 gm of body wt. The animals were killed 2 hr after injection of leucine. [From Drysdale and Munro, *J. Biol. Chem.*, 241: 3630 (1966).]

the question of regulation of iron absorption through the intestinal mucosa, but it does strongly suggest that it is iron that stimulates the formation of ferritin in the cell and that the lability of the iron is related to the saturation of the ferritin. Furthermore, the stability of the protein moiety depends on the presence of the iron, and an *in vitro* study by Crichton (1969) showed tryptic digestion of the protein apoferritin to be 2.5 times that of ferritin.

A corollary to this hypothetical mechanism for the control of iron absorption is the suggestion that the amount of ferritin incorporated into the mucosal cells as "messenger iron" at the time of their generation in the crypts of Lieberkühn is indicative of the iron status of the body (Conrad and Crosby, 1963; Conrad et al., 1964). As these cells migrate up the villus during their 2 to 3 day life span, their ferritin content determines their receptivity to iron from the lumen. Nascent cells that are well stocked with ferritin will not accept more and will take their supply of stored ferritin with them when they are sloughed off from the tip of the villus. This would constitute both a block to absorption and an excretory

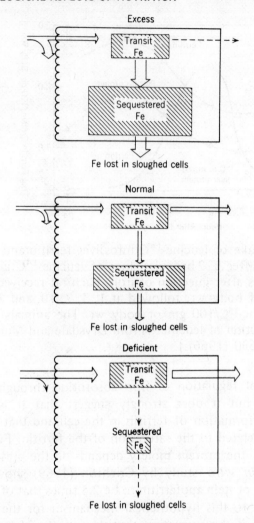

Fig. 6.25 Effects of iron status on transport of iron across intestinal mucosal cells. [From D. Van Campen, *Fed. Proc.*, 33: 103 (1974).]

path. For an interpretation of this mechanism see Van Campen (1974) and Fig. 6.25. In rats with normal iron stores, radioactivity was concentrated in those cells present and absorbing when an oral dose of radioactive iron was given. Less radioactivity appeared in cells that were formed later. The radioactivity remained in the cells until they were sloughed off into the lumen. No radioactivity appeared in the villi of rats that were either iron-depleted or iron-loaded. In the iron-depleted rats the absorbed iron did not remain in the cell but was transported through to the plasma; whereas in iron-loaded rats, no absorption of radioactive iron occurred. After an injected dose of radioactive iron the radioactivity appeared in the cells generated after iron administration in both normal and iron-loaded rats. However, no radioactivity appeared in the villi of iron-depleted rats since all of the injected dose was used to correct the depletion and none was available for use as messenger iron.

One other way of sequestering iron probably is active only when large quantities of iron are present in the lumen. When that occurs, macrophages in the villi will take up some of the excess iron into their lysosomes (see Chapter 14). These iron-filled macrophages are capable of crossing the epithelium to carry this intercepted iron back into the lumen for excretion (Astaldi et al., 1966).

If it is assumed that the ferritin content of the intestinal mucosal cell influences the quantity of iron that can be taken up by the cell from the lumen, there are still many aspects of iron absorption to be resolved. For example, how do conditions in the intestinal lumen influence uptake? How does iron penetrate the mucosal cell membrane? What controls the release of iron to the plasma? These are some of the questions that are pertinent for discussion in this section; aspects of iron metabolism related to hematopoiesis will be discussed in Chapter 16.

There is a wide range in the availability of the iron present in the intestinal lumen and generalizations are misleading. Probably about two-thirds of the iron in the American diet is in the form of the porphyrin iron of hemoglobin and myoglobin with the remaining third coming from cereal grains, primarily white flour that has been fortified with iron salts. In areas of the non-Western world, cereal grains are the major source of iron in the diet. Most studies of iron absorption, however, have measured the availability of various iron salts administered to a fasting subject or animal. Such information can indeed be misleading when applied to absorption under normal intraluminal conditions.

Hemoglobin iron was thought to be unavailable on the basis of animal studies (Weintraub et al., 1965). Although the rat, mouse, and man all digest hemoglobin in the lumen, the released heme polymerizes in the animal lumen and becomes unabsorbable, whereas in man the heme enters the mucosal cell (Callender et al., 1957; Turnbull et al., 1967). In the cell the ring is split and the iron released

(Weintraub et al., 1968; Dawson et al., 1970). It is apparent then that the iron from hemoglobin protected by the porphyrin ring until it reaches the confines of the cell is not subjected to the same hazards in the intestinal lumen as iron from other sources. Indeed, the variety of complexes in which iron is found in food and the risk of its forming insoluble complexes with other foods in the lumen all tend to impede its chances for escaping from the lumen and reaching the cell. A study by Callender and Warner (1968) on subjects who served as their own controls determined iron absorption from a test meal of iron-fortified bread, using two forms of iron commonly used for fortification: ferric ammonium citrate and reduced iron. Both forms of iron in bread were poorly absorbed even by subjects with quite severe iron deficiency and amounted to only one-tenth the amount absorbed from a dose of ferrous iron by the same subjects. Addition of orange juice to the meal approximately doubled absorption of the iron from bread. Comparable results on the enhancement of iron absorption with orange juice were reported by Elwood et al. (1968), and with ascorbic acid by Steinkamp et al. (1955) and Kuhn et al. (1968). The subject of intraluminal effects becomes clouded further by data indicating that egg markedly inhibits absorption of iron salts (Callender et al., 1970), but apparently does not affect the absorption of wheat iron (Elwood et al., 1968). Whereas Moore and Dubach (1951) reported that citrus fruit juice had a beneficial effect on the absorption of iron from egg, Schultz and Smith (1958) reported that less radioiron from egg was absorbed when given with orange juice, toast, and milk than when egg was given alone. Layrisse et al. (1968) interpreted their data on the interaction of vegetable and animal sources of iron to indicate that a certain proportion of animal food enhanced the absorption of iron from vegetable sources; however, less of the iron from the animal source was absorbed when combined with the vegetable source. Although these investigators suggest that the amino acids that are present in the animal food may have been responsible for the better iron absorption and cite the work of Klavins et al. (1959; 1962) as support, Drysdale et al. (1968) have shown that with protein depletion there was no loss in capacity to respond to administered iron with ferritin synthesis. The results of these studies are no doubt sufficiently confusing to emphasize our paucity of knowledge at this time.

An idea evolved for a method believed suitable for measuring iron absorption from a mixed meal at a joint meeting of the International Atomic Energy Agency-World Health Organization (IAEA-WHO). The method was based on the premise that as far as absorption is concerned food iron can be regarded as a two-pool system: heme and nonheme. It is known that an inorganic iron tracer cannot be used to measure heme absorption, but it was reasoned that absorption of an inorganic iron tracer might be a valid measure of the absorption of nonheme iron either because it is bound to compounds that are absorbed in approximately the same amounts as the food iron, or, more likely, because a partial isotopic exchange takes place between the tracer and the food iron. If the latter were true, then mixing of the tracer in the preparation of the food should give a more reliable index of absorption than should administration of the tracer as a drink along with the food. The first report on the validity of the method was recently presented by Björn-Rasmussen et al. (1972). The method involved preparation of a food made from biologically radioactive maize, wheat, or eggs to which a trace amount of an iron salt labeled with another iron radioisotope was added during the food preparation. From the results it was apparent that isotope exchange did indeed occur indicating a common nonheme iron pool. An absorption ratio close to unity, extrinsic isotope/intrinsic isotope, was obtained, where extrinsic refers to isotope added in preparation and intrinsic to isotope biosynthetically incorporated into the food. This indicated that the biosynthetically labeled food iron was completely released and partially bound to various compounds in the food to which the extrinsic tracer was also bound. It was very improbable that such a ratio could be coincidental for all the foods tested especially since the absorption of iron from them differed markedly. These results suggested that absorption studies that showed differences in iron availability in foods may have, in reality, been differences due to noniron compounds in the foods that favored or inhibited iron absorption. Ascorbic acid and other reducing compounds have been shown to favor iron absorption, and phosphates, carbonates, and phytates to inhibit absorption due to the formation of insoluble salts in the lumen. Further studies are planned to measure absorption from both the heme iron pool and the nonheme pool using one isotope as an inorganic salt to label nonheme iron, and the other as biologically-labeled hemoglobin to label heme iron. The prospects of understanding this aspect of iron absorption have become considerably brighter with the work of Björn-Rasmussen et al. (1972).

The next point of concern is how iron crosses the membrane into the mucosal cell. Using everted gut sacs of rat duodenum, Dowdle et al. (1960) demonstrated that the transfer of iron from the mucosa to the serosa was an active process against a concentration gradient and depended on phosphate bond energy. In subsequent in vitro studies by Manis and Schachter (1962; 1964), mucosal uptake and serosal transfer were shown to be distinct sequential processes. Mucosal uptake was more rapid and increased in proportion to the concentration of iron in the medium. Serosal transfer was slower and remained constant and maximal. Although both steps were energy-requiring, they appeared to operate independently. Both in vitro and in vivo work indicated that the second step of serosal transfer had the greater dependence on oxidative metabolism. Similar results were reported in studies on humans (Hallberg and Sölvell, 1960a; 1960b; 1960c). Although both divalent and trivalent iron were shown to be absorbed at the mucosal surface, transfer out of the cell was relatively specific for the divalent form. Some investigators have suggested that iron enters the cell as chelates of sorbitol or fructose (Charley et al., 1963), of porphyrin (Weintraub et al., 1968) or of ascorbic acid and amino acids (Schade et al., 1968). Helbock and Saltman (1967) reported that chelate formation was a necessary step, but Sheehan and Frenkel (1972) found no evidence of a soluble iron-chelating molecule within the mucosal cell.

It has been suggested also that iron transport through the cytoplasm of the cell may be carrier-mediated (Helbock and Saltman, 1967; Sheehan and Frenkel, 1972), but no carrier has been identified. Manis and Schachter (1965) suggested the possibility of amino acid complexes acting in such a capacity, and it is also conceivable that some of the unsaturated ferritin, according to the model of Munro and Drysdale (1970), might escort the iron through the cytoplasm for its release to the plasma.

The question concerning what controls the release of iron to the plasma cannot be answered at this time. There are a few suggestions but no facts. From the work of Manis and Schachter (1962; 1964) in animals, and Hallberg and Sölvell (1960a) in man, it appears that the release of iron by the mucosal cell ferritin for transport in the plasma is an energy-dependent transfer, but what specifically initiates the active transport is not known. It is generally agreed that increased need for iron stimulated by pregnancy, growth, anemia, and hypoxia leads to increased erythrocyte formation and stimulates the sequence of events that leads to iron transfer into the plasma. This, of course, is only a superficial and general statement that does little to camouflage our ignorance.

With the identification of transferrin, the iron-binding protein in plasma (Holmberg and Laurell, 1945), came the suggestion that iron absorption from the mucosa might be regulated by the amount of unsaturated transferrin in circulation (Laurell, 1947). This was supported by the work of Hallberg and Sölvell (1960a; 1960b; 1960c) and Sölvell (1960) who found that saturation of the transferrin in plasma apparently caused cessation of iron absorption. Later studies showed this not to be so (Wheby and Jones, 1963). In fact, transferrin is usually only about 33 percent saturated. The extent to which the plasma takes up iron is termed the *iron binding capacity* and under physiologic conditions all but a very small fraction of the plasma iron is complexed to transferrin. *Total iron binding capacity (TIBC)* of the plasma can be measured as the sum of the plasma iron and the *unsaturated iron binding capacity (UIBC)*; the latter can be measured by radioisotope techniques (Charleton et al., 1965; Herbert et al., 1966). TIBC normally ranges from 280 to 400 μg/100 ml, and plasma iron ranges between 60 and 140 μg/100 ml.

Transferrin in human plasma ranges from about 200 to 300 mg/ 100 ml. It is a glycoprotein associated with the β_1-globulins in plasma. Although it has been obtained in pure form there is not yet general agreement as to the precise molecular weight and the estimates are from 68,000 to 89,000 depending upon the analytical method used. It appears to have two branched chains and contains galactose, mannose, *N*-acetyl galactosamine, and sialic acid and binds two atoms of iron at two separate but identical binding sites (Koechlin, 1952). Synthesis occurs mainly in the liver but possibly at other sites as well. Transferrin, then, is the vehicle that picks iron up where it comes in and takes it to where it goes.

For reviews of iron absorption and transport see Crosby (1970); Katz (1970); Van Campen (1974); Callender (1974).

A derangement in the regulation of iron absorption leading to hemosiderosis has been observed in the Bantus, who consume iron in excess of 100 mg/day. This excessively high dietary iron comes from the iron utensils used in the preparation of both food and beer (Gillman et al., 1959). It appears that it is not the high intake of iron alone but its association with a high maize diet that is responsible for the hemosiderosis. It has been shown that animals fed iron-enriched maize diets develop hemosiderosis whereas those on enriched stock diets consuming twice as much iron do not (Kinney et al., 1949). Changes observed in the intestinal cells included disorganization of the endoplasmic reticulum and swelling of the mitochondria on high iron-high maize intakes. Whether these findings are analogous to those occurring in the Bantus is not known, nor is it known whether disproportionate amounts of other dietary constituents can produce disruption of intestinal mucosal cell structure and function.

Other Minerals. Because of the speed with which radioactive copper appears in the blood after oral administration, it had been suggested that absorption occurred through the stomach or upper duodenum. Absorption of copper from the duodenum has been demonstrated in chicks (Starcher, 1969), and in both *in vitro* and *in vivo* work radioactive copper was bound to a duodenal protein with a molecular weight of approximately 10,000. Zinc, cadmium, and silver competed for and were bound by the same protein in the duodenum. Zinc antagonism to copper had been reported previously by Smith and Larson (1946), and zinc and cadmium antagonism to copper absorption by Van Campen (1966). Theoretical insight into the antagonisms have been offered by Hill and Matrone (1970) who postulated that elements with similar physical and chemical properties will exhibit biological antagonism. Since the valence shells of Zn^{2+}, Cd^{2+}, and Hg^{2+} had the same electronic structure as the cuprous ion, and Ag^{2+} the same as the cupric ion, they proceeded to test their theory using these metals. They were able to confirm that zinc was a copper antagonist, that cadmium was antagonistic to zinc and also to copper, and that silver was antagonistic to copper. Although a significant interaction was observed between copper and mercury, it was not one of antagonism. This is particularly interesting in view of the report of Starcher (1969), who found that zinc and cadmium significantly reduced the binding of copper to the duodenal protein, that silver reduced the binding but to a lesser degree, and that mercury had no effect on the binding of orally administered copper by the duodenum.

Hill and Matrone's (1970) work provides an interesting approach to understanding the biological antagonisms by relating these to similarities in physical and chemical properties. On this basis, observed competition for binding sites on the copper-binding protein in the duodenum becomes more understandable. These investigators conclude that when ions are alike enough, interference with each other's uptake occurs in tissue or organelle membranes.

Little is known about the mechanisms associated with the passage through the intestinal mucosal membrane of the protein-bound copper ion or the ions that compete for the same protein binding site. Copper and zinc both appear in the plasma attached to proteins for transport. From 85 to 95 percent of the copper is tightly bound to the β-globulin ceruloplasmin. In a study on young men and women Henkin (1971) found 90 percent of the copper bound to protein, primarily ceruloplasmin, and 10 percent circulating as free copper. Zinc differs from copper in that 80 percent of it was bound loosely to several different proteins in the plasma and 20 percent circulated free (Henkin, 1971).

The absorption of other trace metals and how they reach the plasma for transport is still pretty much of an enigma. Pollack et al. (1965) suggested that the mechanisms of manganese and iron absorption are similar since manganese absorption is increased in iron deficiency. Mertz and Roginski (1971) studied chromium absorption in *in vivo* and *in vitro* preparations. Although they concede their data are preliminary, they reported that absorption appears to be by passive diffusion and depends on the chemical form in which the chromium is presented.

For greater insight into the difficulties inherent in studies of trace mineral absorption and transport, see Mertz (1970) and Mertz and Cornatzer (1971).

Conclusion

The plasma membrane of the intestinal mucosal cell is only the first of the barriers through which nutrients must pass from the environment of the organism to the environment of its constituent cells. Fig. 6.26 indicates the series of additional membranes and compartments through which passage must occur after leaving the mucosal cell through its lateral or basal plasma membranes, penetrating the

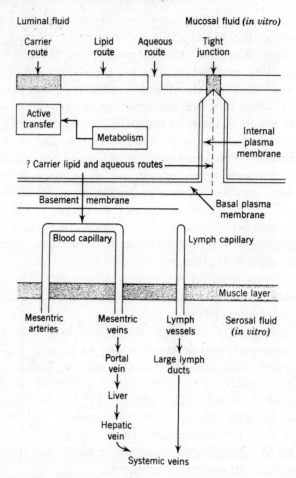

Fig. 6.26 Diagrammatic representation of the gut wall to show the various pathways available to the absorbed nutrients both *in vivo* and *in vitro*. (Adapted from D. H. Smith, *Transport Across the Intestine*, W. L. Burland and P. D. Samuel, eds., Churchill Livingstone, Edinburgh, 1972, p. 3.)

glycoprotein of the basement membrane, and entering the extracellular fluid compartment. This must be followed by passage through the capillary or lacteal wall for eventual delivery to the systemic circulation either by way of the liver or the lymphatics. The following tribute seems a fitting farewell to the small intestine:

THE SUPERBOWEL

I think that I shall never see
A tract more alimentary.
A tube whose velvet villi sway
Absorbing food along the way.
Whose surface folded and striate
Does rapidly regenerate.

A magic carpet whose fuzzy nap
Miniscule molecules entrap.
Then, microvilli with enzymes replete
The last hydrolyses complete.

A tunnel studded with protection
Against abrasion and infection
(Goblet cells their mucus spill
While lymphoid cells the microbes kill).

To top things off, it should be noted,
*This Grand Canal is sugar coated!**

George J. Fruhman

Perspect. Biol. Med., 17: 66 (1973).

FECAL EXCRETION

It seems logical at this point to dispose of the materials that do not pass through the mucosa of the small intestine before following the more extensive course of those that do.

The fluid contents remaining in the ileum are propelled through the ileocecal valve into the cecum and thence to the colon. The total volume constitutes a mere one-twentieth of the secreted and ingested fluid, or 400-500 ml, the remainder having been absorbed through the mucosal membrane higher in the tract. The fluid entering the

---

*The surface coat of the small intestine, also known as the fuzzy coat, is particularly well developed over the microvilli. It is glycoprotein in nature, and gives a positive acid-Schiff reaction.

colon contains sodium and chloride in approximately the same concentrations as extracellular fluid and potassium in somewhat higher concentration. During passage through the colon, water and sodium are absorbed from the lumen but potassium is secreted into it. The 75-170 gm of feces formed per day contain approximately 100 ml of water, 2 to 5 mEq of sodium, and 8 to 13 mEq of potassium. The difficulties in maintaining water and electrolyte balance in any condition that speeds the passage of the intestinal contents, as in severe diarrhea, becomes readily apparent.

Of the organic material in the feces, the undigested food residues constitute but a small part. The remainder is composed of desquamated cells, mucus, digestive secretions and bacteria, yeasts, and fungi.

Much has been written about the influence of the intestinal bacteria on the nutrient economy of the organism. Only in the case of the vitamins, required in such small quantities, could subtraction from or addition to the nutrient intake of the host be of any import. Since bacteria synthesize the vitamins essential for growth, it had been suggested that these products of bacterial synthesis could be absorbed through the intestinal mucosa and provide a convenient source of supply for the host. However, since dietary deficiency of vitamins can produce disorders in laboratory animals and in humans it seems unlikely that the absorption, if it occurs, is of much consequence. Only in the case of vitamin K are we beholden to the intestinal flora. The newborn infant with a sterile tract lacks the vitamin K essential for prothrombin formation until the establishment of flora in the tract, after which synthesis of vitamin K occurs.

Some of the difficulties inherent in a quantitative appraisal of the give and take between bacteria and host are readily apparent, but the development of techniques for growing germ-free animals is helping to elucidate some aspects of the complex role of intestinal flora. Barnes and his group (1963) have shown that the dietary requirements of the rat for the micronutrients can be altered considerably by the synthetic activity of the intestinal bacteria. However, the rat can benefit from intestinal synthesis only if the feces are recycled through the tract. This normally occurs in the rat unless efforts are made to prevent coprophagy. Since the effects on growth rate could be observed only when the feces were consumed directly from the anus, it is presumed that anaerobiosis must be maintained. Daft et al. (1963) have shown that coprophagy is essential to protect against symptoms of pantothenic acid deficiency but that folic acid, which is not normally required in the diet of the rat, is obtained in sufficient amounts from bacteria in the intestinal tract without coprophagy.

Intestinal bacterial synthesis in the rat, under specific conditions, can provide vitamin K and the B-vitamins to the host. However, Levensen and Tennant (1963) found that conventional guinea pigs developed scurvy more quickly than germ-free animals, which suggests that the flora in the intestine may be robbing the host of available tissue ascorbic acid. Early work by Parsons et al. (1945) showed that consumption of live yeast deprived the host of B-vitamins available for absorption. These results raise questions concerning utilization of nutrients by flora in the human tract and the effects this may have in estimating requirements. Are nutritional requirements as they are now studied in the human distorted by the give and take of the bacterial population in the tract? Probably so, but the extent and importance of this intervention to the total organism have yet to be established. Wostmann et al. (1963) suggest that, since the composition of the diet profoundly affects the intestinal microflora, further study could conceivably lead to the establishment and maintenance of a flora which would provide an optimal contribution to the nutrition of the host.

EPILOGUE

Whatever the nutritional potential of a food, its contribution is nonexistent if it does not pass the test of absorption. Those nutrients that have not been transferred through the intestinal mucosal cell to enter the circulation have, for all nutritional intent and purpose, never been eaten. The variety of nutrients from the organism's environment that have been made available by absorption must be transported via the circulatory system to the aqueous microenvironment of the cells. There, they serve their ultimate purpose: participation in the metabolic activities in the cells upon which the life of the total organism depends.

chapter 7

nutrient exchange and homeostatic control

1. Transport to Cells
   a. Plasma Contents
   b. What is Normal?
   c. Metabolic Pools
   d. Storage and Reserves
   e. Control of Plasma Constituents
   f. Compartmentalization of Extracellular Fluid

2. Exchange
   a. Mechanisms of Nutrient Exchange
      1. Ion Distribution
      2. Fluid Movement
   b. Renal Control of Plasma Constituents
      1. Water Balance
      2. Nutrient Conservation
      3. Nitrogen Excretion
      4. Regulation of Plasma pH

3. Coda

"Here, then, is a striking phenomenon. Organisms, composed of material which is characterized by the utmost inconstancy and unsteadiness, have somehow learned the methods of maintaining constancy and keeping steady in the presence of conditions which might reasonably be expected to prove profoundly disturbing."

Walter B. Cannon, *The Wisdom of the Body*, 1939

TRANSPORT TO CELLS

The assortment and concentration of each nutrient in the plasma depend not only on the quantity arriving via the intestinal mucosa but also on the integrated homeostatic mechanisms that are the means of fine adjustment of supply to demand. Despite variation in the nutrient assortment presented to the plasma by the dietary intake, intricate control mechanisms operate to maintain circulating concentrations of many nutrients and synthesized constituents within rather narrow ranges. The enormity of the task and the dynamism inherent in it become evident with the realization that each of the myriad cells is constantly removing from its individual environment all of the nutrients essential for its metabolic needs and returning to this environment both the products of synthesis and catabolism. Homeostasis is maintained despite constant change. If this is interpreted as maintaining the status quo it is the achieving of constancy through rapid, purposeful, orderly change; the maintenance of a steady state by means of rapid flux. The overall logistics are illustrated in Fig. 7.1;

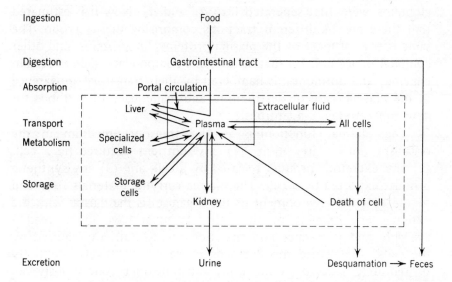

Fig. 7.1 The pathways through which the nutrients in food become available and are transported to the individual cells in man.

it is by means of the plasma and only via this medium that the material of metabolism moves.

Plasma Contents

The plasma is the extracellular fluid of blood in which the cellular constituents are suspended. It constitutes about half the total blood volume from which the cells can be readily separated by centrifugation. Over 90 percent of the plasma is water that readily exchanges with the extracellular (or interstitial) fluid compartments surrounding the cells of all the other tissues in the body. Plasma water functions not only as the solvent for all of the materials transported but also in maintaining the water balance of body compartments. That part of the plasma which is not water—8 to 9 percent—contains, by extremely conservative estimates, from 150 to 200 different kinds of molecules. These include electrolytes, lipids, carbohydrates, organic acids, proteins, amino acids, and other nonprotein nitrogenous molecules, vitamins, hormones, and enzymes (Table 7.1). As methods and instruments improve, more precise separations of components may be made. For example, the plasma globulins were first separated into a_1 and a_2. Now it is estimated that there are 14 different fractions comprising the a_2 group. The same is true of most of the plasma proteins, lipoproteins, and other complex molecules. Estimation of some components, such as certain enzymes and hormones, is hampered by their transitory appearance in the plasma, ease of destruction, and inadequacy of methods for detecting ultramicro quantities.

The plasma, functioning as the transport medium in the organism, must carry in it: (1) any nutrient required by a cell, (2) any excretory product released by a cell, and (3) any synthetic product exported by a cell. The plasma carrying materials from and to the external environment of the organism is the liaison with the external environment of the cells. It must have in it, readily available and in proper concentration, every nutrient required by the cells. And, since the demands of each cell however centrally or remotely located in the body must be met continuously, an extremely sensitive and controlled information system must be in effect to maintain the concentrations of the multitude of constituents in the plasma and tissue fluids within suitable limits. These may vary according to the requirements of specific tissues.

Constituents of the plasma participate in controlled but dynamic exchange with materials in the other extracellular fluid compartments and, ultimately, with all cells including those specialized cells that form the boundary with the organism's external environment: the cells lining the intestinal lumen and those comprising the kidney tubules and lung alveoli. Nutrients that the body cannot accumulate, and products of metabolism that it cannot tolerate, must be transported between the cells and the external environment of the organism unceasingly, as in the case of oxygen and carbon dioxide. Other nutrients or products of metabolism such as vitamin A and fat, both of which can be stored in large quantities will, if and when needed, travel via the plasma between depots and cells. Estimations of plasma level of nutrients therefore, may not be at all indicative of the state of body nutriture since they are the immediate currency for metabolism and will be reduced only when stores and reserves can no longer maintain nutrient levels. The greater the storage of a nutrient, the smaller the chance that plasma levels will fall below the normal range. However, when such a nutrient does fall in the plasma, the situation is likely to be critical.

What Is Normal?

The concept of normality, while comforting, is an illusion arrived at by computation. The definition of normality, while useful, is arbitrary since normality, like beauty, is in the eyes of the beholder. If it is understood and appreciated for what it is, it has meaning; if misunderstood or abused, it may be insidious.

The mass of tables available that catalog and present "normal values" for constituents of plasma, for example, suggest a stability that far exceeds reality and a standard of reference that implies perfection or an ideal. These tables are enormously important and valuable as long as they are properly understood. They are, in fact, a compilation of findings that can be quantitatively measured. They are obtained from a random sampling of a population judged to be representative of a general population and based on the assumption that they fall into a distribution pattern described as a normal curve. In some cases the figure in the table may have been derived from a large and representative sample; in other cases, for a variety of reasons, the sample may have been small and the figure of questionable validity if it is used as a norm for a general population.

Table 7.1 SOME REPORTED PLASMA CONSTITUENTS IN MAN

Minerals	Carbohydrates	Proteins	Lipids
Aluminum	Fructose	Prealbumin	Cephalin
Bicarbonate	Glucosamine	Albumin	Cerebrosides
Bromine	Acetyl glucosamine	α_1 Acid glycoprotein	Cholesterol
Calcium	Glucose	α_1 Glycoprotein	Free
Chloride	Glucuronic acid	α_1 Lipoproteins	Ester
Cobalt	Glycogen	α_2 Glycoproteins	Cholic acid
Copper	Lactose	Ceruloplasmin	Fat, neutral
Fluorine	Pentose	Haptoglobins	Fatty acids
Iodine	Polysaccharides	α_2 Macroglobulins	Glyceride-
Iron	Nonglucosamine	Prothrombin	Phospholipid-
Lead	Protein-bound	β glycoproteins	Saturated
Magnesium		Transferrin	Lecithin
Manganese		β_2 Globulin	Phospholipids
Phosphate		Fibrinogen	Sphingomyelin
Phosphorus		β_1 Lipoproteins	Triglyceride
Inorganic P		β_2 Globulins	
Organic P		γ Globulins	
Adenosine triphosphate P			
Diphosphoglycerate P			
Hexosephosphate P			
Lipid P			
Nucleic acid P			
Potassium			
Rubidium			
Silicon			
Sodium			
Sulfate			
Sulfur			
Tin			
Zinc			

Table 7.1 (Continued)

Nonprotein Nitrogenous Substances	Vitamins	Enzymes	Hormones
Allantoin	Vitamin A	Adenosine poly-	Androgens
Amino acids	Carotenes	phosphatase	Chorionic gonado-
Alanine	Thiamin	Acid	trophic hormone
Aminobutyric acid	Riboflavin	Alkaline	Corticosteroids
Arginine	Nicotinic acid	Aldolase	Conjugated corticoids
Asparagine	Pyridoxine	Amylase	Corticosterone
Aspartic acid	Pantothenic acid	Catalase	Hydrocortisone
Citrulline	Pteroylglutamic	Cholinesterase	17-Hydroxycorticoids
Cysteine	acid	Dehydropeptidase	Epinephrin (adrenalin)
Cystine	Vitamin B_{12}	β-glucuronidase	Estrogens
Glutamic acid	Ascorbic acid	Histaminase	Estradiol
Glutamine	Vitamin D	Lactic dehydrogenase	Estriol
Glycine	Tocopherols	Lipase	Estrone
Histidine	Biotin	Phenolsulfatase	Insulin
Isoleucine	Choline	Phosphatase	Norepinephrin (nor-
Leucine	Inositol	Acid	adrenalin)
Lysine		Alkaline	Progesterone
Methionine		Phosphoglucose	Thyroid hormone (as
1-Methylhistidine		isomerase	protein-bound
3-Methylhistidine		Profibrinolysin	iodine)
Ornithine		Vitamin B_c	
Phenylalanine		conjugase	
Proline			
Serine			
Taurine			
Threonine			
Tryptophan			
Tyrosine			
Valine			
Bilirubin			
Creatine			
Creatinine			
Histamine			
Imidazoles			
Indican			
Urea			
Uric acid			
Ammonia N			
Polypeptide N			

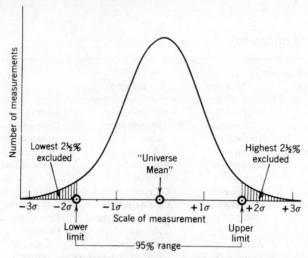

Fig. 7.2 Normal frequency distribution curve. (From *Biology Data Book*, "Introduction," P. L. Altman and D. S. Dittmer, eds., FASEB, 1964, p. xvii.

The figures presented, for example, in the *Biology Data Book* published by FASEB (Altman and Dittmer, 1964) indicate where values for 95 percent of the population would be expected to lie (Fig. 7.2). This excludes the 2.5 percent at either extreme of the normal curve and therefore, by definition, 5 percent of the so-called normal population is outside the limits that are then prescribed as normal. Moreover, the values obtained for any one individual attains a distribution pattern or normal curve established through time; yet the "normal values" for a population are obtained from a compilation of single random values in the continuum of values for the individuals who comprise the randomly derived sample of a population. It becomes clear that there are, in fact, no "normal values" but normal ranges of values, and that even ranges, in some cases, may be too narrow or too wide to be diagnostically useful (McCammon, 1966).

The line between normal and abnormal is an arbitrary one, and what is normal for an individual at a specific moment in time may be abnormal at other times (McCammon, 1962; Thomas, 1966); moreover, what is normal for one individual may be abnormal for others (Widdowson, 1962). Some of the difficulties inherent in establishing normal limits are illustrated by Simonson (1966) and

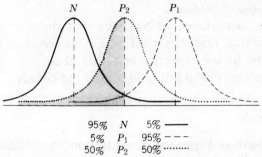

$$
\begin{array}{ccc}
95\% & N & 5\% \text{ ———} \\
5\% & P_1 & 95\% \text{ – – –} \\
50\% & P_2 & 50\% \text{ ········}
\end{array}
$$

Fig. 7.3 Frequency distribution of a hypothetical normal sample (*N*) and two samples of patients (P_1 and P_2) representing two different types of disease for a hypothetical item. The dividing line for 5 percent at the upper end of the normal distribution coincides with that for 95 percent of the patients in group P_1 and for 50 percent (median) in group P_2. The areas of overlap are shaded [From Simonson, *Ann. N.Y. Acad. Sci.*, 134:541 (1966).]

emphasize the fact that the normal limits as they are used are no more than a prediction of the probability of being normal (Fig. 7.3). Only through an understanding of human variation and adaptation can one appreciate why under controlled experimental conditions the minimum requirement for a nutrient, for example, may differ among subjects by 100 percent or more; or why under identical conditions some individuals may develop a disorder and others may not (Boyd, 1966).

The visible aspects of human variation are expected and accepted, and their determinants are both genetic and environmental. Some of the hidden aspects of variation such as individual differences in metabolic response were studied in great detail by Keys and his coworkers (1950). The concept of biochemical individuality was delineated by Williams (1956) who has suggested that each organism possesses a complex and unique metabolic pattern that encompasses every aspect of his biochemistry. Others explored various aspects of physiological individuality (Sargent and Weinman, 1966; Garn, 1966). The relationship between individual genetic and therefore metabolic traits and disease symptomatology has led to special diagnostic procedures (Hsia, 1966; Friedmann, 1971). Pauling (1968) suggests that individual variation in the optimal concentration of specific nutrients for metabolism of specific organs may be considerable and lead to greatly increased requirements for proper metabolic activity in those individuals.

Certainly, acceptance of the idea that there is genetic control of all biochemical reactions must have as its corollary that individual variations are to be expected and that they may be substantial. "Book values" are useful but only if used judiciously.

Metabolic Pools

Early investigators suggested a separation in metabolism of those materials coming from outside, exogenous metabolism, and those of the body substance, endogenous metabolism (Folin, 1905). The revolutionary studies presented by Schoenheimer (1942), now ranked with the classics of biochemical literature, clearly demonstrated that: (1) such segregation does not exist in metabolism; (2) all constituents of living matter, structural and functional, are in a steady state of rapid flux; and (3) fragments derived from complex molecules in the body merge indistinguishably with fragments derived from food sources to form *metabolic pools*. A pool, then, is the quantity of a specific substance that is in a state of active turnover. With techniques available today the pool size can be measured by administering a radioactive isotope and determining its dilution. It should be readily apparent that this kind of pool cannot be located in any one particular place. It is, in fact, illustrated by the two-directional arrows in the box depicting transport, metabolism, and storage in Fig. 7.1. It represents available, labile nutrients in dynamic flux. The size of the pool can be small for some substances and larger for others which may have storage sites. However, in a small pool the turnover can be quite enormous, as it is in the case of ATP which the human produces in an equivalent to his body weight (70 kg) every 24 hours (Karlson, 1968). Steele (1964) has defined a pool of material in steady-state turnover as "a collection of identical molecules from which deletions are made at a constant rate, along with simultaneous addition of new identical molecules at the same rate, the total pool size remaining unchanged." Such turnover was first reported by Schoenheimer (1942), who showed that even adipose tissue was far from static and that 44 percent of an administered tracer dose was in the depots at the end of eight days although the total body fat of the animal had not changed. Similar pool exchanges were observed when labeled amino acids were administered. With these studies Schoenheimer established the concept of the dynamic state of the body's metabolism. Pools are ever-changing and dynamic. They do not constitute storage that, although in a dynamic state, is localized and expendable; but they are fed by and feed into metabolizing cells, storage, and reserves.

Storage and Reserves

Storage, as the term generally applies, is an extra supply of a substance collected in specific cells or tissues that is available when and if needed. Withdrawal from the store in no way interferes with the function of the storage area or with the metabolic activity of the organism. Fat storage is the most obvious and increase or reduction in the quantity stored occurs only when the energy expenditure of the organism is not balanced with intake. Less obvious than fat storage but in most instances far more extensive is the storage in the liver of a well-nourished individual of vitamin A that may be large enough to last for a period of 1 to 2 years. Table 7.2 illustrates the extreme variation in the normal body content of some of the major and minor nutrients with the resulting extremes in survival time that range from 2 days to 20 years.

Reserves for a nutrient such as protein differ from stores in that they do not have a specific locus but are instead all protein tissue that can be reversibly depleted and repleted. The most labile reserves are in the liver and muscle and they will respond most rapidly to changes in nitrogen intake; but all body protein can contribute to the free amino acid pool of each cell. It has been estimated that 20 percent or more of body nitrogen can contribute to essential tissue structures and functions in prolonged stress (Allison et al., 1963). Such contributions, in contrast to those from storage areas, can impair the physiological function of the organism.

Data obtained from liver analyses have indicated that rapid loss in protein reserves is associated with a decrease in the cellular amino acid pool size and that the essential amino acid pool size is correlated with liver and muscle DNA. Fig. 7.4 shows Allison's data relating EAA and DNA for protein-fed animals, animals deprived of protein for three days, and animals starved for three days. These investigators have also shown that RNA of a tissue is closely correlated with protein synthesis and that tissue depletion is related both to a reduction in tissue protein and in the RNA-DNA ratio. The RNA-DNA ratio is believed to be correlated with both a de-

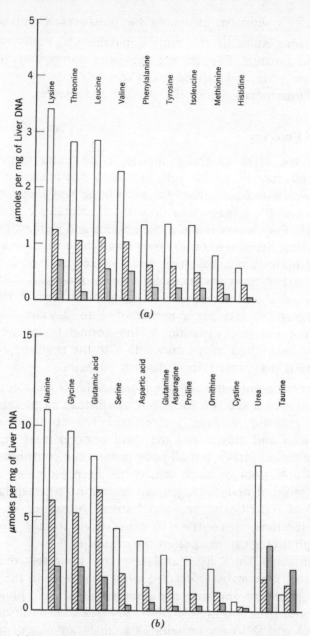

Fig. 7.4 (a) Free essential amino acids in μmoles/mg of liver DNA in rats fed 18 percent of casein (white bars); protein-free diet (slant bars), or starvation (gray bars) for three days. (b) Free nonessential amino acids in μmoles/mg of liver DNA in rats fed diets recorded in (a) for three days.

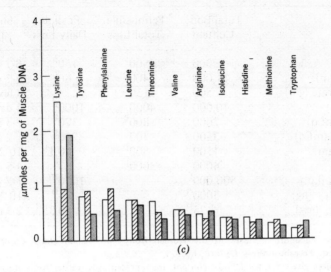

(c)

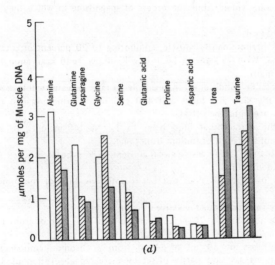

(d)

Fig. 7.4 (continued). (c) Free essential amino acids in μmoles/mg of muscle DNA in rats fed diets recorded in (a) for three days. (d) Free nonessential amino acids in μmoles/mg of muscle DNA in rats fed diets recorded in (a) for three days. [From J. B. Allison, *Fed. Proc.*, 22:1126 (1963).]

Table 7.2 NORMAL STORES OR RESERVES IN THE HUMAN BODY

	Total Body Content	Permissible Total Loss	Possible Daily Loss	Survival Time
Fat (gm)	9000	6500	150[a]	6-7 weeks
Protein (gm)	11,000	2400[b]	60[c]	6-7 weeks
Carbohydrate (gm)	500	150	–	a few hours
Water (gm)	40,000	4000	1000[d]	4 days
Sodium (mEq)	2600	800[e]	320[f]	2-3 days
Potassium (mEq)	3500	300	260[g]	1-2 days
Calcium (gm)	1500	500[h]	0.1[i]	10-20 years
Iron (mg)	4000	3000[j]	23[k]	4-5 months
Vitamin A (i.u.)	500,000[l]		1000[m]	1-2 years
Vitamin B_{12} (μg)	5000[n]		1[o]	10-20 years
Vitamin B_1 (mg)	25[p]		0.35[q]	2-3 months

From R. Passmore, "Stores in the Human Body" in *Human Body Composition*, J. Brozek, Ed., Pergamon Press, Oxford, 1965.

The figures given for total body content are representative values for a normal man living on a good diet. In many parts of the world, where the daily diet is unsatisfactory, the reserves will be much less. The figures for possible daily losses are such as might occur with dietary restrictions or in various diseases as explained in the notes. The figures for survival time may vary greatly, but the orders of magnitude in which they are given are correct.

[a] Equivalent to 1400 kcal.

[b] Wasting of tissue, predominantly muscle, amounting to 20 percent of total protein.

[c] Providing 240 kcal. With 150 gm of fat this will supply 1640 kcal, enough to meet the needs of a starving man.

[d] Under the best possible conditions a man unable to take in water will lose 800 grams by evaporation from the skin and lungs and 400 gm in the urine. Against this about 200 gm of metabolic water must be offset.

[e] A reduction of the extracellular fluid from 15 1. (Na 140 mEq/1.) to 13 1. (Na 123 mEq/1.) and a loss of 300 mEq of sodium from bone.

[f] Sweating at the rate of 4. 1./day with a sweat content of 80 mEq/1.

[g] Severe diarrhea and vomiting.

[h] Assuming clinical osteoporosis does not occur until one-third of the bone mineral is lost.

[i] A substantial figure for a continued negative calcium balance.

[j] A reduction in hemoglobin to 20 percent and a loss of 1 gm of iron, previously stored as ferritin.

[k] Assuming a daily loss of 50 ml of blood from a chronic hemorrhage plus a physiological loss of 1 mg/day and partly offset by increased absorption of 3 mg/day.

[l] A normal content of the liver for the people of the United Kingdom.

[m] A high estimate. Many adults in Southeast Asia live on diets providing much less and with no obvious evidence of vitamin A deficiency.

[n] Almost all in the liver.

[o] This amount of the vitamin will bring about a remission in most patients with pernicious anemia. The daily physiological requirement may be even less.

[p] Assuming about 0.5 μg/gm in skeletal muscle and 1.0 μg/gm in the principal viscera.

[q] Assuming a daily minimum need of 0.7 mg and diet of polished rice providing only 0.35 mg.

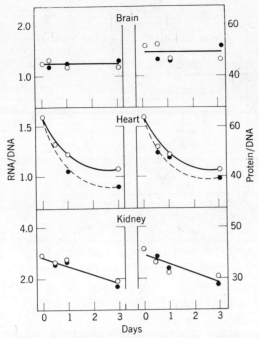

Fig. 7.5 Effect of protein-free diet (open circles) or starvation (closed circles) for various times on the RNA-DNA ratio and protein-DNA ratio of brain, heart, and kidney. [From J. B. Allison, *Fed. Proc.,* 22:1126 (1963).]

crease in the amino acid pool and with decreased protein biosynthesis. Some tissues, such as brain, which are resistant to depletion and do not contribute to the available reserves, do not show a change in the RNA-DNA ratio during protein-free feeding or during starvation, as do both heart and kidney (Fig. 7.5).

Control of Plasma Constituents

The relative constancy of plasma constituents indicates that the nutrients constantly being withdrawn are counterbalanced by like quantities being sent into the plasma. Variability of intake would make that source too precarious to depend on for any real control of supply. When absorption from the small intestine provides more than is required to compensate for current use, the remainder, depending on the nutrient, either is quickly withdrawn to become part of storage or reserves or, for those water-soluble nutrients that do not accumulate, is excreted by the kidney that acts as the regulatory

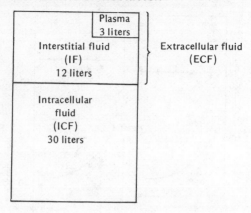

Fig. 7.6 Body fluid compartments.

organ controlling overflow. (Kidney threshholds will be discussed in the section on renal function.) If the quantity of a nutrient being absorbed is too small to compensate for uptake by the tissues, the deficit in plasma content is made up from storage or reserves for as long as these supplies are available.

The plasma, then, operates as a highly effective link between the cellular environment and the distant external environment through which all essentials for both cellular metabolism and its regulation are provided and by means of which all products of metabolism are removed. The moat between the cell and the plasma is the interstitial fluid that, together with the plasma, constitutes the 15 liters of extracellular fluid. Continuous and rapid adjustments made in the composition of a portion of the 3 liters of plasma can maintain the chemical composition of the remaining 12 liters of extracellular fluid (Fig. 7.6). (These changes will be discussed in the section on renal function.) The adjustments in the composition of extracellular fluid are counterpoised by the primary exchanges that take place between the 30 liters of intracellular fluid, the largest fluid compartment of the body, and the immediate external environment of the cell, interstitial fluid. These latter exchanges are considered primary since the very life of the cell depends on the successful exchange of nutrients and metabolites across the cellular membrane into and out of these two interdependent fluid media, intracellular and interstitial fluid. These relationships are illustrated in Fig. 7.7.

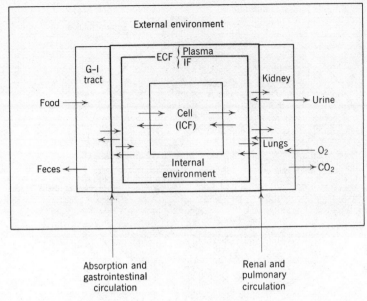

Fig. 7.7 Exchanges of nutrients and metabolites between body fluid compartments showing relationship of the external environment to the internal environment in a complex organism. ECF = extracellular fluid, IF = interstitial fluid, ICF = intracellular fluid.

Compartmentalization of Extracellular Fluids

Body fluid compartments as shown in Fig. 7.6 represent an overall and oversimplified view of volume relationships. It has become quite apparent that the extracellular fluid compartment that contains what is often called interstitial fluid is not a single compartment with a homogeneous fluid but, in all probability, a series of compartments and fluids that vary from tissue to tissue. Neuman (1969) states that the view of three fluid compartments, one plasma, one extracellular fluid, and one intracellular fluid is patently false. He suggests that every organ system may regulate the composition of its own fluid medium and gives as an example the differences observed between extracellular fluid in bone and other extracellular fluid. He suggests that this can be explained only in terms of compartmentalization by a functional membrane that regulates passage between general extracellular fluid and bone extracellular fluid. Similarly, Andersson (1971) discusses compartmentalization of the extra-

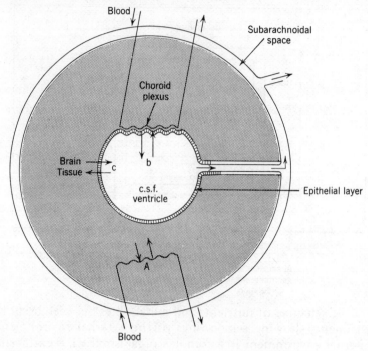

Fig. 7.8 Compartmentalization of extracellular fluid in the brain. (*a*) The blood-brain barrier. (*b*) The blood-cerebrospinal fluid (C.S.F.) barrier. (*c*) The cerebrospinal fluid-brain barrier. [From B. Andersson, *Amer. Sci.*, 59: 408-415 (1971).]

cellular fluids of the brain (Fig. 7.8). The capillaries in brain tissue appear less permeable to solutes and ions than other capillaries. For this reason direct transfer from the plasma to brain tissue is either prevented or delayed. This allows a more stable fluid environment to be maintained. Cerebrospinal fluid (CSF) is secreted by the cells of the choroid plexus and this fluid is different in ionic composition from plasma. The CSF is continuously transported through the ventricles, drained out into the blood in the sub-arachnoid space, but replaced by secretion. A barrier between CSF and brain ECF is created by the epithelial cell layer lining the walls of the brain ventricles thereby delaying exchange between these two fluids despite the fact that in most instances their ionic composition appears to be almost identical. However, Bito (1969) observed that the ECF of mammalian cerebral cortex had lower

K^+ ion and higher Mg^{2+} ion concentrations than were present in the plasma or even the CSF, and he postulated an active transport system across the blood-brain barrier. Because of the barrier to free exchange between plasma and the ECF of brain tissue by the interposition of the CSF compartment, a more stable cellular environment can be maintained. In this way, the brain is protected from variations in plasma composition that might be acceptable to other less discriminating tissues. This could be the explanation for the so-called blood-brain barrier that was postulated and generally accepted but never explained. Similar mechanisms of compartmentalization of ECF appear to be present in other tissues, for example, the humors of the eye and the synovial fluid of joints. An understanding of the controlled environmental conditions of various organs and tissues may yield the clues to better understanding of the way in which they function.

EXCHANGE

Mechanisms of Nutrient Exchange

The basic function of the circulatory system is to bring the blood close enough to each cell to permit rapid exchange of nutrients and removal of products of metabolism. The regulation of inter-compartmental exchange between the cell and its immediate environment involves both active and passive transfer and will be discussed in Chapter 9. Exchange between the plasma and interstitial fluid is a function of both the composition of the fluids and of the controls on blood flow through the capillary beds.

Ion Distribution. Since the protein concentration of the plasma is approximately 7.5 gm/100 ml and the protein concentration of interstitial fluid is only about 1.0 gm/100 ml and apparently due to leakage, an effect is exerted by the plasma protein on the free passage of water and all diffusable ions between the plasma and the interstitial fluid. The distribution occurs according to the *Gibbs-Donnan Equilibrium.* In such an equilibrium the permeating particles are influenced by simple passive forces, and the presence of the protein anion on one side of a membrane (within the capillary) that is permeable to all other ions, will cause the unequal distribution of diffusable ions on the two sides of the membrane. The ionic distribution must satisfy three requirements: (1) the sum of all the cations must equal the sum of all the anions on each side of the membrane; (2) on the side lacking protein, diffusable anions must be present in greater concentrations than on the side containing protein so that electroneutrality is maintained; and (3) osmotic pressure on the side containing protein must be balanced to prevent transfer of fluid and this is effected by the greater hydrostatic pressure in the capillary. The Gibbs-Donnan distribution, then, accounts for the higher concentration of diffusable ions inside the capillary than in interstitial fluid and also accounts for the higher osmotic pressure within the capillary (Fig. 7.9). It becomes apparent why disturbances in ionic distribution occur when plasma protein concentrations are reduced.

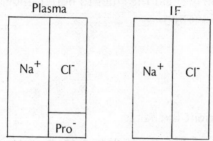

Fig. 7.9 Gibbs-Donnan distribution. Unequal concentration of Na^+ and Cl^- on the two sides of the capillary membrane due to the impermeability of the membrane to the protein anions and the consequently greater concentration of Na^+ in the plasma than in the IF.

Fluid Movement. The movement of fluid from the capillary lumen into the tissue space and back into the capillary was described be Starling (1896). His hypothesis suggested that the higher hydrostatic pressure at the arterial end of the capillary overcomes the osmotic pressure within the capillary due to plasma protein content and forces an ultrafiltrate containing neither particulate matter nor protein into the interstitial space. The hydrostatic pressure falls as the remaining fluid moves through the capillary. At the venous end the osmotic pressure is greater than the opposing hydrostatic pressure; thus the fluid is drawn back into the capillary lumen from the tissue space. The additional small force opposing filtration is

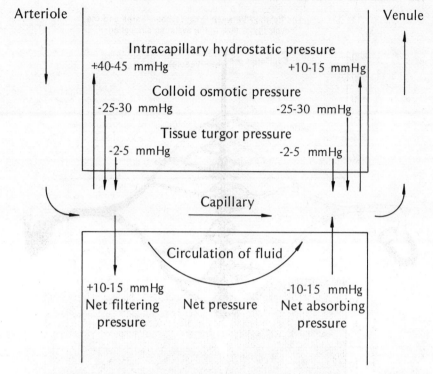

Fig. 7.10 Starling's hypothesis of fluid distribution between plasma and interstitial compartments. (Adapted from R. F. Pitts, *Physiology of the Kidney and Body Fluids,* 2nd ed., Year Book Medical Publishers, Chicago, 1968 p. 39.)

due to the fact that tissue fluid is under turgor pressure. A diagrammatic presentation of Starling's theory is presented in Fig. 7.10.

Starling's hypothesis was based on the assumption that protein molecules do not pass through the capillary walls. Although this theory provides a plausible and simplified scheme of fluid exchange between the blood and interstitial fluid, it appears to be only a partial explanation since some protein does, in fact, move from the lumen to the tissue space. In addition, the quantities of fluid that circulate in this way are far too small to provide for tissue needs. Pappenheimer (see Pitts, 1968, p. 39) calculated that the plasma contained in the capillaries of the forearm exchanges its water, sodium chloride, and glucose at rates of 300, 120, and 40 times per

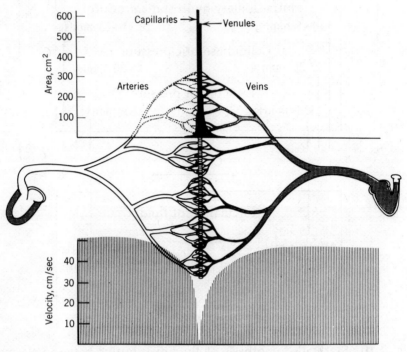

The Relation Between Cross-sectional area and the Velocity of flow in the systemic circulation

Fig. 7.11 At each successive branching of the arterial system, the cross-sectional area increases slightly. The terminal branches of the arterial system greatly increase the total cross-sectional area of the arterioles to some 125 times and capillaries about 600 times that of the aorta. The velocity of blood flow through the vessels diminishes as the cross-sectional area increases. (From R. F. Rushmer, *Cardiovascular Dynamics,* 2nd ed. W. B. Saunders Co., Phila., 1961, p. 5.)

minute, respectively. An alternative to Starling's hypothesis is that all materials in the plasma are exchanged across the capillary wall by diffusion. Since temporary stasis is likely to occur in all capillaries, this would allow all plasma constituents, including protein, to approach diffusion equilibrium. The protein molecules are believed to pass through the walls of the capillary into tissue space by a sieving action. This protein, however, cannot be returned to the capillary. Instead, it enters the terminal lymphatics and, through the lymph ducts, eventually is returned to the blood when the thoracic duct empties into the subclavian vein (see Mayerson, 1963).

Although pressure relationships between capillary and tissue fluid may account for some exchange, a more realistic description of the mechanisms by which the nutrients in the circulatory system are brought close enough to each cell to permit rapid exchange involve branching and local control exerted in the capillary bed. The major vessels in the arterial system branch into smaller and smaller arteries, arterioles, and finally into the extremely large number of capillaries in close association with the individual cells. Since the same volume of blood per minute carried by the aorta under pressure is diverted through capillaries that have 500 to 600 times the cross-sectional area, there is a drastic reduction of pressure and a corresponding reduction in rate of flow when the blood reaches the capillary bed (Fig. 7.11). It is the flow through the capillary bed, or the microcirculation, that is the most important function of the cardiovascular system. Indeed, the primary purpose of the heart and major vessels is to maintain flow through the capillary bed and thereby provide an effective environment for the individual cells. The control of flow through the network of approximately 60,000 miles of capillaries as described by Zweifach (1959) has two specialized components: a thoroughfare channel into which blood flows from the arteriole; and the true capillaries, which form a secondary network connected to the thoroughfare channel. Control of flow is exercised by precapillary sphincters along the channel which open and close periodically, permitting flow through different parts of the microsystem. Closing of the precapillary sphincters restricts blood flow to the thoroughfare channel in what could be considered a short cut to the venous system (Fig. 7.12). The basic characteristics are the same in all tissues: a thoroughfare channel whose muscle cells, though sparsely distributed, control the rate of flow into a secondary network of true capillaries where flow is controlled by precapillary sphincters. So widely spaced are the muscle cells along the thoroughfare channels that they are almost indistinguishable from the true capillaries. The structure or complexity of the network depends on the needs of the tissue. Tissues with changing metabolic needs, such as striated muscle, have a large number of small channels that, when opened, can supply the greatly increased needs of the cells during activity. Secretory cells, with more modest demands, may have few true capillary branches from

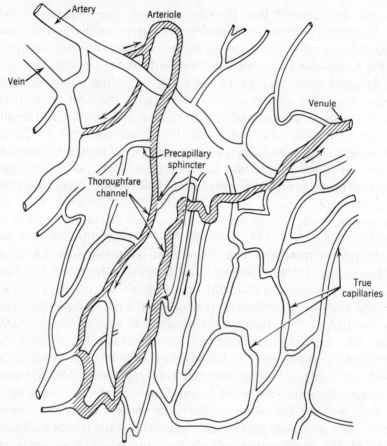

Fig. 7.12 Schematized tracing of capillary bed indicating terminology for different structural components. The preferential pathway for the microcirculation is shaded. Also indicated is a direct anastomosis between a small artery and its adjacent vein. (From B. W. Zweifach, *Functional Behavior of Microcirculation*, Charles C. Thomas, Springfield, Ill., 1961.)

the thoroughfare channels. The dependence of the rapidly metabolizing cell on a correspondingly rapid exchange of nutrients is illustrated by the effects of interruption of blood flow to the brain, which can lead to unconsciousness in about seven seconds.

The control of the muscle cells in the capillary bed is not clear although there are many leads that may eventually be incorporated into a model. There is no obvious or direct innervation that would indicate control through the nervous system. There is, however, direct contact between the sparsely distributed muscle cells and the environment of the tissues they supply and with the metabolic products of the cells comprising that tissue. In addition, the capillary bed exhibits extreme sensitivity to chemical stimuli. These facts suggested to Zweifach (1961) that control might well be maintained jointly by hormonal factors and specific products of tissue metabolism, and he mentioned norepinephrine as a possible candidate for the role of maintaining tone in the microcirculation. The effects of norepinephrine mediated through the action of cAMP have been shown in a variety of tissues (Sutherland, 1972). Triner et al. (1971) have reported that increased formation of cAMP is associated with decreased contractility of vascular smooth muscle; conversely, decreased cAMP leads to increased contractility. The intimate relationship of the capillary muscle cells to the plasma and interstitial fluid of the tissue supplied by the capillary suggests that increased blood flow through the capillary bed may be in response to some factor in cellular metabolism. As either a direct or indirect result, increased adenyl cyclase and cAMP decrease the contractility or tonus of the thoroughfare channel. Cheung (1972) suggests that the action of cAMP might be explained on the basis of a versatile allosteric effector and that the different effects of cAMP could be explained by the kinds of protein with which it interacts. He also indicates how cAMP might act as a unidirectional "off" switch for the effective termination of the action of hormones. If so, the norepinephrine effect might be involved. It almost seems as though the available threads of information about the control of microcirculation involving norepinephrine, cAMP, and the distinctive location of the effector site are just waiting to be woven into whole cloth.

If proper fluid and ionic exchanges occur between the plasma and interstitial fluid, the cell has placed in its immediate environment the nutrients essential for its metabolism. Transfer of a nutrient from interstitial fluid to the cell reduces its concentration in the interstitial fluid and thereby permits more to diffuse from the plasma to the tissue space. Passage of a product of metabolism from the cell into interstitial fluid increases the concentration of that substance in interstitial fluid and causes it to diffuse into the plasma.

The maintenance of cellular function therefore becomes dependent upon the ability of the organism to adjust the plasma concentrations of both essential cellular nutrients and cellular wastes in order to maintain in the cells' immediate environment the proper assortment and concentration of nutrients and to insure removal of the products liberated as a result of metabolism. It is by means of continual adjustment of the plasma passing through the kidneys and lungs that this occurs. (For a more detailed discussion of the dynamics of fluid exchange, see Robinson, 1960).

Renal Control of Plasma Constituents

The kidney provides the chief means whereby the chemical homeostasis of all body fluid is maintained. Each minute approximately 1 liter of blood or 20 percent of the cardiac output courses through the renal circulation. Of this liter, 120 ml/min of ultrafiltrate pass through the glomeruli and into the tubules, which together constitute over 1 million nephrons in each human kidney. This provides a total filtration surface estimated to be well over 1 square meter. If the 120 ml/min of ultrafiltrate escaped into the urine, the extracellular spaces would be drained of everything but protein in 25 minutes, a rapid road to desiccation. Or, if the organism were obliged to replace this catastrophic loss, it would require approximately 173 liters of fluid per day plus adequate quantities of all of the solutes which the filtrate contains: glucose, vitamins, amino acids, electrolytes, hormones, and so forth. Normal kidney function averts the need for such imbibing. Of the original 120 ml/min, only 1 ml/min appears in the bladder as urine, or approximately 1.5 liters per day. It is during the passage through the nephron that the volume and composition of the filtrate are altered, water and essential solutes are returned to the circulation, and end products of metabolism and dietary surplus (exclusive of the calorie-yielding variety) become urinary constituents. It is of more than passing interest that the enormous filtration job performed by the glomeruli requires no energy on the part of the kidney since the requisite energy is imparted by the pressure of the blood entering the glomeruli. However, work is performed in the active reabsorption of the filtrate constituents through the tubular cells for their return to the circulation. The kidneys' job classified on this and other bases is one of conservation and regulation rather than excretion.

The quantitative aspects of the conservation of body water and electrolytes are illustrated in Table 7.3. For details of nephron function the student is referred to Pitts (1968) or Bland (1963).

Table 7.3 ELECTROLYTE AND WATER CONSERVATION: COMPARISON OF LEVELS IN PLASMA, 24-HOUR FILTRATE, AND URINE[a]

Substance	Plasma mEq/liter	Filtered mEq/24 hr	Excreted mEq/liter	Reabsorbed mEq/24 hr	Percent
Sodium	140	25,200	101	25,099	99.6
Chloride	105	18,540	110	18,430	99.4
Potassium	5	900	47	833	92.6
Bicarbonate	27	4860	2	4858	99.9+
Phosphate	2	360	34	326	95[b]
Sulfate	1	180	54	126	70[b]
Water	940 ml/liter	169,200 ml	1200 ml	168,000 ml	99.3

[a]Based on filtration of 180 liters/24 hr.
[b]Varies.

Water Balance. Water is freely diffusable between the intra- and extracellular fluid compartments but cell membranes act as though they are relatively impermeable to Na^+ ions. This, then, makes the relation between the two compartments dependent upon the Na^+ ion concentration in the extracellular fluid that, along with total water content, is maintained within rather narrow limits in the adult mammal. Deviation from the normal distribution stimulates restoration of normal water content through thirst or adjustment in the secretion of antidiuretic hormone (ADH) from the posterior pituitary and through restoration of Na^+ ions mediated by angiotensin and aldosterone. The overall operation of these compensatory mechanisms in adjusting body fluid distribution and composition during negative and positive water and Na^+ ion balances is shown in Fig. 7.13.

The role of the kidney in maintaining the volume and tonicity of the extracellular fluid is accomplished by the coordination of neural and hormonal stimuli with the reabsorptive capacity of the kidney tubules. One model includes the concept of "osmoreceptors" in the brain and was postulated by Verney (1947). He suggested that stimulus to ADH secretion resulted from change in composition

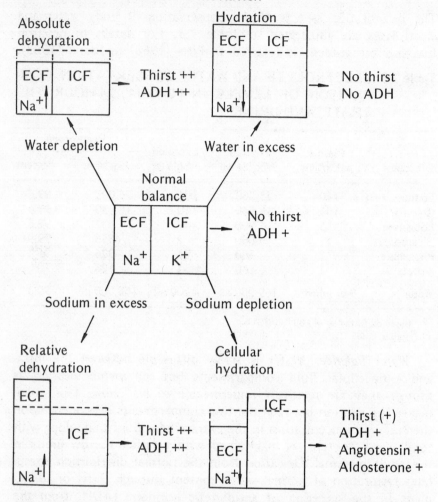

Fig. 7.13 Diagrams of changes in body fluid distribution and composition during negative and positive water and salt balances. ECF, extracellular fluid compartment; ICF, intracellular fluid compartment; ADH, antidiuretic hormone. [From B. Andersson, *Amer. Sci.*, 59: 408 (1971).]

of the ECF leading to cellular dehydration and reduction in volume of the osmoreceptors. It was surmised that both the release of ADH and stimulation of thirst were regulated by the same or similar mechanisms. A later suggestion (Jewel and Verney, 1957) was that the increased tonicity of the blood stimulated osmoreceptors in the hypothalamus and led to both ADH secretion and thirst.

Work in other laboratories indicated that response to tonicity and volume were not the full answer. Stimulation of the renin-angiotensin system was shown to lead to secretion of aldosterone from the adrenal cortex with the consequent increase in Na^+ ion reabsorption by the kidney tubule (Davis, 1971). Fitzsimons (1969) demonstrated that stimulation of the renin-angiotensin system also stimulated the thirst mechanism, and that injection of angio-tensin into the blood produced drinking in the rat (Fitzsimons and Simons, 1969; Epstein et al., 1969). Fitzsimons (1969) suggested therefore that angiotensin either stimulated the brain directly or increased the sensitivity of the receptors in the brain. When Bonjour and Malvin (1970) showed that angiotensin stimulated the release of ADH it was concluded that ECF volume was maintained not only by the effects of the renin-angiotensin system on renal reabsorption of Na^+ ions but also by its effect on ADH secretion and thirst stimulation.

According to Andersson (1971) the central effects of angiotensin seem to be highly dependent upon the Na^+ ion concentration of the cerebrospinal fluid or the brain ECF, rather than changes in cell volume due to osmotic effect. Support for this concept was obtained by Andersson et al. (1967; 1969) who infused hypertonic sodium salts into the third ventricle of the brain and elicited drinking in goats in normal water balance and caused ADH release in hydrated animals. That this was probably due to Na^+ ions and not to osmotic factors was evident when the same effect could not be produced by sugar solutions (Andersson et al., 1967). However, the effect was obtained by infusion of angiotensin, or angiotensin and NaCl (Andersson et al., 1970; Andersson and Westbye, 1970). These authors conclude that Na^+ ion concentration mediates the effect of angiotensin in stimulating the thirst-regulating mechanism and ADH release. The specific manner in which this occurs is not clear, but Andersson (1971) suggests that (1) angiotensin might facilitate transport of Na^+ ions in the immediate environment of receptor cells; (2) angiotensin might increase the sensitivity of receptors to Na^+ ions in the brain ECF; or (3) angiotensin might facilitate passage of Na^+ ions into receptor cells. Which, if any, of these postulates is valid awaits further investigation. Orloff and Handler (1967) have suggested that the mediator of ADH action is cAMP since it was shown to reproduce the effects of ADH in toad bladder.

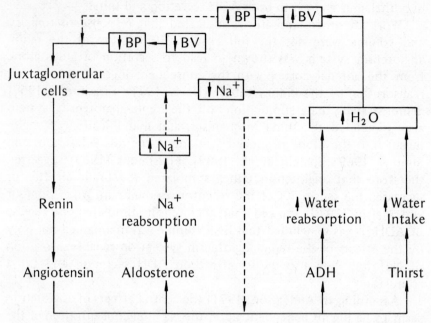

Fig. 7.14 A model of the relationship of angiotensin to regulation of Na^+ and water balance.

A model suggesting how normal water and Na^+ ion relationships are maintained is presented in Fig. 7.14.

Nutrient Conservation. Under normal circumstances all of the nutrients in the filtrate are returned to the plasma by the tubular cell, but the quantity returned varies with both the nutrient and the plasma level. Nutrients that are maintained in the plasma by dynamic regulatory mechanisms such as glucose, amino acids, and sodium have high renal threshholds and are returned completely; whereas those nutrients for which plasma concentrations are a reflection of dietary intake, such as the water-soluble vitamins, have low renal threshholds. For example, plasma levels of water-soluble vitamins reach a maximum point as dietary intake is increased, and any further loading is reflected in markedly increased urinary excretion. Whether this is because of the inability of tissues to store these vitamins or to the inability of the kidney to reabsorb them is an interesting question (see Chapter 15).

The conservation of nutrients by the renal tubule is accomplished primarily by active transport, but water, chloride, and urea are reabsorbed passively. Competition may exist for both transport energy and shared carriers. Glucose, for example, shares a carrier with xylose, fructose, and galactose. Since glucose has the highest affinity for the carrier, its reabsorption takes preference. If the quantity of glucose presented for reabsorption greatly exceeds the carrier capacity or renal threshhold, as it does in uncontrolled diabetes, the excess glucose will appear in the urine.

The amino acids in the plasma and in the tubular filtrate are in dynamic equilibrium with the amino acids in all cells including those of the tubule and thereby constitute a portion of the amino acid pool of the body. Under normal circumstances only negligible amounts of amino acids are likely to appear in the urine since their threshhold is sufficiently high to insure almost complete reabsorption. It is not certain how many different transport mechanisms there are for the amino acids, but it appears that one is responsible for reabsorbing glutamic and aspartic acids; one for lysine, arginine, ornithine, cystine, and possibly histidine; and probably one or more for the other amino acids (Webber et al., 1961). The tubular cells, however, are concerned with more than conservation and transport of amino acids; they are active in transamination, deamination, and urea and ammonia formation.

Nitrogen Excretion. In the process of metabolism the disposal of any carbon, hydrogen, or oxygen as carbon dioxide or water is no problem; nitrogen, however, requires the formation of ammonia, uric acid, or urea. An organism's position on the evolutionary ladder and its habitat give a fair indication of its mode of nitrogen excretion. The toxicity of ammonia makes it a suitable excretory product only for marine animals who have no trouble diluting it and losing it in a watery environment. To embryos that develop within hard shells ammonia would be lethal; these organisms excrete uric acid, which is quite insoluble and therefore harmless. This change during evolution appears to have been an adaptation to land life. Although mammals excrete some uric acid, the major means of eliminating nitrogen is by the formation of urea which has the virtue of being nontoxic and soluble. The formation of urea will be described in Chapter 15. Its presence in the plasma and therefore in the tubular filtrate is directly related to the quantity of protein consumed and the rate of protein catabolism. Tubular reabsorption of urea is passive and closely proportional to the amounts filtered; approximately 60 percent remains in the tubule to be excreted in the urine. The level of urea in the plasma is dependent, then, not only upon its rate of synthesis but also upon the ability of the kidney to excrete a suitable proportion of the quantity presented to it.

One product of metabolism present in the tubular filtrate and rejected completely by the tubular cells for reabsorption is creatinine, the end product of creatine metabolism. The amount of creatinine appearing in the 24-hour urine of a given individual remains remarkably constant and will identify a cheating or forgetful research subject every time!

The renal functions that have been discussed are regulatory in the sense that they operate to adjust and maintain the chemical composition of the plasma and thereby the chemical composition of the extracellular environment in the entire organism. In this sense, the excretory functions of the kidney are also regulatory in that they insure the removal from the body fluids of molecules present in excess of the body's need or beyond its capacity to manage. A prerequisite for renal disposal of such a plethora is, of course, its presence in the glomerular ultrafiltrate. This prerequisite explains the inability to excrete iron or lipids in the urine. Since iron is present in the plasma as transferrin and lipids as lipoproteins, they, along with all other plasma proteins, never get through to the renal tubule.

Regulation of Plasma pH. Related to the renal control of water balance and nutrient conservation, is the control of blood pH and, thereby, the pH of all body fluids. The maintenance of near neutrality of the blood is accomplished by the buffering systems of the blood itself, by respiratory exchange in the lungs involving regulation of carbonic acid, and by regulation of the bicarbonate ion by the kidney tubules. Only the renal control will be discussed here.

The kidney can increase or decrease blood pH by stabilizing the bicarbonate level of the plasma. This involves almost complete reabsorption of the quantities normally filtered. If an excess of bicarbonate gains entrance to the body, its excretion will be controlled by the tubules. Depletion of bicarbonate reserves is arrested by excretion of titratable acid and ammonia. In the formation of titratable acid, hydrogen ions are exchanged for sodium; in the formation of ammonia, the amino group from the deamination of

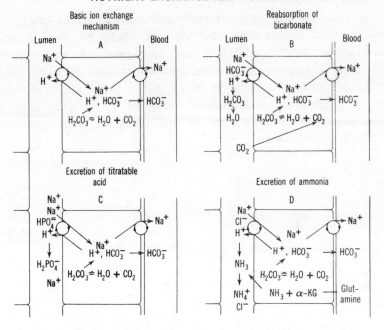

Fig. 7.15 Role of the exchange of cellular H^+ ions for Na^+ ions of tubular fluid in the reabsorption of bicarbonate and in the urinary excretion of titratable acid and ammonia. [From R. F. Pitts, *Physiology of the Kidney and Body Fluids*, p. 210.]

amino acids or deamidation of glutamine diffuses into the tubule and is trapped as the ammonium ion. The operation of this ion exchange is illustrated in Fig. 7.15. (For a more complete discussion see Pitts, 1968.)

CODA

The complex of processes by which food is digested and its constituent nutrients enter the body and reach the locus for metabolic activity is dependent upon the coordinated and synchronized activities of the total organism. Just as in music it is the integration of the composer's score, the musician's skill, and the conductor's interpretation that expresses in totality what no one of them could convey alone, so, too, is understanding and appreciation of the physiological aspects of nutrition (which only to some may be more mundane than a symphony) an exquisite blend of written description of fact, skillful interpretation, and knowledgeable integration. Pathways and mechanisms are not just roadmaps; they must be linked, combined, coordinated, and developed into the metabolic scheme. By seeing individual roles, meaning is imparted to the whole; but the symphony, too, is far more than a sequence of individual themes. Breakdown and analysis followed by interpretation and resynthesis serve equally well in understanding and appreciating symphonies and science.

part three
the cell

Chapter 8   Orientation to Cellular Nutrition
Chapter 9   The Plasma Membrane
Chapter 10   The Nucleus
Chapter 11   The Cytoplasmic Matrix and Endoplasmic Reticulum
Chapter 12   The Golgi Apparatus
Chapter 13   The Mitochondria
Chapter 14   The Lysosomes and Microbodies

Cells are highly individual. There are infinite variations not only in unicellular life, but in the variety of cells that make up complex organisms. However, all cells have certain structural constituents in common; and since these constituents are orderly, interrelated arrangements of macromolecules, and the macromolecules have various constituent molecules in common, these points of likeness have given rise to the concept of the *typical cell.* The typical cell, like the so-called average man, is an image arrived at by extrapolation, a statistical creation that does not actually exist. Nevertheless, it is a convenient point of departure and, if accepted n that sense, provides the Utopian norm; visionary, nonexistent, ınd impossibly ideal.

chapter 8
orientation to cellular nutrition

1. Rationale
2. Historical Aspects
3. Instruments and Techniques
   a. Microscopy
      1. Light Microscopy
      2. Electron Microscopy
      3. Scanning Electron Microscopy
      4. Freeze-Etch Electron Microscopy
      5. Phase-Contrast Microscopy
      6. Radioautography
      7. Low Temperature Ultramicroincineration
   b. Biochemical and Physical Methods
      1. Differential Ultracentrifugation
      2. X-Ray Diffraction
   c. Tissue Culture
   d. Summary
4. Problems Inherent in Studying Cells
5. Rewards Resulting from Studying Cells
6. Geography of the Cell

"...Exploration (of cells) used to be dominated by the micro-scopic study of fixed and stained tissue specimens. Cells were dis-tinguished by the visual appearance of their embalmed mummies, which contributed neither less nor more to the understanding of the living cell than does the study of the ruins of an ancient city tell of the life of its people. Life is process in time. No static image can reflect that time dimension. Microscopic anatomy thus tended to freeze our concepts of the cell: the cell's incessant variation in response to a continuously changing environment escaped attention. Knowledge was hemmed in by limitations of technique. In order to enlarge the scope and content of our knowledge, we must rely on the technical advances."

Paul A. Weiss, "A Cell Is Not an Island Entire of Itself,"
Perspect. Biol. Med., 14: 182-205 (1971)

"Thus the things of our world are simple or complex, according to the techniques that we select for studying them. In fact, func-tional simplicity always corresponds to a complex substratum. This is a primary datum of observation, which must be accepted just as it is."

Alexis Carrel, *Man the Unknown*, 1935, p. 104

RATIONALE

Understanding biological activity depends on an understanding of the fundamental unit of activity: the cell. According to Ham (1969), "a cell is the smallest organized unit of living material capable of existing independently in a suitable nonliving environment, replacing its own substance as necessary by synthesizing new components from nutritives absorbed from its environment." It becomes apparent that proper nutrition is a primary requisite for the existence of the cell. The nutrients are the source of the cell's energy and of the materials for its syntheses. Without suitable nutrient supplies the cell cannot exist.

To understand this fundamental biological unit, its structural composition and molecular organization must be related to its functions. Operations within any of its subunits are related to the operation of the unit as a whole, to other units with which it is associated and, in a coordinated complex of cells, to the total organism and the environment in which it exists. The cell can be viewed from the outside looking in or from the inside looking out; but any attempt to extrapolate what might occur at one level of operation from observations at another level can be hazardous. The behavior of a molecule in solution in a test tube is not the same as its operation in an intact organism; but the *in vitro* behavior can give important information on how it *might* behave *in vivo*. Similarly, organelles in isolation do not operate as they do in cells; however, observations of both structure and function can give insight into their likely activities when they are subjected to the interrelated and coordinated functions of other organelles within the cell. Nor do cells in culture function as they do in an intact organism where they are subjected to the influence of other cells and organs; but cell cultures give some indication of specific capabilities and attributes of the constituent cells.

HISTORICAL ASPECTS

All the spectacular advances of today are completely dependent upon and inseparable from the advances made all through the long history of science. The hesitating steps and wrong turns, as well as the great leaps, have added to our scientific knowledge. Today's hindsight can thoughtlessly tarnish or spoil the brilliance of yesterday's foresight, but without the discoveries of all of the yesterdays, today's world, its aspirations and dreams, its science and technology would not exist. We could not be studying cell organelles had not the powerful electron microscope been developed; nor cells without the light microscope; nor microscopes if Galileo and those before him had not been interested in lenses; nor lenses had not the ancient Egyptians discovered how to make glass. To paraphrase Macbeth, all our yesterdays have lighted men the way to the scientific creativity of today.

An unknown and miniature world came into view with the construction of the first compound microscope by Zacharias Janssen in 1590. In 1665 Robert Hooke, observing cork through a microscope, used the word cell for the first time as a biologically descriptive term. He described cork as a tissue which was made up of "little boxes or cells." This may have been an accurate description for cork tissue as Hooke observed it, but this word, carried over from the descriptions of the seventeenth-century botanists, came into use to designate the ultimate particle of living matter. For the seventeenth century, this *was* the ultimate unit of structure; nothing smaller could be seen or, perhaps, imagined. It was during that century, too, that the atom was described as a body so small as to be incapable of further division, and it was assumed to be the ultimate particle in which matter existed. For both the cell and the atom, technology eventually provided the means for going beyond what was thought then to be ultimate. Ferreting out and understanding the substructure within the cell is the biological counterpart of the physical study of atomic particles.

INSTRUMENTS AND TECHNIQUES

The sophisticated methods employed in studying cellular morphology and physiology are the direct outgrowth of an increasingly sophisticated technology. Advances in biological probing, like advances in atomic or cosmic probing, have been closely tied to progress in optics, electronics, and engineering. Many similar laboratory instruments are employed today in studying the nutrition of the cell, the composition of moon rocks, and the identity of atmospheric pollutants. The hands and senses of the nutritional scientist are probably limited more often by his own vision than by the availability of instrumental means. The acceleration of analytical work, recording, and calculating are the combined contributions of automation and computer science.

Microscopy

Twenty years after Hooke's observations on cork, Anton van

Leeuwenhoek ground and polished high power lenses that enabled him to see objects 100 times smaller than could be observed by the naked eye. He was the first to observe the existence of unicellular life. Today's *light microscopes* can magnify 1000 times or more and permit observation of some cellular detail.

Electron Microscopy. More specific knowledge of cell structure and the structure of organelles within the cell is the result of the development of the *electron microscope* by Knoll and Ruska in 1933. This instrument, which became available for general research about 1940, permits magnifications of 150,000 to 300,000 times and greater, revealing intimate details of cell structure. Electron microscopy has permitted visualization of cellular structures down to molecular dimensions. It has revealed that macromolecules are arranged in strict and orderly patterns and constitute the substructures or organelles of the cell.

The transparence of tissues in visible light makes it necessary to utilize techniques to increase contrast. For light microscopy, biological stains that react with specific molecules in the cell are used. In electron microscopy, heavy atoms such as lead and osmium form dense derivative compounds with cellular material and, in effect, are electron stains. The use of any foreign material reacting with the molecular material of the cell can, and does, produce artifacts. Cytologists suggest that some of the details clearly observed in electron microscopy may, in fact, be the result of such interactions between the molecular components of the cell and the heavy atoms rather than actual details of cell structure.

Scanning Electron Microscopy. The scanning electron microscope uses secondary electrons produced by the scanning beam to give a life-like, almost three-dimensional image of the surface of the specimen being scanned. The magnification can be from 10 to 100,000 times or more which means that it overlaps the hand lens, the light microscope and the electron microscope. In addition to the wide range of magnification, it also extends the range and quality of the electron micrograph. The image is not only larger than life, but it seems twice as real. The scanning electron microscope permits in depth visualization of microfeatures, a topological picture, giving actual spatial relationships (see Fig. 20.1).

Freeze-Etch Electron Microscopy. This permits study of membranes and organelles from unfixed cells. Tissue is frozen in liquid nitrogen and then fractured under vacuum along natural cleavage planes with a sharp blade. The splintered preparation is etched by sublimation. Platinum and carbon are deposited along the fracture surface. This replica is then mounted for electron microscope study. It is believed that electron micrographs prepared in this way give images of cell structures that closely approximate the normal condition since no chemical fixatives and dehydrating agents are used. Due to the etching and shadowing the view is somewhat three dimensional (Fig. 8.1).

Phase-Contrast Microscopy. Development of special optical techniques has permitted the study of living cells. Use of *phase contrast* and *interference microscopy* are based on the fact that biological structures, which are highly transparent to visible light, can cause phase changes in transmitted radiations. These result from small differences in the refractive index and thickness of different parts of the structure. Phase microscopy has permitted study of living cells using time-lapse motion pictures to record cell division, phagocytosis, formation of membranes, and other structure-related processes of living. Interference microscopy, based on the same principles as phase microscopy can, in addition, give quantitative data; for example, simultaneous determination of the thickness of an object, concentration of dry matter, and water content.

Radioautography. A radioactive label incorporated into metabolizing tissue can be detected after the tissue is fixed and prepared for microscopy since the radioactive products in the section emit electrons that affect photographic emulsions. The prepared slides are permitted to develop in a light-proof box for a period of time during which each minute amount of isotope is a source of radiation hitting the photographic emulsion. After a suitable period of time, the preparations are developed just as photographic negatives are developed. In the developed radioautographic preparation areas of radiation in the tissue below show as black dots indicating where the administered isotope was incorporated into the cell. Isotopic labels attached to specific molecules used in cellular syntheses can be traced into final products through radioautography. Through the use of suitable techniques, tissue can be prepared for study by either light or electron microscopy.

Low Temperature Ultramicroincineration. A technique of chemical incineration at the electron microscope level, this process per-

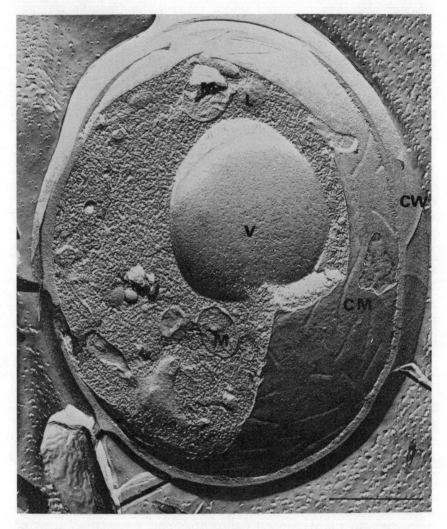

Fig. 8.1 Freeze-etch electron micrograph of yeast cell, *Saccharomyces cerevisiae*, showing cell wall (CW) and cell membrane (CM), mitochondria (M), lipid granule (L) and large cytoplasmic vacuole (V). Marker bar = 1µ. Shadow direction from bottom to top. Magnification 32,500. (Courtesy of Thomas E. Rucinsky).

mits visualization of metallic substances within cells. Organic matter is selectively removed with a stream of very reactive, excited oxygen. The remaining ash represents the mineral/metallic ultrastructure of cells (Hohman and Schraer, 1972). This technique holds promise for localizing and identifying minerals within the cell.

Biochemical and Physical Methods

Whereas structural patterns can be observed visually, the function of the organelles and of their constituent chemical components is dependent upon the development and use of other instruments and techniques. Svedberg's interest in colloids led him to develop the first centrifuge to give quantitative data on sedimentation rates. This instrument, developed in 1924, whirled at 10,000 rpm and produced a centrifugal force 5000 times gravity. Ultracentrifuges are now obtainable that spin at 60,000 rpm. The ultracentrifuge permitted the estimation of molecular weights and confirmed the existence of giant molecules.

Differential Ultracentrifugation. This permits biochemical study of organelles and of their functional attributes. Cells placed in a suitable medium, usually sucrose, are disrupted mechanically or sonically, and the homogenate is subjected to successive centrifugations (Fig. 8.2). The size, density, and shape of the particles determine their movement in the centrifugal field, and this forms the basis for differential ultracentrifugation. At a given force, large, heavy, and dense structures sediment most rapidly and, with increasing force, successive fractions are obtained. Some organelles, nuclei, and mitochondria, for example, come down essentially intact; however, the fraction designated as the microsomes is composed mostly of fragmented bits of endoplasmic reticulum and plasma membrane. There are, of course, no organelles called microsomes. Isolated cell fractions can be subjected to full biochemical and physical analyses.

Various refinements in technique and use of the analytical ultracentrifuge permit further separation of materials into macromolecular layers. In this way, the relationship of the structural units, or organelles, of the cell can be related to molecular constituents and to function.

X-Ray Diffraction. This technique has wide application in the study of the configuration of molecules. Collimated X-rays traverse the material to be analyzed, and the diffraction pattern is recorded on a photographic plate. Through a complex mathematical process a three-dimensional representation of the object can be constructed.

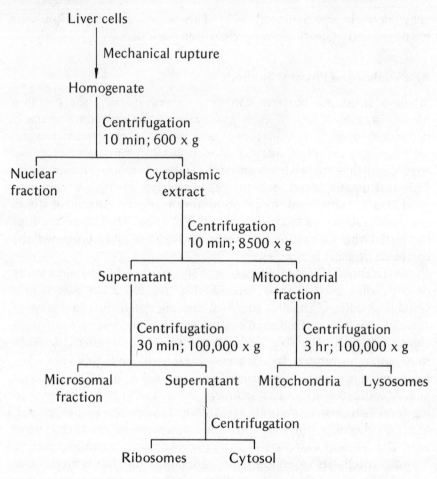

Fig. 8.2 Differential ultracentrifugation.

Tissue Culture

Tissue culture techniques permit the study of living cells grown in a suitable medium that contains the nutrients and oxygen essential for growth. Nutritional requirements of specific cells and organs can be studied under a variety of experimental conditions. Tissues in culture will grow and divide behaving to some degree as they do in the total organism. They are of value also in studying particular attributes of cell membranes in a living cell through the use of phase microscopy.

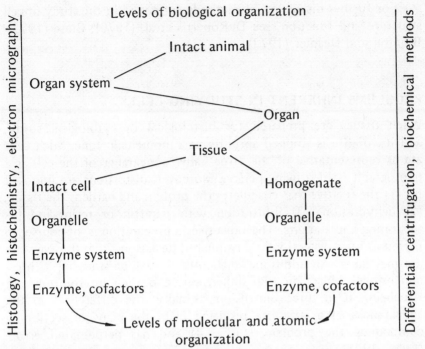

Fig. 8.3 Levels of biological organization. Morphological and biochemical studies of the cell complement each other, and events at any level may be involved in observations at any other level. (Adapted from J. Tepperman, *Metabolic and Endocrine Physiology*, 2nd ed., Year Book Medical Publishers, Chicago, Ill., 1968.)

Synthetic media have also been developed for organ culture permitting the study of growing bone and endocrine glands under a variety of experimental conditions.

Summary

Neither biochemical nor morphological studies of cells tell the full story, but they complement each other in providing an understanding of relationships of structure to function and in suggesting mechanisms of operation within the living cell. Furthermore, knowledge of the living cell suggests mechanisms of operation and understanding of relationships existing in the total organism. The complementary effects of various avenues of study at any level of biological organization is illustrated in Fig. 8.3.

For further discussion of methods employed in the study of cell structure and function, see DeRobertis et al. (1970); Giese (1973); Branton and Deamer (1972).

PROBLEMS INHERENT IN STUDYING CELLS

When tissues are prepared for histological or cytological study, activity or life is stopped abruptly at a moment in time. Such cells are as representative of the "true" alive appearance of the cell as a photograph is of a living person. Moreover, distortions are imposed by (1) the fixative that coagulates the protein and hardens the tissue; (2) dehydration; (3) infiltration with paraffin or resin; and (4) sectioning and staining. The objective in preparation is, of course, to permit as little distortion as possible but deviations from the live state are inevitable. An additional difficulty is that of studying a three-dimensional object in two dimensions and then interpreting and visualizing it in three dimensions. Finally, the differences in the appearances of a structure resulting from the plane of sectioning compounds the problem (Fig. 8.4) and has perpetuated errors (Elias, 1971).

Preparative methods for biochemical studies of cellular organelles involve procedures as drastic as those in microscopy. Maceration of the tissues prior to centrifugation permits loss of soluble enzymes and enzyme systems from specific loci in the cell to the cytosol. Fractions that contain only one organelle are extremely difficult to obtain and must be checked by electron microscopy. The cytosol which contains what is referred to as the soluble fraction has in it enzymes and enzyme systems that were originally in, but pulled from, organelle fractions.

REWARDS RESULTING FROM STUDYING CELLS

The instruments and methods developed during the last decade or so have provided the means for the essential communication between cytologist and biochemist. Previously the cytologist was restricted to studying static images of the living cell through fixed and stained preparations, and the biochemist was limited to studying composition and chemical activity in disrupted cell fragments. The cytologist

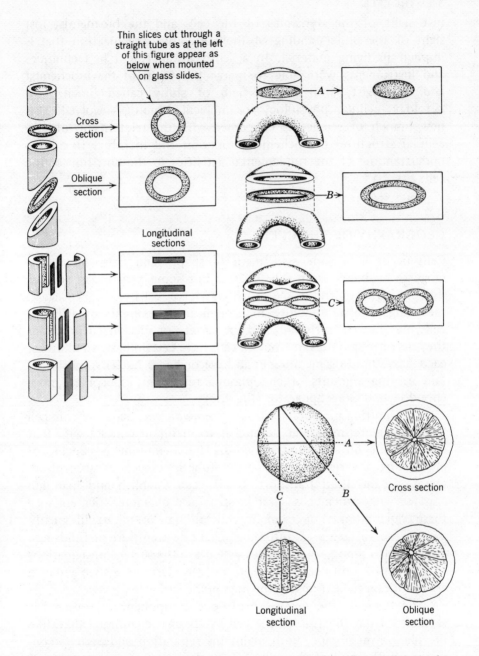

Fig. 8.4 Diagrams showing different appearances of sections cut in different planes. (From A. W. Ham, *Histology*, 6th ed., J. B. Lippincott Company, 1969 p. 29.)

347

lost sight of the dynamics of the cell, and the biochemist lost sight of the understanding of the correlative organization that is implicit in living material. In a sense, advancement in techniques and instruments were able to merge the focus of the biochemist and cytologist, and a new field of study—called biochemical cytology, cellular physiology, or molecular biology—evolved. This new branch of science is concerned with the relationship of sub-cellular structure to biochemical function and therefore to a basic understanding of the fundamental activities in the nutrition of the cell.

GEOGRAPHY OF THE CELL

Cells occur in a wide assortment of shapes and sizes. Most cells range in diameter from 0.5 to 20 μ but some may be as huge as the ostrich egg; and some, such as nerve cells, may be several feet long. The architecture and chemical components of different cells may be very different, and the variety of specialized functions they perform quite diverse, but all cells have certain basic similarities: each has a limiting membrane; all have or had a nucleus; most con-tain varying amounts of endoplasmic reticulum, ribosomes, mito-chondria, and Golgi apparatus (Fig. 8.5).

The limiting membrane, or *plasma membrane,* separates the cell from its environment yet permits it to maintain contact with that environment on which it depends. The membrane is capable of performing a variety of specialized functions such as absorption, secretion, and fluid transport. It also can establish and maintain contact with other cells. Certain structural characteristics enhance these capabilities. For example, outfoldings or microvilli greatly extend the surface area; infoldings facilitate transport of fluids and develop into pinocytotic vesicles which are the surface invaginations that pinch off and become free in the cytoplasm. Flagellae and cilia are motile specializations on the membrane surface.

The *nucleus,* the most conspicuous component of the cell, is separated from the rest of the cell by its own membrane that, like the plasma membrane, both maintains separation and permits con-tact with the rest of the cell. The nucleus contains practically all of the cell's DNA and is the site of both replication of DNA and its transcription to RNA. The DNA because of its affinity for biological

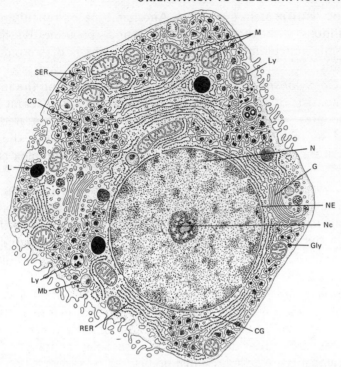

Fig. 8.5 Drawing showing fine structure of hepatocyte. PM, plasma membrane; M, mitochondrion; Ly, lysosome; SER, smooth endoplasmic reticulum; RER, rough endoplasmic reticulum; N, nucleus; NE, nuclear envelope; Nc, nucleolus; G, golgi complex; Mb, microbody; CG, cisternae of endoplasmic reticulum; L, lipid droplet; Gly, glycogen. (From T. L. Lentz, *Cell Fine Structure*, W. B. Saunders Company, Phila., 1971.)

stains was originally called chromatin, and the concentrated areas of RNA are referred to as *nucleoli*. The nuclear membrane is continuous with the endoplasmic reticulum of the cell.

The *endoplasmic reticulum*, an interconnected system of membraneous channels, appears to be a means for channeling substances through the cell. The rough endoplasmic reticulum is studded with *ribosomes* that are composed of RNA and protein which complex with messenger RNA to form polysomes. Protein synthesis takes place on the polysomes, and the proteins enter the channels of the endoplasmic reticulum to be transported to different parts of the cell. Some ribosomes are free in the cell matrix and these, too, are concerned with protein syntheses. Another type of reticulum that is continuous with the rough endoplasmic reticulum is smooth endoplasmic reticulum. It is involved in synthesis of steroids and other lipids.

The *Golgi apparatus,* usually between the nucleus and the apex of the cell consists of a stack of flat sacs and vesicles of different sizes. It is the area where synthesized materials are concentrated and packaged in membrane-limited vesicles for export from the cell. The Golgi are also responsible for the synthesis of complex carbo-hydrates.

Mitochondria are the site of cellular respiration. Cells that are metabolically active may contain as many as 1000 mitochondria; other cells may contain only a few. They are usually located in the region of the cell's greatest metabolic activity. Some non-nuclear DNA is contained in mitochondria and is probably responsible for coding for specific mitochondrial proteins.

Lysosomes are membrane-limited bodies that contain a variety of hydrolytic enzymes that function in the breakdown of materials taken into the cell by phagocytosis. Because of their function, their appearances are quite diverse. Some lysosomes containing indi-gestible remnants are called residual bodies.

Cell inclusions are the inactive storage forms of cell products and include lipid droplets, glycogen granules, and pigment granules.

The *cytoplasmic matrix* has embedded in all of the structures and organelles of the cell. It also contains water, ions, soluble enzymes, and proteins. At present the matrix is thought to be structureless, but instruments providing greater magnification and resolution may in the future disclose some structural character-istics.

The aim of this overview of the cell and its contents is only to provide some points of reference. Detailed study of structure and function of the organelles in the chapters that follow then can be understood as part of the integrated whole.

chapter 9
the plasma membrane

1. Role
2. Structure
   a. Early Studies
   b. Development of the Unit Membrane Concept
   c. Modification of the Unit Membrane Concept
   d. Current Membrane Models
   e. Membrane Integrity
   f. Other General Structural Characteristics
      1. Glycocalyx or Cell Coat
      2. Membrane Pores
      3. Cell Junctions

3. Function
   a. General Characteristics
   b. Transport
      1. Passive Transport
         a. Simple Diffusion
         b. Facilitated Diffusion
         c. Exchange Diffusion
      2. Active Transport
      3. Bulk Transport
   c. Communication Between Cells
   d. Specialization and Control
4. Summary

All cells are units separated from their environment by a membrane. This is a barrier whose presence determines the shape and encloses the substance of the cell. Despite the variability and potential hostility of the outside environment, it is the membrane upon which the constancy of the internal chemistry of the cell is dependent. The discharge of this responsibility is made possible by the ability of the membrane to discriminate among those organic and inorganic molecules in the surrounding medium, permitting entrance to some and rebuffing others. This is a truly vital task since either mass invasion of potentially toxic materials or rejection of essential nutrients can lead to cellular death by asphyxiation, hydration, desiccation, poisoning, starvation, or other equally effective means. The cell, thus dependent upon the external environment for all the raw materials from which it is made and with which it operates, by means of the membrane barrier and its fastidious selectivity can enjoy a distinct and separate existence.

A cell in equilibrium with its environment is a dead cell. One of the fundamental attributes of a living cell therefore is the ability to prevent the establishment of an equilibrium between its cytoplasm and the extracellular fluid. The differences in concentration of ions and molecules between these two compartments are maintained by the diligent and persistent management of movement through a barrier. The specific barrier is the innermost section of the cell membrane, the *plasma membrane.* Many cells may have protecting or supporting membranes exterior to the plasma membrane, but it is this innermost section of the membrane that exerts the dominant role in the viability of the cell and maintains the dynamic relationship between the cell and its environment. To achieve such a relationship, selected nutrients must constantly flow in and reaction products must flow out through the boundary of the system in a controlled manner. A congested or ungoverned traffic pattern would be as devastating to the cell as it would be to a busy highway.

Incoming nutrients provide the materials upon which the life of the cell and its substance depend: carbohydrates, protein, lipids, minerals, and vitamins. These nutrients are of value to the living cell, whether it be a protist or each of the millions in a complex organism, only after they have passed the hurdle of the plasma membrane. Once inside the cell, the nutrient may play any of its defined roles. In this fundamental way the unicellular and multicellular organisms in both the plant and animal kingdoms are identical. The hurdles leading up to the final barrier of the plasma membrane may range from a simple protective membrane in a free-living cell to the complexities of mammalian digestive and transport systems through which nutrients must pass. In the long voyage to each of the cells, membranes must be traversed: from the lumen of the digestive tract into and out of the cells of the intestinal mucosa and then into and out of the vascular system. Finally, the nutrients can be presented to the plasma membranes of each of the individual cells in the complex multicellular organism. After passing this final barrier, the nutrients can participate in the metabolic processes which release energy and provide the constituents for synthesis of both the cell's own substance and its secretory or other products. *It is for these purposes, and at this level of organization, that food is essential for life.*

ROLE

The complex processes involved in the acceptance and utilization of nutrients presented to the cell are dynamic, interrelated, and cyclic. The presentation of nutrients to the outer surface of the plasma membrane is but the first step and does not insure passage. If cellular work is required to transport the molecules across the membrane, this work is supported by energy provided by nutrients previously admitted to the cell. Essential nutrients supplied by the environment, transmitted through the membrane, and presented to the cellular organelles, permit the synthetic processes and the supporting energy-yielding catabolic activities to be carried on. A cell, any cell, deprived of nutrients to yield the energy to synthesize its substance cannot survive.

Whereas any starting point is arbitrary in describing as cyclic an activity as cellular nutrition, life begins—or ends—with the capacity of the plasma membrane of an existing and functioning cell to perform properly its specific functions. Molecular pathologies may arise, however, that interrupt membrane function. For example, in the untreated diabetic, glucose present in the interstitial fluid cannot penetrate the plasma membrane because of an insulin lack. Normal carbohydrate metabolism is therefore interrupted and the classic symptoms of diabetes develop.

The exact manner in which the plasma membrane discharges its fundamental responsibility remains an enigma. Some of the details of the membrane architecture have been revealed, others are conjectural. What is known is that the intracellular environment is meticulously maintained and this, presumably, is effected by the systematic arrangement and functional capabilities of the macromolecules synthesized by the cell. However, the performance of the plasma membrane is dependent not only upon its own capabilities and the supporting cellular activity but also upon the degree of stress imposed upon it by its environment.

STRUCTURE

The cell membrane is actually a group of membranes, only one section of which, the boundary or *plasma membrane*, is essential for the life of the cell. Damage to the plasma membrane is as lethal to the cell as damage to the nucleus itself. The plasma membrane lies closest to the cytoplasm and the layers exterior to it are supporting or protecting membranes.

Early Studies

The structure of the plasma membrane was first described decades before it was ever seen. Using a light microscope, one could easily see the discrete cell distinct from its environment. However, the nature of the demarcation between the cytoplasm of the cell and the extracellular sphere under such magnification could only be deduced from knowledge of its functional role. As early as 1895 Overton suggested that the cell was covered with lipid since it was preferentially permeable to lipid-soluble substances. Knowledge of the manner in which fatty acid molecules behave at a water interface provided a basis for defining membrane structure and permeability behavior (Fig. 9.1). The reason for the tidy alignment of fatty acid molecules resides in the properties of the molecules themselves. Fatty acids contain a carboxyl group that is *hydrophilic*, or freely miscible in water, and a hydrocarbon chain that is *hydrophobic*, or incompatible with water. It is for this reason that fatty acids orient themselves at an oil-water interface so that the hydrocarbon chain is in the oil and the carboxyl or *polar* group is in the water.

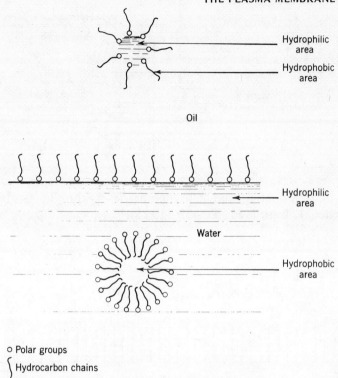

Oil

Hydrophilic area

Hydrophobic area

Hydrophilic area

Water

Hydrophobic area

○ Polar groups

) Hydrocarbon chains

Fig. 9.1 Model of polar lipids at oil-water interface. [From V. Luzzati, H. Mustacchi, and A. Skoulios, *Farad. Soc. Disc.*, No. 25, 43 (1958).]

The polar, or charged, groups are freely miscible in water because they dissociate and form hydrogen bonds to water molecules. Such molecules are called *amphipathic*, that is, they are structurally asymmetric with one highly polar and one nonpolar end. The lipid portions of living membranes are made up of phospholipids, cerebrosides, and cholesterol. The hydrocarbon chains of these lipids are the hydrophobic groups. The polar groups, in the case of the phospholipids, are the charged phosphate and various other ionic groups characteristic of phospholipids (Chapter 2). The single hydroxyl group of cholesterol makes it weakly hydrophilic.

Development of the Unit Membrane Concept

Lipid extracted from red blood cell membranes indicated that there

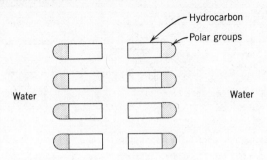

Fig. 9.2 Model of red cell membrane. [From E. Gorter and F. Grendel, J. Exp. Med. 41:439 (1925).]

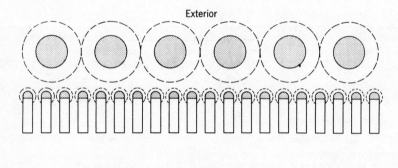

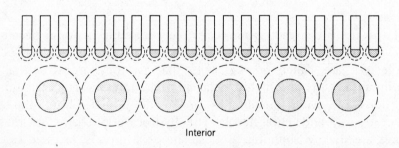

Fig. 9.3 Conception of cell membrane structure according to Danielli and Davson (*J. Cell. Comp. Physiol.*, 5:495, 1935). The membrane is represented by a layer of lipoid of indefinite thickness with polar surfaces oriented toward both the exterior and interior of the cell. These polar surfaces are shown covered by monolayers of globular protein molecules. [From J. D. Robertson, *Prog. Biophys. and Biophys. Chem.*, 10:343 (1960).]

was enough lipid for a double layer (Gorter and Grendel, 1925). Since both the internal and external environments of the cell are aqueous and since the membrane is freely permeable to lipid-soluble substances, it was reasonable to postulate a double layer of lipid, oriented so that polar groups formed the inner and outer boundaries with the two rows of hydrocarbon forming the core (Fig. 9.2). Such reasoning and knowledge of the physiological properties of membranes led to the deductions made by Danielli and Davson (1935). They based their structural model on certain fundamental properties of cell membranes: preferential permeability to lipid-soluble substances, existence of a low surface tension, and high electrical resistance. From these properties they deduced that there must exist a continuous layer of lipid molecules, such as phosphatides, sterols, and fats, with their polar groups oriented toward both the exterior and interior of the cell, and that on these polar surfaces were adsorbed a single layer of protein molecules (Fig. 9.3). They suggested that the protein layer consisted of polypeptide chains, or meshworks of such chains, lying in the plane of the interface with the hydrocarbon portions of the amino acid residues dissolved in the lipid layer and the polar groups in the aqueous phase. The elasticity and the relatively great mechanical strength of the membrane were attributed to the polypeptide chains.

Twenty-five years after the Danielli and Davson proposal, during which time membranes were studied by electron microscopy, X-ray diffraction, and chemical techniques, Robertson (1959) presented a model of the *unit membrane* that corresponded to the one proposed by Danielli and Davson although it was based on different lines of evidence. Robertson described the structure as a central core of a bimolecular leaflet of lipid bounded on either side by protein or other hydrophilic monolayers of nonlipid material (Fig. 9.4). Examination of cell membranes from a great variety of tissues from many species of plants and animals led Robertson (1960) to postulate that this structure was probably universally present in all animal and possibly all plant cells, and it was for this reason that he called it the unit membrane. The unit membrane was thought to be not only the barrier between the cell and its environment but also between the cell organelles and the cell matrix.

Modifications of the Unit Membrane Concept

The concept of the universality of the unit membrane was later

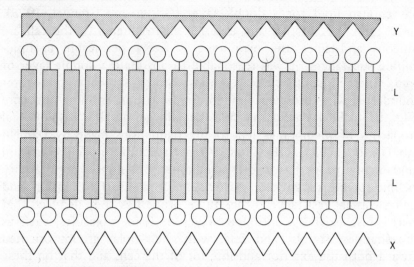

Fig. 9.4 Model of unit membrane. A highly schematic diagram of a unit membrane showing two monolayers of lipid molecules (L) and two fully spread monolayers of nonlipid designated by the letters X and Y. Different letters are used for the nonlipid monolayers to indicate that they are chemically different, even though the exact nature is as yet unknown. X borders cytoplasm. [From J. D. Robertson, *Ann. N. Y. Acad. Sci.*, 94:339 (1961).]

amended on the basis of evidence that all plasma membranes were not symmetrical structures and that the layers on either side of the lipid core differed in chemical reactivity. Information obtained from the use of a variety of fixatives in the preparation of sections for electron microscopy led Robertson to suggest that the lipid core might be bounded on one side by a protein monolayer and on the other side by a carbohydrate-containing monolayer.

Objections to the concept of a unit membrane common for all structures were based on the fact that Robertson's theory was derived from the study of myelin (Fig. 9.5), and generalizations drawn from such a specialized membrane seemed unwarranted (Korn, 1966; 1969). Furthermore, the unit membrane theory presupposed sufficient lipid to cover the surface area of the membrane with a bimolecular leaflet. This idea was based on data from the erythrocyte membrane and seemed reasonable at the time. However, protein-lipid ratios of membranes have since been shown to vary,

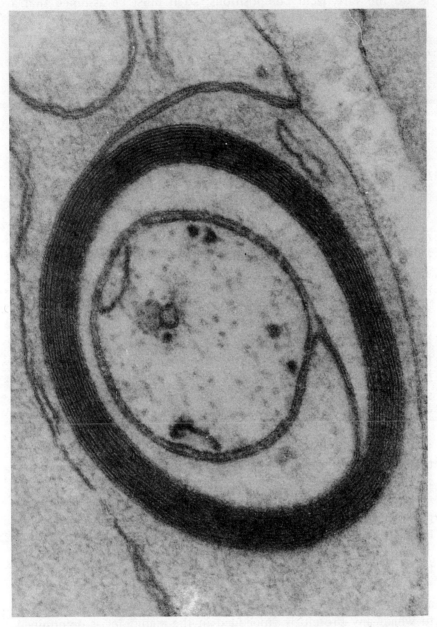

Fig. 9.5 Concentric organization of unit membranes forming a myelin sheath. Mouse sciatic nerve. Magnification 135,000. (Courtesy of Dr. J. David Robertson.)

as do the fatty acid compositions, so it must be assumed that a wide spectrum of membrane components exists with myelin at one end of the spectrum. Although there is reasonable but not conclusive evidence to support the bimolecular leaflet of phospholipid and protein as the structure of myelin, there is little basis for extending this concept to biological membranes in general (Korn, 1966; Sjöstrand, 1968). The specialized function of myelin is that of an electrical insulator for which it is well adapted with its repeating layers of lipids. However, the diversified functions of membranes suggest that such a single structure is rather unlikely. (For further discussion of myelin see Chapter 19.)

Current Membrane Models

Other investigators proposed models with globular micelles of lipid in dynamic equilibrium with the bimolecular leaflet and indicated either globules of proteins to account for the enzymes known to be in membranes (Lucy, 1968) or repeating globular lipoprotein subunits associated to form a two-dimensional membrane (Benson, 1966; Green and Tzagoloff, 1966). A model proposed by Lenard and Singer (1966), and subsequently extended (Glaser and Singer, 1971; Singer, 1971; 1972), has the formidable name of the *lipid-globular protein mosaic*. This model has a great number of adherents. It shows the lipid arranged in a discontinuous bilayer alternating with the globular proteins. The interspersed proteins are arranged with their ionic and highly polar groups exposed at the exterior surfaces of the membranes. Singer and Nicolson (1972) suggest that it can be best thought of as a two-dimensional oriented viscous solution, in other words, a *fluid mosaic* as it is sometimes called. A schematic cross-sectional view is presented in Fig. 9.6. The folded polypeptide chains of the globular proteins may be partially embedded in the phospholipid bilayer or may extend through the bilayer protruding from each surface and maintaining contact with the aqueous solvent on both sides of the membrane. In each case, the ionic residues of the protein are on the protruding surfaces and the nonpolar residues are in the embedded parts. The extent to which any protein is embedded in the membrane is determined by the size and structure of the molecule. The fact that different proteins can be integral parts of the membrane helps to explain the

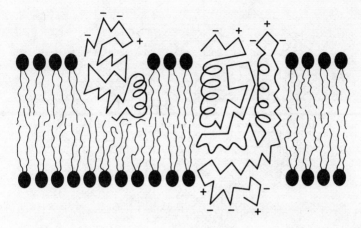

Fig. 9.6 The lipid-globular protein mosaic model of membrane structure: schematic cross-sectional view. The phospholipids are arranged as a discontinuous bilayer with their ionic and polar heads in contact with water. The integral proteins, with the heavy lines representing the folded polypeptide chains, are shown as globular molecules partially embedded in, and partially protruding from, the membrane. The protruding parts have on their surfaces the ionic residues (– and +) of the protein, while the nonpolar residues are largely in the embedded parts; accordingly, the protein molecules are amphiphathic. The degree to which the integral proteins are embedded and, in particular, whether they span the entire membrane thickness depend on the size and structure of the molecules [From S. J. Singer and G. L. Nicolson, *Science*, 175: 720 (1972).]

variety of functional membranes. The three-dimensional model of the lipid-globular protein mosaic (Fig. 9.7) shows the large irregular globular proteins embedded to various degrees in the phospholipid matrix. The embedded proteins are the *intrinsic* or *integral* proteins of the membrane. They may extend partly or all the way through the lipid bilayer thereby forming an integral part of the membrane continuum. The *extrinsic* or *peripheral* proteins are associated with the exposed surfaces of the membrane and can be easily dissociated from the membrane as molecularly intact proteins free of lipid and relatively soluble. The extrinsic proteins are not critical to the structural integrity of the membrane (Singer and Nicholson, 1972; Capaldi, 1974). Although no proteins or polypeptide subunits in the membrane serve purely structural purposes, proteins unique

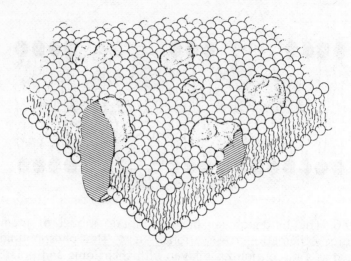

Fig. 9.7 The lipid-globular protein mosaic model with a lipid matrix (the fluid mosaic model); schematic three-dimensional and cross-sectional views. The solid bodies with stippled surfaces represent the golbular integral proteins, which at long range are randomly distributed in the plane of the membrane. At short range, some may form specific aggregates, as shown. [From S. J. Singer and G. L. Nicolson, *Science,* 175: 720 (1972).]

to particular membranes and associated with their functions can also serve a structural role (Dreyer et al., 1972). In fact, membrane function depends on how the membrane proteins are linked in the membrane structure.

The matrix in which the protein is embedded is fluid under physiological conditions and therefore dynamic: that is, the membrane appears to be a two-dimensional viscous solution that permits the protein components to maintain mobility and enables carrier mechanisms to operate. The fluidity of the phospholipid matrix is determined by the structure and relative proportion of the unsaturated fatty acids and on ambient temperature (Fox, 1972). At body temperature phospholipids with only saturated fatty acids are arranged in an orderly and rigid crystalline fashion. Mixtures of saturated and unsaturated fatty acids provide a less orderly arrangement and are, therefore, more fluid. This occurs because the double

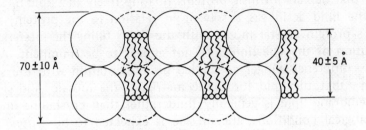

Fig. 9.8 The protein crystal model for membranes. The large circles represent proteins; the dashed circles are understood to be proteins behind the plane of the section. The small circles represent the polar lipid heads and the wavy lines the nonpolar lipid tails [From Vanderkooi and Green, *Proc. Natl. Acad. Sci.*, 66: 615 (1970).]

bonds lead to structural deformation and disturb ordered stacking. The greater the degree of unsaturation of the fatty acids in the phospholipids, and the greater the proportion of unsaturated to saturated fatty acids, the more fluid the membrane.

Mammalian cell membranes contain a considerable portion of unsaturated fatty acids and, therefore, the melting temperature for the lipid bilayer is below normal mammalian body temperature permitting relatively free movement of the fatty acid tails. The combination of unsaturation and temperature gives the whole lipid bilayer the consistency of a light oil, and the lipid and protein molecules are free to move, mostly from side to side (Capaldi, 1974). Independent movement of the lipid and protein molecules has also been demonstrated in red cell membranes by Glaser et al. (1970), adding support to the suggestion for organization in a mosaic.

In still another membrane model, postulated by Green's group (Vanderkooi, 1972), it is suggested that the proteins form the backbone and are arranged in crystal-like structure with the lipids filling the interstices (Fig. 9.8). The intrinsic proteins according to this version are linked into sets by hydrophobic bonding to form functional units and the functional units are linked together by electrostatic forces. Green contends that such a structural arrangement is essential to transfer a sequence of changes through a membrane and that this could not occur in a lipid sea such as Singer suggests.

There are currently two major schools of thought concerning the dominant structural element of membranes: Singer's fluid mosaic model that depicts intrinsic proteins floating freely in a lipid bilayer with the lipid acting as a solvent in relation to the protein, and Green's protein crystal model with the lipids filling the interstices. Resolution of the question does not appear to be imminent. At a recent conference Singer concluded his presentation with the suggestion "that the lipid forms the matrix of the mosaic, and since the membrane lipid is generally fluid rather than crystalline under physiological conditions, the mosaic is expected to be a *dynamic* one. That is, the membrane appears to be a two-dimensional viscous solution, with its components able to undergo translational diffusion in the plane of the membrane" (Singer, 1972). Green stated just as positively (Green, 1972): "Judging from the increasing frequency with which crystalline membranes are being reported, it is a reasonable presumption that *under the right conditions* all biological membranes will show a crystalline character when examined by negative staining. The recurrence of these crystalline patterns suggests that the regular alternation of protein and lipid domains is a constant feature of biological membranes."

Membrane Integrity

The lipid-protein complexes that form the plasma membranes, and the complexes with a relatively greater amount of phospholipid containing polyunsaturated fatty acids that form the membranes of organelles, are particularly susceptible to peroxidation. The manner in which the membrane containing unsaturated fatty acid tails is predisposed to disruption through the chain reactions associated with the generation of free radicals is illustrated in Fig. 9.9. Demopoulos (1973) indicates that drastic effects should be expected also on membrane proteins and membrane-associated structures such as attached ribosomes, surface glycoproteins, and various complex receptor sites as a result of lipid peroxidation. Such peroxidative changes undoubtedly play a significant role in cellular pathology (Pryor, 1973). Often, powerful catalysts that initiate lipid peroxidation such as coordinated iron and hemoproteins, are located in close proximity to polyunsaturated membrane lipids. The damage that ensues involves changes in the membrane proteins resulting from polymerization, polypeptide chain scission, and chemical changes in individual amino acids (Tappel, 1973). The polymerization or

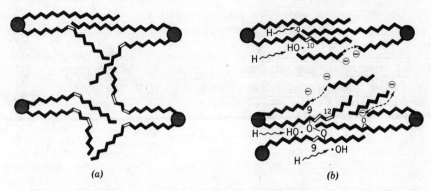

Fig. 9.9a Schematic representation of bimolecular leaflet of phospholipid molecules, forming the skeleton of a plasma membrane. The circles are the glycerophosphate head groups, which are polar, while the zigzag fatty acid tails extend into the hydrophobic midzone. In the normal membrane there is a saturated carbon separating the two carbons that have unsaturated bonds. These are unconjugated double bonds. The saturated carbon in between is partly activated and can lose one of its hydrogens quite readily.

Fig. 9.9b Schematic of free radical peroxidative damage to the fatty acids that formed the hydrophobic midzone seen in (a). Most of the double bonds are now in the nonbent transconfiguration; a saturated carbon no longer separates the carbons with unsaturated bonds and this is referred to as conjugation; alkoxy radicals, RO·, are present and react to form peroxides, ROOR, thereby joining two adjacent fatty acids in an abnormal bond; mobile ·OH radicals are shown as the result of hydroperoxide schism; hydrogens are shown being abstracted by ·OH, possibly from adjacent lipid and protein molecules; abstracted hydrogens react with hydroxyls to form water in the hydrophobic midzone; fragmentation of fatty acid tails is shown with eventual production of negatively charged carboxylic acid groups, represented as a minus sign inside an oval mark. The numerals, 9, 10, 12, signify the carbon atom number in the carbon chain that makes up the fatty acid. [From H. B. Demopoulos, *Fed. Proc.*, 32: 1859 (1973).]

cross-linking of enzymes can wreak particular havoc to a cell and its organelle membranes completely disrupting the precise arrangement of molecules responsible for the integration of structure and function. Among the amino acids most readily susceptible to the effects of lipid peroxidation are methionine, histidine, cystine, and lysine

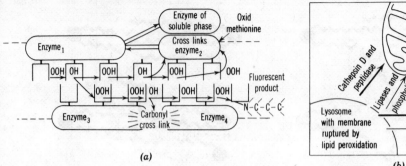
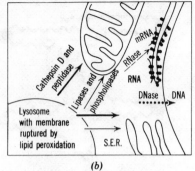

(a)

(b)

Fig. 9.10a Schematic drawing of a biomembrane in cross section showing propagation of peroxidation of the polyunsaturated fatty acids in the phospholipids. Shown are some of the various types of molecular damage to membrane components as a result of the peroxidation reaction.

Fig. 9.10b Schematic illustration of the concept of amplification of lipid peroxidation damage through the release of lysosomal hydrolytic enzymes. The released enzymes initiate random hydrolysis of subcellular structures and components. [From A. L. Tappel, *Fed. Proc.*, 32: 1870 (1973).]

(Tappel, 1973). Various effects of lipid peroxidation on membrane components are illustrated in Fig. 9.10. If the membrane subjected to lipid peroxidation and rupture is a lysosomal membrane, the release of the enzymes normally contained within the confines of the organelle initiates random hydrolyses within the cell further damaging structure and function.

The generally accepted mechanism of peroxide formation involves the formation of a free radical ($R^{\cdot}$) by a polyunsaturated fatty acid (RH), followed by the addition of oxygen to form a peroxide ($ROO^{\cdot}$):

$$RH \longrightarrow R^{\cdot} + H^{+}$$

$$R^{\cdot} + O_2 \longrightarrow ROO^{\cdot}$$

$$ROO^{\cdot} + RH \longrightarrow ROOH + R^{\cdot}$$

A chain is propagated by the reaction of the peroxide with another polyunsaturated fatty acid to produce another free radical (see Uri, 1961). A chain reaction such as this can be inhibited either by replacing or depleting one of the substrates.

Vitamin E exerts a protective action in preventing lipid peroxidation and in so doing is fundamental to the structural and functional integrity of cell membranes and, therefore, the cell itself. It should come as no surprise that the function of vitamin E in membrane protection is closely related to its position in membrane structure. Vitamin E interdigitates with the phospholipids, cholesterol, and triglycerides in the plasma membrane and in the membranes of the mitochondria, lysosomes, and endoplasmic reticulum. In mitochondrial membranes, the ratio of vitamin E to the polyunsaturated fatty acids in membrane phospholipids, whose unsaturated state the vitamin E protects, is about 1:1000. From its vantage point within the membrane structure, vitamin E is in an ideal position to capture free radicals.

Vitamin E functions as an antioxidant (AH) by replacing a fatty acid as substrate for the oxidation and thereby breaking the chain of free radical formation. This mechanism is referred to as hydrogen abstraction:

$$ROO^. + AH \longrightarrow ROOH + A^.$$

Thus, the close association of vitamin E and fat *in vivo* is propitious. (However, the relationship can present a problem to the investigator who wishes to prepare a vitamin E-free ration since the vitamin E must be stripped from fats or oils.) Tappel and Zalkin (1959; 1960) showed *in vivo* lipid peroxidation in the mitochondrial and microsome fractions from livers of vitamin E-deficient rabbits. Zalkin and Tappel (1960) concluded that vitamin E functions solely to stabilize cellular unsaturated lipids against oxidative deterioration, thereby maintaining structural and functional integrity at the subcellular level. Vitamin E functions in maintaining membrane integrity by interacting with free radicals that are generated during certain types of oxidoreductase activities (McCay et al., 1972). In the process, a-tocopherol is converted to a polar lipid. Inadequate membrane protection may be the explanation for the fragility of erythrocyte membranes and for alterations in the structure of hepatocyte membranes in vitamin E deficiency (Machada et al., 1971). The hemolytic anemia that occurs in premature infants also appears to be due to vitamin E deficiency. In this instance, fragility of the erythrocyte membranes is due to inadequate absorption of the vitamin through the immature intestinal mucosal cells (Gross and Melhorn, 1972). It is probable that the fragility and spontaneous hemolysis of blood stored in blood banks for periods longer than 2 to 3 weeks are due to peroxide generation from red cell lipid, which is enhanced by heme and produces a reduction of vitamin E in the erythrocyte. György (1962) suggests that vitamin E repeatedly added to blood might permit longer storage.

In addition to vitamin E, small amounts of sulfhydryl compounds such as glutathione, sulfhydryl proteins, and cysteine and methionine also react as free radical scavengers and peroxide decomposers (Tappel, 1973).

Other General Structural Characteristics

Glycocalyx or Cell Coat. What originally was thought to be an extraneous coat or "fuzz" covering the plasma membrane has recently been shown to have fine structure and histochemical properties to indicate that it is synthesized by the cell whose free surface it covers. This cell coat or *glycocalyx* is an integral part of the membrane and glycoprotein in nature. It appears to be a dynamic surface component and requires the intact cell not only for its synthesis but also for its maintenance (Ito, 1969). It appears to be filamentous and inseparable from the cell as long as the cell maintains its integrity; however, the fine structure of the glycocalyx tends to vary with different preparative procedures.

The functions of the glycocalyx will be discussed in a subsequent section, and its synthesis by the Golgi apparatus in Chapter 12.

Membrane Pores. A characteristic of membrane structure, postulated by some investigators as perhaps fundamental to certain aspects of permeability, is the presence of membrane pores. Danielli first suggested that groups of protein molecules oriented radially with their polar groups directed toward the interior formed pores that he called *polar pores* (Fig. 9.11). Solomon (1960) suggested that a large part of the traffic through the membrane travels via holes in the walls. He postulated that there is probably a uniform number of such pores and that they do not exist as fixed canals but act in response to conditions both outside and inside the cell that cause some pores to open and others to close. An interesting analogy that he used likened the membrane to a "bowl of spaghetti shaken continually, opening up new pores or passages in one place and closing them somewhere else" (ibid).

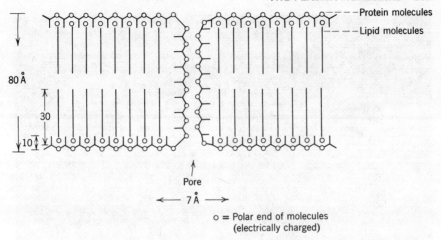

Fig. 9.11 Model of cell membrane with polar pore. (After Danielli).

The pore as a dynamic or temporary channel appears to be a more realistic version if the membrane is conceived as a fluid mosaic. The constant movement of the molecules in the membrane might result in a transient realignment in order to create a temporary channel through which passive diffusion might occur.

Cell Junctions. Membranes of adjacent cells in a tissue may run straight and parallel to each other or may have tortuous interdigitations (Fig. 9.12). Not only does the membrane form the boundary for the individual cell but it also participates in the formation of specialized junctions between cells that are important in cell to cell transport mechanisms. Cell junctions are composed of three elements that, according to the terminology of Farquhar and Palade (1963), are the *zona occludens* or *tight junction, zona adherens* or *intermediate junction,* and the *macula adherens* or *desmosome.* These zones appear structurally distinguishable and functionally distinct. Fig. 9.13 illustrates the junctional complex in intestinal epithelial cells. The *zona occludens* begins close to the lumen at the junction of neighboring cells where the surface plasma membrane is deflected inward. There is fusion of the two straight and parallel adjacent plasma membranes and no intercellular space. This area encircles the cell in a ribbonlike fashion, thereby sealing off the lumen from the rest of the intercellular space. The membranes then diverge and are separated by an intercellular space to form the *zona adherens.* This area, too, runs around the perimeter

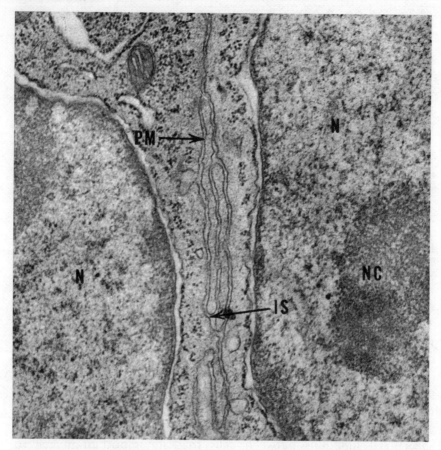

Fig. 9.12 Interdigitating plasma membranes (PM) with intercellular space (IS) between. N = nucleus, Nc = nucleolus. Gland cells of uterine mucosa of Japanese quail. Magnification 40,000. (Courtesy of Dr. Harald Schraer.)

of the cell. The area between the membranes is filled with a material of low electron density and may be glycocalyx material. Dense patches of fine filaments are arranged on the cytoplasmic sides of the membranes. The desmosome is the most complex region (Fig. 9.14). It is extremely dense in electron micrographs where an ordered system of cytoplasmic fibrils converge on the cytoplasmic sides of the two cells to form a supporting structure. The cells appear neither to be fused nor in direct contact. The dark line in the center of the area is thought to be merged glycocalyx from the

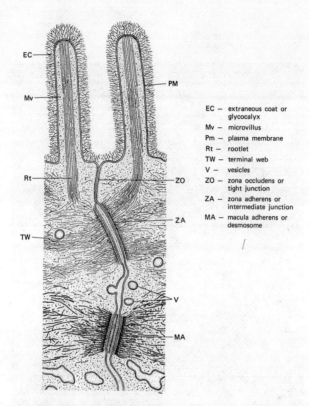

EC — extraneous coat or glycocalyx
Mv — microvillus
Pm — plasma membrane
Rt — rootlet
TW — terminal web
V — vesicles
ZO — zona occludens or tight junction
ZA — zona adherens or intermediate junction
MA — macula adherens or desmosome

Fig. 9.13 Junctional complex in intestinal epithelial cells. (From T. L. Lentz, *Cell Fine Structure*, W. B. Saunders Co., Phila., 1971.)

two cells. The desmosomes are not continuous around the cell but occur only at discrete points.

The role of the junctional complex in the attachment of cells to each other in tissue and in cell to cell transport mechanisms will be discussed in the section on function.

For reviews of membrane structure see Bretscher (1973) and Capaldi (1974).

FUNCTION

The concept of diversity in structure is consonant with the diversity in function that is known to exist. The capacity of the cell mem-

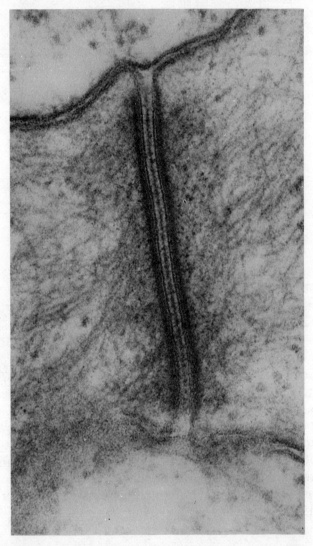

Fig. 9.14 Desmosome from the skin of the frog, Rana pipiens. Magnification 120,000. (Courtesy of Dr. Joan Borysenko).

brane to act as both barrier and gateway is undoubtedly a function of its molecular structure and of the size and character of the molecules seeking passage. Above and beyond the preferential admission of nutrients to the cell, membranes exert a selectivity leading to localization and concentration of specific nutrients in certain organelles, cells, and tissues. Such selectivity is inextricably related to specialized function. That the membrane is not a static barrier will be apparent: neither size nor concentration gradient nor chemical resemblance is itself sufficient to insure acceptance of unwanted molecules. It is reasonable to suspect that the physiological diversities may be attributable to (1) the assortment of lipid constituents, (2) the character of the globular proteins interspersed in the lipid matrix, and (3) the chemical specificity of different sections of a continuous membrane and its glycocalyx.

General Characteristics

All membranes have in common the characteristic of *selective permeability*. A membrane that is selectively permeable permits one material to pass more easily than another; this is different from a semipermeable membrane that is permeable to the solvent only. The characteristic of selective permeability enables the membrane to maintain a balance between the osmotic pressure of the intracellular fluid and that of the interstitial fluid. It also enables a difference in the ionic concentration between the cell and extracellular fluid to be maintained, and this leads to an electrical potential across the membrane. These characteristics associated with diffusion, plus the mechanisms which require energy generally described as active transport, account for the major exchanges across membranes.

The structure of the membrane also contributes to its characteristic of selective permeability. Whereas it is practically impermeable to intracellular protein and related anions, it is freely permeable to water and to sodium, potassium, and chloride. These differences in permeability create the chemical and electrical gradients existing between the cell and its environment. The cell maintains a high concentration of potassium along with a high concentration of protein and related anions. It has a low concentration of sodium and chloride. The environment surrounding the cell on the other side of the membrane has a low concentration of potassium and a high concentration of sodium. Unrestrained cation movement would be along the gradient: sodium moving into the cell and potassium moving out. It is obvious that such movement along the concentration gradients is either counterbalanced or impeded since all cells maintain high ratios of potassium to sodium in an environment with a reverse ratio. Sodium does diffuse into the cell and potassium does diffuse out, but the passive diffusion along the concentration gradients are counterbalanced by active transport. In effect, the emigrating potassium ions are returned to the cell and the emigrating sodium ions to the environment. Current hypotheses explaining this mechanism will be discussed in detail in a later section.

The counterbalancing effect of ion diffusion is supported by the favorable electrical gradient which tends to retain potassium within the cell. The concentration of anions within the cell attracts and holds the positively charged potassium creating an electrical gradient from the outside in. Disruption of this favorable electrical gradient by chloride, which diffuses freely, is prevented because the chloride ions that enter are repelled by the concentration of anions within the cell. A balance is thus achieved with more potassium ions inside the cell and more chloride outside. The active extrusion of sodium is also a major factor in the maintenance of this potential difference. Because some potassium does passively diffuse out of the cell and some chloride in, an electrical potential is created across the membrane. The membrane is said to be polarized with the cytoplasm negative to the extracellular fluid. In other words, there are more positive charges on the outer surface and more negative charges along the inner surface. This is true of most membranes. The transient reversal of this state of polarization in nerve and muscle cells explains their physiological action and will be discussed in Chapters 18 and 19.

Transport

Passive Transport. There are three major categories of passive transport: *simple diffusion, facilitated diffusion,* and *exchange diffusion.* Although these will be discussed individually, it will become apparent that these mechanisms are not rigidly defined and, in fact, do overlap.

Simple Diffusion. Simple diffusion along a concentration gradient or an electrical gradient occurs from a high concentration or potential to a lower one. It is always in a downhill direction, and no energy is required for the process (Fig. 9.15). However, in some

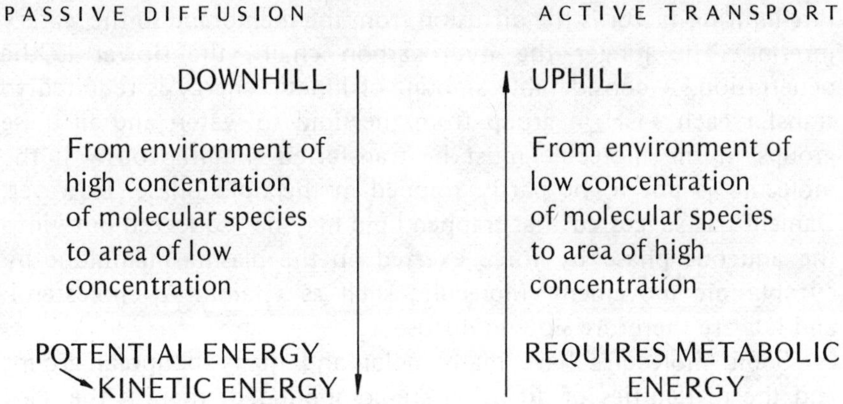

PASSIVE DIFFUSION   ACTIVE TRANSPORT

DOWNHILL | ↑ UPHILL

From environment of | From environment of
high concentration | low concentration
of molecular species | of molecular species
to area of low | to area of high
concentration | concentration

POTENTIAL ENERGY | REQUIRES METABOLIC
↘KINETIC ENERGY ↓ | ENERGY

Fig. 9.15 Contrast of passive diffusion and active transport.

instances, a revolving door policy is established and an intruding molecule that has diffused in may be escorted out again. The planned exit is an active, energy-requiring process against the gradient and is discussed in the section on active transport. Passive diffusion, of course, could not be the only mechanism in the maintenance of the relationship between the cell and its environment since, unrestricted and unchecked, an equilibrium would ultimately be established leading to the death of the cell.

The major deterrent to penetration by diffusing molecules is in the lipoprotein character of the membrane itself. Brown and Danielli (1964) suggest that the membrane resistance is tripartite: (1) resistance encountered in passing from the aqueous phase of the environment into the membrane; (2) resistance encountered in diffusing through the membrane; and (3) resistance encountered in passing from the membrane into the watery milieu of the cell's interior. Each of these may be the limiting step, depending on the diffusing molecule.

If a molecule is passing from the water phase of the environment into the membrane, all the hydrogen bonds to the water must be broken simultaneously if entrance into the lipid phase is gained. If there are three or more polar groups in the molecule, this step is likely to be the one that limits the rate of entry. Predominantly polar molecules such as sugars, glycerol, and glycogen would therefore be slow.

If the molecule seeking entrance is predominantly nonpolar, the rate-limiting factor is the diffusion from the membrane to the watery interior. The longer the hydrocarbon chain, the slower is the penetration. A considerable amount of kinetic energy is required to transfer each $-CH_2-$ group from the lipid to water, and all these groups in the molecule must be transferred simultaneously if the molecule is not to be partly trapped in the lipid phase. However, Danielli has suggested that trapped lipid may be "squeezed out" into the aqueous phase by force exerted on the plasma membrane by cytoplasmic movement. Molecules such as vitamin A, cholesterol, and fats are therefore slow to diffuse.

Some molecules have many polar and many nonpolar groups and the difficulties of diffusion are compounded: there is the need to break the hydrogen bonds for entry into the lipid phase followed by the movement of the nonpolar groups from the lipid to the water phase. Diffusion would therefore be slow for proteins and is probably an unlikely means of passage.

Studies of the kinetics of diffusion indicate that many different nonelectrolytes, as indicated above, can penetrate a lipoprotein membrane by simple diffusion. However, it is evident that other more selective and rapid means of entry into a cell must occur if the required broad assortment of nutrients are to enter and if the cell is to maintain its discriminating position in an environment on which it is totally dependent.

Facilitated Diffusion.   One means of facilitating the passage of solutes across the plasma membrane is by the provision of a carrier to link with the solute and carry it across. This type of transport, *facilitated diffusion,* does not require an expenditure of energy by the cell and proceeds downhill along the concentration gradient. The molecule being transported is temporarily bound to a membrane constituent at one surface of the membrane, diffused through as a complex, and released at the opposite side. Presumably the carrier returns to pick up another molecule or ion (Fig. 9.16). This type of diffusion can proceed as long as carriers are available; that is, up to the point where the carrier system becomes saturated. The differential rates of sugar transport, for example, are probably due to

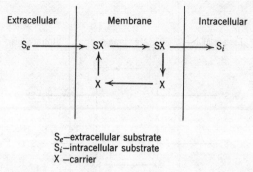

S_e—extracellular substrate
S_i—intracellular substrate
X —carrier

Fig. 9.16 Model of facilitated diffusion.

competition for carrier molecules. The order of decreasing affinities to transport—glucose, mannose, xylose, galactose, arabinose, sorbose, fructose—suggests that success in competition for a position on the carrier is affected by the configuration of the molecule (see Chapter 6.)

Facilitated diffusion does not alter the final equilibrium that could be attained even if the carrier were not present; but it does alter the speed with which the equilibrium is attained.

Exchange Diffusion. Another type of carrier-dependent transport that has been shown to operate in the passage of certain ions and amino acids is *exchange diffusion.* For each molecule transported through the membrane in one direction, a similar molecule must be transported on the return trip (Fig. 9.17). Because of the dependence on the carrier molecule, the rate of transport is independent of the solute concentration but limited by the number of carrier molecules. This type of diffusion is responsible for the major exchange of labeled for nonlabeled ions and amino acids. A sodium for a sodium or a glycine for a glycine is termed auto-exchange. What purpose this type of equal exchange may serve is not clear. Some heteroexchange may also take place but is very specific for carrier substrates.

Active Transport. When a substance must be moved against a concentration or electrochemical gradient, work is required. The source of the energy for this work is metabolically derived and the movement is called *active transport.* Active transport is carrier-mediated, and the carrier is a specific transport protein that is an integral part of the membrane to be traversed. A carrier works by binding the substance, carrying out translocation, and then releasing

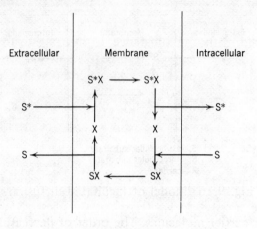

Fig. 9.17 Model of exchange diffusion. (Adapted from D. B. Tower, S. A. Luse, and H. Grundfest, *Properties of Membranes*, Springer Publishing Co., N. Y., 1961.)

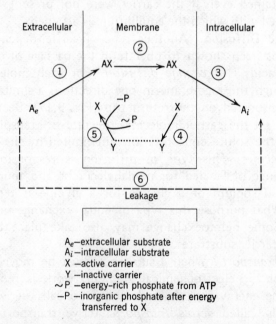

Fig. 9.18 Model of active transport. [Adapted from E. Heinz and P. M. Walsh, *J. Biol. Chem.*, 233:1492 (1958).]

it (Pardee, 1968). Carriers involved in any type of transport can become saturated with the substance to be transported; each has specificity for the substance it transports; and each is subject to specific inhibition by molecules that can compete for the specific binding site.

An early model of active transport (Fig. 9.18) incorporated the characteristics of the simpler transport systems with the addition of an energy-rich phosphate from ATP to activate the carrier. The model proposed that the activated carrier released the molecule it transported, reverted to an inactive form, and subsequently was reactivated by ATP as it returned through the membrane. Since active or energy-dependent transport was often compared to a pumping system, such as that required to carry water from a lower to a higher level, models appeared that described the active transport of sodium and were referred to as the *sodium pump*. Energy derived from cellular metabolism was depicted as driving the pump or, more specifically, of energizing the carrier to transport sodium out of and potassium into the cell. The release of the sodium to the outside was presumed to convert the carrier by enzymatic action to one which carried potassium to the inside. Net transport of the two ions results because the rate. of active transport exceeds the rates of leakage along the gradients in the opposite direction.

Isolation of an enzyme system activated by sodium and potassium ions and dependent upon the presence of both ATP and Mg^{2+} was shown to be capable of hydrolyzing ATP at a rate that depended on the concentration of sodium inside the cell and of potassium outside (Skou, 1965). The enzyme, Na,K-adenosine triphosphatase (Na,K-ATPase), was shown to be in the membranes of all cells that had a coupled transport mechanism for sodium and potassium. It was suggested that this enzyme system was the one involved in the active transport of sodium and potassium across cell membranes.

Increased insight into membrane structure and the isolation of this enzyme system led to intensified work on the nature and operation of the sodium-potassium pump. It has been shown that the cation that activated the ATPase is on the side of the membrane from which it is transported; that is, the concentration of sodium activates from the inside and the concentration of potassium from the outside. The hydrolysis of the substrate Mg-ATP takes place inside the cell and the rate of active transport and the rate of enzyme activity regulate each other. Whittam (1967) has summarized some of the facts: (1) ATP is hydrolyzed in such a way that the products of hydrolysis stay inside the cell; (2) the splitting occurs only when sodium is on the inside and potassium on the outside; (3) the ions are moved as part of the vectorial reaction[1]; (4) sodium is required to permit the substrate, MgATP, to attach to the enzyme; (5) a phosphate intermediate is formed and then broken down by the potassium on the outside. Based on these and other data, it is suggested that the enzyme, Na,K-ATPase, in the membrane can assume two conformations: one shape when sodium facilitates attachment of MgATP to the enzyme forming a phosphate intermediate; the other after hydrolysis occurs as a result of the external potassium. This second change is associated with the movement of the ions, and the enzyme reassumes its original conformation. This type of enzyme is *allosteric*, one with two or more distinct binding sites where the binding to one site affects the conformation of the protein and, therefore, the binding to the second site. According to Whittam (1967) the concept that transport of cations is dependent on the conformation of molecules in the cell membrane is entirely compatible with all facts known thus far and might well be the mechanism of active transport. The model he proposed is shown in Fig. 9.19.

According to the internal transfer model proposed by Stein et al. (1974) the Na,K-pump is a tetrameric protein embedded in the membrane. Each unit of the tetramer is capable of existing in either a high- or low-affinity state for the binding of sodium. In the operation of the pump each unit successively assumes each state. The model illustrated in Fig. 9.20 shows high affinity for sodium associated with low affinity for potassium; while low affinity for sodium is associated with high affinity for potassium. The flipping from one form to the other (A to A') allows transport to occur to the center cavity formed by the two upper subunits of the tetramer. The ions then redistribute since the affinity of the subunits for the ions has changed. The tetramer then flips back to the first conformational state, and the sodium is expelled into the external medium and the potassium into the cell interior. The process repeats from the beginning. The two lower subunits func-

[1] A vectorial reaction is one that is directional because one of the components (ATPase) is fixed in space (the membrane), and the two sides can be distinguished (either Na or K affinity).

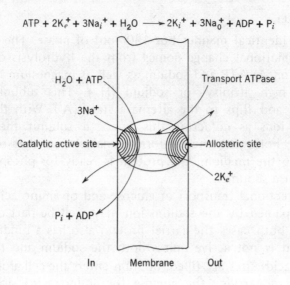

$$ATP + 2K_e^+ + 3Na_i^+ + H_2O \longrightarrow 2K_i^+ + 3Na_0^+ + ADP + P_i$$

Fig. 9.19 Net enzyme reaction of active transport. (From R. Whittam, *The Neurosciences*, Rockefeller Institute, N. Y., 1967, pp. 313.)

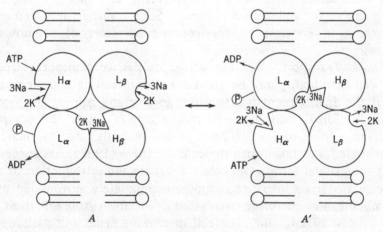

Fig. 9.20 The internal transfer model of cation transport. The enzyme is represented as a tetramer, each subunit having the potential to exist in either a high- or low-affinity state for the binding of sodium and assuming such high- and low-affinity states successively. *A* represents the initial high-affinity (Ha) and low-affinity (La) states for sodium that flip to *A'*, low-affinity (La) and high-affinity (Ha). For more detailed description of the model, see text. [From Stein et al., *Ann. N. Y. Acad. Sci.*, 227: 328 (1974).]

tion in an identical manner but 180° out of phase. The energy for the conformational change comes from the hydrolysis of ATP. In conformation A, ATP and sodium as well as magnesium bind to the unit with high affinity for sodium (H_a). This subunit is phosphorylated and flips to the alternate state (A'). With the internal potassium ions as cofactors this upper a subunit then dephosphorylates. Following the conformational change that releases the cations into the medium, the protein is ready for phosphorylation at the lower a subunits.

The directional transport of glucose and of amino acids into the cell accompanied by the sodium ion may well be part of a similar system. In both cases the carrier protein also has a binding site for sodium and is not active unless both the sodium and the glucose (or amino acid) sites are filled. Sodium enters the cell along a downward gradient carrying the glucose (or amino acid) along with it against their respective gradients. The downward gradient of sodium is maintained by its active extrusion from the cells it has thus entered. According to Crane (1965) the sodium and glucose entry and the sodium extrusion are independent, and this is thought to be true also for amino acid transport. Such transport is *noncoupled transport* in contrast to the *coupled transport* of sodium and potassium.

Bulk Transport. Whereas active or passive transport through the cell membrane may be viewed as polite tasting and sipping of what the environment has to offer, gorging and gulping also occur. A distinction is made between the gorging of solids, *phagocytosis,* and the gulping of liquids, *pinocytosis.* In both cases the material is encircled and taken into the cell. De Duve (1963a) has suggested that the general term *endocytosis* designate the introduction of any foreign materials into the cytoplasm completely surrounded by a membrane and therefore segregated from the cytoplasm itself. In the process of engulfing, the cell membrane sends out pseudopod-like projections that surround and trap the desired material. The encircling membrane then separates from the inner surface and becomes a small membrane-enclosed vesicle within the cell, called a phagosome or a pinosome. The phagosome may be one of the precursors of the lysosome, the cellular digestive system to be discussed in Chapter 14. The plasma membrane removed from the surface in the formation of a phagosome must be replaced, but just how this occurs is not known. A recent suggestion (McKanna, 1973) from work on amoeba and mammalian secretory cells is that the membrane recycles as membrane and is not broken down into molecules or micelles except in digestive or autophagic vacuoles (see Chapter 12).

It is not clear whether endocytosis is a characteristic of all cells, but it would appear to be a rather general phenomenon and probably retained in most, if not all, animal cells. Classic examples of mammalian cells generally involved in endocytosis are the granular leucocytes, the macrophages of the reticuloendothelial system and the endothelial cells lining the sinusoids of the liver, among others.

The amoeba, which is both accessible and photogenic, suggests that endocytosis is discriminatory and that there is something of the gourmet about cells that partake in this way. The amoeba will not drink plain water or water to which sugar or other carbohydrate has been added, but when given protein, or amino acids and salts, all restraint is lost. The amoeba becomes an unabashed glutton, drinking to exhaustion and consuming within 30 minutes an amount equivalent to 25 percent of its total mass. The exhaustion is not fatigue on the part of the cell but rather the depletion of available membrane for invagination (Holter, 1961). The ability of certain substances to induce endocytosis, or the predilection of the membrane for these substances, may be presumed to be due to an affinity or binding between the substance and the membrane. This first step appears to be the essential prelude to consumption and may, indeed, be an important *mechanism of cell nutrition* as suggested by Lewis in 1931 when he first observed the process and coined the term *pinocytosis* to describe it.

Bulk transport occurs also in reverse, not into but out of cells. Evidence is accumulating that secretion from endocrine as well as exocrine and nerve cells occurs by the process called *exocytosis* or *emiocytosis*. Morphological evidence for this process was difficult to obtain in thin electron micrograph sections, but recently use of the freeze-fracture technique has shown the extent of exocytosis in stimulated cells of the adrenal medulla. Visual evidence of attachment and fusion to the plasma membrane followed by extrusion of vesicle contents and retrieval of vesicle membrane has been obtained (Smith et al., 1973). A similar series of events on the cell surface of the stimulated β cells of the pancreas has indicated that this is also the means for insulin release (Orci et al., 1973), although the authors do not rule out the possibility of other mechanisms as well leading to concomitant release of the hormone.

An important step beginning to be investigated is the mechanism that permits fusion between pinocytotic vesicles and plasma membrane but prevents fusion between intracellular membrane-bound organelles and the membrane. This mechanism is being studied in endothelial cells and applies also to exocytotic vesicles. Dempsey et al. (1973) present evidence which suggests that the polarity of the vesicle membrane may lead to its preferential fusion with the plasma membrane. Some means of recognition of the desired direction of membrane traffic is, of course, of fundamental importance to the cell and the organism of which it is a part.

Communication Between Cells

Cells functioning together as part of an organized tissue are joined through the membrane junctional complexes described under the section entitled "Structure." The junctional complexes were originally thought to be solely for the purpose of adhesion and organization of the independent cellular units, areas containing the hypothetical intercellular cement. The junctional complexes are, instead, important functional areas in a tissue. Sections of the junctional complex have been found to effectively seal off certain areas of membrane and to provide a means for intercellular communication through other areas.

The *zona occludens* (see Fig. 9.13) provides a strong and effective seal between adjacent cells and between the lumen and the intercellular space. In the intestinal tract this zone effectively seals off the lumen and prevents its contents from mixing with the intercellular fluid. It provides high resistance to water flow but very low resistance to the lateral flow of ions and, therefore, does not act as a barrier to electrical potential. In fact, the lack of polarization and the low resistance to the lateral flow of ions at these tight junctions causes the cells to be electrically coupled (Loewenstein and Kanno, 1964; Loewenstein et al., 1965). As far as electric charges are concerned, the connected cells in the tissue act like one huge cell whose exterior is the membrane of the entire group of cells except where they are coupled at the tight junction sites. This means of coordinating the cells and transmitting the action potential from cell to cell by an electrical coupling becomes extremely important in the function of certain tissues such as cardiac muscle. In the absence of these tight junctions, cell membranes are polarized and insulated from one another as far as electrical currents are concerned. Bennett (1973), however, suggests that neither the desmosome nor the *zona occludens* are responsible for electrical coupling between cells. He suggests that intercytoplasmic channels form in junctional regions and that formation and separation of the junctions are physiological processes under cellular control.

The desmosome that is separated from the *zona occludens* by the *zona adherens* forms another seal. This one, however, provides only localized restriction to diffusion. The cells at this point are not in direct contact although there is the suggestion that fibril bridges may cross the intercellular space to permit some ion communication as in the *zona occludens.* The function of the desmosome appears to be primarily to promote strong adhesion.

The area that permits real communication of cell contents among the cells comprising the epithelial tissue is the *zona adherens* or the intermediate zone. Molecules at this part of the junctional complex pass from cytoplasm of one cell to that of the next. Each individual cell functions along with all the others as a unit. As described by Palay (1967): "The cells, more or less alike and bound together by the junctional complexes...carry out similar functions, each unit repeating what its neighbors do with the monotonous regularity required by the functions of the epithelium as an organ." This means of communicating makes the group of cells a coordinated tissue rather than a collection of isolated and individual units.

An interesting observation reported by Loewenstein and Kanno (1967) was that growth-controlling substances appeared to be transmitted through junctions in normal tissues but that no communication was detectable among certain types of cancer cells or between cancer and normal cells. This suggests that communication through junctional complexes has an unusual potential in developmental processes where information concerning a cell community's finite number, shape, and position of cells must be conveyed (Loewenstein, 1970). Currently, the production of defective junctional connections with the consequent noncoupling and uncontrolled growth as a result of a genetic defect is being investigated (Loewenstein, 1973).

Although the mechanisms of junctional communication are far from clear, the concentration of calcium ions appears to play a role. Junctional communication appears to be due to the high concentration of calcium ions in the extracellular fluid and the low concentration of calcium ions in the cytoplasm (Loewenstein, 1970). An increase in permeability at a junction is associated with the removal of the normal calcium gradient between the outer and inner surfaces of the membrane at the junction site since the outer surfaces of the two opposing membranes are no longer in contact with the extracellular fluid.

Specialization and Control

Function in all cell membranes depends on the structural characteristics that determine the selectivity of the membrane. The passage of materials into and out of the cell is coordinated with the activity of the cell and of the organelles within it. For example, specialized membrane receptors provide the thyroid cell with a special affinity for iodine; liver and fat cells for insulin; ileal cells for the vitamin B_{12}-IF complex. In the lumen of the small intestine the glycocalyx of cell membranes is provided with disaccharidases, dipeptidases, and a variety of other enzymes synthesized within the cell that are important in the membrane phase of digestion (see Chapter 6). In other words, the membrane structure and function depend on the synthetic capacities of the cell, and the synthetic capacities of the cell, in turn, depend on membrane structure and function. Understanding of the interrelated dependence of cellular function and membrane integrity helps to clarify the far-reaching effects of specific nutrients.

Cells that are sensitive to and respond to stimuli evoked by hormones, metallic ions, or other specific molecules must be recognized by the stimulatory agent and then must interact with it to initiate a specific sequence of events. In the case of insulin, the "receptor" is comprised of molecules not only capable of recognizing insulin but also possessing the ability to convey the existence of the "recognition" to other structures and thereby eliciting a biologically significant event (Cuatrecasas, 1973). Such a receptor for insulin has been located on the surface of the membranes of both liver and fat cells. This receptor responds to insulin exclusively and leads to the specific insulin effect evoked in that cell. The precise effect

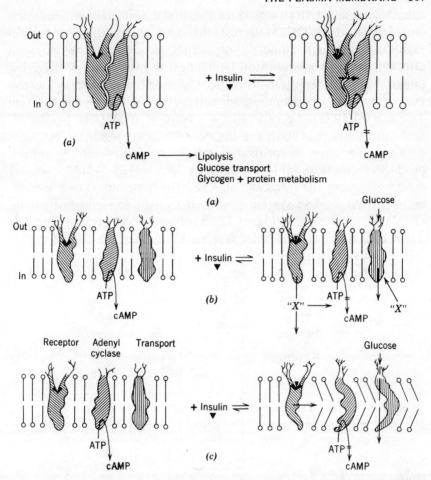

Fig. 9.21 Schematic representation of three possible mechanisms by which insulin exerts its effects on (*a*): adenylate cyclase activity (changes in adenyl cyclase basic to all metabolic effects); (*b*): transport processes, production of chemical mediator "*X*" (from endogenous membrane substrates or ATP, can modulate different processes); and (*c*): other metabolic events in the cell (many membrane-localized functions modified independently). [From P. Cuatrecasas, *Fed. Proc.*, 32: 1838 (1973).]

is suggested to be the result of conformational changes in membrane molecules brought about by the interaction of insulin and receptor. Fig. 9.21 suggests three ways in which insulin at the receptor site leads to a change in membrane conformation which, in turn, influences adenyl cyclase activity to produce the effect. Similarly, evidence presented by Rodbell (1973) suggests that a membrane receptor for glucagon acts through allosteric regulation to produce the glucagon effect. The hormone-receptor interaction is envisioned as triggering one or more allosteric transformations of membrane proteins thereby leading to the activation of adenyl cyclase in the membrane (see Tepperman, 1973). According to the concept enunciated by Sutherland and Robison (1966), the hormone, or first messenger, interacts with a membrane receptor to stimulate adenyl cyclase which, in turn, produces an increase (or in some cases a decrease) in cAMP, or second messenger, from the intracellular ATP. The basic model of the membrane adenyl cyclase system proposed by Robison and Sutherland (1971) is presented in Fig. 9.22. Receptors incorporated into the plasma membrane on its outer face are subunits of the adenyl cyclase enzyme system. The associated catalytic subunit extends to the inner surface of the membrane. These two subunits, the regulator and the

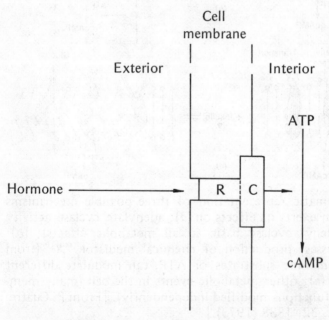

Fig. 9.22 Model of the membrane adenyl cyclase system showing the relationship between the regulatory (R) subunit and the catalytic (C) subunit of the protein component. [From G. A. Robison and E. W. Sutherland, *Ann. N. Y. Acad. Sci.*, 185: 5 (1971).]

catalyst, provide a model for the multitude of regulatory functions performed by cAMP and provides also for the diversity of these functions from tissue to tissue and cell to cell. The effect elicited depends not only on the hormone that initiates the response by interacting with the membrane receptor but also on the effect that such an interaction propagates through the membrane that determines the cAMP response within the cell. For a review of the versatility of responses evoked by cAMP, see Jost and Rickenberg (1971); Robison et al. (1971).

It is the fluid, dynamic, ever-changing membrane that has the capacity to retain its own integrity, specificity, and unique characteristics that is responsible not only for the cell it surrounds but also for the widespread effects that radiate to the total organism. In some cases an obvious relationship exists: a membrane enzyme such as lactase is defective or missing from the intestinal mucosal cell membrane; or an unresponsive insulin receptor in the fat cell membrane prevents glucose entry into the cell (see Chapter 20). In other cases the relationship may be less clear, perhaps merely suspected; in still other instances, not even suspected. However, it is obvious that a nutrient or metabolite cannot influence the course of cell metabolism nor the cell influence the metabolism of the total organism if the gates to the arena are barred.

SUMMARY

The discriminatory role the plasma membrane plays is not only the basis for the very existence of the cell, its uniqueness and individuality, but for whatever specialized capabilities it may possess. The membrane is, of course, a product of the genetic endowment of the cell: its structure depends on molecular syntheses within the cell, its function on the specificity of the carriers it synthesizes. The exquisitely engineered membrane becomes dynamic only by being coordinated with intracellular activity. An adequate supply of nutrients in the environment of the cell insures adequate nutrition only if the molecules presented to the membrane can be selectively transported. The selectivity demands syntheses that fall within the scope and control of nuclear and ribosomal activity and availability of high energy phosphate that the mitochondria have trapped in

ATP in the course of intermediary metabolism. The integration of structure and function and of syntheses and degradations in the single-celled independent organism or in a single cell of the liver, intestine, muscle, or gland of a complex mammal are all inextricably linked to the plasma membrane.

chapter 10
the nucleus

1. **Structure and Composition**
   a. Nuclear Membrane or Nuclear Envelope
   b. Nucleolus
   c. Chromatin
   d. Nuclear Matrix

2. **Function**
   a. Replication
      1. Mutation
      2. Repair Synthesis
   b. Transcription
      1. Regulation of Gene Action
      2. RNA Synthesis
   c. Reverse Transcription
   d. Nuclear Protein Synthesis

3. **Conclusion**

The nucleus is the keeper of the keys to the cell's genetic archives. It is within the nucleus that the plans for construction of all of the cell's proteins are filed in the form of deoxyribonucleic acid (DNA), which the nucleus can duplicate for the endowment of daughter cells and for the continuity of the species. It can also transcribe this genetic information into ribonucleic acids (RNA) that, acting as emissaries from the nucleus, appear in the cell matrix and translate the message into cell protein. Since all cellular function depends on enzyme systems, and since enzymes are proteins, it is obvious that the life of the cell and of the species depend on this nuclear capability.

When the nucleus was first observed by early cytologists, the christening was probably easy since it was usually in the central part of the cell, surrounded by the rest of the cellular material. As observations on the cell became more detailed, the early cytologists as well as today's molecular biologists surely agree that the name *nucleus* was prophetic. As we observe it today, the nucleus may not fulfill the original geometric conditions of location; but of far more consequence is the applicability of the name to the central and coordinating role played by the nucleus in the organization, operation, and perpetuation of the cell. The nucleus is, indeed, the central part of the cell and, as such, central to its life. The cell without a nucleus is in even worse straits than the proverbial ship without a rudder. At least the ship can survive, albeit without direction, if the environmental conditions are favorable. The cell without a nucleus, in the most favorable of environments, will slow down and die.

The nucleus of the cell was at first thought to contain all of the DNA which was replicated during cell division, thereby insuring continuation of its kind. It is now apparent that some genetic material resides in the mitochondria as mitochondrial DNA. The significance and function of this DNA which apparently is specific for certain mitochondrial coding will be discussed in Chapter 13. Nuclear DNA however can still be considered the repository for the information required for the preponderance of protein syntheses. It is protein synthesis upon which, ultimately, all other cellular reactions depend, since cellular reactions require enzymes, and enzymes are proteins. The coded information in DNA reproduced in the form of RNA for transmission to the cytoplasm is the prerequisite of protein synthesis. The miniaturization of the mechanism is apparent from the calculation that the DNA containing all of the genetic information of mankind would weigh roughly 20 mg (Dobzhansky, 1964).

The replication of DNA and its transcription into RNA require, in addition to specific enzymes, the presence of the nucleotide components of these complex, yet so simple, polymers. The cell can synthesize the fundamental ring structure of the purines and pyrimidines from simple sources of carbon and nitrogen. These are joined with the sugar and phosphate to make the nucleotides of the nucleic acids. It is this stroke of synthetic genius that permitted life to evolve on this planet.

STRUCTURE AND COMPOSITION

The structure of the nucleus refers to what can be seen; the composition to what can be separated out and analyzed. Integration of these procedures at micro- and ultramicrolevels has been the means of probing into the nucleus.

The size of the nucleus varies with cell type and function. For example, the nucleus of liver cells constitutes 10 to 18 percent of cell mass, whereas the nucleus of the sperm cell is almost the entire cell. The nucleus also varies with the stage in the cell's life cycle. Every cell has essentially two periods: *interphase,* the period of nondivision; and *division,* which produces two daughter cells. The cycle is repeated each cell generation, but the length of the cycle varies greatly among cells. Some cells such as the intestinal mucosal cells have a very short life span and others, like the nerve cell, may have a life span that matches that of the organism. For details of the changes that occur in nuclear structure and composition during division, see DeRobertis et al. (1970); Geise (1973).

Most cells are mononucleate, but there are binucleated cells such as some liver and some cartilage cells, and polynucleated cells such as the osteoclasts (see Chapter 17). Certain tissues appear as a large protoplasmic mass called *syncytium* in which cell boundaries are not apparent and the nuclei are extremely abundant. Striated muscle is such a tissue (see Chapter 18). The location of the nucleus in the geometric center of the cell occurs only in embryonic cells. As differentiation takes place, the nucleus assumes a characteristic position for the type of cell; in gland cells, for example, the nucleus is located in the basal portion of the cell.

The structures visible in the nucleus vary with the type of cell, the preparation of the specimen and the magnification. Generally, in electron micrographs the following are visible: (1) A *nuclear membrane* or *nuclear envelope,* which provides a clear demarcation on both the nuclear and cytoplasmic sides. (2) *Nucleoli,* which are spheroidal bodies, often quite large, and often multiple, which are regions of condensed chromatin that vary in ribonucleoprotein content and, therefore, in prominence in stained preparations.

(3) *Chromatin*, which is in the form of filaments distributed throughout the nuclear sap and in clumps near the nuclear envelope in the interphase nucleus. It is composed of deoxyribonucleoproteins and is the material that forms the chromosomes during division. (4) The *nuclear sap* or *nuclear matrix*, which fills the space between other nuclear components.

Nuclear Membrane or Nuclear Envelope

The nuclear envelope is revealed through electron microscopy as two concentric membranes separated by the perinuclear space. Most descriptions of the membranes have indicated their similarity to other cellular membranes (Franke, 1966). Many electron micrographs suggest a globular organization of the membranes that can be understood in terms of current membrane theories (Hendler, 1971). The membranes that make up the nuclear envelope appear to be dynamic structures intimately involved in exchange of information between nucleus and cytoplasm. The arrangement provides continuity of the channel between the two nuclear membranes with those of the endoplasmic reticulum (see Chapter 11). In this way, materials in the extracellular environment can enter, pass through the channels of the endoplasmic reticulum, and reach the envelope surrounding the nucleus. It would therefore be possible to obtain entry to the nucleus without passing through the cytoplasmic matrix. It is conceivable that certain materials denied transport through the plasma membrane may reach and be selectively absorbed through the specialized nuclear membrane.

Fusion of the inner and outer membranes of the nuclear envelope occurs at irregular intervals forming *nuclear pores*. The number of pores varies with the species and cell type and may account for 10 to 30 percent of the envelope. According to Franke and Scheer (1970a; 1970b) a universal structure exists for the pore complex (Fig. 10.1). This pore complex model consists of a ringlike structure, the *annulus*, plus the pore itself around which are spaced eight or nine granules on both the nuclear and cytoplasmic sides. One to three central granules of variable shape and dimensions appear to be in the process of going through the pore, and Franke (1970) has interpreted this to mean that the central granules are ribonucleoprotein particles and, if so, are not structural components of the

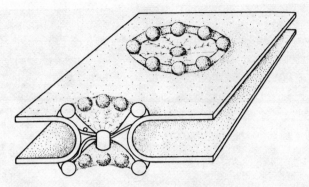

Fig. 10.1 Diagrammatic representation of the pore complex. [From W. W. Franke, *A. Z. Zellforsch.*, 105:405 (1970) in C. M. Feldherr, *Adv. Cell Molec. Biol.*, 2:273 (1972).]

nuclear pore. Models of the pore complex have also been proposed by Gall (1967) and Vivier (1967) among others.

The suggestion has been made that the pores do not provide for free communication between the nucleus and cytoplasm and Afzelius (1955) suggested that the annulus might function as a diaphragm. The presence of a structural element on the inner surface of the nuclear envelope led Fawcett (1966) to suggest that this was a lid or diaphragm with an easily discernible flange (Fig. 10.2). Such covered pores would not act as fixed canals but, it is presumed, would react to conditions on either side of the membrane and thus be involved in nucleocytoplasmic exchanges. The dense areas of chromatin near the nuclear envelope with distinct interchromatin channels leading to the nuclear pores also suggest an arrangement for exchange between the nucleus and the cytoplasm.

For further details on the nuclear envelope, see Feldherr (1971) and Wischnitzer (1974).

Nucleolus

The nucleolus is readily observable, even by light microscopy, as a dense area within the nucleus. However, there was little information assembled concerning the nucleolus until the 1960s when improved fixation and embedding techniques permitted better preservation of ultrastructure and analysis of nucleolar organization. It was found

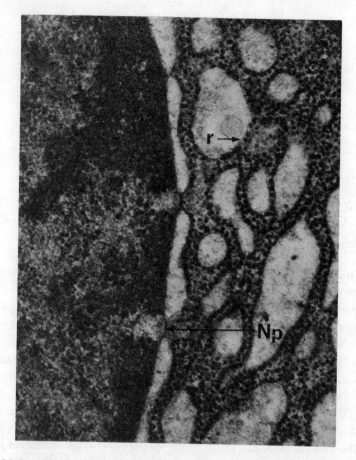

Fig. 10.2 Nuclear pores (Np) between nucleus and endoplasmic reticulum containing ribosomes (r). Pancreatic acinar cell from rat. Magnification 59,000. (Courtesy of Dr. Harald Schraer).

that the architecture of the nucleolus varied with the physiological state of the cell and with cell type. Detailed observation with the electron microscope reveals that this dense structure has no membrane to separate it from the rest of the nucleus (Fig. 10.3). There is therefore no barrier limiting the interactions between the nucleolus and the other nuclear material.

The nucleolus is not visible during certain stages of cell division but, when division is completed, it is reformed by an organization of materials that appear to be closely associated with the chromo-

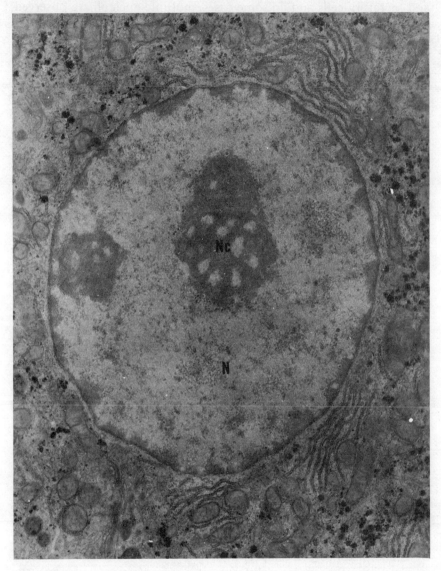

Fig. 10.3 Dense area of nucleolus (Nc) within the nucleus (N). Nuclear membrane separates nucleus from cytoplasmic material but no membrane separates nucleolus from the rest of the nucleus. Mouse liver cell. Magnification 11,600. (Courtesy of Dr. Harald Schraer.)

somes. It is conspicuous in highly active cells such as nerve cells and secretory cells and, in some cases, multiple nucleoli are observed. The nucleolus contains fine coiled material in an amorphous background.

Four principal components of the nucleolus have been recognized: (1) a network of closely packed fibrils, (2) granules along and between the strands of the fibrillar network, (3) amorphous matrix material, and (4) nucleolar-associated chromatin surrounding the nucleolus (see Bernhard and Granboulan, 1968). It was shown that the nucleolar fibrils and granules contained RNA, and that these RNA fibrils represented the origin of the ribonucleoprotein (RNP) granules, precursors of ribosomal RNA (rRNA). The actual migration of RNP particles into the cytoplasm has not generally been observed in the pores although Franke (1970) suggested this as part of his model. Nucleolar proteins make up the amorphous matrix within the nucleolus, and studies with ^{3}H-leucine indicate that the synthesis of these proteins takes place in the nucleolus. Their chemical nature, however, has not been clarified. The nucleolar-associated chromatin and the intranucleolar chromatin form a single system, and the indications are that a very large quantity of nucleolar DNA could operate as a template for nucleolar RNA synthesis. All biochemical, genetic, and cytological findings agree that the nucleolar RNA is the precursor of the rRNA; and it is generally believed that the nucleolus is the locus where very active RNA synthesis from a DNA template takes place with the resulting accumulation of ribosomes as a visible electron-dense mass.

Chromatin

Chromatin is a complex structure that contains, in addition to DNA, large amounts of histone and nonhistone proteins and small amounts of RNA (Stein et al., 1974). It is packaged as distinct bodies in the nucleus called chromosomes. (For a review of the structure of both DNA and histones, see Chapter 2.)

The total chromosomal DNA of any cell is its *genome*. The amount of DNA is constant in all diploid cells of the individual and for the species since the DNA is related to the number of chromosome sets in the nucleus. Therefore, determination of the total DNA content permits calculation of the number of nuclei in a

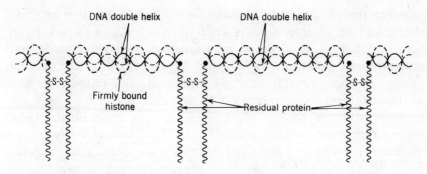

Fig. 10.4 Schematic diagram of model proposed for structure of chromosomal fibers. The number of peptide chains in residual protein is not known; the minimal requirement of 2 is shown in this diagram. [From A. L. Dounce and C. A. Hilgartner, *Exper. Cell Res.*, 36: 228 (1964).]

given tissue (see Chapter 21). This calculation does not hold for cells containing two or more nuclei; in most cases, however, it can be used for the number of cells. The weight of the nucleus can be calculated from the total weight of the tissue divided by the number of nuclei. The weight per nucleus varies with cell size and can be used, therefore, as a means of distinguishing *hypertrophy*, increase in cell size, from *hyperplasia*, increase in cell number.

The *genes* are functionally defined segments of the DNA molecule that code for specific polypeptide chains. Most genes contain from 600 to 1800 nucleotides which would code for 200 to 600 amino acids in a polypeptide chain. In a chromosome, the distance between one gene and the next may be very short, perhaps only a few nucleotides. The evidence is strong that adjacent genes in a chromosome are related in function; however, they are not necessarily arranged according to the order in which the respective enzymes participate in a biosynthetic pathway.

The proposed model for the chromosome fiber (Fig. 10.4) according to Dounce and Hilgartner (1964) depicts units of residual protein alternating with units of DNA. The *residual protein* is what is left in the nucleus after removal of globulins and loosely bound histones. Each unit of DNA is attached at both ends to the residual protein except where a DNA unit might happen to lie at the end of the structure (Hilgartner, 1968). The DNA-residual *linkers* join together the cellular chromosomes into a long chain forming fibers that could be of super lengths when uncoiled. Dounce's linker concept is based on evidence of gel formation by isolated nuclei and chromosomes (Dounce, 1971), and he suggests that the residual protein is responsible for the gel formation. The residual proteins of Dounce and Hilgartner (1964) are also referred to as *acidic proteins* or *nonhistone chromosomal proteins.* Stein et al. (1974) suggest that these proteins interact with DNA and are the regulators of gene expression (see below). This protein component may account for 5 to 10 percent of the total protein content of the nucleus, and one of its striking properties is the extensive phosphorylation that it undergoes. More than 90 percent of the nuclear protein-bound phosphorus is associated with these nonhistone chromosomal proteins (Stein et al., 1974). The phosphorus is present mainly as the phosphorylated amino acid phosphoserine, which accounts for 20 percent of the amino acid residues (Kleinsmith and Allfrey, 1969).

Nuclear Matrix

Completely filling the space between the other components of the nucleus is what had been referred to as the nuclear sap or nucleoplasm. These are old terms that appear to have outlived their usefulness. They were a means of acknowledging that the space was occupied by a clear fluid or transparent gel in which the stainable portions of the nucleus were suspended. *Nuclear matrix* is probably a better term to identify this area that is occupied by dispersed chromatin and all the other soluble and insoluble materials essential for the activity of the nucleus. A great deal of activity must go on in this matrix, and it must account for the nuclear constituents revealed in chemical analysis that have not been assigned to known nuclear sites. For example, in addition to the residual protein that appears to be part of the chromosome structure, there are the enzymes that are also nonhistone proteins as well as loosely bound histones and other proteins. There is evidence that the nucleolus is implicated in histone synthesis (Birnsteil and Flamm, 1964), and that would necessitate the presence of specific enzymes as well as the essential substrates. A variety of enzymes have, in fact, been identified in the nucleus, and these could be components of the colloid matrix and participate in many of the nuclear synthetic activities. There are DNA polymerases, RNA polymerases, exonucleases, ligases, NAD synthetase, nucleoside triphosphatases, and various other enzymes concerned with purine and nucleoside metabolism as well as with protein metabolism.

In many of the types of nuclei studied, all of the enzymes necessary for glycolysis were present suggesting that the nucleus uses glycolysis as the main source of energy. Two substrate-linked oxidative phosphorylations that provide a source of nuclear ATP were identified, and a great increase in nuclear glycolysis was noted when nuclear activity increased. An unsuspected finding was a complete TCA cycle in calf thymus nuclei. Several enzymes and substrates in the TCA cycle also have been isolated from nuclei of liver, kidney, and brain cells. Further, there is a high concentration of the pyridine nucleotide coenzymes, and the nucleus is the main site of NAD biosynthesis. In thymus nuclei, electrons are transferred from NADH or (NADPH) to flavin coenzymes. These cells appear to contain a complete cytochrome sequence and are also capable of aerobic phosphorylation. Evidence has been obtained as well for the presence of enzymes of the hexose monophosphate shunt (see Allfrey, 1970).

There is some speculation that ATP is transferred into the nucleus from the mitochondria since mitochondrial membranes and nuclear membranes have often been observed in very close proximity to each other. However, the ability of the nucleus to synthesize some of its own requirements locally is accepted.

Calcium and magnesium are both present in the nucleus. Calcium is firmly held to the protein, and magnesium appears to be bound to both DNA and a mononucleotide, probably at the phosphate groups. Sodium was thought at one time to be higher in concentration in the nucleus than in the cytoplasm (Naora et al., 1962) and to be actively transported across the nuclear envelope (Goldstein, 1964). However, recent evidence indicates that sodium concentration is higher in the cytoplasm than in the nucleus (Riemann et al., 1969; Century et al., 1970). It is generally assumed that the sodium in the nucleus enters as part of the active transport of amino acids through the nuclear membrane, a process that also requires ATP. The concentration of potassium also is higher in the nucleus than in the cytoplasm and may be related to a higher concentration of nuclear water (Horowitz and Fenichel, 1970). The high phosphate content of the nucleolus suggests that it may serve as the precursor of the RNA phosphorus (Tandler and Sirlin, 1962).

FUNCTION

It is fast becoming axiomatic that the replication of DNA in cell division is the basis for the continuity of the species. On cursory examination DNA replication does not appear to be of any concern to the nutritionist, although it is, of course, of primary concern to the species. Lederberg (1960) stated in his Nobel lecture, "If species are delimited by their genes, then genes must control the biosynthetic steps which are reflected in nutritional patterns." These nutritional patterns therefore reflect the limitations of the biochemical capability of the cell. In other words, genes dictate which substances the cell can synthesize for itself and which substances it must obtain from its environment as food. For example, all mammals with the exception of man, monkey, and the guinea pig have the capacity for synthesizing ascorbic acid and therefore do not require a dietary source. Man, monkey, and the guinea pig, in the course of evolutionary development, have lost this capability and, for them, ascorbic acid is an essential nutrient.

Of extraordinary interest is the fundamental similarity in nutrient needs among all living cells, and this similarity far overshadows the differences. But, as for all characteristics and attributes, the differences among species and individuals provide the spice. It was the observation and study of the differences in nutrient needs of strains of red bread mold, *Neurospora*, that opened up the entire field of biochemical genetics. Whereas nutritionally speaking, there is little difference among molds and mice and men, both scientist and layman, for diverse reasons, can say *vive la difference!*

Biologists have long known that the nucleus contains the chromosomes and that the chromosomes contain the genes. It has also been known that there is a linear splitting of the chromosomes during cell division, providing each daughter cell with identical halves of the chromosome material. These established facts are compatible with more recently accumulated data and accompanying theory.

The ability of the double-stranded DNA polymer to replicate provides the way that the genetic information encoded in the cell

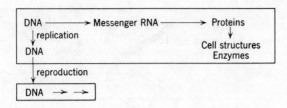

Fig. 10.5 Functions of DNA. (From A. Kornberg, 38th Priestley Lecture, p. 3.)

is divided and passed on to daughter cells during cell division, thereby providing for continuity of a species. However, this equal division of the parental genetic legacy is negotiable only if the coded message it contains can be transcribed into a form that can be used in protein synthesis. The transcription is carried out in the nucleus through the synthesis of the several forms of RNA: messenger RNA (mRNA), ribosomal RNA (rRNA) and transfer RNA (tRNA). These molecules leave the nucleus for the endoplasmic reticulum where they are finally translated into polypeptide chains (see Chapter 11). Fig. 10.5 indicates these fundamental functions of DNA.

Replication

The Watson-Crick model of the double helical structure of DNA provided a neat means of postulating replication since the two strands were complementary; separation of the strands would permit each to attract a complementary strand resulting in two daughter DNA molecules (Fig. 10.6). Each of the new molecules would then contain one of the parental strands. This is referred to as *semiconservative replication*, and was proved to be the means of replication by Meselson and Stahl (1958). One would assume that this was what occurred in mitosis when each of the chromosomes was observed to split longitudinally to form two chromatids, which in turn became the chromosomes in the daughter cells, each identical to the parental chromosomes.

Several problems arise concerning the mechanism of replication. The manner in which the parent strands go through the process of sequential unwinding and rewinding of the helix about each other during replication is still not clear. DuPraw (1970b) has estimated

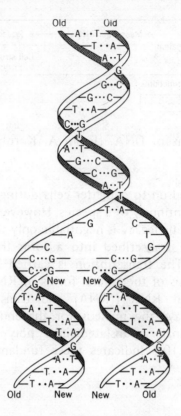

Fig. 10.6 The replication of DNA. (From J. D. Watson, *Molecular Biology of the Gene,* 2nd ed., W. A. Benjamin, N. Y. 1970, p. 267.)

that the 1000 μ-long DNA molecule of *E. coli* has approximately 300,000 twists, and since it replicates in 30 minutes it must participate in an untwisting process that can operate continuously at 10,000 rpm! Evidence to date appears to indicate that the unwinding of the parent strands and the rewinding of the daughter strands occur simultaneously forming a *replication fork* in which all three strands are spinning rapidly along their own axes, the unwinding in front and the rewinding following.

A problem in DNA replication not covered by the Watson-Crick model arose from the fact that DNA polymerase functions in polymerization only in one direction, from the 5′ end to the 3′ end. When the strands unwind, the 5′ end of one is opposite the 3′ end of the other, and the question of how both chains could be replicated simultaneously presented a problem. The observation of numbers of DNA fragments in rapidly growing *E. coli* cells suggested a means of simultaneous replication of the two anti-parallel strands (Okazaki, 1968). According to this model, one strand of the double helix is synthesized continuously in a 5' to 3' direction, but the other strand is synthesized in short segments that are later linked together. Support for this idea was provided by Sugimoto et al. (1968) who found that fragments accumulated in a mutant *E. coli* that had defective polynucleotide ligase. These findings, along with those of Kornberg (1969) that DNA polymerase binds duplex DNA only at nicks, led to the following model for DNA replication (Fig. 10.7) that involves three enzymes, DNA polymerase, DNA ligase, and an endodeoxyribonuclease, which operate as follows:

1. Replication starts when a nick is made in one strand of the duplex DNA by the action of the endonuclease.

2. DNA polymerase then catalyzes the addition of successive nucleotides to the one strand growing from the 5' to the 3' direction. The other antiparallel strand peels away.

3. After the DNA polymerase has catalyzed the addition of a number of nucleotides to the one chain it switches, or jumps, to the other strand at the fork where the two strands separate. The enzyme then proceeds to add nucleotides in the 5' to 3' direction down this strand until it is replicated.

4. The endonuclease then nicks the newly formed strand at the fork, and the polymerase proceeds up along the one strand and down the other as before.

5. A ligase joins the newly formed broken fragments on the loose template.

6. The entire process starts again with the endonuclease cleaving at the fork.

In this manner with three enzymes—an endonuclease, a polymerase, and a ligase—the DNA is replicated in successive stages, always in the 5' to 3' direction, first up along one strand and then down the other in repeating cycles.

For discussion of some of the complexities of the multienzyme systems involved in replication, see Schekman et al., (1974).

Mutations. Any mistake in the sequence of base pairing would be carried to the daughter cells and, if it were not a lethal mistake, would appear in all progeny. This is a mutation. Gene mutations

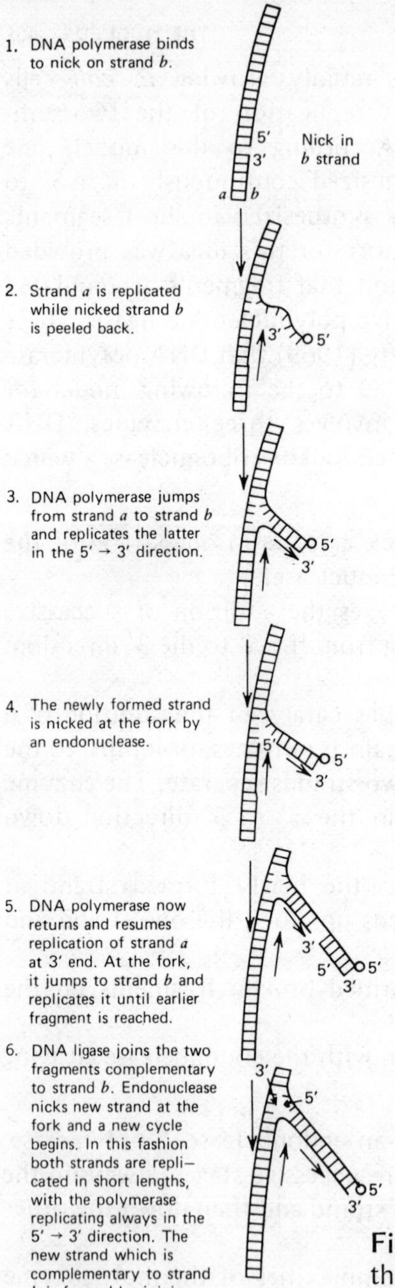

1. DNA polymerase binds to nick on strand *b*.

5'
3'   Nick in *b* strand
a   *b*

2. Strand *a* is replicated while nicked strand *b* is peeled back.

3'   5'

3. DNA polymerase jumps from strand *a* to strand *b* and replicates the latter in the 5' → 3' direction.

5'
3'

4. The newly formed strand is nicked at the fork by an endonuclease.

5'
5'
3'

5. DNA polymerase now returns and resumes replication of strand *a* at 3' end. At the fork, it jumps to strand *b* and replicates it until earlier fragment is reached.

3'
5'   5'
3'

6. DNA ligase joins the two fragments complementary to strand *b*. Endonuclease nicks new strand at the fork and a new cycle begins. In this fashion both strands are repli- cated in short lengths, with the polymerase replicating always in the 5' → 3' direction. The new strand which is complementary to strand *b* is formed by joining the fragments through the action of DNA ligase.

3'
5'
5'
3'

Fig. 10.7 Hypothesis of Kornberg for the replication of both strands of anti- parallel duplex DNA by DNA polymer- ase. (From A. L. Lehninger, *Biochem- istry*, Worth Publishers, 1970 p. 674.)

Normal sequence

Substitution of base pair

Deletion of base pair

Insertion of base pair

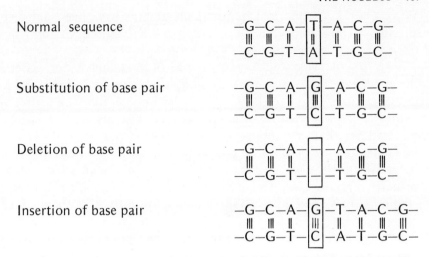

Fig. 10.8 Development of mutations due to changes in sequence of base pairing.

can also occur by substitution of nucleotide pairs, by deletion of one or more units, or by insertion of units (Fig. 10.8). In this way, the so-called inborn errors of metabolism arise and are transmitted.

Since the genetic code is read linearly starting from one end, either deletion or insertion of one or more nucleotides generally leads to completely nonfunctional genes. However, if there is substitution of a single nucleotide in the sequence, the result is referred to as a "leaky gene" in which the resultant mutant protein has partial enzymatic activity. There is no reason to believe that all nucleotide substitutions result in functional changes in the corresponding proteins (Yanofsky, 1967). It is the location of the substitution and consequently of the amino acid in the synthesized polypeptide that determines the effect. If the aberrant amino acid is at a critical point in the molecule, the resulting change in the properties of the polypeptide chain could lead to complete interference with the activity. Such a single nucleotide change resulting in the substitution of valine for glutamic acid in one of the chains of hemoglobin is responsible for sickle cell anemia. In this condition the characteristics of the molecule are so altered that the entire erythrocyte form is changed, and it is much less effective in transporting oxygen. Other changes in polypeptide sequence resulting from substitution of a single nucleotide in the gene coding for hemoglobin chains may or may not give rise to pathological conditions. Over 120 abnormal human hemoglobins have been detected through electrophoretic analysis but many show no deviation from normal functional properties.

All of the so-called inborn errors of metabolism, or genetic disorders, are the result of mutation, a change in the nucleotide sequence that is reflected in a changed polypeptide chain that is expressed as a defective or nonfunctional enzyme. It is a change at this level that is responsible for the occurrence of phenylketon-uria, hemophilia, albinism, and other known, inherited enzyme defects, as well as other disorders with heritable tendencies such as diabetes, certain cardiovascular disorders, pernicious anemia, hemo-globinopathies, and others. Spontaneous mutations probably take place frequently in all living cells, but only the indifferent or superior ones are likely to be retained. Stable inferior mutations are lost in natural selection, some being lethal mistakes. In addition, mutations may also occur as the result of high energy radiation and a variety of chemical agents that react with DNA (Auerbach, 1967).

Repair Synthesis. The chances that a mutation will occur are not nearly as impressive as the apparent stability of the DNA molecule. However, it is clear that changes in DNA have occurred that, along with natural selection, have led to evolutionary change. Without mutagenesis, evolution could not have occurred, and such a contingency would have eliminated this discussion. Genetic stability, then, is not the result of infallibility but the result of a fallible error-correcting mechanism, one that has permitted some "mistakes" to remain while others were corrected.

According to Hanawalt (1972), there are three ways in which an organism can respond to damaged DNA: (1) repair the damage *in situ;* (2) replace the damaged portion; or (3) bypass the damage. A specific type of repair process was discovered by accident follow-ing ultraviolet irradiation of bacteria. Ultraviolet light causes thymine dimers to be produced; that is, it causes fusion of two adjoining thymine molecules in the nucleotide chain. The discovery of a bacterial strain that was resistant to ultraviolet irradiation was the first inkling of a molecular mechanism for repair. Setlow and Carrier (1964) found that the resistant strain was able to release the dimers and this led to the repair model suggested by Pettijohn and Hanawalt (1964) called *excision repair* or, more familiarly, *cut and patch.* A model of the postulated steps in excision repair (Fig. 10.9)

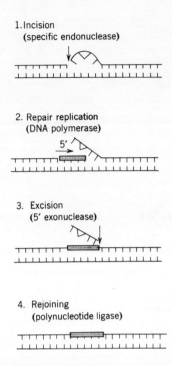

1. Incision
   (specific endonuclease)

2. Repair replication
   (DNA polymerase)

3. Excision
   (5′ exonuclease)

4. Rejoining
   (polynucleotide ligase)

Fig. 10.9 The postulated steps in excision repair. The repair patch is shown as a heavy line. The vertical arrows indicate the locations of nuclease cuts in the damaged parental strand and the horizontal arrow indicates the direction of repair replication, beginning at a 3′OH end of the parental strand. [From P. C. Hanawalt, *Endeavor*, XXXI(113): 83 (1972).]

involves a specific endonuclease, DNA polymerase I, and polynucleotide ligase, functioning as follows:

1. Upon recognition of the damaged DNA strand, a specific endonuclease makes an incision in the parent DNA strand.

2. DNA polymerase I, which possesses a 5′ to 3′ exonuclease activity, specifically releases the damaged or mismatched sequence from the DNA while concurrently adding nucleotides complementary to the good strand at the initial incision (Kelly et al., 1969).

3. Polynucleotide ligase forms the last 3′ to 5′ phosphodiester bond. (For discussion of the structure and function of DNA ligase in repair as well as replication see, Lehman (1974)).

1. Replication

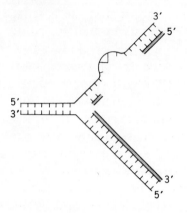

2. Recombination

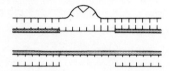

3. Gap filling
   (DNA polymerase and ligase)

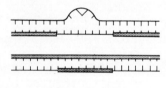

4. Result of next replication

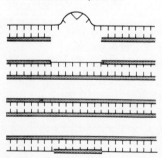

Fig. 10.10 A postulated model for postreplication recombinational repair. Normal replication proceeds, but leaves gaps opposite distorted regions of the parental strand. After replication the other parental strand provides the missing nucleotide sequence to fill the gaps. A DNA polymerase fills in gaps remaining opposite undamaged strands of either parental or daughter strands. Some of the double-strand templates for the next round of normal replication contain no damage. The damaged DNA strands are gradually "diluted out," but the damage is never removed from those strands. [From P. C. Hanawalt, *Endeavor,* XXXI (113): 83 (1972).]

Therefore, under the aegis of three enzymes, the damage is located, excised, and repaired. Cleaver (1968) has shown that the absence of the normal repair system in skin fibroblasts in man following ultraviolet irradiation is responsible for a type of skin cancer.

Another type of repair system, *genetic recombination,* was proposed by Rupp and Howard-Flanders (1968). This model suggests that gaps are left in daughter strands where dimers occur and replication proceeds again after the interruption. This leads to smaller strands (Fig. 10.10). The gaps are filled subsequently with the correct nucleotides "borrowed" from the other parental strand. These nucleotides join the smaller broken strands (Rupp et al., 1971). The dimer is not removed from the parent strand, and a similar correction is required each time around, but the corrected daughter strand each time serves as the template for replication. Hanawalt (1972) suggests that the same DNA polymerases may be used as in the excision-repair process.

Another type of repair that is rather like a "quality-control" has been postulated by Brutlag and Kornberg (1972). This may have an editing role *in vivo* by correcting base pairing errors produced in the course of normal replication. This repair mechanism has a 3' to 5' exonuclease that removes mismatched nucleotides from the 3' OH end of a growing DNA strand.

Transcription

The genetic information replicated by DNA to insure continuation of the species contains all of the specific information required by the cell for the synthesis of proteins. Since cell activity can function only in the presence and under the influence of the protein enzymes, the existence of the cell is dependent upon the transcription of the genetic code to a form that can direct protein synthesis. The formation of RNA fulfills this second fundamental function of the nucleus. The discharge of this function is dependent upon the translation of the four-letter code of polynucleotides into the 20-odd unit language of proteins. In this way RNA provides the link between the information coded in the DNA in the nucleus and the protein synthesis that takes place in the cytoplasm. The regulation and separation of the two kinds of DNA template activity is undoubtedly under the control of specific mechanisms, since they must and do occur at different times and therefore, one would guess, under different auspices. Only precise control, suavely administered, could prevent schizophrenic DNA.

The chemical similarity of RNA to DNA has been discussed in Chapter 2. Despite the differences that do exist, RNA molecules are also capable of forming complementary helical structures similar to those formed by DNA; however, most RNA exists as single polyribonucleotide strands. In mammalian cells about 10 percent of the cellular RNA is in the nucleus. Of this, about 20 percent is present in the dense nucleolar material and the remainder in the nucleoplasm or matrix. However, the quantity in a cell varies markedly with the condition of the cell and its nutritional state. For example, during starvation, when catabolic processes take precedence and protein synthesis is limited, nuclear RNA may be drastically reduced. This apparently is a result of the depressed activity of RNA polymerase observed in starvation (Onishi, 1970). It is generally found that cells active in protein synthesis have RNA-rich nuclei and those performing little synthetic activity have RNA-poor nuclei. Nuclear RNA has a high turnover rate and except for what is needed for the synthesis of nuclear protein, all the RNA molecules synthesized in the nucleus migrate to the cytoplasmic matrix.

Regulation of Gene Action.   Since the DNA of each cell in a multicellular organism appears to be the same, this means that various cell types use the information contained in this DNA differently. In fact, most of the DNA in the nucleus does not function in transcription, and much of the cell RNA is coded by less than one percent of the genome or chromosomal DNA. This includes both the rRNA and tRNA The amount of DNA that codes for mRNA and for other types of nuclear and cytoplasmic RNAs amounts to less than 5 percent of the cellular DNA. Therefore, most of the DNA of the genome is nonfunctional at a given time. Specific regulatory mechanisms must, therefore, be available for activating and inactivating particular regions of the genome for RNA synthesis depending on the requirements of the cell.

A model to explain the mechanism that promotes DNA transcription to a specific mRNA for subsequent protein synthesis

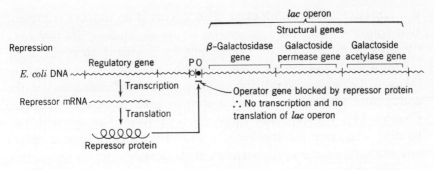

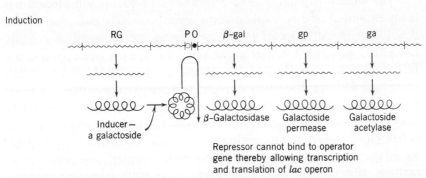

Fig. 10.11 Regulation of gene action as postulated by Jacob and Monod, illustrating repression and induction of enzyme synthesis by the lactose operon in E. coli. (From E. E. Conn and P. K. Stumpf, *Outlines of Biochemistry*, 3rd ed., Wiley, N. Y., 1972 p. 481.)

was proposed by Jacob and Monod (1961) and earned its originators a Nobel Prize in 1965. It is based on the concept of the *operon* that, together with a *regulatory gene,* an *operator,* and a *repressor protein,* can explain both induction and repression of mRNA synthesis (Fig. 10.11). The operon according to this model is a section of DNA consisting of adjacent and related genes that function together. These structural genes are responsible for transcription to mRNA and are under joint control of the operator and a regulatory gene. According to this model, the regulatory gene codes for the mRNA that is the template for the repressor protein. The repressor protein blocks the operator gene to prevent transcription of the structural genes. For induction of mRNA synthesis by the structural genes (leading, in turn, to induction of enzyme synthesis) the repressor must be blocked. This occurs if an inducer is present that combines with the repressor at a specific binding site to form a *repressor-inducer complex.* This complex is unable to bind to the operator and, therefore, transcription of the structural genes takes place and is normally followed by their migration to the endoplasmic reticulum for translation to specific polypeptides (see Chapter 11). The repressor molecule is envisioned as one with two binding sites, one for the inducer and one for the operator. When one site is filled, the other becomes inoperable.

The operon-regulator gene hypothesis of Jacob and Monod has been extended also to explain some aspects of differentiation during development. All cells of higher organisms are believed to contain the entire genome for that organism; that is, each cell contains the full book of genes, but much of the genome in any one cell is repressed. Differentiation is thought to take place by what is termed *programmed derepression* of different operons. This area of study has been named *epigenetics.* An example of programmed derepression is the rapid rise in lactase activity in the intestinal mucosa just prior to birth. Its fall in postweaning years is coupled with the rise in maltase and sucrase (see Chapter 6). The shift from the prenatal hemoglobin, Hb-F, to the adult form, Hb-A, is another example of programmed derepression. Each of the hemoglobin chains is under separate genetic control. During recovery from some types of anemia, there is temporary induction of Hb-F synthesis followed by its repression and the induction of Hb-A (see Chapter 16).

The mechanism for control in the regulation of transcription in the Jacob and Monod model is still largely conjectural. Histones have been reported to inhibit the ability of DNA to serve as a template for RNA synthesis (Huang and Bonner, 1962; Allfrey et al., 1963). The histones in the cell nucleus, present in the form of deoxyribonucleohistone complexes, have been implicated in the more permanent type of repressor in the nucleus that undergoes derepression primarily during differentiation. The fact that histones are not present in cells that do not differentiate and are conspicuous in cells that do, has suggested their implication in this process. Langan (1971) has suggested that a change in histone configuration is produced by its phosphorylation and this change is involved in the release of the histone from the DNA template followed by a

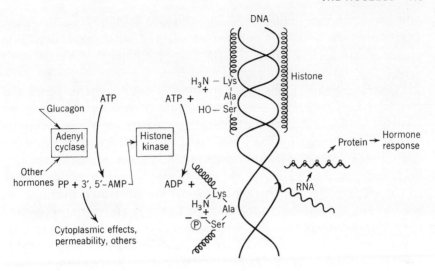

Fig. 10.12 Scheme for hormonal induction of RNA and protein synthesis. [From T. A. Langan, *Ann. N. Y. Acad. Sci.,* 185: 166 (1971).]

release in the repression it exerts. This, then, is followed by mRNA synthesis (Fig. 10.12).

There is also provocative evidence suggesting the intervention of nonhistone chromosomal proteins in the regulation of specific gene transcription. These proteins are made in the cytoplasm (Stein and Baserga, 1971) and are more actively synthesized and turned over than histones (Hancock, 1969; Holoubek and Crocker, 1969). Synthesis of specific classes of these nonhistone proteins is associated with the induction of gene activity (Teng and Hamilton, 1969). It has been established also that nonhistone chromosomal proteins interact with DNA and modify transcription in a way that is characteristic of the tissue from which they have been derived (Stein et al., 1974). They are highly heterogeneous and possess both tissue and species specificity. It was speculated originally that nonhistone chromosomal proteins displaced the inhibitory histones from the DNA-histone complex thereby permitting the DNA to become active as a template for RNA synthesis in a manner similar to the suggested role of phosphorylation of histones in the Langan model. More recently, it has been shown that histones stimulate the phosphorylation of the nonhistone chromosomal proteins (Kaplowitz et al., 1971). Stein et al. (1974) suggest that this could release histone from the DNA double helix thereby allowing gene transcription to take place.

One important unresolved question is how specific genes are recognized. A suggested possibility is that phosphorylation may be involved in the recognition of the promoter site for transcription, a function performed by the sigma factor associated with RNA polymerase (see following section on RNA synthesis). Sigma factor can be phosphorylated (Stein et al., 1974), but whether this is related to or dependent on the phosphorylation of either histones or nonhistone chromosomal proteins, or both, is entirely speculative. Nevertheless, it appears that the nonhistone chromosomal proteins play a role in the regulation of gene activation and that phosphorylation is somehow involved. What the specific mechanism is that initiates, modifies, or augments the transcription of specific mRNA molecules encoded in the cell's DNA is still far from clear. If phosphorylation does regulate transcription, then a major question is, what regulates the phosphorylation?

Mechanisms involving induction of enzyme systems at the level of mRNA translation into protein are discussed in Chapter 11.

RNA Synthesis. Synthesis of RNA is fundamentally very similar to the synthesis of DNA. Nucleotide triphosphates are the precursors, and the synthetic reaction is catalyzed by a single enzyme, RNA polymerase in the presence of Mg^{2+}, for all four possible nucleotides. Although only one of the two DNA strands is transcribed, double-stranded DNA is required as the template, and the synthesis of many RNA chains takes place simultaneously from a single gene. The base composition of the RNA is complementary to the DNA template with uracil as the complement to adenine instead of thymine as in DNA. RNA transcription is probably as accurate as DNA replication. However, if errors occur there is no need for correction since the mistake dies with the molecule; RNA is not self-replicating (see below for exception).

RNA polymerase, responsible for the synthesis of RNA from the DNA template, is a much more complicated enzyme than is DNA polymerase, which is a single polypeptide chain. RNA polymerase contains five different polypeptide chains with a molecular weight of over 500,000. For RNA polymerase to function properly

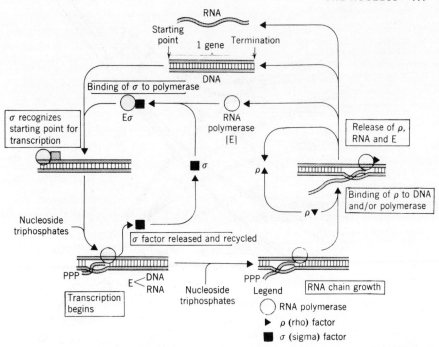

Fig. 10.13 RNA synthesis—outline diagram. (From J. D. Watson, *Molecular Biology of the Gene,* 2nd ed., W. A. Benjamin, 1970 p. 351.)

it must have associated with it the sigma (σ) factor. This factor is one of the polypeptide chains that readily dissociates from the rest of the enzyme after it has recognized the specific nucleotide sequence for starting an RNA chain. Speculation of how this recognition takes place was discussed in the preceding section. The released σ repeats its function with another core RNA polymerase. Synthesis of all chains starts with either adenine or guanine depending on the start signal in the DNA template. As in replication, transcription proceeds in the 5′ to 3′ direction. A stop signal at a specific nucleotide sequence identifies the conclusion of the chain that always ends with a triphosphate group. The stop signal is not part of RNA polymerase but is a separate factor called the rho (ρ) factor. How this factor operates also is not at all clear. A summary of RNA transcription is illustrated in Fig. 10.13.

It appears that there is but a single DNA-directed RNA polymerase for the synthesis of mRNA, rRNA and tRNA. These three RNAs

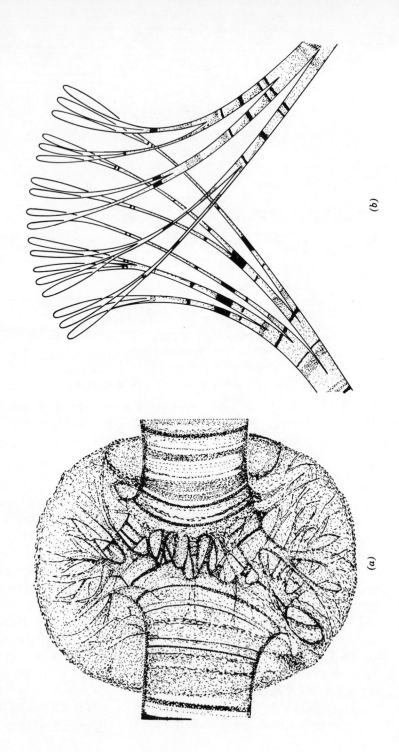

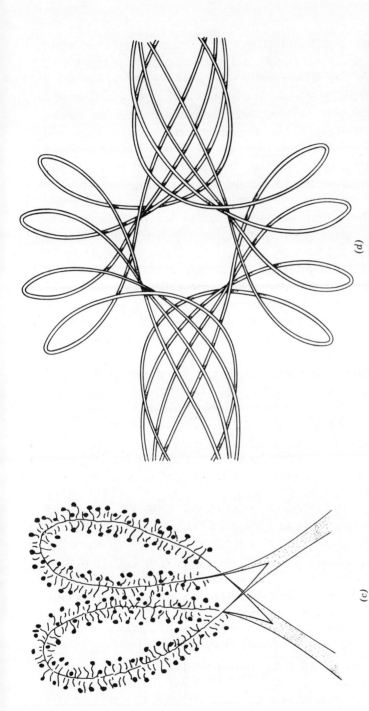

(c)

(d)

Fig. 10.14 (a) Structure of a large puff is diagramed. (b) A few of the fibrils at very high magnification in the light microscope. (c) The much greater magnification provided by the electron microscope shows two puff fibrils with granules that are believed to be messenger RNA produced by the genes. (d) Schematic representation of a large puff with fibrils untwisted. Those untwisted here are tightly coiled when in the form of bands. [Redrawn from W. Beerman and V. Clever, *Sci. Amer.*, 210: 4 (1964).]

are in reality three different classes of RNA since there are three types of rRNA, about 60 tRNAs and an extremely large number of mRNAs in every cell. Ribosomal RNAs, composed of a large and a small RNA molecule associated in the ribosomes with protein chains, contain approximately 6000 nucleotides compared to the tRNAs, which are the smallest of the natural nucleic acid molecules and contain some 80 nucleotides. Each of the tRNAs has a specificity for a given amino acid, and there is a similarity of structure and dimensions, the advantage of which becomes readily apparent as these molecules participate in protein synthesis. Messenger RNA, which carries the information from nuclear DNA to the protein-synthesizing ribosomes, is extremely variable in length since it takes three nucleotides for each of the amino acids in the chain to be synthesized. Rarely do polypeptide chains contain fewer than 100 amino acids, which means that mRNA molecules must contain at least 300 nucleotides and may contain far more. In addition, one mRNA frequently codes for the synthesis of several different poly-peptide chains with related functions, and the nucleotide count may go beyond 10,000.

The structural characteristics of each of the classes of RNA will be discussed in relationship to their function in Chapter 11.

Visualization of the process of RNA formation is possible in the giant chromosomes located in the giant cells of the salivary glands of the fruit fly Drosophila. These chromosomes are almost 100 times thicker and 10 times longer than chromosomes of typical cells. Beerman and Clever (1964) found puffs scattered along these chromosomes and found that puffing was associated with RNA production (Fig. 10.14). Edstrom and Beerman (1962) demonstrated that different puffs produced different kinds of RNA and that the RNA produced represented the activity of only one of the DNA strands. The biochemical activities associated with puff formation were studied through cytochemical and autoradiographic techniques. A clear association was established between a puff and a specific cellular product thus demonstrating that a definite relation exists between certain puffed genes and certain cell functions. Swelling or looping out of the puff appeared before RNA synthesis (Berendes, 1968) and was associated with the accumulation of acid proteins that were not synthesized in the puff. Later Stein and Baserga (1971) showed that synthesis of these proteins occurred in the cytoplasm. With the increase in acidic protein there was a relative fall in the basic histone although the ratio of histone to DNA remained constant. When RNA synthesis started, the puff attained maximum size. In some instances, the puff size was related to the amount of RNA that was synthesized.

The puffing of one strand of the DNA is interpreted as reasonable and visible evidence of mRNA synthesis (Beerman, 1964) since only one of the two possible RNA copies of the double-stranded DNA serves as a template. Movement of particles in the nuclear matrix has been observed. It is presumed that the particles carrying mRNA pass through the nuclear pores and, in association with the ribosomes that also are synthesized in the nucleus, participate in protein synthesis.

Reverse Transcription

The *central dogma* of molecular biology first formulated by Crick (1970) states that once information has passed into protein it cannot get out again; that is, genetic information can be transferred from DNA to DNA or from DNA to RNA to protein, but the reverse cannot take place. Work reported by Temin (1972) indicates that what had been referred to as *reverse transcription* can take place. Information can be transcribed from RNA into DNA. This occurs under the influence of *RNA-directed DNA polymerase.* The suggestion is that all DNA polymerases are capable, under appropriate conditions, of transcribing information from RNA into DNA. Temin (1972) suggests that this may occur in normal cellular processes such as those involved in embryonic differentiation of cells. He calls this the *protovirus hypothesis,* which states that there are regions of DNA in normal cells that serve as templates of RNA and that this RNA, in turn, serves as a template for the synthesis of DNA, which then becomes integrated with the cellular DNA. By this process certain portions of DNA become amplified and changes introduced into the DNA of some cells can be different from the DNA of other cells. This has been shown to occur in tumor-causing viruses but may have far greater implications.

Nuclear Protein Synthesis

In addition to the synthesis of DNA and the RNAs, the nucleus also synthesizes ATP and other nucleotide triphosphates, ribonucleoprotein, and various other proteins and enzymes. The histones, for example, which represent up to 32 percent of the nucleolar proteins, are reported to be synthesized in the nucleolus (Birnsteil and Flamm, 1964). In the sperm cell protamines are substituted for histones and these, too, may be synthesized in the nucleus. The details of protein synthesis will be discussed in Chapter 11 since the major portion of cellular protein synthesis occurs in the endoplasmic reticulum and the mechanisms in the nucleus are believed to be comparable.

CONCLUSION

The nucleus, separated from the cytoplasm of the cell by a double membrane, is the repository of the cell's genetic information, DNA. Replication of DNA is a prerequisite to cell division for it is only in this way that the encoded information which determines all the nuclear and cytoplasmic characteristics of the cell is made available to daughter cells for continuity of the cell species. Transcription of DNA to RNA translates the code to forms usable for protein synthesis in the cytoplasmic portion of the cell. The control over what the cell can synthesize determines what nutrients must be acquired from the environment.

The activities of the nucleus are continually dependent upon and responsive to the activities of the other organelles in the cell and upon the demands of the total organism and its environment. Allfrey (1970) points out that the scope of nuclear involvement and responsibility is slighted when it is simplistically stated that the nucleus is responsible for the DNA that makes RNA that makes protein.

chapter 11

the cytoplasmic matrix and endoplasmic reticulum

1. The Cytoplasmic Matrix or Ground Substance
2. Endoplasmic Reticulum
   a. Structure
   b. Composition
   c. Function
      1. Mechanical Support
      2. Transport and Exchange
      3. Protein Synthesis
         a. Genetic Code
         b. Punctuation
         c. The Adaptor Hypothesis
         d. The Ribosomes
         e. Building a Polypeptide

4. Regulation of Protein Synthesis
   a. Inhibition of Protein Synthesis
   b. Product and Feedback Inhibition
   c. Repression of Protein Synthesis
5. Glycolysis
6. Pentose Phosphate Shunt
7. Glycogenesis
8. Fatty Acid Synthesis
9. Synthesis of Unsaturated Fatty Acids
3. Conclusion

The endoplasmic reticulum is the complicated and organized system of membranes in the cytoplasmic area of the cell. It is sometimes called the "cytoskeleton" since it appears to be a structural arrangement providing a means of equilibration among the various parts of the cell and the genetic material of the nucleus. The cytoplasmic matrix, like a sea, is the continuous phase of the cell and holds within it or surrounds all the membrane-enclosed bodies in the cytoplasm including the endoplasmic reticulum, the mitochondria, lysosomes, and nucleus. In addition, there are lipid droplets, vacuoles, and the many dense particles rich in RNA, the ribosomes, which are closely associated with the continuous membranes of the endoplasmic reticulum. The endoplasmic reticulum and the surrounding matrix are not only areas for specific metabolic activities, but they also provide the means of communication among the external, nuclear, and organelle environments.

Light microscopy could give only the barest hints of the organization that was present in the cytoplasmic area of the cell. Although some structures had been identified, such as the Golgi apparatus and the mitochondria, the revelation of the complex organization of the cytoplasmic components of the cell awaited the development of the electron microscope. The reticular character of the endoplasmic portion of the cell was first noted by Porter et al. (1945) and they proposed that it be called the *endoplasmic reticulum.* Palade defined the endoplasmic reticulum and discovered the ribosome, the particle associated with it. For this work and his identification of the ribosome with protein synthesis, he was a Nobel prize recipient in 1974. This ramification of channels constituting the endoplasmic reticulum extends through the cell and is separated by the channel membrane from the continuous phase of the cell, the *cytoplasmic matrix* or *ground substance.* The cytoplasmic matrix is the environment that surrounds all of the organelles within the cell; it is the colloidal sea which supports them.

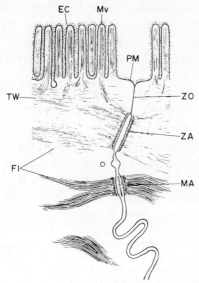

Fig. 11.1 Diagram of portion of cell showing fibrils in cytoplasmic matrix. EC, external coat; Mv, microvilli, PM, plasma membrane; TW, terminal web; Fl, filaments; ZO, zona occludens; ZA, zona adherens; MA, macula adherens. (From T. L. Lentz, *Cell Fine Structure*, W. B. Saunders Company, Philadelphia, 1971.)

THE CYTOPLASMIC MATRIX OR GROUND SUBSTANCE

The cytoplasmic matrix, the continuous phase of the cytoplasm, is the true internal environment of the cell. It appears homogeneous or finely granular, but the apparent lack of fine structure may be due only to the limitation of instruments and techniques. Light microscopy led to suggestions that the matrix contained filaments that showed parallel organization; these show plainly in electron micrographs. Such fibrillar structures appear to provide internal support for the cell and, according to Ham (1969, p. 182), could be an organelle, the *cell web*. The arrangement of the cell web varies with the cell, and in the intestinal epithelial cells appears to form a lacework of fine fibrils at the free border of the cell called the terminal web. The web seems to connect with the cell membrane all around the circumference of the cell. Intestinal epithelial cells also have long parallel arrays of fibrils in the terminal web (Fig. 11.1), and there is fibrillar material in the desmosomes and in other regions of the cell junctions. These fibrils all appear to be part of the internal support system in the cytoplasmic matrix and probably offer tensile strength. The fibrils associated with cell junctions are thicker and denser than those in either the microvilli or the terminal web.

Microfibrils also appear in many of the cells of the nervous system. In neurons they are seen in the cell body and coursing down into the axon in parallel clusters (see Chapter 19). The microfibrils appear to function as structural polypeptide chains that are held together by various cross-linkages. Changes in the characteristics of the chains and the linkages cause changes in the sol-gel relationships of this cytoplasmic colloid. For example, in the sol only loose and temporary bonds are formed and it is, therefore, liquid; whereas the gel is characterized by numerous stronger linkages between the polypeptide chains. Geise (1968, p. 102) suggests that the paradox of cytoplasm behaving like a liquid while displaying the structural properties suggestive of a solid scaffolding is best explainable on the basis of its being a colloid.

Intracellular movement or cytoplasmic streaming is part of the activity of all cells but to varying degrees. Endocytosis involves cytoplasmic movement, as does exocytosis; macrophages move with amoeboid motion; lysosomes and vacuoles approach and merge with each other. All these are examples of movement within the cell and within the cytoplasmic matrix. The microfibrils in the matrix are believed to be implicated in these and other kinds of movement. Contractile fibers are responsible for localized movement in the matrix; they are organized for the movement of cilia. Organization and specialization of microfibrils on a grander scale are observed in skeletal muscle (see Chapter 18).

The cytoplasmic matrix contains water, ions, and all the soluble nutrients, enzymes, and other proteins of the cell and, in addition, there are the inclusions containing stored nutrients such as glycogen and lipid. Since the density of the matrix from different cells is different, one can only conclude that the composition of the matrix varies and is related to the specialized structure and function of the cell. The cytoplasmic matrix, then, is the true internal milieu of the cell. It carries on its share of glycolysis and of biosyntheses and, in addition, provides the intimate environment of the channels and cellular organelles immersed in it.

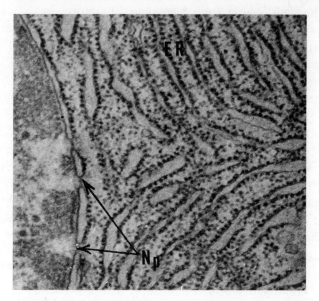

Fig. 11.2 Rough or granular endoplasmic reticulum (ER) showing dense granules of uniform size, the ribosomes, adhering to the outer surface. Continuity of the nuclear envelope with endoplasmic reticulum is clearly shown. Ribosomes also adhere to outer membrane of nuclear envelope. Pancreatic acinar cell from rat. Magnification 41,500. (Courtesy of Dr. Harald Schraer.)

ENDOPLASMIC RETICULUM

The channels comprising the endoplasmic reticulum (Fig. 11.2) are, in reality, part of the larger cytoplasmic vacuolar system that includes the nuclear envelope (see Chapter 10 and below) and the Golgi complex (see Chapter 12). This system, divided into compartments that can function independently, is a continuous system that synthesizes, circulates, and packages materials absorbed by the cell or synthesized within it.

The membranous channels constituting the endoplasmic reticulum occur in all cells of higher plants and animals with the exception of the mature erythrocyte, which has neither a nucleus nor endoplasmic reticulum. The complexity of the reticulum appears to vary directly with the degree of protein synthesis which takes place within the cells, being well developed, therefore, in secretory cells particularly in those secreting a protein-rich product. The absence of both the nucleus and endoplasmic reticulum in the erythrocytes readily explains the inability of these cells to synthesize enzymes since, with the lack of nuclear RNA and of the endoplasmic reticulum, both management and assembly line for protein synthesis are missing (see Chapter 16). The liver cell, in contrast, has a well-developed endoplasmic reticulum. The total surface of the endoplasmic reticulum contained in 1 ml of liver tissue has been calculated by Weibel et al. (1969) to be approximately 11 m^2, two-thirds of which is granular and one-third smooth (see Chapter 15).

Granular or *rough endoplasmic reticulum,* abundant in growing cells and in others engaged in protein synthesis, is easily recognized. Along the outer surfaces of the membranous channels facing the cytoplasmic matrix are dense particles of uniform size, the *ribosomes.* These may be arranged in close proximity to each other or may be spread out along the surface. The greater the protein synthetic activity, the denser the ribosomal population. It is this type of reticulum that forms the outer membrane of the nuclear envelope.

Agranular or *smooth endoplasmic reticulum,* as the name implies, does not have the ribosomal studding along the outer membrane and therefore gives a smooth appearance. In other respects it appears similar to the granular form and is continuous with it and with the Golgi complex. It is found (1) in cells that synthesize steroids, (2) in liver cells where it is associated with detoxification functions and with lipid and cholesterol metabolism, (3) in the small intestine where it is associated with lipid absorption and transport, and (4) in skeletal muscle where it participates in excitation-contraction coupling. The specialized endoplasmic reticulum in skeletal muscle is called sarcoplasmic reticulum and will be discussed in Chapter 18.

Structure

The endoplasmic reticulum is a membranous system of channels that leads from the plasma membrane to the nuclear membrane (Fig. 11.2). In a sense, it provides an extracellular environment deep within the structure of the cell and surrounding the nucleus, thereby providing a means of communication between the extracellular and intranuclear environments.

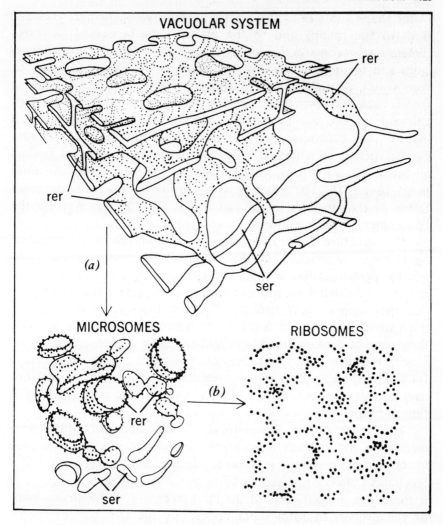

Fig. 11.3 Diagram of the vacuolar system with the granular (rer) and agranular reticulum (ser). (*a*) Microsomes, produced by homogenation; (*b*) free ribosomes, after membranes are lysed by detergent action. (From E. S. P. DeRobertis, W. W. Nowinski, and F. A. Saez, *Cell Biology*, 5th ed., W. B. Saunders Company, Philadelphia, Pa., 1970, p. 184.)

A three-dimensional view of the continuously folded membranous channels shows cavities of varying sizes and shapes appearing as vesicles and tubules and flattened sacs (Fig. 11.3). The variety in the shape and size of the areas enclosed by the membrane is due both to the folding and to the plane of the sectioning. A three-dimensional reconstruction of serial sections reveals the interconnections and tortuous winding of the channels. This should be easy to reconstruct mentally if one imagines a long piece of rubber tubing folded back and forth and placed in a box which is then cut through the middle. The cut tubing would appear as circles, ellipses, and long tubules, depending on the angle of the cutting edge. The picture can be further complicated by enclosing several lengths of tubing, all folded but all with one end at the edge of the box and the other in the center. This latter picture would probably be a closer representation of the channels in the cell and a better explanation for the appearance of tissue sections.

The structure of the endoplasmic reticulum can only be studied by electron microscopy of the intact cell. It cannot be separated out by centrifugation and subsequently studied as can certain of the other organelles because centrifugation breaks up the membranes and they appear as fragments. This fraction referred to as the microsomal layer is an artefact of homogenization and includes fragments of the endoplasmic reticulum, Golgi complex, and of the plasma membrane. In some cases the ribosomes are also part of the fraction although they can be separated out. Such preparations have been used extensively for biochemical studies of both composition and function.

The membrane of the endoplasmic reticulum, like the plasma membrane and all other membranes of the cell, was first described in terms of the unit membrane theory of Robertson (1959). Sjöstrand (1964) suggested that functional advantages would accrue if there was discontinuity in the lipid layer and in the arrangement of the protein to form septa connecting the two surface layers. Despite the teleological overtones, the discussion of membrane structure in Chapter 9 indicates that current models of membranes suggest such arrangements of the protein and lipid constituents. In the chapter on the Golgi complex, the membraneous system within the cell will be presented as a product of its own synthesis. It is subjected to modifications in composition and structure during the process of membrane flow (see Chapter 12).

In tissue sections the *nuclear envelope* appears as a large cisternal unit of the granular endoplasmic reticulum that sur-

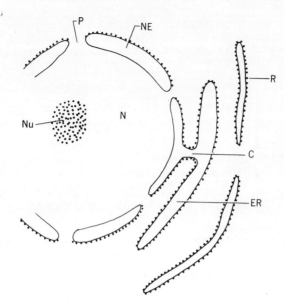

Fig. 11.4 Nuclear envelope (NE) showing nucleolus (Nu), pores (P), granular endoplasmic reticulum (ER) with ribosomes (R) attached, and channel (C) from nucleus (N) to ER. (Adapted from G. H. Haggis et al., *Introduction to Molecular Biology*, Wiley, N. Y. p. 145.)

rounds the nucleus and is separated from the nuclear membrane by a space that, according to Porter (1961b), resembles a moat. At intervals the inner and outer membranes are joined, forming pores (see Chapter 10) that are continuous with the cytoplasmic phase of the endoplasmic reticulum (Fig. 11.4). Some investigators suggest that the pore is an open structure permitting passage of molecules from the nuclear contents to the cytoplasmic matrix (Moses, 1964); and others, that it is plugged or covered (Merriam et al., 1961), but, one would presume, opened when traffic warranted. In the discussion on protein synthesis which follows, it is evident that mRNA, tRNA, and ribosomes must pass from within the nucleus to the cytoplasmic matrix. In the case of these and other macromolecules, the pores in the nucleus are likely to be the only pathway to the cytoplasm. Feldherr (1972) suggests that the annular material of the pore complex is able to limit the size of the particles that can penetrate and can also select and concentrate substances for passage. There is the possibility that this may be an energy-requiring process since Klein and Afzelius (1966) found that the pore complex material contained ATPase activity.

In addition to the emigration of molecules from the nucleus to the cytoplasmic phase of the cell, there would have to be passage of all of the nutrients required to support the major biosynthetic activities that occur in the nucleus from both the extra- and intracellular environments (see Chapter 10).

The channels of the endoplasmic reticulum from the plasma membrane to the nuclear envelope provide contact with the extracellular environment; the nuclear pores provide continuity with the cytoplasmic matrix. One must assume that two-way traffic prevails on both routes.

The suggestion has been offered that the endoplasmic reticulum may develop by evagination from the nuclear envelope (Porter, 1961b); however, there is evidence that the converse actually occurs, that the nuclear envelope is reformed after cell division by the vesicles of the endoplasmic reticulum (Barrer et al., 1959). Cytochemical study suggested the identical composition of these two membranes (Essner and Novikoff, 1962) but recent biochemical analyses indicate that despite general similarity, specific differences are apparent in lipid content (Kleinig, 1970), protein content (Franke et al., 1970), and enzymatic activity (Franke et al., 1970; Kasper, 1971). Kasper (ibid) suggests that the outer leaflet of the nuclear envelope may represent an undifferentiated segment of the endoplasmic reticulum. This is consonant with the findings of Morré and his group (see Chapter 12) who showed the direction of development to be from the nuclear membrane to the plasma membrane.

Composition

In the fractionation of cell homogenates, the microsomal fraction usually constitutes about 15 to 20 percent of the cell. The protein component of the fraction is 40 to 60 percent, the lipid from 30 to 50 percent, and there is some RNA even after the ribosomal portion is removed. Siekevitz (1963) found that the RNA content after ribosomal removal still constituted about 10 percent of the total dry weight of the membranes. The protein has been described as partly structural and partly enzymatic, but there is question concerning such distinctions and the suggestion is that the enzymatic protein component of membrane performs a dual role (see Chapter 9). The lipid is predominantly phospholipid, most of which is lecithin, but there are also cephalins, inositides, and cholesterol and its esters. The enzyme composition reflects the variety of metabolic activities (Table 11.1), some of which will be discussed in a later section.

Table 11.1   SOME MICROSOMAL ENZYME ACTIVITIES

Synthesis of glycerides
  Triacylglycerols
  Phosphatides
  Glycolipids and plasmalogens
Metabolism of plasmalogens
Fatty acid synthesis
Steroid biosynthesis
  Cholesterol biosynthesis
  Steroid hydrogenation of unsaturated bonds
$NADPH_2 + O_2$-requiring steroid transformations
  Aromatization
  Hydroxylation
$NADPH_2 + O_2$-requiring drug detoxification
  Aromatic hydroxylations
  Side-chain oxidation
  Deamination
  Thio-ether oxidation
  Desulfuration
L-Ascorbic acid synthesis
UDP-uronic acid metabolism
UDP-glucose dephosphorylation
Aryl- and steroid-sulfatase

Modified from J. Rothschild, "The Structure and Function of the Membranes and Surfaces of Cells," *Biochem. Soc. Symp.*, 22: 4, Cambridge University Press (1963).

Function

The specialized functions of the endoplasmic reticulum are localized among the various structural subdivisions. There are, however, the general functions such as mechanical support, transport, and exchange.

Mechanical Support. By compartmentalizing the intracellular fluid, the complex membraneous channels provide supplementary mechanical support for the colloidal structure of the cytoplasmic matrix. This, undoubtedly, is of great importance since the integration of structure and function presumes a complex organization of molecules in space as prerequisite to organization of function.

Transport and Exchange. It is evident that both nutrients and products of metabolism move not only in and out of the cell but also from one area of the cell to another. A molecule of glucose that enters the cell and is phosphorylated may be metabolized to pyruvic acid in the cytoplasmic matrix, may become a part of the TCA cycle in the mitochondria, and through oxidative phosphorylation may have its potential energy trapped in ATP. Some of the trapped ATP in the mitochondria must be released into the matrix for activation of the amino acids transported there for protein synthesis. Some of the synthesized proteins are the enzymes which participate in all of the foregoing processes, and they therefore must be transported to their sites of action through the various membranes along the route. All aspects of membrane transfer discussed in Chapter 9 are pertinent for the membranes of the endoplasmic reticulum and other organelles.

A further complicating factor is the change of locus during synthesis of a particular metabolite that may involve shuttling of intermediates through membranes from organelles to matrix and back again in varying orderly pathways. Following the synthetic pathway of one protein or one steroid hormone can be fascinating and will be presented later in this chapter; following the concurrent activities within the cell becomes too staggering to comprehend. Inability to comprehend, however, should not preclude our attempts to apprehend the complexity of a problem that future students may be expected to grasp.

Protein Synthesis. A general acceptance of the idea that genes controlled protein and, therefore, enzyme synthesis developed early in the twentieth century with the work of Garrod (1902) who described alkaptonuria as an "inborn error of metabolism", that is a defect in biochemical function due to a defective gene. The work of Pauling et al. (1949) provided clear evidence that a gene determines the structure of a protein, and it soon was demonstrated that it is the single polypeptide chain that the gene controls. How the genes exert such control was not known but with the announcement of the Watson-Crick model of DNA (Watson and Crick, 1953) came the tremendous impetus in research into the mechanism of genetic control of polypeptide synthesis.

Genetic Code. Crick et al. (1961) set forth a group of assumptions based on the then current thought and slim empirical evidence. They asserted that the genetic code was in the form of nucleotide triplets; was not overlapping; was read from a fixed starting point with no special "commas"; and was probably degenerate, that is, one amino acid could be coded by several triplets. Crick and his colleagues then proceeded to put these assumptions to experimental test. Perhaps this group was prescient since other groups were arguing in favor of either two letter (Sinsheimer, 1959) or four letter codes (Gamow, 1954), overlapping codes (Wall, 1962) as well as other variations, all of which were being tested by statistical and other means. Just about this time, Nirenberg and Matthaei (1961) reported that they had induced the synthesis of polypeptides by adding ribonucleic acid to a cell-free system. They had synthesized a nucleotide containing only uridylic acid, poly U, which led to the production of a monotonous polypeptide containing only phenylalanine units. They found also that poly C, or CCC, carried the message for proline. This work, together with the work from Crick's laboratory, was taken to mean that the triplet UUU was the code or *codon* signifying phenylalanine and CCC, proline. This development was a major landmark in accelerating the understanding of the genetic code and protein synthesis since it provided an *in vitro* system for investigating what otherwise would have to be studied by genetic methods involving the effects of amino acid replacements and the effects of mutagenic agents, a far more tedious and time-consuming procedure.

Nirenberg et al. (1962) next showed that phenylalanine-tRNA was an intermediate in the synthesis of polyphenylalanine and then that poly U associated rapidly with ribosomes (Barondes and Nirenberg, 1962). These findings were in accord with the concept that had been proposed by Jacob and Monod (1961) that RNA was an intermediate in the transfer of information from DNA to protein and that this "messenger RNA" had a short half-life. Soon, other investigations indicated that the code for lysine was AAA (Ochoa, 1963). This work was followed by the use of polynucleotides having more than one kind of base. Most of the work on coding was carried on in the laboratories of Nirenberg and of Ochoa and within a year 54 random codons were assigned, all but 8 of which were correct (Nirenberg, 1963). From this work it became fully apparent that the code was indeed a triplet code and that it was degenerate (two or more codons coding for the same amino acid).

The now completed dictionary of accepted codon assignments is shown in Table 11.2. Several features are apparent: all codons are triplets and the code is highly degenerate, but the degeneracy has a pattern, one that was first deduced by Eck (1963). The codons for each amino acid consist of two bases that are characteristic of the amino acid; and the third base is read only as a purine, a pyrimidine, or merely as a base. Three exceptions—leucine, serine, and arginine—

Table 11.2   RNA-AMINO ACID CODE

		Second Base of Codon				
		U	C	A	G	
First Base of Codon	U	UUU UUC } Phe UUA UUG } Leu	UCU UCC UCA UCG } Ser	UAU UAC } Tyr UAA UAG	UGU UGC } Cys UGA UGG Try	U C A G
	C	CUU CUC CUA CUG } Leu	CCU CCC CCA CCG } Pro	CAU CAC } His CAA CAG } GluN	CGU CGC CGA CGG } Arg	U C A G
	A	AUU AUC AUA } Ileu AUG Met	ACU ACC ACA ACG } Thr	AAU AAC } AspN AAA AAG } Lys	AGU AGC } Ser AGA AGG } Arg	U C A G
	G	GUU GUC GUA GUG } Val	GCU GCC GCA GCG } Ala	GAU GAC } Asp GAA GAG } Glu	GGU GGC GGA GGG } Gly	U C A G

(Right margin label: Third Base of Codon)

From Spirin and Gavrilova, *The Ribosome*, Springer Verlag, N. Y., 1969, p. 9.

have two sets of base pairs that are characteristic for them. Methionine and tryptophan have only one set, or a single codon. Two nonsense codons, not assigned to any amino acid appeared to act as punctuation.

The universality of the code, at least for bacteria and protozoa at first, became evident from detailed consideration of the relations between DNA and protein compositions (Sueoka, 1961a; 1961b). Studies of amino acid replacements due to single base changes in the code were next studied in a plant virus, bacterium, and mammal. The discovery of sickle cell hemoglobin by Pauling et al. (1949) had been shown to be due to substitution of a normal valine by a glutamic acid in one position in the β chain of hemoglobin (Ingram, 1957; Hunt and Ingram, 1959). Other human abnormal hemoglobins also had been shown to be due to single amino acid replacements. All the amino acid replacements in the hemoglobin mutations proved to be compatible with the code (Table 11.3).

Table 11.3 EXAMPLES OF POSSIBLE CODON CHANGES UNDERLYING SOME AMINO ACID REPLACEMENTS IN THE MUTANT HEMOGLOBINS

Amino Acid in Normal Hemoglobin		Amino Acid in Mutant Hemoglobin	
Lysine (AAA)	⟶	Glutamic acid (GAA)	A ⟶ G
Glutamic acid (GAA)	⟶	Glutamine (CAA)	G ⟶ C
Glycine (GGU)	⟶	Aspartic acid (GAU)	G ⟶ A
Histidine (CAU)	⟶	Tyrosine (UAU)	C ⟶ U
Asparagine (AAU)	⟶	Lysine (AAA)	U ⟶ A
Glutamic acid (GAA)	⟶	Valine (GUA)	A ⟶ U
Glutamic acid (GAA)	⟶	Lysine (AAA)	G ⟶ A
Glutamic acid (GAA)	⟶	Glycine (GGA)	A ⟶ G

From J. D. Watson, *Molecular Biology of the Gene*, 2nd ed., W. A. Benjamin Inc. New York, 1970 p. 418.

Punctuation. Since the code is read sequentially, the matter of punctuation, or where to start and where to stop, is crucial. Using three of the simplest codes—poly U, poly A, and poly C—it will become obvious that a wrong start drastically changes the meaning. Fig. 11.5 shows how a one-nucleotide shift in the starting position changes the codons and, therefore, designates a different sequence of amino acids providing, of course, that the codons are valid. Crick (1963) showed that the message is read starting with a constant fixed point at one end of the nucleotide chain and reading in successive triplets from there.

UUUAAACCCUUUAAACCC   =   UUU AAA CCC UUU AAA CCC
↑

UUUAAACCCUUUAAACCC   =   UUA AAC CCU UUA AAC
  ↑

UUUAAACCCUUUAAACCC   =   UAA ACC CUU UAA ACC
   ↑

Fig. 11.5 How a one-nucleotide shift in the initiation point changes the code.

If the triplet sequence in mRNA contains the message or the template for the construction of a polypeptide chain, the next big question was how the amino acids recognized their codes or call numbers. It certainly was not a random, hit-or-miss, come-when-you-can invitation to the amino acids. If the message is read as Braille from one end to the other without interruption, then the required amino acids must be delivered into their proper positions sequentially. The direction of the assembly of ribonucleotides by addition to the 3'-OH group of the end ribonucleotide was established in an *in vitro* system of RNA polymerase primed with DNA (Maitra and Hurwitz, 1965). The initial residue remained as a triphosphate. The assembly of protein was clearly demonstrated to be sequential (Dintzis, 1961; Naughton and Dintzis, 1962). Tritium-labeled leucine was added to suspensions of reticulocytes that were actively synthesizing hemoglobin but that were being retarded by low temperature. Samples were taken at intervals and plotted to show the specific activity of the leucine-containing peptides whose

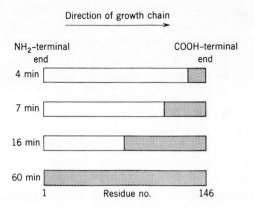

Fig. 11.6 Addition of labeled leucine residues to the COOH-terminal end of a polypeptide chain. The dark portions of the bars indicate the relative radioactivity of leucine residues along the a chain of hemoglobin following addition of ^{3}H-leucine to reticulocytes. At 4 minutes only a few leucine residues at the COOH-terminal end were labeled; by 60 min the entire chain was labeled. (From H. M. Dintzis, *Proc. Natl. Acad. Sci. U. S.*, 47: 247 1961.)

positions were known in the hemoglobin chain. In the first samples, only the leucine-containing peptides from the COOH-terminal ends of the a and β chains were labeled. Longer exposure to the ^{3}H-leucine led to a gradual increase in the number of labeled peptides proceeding toward the NH$_2$ terminus. After 60 minutes all were labeled (Fig. 11.6). Clearly, polypeptides grow by stepwise addition of single amino acids starting with the amino terminal and ending with the carboxyl terminal. Any interference in the continuity of assembly for lack of a required amino acid halts synthesis completely and the polypeptide chain is not formed. (Here is the fundamental explanation for the dictum established by nutritionists over two decades ago: *the time factor in protein synthesis.* On the basis of animal feeding experiments it was established that protein synthesis could take place only if all of the necessary amino acids were present in the proper amounts at the same time (Geiger, 1950). The mechanisms involved in protein synthesis worked out jointly by geneticists and biochemists now explain why.)

The need for punctuation that had been postulated became even more apparent when Jacob and Monod (1961) reported that one mRNA carried the code for a series of separate proteins. The codons signifying *N*-terminal punctuation, or the starting amino acid, *N*-formyl methionine in bacterial systems and methionine in animal systems (Petermann, 1971), turned out to be AUG and GUG. These are ambiguous codons in the sense that they can be read both as internal amino acids and as *N*-terminal methionine. The way they are read depends upon whether they are preceded by *C*-terminal punctuation or the codon for another amino acid. The *C*-terminal punctuation appears to be provided by nonsense codons, that is, codons that do not specify any amino acid. The nonsense codons, UAA, UAG, and UGA, in the sequence of nucleotides indicate the *C*-terminal, or stop signal. The details of *how* this works are not entirely clear; but there is substantial evidence to support the fact that it *does* work. The suggestion is that these codons are read by specific proteins, the release factors (see below).

The Adaptor Hypothesis. In order for the code to be translated into amino acids, there must be some means whereby amino acids recognize specific codons. It became apparent early that RNA could not be a direct template and Crick (1966a), in reviewing early history, reports his suggestion in 1957 of an RNA molecule acting as an adaptor between the template and the amino acid. It soon became evident that the adaptors were the relatively small molecules of transfer RNA (tRNA). Like all other cellular RNA, tRNA is specified by a base sequence in DNA. The tRNAs for the 20 different amino acids are different, yet alike in certain respects. Each contains approximately 80 nucleotides in a single chain, the 3' end of which always reads CCA and the 5' end is usually an unpaired guanine.

Alanine-tRNA (Fig. 11.7) was the first to have its nucleotide sequence worked out (Holley et al., 1965). Only after the nucleotide sequences in several other tRNAs had been determined was it realized that there were certain sequences common to all; the

Fig. 11.7 Schematic representation of three conformations of the alanine RNA with short, double-stranded regions. [From R. W. Holley et al., *Science*, 147:1462 (1965).]

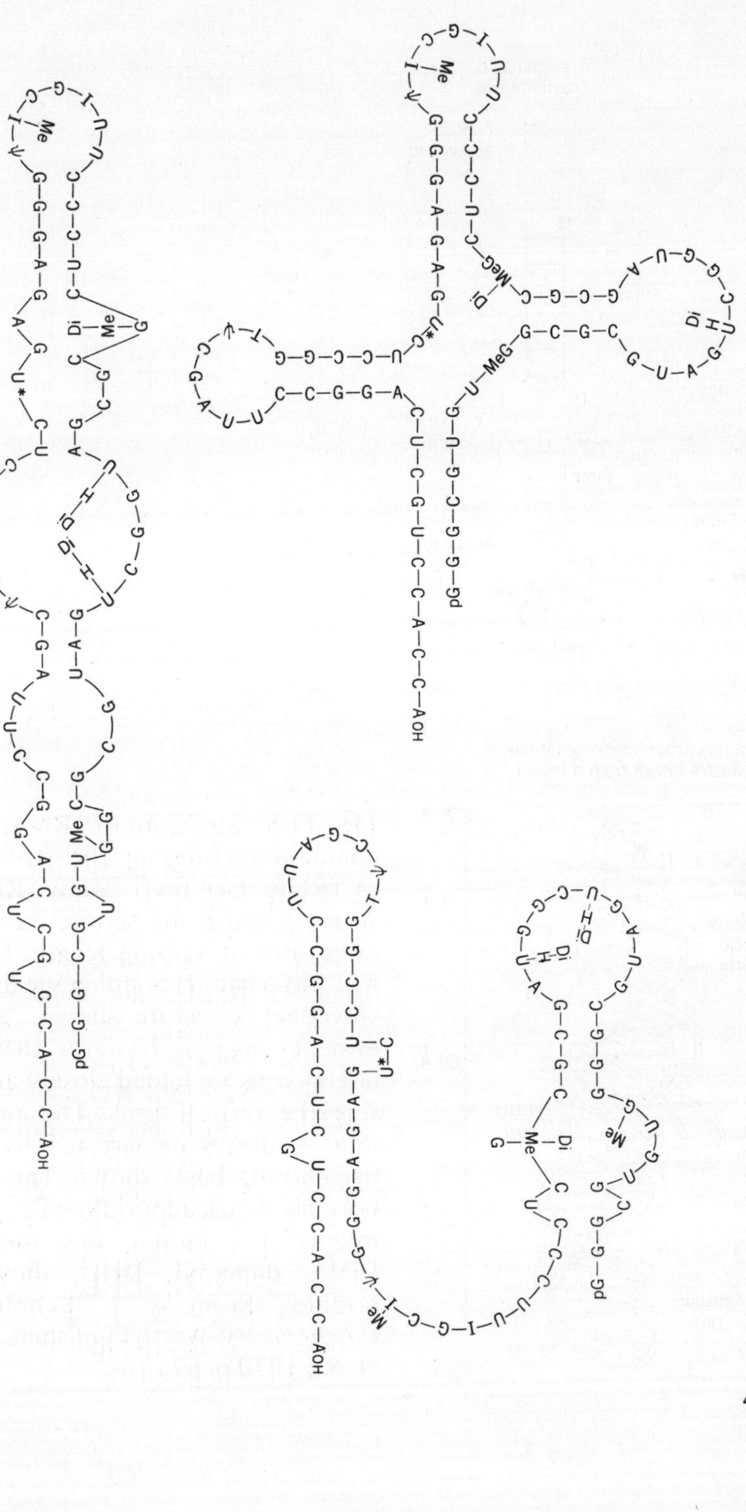

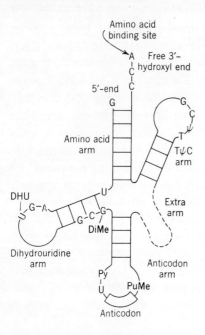

Amino acid binding site

A — Free 3'- hydroxyl end
C
C

5'-end   C
G

Amino acid arm

Amino acid arm

DHU
G—A
G—C—G
DiMe

Dihydrouridine arm

G
C
T
TψC arm

Extra arm

Anticodon arm

Py
U   PuMe

Anticodon

The three-dimentional conformation
of DNA drawn from a model

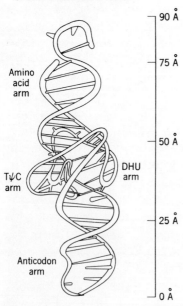

Amino acid arm

TψC arm

DHU arm

Anticodon arm

90 Å
75 Å
50 Å
25 Å
0 Å

Fig. 11.8 Structure of tRNA. The common features in the structure of tRNAs (see text). Some tRNAs, such as those for serine, have an extra arm of varying length. Maximal intrachain H-bonding yields the cloverleaf structure shown. X-ray evidence suggests, however, that the lateral arms are folded closely alongside the vertical arms. The anticodon is always demarcated by the neighboring bases shown. The symbols are ψ, pseudouridine; Py, pyrimidine; Pu, purine; Me, methyl; DiMe, dimethyl; DHU, dihydrouridine. (From A. L. Lehninger, *Biochemistry*, Worth Publishers, Inc., N. Y., 1970 p. 695.)

configurations that led to the maximal number of base pairings led to a common shape, that of the cloverleaf (Fig. 11.8). Each tRNA has its characteristic *anticodon* that pairs with the codon on the template mRNA. The anticodon is antiparallel, that is, it reads in the 3' to the 5' direction. When it became evident that a highly purified specific tRNA could recognize several codons, and that inosine often replaced one of the four common bases in the anticodon, Crick (1966b) proposed the *wobble hypothesis*. Since the third base in a codon could vary without changing meaning, he suggested that this might occur also in the anticodon with the two bases at the 3' end of the anticodon quite specific for an amino acid, but the one at the 5' end not as confined spatially, that is, it could wobble and form hydrogen bonds with bases other than those in standard base pairs.

The evidence was clear that the adaptor was tRNA and that this nucleotide was the intermediary through which the code was translated into amino acids. For more details on tRNA, see von Ehrenstein (1970).

A recitation of the rapid rate of discoveries leading to an understanding of the genetic code and its translation has the advantages bestowed by hindsight. The literature from 1961 on is filled with reports on all conceivable aspects of the coding problem and of attempts to arrive at a solution. Various systems of coding were postulated and became dogma, only to be discarded. For an extensive and thorough history of biological coding, see Yĉas (1969). For briefer views, see Woese (1967) and Nirenberg (1970).

The Ribosomes. The ribosomes are the ribonucleoprotein particles in which the protein synthesis takes place. They consist almost entirely of ribosomal RNA and ribosomal protein. The RNA molecules during synthesis in the nucleolus are complexed with protein that is synthesized in the cytoplasm and transported into the nucleus (Miller, 1973). The ribosome is synthesized as a large precursor molecule that is cleaved in the nucleolus to form the two subunits that leave the nucleus. The subunits reassociate in the cytoplasm (but not necessarily as units from the same precursors) to form the complete ribosome. In bacteria the ribosome has a sedimentation coefficient of 70 Svedberg units and is commonly referred to as the 70S ribosome, with a 30S and 50S subunit (Tissiers and Watson,

1958). In higher plants and animals the ribosome is 80S (Tashiro and Siekevitz, 1965) with subunits of approximately 60S and 40S. Since the bacterial ribosome has been studied much more extensively, reference here will be mostly to the 70S ribosome and its component parts.

The 30S subunit contains about 20 different proteins each of which appears to have an individual role in the structure or function of the ribosome (Nomura, 1970); the 50S subunits contain 30 to 36 individual proteins (Petermann, 1971). The association of the subunits into the ribosome is stable only in solvents that contain enough Mg^{2+} to saturate the RNA phosphate groups. When the Mg^{2+} is reduced and two-thirds dissociates from the ribosome, the two subunits of the ribosome separate. In some cases Ca^{2+} has also been found associated with the ribosome (Ts'o, 1958) and has been shown to be able to replace Mg^{2+} to some degree (Chao, 1957; Elson, 1959; 1961). Stabilizing roles have also been attributed to Mn^{2+} and Co^{2+} (Lyttleton, 1960; 1962; Abdul-Nour and Webster, 1960).

Under physiological conditions, ribosomes bound to endoplasmic reticulum membranes in the cell are in the form of polysomes, that is, groups of ribosomes. The binding of the mRNA to the ribosome involves the small subunit; whereas the binding of the ribosome to the membrane involves the large subunit (Sabatini et al., 1971). Each 70S or 80S ribosome contains two sites into which tRNA can be inserted: The peptidyl or *P site*, and the aminoacyl or *A site*. These ribosomal sites can accept any aminoacyl tRNA since the ribosome binds to an unspecific part of the tRNA molecule. It is only the codon-bound surface of the tRNA that is specific. The growing polypeptide chain is always terminated by a tRNA and it is the binding of this terminal tRNA to either the P site or the A site of the ribosome that is the main force holding the growing chain to the ribosome.

Electron microscopic observations on isolated membrane from microsomal fractions (Sabatini et al., 1966; Florendo, 1969) show that the groove separating the ribosomal subunits of a membrane-bound ribosome lies parallel to the membrane surface (Fig. 11.9). Sabatini et al. (1966) have shown with experimental dissociation of the ribosomal subunits that nascent polypeptides remain attached to the large subunit which remains attached to the membrane. These

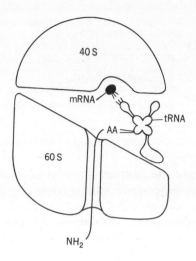

Fig. 11.9 Diagram of a ribosome showing the two subunits and the probable position of the messenger RNA and the transfer RNA. The nascent polypeptide chain passes through a kind of funnel within the large subunit. (From E. D. P. DeRobertis, W. W. Nowinski, and F. A. Saez, *Cell Biology*, 5th ed., W. B. Saunders Company, Phila., 1970 p. 401.)

investigators suggest that nascent polypeptides are involved in maintaining the ribosome-membrane interaction. A model of ribosome-membrane interaction derived from the work of Sabatini et al. (1971) depicts the individual ribosomes of the polysome attached to the membrane through their large subunits (Fig. 11.10). The nascent polypeptide chains grow within these subunits, protected from proteolytic enzymes, in a space that is or can become continuous with the lumen of the endoplasmic reticulum via a passageway in the membrane. This passageway is at or very near the binding site and serves to direct the exposed segment of the growing polypeptide into the endoplasmic reticulum cavity. In this way the product of synthesis has no way of entering the cytoplasmic matrix. This mechanism operates in cells synthesizing protein such as hormones, milk, and certain enzymes for export. Passage through the channels of the endoplasmic reticulum is followed by packaging in the Golgi complex prior to discharge (see Chapter 12). Proteins that are synthesized for internal use are synthesized by the free

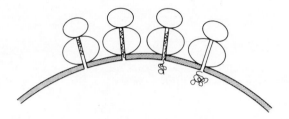

Fig. 11.10 A model indication how structural features of the ribosome-membrane junction could account for the vectorial discharge of nascent polypeptides from attached ribosomes to the lumen of the endoplasmic reticulum. [From D. D. Sabatini, G. Blobel, Y. Nonomura, and M. R. Adelman, *Adv. Cytopharmacol.*, 1: 119 (1971).]

polysomes in the cytoplasmic matrix. In this category are the enzymes maintained in the cytoplasmic matrix for cellular metabolism as well as those required for such specialized protein syntheses as hemoglobin in the erythrocyte.

For more detailed reviews on ribosomes, see Spirin and Gavrilova (1969); Nomura (1969); Peterman (1971); Miller (1973).

Building a Polypeptide. For polypeptide synthesis to take place in the endoplasmic reticulum, the mRNA, rRNA and ribonucleoproteins, tRNAs and the required enzymes must be assembled in the cytoplasmic matrix where the amino acids, cations, and energy sources are all simultaneously available.

Several other factors that play specific roles in the synthetic process have been identified: Three specific protein-initiation factors identified as F1, F2, and F3 were isolated and characterized in Ochoa's laboratory (Thach et al., 1966; Iwasaki et al., 1968; Revel et al., 1968). These appear to interact with and stabilize the 30S subunit complex. Peptidyl transferase factors, TF1 and TF2, active in the elongation of the polypeptide chain, were isolated in Lipmann's laboratory (Nishizuka and Lipmann, 1966; Ertel et al., 1968). TF2 is sometimes referred to as translocase.

For protein synthesis to proceed, there first must be activation of the amino acids through formation of an amino acid adenylate

(Hoagland, 1955; Hoagland et al., 1956):

1. AA + ATP - - - ► AMP ∼ AA + PP

followed by transfer, or transacetylation of the amino acids to tRNA (Hoagland and Zamecnik, 1975; Allen et al., 1960):

2. AMP ∼ AA + tRNA - - - ► AA ∼ tRNA + AMP

Steps 1 and 2 are both catalyzed by the same enzyme, aminoacyl synthetase. The amino acids are transferred to the terminal adenylic acid of tRNA, each of which has a 3′ terminus reading CCA.

Since the same activating enzyme binds to a given amino acid and to its tRNA, the enzyme must have two different binding sites. Each tRNA also must have two binding sites, one for the activating enzyme, and the other for a specific group of template nucleotides. This latter site carries the anticodon for each of the amino acids and, therefore, determines the specificity of the tRNAs for the various amino acids (Berg and Ofengand, 1958).

The process of polypeptide synthesis can be divided into three steps: *initiation, elongation,* and *termination.* In the initiation step, a free 30S ribosomal subunit binds to the mRNA at the specific initiation site that reads AUG. Protein factor F3 is required for the binding. The 30S-mRNA complex binds the starting aminoacyl tRNA, which is met-tRNA in animals and F-met-tRNA in bacteria. [An amino peptidase has been identified that subsequently removes the terminal methionine from many of the completed chains (Clark and Marker, 1968).] The 50S-ribosomal subunit joins the complex. Whether entry of the met-tRNA complex to the 50S-ribosomal subunit is made at the amino acid site (A site) or directly to the peptidyl (P) site is not known, but with the starting complex at the P site, the ribosome becomes functional. Fig. 11.11 illustrates the geography of a functional ribosome with the starting aminoacyl-tRNA in place.

A second aminoacyl-tRNA with an anticodon that complements the second codon on the mRNA joins the complex and occupies the A site on the 50S ribosome. Peptide bond formation then occurs by a reaction between the amino group of the aminoacyl-tRNA and the carboxylic group of the peptidyl-tRNA. This

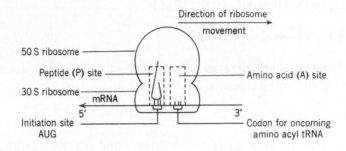

Fig. 11.11 Geography of a functional ribosome with starting aminoacyl-tRNA in place.

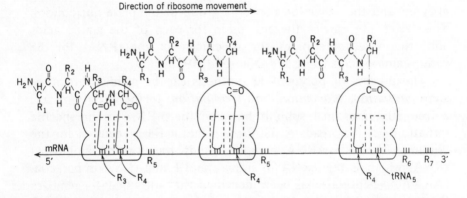

Fig. 11.12 Peptide bond formation between the carboxyl group of the peptidyl-tRNA and the amino group of the aminoacyl-tRNA followed by translocation of the aminoacyl-tRNA carrying the polypeptide chain to the P site.

reaction is catalyzed by the enzyme peptidyl transferase and requires GTP (Fig. 11.12).

After the formation of the peptide bond, the peptidyl-tRNA and the now-elongating chain are part of the complex on the A site and must be translocated to the P site before the next aminoacyl-tRNA can bind at the A site. Simultaneously, the deacylated tRNA leaves the P site, and the mRNA moves along three nucleotides so

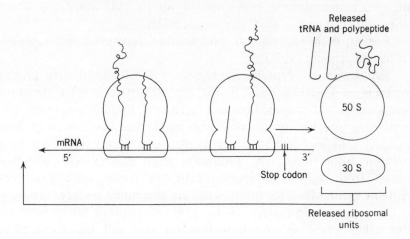

Fig. 11.13 Termination of polypeptide chain by the stop codon. The polypeptide release is accompanied by release of tRNA and the dissociated ribosomes that are available for reuse.

that the next nucleotide triplet codon is in the correct position at the A site.

After the full complement of amino acids is thus added, termination of the chain is activated by the stop codons, UAG, UAA, UGA. The stop or nonsense codon causes termination of the chain with the amino acid on the codon just prior to it. The stop codon apparently is read by the protein release factors that act enzymatically splitting off the terminal tRNA (Siekevitz and Palade, 1960). The polypeptide that has probably assumed its three-dimensional configuration is released directly into the channel of the endoplasmic reticulum if it is a secretory protein, or into the cytoplasmic matrix by free polysomes. The released ribosome is dissociated into the 30S and 50S subunits that become available for reuse, as does the free tRNA that delivered the carboxyl terminal amino acid (Fig. 11.13).

The synthesis of many polypeptide chains occurs on the succession of ribosomes that form the polysome associated with one mRNA. Each ribosome functions independently of the others and a relatively short mRNA may be read simultaneously by six or so ribosomes constituting the polysome; whereas an mRNA that codes for a long polypeptide chain of perhaps 1500 amino acids might accommodate a polysome of up to 100 ribosomes simultaneously reading the 4500 nucleotide m RNA tape.

For further reading on polypeptide synthesis, see Lipmann (1969); Nirenberg (1970).

Regulation of Protein Synthesis. All cells synthesize protein for their own internal need: that is, complex molecules for structural components and enzymes for cell functions. In addition, many cells synthesize specific products for export: digestive enzymes from mucosal cells and pancreatic cells, plasma proteins from liver cells, collagen from fibroblasts, antibodies from plasma cells, and hormones from various endocrine cells, to name some examples. Proteins synthesized for internal use are assembled on free ribosomes in the cytoplasmic matrix. (Some protein synthesis for internal use also takes place in the mitochondria and will be discussed in Chapter 13.) The protein for export, as indicated earlier, is released directly into the channels of the endoplasmic reticulum and passes through the Golgi apparatus for additions of complex carbohydrate, lipid, sulfate or other molecules prior to concentration, storage, and release.

Since all metabolic processes depend on enzyme action, and since all enzymes are proteins, the life of the cell depends on its protein synthetic capacity. The only cell deprived of the ability to synthesize protein is the mature erythrocyte since it loses its nucleus during maturation and therefore loses the required DNA for RNA production. This cell exists and functions only as long as its RNA and package of enzymes lasts (see Chapter 16). When these have been used up, since they cannot be replaced, the erythrocyte life span is completed. In other cells, if the DNA in the nucleus is induced to produce the requisite RNA and if the necessary nutrients for synthesis are available, the cell will synthesize the enzymes or other proteins it requires for its structure and function.

There is a constant turnover of cellular protein; that is, synthesis and degradation within the cell. The turnover rates vary not only among cells but also among organelles and specific proteins within the cells. For example, the half-life of the protein of the endoplasmic retidulum is approximately 2 days, whereas that of mitochondria is almost 7 days. Some enzymes have a half-life of 2 to 4 days and others just a few hours.

The protein production schedule for any cell must, of necessity, be very carefully organized and controlled if the proper amounts of each of the multitude of enzymes required for cell function are to come off the assembly line at the proper time. In addition, there must be careful allocation and precise regulation of the common precursors, as well as energy, necessary for the cell's countless functions. Syntheses must be started, and they must be stopped, and both the initiation and termination of each synthesis is part of the overall program. The surviving cell is proof of successful regulation.

Initiation of the synthesis of a protein involved in a metabolic reaction in the cell may occur when the substrate is introduced. This is called *enzyme induction* and the enzymes themselves are said to be *inducible enzymes.* This type of response has been studied in bacterial cultures but is also implicated as a type of control in mammalian metabolism. For example, introduction of lactose as the sole source of carbon to bacterial culture will induce the synthesis of β-galactosidase that will continue as long as lactose is the carbon source. If glucose is provided, the enzyme β-galactosidase will no longer be induced. Some investigators have suggested that a similar type of enzyme induction might be the mechanism responsible for the lactose tolerance observed in adult Caucasians (see Chapter 6).

Inhibition of Protein Synthesis. From what has been discussed in Chapter 10 it is evident that DNA transcription is normally believed to be in an "off" position. According to the Jacob and Monod model, the regulatory gene codes for the mRNA that is the template for the repressor protein. The repressor protein generally functions to block the operator gene so that transcription does not take place. However, when the inhibition is counteracted by an inducer that combines with the repressor to form a repressor-inducer complex, transcription to mRNA occurs leading to protein synthesis. Once started, however, there must be ways to get it stopped, and several mechanisms have been suggested to explain what the procedure might be.

Product and Feedback Inhibition. If a cell is supplied with a product it normally synthesizes, it will frugally cut off its own production by repressing synthesis of the enzymes involved. Such a cutoff stimulated by the end product is called *product inhibition* or *enzyme repression* and is usually the result of a mass action effect.

When the synthesis of a product is the result of a series of enzyme actions, accumulation of the end product triggers a regulating mechanism that sets up the inhibition at the point of the first

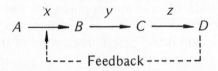

Fig. 11.14 Feedback inhibition. Accumulation of product *D* inhibits enzyme *x* required for reaction A → B.

enzymatic reaction in the chain, thereby preventing further production of that metabolite and of its immediate precursors in the synthetic pathway. This is called *feedback inhibition* and is one of the common means of controlling metabolic pathways (Fig. 11.14). In feedback inhibition, the enzyme responsive to the block is also referred to as the *pacemaker* or *regulatory enzyme.* Enzymes exerting this type of regulation are usually allosteric; that is, they will have one site promoting the reaction and another site responsive to the end product leading to inhibition of the reaction. Through this type of regulation there can be continual adjustment in the rate of enzyme synthesis to fulfill the demands of the cell. Increased demand delays both product and feedback inhibition; whereas a decrease in demand leads to a cut-off in synthesis. Many variations of feedback inhibition have been described to account for control of metabolic pathways of varying complexities (see Conn and Stumpf, 1972, p. 471).

Repression of Protein Synthesis. The model of Jacob and Monod accounts for the repression exerted by the biosynthetic end product by postulating that the repressor molecule does not act by itself in a feedback inhibition but must have a *corepressor.* The corepressor is usually a small molecule that may be an end product in the metabolic pathway. It becomes the repressing metabolite and forms the *repressor-corepressor complex,* which then combines with the operator gene to prevent transcription.

Several other types of data have been forthcoming to provide support for the Jacob-Monod hypothesis. Two repressor proteins have been isolated: the galactosidase repressor (Gilbert and Müller-Hill, 1966) and the repressor protein for the *lac* operon (Ptashne, 1967). It was mentioned previously that lactose supplied as the only source of carbon for *E. coli* induced synthesis of enzymes for its metabolism. The repression of these enzymes effected by the

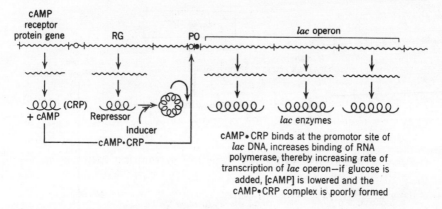

Fig. 11.15 Catabolite repression indicating effect of cAMP. (From E. E. Conn and P. K. Stumpf, *Outlines of Biochemistry*, 3rd ed., Wiley, N. Y., 1972 p. 483.)

addition of glucose is called *catabolite repression,* and its action has recently been linked to cAMP. Pastan and Perlman (1969) have demonstrated that the mechanism involved binding of cAMP to the *receptor protein* followed by association of *cAMP-receptor protein* with a specific binding site in the *lac* genome. This promotes the binding of RNA polymerase to DNA thereby increasing the rate of synthesis of the enzymes essential for lactose metabolism. The addition of glucose to the medium decreases the concentration of cAMP and interferes with this binding (Fig. 11.15).

The presence of receptor sites in plasma membranes that operate through an associated adenyl cyclase site to stimulate the formation of cAMP was discussed in Chapter 9. Similarly associated receptor and adenyl cyclase sites are present in the membranes of the endoplasmic reticulum and mitochondria. Several mechanisms involving selective induction of enzyme synthesis by cAMP have been proposed.

The exquisite sensitivity with which the selective induction of hepatic enzymes occurs following stimulation by various hormones has been attributed to cAMP (Wicks, 1971; 1974). In both glycogenesis and glycogenolysis there is elegantly coordinated control of the involved enzymes that is mediated by hormones through cAMP. The biochemical pathways will be discussed in subsequent sections; the mechanisms of enzyme activation and control are pertinent here.

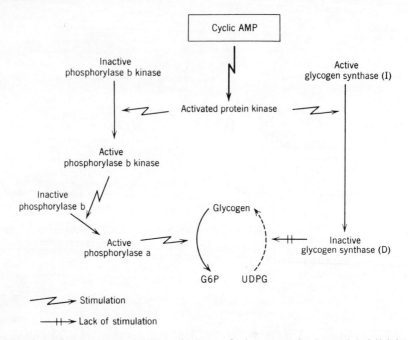

Fig. 11.16 Coordinate stimulation of glycogenolysis and inhibition of glycogenesis. (From J. Tepperman, *Metabolic and Endocrine Physiology*, 3rd ed., Year Book Medical Publishers, 1973, p. 28.)

The same cAMP-dependent protein kinase controls *phosphorylase activation* and *glycogen synthetase inactivation*. This clearly permits the right hand to know what the left hand is doing in making glucose available or sequestering it as glycogen. The action of cAMP in activating protein kinase simultaneously converts inactive phosphorylase b kinase to the active form and active glycogen synthetase to the inactive form. This leads through a cascade of events to the stimulation of glycogenolysis and the inhibition of glycogenesis (Fig. 11.16).

Garren et al. (1971) have postulated that ACTH acts through cAMP to regulate adrenal function by modulating protein synthesis at the level of translation of mRNA. They propose that the binding of cAMP to the inhibitory receptor protein causes it to dissociate from the protein kinase activating the enzyme. The activated enzyme then catalyzes the transfer of phosphate from ATP to ribosomal protein. This action of cAMP, releasing the inhibition of the protein

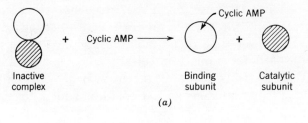

(a)

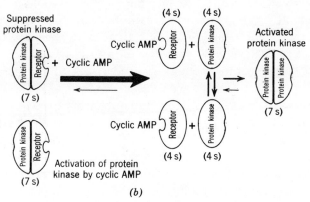

(b)

Fig. 11.17 Two models of protein kinase activation by cAMP. (a) A model for the mechanism of activation of kinase 1 by cyclic AMP. [From M. Tao, *Ann. N. Y. Acad. Sci.*, 185: 227 (1971).] (b) Hypothetical model for the activation of protein kinase by cAMP. [From T. A. Langan, *Ann. N. Y. Acad. Sci.*, 185: 166 (1971).]

kinase, appears to be a general phenomonon and not limited to the adrenal cortex. Tao (1971) reported a similar mechanism in rabbit reticulocytes and Kuman et al. (1970) in liver. These observations are consistent with the finding that protein kinase is composed of two subunits that together form an inactive enzyme. By binding with one subunit, cAMP causes the release of the other subunit, which is the active kinase. Two suggested models are depicted in Fig. 11.17.

It may well be that the general mechanism of hormone action starts with the activation of adenyl cyclase in the cell membrane leading to formation of cAMP, the second messenger, that in turn releases active protein kinase. Protein kinase may be involved in most of the effects of cAMP (Sutherland, 1972). It may activate another enzyme and produce a rapid response; or, it may influence the binding of RNA polymerase and thereby the rate of transcription and enzyme synthesis in the slower type of hormone response. Cheung (1972) suggests that cAMP functions as a versatile allosteric effector and that the different effects of cAMP are explained by the kinds of proteins with which it interacts and, it could be added, by the kind of proteins it represses or induces.

Glycolysis. A fundamental role of the cytoplasmic matrix is the preparatory degradation of carbohydrate units to pyruvic acid which enters the mitochondria and there is further oxidized for the release of energy. *Glycolysis* is the term used to describe this initial stage of carbohydrate metabolism and refers to the breakdown of glucose or glycogen to pyruvic acid.

Glucose enters the cell from the interstitial fluid in the free state and is actively transported across most cell membranes under the influence of the hormone insulin. The membranes of some cells, however, such as intestinal mucosa and brain do not require insulin for glucose transport. This function of insulin accounts for many of the aberrations in carbohydrate metabolism observed in the diabetic state but is not sufficient to explain other apparently direct effects of the hormone, such as the effects on fatty acid and protein synthesis.

Free glucose cannot enter into cellular metabolic activity; thus, upon entrance into the cell, it is immediately phosphorylated, a process that requires ATP and which results in the formation of glucose-6-phosphate. Three chief pathways are open to the phosphorylated glucose: glycolysis, glycogenesis (formation of glycogen) or metabolism by way of the pentose phosphate shunt. The pathway followed is determined by the metabolic state existing within the cell; primarily, the available amounts of glucose, ATP, NADP, and oxygen determine the pathway of glucose degradation.

Glycolysis has been studied most in muscle and nerve tissues but occurs actively in liver cells and undoubtedly occurs in cells of all tissues. The metabolic scheme is known as the Embden-Meyerhof glycolytic pathway in honor of two of the scientists whose work contributed most to elaboration of the reactions involved. Glycolysis may proceed from either free glucose or glycogen, but in either instance the formation of the active metabolite, glucose-6-phosphate, is essential. Phosphorylation of free glucose, however, requires the high energy of ATP, whereas phosphorylation of a glucose unit from glycogen is accomplished by phosphorolysis, a reaction utilizing inorganic phosphate and which, therefore, does not require the expenditure of high energy. The difference in initial energy expenditure obviously affects the final net yield of energy from glycolysis depending on whether the starting point is glucose or glycogen.

The principle reactions involved in the Embden-Meyerhof scheme are shown in Fig. 11.18 and are described in the following:

1. Glucose-6-phosphate is formed either by phosphorylation of free glucose that has just entered the cell or phosphorolysis of glycogen with glucose-1-phosphate as an intermediate.

2. Glucose-6-phosphate is isomerized to the phosphorylated keto hexose, fructose-6-phosphate.

3. Fructose-6-phosphate is further phosphorylated by ATP at the first carbon to form fructose-1,6-diphosphate. The reverse reaction occurs by means of a phosphatase, but does not utilize ATP.

4. Fructose-1,6-diphosphate is split into two molecules of triosephosphate, glyceraldehyde-3-phosphate, and dihydroxyacetone phosphate under the influence of the enzyme, triose phosphate isomerase. Dihydroxyacetone phosphate may be converted to the glycerol fraction of neutral fat and thus provides a link between carbohydrate metabolism and fat metabolism. From this point, carbohydrate metabolism proceeds from glyceraldehyde-3-phosphate, but, because this compound and dihydroxyacetone phosphate are interconvertible, in effect, two molecules of glyceraldehyde are formed from one hexose unit.

5. The first step in the triose stage of glycolysis is the oxidation of glyceraldehyde-3-phosphate to glyceric acid-1,3-diphosphate. The hydrogen thus released is taken up by NAD, which may be re-oxidized by the mitochondrial electron transport system leading to the synthesis of three moles of ATP (see Chapter 13). In the absence of oxygen (anaerobic glycolysis), NADH is utilized in the formation of lactic acid (reaction 9).

6. Glyceric acid-1,3-diphosphate reacts directly with ADP to form ATP and glyceric acid-3-phosphate. (This reaction and others of this type are known as *substrate level phosphorylations* as distinguished from oxidative phosphorylation to be discussed in Chapter 13 on the mitochondria. At the substrate level only one

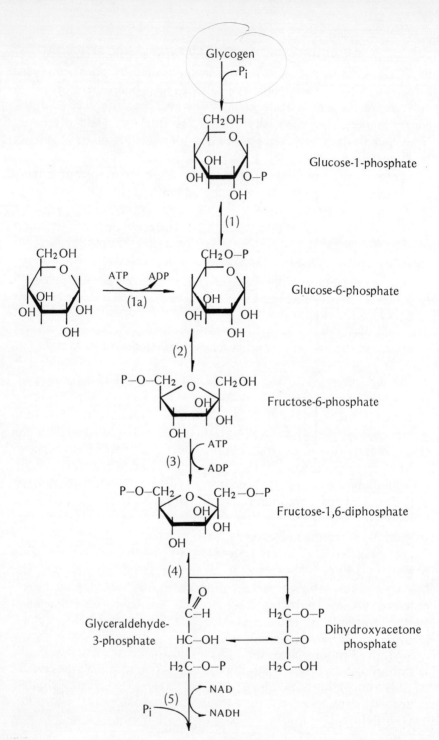

Glucose-1-phosphate

Glucose-6-phosphate

Fructose-6-phosphate

Fructose-1,6-diphosphate

Glyceraldehyde-3-phosphate

Dihydroxyacetone phosphate

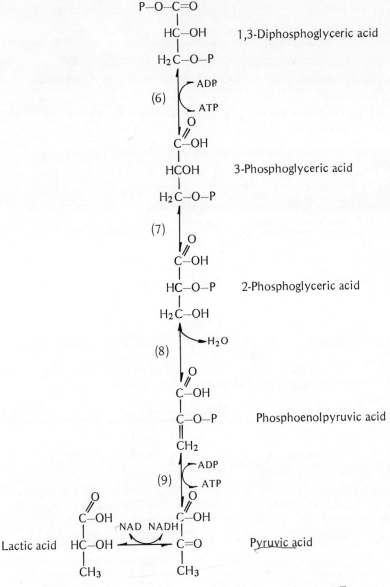

Fig. 11.18 Embden-Meyerhof glycolytic pathway. Enzymes are
(1) phosphoglucomutase, (1a) glucokinase, (2) phosphoglucoisomer-
ase, (3) phosphofructokinase, (4) aldolase, (5) glyceraldehyde-
3-phosphate dehydrogenase, (6) phosphoglyceryl kinase, (7) phospho-
glycerol mutase, (8) enolase, and (9) pyruvic kinase.

mole of ATP is synthesized in contrast to three moles produced by oxidative phosphorylation.)

7. Glyceric acid-3-phosphate is converted to glyceric acid-2-phosphate, essentially a migration of the phosphate group.

8. Glyceric acid-2-phosphate is dehydrated to form phospho-enolpyruvic acid.

9. Phosphoenolpyruvic acid reacts with ADP, another *substrate level phosphorylation*, to form pyruvic acid and ATP.

Pyruvic acid, thus formed, enters the mitochondrion for further oxidation. When the oxygen supply is low, as in prolonged muscular activity, pyruvic acid may be used to oxidize NADH, forming NAD and lactic acid. The reaction is catalyzed by the enzyme lactic dehydrogenase (LDH) and is coupled with the NADH-forming reaction between glyceraldehyde-3-phosphate and 1,3-diphospho-glyceric acid as shown below.

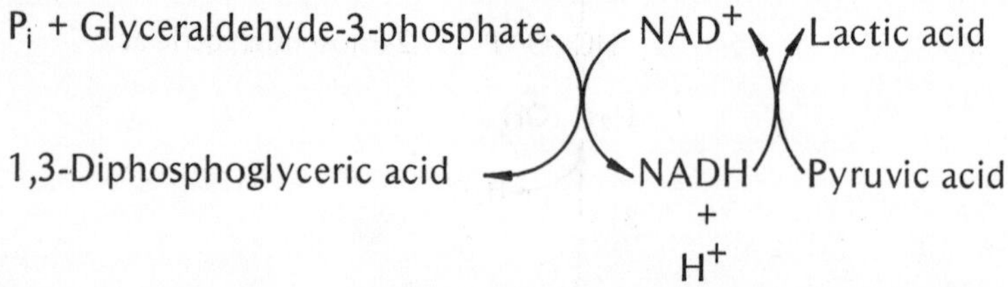

P_i + Glyceraldehyde-3-phosphate $\quad$ NAD$^+$ $\quad$ Lactic acid

1,3-Diphosphoglyceric acid $\longleftarrow$ NADH $\quad$ Pyruvic acid
$+$
H^+

Lactic dehydrogenase occurs in several molecular forms, or isozymes. At least five different isozymes are known to occur in animal tissues. The enzyme in heart (H_4) and the enzyme in skeletal muscle (M_4) have been shown to have very different kinetic properties that are, however, beautifully consistent with the functions of the two tissues. The heart enzyme is inhibited by pyruvate and is active only at low levels of pyruvate. This property assures a steady supply of necessary energy from the complete oxidation of pyruvate via the TCA cycle. In contrast, muscle LDH does not operate at maximum rate until pyruvate concentrations are quite high and, unlike the heart, energy demands can be supplied for short periods of time by anaerobic glycolysis in which ATP is generated (see Fig. 11.18, reactions 6 and 9). Thus LDH isozymes may operate in highly aerobic (H_4) or anaerobic (M_4) environments. Other forms of LDH (M_3H_1, M_2H_2, and M_1H_3) occur in tissues in which the metabolic activity is intermediate between these two extremes.

Furthermore, when the oxygen supply is low and large amounts of lactic acid are formed, the lactic acid, so produced, is transported to the liver for resynthesis to glycogen (see Chapter 15). This step is necessary since there is no enzymatic mechanism in muscle cells for the conversion of lactic acid to glycogen. The cycling of lactic acid formed from anaerobic glycolysis in muscle to the liver for glycogen synthesis was first described by Carl and Gerti Cori and is known as the Cori Cycle (see Cori, 1931).

Although glycolysis may proceed in the presence or absence of oxygen, from the standpoint of energy yield to the cell, aerobic glycolysis is the more efficient mechanism. The energy yield of anaerobic glycolysis obviously is low. Two ATP are formed in the substrate level phosphorylation of reactions 6 and 9, a total of four ATP from one hexose unit yielding two triose units. Assuming glucose as the starting point, two ATP are used up in the phosphorylation of glucose and of fructose-6-phosphate and therefore must be subtracted from the total ATP produced. The net gain in ATP thus is only 2 moles.

When the oxygen supply is high, lactic acid is not formed and NADH synthesized in reaction 5 may be oxidized via the mitochondrial electron transport system. Six additional moles of ATP then are formed, three for each pair of electrons, assuming two triose units for each hexose. The total energy yield for aerobic glycolysis thus is eight ATP, exactly four times that of anaerobic glycolysis (Chapter 13).

If the starting point of glycolysis is glycogen rather than free glucose, which requires high energy phosphate, the energy yield is increased by one ATP for either aerobic or anaerobic glycolysis.

Pentose Phosphate Shunt. The pentose phosphate shunt, sometimes called the hexose monophosphate shunt or phosphogluconate pathway, is a significant alternative pathway for glucose oxidation. In contrast to the Embden-Meyerhof glycolysis, oxidation of glucose via the pentose phosphate shunt does not require ATP and therefore may proceed under conditions that would seriously retard glucose degradation by the glycolytic route. About 30 percent of glucose metabolism in liver cells occurs by way of the pentose phosphate shunt and an even larger proportion of glucose oxidation proceeds via the shunt mechanism in the mammary gland, testis, adipose tissue, leukocyte, and adrenal cortex. This pathway, however, is of little or no importance in striated muscle, and apparently in this tissue glucose degradation proceeds entirely by anaerobic glycolysis and the TCA cycle.

The outline shown in Fig. 11.19 is simplified and is intended chiefly to point up reactions of special interest and significance in the total metabolic scheme. Six moles of glucose-6-phosphate enter into the chain of reactions during which 1 mole of glucose is oxidized completely by the shunt mechanism. The oxidation is accomplished entirely in reactions 1-3 in which $NADP^+$ is reduced to NADPH, CO_2 is released, and 6 moles of ribulose-5-phosphate are formed. The rest of the series results in the rearrangement of molecules to form compounds with 5, 7, 3, 4, and 6 carbon atoms in the chain leading ultimately to the final formation of 5 moles of glucose-6-phosphate, which can then reenter the cycle.

The overall reaction may be written as follows:

6-Glucose-6-phosphate + 12 $NADP^+$ $\longrightarrow$

5-Glucose-6-phosphate + 6 CO_2 + 12 NADPH + 12H^+ + P_i

The individual reactions are shown in Fig. 11.19 and are described below.

Reaction

1 and 3. In two separate oxidation steps, NADP is hydrogen acceptor. NADPH, thus formed, may be oxidized by way of the electron transport system after passing on its electrons to NAD (Chapter 13). There is no built-in system in this series of reactions for reoxidation of NADPH, such as occurs when NADH is reoxidized in the formation of lactic acid in the Embden-Meyerhof pathway. Highly significant, however, is the specific

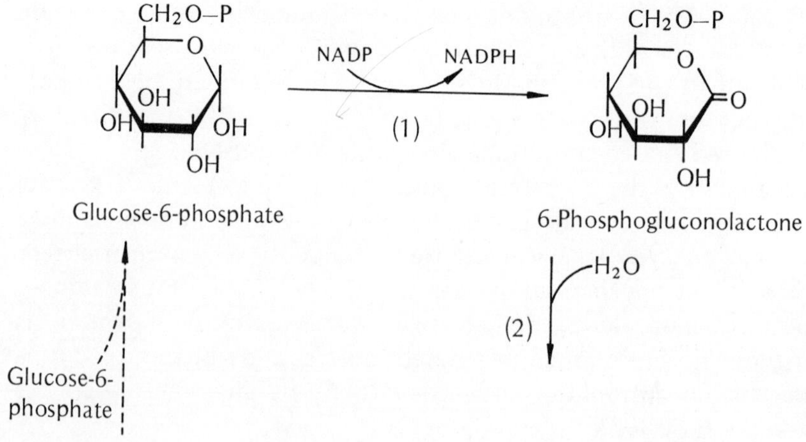

Glucose-6-phosphate

6-Phosphogluconolactone

Glucose-6-phosphate

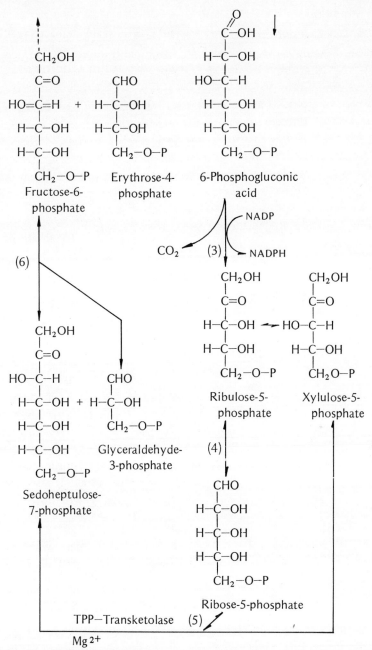

Fig. 11.19 Pentose phosphate shunt. Enzymes are (1) glucose-6-phosphate dehydrogenase, (2) 6-phosphogluconic acid dehydrogenase, (4) phosphoriboisomerase, (4*a*) phosphoketopentoepimerase, (5) transketolase, and (6) transaldolase.

requirement for NADPH in certain cellular reactions such as synthesis of fatty acids and cholesterol, conversion of phenylalanine to tyrosine, and reduction of dihydrofolic acid to tetrahydrofolic acid. These specific requirements are met in large part by the pentose phosphate shunt production of NADPH.

4. Ribose formed by isomerization of ribulose-5-phosphate may be utilized directly in synthesis of ribonucleic acid and nucleotides such as NAD, ATP, and UTP.

4 and 5. Ribulose-5-phosphate may also isomerize to form the 5-carbon keto sugar, xylulose-5-phosphate, which, in turn, may react with ribose-5-phosphate, an aldo sugar, to form the 7-carbon sedoheptulose and the 3-carbon glyceraldehyde-3-phosphate. The reaction is one of a general group catalyzed by the enzyme, *transketolase,* which catalyzes the transfer of a ketol grouping

$$\left(\begin{array}{c} CH_2-OH \\ | \\ C=O \\ | \end{array}\right) \text{ to an aldehyde acceptor } \left(\begin{array}{c} H \\ | \\ C=O \\ | \end{array}\right) \text{ and}$$

which requires TPP and Mg^{2+} as cofactors. The transketolase enzyme may also catalyze the transfer of a ketol group from xylulose-5-phosphate to erythrose-4-phosphate to form fructose-6-phosphate and glyceraldehyde-3-phosphate (not indicated in Fig. 11.19). The importance of the transketolase reaction in the study of thiamin deficiency will be dealt with in a later section (Chapter 24).

It is significant that reaction 6 between sedoheptulose and glyceraldehyde is not a transketolase reaction but is catalyzed by a transaldolase enzyme involving the transfer of a dihydroxy-

$$\text{acetone grouping } \left(\begin{array}{c} CH_2\,OH \\ | \\ C=O \\ | \\ HO-C-H \\ | \end{array}\right) \text{ to an aldose acceptor. This}$$

reaction does not require TPP as coenzyme.

The pentose phosphate shunt offers certain advantages over the glycolytic route: its lack of dependence upon ATP as a starting mechanism, the production of NADPH requisite for lipid synthesis, and the synthesis of ribose, an essential nucleotide component. Without delving further into the many intricacies of the system, clearly this alternative pathway for glucose metabolism plays a fundamental role in total cellular activity.

Glycogenesis. The formation of glycogen, *glycogenesis*, involves the addition of a glucose unit to an already existing glycogen chain. Since the glycogen molecule is not a stable structure but constantly changes as glucose units are added or removed, for convenience, glycogen may be designated as comprised of n glucose units. The key metabolite in the formation of glycogen, as in its degradation, is glucose-6-phosphate. This compound is readily converted to glucose-1-phosphate. The glucose-1-phosphate, thus formed, reacts with a nucleotide, uridine triphosphate (UTP), to yield inorganic pyrophosphate (PPi) and uridine diphosphate glucose (UDPG). UDPG reacts with the preexisting glycogen molecule containing n glucose units to form UDG and glycogen now containing $n + 1$ glucose units. In other words, the glycogen molecule is now larger by one glucose unit. These reactions are depicted in Fig. 11.20.

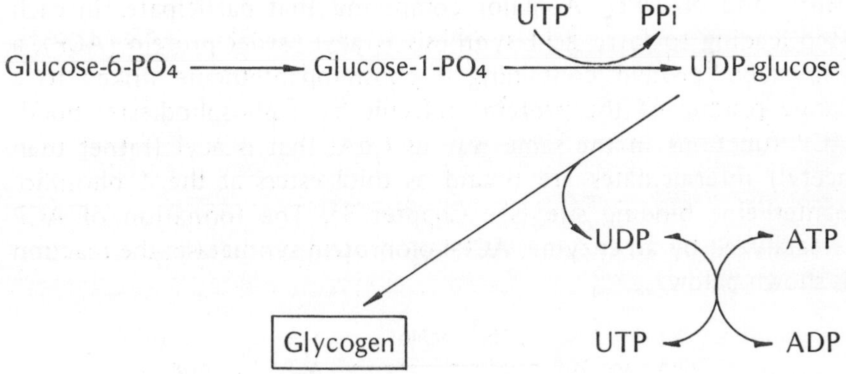

Fig. 11.20 Glycogenesis.

Glycogenesis thus proceeds by a route different from glycolysis and involves a different set of enzymes. The independence of the two sets of reactions is clearly advantageous to cellular activity, since an accelerator or inhibitor of one set of reactions will not affect the other in the same direction.

An interesting departure in glycogenesis is the source of high energy phosphate. Most synthetic reactions require ATP as a source of high energy, whereas, in the formation of glycogen, UTP is the high energy nucleotide utilized. ATP enters into the reaction indirectly, however, by providing the high energy phosphate for the conversion of UDP to UTP.

Fatty Acid Synthesis. Fatty acids may be synthesized by at least two pathways: (1) elongation of existing fatty acid chains by addition of two-carbon acetyl CoA units, such as the conversion of palmitic to stearic acid and (2) *de novo* synthesis from acetyl CoA, that is, the formation of a fatty acid from two-carbon units only. The former pathway is a function of the cytoplasm and the mitochondria (see Chapter 13); the latter pathway appears to be limited to the soluble fraction of the cytoplasm.

The key compound in *de novo* synthesis of fatty acids is not acetyl CoA but a compound derived from the acetyl unit, malonyl CoA. The discovery by Wakil (1958) of malonyl CoA as an intermediate in fatty acid biosynthesis was a major contribution to the understanding of the process involved. *De novo* synthesis is referred to as the palmitate-synthesizing system and converts acetyl CoA to long chain fatty acids. The reactions involved require ATP, CO_2, Mn^{2+} and NADPH. A major compound that participates in each step leading to fatty acid synthesis is acyl carrier protein (ACP), a heat-stable protein containing 4'-phosphopantetheine linked to a serine residue of the protein molecule by a phosphodiester bond. ACP functions in the same way as CoA, that is acyl (rather than acetyl) intermediates are bound as thiol esters at the 4'-phosphopantetheine binding site (see Chapter 3). The formation of ACP is catalyzed by an enzyme, ACP-holoprotein synthetase; the reaction is shown below.

$$CoA + \text{apo-ACP} \xrightarrow{Mg^{2+} \text{ or } Mn^{2+}} ACP + 3',5'\text{-ADP}$$

The first step in fatty acid synthesis is the formation of malonyl CoA from acetyl CoA, bicarbonate, and ATP, a CO_2-fixation reaction that is catalyzed by acetyl CoA carboxylase, a biotin-containing enzyme and one that requires Mn^{2+}. The reaction is shown below.

$$\underset{\text{Acetyl CoA}}{CH_3\overset{O}{\overset{\|}{C}}-SCoA + HCO_3^- + ATP} \underset{}{\overset{Mn^{2+}}{\rightleftharpoons}} \underset{\text{Malonyl CoA}}{ADP + P_i + HOOCCH_2\overset{O}{\overset{\|}{C}}-SCoA}$$

In the conversion of malonyl CoA to palmitic acid seven molecules of CoA and one molecule of acetyl CoA are utilized. ACP is involved in every step and, as shown below, it is acyl ACP rather than acyl CoA that is incorporated into the long chain fatty acids. The reactions are summarized below.

$$AcetylSCoA + HSACP \rightleftharpoons acetylSACP + HSCoA \tag{1}$$

$$AcetylSACP + HSEnz \rightleftharpoons acetylSEnz + HSACP \tag{1a}$$

$$MalonylSCoA + HSACP \rightleftharpoons malonylSACP + HSCoA \tag{2}$$

$$MalonylSACP + acetylSEnz \rightleftharpoons acetoacetylSACP + EnzSH + CO_2 \tag{3}$$

$$AcetoacetylSACP + NADPH + H^+ \rightleftharpoons D(-)\beta\text{-}hydroxybutyrylSACP + NADP^+ \tag{4}$$

$$D(-)\beta\text{-}HydroxybutyrylSACP \rightleftharpoons crotonyl SACP + H_2O \tag{5}$$

$$CrotonylSACP + NADPH + H^+ \rightleftharpoons butyrylSACP + NADP^+ \tag{6}$$

$$ButyrylSACP + malonylSCoA \rightleftharpoons \beta\text{-}ketocaproylSACP + HSCoA + CO_2, \text{etc.} \tag{7}$$

The series of reactions then continues from reaction 4 (acetoacetylSACP), and the chain is lengthened by two carbon atoms with each cycle resulting in the formation of even-numbered fatty acids. These reactions and the enzymatic machinery involved are shown in Fig. 11.21.

Odd-chain fatty acids are synthesized to a limited extent in mammalian tissues. The synthesis differs from that described above only in that propionyl CoA replaces acetyl CoA in the initial condensation reaction.

Synthesis of Unsaturated Fatty Acids. Of the various unsaturated fatty acids present in animal tissues only one series of compounds can be synthesized in the animal body. These unsaturated fatty acids contain double bonds only between the carboxyl group and the seventh carbon from the terminal methyl group (Chapter 2) and derive from the palmityl synthesizing system. The various fatty acids are subsequently produced by alternate desaturation and elongation of the carbon chains (Fig. 11.22). The latter reactions

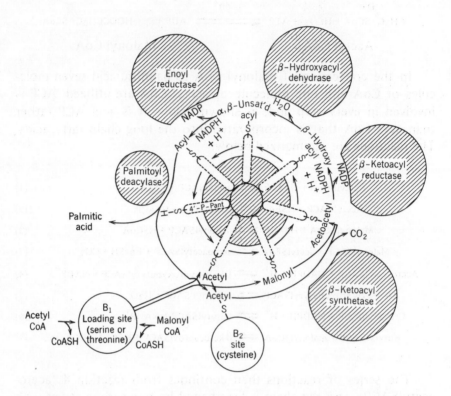

Fig. 11.21 Proposed mechanism of fatty acid synthesis. The cycle begins with the acetyl group of acetylSCoA being first transferred to a hydroxyl group of a serine or threonine residue at the B_1 loading site, then to the SH of ACP (Reaction 1) and then to a cysteine residue site. The malonyl group from malonylSCoA is then transferred to ACP (Reaction 2). Formation of acetoacetylSACP occurs on the ACP site (Reaction 3) and the carbon chain remains on this site. Reactions 4, 5, and 6 then continue as the bound compound attached to the rotating 4'-phosphopantetheine group of the ACP is subjected to the successive enzymes catalyzing the two reductions and the dehydration reactions to form butyrylSACP. Reaction with malonylSCoA and repetition of the cycle six more times yields palmitoylSACP. Palmitic acid is liberated by the action of palmitoyl deacylase. [From G. T. Phillips, J. E. Nixon, J. A. Dorsey, P. H. W. Butterworth, C. J. Chesterston, and J. W. Porter, *Arch. Biochem. Biophys.*, 138:380, (1970).]

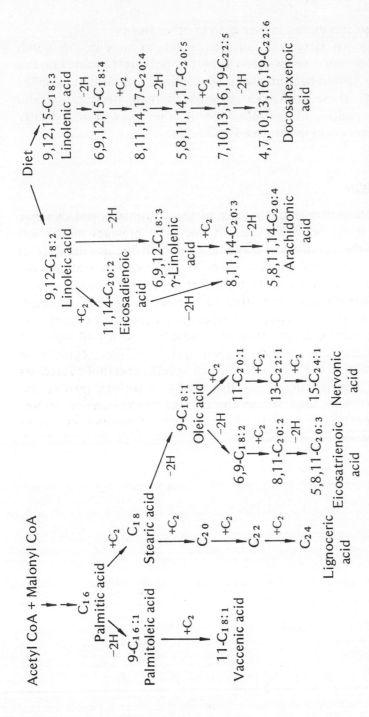

Fig. 11.22 Biosynthesis of some fatty acids in mammals. The numbers in boldface indicate the position of the double bonds; the subscripts indicate the number of carbon atoms, with the number of double bonds to the right of the colon. (From A. White, P. Handler, and E. L. Smith, *Principles of Biochemistry*, 5th Ed., McGraw Hill, New York, 1973, p. 567.)

occur to a greater extent in liver than in other tissues.

The essential fatty acids all contain one or more double bonds within the terminal seven carbons of the fatty acid chain. For this reason they cannot be synthesized by the body and must be supplied in the diet. These acids also undergo alternate desaturation and elongation resulting in the formation of other more saturated fatty acids of longer chain length (see Fig. 11.22).

CONCLUSION

The endoplasmic reticulum is part of the continuous and dynamic membrane structure of the cell. It not only provides mechanical support for the cytoplasmic contents of the cell but also provides its transport lanes. The concentration of membranous endoplasmic reticulum varies with the synthetic activity of the cell, sparse in those cells in which synthesis is limited to internal needs, and extremely dense in those that are active in synthesizing proteins for export. The cytoplasmic matrix is the transport medium in which all nutrients and metabolites are carried on their way from one organelle to another. It also is the medium in which specific metabolic reactions take place. The reticulum and the matrix, therefore, provide the lanes of communication within the cell and to the exterior. In this way, they contribute both to the movement of metabolites and to their temporary sequestration.

chapter 12
the golgi apparatus

1. Structure
2. Function
   a. Membrane Flow
   b. Cell Surface Materials
   c. Secretion
   d. Lysosome Formation
   e. Phospholipid Formation
   f. Lipoprotein Synthesis
   g. Hormone Synthesis and Secretion
   h. Milk Synthesis
3. Conclusion

The Golgi apparatus was barely mentioned in the first edition of this book beyond noting its presence and indicating its function. Details of how it performed its suggested assembly-line function of packaging synthesized products for export were not sufficiently deciphered to warrant more extended treatment. Now the status of the Golgi apparatus as an organelle of consequence is fully established. No longer are there disbelievers in its existence. It is known to occupy a key position in the transport system of the cell and, according to Northcote (1971), "acts like a valve in controlling the distribution of cellular material".

In 1898 Golgi discovered a structure in the cell close to the nucleus that he called the internal reticular apparatus. Many cytologists thought this was an artifact attributable to his staining technique since it could not be seen in the living cell nor with routine stains. Not until the 1950s and the advent of the electron microscope was it finally established that, skeptics notwithstanding, such an organelle did exist as Golgi had indicated. Further, this organelle, now called the *Golgi apparatus* or *Golgi complex,* can be found in almost all mammalian cells. In fact, it has come to be one of the readily identifiable components of the cell in electron micrographs. (Fig. 12.1).

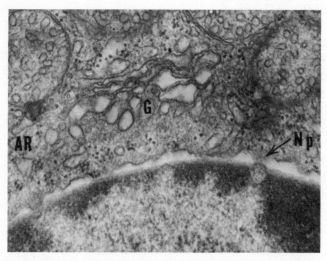

Fig. 12.1   Golgi complex (G) showing flattened sacs and clusters of vacuoles. The reticulum (AR) is the smooth or agranular type. Mitochondria (M) show the tubular cristae seen in adrenal cortical cells. N = nucleus, Np = nuclear pore, Ly = lysosomes. Adrenal cortex of rat. Magnification 56,800. (Courtesy of Dr. Harald Schraer.)

STRUCTURE

The Golgi complex consists mainly of smooth surfaced membranes that, in electron micrographs, appear as a stack of more or less flattened vesicles that are variously called *cisternae, lamellae,* or *saccules.* These stacks may appear singly or, in secretory cells,

Secretory vesicles
leaving mature face

Saccule

Transfer vesicles
reaching forming face

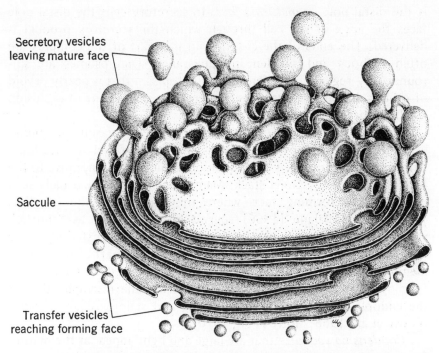

Fig. 12.2 Drawing depicting the Golgi apparatus of a secretory cell in 3 dimensions. The transfer vesicles shown below are in this instance small enough to be termed microvesicles, but in some kinds of cells they are larger. The transfer vesicles bud off from rough-surfaced endoplasmic reticulum, which would be below. The secretory vesicles that bud off from saccules on the mature face become, in the instance of acinar cells, the so-called zymogen granules. (From A. W. Ham, *Histology*, 6th ed., Lippincott, Phila., 1969, p. 141.)

several may appear together. They vary in size and usually contain from five to eight lamellae but may contain many more in a slightly curved stack (Fig. 12.2). The stack is the *dictyosome.* The location and size of the dictyosome varies among cell types and also with the physiological state of the cell. Generally, the dictyosomes are polarized so that one pole is associated with the endoplasmic reticulum or the nuclear envelope. This is the proximal pole and is the *forming face* or *immature face.* These cisternae are usually flat and appear empty, and the membranes are similar in structure and enzyme composition to those of the endoplasmic reticulum. The opposite pole is concave and is closer to the plasma membrane. This is the distal pole or *maturing face*. In secretory cells the distal pole faces the apex of the cell through which the secretory product is delivered. The ends of the cisternae in this part of the complex are often bulbous and swollen in appearance. Dictyosomes are surrounded by regions of differentiated cytoplasm that is nearly devoid of other cell components. This is referred to as the zone of exclusion (Mollenhauer, 1965).

Transfer vesicles bud off from the rough endoplasmic reticulum, lose the attached ribosomes and, as smooth surfaced vesicles filled with protein synthesized by the endoplasmic reticulum, move to the forming face of the Golgi stack. Many small vesicles are usually seen close to the forming face where they fuse with the lamellae. Jamieson and Palade (1966) suggest that they act as "shuttle" vesicles. The protein carried within the vesicle is transferred to the saccule and the membrane of the vesicle becomes part of the saccule membrane. In this way, membrane is continuously added to the forming face of the Golgi stack. This membrane resembles that of the endoplasmic reticulum in thickness and staining characteristics (Grove et al., 1968; Morré et al., 1970).

Condensing vacuoles that are large and light appear at the mature face of the stack. These, like the transfer vesicles, sometimes appear to be continuous with the lamellae. The vacuoles pinch off from the ovoid, swollen ends of the lamellae and carry away the secretion. After becoming progressively smaller and denser, they are often called *zymogen granules*. They move toward the plasma membrane or apex of the secretory cell and discharge their contents by exocytosis. In the process, the membrane of the vacuole, which by now resembles the plasma membrane in thickness and staining intensity fuses with it, (Dalton, 1961; Grove et al., 1968; Morré et al., 1970). This membrane leaving the stack balances that brought to the forming face by the transfer vesicles.

The entire membranous complex of the Golgi apparatus is in a dynamic state, constantly being renewed. The vesicle merges with the lamellae at the forming face and the vacuole pinches off or "blebs" at the mature surface to migrate to the plasma membrane (Morré et al., 1971b). This renewal is part of a larger system of renewal designated as membrane flow that will be discussed in the section on function.

From work on Golgi lamellae in tissue culture cells, Takagi et al.

(1965) found that these were flexible and elastic structures. The gradient they exhibit in morphology from endoplasmic reticulum-like to plasma membrane-like results from either difference in chemical composition or the arrangement of molecules within the membrane (Morré et al., 1971a). In the transformation of endoplasmic reticulum membrane into Golgi membrane, enzymatic activities and prosthetic groups are progressively lost. The lecithin content of Golgi membranes and the chemical lipoprotein composition is intermediate between that of endoplasmic reticulum and plasma membrane (Keenan and Morré, 1970; Yunghans et al., 1970). Gel electrophoresis patterns are intermediate between plasma membrane and endoplasmic reticulum as far as appearance and number and position of the bands but resemble more closely the pattern of endoplasmic reticulum (Yunghans et al., 1970).

Concentrated in the Golgi complex are ADPase, $Mg^{2+}ATPase$, CTPase, TPPase, and acid phosphatase. In addition, there are high concentrations of UDP-N-acetylglycosamine transferase and galactosyl transferase, but glucose-6-phosphatase, which is characteristic of the endoplasmic reticulum, is in low concentration in the Golgi complex (DeRobertis et al., 1970). Enzyme activities change when endoplasmic reticulum membranes are incorporated into Golgi saccules (Novikoff et al., 1962). In cells where TPPase is not present in the endoplasmic reticulum, the Golgi membrane acquires it or, if the endoplasmic reticulum had such activity, it becomes higher in the Golgi. Then, when the vacuoles leave the Golgi complex, they lose the TPPase activity (Novikoff, 1963b). Another change observed is the loss of nucleoside diphosphatase activity from the endoplasmic reticulum to the saccule (Novikoff, ibid).

How the Golgi complex originates has not been established. It is clear that it multiplies in some way since there is no decrease in number after cell divisions (Morré et al., 1971b). How multiplication occurs is far from clear but over the years, several suggestions have been made including *de novo* formation (Flickinger, 1969); derivation from preexisting Golgi material by division (Whaley, 1966) or fragmentation (Mollenhauer and Morré, 1966); and derivation from another membrane system of the cell (see Beams and Kessel, 1968). The arguments are not strong for *de novo* synthesis and studies of dividing cells have shown fragmentation of the Golgi complex followed by a quantitative separa-

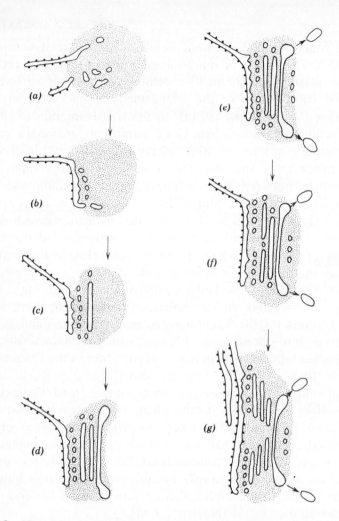

Fig. 12.3 Hypothetical scheme relating observations concerning the origin and continuity of Golgi apparatus. $(a \rightarrow d)$. In the absence of preexisting dictyosomes, cisternae are presumed to arise from small groups of vesicles associated with the endoplasmic reticulum or nuclear envelope. Further differentiation gives rise to flattened platelike cisternae. Additional cisternae form by multiplication of this process. $(e \rightarrow g)$ Multiplication of Golgi apparatus suggested by formation of two sets of shorter cisternae where there was previously one longer cisterna. Continued separation leads to formation of two daughter stacks. (From D. J. Morré, H. H. Mollenhauer, and C. E. Bracker, *Origin and Continuity of Cell Organelles,* Vol. 2, Springer-Verlag, N. Y., 1971c, p. 82.)

tion between the two daughter cells. Opinion concerning division has not changed in the last 50 years since Bowen (1926) stated that the Golgi complex maintained itself through a process of mass division that was much like fragmentation and had nothing in common with the precise division observed for nuclear material.

According to Morré et al. (1971c) the Golgi apparatus appears to be formed from dictyosomes that arise one cisterna at a time. Fig. 12.3 summarizes the series of postulated stages leading up to dictyosome formation, one cisterna at a time, by what appears to be fusion of vesicles in a cytoplasmic zone of exclusion.

FUNCTION

Membrane Flow

An important function of the Golgi complex alluded to in the section on structure is the role it plays in *membrane flow*. Biochemical and morphological studies both indicate that plasma membranes are derived from the nuclear membranes or endoplasmic reticulum via the Golgi complex, and that this occurs through a process of membrane flow and differentiation. Morré et al. (1971b) describe this concept as one in which membranes move along a chain of cell components that serve as a developmental pathway. As the membranes move along this path they are transformed. This membrane flow and change is apparent from the endoplasmic reticulum to the plasma membrane via the Golgi apparatus.

Kinetic evidence of membrane flow was obtained from short-time labeling studies with rat liver cells (Morré et al., 1971a). Fractions obtained from liver cells of rats injected with ^{14}C-arginine were assayed for the marker. The order of the labeling was endoplasmic reticulum or nucleus, Golgi apparatus, and plasma membrane. Radioactivity increased steadily in the plasma membrane and decreased rapidly in the endoplasmic reticulum and Golgi apparatus. Morré et al. (1971a) conclude that membrane differentiation coupled with membrane flow account for the origin of the plasma membrane from the endoplasmic reticulum with the Golgi apparatus acting as the mediator (Fig. 12.4).

Membranes of secretory vesicles are morphologically similar to

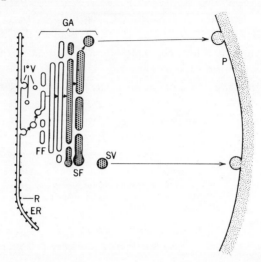

Fig. 12.4 Diagrammatic representation of Golgi apparatus functioning in membrane flow and differentiation. ER, endoplasmic reticulum; R, ribosome; GA, Golgi apparatus; FF, forming face; SF, secreting face; I°, primary vesicle; SV, secretory vesicle; PM, plasma membrane. Direction of membrane flow and vesicle migration denoted by arrows. (From D. J. Morré, W. W. Franke, B. Deumling, S. E. Nyquist, and L. Ovtracht, Biomembranes, Vol. 2, Plenum Press, N. Y., 1971a, p. 95.)

plasma membranes and fuse with plasma membranes when the product is extruded (Sjöstrand, 1963; Helminen and Ericsson, 1968). Jamieson (1972) suggests that the cell probably reuses its intracellular membranes extensively during the course of transport and discharge of secretory proteins. In addition, the discharge of the secretory product requires respiratory energy, and this may be related to the membrane fusion process involved in zymogen discharge. Similarly, the membrane of a phagocytosed particle is plasma membrane, and this is replaced by flow through the synthetic assembly maintained by the Golgi complex.

There are suggestions, also, that the Golgi complex may function in the formation of "new" membrane since the assembly of lamellae or cisternal envelopes increases substantially under some conditions, and the Golgi apparatus is the logical place for this activity to occur (Whaley et al., 1971). Fawcett (1962) postulated that membrane components might be withdrawn from the plasma membrane and

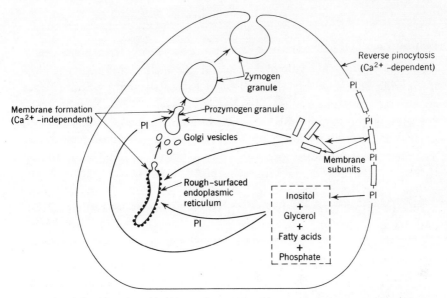

Fig. 12.5 A possible mechanism of membrane circulation based on subunit relocation. Membrane added to the plasma membrane following coalescence of a zymogen granule is broken down into subunits and released back into the cytoplasm. The breakdown into subunits possibly is due to hydrolysis of phosphatidylinositol (PI) postulated to link subunits together. In this way, membrane lost from the endoplasmic reticulum and Golgi apparatus in the formation of zymogen granules is replaced by reassembly of subunits in these organelles through the resynthesis of phosphatidylinositol to join them together. [From C. E. Hokin, *Internatl. Rev. Cytol.*, 23: 187 (1968).]

then reassembled in the Golgi region. Hokin (1968) has suggested that membrane subunits are transferred to the endoplasmic reticulum and to the Golgi complex for reassembly (Fig. 12.5). In either case, on leaving the Golgi complex the membrane may function as plasma membrane, membrane bounding vesicles, vacuoles, or some other intracytoplasmic membrane system. There is no doubt that an important function of the Golgi complex is in the assembly of membrane, its differentiation in both structure and enzyme constituents, and its transfer to other membrane-bound organelles such as lysosomes (Whaley, 1968). In order to function in this manner, it is clear that there must be integration of function among cellular organelles and recycling of the membrane constituents.

Cell Surface Materials

Associated with the role of the Golgi apparatus in membrane flow is its role in providing the cell with materials that confer surface specificity to membranes. These materials are either on the outer surface of the membrane, the *cell coat (glycocalyx)*, components of the plasma membrane itself, or cell surface-associated materials. The surface specificity provides for selective uptake of materials through adhesion characteristics, receptor sites, ion permeability, antigen specificity, and the like. Such cell surface information plays a role in interactions between cells and between an individual cell and its environment; in gamete recognition; in cell differentiation during development; in development of tissue structure; in specialized function of intestinal microvilli including enzyme content and specific receptor sites; and other similar functions dependent on recognition phenomona. Many of the macromolecules that confer such specificity have carbohydrate moieties, and it is the Golgi apparatus that functions in the synthesis of these polysaccharides and attaches them to the protein moiety in the formation of glycoproteins, mucopolysaccharides, and like substances. Genetic control is exerted through the enzymes present in the membranes of the Golgi complex for the synthesis of the particular carbohydrate components. It is the specific carbohydrate component linked to the specific protein material that provides the informational properties. Through membrane flow and recycling of the surface materials, changes in information can be provided (Whaley et al., 1972).

The relationship between the polysaccharide synthesis in the Golgi complex and its localization at the cell surface has been established through a variety of staining procedures (Rambourg and Leblond, 1967; Rambourg et al., 1969). Further evidence has been obtained through radioautographic techniques indicating the uptake of labeled sugars directly into the Golgi complex and their subsequent secretion as part of a surface macromolecule (Ito, 1969; Bennett, 1970; Bennett and Leblond, 1970). Revel and Ito (1967) postulated that this mechanism is similar to other secretory mechanisms except that the Golgi-synthesized material remains attached to the membrane when the membrane is exteriorized.

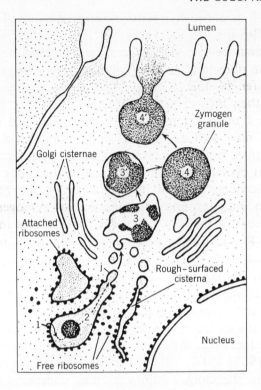

Fig. 12.6 Diagram summarizing events in elaboration of the enzyme secretion in the pancreatic acinar cell. (1) Synthesis of the secretory protein on the ribosomes and into the channel of the endoplasmic reticulum. (2) Transfer of the nascent protein out of the endoplasmic reticulum into transfer vesicles formed by blebbing of the wall. (3) Fusion of isolated vesicles with condensing vacuoles of Golgi complex. (4) Conversion into zymogen granules and release from cell. (From G. E. Palade, P. Siekevitz and L. G. Caro, *Ciba Foundation Symposium on Exocrine Pancreas, Normal and Abnormal Functions*, A. V. S. Rueck and M. P. Cameron, eds., Churchill, London, 1962, p. 23.)

Secretion

The Golgi apparatus is highly developed in secretory cells, especially those cells secreting protein or complex polysaccharides. The secretory mechanism in each case has been followed by autoradiography as well as through fractionation procedures. Using leucine-^{14}C and following its incorporation into chymotrypsinogen by pancreatic acinar cells, Siekevitz and Palade (1958) observed rapid uptake by the ribosomes and endoplasmic reticulum, followed later by the transfer of the label to the Golgi apparatus and related vesicles and then into zymogen granules for export from the cell. From this ar other related studies they described the secretory cycle that is now well defined: (1) incorporation of amino acids into polypeptides by the rough endoplasmic reticulum; (2) transfer of the nascent proteins into the cisternae of the endoplasmic reticulum; (3) intracellular transport to the Golgi apparatus for packaging into zymogen granules; and (4) migration of zymogen granules in the vacuoles toward the apex of the cell for discharge into the lumen of the gland (Fig. 12.6). The procedure is rapid, and Caro and Palade (1964) showed with the use of leucine-^{3}H that within 5 minutes after injection the label appeared in the rough endoplasmic reticulum; by 20 minutes, in the Golgi complex; and after one hour the label was in the zymogen granules. It has since been established that the smooth surfaced vesicles are the means of transport from the rough endoplasmic reticulum to the Golgi complex (Jamieson and Palade, 1965; 1966; 1967a; 1967b); that the secretory protein is carried from the Golgi complex by the condensing vacuoles; and that progressive concentration occurs in the vacuoles in the formation of zymogen granules.

In many cells the synthesis of complex carbohydrates, such as glycoproteins, mucopolysaccharides, and glycolipids, takes place in the Golgi complex. This was demonstrated in the mucus-secreting goblet cells of rat colon. Using radioautographic techniques, Neutra

---

Fig. 12.7 (*a*) Diagram illustrating the relationship of the Golgi complex and mucigen granules in colonic goblet cells. (Courtesy of Dr. C. P. Leblond.) (*b*) Illustrates the activity within the goblet cell based on the radioautographic studies of Neutra and Leblond (1966). This diagram indicates the entrance of amino acids into the goblet cells from a capillary where they are synthesized into protein in association with the endoplasmic reticulum. The newly synthesized proteins are transported to the Golgi complex which synthesizes carbohydrate. The carbohydrate is added to the incoming protein, both materials being packaged in the Golgi region and released. The mucigen granules then migrate to the apical end of the cell and are released to the exterior. (Courtesy of Dr. C. P. Leblond.)

and Leblond (1966) found that 5 minutes after the injection of
^{3}H-glucose the label was in the cisternae of the Golgi complex; at
20 minutes both the cisternae and mucinigen granules were labeled;
by 40 minutes all the label was in the mucinigen; and within one to
four hours the labeled granules had migrated from the region of the
Golgi complex to the apex of the cell for extrusion. From this it
was concluded that the Golgi complex is the area for the synthesis

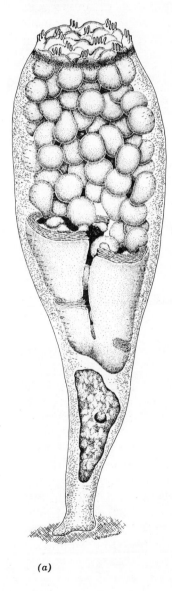

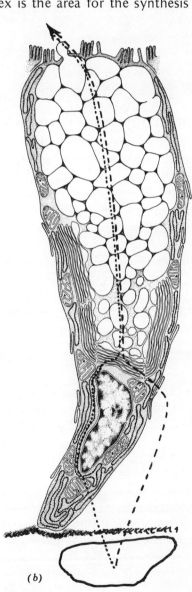

(a)   (b)

of the complex carbohydrate that is joined to protein delivered to it from the endoplasmic reticulum to form the glycoprotein of the mucus (Fig. 12.7). Neutra and Leblond (1966) estimated that one distended saccule was transformed into mucigen granules and released by each Golgi stack every 2 to 4 minutes. This is indicative of a rapid renewal of the Golgi stack by addition to the immature face. The entire Golgi apparatus in the mucus-secreting goblet cells of the colon was estimated to be formed and re-formed within 20 to 40 minutes.

The Golgi complex is also the site of sulfonation of the carbohydrates of mucus (Berlin, 1967) and for the addition of sulfate to chondroitin in collagen formation (Neutra and Leblond, 1969).

Many cell products are known to be packaged and transported through the Golgi apparatus and its associated vesicles. Many of these are polysaccharides, or they are proteins or lipids that acquire carbohydrate moieties to become glycoproteins or glycolipoproteins in the membranes of the Golgi apparatus. In fact, Northcote (1971) speculates that conjugation with carbohydrate may be a prerequisite for subsequent transport of materials across the plasma membrane. If, indeed, this is so, the role of the Golgi apparatus takes on even greater significance.

Only the complex carbohydrates attached to protein and destined for secretion are synthesized in the Golgi complex. Glycogen is not synthesized there but in the cytoplasm instead (see Chapter 11).

For further discussion of Golgi complex involvement in the synthesis of complex carbohydrate, see Neutra and Leblond (1969).

Lysosome Formation

The formation of lysosomes by the Golgi apparatus is analogous to the synthesis of protein secretion granules and is discussed in detail in Chapter 14. This role of the Golgi apparatus may be considered synthesis of catabolic agents; that is, synthesis of enzymes into vesicles whose membranes have the capacity to fuse with endocytotic vesicles or the plasma membrane itself for catabolic purposes. The informational characteristics of the lysosomal membrane, incorporated into it in the Golgi complex during synthesis, endow it with the capacity to ferret out only specific membranes with which to merge and to shun all others.

Phospholipid Synthesis

Membrane phospholipids may be synthesized by a variety of cell components including both rough and smooth endoplasmic reticulum (Stein and Stein, 1969). However, if the Golgi complex is implicated in changing endoplasmic reticulum-like to plasma membrane-like membranes, this involves a change in lipid composition (Morré et al., 1971b). In the transition toward the plasma membrane type, there is an increase in the proportion of sphingomyelin and sterols with a corresponding decrease in the proportion of phosphatidyl choline (lecithin). In Golgi apparatus fractions from rat liver, Morré et al. (1970) found choline kinase and phosphorylcholine-cytidyl transferase, important in lecithin and sphingomyelin metabolism.

Lipoprotein Synthesis

The synthesis and transport of lipoprotein particles in liver cells studied by Morré and his group (Morré et al., 1971b) illustrates the multistep, continuous process in which lipids, sterols, and polysaccharides are added to the protein component (Fig. 12.8). During the process the protein particles migrate from their area of origin in the rough endoplasmic reticulum through what appears to be smooth endoplasmic reticulum to the transfer vesicles of the Golgi complex. The integration of structure and function is apparent from the associated changes in membrane type with change in activity as the synthetic process proceeds through the cisternal channels to the secretory vacuoles. The enzyme complement in the Golgi complex membranes may well serve both in the synthesis of membrane components and of products synthesized for export.

Nyquist et al. (1971) have suggested that the involvement of the Golgi apparatus of liver cells in lipoprotein transport may be but one aspect of a broader function that could include the fat-soluble vitamins, particularly vitamin A. The vitamin A content of the Golgi complex fraction of liver cells was found to parallel the vitamin A status of the animal, and no vitamin A was detected in the fraction

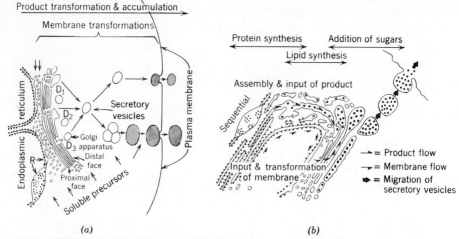

(a) *(b)*

Fig. 12.8 Summary of the structural and functional relationships among Golgi apparatus, endoplasmic reticulum, secretory vesicles and the plasma membrane. The common function of the Golgi complex in the different cell types appears to be the transformation of membranes from endoplasmic reticulum-like to plasma membrane-like. *(a)* In polysaccharide- or mucopolysaccharide-secreting cells, product formation is associated with progressive changes in both cisternal and vesicle contents. *(b)* In hepatocytes the synthesis and transport of lipoprotein particles (solid black dots) is visualized as a continuous multistep process with the addition of lipids, sterols and polysaccharides to the protein component. At the same time the particles migrate from the point of origin to the secretory vesicles. (From D. J. Morré, H. H. Mollenhauer, and C. E. Bracker, *Origin and Continuity of Cell Organelles,* Vol. 2, Springer-Verlag, N. Y., 1971b, p. 82.)

from vitamin A-deficient rats. A role for the Golgi complex in the mobilization and transport of vitamin A compounds was suggested. Alternative, or possibly additional, roles of vitamin A might be related to its function in changing the properties of cytoplasmic and lysosomal membranes (Dingle and Lucy, 1965), and in mucopolysaccharide synthesis.

Hormone Synthesis and Secretion

In general, the Golgi complex in cells of endocrine glands secreting protein and peptide hormones is the area where the product is concentrated and formed into droplets enclosed in a membrane. Usually after a period of storage the secretory product is released through the plasma membrane through exocytosis.

The role of the Golgi complex in the thyroid gland is somewhat different since there is no storage of the secretion within the cell. Instead, the secretion is stored in a follicle as the colloid thyroglobulin. It is believed that the carbohydrate moiety of thyroglobulin is added to the secretion before it is transported into the follicular lumen for storage. When the gland is stimulated to secrete, the colloid is taken from the follicle into the cell by endocytosis, and the hormone is released through lysosomal action (see Chapter 14). Since the lysosomes originate in the Golgi apparatus, this is another aspect of the role of this organelle in thyroid function. The lysosomes release thyroxine from thyroglobulin prior to its secretion from the cell into the perifollicular capillaries.

Steroid-secreting cells have prominent Golgi complexes that become enlarged when the cells are stimulated. The role of the Golgi apparatus is baffling since storage granules that would indicate involvement in packaging are not visible in the cells. Sulfation of protein-polysaccharide complexes is known to take place in the Golgi complex and, since it is believed that steroids are secreted as sulfates, Fawcett et al. (1969) suggest that steroid sulfates may be formed in the Golgi prior to release.

The catecholamines, epinephrine and norepinephrine (secreted by the cells of the adrenal medulla), and other neurosecretory hormones held in synaptic vesicles (see Chapter 19) are packaged in granules enclosed by a smooth-surfaced membrane. This suggests involvement of the Golgi complex.

For further discussion of Golgi complex function, see Jamieson (1971), Whaley et al. (1972) and Dauwalder et al. (1972).

Milk Synthesis

Lactogenesis, or the synthesis and secretion of milk, depends on hormonal action for its initiation. Before synthesis can take place, changes occur in the mammary cells and their constituent organelles. These are induced by estrogen and progesterone as well as by prolactin, the lactogenic hormone from the pituitary. The Golgi apparatus is specifically involved in the secretion of prolactin in the pituitary cells. Smith and Farquhar (1970) have shown, in addition, that enzymes—primarily phosphatases derived from the Golgi—are packaged in the secretory granule containing prolactin.

In the mammary cells there is extensive proliferation of the rough endoplasmic reticulum in the basal portion of the cell for the synthesis of milk protein. The protein is delivered in transfer vesicles to the saccules on the forming face of the Golgi apparatus located on the lumen side of the cell. Passage of the secretory product through the Golgi apparatus in the mammary cell is probably similar to that of other secretory cells such as the exocrine pancreas. According to Patton (1969), it is reasonable to assume that a-lactalbumin, the B protein of lactose synthetase, joins the A protein in the Golgi apparatus. This allows the synthesis of lactose to take place in the Golgi prior to the packaging of the lactose, milk protein, and other constituents of milk serum for secretion. The protein in the vacuoles of the Golgi has the appearance of casein micelles in electron micrographs. Patton (1969) suggests that other proteins may be present also and that the vacuoles must carry some of the fluid of milk and may provide the vehicle for the secretion of milk serum constituents such as lactose.

In mammary cells, as in other cells, the lipid is synthesized in the cytoplasmic matrix. The lipid droplets are extruded from the cell into the lumen by what appears to be reverse pinocytosis.

CONCLUSION

Despite the list of functions attributed to the Golgi complex, it should be apparent that these could be consolidated into two categories: (1) membrane synthesis and recycling and (2) compartmentalization of synthesized products. One could even suggest the single all-encompassing function of membrane synthesis since compartmentalization can occur only if membrane boundaries are established. Membranes are, without doubt, primary and indispensable units of biological structure and function. It would seem, therefore, that the membranes that synthesize membranes should occupy a position of prestige in the hierarchy of organelles. However, the Golgi complex as the synthesizer of membranes performs only one role in the closely integrated collaboration controlling the dynamic yet disciplined character of cellular function. Only the most shortsighted view would suggest an inequality of roles among the organelles. In the long view, each shares equally in the ultimate responsibility for the life or death of the cell, a responsibility that can be fulfilled successfully only when assured by the nutrient content of the extracellular environment.

chapter 13
the mitochondria

1. Location and Number
2. Structure
3. Composition
4. Mitochondrial Compartments
5. Conformational Changes

6. Function
   a. Oxidation of Fatty Acids
   b. Oxidation of Pyruvic Acid
   c. Tricarboxylic Acid Cycle (Krebs cycle, citric acid cycle)
   d. Oxidation of Amino Acids
   e. Electron Transport and Oxidative Phosphorylation
   f. Energy Yield
      1. Oxidative Phosphorylation
      2. Complete Oxidation of Glucose
      3. Fatty Acid Oxidation
   g. Synthesis
      1. Fatty Acids
      2. Protein
   h. Calcium Transport
7. Biogenesis of Mitochondria
8. Conclusion

The mitochondrion is the "powerhouse of the cell" and is responsible for transforming the chemical bond energy of nutrients into the high energy phosphate bonds of ATP. There may be 50 to 2500 of these organs of respiration in a single cell, each containing 500 to 10,000 complete sets of oxidative enzymes. Each enzyme assembly contains 15 or more active molecules in a highly ordered arrangement which is an integral part of the organelle structure. All the activities of the cell which are necessary for its survival are completely dependent upon the ability of the mitochondria to release the potential energy in a nutrient molecule and transduce that energy into a form of cellular work: osmotic, mechanical, electrical, chemical.

The development of molecular biology probably received its greatest impetus when the granules that the cytologists called mitochondria were first isolated by differential centrifugation and found by the biochemists to be capable of carrying out the oxidation of all the Krebs tricarboxylic acid (TCA) cycle intermediates. The transformations of energy that are accomplished by this series of integrated enzymatically controlled reactions end in a chemical trap: the formation of ATP, the universal intracellular carrier of chemical energy. The locus for this activity in all cells, from the single cell of the protist to each of the myriad cells in the complex organism, is the mitochondrion. It is the discharge of this function upon which the continuing supply of energy for all other mitochondrial and cellular functions depend. There are other mitochondrial functions that may vie with, but can never overshadow, the primacy of this process of oxidative phosphorylation. This should in no way depreciate the ability of the mitochondrion to synthesize fatty acids, synthesize and catabolize proteins, form amino acids, perform carboxylations, participate in ionic regulation in the cell, and change the permeability of its membranes to make new substrate available. Nor can the presence of the only extranuclear supply of DNA so far discovered be easily subordinated. However, these processes could not progress far without the requisite energy that the mitochondrion releases for itself and for all the activities of the organelles of the cell.

LOCATION AND NUMBER

Mitochondria are found in all aerobic respiring cells except bacteria. Although they appear to be distributed rather generally throughout the cytoplasmic matrix, their locations within the cell are related to their function. Often they are located close to the source of fuel and in liver cells of fasting rats have been found draped around lipid droplets. More often, according to Lehninger (1967), they are found near the structure that will receive their end product, the ATP molecules. The locations in different cell types is frequently characteristic: in muscle cells, they are aligned in rows along the sarcomeres; in axon endings, near where transmitter substances are synthesized (see Chapters 18 and 19); in acinar cells of the pancreas, they are in and near the rough endoplasmic reticulum where active enzyme synthesis is taking place. Generally, in secretory cells their orientation is along the secretory axis.

The number of mitochondria in a cell varies enormously with the cell type. Liver cells may contain 1 to 2000 and renal tubule cells about 300. Sperm cells have as few as 20 mitochondria and, never underestimate the power of the female, oocytes may contain up to 300,000 mitochondria per cell (Lehninger, 1964; 1967).

STRUCTURE

The first truly collaborative efforts of the cytologist and biochemist derived from observations of the mitochondrial fragments that carried the enzymes essential for oxidative phosphorylation. In suspensions of disrupted mitochondria Kennedy and Lehninger (1949), Schneider and Potter (1948), and Green et al. (1948) identified the enzymes of the Krebs cycle in the soluble portion, and the electron transport mechanism in the lipoprotein moiety of the cristae membrane. All efforts to separate the enzyme activity from the membrane were unsuccessful and it became evident that the enzymes were, in fact, an integral part of the membrane structure.

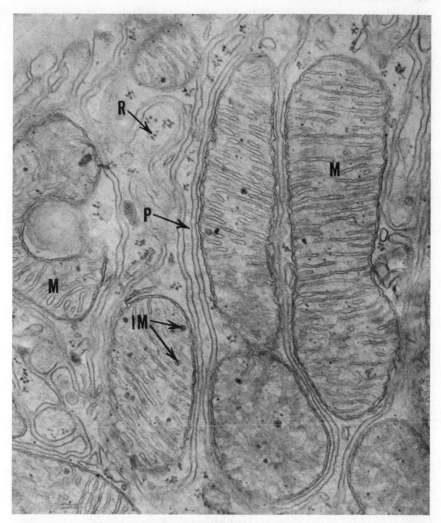

Fig. 13.1 Mitochondria (M) showing double membrane structure and transverse cristae. IM = intramitochondrial granules, P = plasma membrane, R = ribosomes. Rat kidney proximal tubule. Magnification 42,000. (Courtesy of Dr. Harold Schraer.)

There is a striking similarity in the fundamental structure of mitochondria found in all forms from protozoa to primates. Palade (1952) was first to describe the complex and highly differentiated ultrastructure of the mitochondrion revealed by the electron microscope (Fig. 13.1). From his early description and from later more detailed studies, the mitochondrion was revealed as a double-membraned structure, one sac enclosing another (Fig. 13.2).

The two membranes are quite different in structure and in their biochemical and physical properties. The outer membrane is smooth and the inner one has infoldings or invaginations that extend into the lumen. These are the *cristae* or *mitochondrial crests.* The number of cristae and the surface area of their membranes vary directly with the respiratory activity of the cell. In some cells the cristae may be short and relatively few in number whereas in cells having

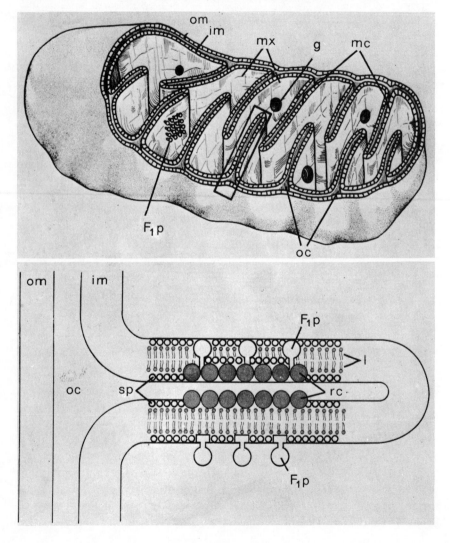

intense activity they are very numerous and regularly arranged. For example, in a cell with a moderate rate of respiration such as the liver cell, the area has been estimated to be 40 m^2/gm protein (Mitchell, 1966), but muscle mitochondria may comprise 10 times that area. A most complex arrangement of cristae, which is practically a crystalline-like lattice, has been found in the heart muscle of the canary, which beats at a rate of 1000 per minute (Slautterback, 1965).

The outer membrane is separated from the inner membrane by a space that is referred to as the outer compartment. The inner membrane bounds the inner compartment, which is the larger of the two chambers, and contains the mitochondrial matrix. The matrix is gel-like, appears granular and generally homogeneous, but filaments have been observed (DeRobertis and Franco Raffo, 1957). Electron-dense granules are observed in the inner compartment, free in the matrix, and often close to the inner membrane. Barnard and Afzelius (1972) suggest that these inclusions represent stores of phospholipid destined for incorporation into the inner membrane. Most descriptions of the mitochondria indicate that the inner and outer membranes are completely separated, but Novikoff (1961a) suggested that there is probably continuity of the inner membranes and the external surface. Only recently, Hackenbrock (1968) reported that as many as 100 contact points exist between the membranes in rat liver mitochondria, and that these may be analogous to the tight

---

Fig. 13.2 Diagram of the ultrastructure of a mitochondrion. Above, a three-dimensional diagram of a mitochondrion showing: the outer membrane (om), the inner membrane (im), the mitochondrial matrix (mx), the mitochondrial crests (mc), granules (g) present in the matrix and containing calcium and magnesium. The outer chamber (oc), between the membranes, and the F_1 particles (F_1p) are also indicated. Below, the molecular organization of a mitochondrial crest. (This portion corresponds to the inset in the upper figure.) Notice that the respiratory chains (rc) are disposed in the outer edge of the inner membrane. The F_1 particles are probably within the membrane in the intact mitochondria, but they become exposed (lower part) with osmotic treatment and negative staining; lipid layer (l); structural protein (sp). (Lower portion of the figure courtesy of A. L. Lehninger.) (From De Robertis et al., *Cell Biology*, 5th ed. W. B. Saunders Co. Phila., 1970, p. 203.)

junctions of plasma membranes (see Chapter 9). These contact areas, according to Winkler (1969), may be the points at which the ATP transport carriers are located.

The morphological difference between the outer and inner mitochondrial membranes has long been the subject of controversy. The inner surface of the inner membrane appeared to be covered with thousands of small particles that were referred to by Green and Hatefi (1961) as the electron transport particles. Fernandez-Moran (1962) called them elementary particles and his electron photomicrographs showed them connected by narrow stalks to the core of the membrane. Smith (1963) estimated that there were about 4000 particles/μ^2 of membrane surface. These elementary units according to some investigators (Blair et al., 1963; Green, 1964) were the respiratory assemblies that carry out the metabolic activity of the mitochondrion. Green and Perdue (1966) suggested that the elementary particles are not projections from the inner membrane of the mitochondrion but that the particles are tripartite and that the base portion forms the membrane. Attached to each of the fused base particles is a stalk and detachable knob (Fig. 13.3). They suggest that the repeating units in the same membrane have the same form and size but that they differ with respect to chemical composition and enzyme activity. This model differs significantly from that of Lehninger (1965), who postulated that the enzyme assemblies in the mitochondrial membrane are not knob-like particles protruding from the surface

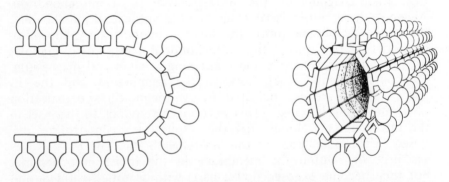

Fig. 13.3 Diagrammatic representation of the inner membrane of the mitochondrion as a fusion of the elementary particles. [From D. E. Green and J. F. Perdue, *Ann. N. Y. Acad. Sci.*, 137:667 (1966).]

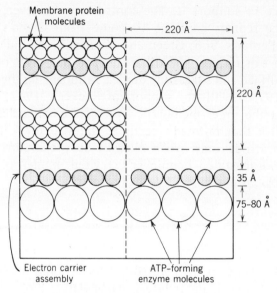

Schematic representation of surface of inner
mitochondrial membrane (to scale)

Fig. 13.4 Schematic representation of structure of inner mitochondrial membrane. [From A. L. Lehninger, *Adv. Cytopharmocol.,* 1: 199 (1971).]

but are embedded in the protein layer of the membrane. Stoeckenius (1963; 1966) suggested that the particles of Fernandez-Moran
(1962) and of Green (1964) might be large ATPase molecules. In
preparations of submitochondrial fractions studied biochemically
and electron microscopically, Racker (1967; 1968) reported that the
so-called elementary particles do not represent the electron transport enzymes since rapid oxidation of DPNH occurred in the absence
of the particles. A subsequent report from Racker's (1970) laboratory indicated quite clearly that the membrane spheres are ATPase
molecules that are not protrusions from the membrane, as Green
and his colleagues contended, but are embedded in the membrane
structure as had been suggested earlier by Lehninger (1965a).
The knob-like appearance on the membrane surface was thought to
be an artifact following the preparatory procedures. Stoekenius
(1970) has reviewed the evidence presented to support the presence
of the subunit particles on the mitochondrial membranes and concluded that the model proposed by Green is unsatisfactory and has

little evidence to support it. The controversy, however, is far from resolved since reports continue to come from Green's laboratory (Green and Perdue, 1966; Green and Young, 1971) indicating their belief in the existence of the tripartite repeating units on the inner membrane surface and suggesting models rationalizing their function. Lehninger (1971a), with the support of Racker's (1967; 1970) data, reasserts that the inner membrane spheres are molecules of the F1 coupling factor that normally occur as flat structures in the membrane and protrude only when released by preparatory treatment with phosphotungstate. Lehninger's revised model of the inner membrane structure is shown in Fig. 13.4.

COMPOSITION

The exquisite precision with which the mitochondrion performs the intricate biochemical procedures, particularly those involved in oxidative phosphorylation, implies a corresponding precision in organization. Such coordinated and efficient function could not occur by random meeting of enzymes and substrates.

In cells with high mitochondrial counts, the mitochondria may account for over 20 percent of the cytoplasmic volume and for 30 to 35 percent of the total protein of the cell. Of the mitochondrial protein, approximately 4 percent is in the outer membrane, 21 percent in the inner membrane, and 67 percent accounted for by the matrix, with the remainder in the intermembrane space (Sottocasa et al., 1967; Schnaitman and Greenawalt, 1968). There are many different species of membrane protein (Schnaitman, 1969) with at least 25 percent of that in the inner membrane made up of catabolically active proteins. There is no answer yet about whether there is a division between structural and functional proteins or whether the individual proteins comprising the membrane share both responsibilities.

Although a contractile protein similar to myosin had been reported by Ohnishi and Ohnishi (1962a; 1962b), and Lehninger (1962; 1964) also referred to a mitochondrial actomyosin, Conover and Bárány (1966) have since suggested that such a factor was due to contamination. Bemis et al. (1968) report that mitochondria do not contain a contractile protein and that change in shape is due to the flexibility of the membranes and the passive consequence of ion-pumping coupled to electron transport.

Glycoproteins have been identified in liver mitochondria (Sotto-casa et al., 1972) and appear to be located in the outer compartment. Swelling of the mitochondria leads to the release of some 30 percent of the total mitochondrial protein. Involvement of glycoprotein in calcium transport has been suggested (Lehninger, 1971b; Carafoli et al., 1972).

The lipid content of all mitochondria is approximately the same, 27 percent, with phospholipid accounting for 90 percent of the lipid fraction (Fleischer et al., 1967). The phospholipids present in all mitochondria are phosphatidyl choline, phosphatidyl ethanol-amine, and cardiolipin. Phosphatidyl choline and phosphatidyl ethanolamine are present in approximately equal amounts comprising 76 to 78 percent of the total phospholipid present, and cardio-lipin 20 percent. There is a very high degree of unsaturation found in the fatty acyl chains, but chain length and chain unsaturation vary within wide limits among both species and organs and are thought to be influenced by both dietary and environmental factors (Chapman and Leslie, 1970). A comparative study on the effect of diet on mitochondrial lipid patterns (Richardson et al., 1961; 1962) showed a higher degree of unsaturation in fish and fish-eating animals, but whether this is due to possible dietary or environmental temperature effects among the species could not be ascertained. Fish mitochondria were found to have little or no linoleic, linolenic, and very little arachidonic acid in contrast to those of the rat. Richardson and Tappel (1962) suggest that some of the very highly unsaturated lipids (22:5 and 22:6) in fish mitochondria are associated with their ability to function at lower temperatures. Vos et al. (1972) found that the total number of membrane-bound fatty acyl chain double bonds was lowered in vitamin E deficiency and that the effect was much more obvious in the inner mitochondrial membranes than in the microsomal membranes.

Recently, separation of the inner and outer mitochondrial membranes has been effected by exposing mitochondria to swelling agents or detergents and subjecting them to density centrifugation (Sottocasa et al., 1967; Schnaitman and Greenawalt, 1968). This has permitted a clear demonstration that the two membranes differ in chemical composition, enzyme content, and ultrastructure (Table

Table 13.1 LOCALIZATION OF SOME LIVER MITOCHONDRIAL ENZYMES

Outer Membrane	Intermembrane Space	Inner Membrane	Matrix
Rotenone—insensitive NADH-Cyt b_5 reductase	Adenylate kinase[a]	Cytochrome b, c, c_1, a, a_3	Malic dehydrogenase
	Nucleoside diphosphokinase	β-Hydroxybutyrate dehydrogenase	Isocitric dehydrogenase
Monoamine oxidase[a]		Ferrochelatase	Glutamic dehydrogenase
Kynurenine hydroxylase		δ-Amino levulinic synthetase	Glutamic-aspartic transaminase
ATP-dependent fatty acyl CoA synthetase		Carnitine palmityl transferase	Citrate synthase
Glycerophosphate acyl transferase		—	Aconitase
Lysophosphatidate acyl transferase			Fumarase[a]
		Fatty acid elongation enzymes	Pyruvic carboxylase

500

Lysolecithin acyl transferase	Respiratory chain-linked phosphorylation enzymes	Protein synthesis enzymes
Phosphocholine transferase	Succinic dehydrogenase	Fatty acyl CoA dehydrogenase
Phosphatidate phosphatase	Cytochrome a_3 oxidase[a]	Nucleic acid polymerases
Nucleoside diphosphokinase	Mitochondrial DNA polymerase	ATP-dependent fatty acyl CoA synthetase
Fatty acid elongating system C_{14} - C_{16}		GTP-dependent fatty acyl CoA synthetase

Adapted from L. Ernster and B. Kuylenstierna, *Membranes of Mitochondria and Chloroplasts*, E. Racker, ed., Van Nostrand Reinhold Co., N. Y., 1970, p. 196.

[a]Marker enzymes.

13.1). The most distinguishing feature is the lipid distribution between the inner and outer membranes (Stoffel and Schiefer, 1968). The inner membrane is 80 percent protein and only 20 percent lipid. These relative proportions are very different from the outer and most other membranes, which are approximately 60 percent protein and 40 percent lipid. Qualitative differences in the phospholipid composition are striking particularly with respect to cardiolipin, which is predominantly, if not exclusively, in the inner membrane and phosphatidyl inositol, which is mostly in the outer membrane (see Ernster and Kuylenstierna, 1970). In both cases, the outer membrane of the mitochondrion resembles that of endoplasmic reticulum. Most of the cholesterol is in the outer membrane giving a molar ratio of cholesterol to phospholipid of 1:9, whereas the ratio for the inner membrane is 1:53 (Levy and Sauner, 1968). The presence of any cholesterol in the inner membrane of liver mitochondria is questioned by Neupert et al. (1972), but they do suggest that sterols in general are essential components of the outer mitochondrial membranes; in *Neurospora* there is an extremely high concentration of ergosterol; in liver, it is cholesterol.

With improved biochemical techniques that permit analysis of each of the membranes, coupled with electron microscopic analyses, a molecular picture of the organization of the inner membrane has been formulated (Klingenberg, 1967). Even though the actual structural organization within the membrane may be the subject of controversy, enzymatic studies have shown that all of the flavoproteins and cytochromes are located in the inner mitochondrial membrane along with all the enzymes required to regenerate ATP from ADP and Pi. In a single liver mitochondrion there are estimated to be about 15,000 electron carrier molecules and about 50,000 in a heart mitochondrion. Calculations indicate that one respiratory assembly occupies a square 200 Å on a side with the inner spheres occupying a large part of this area (see Fig. 13.4). There are three to five spheres per respiratory assembly according to the model suggested by Lehninger (1971a), and all types of mitochondria in all species follow this pattern with the result that there is a proportionality between the number of respiratory assemblies per mitochondrion and the area of the inner membrane.

Metabolic exchanges across the mitochondrial membranes

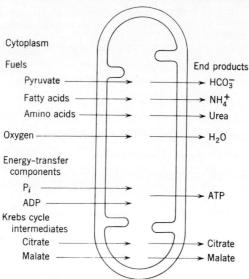

Fig. 13.5 The metabolic traffic across the mitochondrial membrane. [From A. L. Lehninger, *Adv. Cytopharmacol.*, 1: 199 (1971a).]

MITOCHONDRIAL COMPARTMENTS

Most of the important metabolic activities for which the mitochondrion is responsible take place within the inner compartment. The outer membrane is freely permeable to water, simple electrolytes, sucrose, and even some polypeptides. The inner membrane is permeable to water, to certain small molecules such as urea, glycerol, and short chain fatty acids. However, it is not permeable to the flavoproteins, to the nucleoside mono-, di-, or triphosphates or to CoA and its esters. This means that the inner compartments of mitochondria contain an internal pool of these molecules that is separate and distinct from the cytoplasmic pool. All of the respiratory substrates must enter the inner compartment for oxidation; ADP and phosphate must enter if ATP is to be formed and, of course, the ATP must be able to cross the membrane to leave the mitochondrion. A diagram of the metabolic traffic is shown in Fig. 13.5. The mechanisms controlling the mitochondrial membrane traffic are of considerable interest. Two mechanisms that appear to be involved are (1) substrate-specific carrier systems that are probably membrane proteins or lipoproteins; and (2) shuttle systems that employ mobile, low molecular weight molecules as carriers.

Specific carriers in the inner mitochondrial membrane are believed to function by facilitated diffusion. There is strong evidence for the presence of a specific carrier for ATP and ADP (Winkler et al., 1968; Winkler and Lehninger, 1968), which works in close conjunction with the phosphate carrier system. The ATP-ADP carrier works on an exchange basis and a molecule of ADP can enter the inner compartment only if a molecule of ATP leaves. There is strong evidence that carriers exist for succinate or malate, isocitrate, glutamic acid, and bicarbonate (Lehninger, 1971b). Lehninger (1969) has also presented evidence of a carrier specific for Ca^{2+}, Mn^{2+}, or Sr^{2+}. Since the electrical charge must be balanced on either side of the membrane, Pfaff and Klingenberg (1968) suggest that the carriers are electrically integrated. Carbonic hydrase which has been found in the inner membrane (Rossi, 1968) appears to be able to function as a bicarbonate or CO_2 carrier.

The Ca^{2+} carrier has been studied by Lehninger's group (Reynafarje and Lehninger, 1969; Lehninger and Carafoli, 1969) who have found that it is a protein which is different from the calcium-binding protein found in the intestine (Wasserman et al., 1968a). They suggest that this carrier may be involved in rapid reversible segregation of ionic Ca^{2+} in mitochondria during muscular activity as well as during calcification changes in bone (see Chapters 17 and 18). Carafoli et al. (1972) have isolated mitochondrial fractions capable of binding Ca^{2+} and have found that a component common to the binding factors is sialic acid and that the purified glycoprotein also contains hexosamines and neutral sugars.

Two mitochondrial shuttle systems of importance are the a-glycerophosphate shuttle of liver and muscle and the acylcarnitine transferase system. The latter system enables transfer from extramitochondrial CoA to intramitochondrial CoA (Tubbs and Garland, 1968). These systems will be discussed in a subsequent section.

CONFORMATIONAL CHANGES

The ability of the mitochondrial membrane to swell or to contract was observed and was believed to depend on the oxidation-reduction state of the enzymes in the membranes (Lehninger, 1962). Swelling was observed when respiration was occurring in the absence or deficiency of ATP. Contraction with the extrusion of water occurred with the addition of ATP, and Lehninger (1964) postulated that the electron carriers or ATP-forming enzymes underwent con-

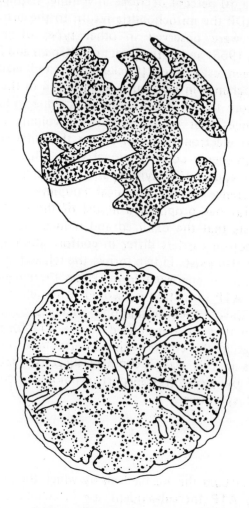

Fig. 13.6 The conformation states of rat liver mitochondria. Top: orthodox conformation observed in absence of ADP. Bottom: condensed conformation observed in presence of ADP. [From A. L. Lehninger, *Adv. Cytopharmocol.*, 1: 199 (1971a).]

formational changes. It has since been demonstrated through electron microscopy (Hackenbrock, 1966; 1968) that liver mitochondria reversibly oscillate between two states: the classical or *orthodox* state observed in the absence of ADP, and the *condensed* state that occurs with the addition of ADP and the stimulation of respiration (Fig. 13.6). In the condensed state the inner compartment is contracted with a 50 percent decrease in volume. With phosphorylation of all the ADP the mitochondria return to the orthodox state. Similar changes were observed in other types of mitochondria (Penniston et al., 1968) and in the intact cell (Green and MacLennan, 1969). It has been established (Hackenbrock and Gamble, 1969) that there is no change in osmolar concentration in the inner compartment, therefore the change in state is not due to ion transport or osmotic changes that would produce a volume change. The suggestion is that electron transport causes the inner compartment to go into a high-energy conformational state. This is used as the driving force to cause ATP synthesis. This concept is generally favored in preference to the chemical coupling hypothesis, and Lehninger (1971a) has proposed a model of the mechanism (Fig. 13.7). He suggests that the oxidized and reduced forms of certain or all of the electron carriers differ in conformation and the ATP-forming enzyme also exists in two forms: the relaxed or energy-poor form and the taut or energized form. When the enzyme is in the energized form, ATP formation is favored. When electron transport takes place, a wave of conformational changes occur down the respiratory chain that are transmitted to the ATP-forming enzyme through a change in the conformation of structural proteins in the membrane. It is in this way, Lehninger suggests, that mechanical change induced by electron transport promotes chemical change leading to ATP synthesis.

FUNCTION

In order to understand the mechanisms by which the mitochondrion traps energy in ATP for subsequent use in cellular processes and becomes, thereby, the powerhouse of the cell, many accepted generalities, scientific clichés, and terms of convenience must be unveiled and then scrutinized, comprehended, and redefined. Only

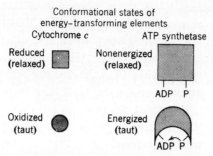

Fig. 13.7a A schematic representation of the conformational states of a respiratory carrier (cytochrome c) and the ATP synthetase.

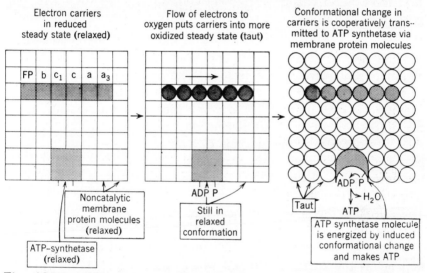

Fig. 13.7b Schematic representation of conformational coupling. A conformational state induced by onset of respiration is sterically and cooperatively transmitted to the ATP synthetase molecule, energizing it to form ATP. [From A. L. Lehninger, *Adv. Cytopharmocol.*, 1: 199 (1971a).]

then will the scientific colloquialisms acquire meaning and the concepts become lucid.

The law of conservation of energy can be mouthed by almost any schoolboy. What concepts does it encompass? Does it include the utter dependence of animal life upon the photosynthetic trap in the chloroplasts of the plant cell? Does it point to the uniqueness of the photosynthetic process in utilizing quanta of light as the energy source? Does it recognize that only the plant cell of all living things possesses the capacity to absorb solar energy[1] and to convert and trap it as chemical energy? Does it clarify why plant life had to precede animal life on this planet? Does it explain why food for all animal cells comes ultimately from plants and that food is the sole source of energy upon which animal life depends? Does it humble sophisticated man who comes to realize his complete subordination to the genius of the grass upon which he treads?

The foodstuffs, carbohydrate, protein, and fat, are the fuel that the animal cell is capable of converting into mechanical, chemical, electrical, osmotic, sonic, light, or heat energy. The measurement or quantitation of these forms of energy can be made in any convenient unit and the unit may vary with the kind of energy measured and the ease of measurement: ergs, electron volts, kilowatt hours, millimeters of mercury, or decibels. The potential energy of foodstuffs is measured as heat and, since other forms of energy are easily expressed in heat units, the *kilocalorie* (kcal) has until recently been the accepted unit of measurement in nutritional studies. A kilocalorie is defined as the amount of heat required to raise the temperature of one kilogram of water from 14.5 to 15.5°C. (The kilocalorie is to be distinguished from the calorie that is used later in this chapter in calculating the energy yield of metabolic oxidation. The calorie is the amount of heat required to raise the temperature of one gram of water from 14.5° to 15.5°C.)

The kilojoule (kJ) is now the international unit of energy and is defined as the energy expended when one kilogram is moved one meter (m) by a force of 1 newton (N). Conversion of kilocalories to kilojoules is accomplished by multiplying by a factor of 4.2. (Because of the large amounts of energy involved in some nutritional calculations, the megajoule (mJ) is sometimes preferred.) The kilojoule has not yet been accepted in the United States, and arguments have been presented for (Ames, 1971; Harper, 1971) and against (Kleiber, 1972) its adoption. For purposes of comparison some of the data presented in Chapter 23 will be expressed in terms of both kilocalories and kilo- or megajoules.

[1]We do not intend to ignore, or even minimize, the capacity of photoreceptor cells, such as those found in the retina, to absorb light energy nor the photoactivation of 7-dehydrocholesterol in the cells of the skin. However, except in these specialized cases, the capacity to use light energy appears to be nonexistent in animal cells.

The conversion, then, of the potential energy supplied by the cell's food to chemical bond energy in ATP is measured in calories. This conversion is the primary function of the mitochondria. The manner in which the mitochondria accomplish this ultimate goal involves a series of reactions in which intermediary products in the metabolism of carbohydrates, fats, and proteins are broken down in a succession of steps and merge in a common oxidative pathway, the TCA cycle. This oxidative pathway leads to the release of carbon dioxide and hydrogen. The carbon dioxide is quickly removed from the cell as a noxious and potentially dangerous waste product. The hydrogen (H+ and electron) is carried along a chain of reactors, eventually combining with molecular oxygen to form water. In this process, the energy released by the transfer of electrons along the respiratory chain is captured by ADP and inorganic phosphate to form ATP. This coupling of the oxidation of foodstuffs with the formation of ATP, aptly described by Szent-Györgyi as the *energy currency* of the cell, is known as *oxidative phosphorylation.* Oxidation in a living cell thus proceeds in an orderly step-by-step fashion, enabling the cell to harness efficiently the energy released from food, the energy requisite for its existence.

Carbohydrates, fats, and proteins enter the mitochondria as their breakdown products: pyruvic acid, fatty acids, and amino acids. The general pathway of these metabolites to their common oxidative fate, the TCA cycle, is depicted in Fig. 13.8. Pyruvic acid and fatty acids are degraded to the two-carbon acetate and

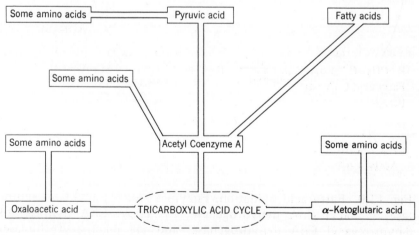

Fig. 13.8 Oxidation of foodstuffs in mitochondria.

enter the cycle joined to the pantothenic acid-containing CoA. Amino acids undergo a variety of changes: some are converted to pyruvic acid, some to acetyl CoA, and others to the TCA cycle intermediaries oxaloacetic acid and α-ketoglutaric acid. This diagrammatic representation is, of course, grossly oversimplified. Each step involves a series of reactions and requires a number of enzymes,

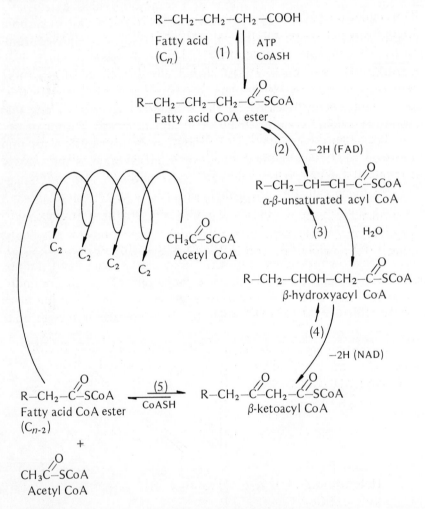

Fig. 13.9 Fatty acid oxidation. Enzymes are: (1) acyl CoA synthetase, (2) acyl CoA dehydrogenase, (3) enoyl CoA hydrase, (4) β-hydroxyacyl CoA dehydrogenase, and (5) β-ketoacyl thiolase.

coenzymes, and other factors. The purpose of the following sections is to add to a general understanding of these processes. No attempt will be made to present the detailed intricacies of the enzymatic machinery involved.

Oxidation of Fatty Acids

The oxidation of fatty acids to acetyl CoA involves a series of reactions by which two-carbon fragments are split off a fragment at a time. This process is often depicted as a spiral (Fig. 13.9). The loss of each two-carbon fragment involves five separate reactions in which CoA-acyl derivatives are formed. The oxidation of stearic acid (C_{18}), for example, would necessitate at least 45 separate reactions leading to the formation of nine moles of acetyl CoA.

The steps in the oxidation of fatty acids are given below and correspond to the numbers in Fig. 13.9. ATP is required to prime the reaction, to provide the energy of activation.

1. Activation of the fatty acid by formation of a corresponding fatty acid CoA ester. ATP is required as the source of energy. The products are fatty acid CoA ester, AMP, and inorganic pyrophosphate (PP_i), which may be further degraded to the monophosphate (P_i).

$$R-CH_2-CH_2-COOH + ATP + CoA \xrightarrow{Mg^{2+}K^+} R-CH_2-CH_2\overset{O}{\overset{\|}{C}}-SCoA + AMP + PP_i$$

2. Dehydrogenation of the fatty acid CoA ester to form the a-β-unsaturated acyl CoA. The enzymes involved in this reaction contain FAD and Cu or Fe.

$$R-CH_2-CH_2\overset{O}{\overset{\|}{C}}-SCoA \underset{+2H+}{\overset{-2H+}{\rightleftharpoons}} R-CH=CH\overset{O}{\overset{\|}{C}}-SCoA$$

3. Hydration of the a-β-unsaturated acyl CoA ester to form β-hydroxyacyl CoA.

$$R-CH=CH\overset{O}{\overset{\|}{C}}-SCoA + H_2O \rightleftharpoons R-CHOHCH_2\overset{O}{\overset{\|}{C}}-SCoA$$

4. Dehydrogenation of the β-hydroxy acyl CoA to form β-keto acyl CoA. NAD is the hydrogen acceptor.

$$R-CHOHCH_2\overset{O}{\overset{\|}{C}}-SCoA + NAD \rightleftharpoons R-\overset{O}{\overset{\|}{C}}-CH_2-\overset{O}{\overset{\|}{C}}-SCoA + NADH_2$$

5. Thiolytic cleavage of the β-keto acyl CoA to yield acetyl CoA and a fatty acyl CoA having 2 fewer carbon atoms.

$$R-\overset{O}{\overset{\|}{C}}-CH_2-\overset{O}{\overset{\|}{C}}-SCoA + CoASH \rightleftharpoons R-\overset{O}{\overset{\|}{C}}-SCoA + CH_3\overset{O}{\overset{\|}{C}}-SCoA$$

The cycle, then, is repeated as indicated by the spiral representing subsequent removal of two carbon fragments as acetyl CoA.

Oxidation of Pyruvic Acid

Pyruvic acid, the converging point for the oxidation of glucose and of the amino acids alanine, serine, and cysteine, enters the TCA cycle as acetyl CoA. The oxidation of pyruvate to acetyl CoA is an oxidative decarboxylation and involves a sequence of reactions requiring TPP, lipoic acid, CoA, NAD, Mg^{2+}, and a large complex of enzymes known as pyruvic oxidase. Four vitamins, thiamin, pantothenic acid, riboflavin, and nicotinic acid, thus participate in pyruvate oxidation. The over-all reaction may be summed up briefly as:

$$\text{Pyruvate} + \text{CoA} + \text{NAD} \xrightarrow[\text{Lipoic acid}]{\text{TPP}} \text{Acetyl CoA} + CO_2 + NADH_2$$

A more detailed but still incomplete representation (Fig. 13.10) illustrates one way in which these four vitamins virtually control a key reaction in cellular metabolism. Each acts independently; yet a lack of any one of these vitamins will interfere with the coordinated flow of the reaction.

The steps in pyruvate oxidation are as follows:

1. Pyruvic acid is decarboxylated to a two-carbon aldehyde and becomes attached to the thiazole ring of TPP. This reaction also requires Mg^{2+}.

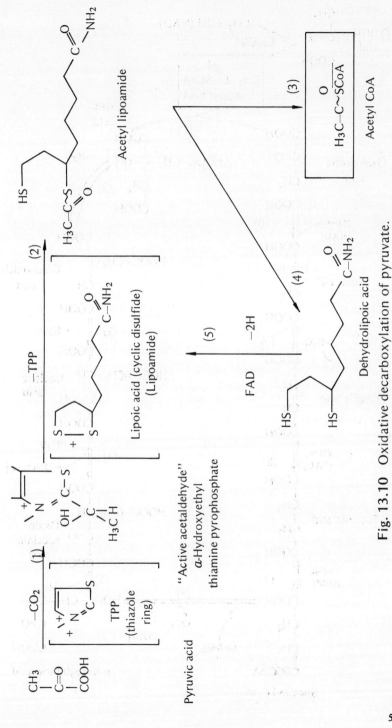

Fig. 13.10 Oxidative decarboxylation of pyruvate.

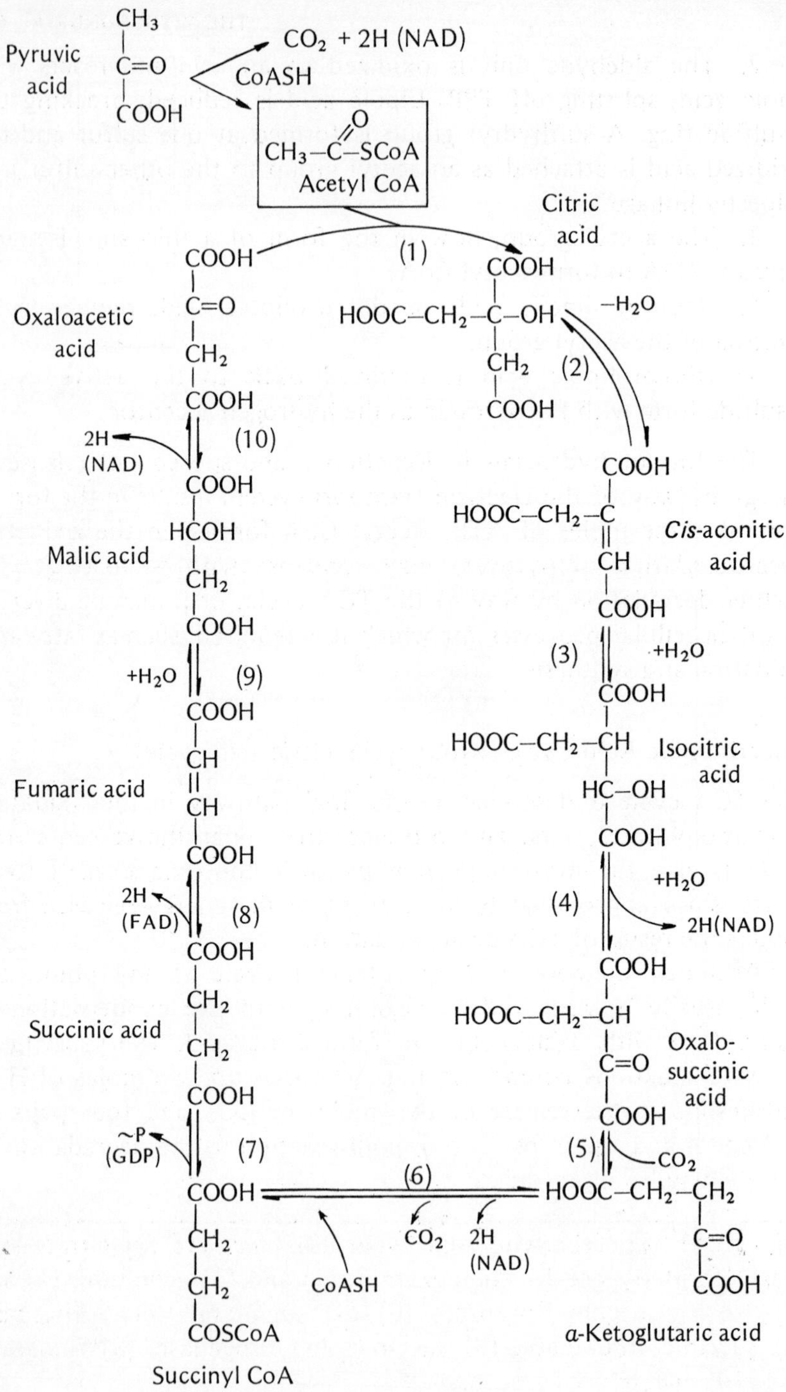

Pyruvic
acid

$$CH_3$$
$$C=O$$
$$COOH$$

$$CO_2 + 2H\ (NAD)$$
CoASH

$$CH_3-\overset{O}{\overset{\|}{C}}-SCoA$$
Acetyl CoA

(1)

Citric
acid

$$COOH$$
$$HOOC-CH_2-\overset{|}{\underset{|}{C}}-OH$$
$$CH_2$$
$$COOH$$

$$-H_2O$$

(2)

Oxaloacetic
acid

$$COOH$$
$$C=O$$
$$CH_2$$
$$COOH$$

2H
(NAD)

(10)

$$COOH$$
$$HCOH$$
$$CH_2$$
$$COOH$$

Malic acid

$$COOH$$
$$HOOC-CH_2-\overset{|}{C}$$
$$CH$$
$$COOH$$

Cis-aconitic
acid

(3)

$$+H_2O$$

$$COOH$$
$$HOOC-CH_2-\overset{|}{C}H$$
$$HC-OH$$
$$COOH$$

Isocitric
acid

+H_2O

$$COOH$$
$$CH$$
$$CH$$
$$COOH$$

Fumaric acid

$$+H_2O$$

(9)

(4)

$$+H_2O$$

2H(NAD)

2H
(FAD)

(8)

$$COOH$$
$$CH_2$$
$$CH_2$$
$$COOH$$

Succinic acid

$$COOH$$
$$HOOC-CH_2-\overset{|}{C}H$$
$$C=O$$
$$COOH$$

Oxalo-
succinic
acid

~P
(GDP)

(7)

(5)

$$CO_2$$

$$COOH$$
$$CH_2$$
$$CH_2$$
$$COSCoA$$

Succinyl CoA

(6)

$$CO_2$$ 2H
(NAD)

CoASH

$$HOOC-CH_2-CH_2$$
$$C=O$$
$$COOH$$

α-Ketoglutaric acid

514

2. The aldehyde unit is oxidized to an acid and reacts with lipoic acid, splitting off TPP. Lipoic acid is reduced, breaking the disulfide ring. A sulfhydryl group is formed at one sulfur and the oxidized acid is attached as an acetyl group to the other sulfur in a thioester linkage.

3. The acetyl group, now in the form of a thioester, is transferred to CoA to form acetyl CoA.

4. Reduced lipoic acid, or dihydrolipoic acid, remains after removal of the acetyl group.

5. Dihydrolipoic acid is oxidized back to the active cyclic disulfide form with flavoprotein as the hydrogen acceptor.

The loss of hydrogens in Reaction 5 and subsequent release of energy by way of the electron transport system results in the formation of three moles of ATP. Acetyl CoA formed in the oxidative decarboxylation of pyruvate may condense with oxaloacetate for further degradation by way of the TCA cycle, or it may be diverted to other cellular processes for which it is required, such as fatty acid oxidation and synthesis.

Tricarboxylic Acid Cycle (Krebs cycle, citric acid cycle)

The TCA cycle is described as the final pathway in the oxidation of carbohydrates, fats, and proteins. In a quantitative sense, this cycle is also the most important phase in the oxidation of foodstuffs, since approximately 90 percent of the energy released from food is the result of TCA cycle oxidation.

Although metabolites may enter the cycle at any point, the cycle usually is visualized as beginning with the condensation of acetyl CoA with oxaloacetate to form citric acid. The subsequent series of reactions comprising the cycle uses up two moles of H_2O and results in the release of two moles of CO_2 and four pairs of hydrogens and electrons. The over-all reaction in the degradation of acetate may be expressed as:

Fig. 13.11 Tricarboxylic acid cycle. Enzymes are (1) citrate synthase (formerly condensing enzyme), (2) and (3) aconitase, (4) and (5) isocitrate dehydrogenase, (6) α-ketoglutarate dehydrogenase, (7) succinic thiokinase, (8) succinic dehydrogenase, (9) fumarase, and (10) malate dehydrogenase.

$$CH_3COOH + 2H_2O \longrightarrow 2CO_2 + 8H+$$

The individual reactions are depicted diagrammatically in Fig. 13.11. A description of the reactions corresponding to numbers in the diagram follows:

CO_2 and H+ released	Reaction	
	1.	Condensation of oxaloacetate and acetyl CoA to form citrate. CoA is split off hydrolytically in the process.
	2 and 3.	Isomerization of citrate to yield isocitrate. *Cis*-aconitate may be formed as an intermediary. Water assists in the isomerization but is not used up in the process.
2H+	4.	Dehydrogenation of isocitrate to form oxalosuccinate. NAD or NADP may serve as hydrogen acceptor.
CO_2	5.	Decarboxylation of oxalosuccinate to a-ketoglutarate. Loss of CO_2 results in first shortening of the carbon chain.
CO_2 2H+	6.	Oxidative decarboxylation of a-ketoglutarate to form succinyl CoA. This reaction requires TPP, Mg^{2+}, NAD, FAD, lipoic acid, and coenzyme A as cofactors and is analogous to the oxidative decarboxylation of pyruvate. NAD is the hydrogen acceptor. The loss of a second CO_2 molecule results in a four-carbon chain.
	7.	Utilization of high energy bond from succinyl CoA to form succinic acid and donation of high-energy phosphate bond to GDP to form GTP. The high-energy phosphate is transferred to ADP to form ATP.
2H+	8.	Dehydrogenation of succinate to form fumarate. FAD is the hydrogen acceptor.

9.   Addition of water to fumarate to form malate.

2H+   10.   Dehydrogenation of malate to form oxaloacetate.

Oxaloacetate now is available to condense with another mole of acetyl CoA and thus to repeat the cycle. This is not an obligatory reaction, however. Oxaloacetate can contribute to other cellular processes such as synthesis of glucose and certain amino acids by the loss of carbon dioxide and formation of phosphoenolpyruvate. The reverse of this reaction is a means of providing oxaloacetate when the supply is limited. Decreased formation of oxaloacetate might occur, for example, if TCA cycle intermediates are diverted to other reactions and, in a very loose sense, leave the cycle.

Acetyl CoA arises through the degradation of fatty acids and certain amino acids as well as from carbohydrate, and its oxidation is dependent upon a ready supply of oxaloacetate. The oxidation of acetyl CoA produces no *net* increase in oxaloacetate or other cycle intermediaries; therefore if additional oxaloacetate is needed, it must be provided from other sources. One such source is the conversion from phosphoenolpyruvate. Pyruvate also may give rise indirectly to oxaloacetate; this reaction involves the addition of carbon dioxide to form malate which then is dehydrogenated to oxaloacetate. The conversion of carbohydrate metabolites to oxaloacetate may account, in part, for the ameliorative effect of carbohydrate feeding when ketosis develops as a consequence of a predominantly fatty acid metabolism as, for example, occurs during fasting.

All of the enzymes and coenzymes necessary for TCA metabolism are located either in the inner membrane or in the inner matrix of the mitochondrion. As indicated in Chapter 11, pyruvate produced by anaerobic metabolism of carbohydrate in cytoplasm must enter the mitochondrion to be oxidized via the TCA cycle.

Certain other TCA cycle intermediates also permeate the mitochondrial membrane in either direction by an exchange mechanism involving other compounds within or outside the mitochondrion (Fig. 13.12). Malate, succinate, citrate, and isocitrate enter in exchange for an equivalent amount of inorganic phosphate. Alpha-ketoglutarate does not cross the mitochondrial membrane as such

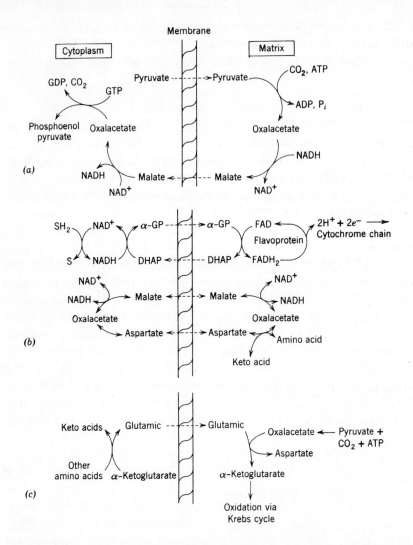

Fig. 13.12 Four shuttle systems operating across the mitochondrial inner membrane. (*a*) System required to convert pyruvate (or lactate) to phosphoenolpyruvate in gluconeogenesis. (*b*) The unidirectional *a*-glycerol phosphate (*a*-GP) and dihydroxyacetophosphate (DHAP) shuttle that transports reducing equivalents only into the mitochondrial matrix. The reversible malate-oxalate-aspartate shuttle for reducing equivalents is also given. (*c*) The glutamate shuttle for transport of amino nitrogen. (From E. E. Conn, and P. R. Stumpf, *Outlines of Biochemistry*, 3rd ed., Wiley, N. Y., 1973, p. 335.)

but is first converted to glutamate that, after traversing the membrane barrier, is reconverted to the keto acid. Fumarate and oxaloacetate, however, cannot cross the mitochondrial membrane in either direction.

Oxidation of Amino Acids

Although some synthesis of protein apparently takes place in the mitochondrion, it is generally believed that amino acids traverse the mitochondrial membrane chiefly to be oxidized via the TCA cycle. In order for oxidation to take place, an amino acid first must lose its amino group. The keto acid so formed may be oxidized through the cycle or converted by a series of reactions to an oxidizable substrate.

Fig. 13.13 indicates that amino acids enter the TCA cycle through at least three avenues: pyruvic acid, TCA cycle intermediaries, and acetyl CoA. The term *glycogenic* sometimes is used to designate amino acids that give rise to TCA cycle intermediates or pyruvate and therefore are on the general pathway to carbohydrate synthesis. *Ketogenic* refers to amino acids that give rise to acetyl CoA and consequently are potential fatty acid and acetoacetate producers. The two terms, however, tend to be confusing. In view of the labyrinth of interrelated metabolic reactions, the terms glycogenic and ketogenic probably should be discarded as obsolete nomenclature.

The diagrammatic representation in Fig. 13.13 obviously is oversimplified. Only three amino acids—alanine, aspartic acid, and glutamic acid—are converted directly to keto acids that are intermediaries in the main oxidative scheme. These keto acids are pyruvate, oxaloacetate, and a-ketoglutarate. Other amino acids must undergo a series of reactions before they are converted to substances that can be oxidized through the TCA cycle. In the degradation of phenylalanine and tyrosine, for example, the molecule splits, forming two oxidizable substances: fumarate and acetoacetate. The mechanisms by which amino acids are degraded vary in complexity, depending upon the amino acid involved. All, however, share the initial step; that is, removal of the amino group.

The most common method for biological removal of amino groups is *transamination*. This reaction requires both an amino acid

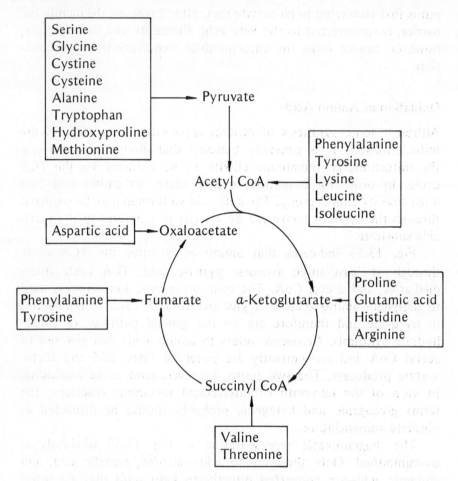

Fig. 13.13 Oxidative pathways of amino acids.

and an α-keto acid. The amino and keto groups are exchanged, forming a new amino acid and a new keto acid. Transamination requires the vitamin B_6 coenzyme, pyridoxal phosphate, and a variety of specific enzymes known appropriately as transaminases.

The classic examples of transamination are the alanine-pyruvate, aspartate-oxaloacetate, and glutamate-α-ketoglutarate systems. However, all amino acids participate in transamination; and, with the exception of lysine and threonine, the reactions are reversible. In most or in all transaminations, glutamate and α-ketoglutarate are involved. A typical example is as follows:

| Tyrosine | α-Ketoglutaric acid | Phenylhydroxy pyruvic acid | Glutamic acid |

Another method for removing amino groups is *oxidative deamination*. Although theoretically all amino acids may be deaminated by this method, apparently the only such reaction of physiological importance is that involving glutamic acid. The initial reaction is a dehydrogenation with NAD or NADP as hydrogen acceptor, followed by hydrolysis yielding α-ketoglutarate and ammonia. This reaction also requires pyridoxal phosphate as a coenzyme.

$$\text{Glutamic acid} + \text{NAD} + H_2O \longrightarrow \alpha\text{-Ketoglutaric acid} + NH_3 + NADH_2$$

Deamination of glutamate is significant chiefly as a means of disposing of amino groups transferred from other amino acids to α-ketoglutarate in transamination reactions. Ammonia formed by this process may be converted to urea.

Electron Transport and Oxidative Phosphorylation

The oxidation of carbohydrates, fats, and proteins via the TCA cycle is the common pathway in the conversion of the energy of foodstuffs to a form that the cell can use. This usable form of energy, the *currency of the cell*, is ATP. The energy-yielding system is the electron transport system or respiratory chain that couples the oxidation of TCA cycle substrates with the formation of ATP, thus transforming the energy of oxidation into the phosphate bond energy necessary for cellular processes.

The components of the electron transport system are substances capable of alternate reduction and oxidation. A general scheme showing carriers and apparent sites of ATP formation is shown in Fig. 13.14.

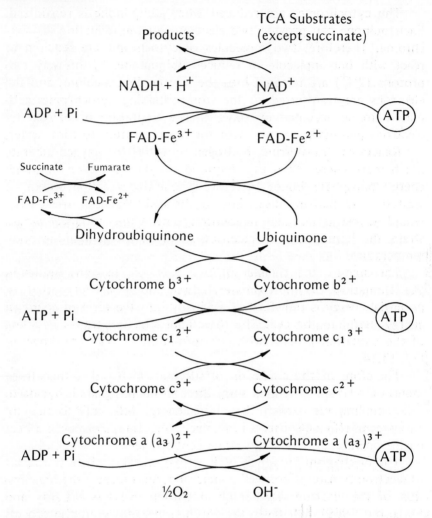

Fig. 13.14 Electron transport and oxidative phosphorylation.

Electrons from oxidized TCA substrates, with the exception of succinate, are transferred to NAD. Electrons are also donated to NAD from pyruvate and α-ketoglutarate dehydrogenase by way of the flavoproteins associated with these enzyme complexes. Electrons from succinate oxidation are donated to FAD. Evidence suggests that ubiquinone serves as the carrier between the flavoproteins and the cytochromes.

The cytochromes are reduced when ubiquinone is reoxidized. Each quinone can provide two electrons for the reduction of cytochrome. Therefore, two molecules of cytochrome are required to react with one molecule of reduced ubiquinone. In this way two protons ($2H^+$) are released into the surrounding medium, and the electrons are transferred to the iron-containing cytochromes ultimately to be accepted by oxygen. The excitation of oxygen by electrons permits it to join with the hydrogen ions to form water.

Reactions transferring hydrogen directly to oxygen liberate much more energy than that required for the formation of a high energy phosphate bond; therefore a one-step reaction would be wasteful and perhaps disastrous to the cell. Much of the energy would be lost as heat that, in addition to being uneconomical, would strain the homeostatic mechanisms involved in maintaining body temperature.

The step-by-step transfer of two pairs of electrons results in the formation of approximately three moles of ATP; that is, potential energy is transformed gradually into the form of chemical energy useful to the cell. The three approximate sites for coupling of the oxidation process with the formation of ATP are shown in Fig. 13.14.

Therefore in the oxidation of succinate two rather than three moles of ATP are generated since the first coupling site is bypassed. The coupling mechanism that traps energy into ATP is roughly 60 percent efficient. This is a relatively high rate, since even a heat engine operates at only about 30 percent efficiency.

The mechanism by which ATP formation takes place as a result of electron transfer is not well understood, nor indeed is the organization of the electron transfer chain entirely clear (see Lardy and Ferguson 1969). Whatever the mechanisms, however, the process of *oxidative phosphorylation* is not only the primary goal of mitochondrial activity, but it is also the fundamental device at the command of the cell for trapping energy in a manner compatible with life and in a form which can be utilized efficiently by the cell.

Energy Yield

Oxidative Phosphorylation. The energy yield from TCA cycle oxidations can be estimated from the moles of ATP produced

Table 13.2 ENERGY YIELD FROM PYRUVATE OXIDATION VIA THE TCA CYCLE

Reaction	Coenzyme	ATP Yield
Pyruvate → acetyl CoA	NAD	3
Isocitrate → α-ketoglutarate	NAD	3
α-Ketoglutarate → succinyl CoA	NAD	3
Succinyl CoA + ADP + P_i → succinate + ATP	GDP	1
Succinate → fumarate	FAD	2
Malate → oxaloacetate	NAD	3
		15

(Table 13.2). Those reactions giving rise to NADH lead to the formation of 3 moles of ATP and include all but two of the energy-yielding reactions of the cycle. An additional high-energy phosphate is formed from the conversion of succinyl CoA to succinate in a complex reaction involving the enzyme succinate thiokinase in which the coenzymes are guanosine di- and triphosphate. The oxidation of succinate to fumarate by-passes the NAD step and therefore yields only 2 moles of ATP. The total yield in high-energy phosphate from the TCA cycle totals the equivalent of 15 moles of ATP.

Similarly the high-energy phosphate yield from the complete oxidation of glucose also can be estimated. The degradation of glucose to pyruvate results in the formation of two moles of ATP from substrate level phosphorylations (see Chapter 11). Since one mole of glucose yields 2 moles of pyruvate, the total via the TCA cycle then is 30 moles of ATP. The total yield from the oxidation of 1 mole of glucose then is at least 32 moles of high-energy phosphate. In addition approximately 6 moles of high-energy phosphate may be added to the total of 32 moles of ATP if pyruvate is not reduced to lactate. In this case, 2 moles of NADH remain in the cytoplasm to be accounted for and, although oxidation is not obligatory, in tissues actively oxidizing glucose completely to CO_2 and H_2O these two molecules could be oxidized by the electron transport chain to produce 6 moles of ATP. Thus, a total of 38 moles of ATP conceivably could be produced from the complete oxidation of glucose.

Complete Oxidation of Glucose. As noted in the previous section, the efficiency of energy transformations in biological systems is approximately 40 percent. The theoretical yield for oxidation of glucose from calorimetric data is -686,000 cal. If there were no mechanism for harnessing this energy, all of it would be lost as heat. In biological systems, however, the coupling of energy released to ATP formation conserves the amount of energy equivalent to a maximum of 38 moles of ATP. Since each mole of ATP is equivalent to -7300 cal, the total amount of energy conserved is -277,000 cal (38 x -7300). The efficiency of the total reaction, thus, is 40 percent (-277,000/-686,000 x 100).

Fatty Acid Oxidation. The oxidation of fatty acids yields acetyl CoA and the reduced coenzymes, NADH and $FADH_2$. The latter are oxidized by the electron transport system to yield 5 moles of ATP for each mole of oxygen used for the production of acetyl CoA. Oxidation of acetyl CoA via the TCA cycle yields another 12 moles of energy-rich phosphate for each mole of acetyl CoA. As an example, the β-oxidation of stearate yields 148 moles of high-energy phosphate. Stearate yields 9 acetyl CoA (9 x 12 = 108). Eight moles of O_2 are required since the terminal acetyl does not require oxygen. Thus, NADH and $FADH_2$ give rise to an additional 40 moles of high-energy phosphate. Assuming an energy worth of -7300 cal/mole of ATP under physiological circumstances, this represents a yield of about 1,080,400 cal, which is about half the energy released when 1 mole of stearate is oxidized in a bomb calorimeter.

Synthesis

Fatty Acids. Although fatty acid synthesis apparently proceeds more efficiently in cytoplasm and the endoplasmic reticulum (Chapter 11), mitochondria contain an enzyme system capable of catalyzing the elongation of preformed saturated or unsaturated fatty acids by the successive additions of acetyl CoA. The mitochondrial system requires both NADH and NADPH. The fatty acids formed are primarily C_{18}, C_{20}, C_{22}, and C_{24} fatty acids.

The mitochondrial system does not require CO_2 fixation and the reactions leading to elongation of existing fatty acids apparently are at least partially a reverse of β-oxidation.

Protein. Until quite recently it was believed that the cell's entire complement of DNA was in the nucleus. When small amounts of DNA appeared in mitochondrial fractions it was ascribed at first to contamination. However, Nass and Nass (1963) showed that the fiberlike inclusions in the mitochondria of normal chick embryos were DNA by specifically removing them from ultra-thin sections with DNAase. When it was shown that the DNA in intact mitochondria was not susceptible to DNAase, the intramitochondrial locus of DNA was substantiated (Luck and Reich, 1964).

Mitochondrial DNA differs from the nuclear DNA in the same cell in size and base composition. Like the DNA of certain viruses, it is a circular and hypertwisted double strand (Van Bruggen et al., 1966). A typical mitochondrial DNA molecule from an animal cell has a molecular weight of approximately 11 million, enough DNA to represent about 10 to 25 average-sized genes (Goodenough and Levine, 1970). Each mitochondrion may contain 2 to 6 DNA circles. It is estimated that the DNA in a single bovine heart mitochondrion can maximally code for about 70 polypeptides (Schatz, 1970). The genetic role for mitochondrial DNA is supported by the fact that both RNA synthesis and amino acid incorporation are blocked by actinomycin, which is a specific inhibitor of DNA transcription.

Mitochondrial DNA does not carry a sufficient amount of genetic information to code for all the proteins and enzymes present in the mitochondrion, and it is generally believed that it codes for some of the structural protein and that synthesis of other mitochondrial proteins are directed by nuclear DNA (Nass, 1969). Beattie (1971) estimates that less than 10 percent of total mitochondrial protein is directed by mitochondrial DNA and that most of it is localized in the inner membrane. The remainder of the protein in the inner membrane, and the protein of the outer membrane and the matrix are synthesized outside the mitochondrion and transferred in.

The protein synthesis within the mitochondrion presumes both a transcription and translation system. Conclusive proof of mitochondrial tRNA distinct from cytoplasmic tRNA has been reported by Barnett and coworkers (Barnett and Epler, 1966; Barnett and Brown, 1967; Barnett et al., 1967). Mitochondrial ribosomes that are smaller than cytoplasmic ribosomes have been identified by André and Marinozzi (1965). Mitochondrial rRNA is unquestionably coded for in the mitochondrion yet most if not all of the ribosomal proteins are coded for by the nucleus and synthesized on cytoplasmic ribosomes. However, an apparently irreducible part is coded for by the mitochondrial genome. Mitochondrial ribosomal proteins are quite distinct from cytoplasmic ribosomal proteins (Raff and Mahler, 1972).

The presence of a mitochondrial mRNA has not been definitively established, but it would be difficult to argue for the transport of mRNA across the mitochondrial membranes. Despite the fact that Wheeldon and Lehninger (1966) reported that mitochondria are completely self-contained units with respect to protein synthesis, and that it is necessary to supply them with only ATP and an ATP-generating system, inorganic phosphate and Mg^{2+}, Raff and Mahler (1972) indicate that interference with mitochondrial protein synthesis prevents the formation of mitochondria capable of respiration.

For an extensive review of mitochondrial protein synthesis, see Schatz (1970).

Calcium Transport

Mitochondria have the capacity to accumulate Ca^{2+}. *In vitro* studies have indicated that the accumulation can be quite massive and can progress to the extent that no Ca^{2+} is left in the reaction medium (Vasington and Murphy, 1962). De Luca and Engstrom (1961) and De Luca et al. (1962) reported similar results. This uptake of calcium and of other divalent cations (Mn^{2+}, Mg^{2+} and Sr^{2+}) were shown to be coupled with electron flow and will be discussed in a subsequent section. However, about 50 percent of the total calcium transport in mitochondria is energy-independent and of considerable physiological interest (Carafoli and Rossi, 1971).

The data assembled by Carafoli and his colleagues (Patriarca and Carafoli, 1968; Carafoli et al., 1969) indicate the role of mitochondrial calcium transport in the contraction and relaxation of the heart. Heart muscle, in contrast to skeletal muscle, is rich in mitochondria and the segregation of Ca^{2+} in the mitochondria instead of the sarcoplasmic reticulum returns the muscle to the resting state. In an *in vitro* study on energy-linked calcium transport in hearts from genetically myopathic hamsters with advanced degree of heart failure, Sulakhe and Dhalla (1973) demonstrated a decrease in calcium binding and uptake by the mitochondrial and heavy microsomal fractions of hearts. Their results suggest alterations in the membranes of cardiac mitochondria in heart failure. The reduced ability of the subcellular particles from the failing heart to bind and accumulate calcium was conceived to interfere with the process of relaxation of the cardiac muscle. Such impairment is considered to result in decreasing the intracellular stores of calcium thereby making less calcium available for release on depolarization of the failing heart cell.

Carafoli and Rossi (1971) suggest that many other cellular reactions may depend on mitochondrial calcium transport. There have been suggestions of mitochondrial intervention in biological mineralization and demineralization. Gonzales and Karnowski (1961) observed many electron-dense masses in mitochondria of osteoclasts in healing bone fractures, and De Luca et al. (1962) reported that calcium uptake by mitochondria was influenced by parathyroid hormone. Rasmussen and Nagata (1970) reported a rise in free plasma calcium concentration after parathyroid hormone administration; and Borle (1973) suggests that mitochondria respond also to the influences of calcitonin and vitamin D. In vitamin D-deficient rats complete disappearance of calcium granules in the mitochondria of the intestinal cells was reported (Sampson et al., 1970). This was followed by an immediate and dramatic increase in number and density of granules after vitamin D administration. Borle (1973) postulates that mitochondria may be the main regulators of cytoplasmic calcium activity and calcium transport. His suggestion is that mitochondria function as an ion buffer, as a calcium trap, and as the main regulator of the concentration of free calcium in the cytoplasm. He further suggests that vitamin D may be essential for the uptake of calcium by mitochondria and that mitochondria control cell calcium metabolism. In vitamin D deficiency the mitochondrial buffer system would be slowly depleted and cease to function, the calcium activity of the mitochondria and consequently the free calcium in the cytoplasm would fall, leading to a decreased efflux and transport of calcium across the intestinal epithelium.

Investigations reported by Schraer et al. (1973) on both *in vivo* and *in vitro* response to calcium by the mitochondria of avian shell gland and liver strongly support the concept that the mitochondrion is involved in the cellular transport of calcium. The propensity for mitochondria to accumulate calcium led to speculation about their role in biological calcification. In the shell gland of the hen the observation was made that there was more calcium in the endoplasmic reticulum than in the mitochondria when calcification was taking place; but there was more in the mitochondria when calcification was not taking place (Hohman and Schraer, 1956). This was interpreted to mean that during shell formation calcium moved from the mitochondria through the endoplasmic reticulum to the cell exterior for deposition as calcium carbonate. When shell formation was not occurring, calcium moved into the mitochondria from the cytoplasm with the consequent decrease in the endoplasmic reticulum. Similarly, Lehninger (1970) has postulated that during bone calcification calcium moves through the mitochondrial membrane to the cytosol and then to bone matrix. However, the evidence implicating mitochondria in bone calcification is less clearly established than in shell gland.

For further discussion of the interrelated roles of parathyroid hormone, calcitonin and vitamin D on calcium metabolism, see Chapter 17.

BIOGENESIS OF MITOCHONDRIA

The origin of mitochondria with their full complement of enzymes has been the subject of both speculation and investigation. Three major hypotheses have been presented concerning their biogenesis: (1) formation from other intracellular structures, (2) de novo formation, and (3) growth and division of preexisting mitochondria.

Almost every cellular organelle has been implicated at one time or another in mitochondrial biogenesis. It has been suggested that they are formed from the existing plasma membrane (Robertson, 1961), the nucleus (Hoffmann and Grigg, 1958), the nucleolus (Ehret and Powers, 1955) and the Golgi complex (Lever, 1956a; 1956b). As techniques improved in electron microscopy and these were correlated with biochemical procedures, some of the apparent similarities in structure and composition gave way to obvious differences. With the identification of DNA in mitochondria (Wildman et al., 1962; Luck 1963a, 1963b; Gibor and Granick, 1964) and the presence of RNA (Rendi, 1959) it became more and more difficult to postulate mitochondrial origin from other cellular organelles. However, it is apparent that the endoplasmic reticulum does synthesize most of the mitochondrial proteins (Beattie, 1971) and probably some of the lipids but this occurs also for other organelles and their membranes.

The data that have recently been assembled provide evidence of the existence of a specific mitochondrial genetic system and make it difficult to support the suggestion that *de novo* synthesis occurs. It is unlikely that there are many who are willing to strongly support such an hypothesis.

The formation of mitochondria by growth and division of existing mitochondria has for a long time been intriguing to many investigators. Observations of dumbbell-shaped mitochondria in many tissues were presented as evidence of incipient division (Lafontaine and Alfard, 1964; Fawcett, 1955). When Luck (1963b) incorporated labeled choline in phosphatidyl choline of mitochondrial membranes of *Neurospora,* and observed that when the number of mitochondria increased all contained labeled phospholipid, he concluded that most, if not all, of the mitochondria formed had arisen by growth and division of preexisting mitochondria. Gibor and Granick (1964) postulated that a DNA unit that is self-duplicating and serves as a code for RNA is the basic hereditary unit of each mitochondrion. Current evidence is strong enough to no longer question the fact that mitochondria are capable of growth and division and that this is probably the manner in which mitochondrial multiplication occurs. There are interactions between mitochondria and other cytoplasmic organelles and substantial evidence that some of the mitochondrial protein arises through synthesis by the endoplasmic reticulum. This suggests that mitochondria are biochemically integrated with other organelles in the cell. Probably most of the outer membrane and many of the enzymatically active proteins are synthesized extramitochondrially (Neupert et al., 1972) and under the direction of nuclear DNA. However, the mitochondrion is unique, as far as is now known, in that it does contain genetic capability, even though somewhat limited, that permits it to synthesize a small portion of its own substance. Many investigators have drawn analogies between mitochondria and chloroplasts and between these organelles and procaryotic organisms and suggest that these organelles had their origins as independent organisms (Raven, 1970; Goodenough and Levine, 1970; Raff and Mahler, 1972).

For a more detailed presentation on the origin of mitochondria, see Wagner (1969); Schatz (1970); Baxter (1971); Raff and Mahler (1972).

CONCLUSION

The exquisite precision with which the mitochondrion performs its intricate biochemical procedures implies a corresponding precision in organization. Such coordinated and efficient function could not occur by random meeting of enzymes and substrates; it could only occur with an architectural design elegantly integrated with function. It is quite apparent now that the mechanisms of energy transfer associated with respiration and oxidative phosphorylation are but one facet of the functional capability of the mitochondrion. However, it is the ATP made available by mitochondrial activity that provides the power for all the energy-requiring activities of the cell: synthesis of large molecules, mechanochemical work of contraction, and osmotic work involved in active transport.

The nutritionist ascertaining the energy expenditure or metabolic rate of the whole organism is, in effect, estimating very indirectly the total amount of ATP trapped by the infinite number of mitochondria that function at quite disparate rates in oxidizing the cells' food. The metabolic rate of the whole organism is, in reality, the sum of the metabolic rates in the incomprehensively large total mitochondrial population of its constituent cells.

chapter 14
the lysosomes and microbodies

1. Identification of Lysosomes
2. Structure of Lysosomes
   a. Membrane Characteristics
   b. Membrane Stabilizers and Labilizers
3. Origin, Development, and Fate of Lysosomes
4. Function of Lysosomes
   a. Lysosomes and Kidney Function
   b. Macrophages and Other Phagocytes
   c. Hormone Secretion and Regulation
   d. Bone Resorption
   e. Cellular Autophagy
   f. Lysosomes and Disease
      1. Storage Diseases
      2. Muscular Dystrophies and Vitamin E Deficiency
      3. Rheumatoid Arthritis
5. Microbodies or Peroxisomes
6. Conclusion

The lysosome is the cell's cup of hemlock or, as de Duve described it, the "suicide bag," a term that he deplores now as "unfortunately catchy," since the lysosome's active role in cell life is of greater import than its role associated with cell death. This organelle is present in cells in varying numbers, being particularly large and abundant in cells that perform digestive functions such as the macrophages and white blood cells. It is a membrane enclosing three dozen or so powerful enzymes capable of breaking down complex nutrients. As long as the membrane remains intact, the lysosome can and does function as the digestive organ of the cell. However, disruption of the membrane frees the enzymes and the cell then digests itself. The disruption of a cell by a lysosome is obviously catastrophic in the life of a single cell organism but in complex organisms, the death of individual cells and their replacement by new young cells occur in the normal course of events and is characteristic of certain tissues.

IDENTIFICATION OF LYSOSOMES

The *lysosome* was identified and named by de Duve (1955). The relatively tardy recognition of its existence was undoubtedly due, in part, to its heterogeneity in appearance and its small size when seen in electron photomicrographs. The lack of structural conformity made it extremely difficult for cytologists to identify lysosomes as specific organelles on the basis of appearance and their recognition was the result of the complementary efforts of cytologists and biochemists. Collaborative studies revealed that certain cytoplasmic particles appeared to be associated with a group of hydrolytic enzymes, all of which showed an acid pH optimum. This association of the particles and enzymes led de Duve to suggest the name lysosome, which means lytic body. For his work on the identification of lysosomes, de Duve was one of the recipients of a Nobel prize in 1974.

Lysosomes are present in greatest number in kidney cells, certain white blood cells with macrophagic function, thymus, and spleen, but they occur in all animal cells except red blood cells. The high concentration of lysosomes in the macrophages as associated with the phagocytic function of these cells since one aspect of lysosomal function is the role it plays in the processing and digestion of extracellular materials.

Some of the difficulties encountered in the isolation and identification of lysosomes were due to the fact that early methods of centrifugal fractionation put the particles containing the hydrolases in both the mitochondrial fraction and in the fraction containing microsomes, the fragmented portions of the endoplasmic reticulum. It was through de Duve's critical standardization of fractionation techniques that the lysosomal fraction was separated from other cell fractions (see Chapter 7), and the morphological studies of Novikoff et al. (1956) that led to the lysosomal concept. Novikoff identified the so-called dense bodies, surrounded by a single lipoprotein membrane, as the structures containing the histochemically detectable acid phosphatase, one of the characteristic lysosomal enzymes. This was the first time that such a sequence in the identification of an organelle, first biochemical and then visual, had occurred.

The lysosomes were first described as membrane-bound granules containing five acid hydrolases in latent form (de Duve et al., 1955). The list of enzymes increased to 12 and is now thought to be approximately 36 separate hydrolytic enzymes (Tappel, 1969), all acting in an acid pH, capable of splitting important biological compounds such as proteins, nucleic acids, polysaccharides, and phospholipids. Such a powerful arsenal is potentially lethal to the cell unless it is contained, controlled, and channeled for proper use. The existence of such a stockpile of potential danger in a functioning cell indicates that some barrier must exist to unrestrained hydrolytic activity. Yet if these enzymes perform a digestive function for the cell, the substrates for their activity must be presented within the confines of the organelle barrier. This line of reasoning led de Duve to present a model of the lysosomes as a biochemical concept (Fig. 14.1) that visualizes the intact lysosome surrounded by a lipoprotein membrane making the enzymes inaccessible to the rest of the cell. Injury to the membrane, however, by known abnormal situations such as freezing and thawing, sonic vibrations, fat solvents, and

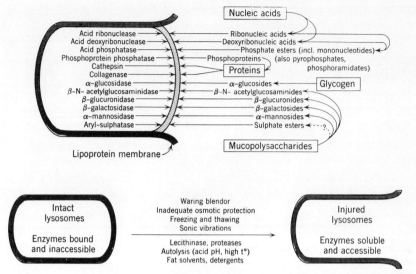

Fig. 14.1 Lysosomes as a biochemical concept. The model shown applies to rat liver lysosomes. Additional enzymes identified in lysosomes include lysozyme, phospholipase, phosphatidic acid phosphatase, esterases, and hyaluronidase. (From C. de Duve, "The Lysosome Concept" in *Ciba Foundation Symposium on Lysosomes*, A. V. S. de Rueck and M. P. Cameron, eds., Little, Brown and Co., Boston, Mass., 1963 p. 2.)

detergents or by inadequate osmotic protection or drastic changes in cellular pH or temperature, could liberate the contained enzymes into the cell contents. The meeting of lysosomal enzymes and the substrates within the cell would lead to the digestion of the cell. Such a seemingly catastrophic situation might be the sequence in a normal developmental process or in a pathological situation. Examples of both processes will be discussed.

For an interesting view of the lysosome in retrospect and the work leading to the current concept of the lysosome as part of a cell system, see de Duve (1969).

STRUCTURE

The heterogeniety of lysosomes with respect to size, form, function, and origin can be more readily understood now that lysosomes have

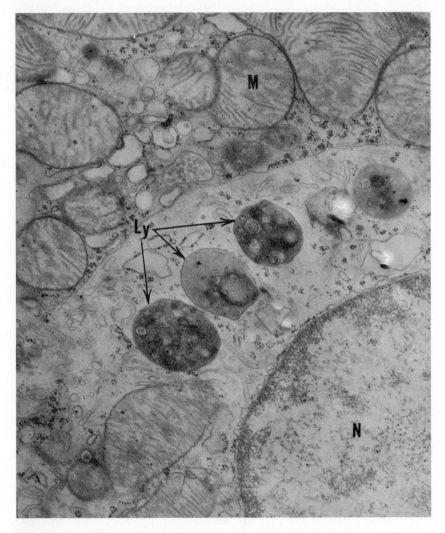

Fig. 14.2 Variations in the fine structure of lysosomes in a cell from rat kidney proximal tubule. Ly = lysosomes, N = nucleus, M = mitochondrion. Magnification 21,200. (Courtesy of Dr. Harald Schraer.)

been identified as part of a complex system of great importance to the physiology of the cell, rather than merely as a digestive and waste-disposal system.

Lysosomes are so varied in structural appearance and so lacking in unique morphological characteristics that their identification without combined biochemical or cytochemical methods is extremely difficult. They possess no aspects of fine structure that could categorize them unmistakably as do the constant features found in mitochondria, nuclei, or endoplasmic reticulum (Fig. 14.2). The appearance of lysosomes depends on their functional state. There are, however, certain characteristics that they have in common. They have a single limiting membrane that, like the membrane of the Golgi vesicles, is 25 percent thicker than the membranes of mitochondria, rough endoplasmic reticulum, and Golgi lamellae (Yamamoto, 1963). Another characteristic of lysosomes is the *halo,* a clear electron-lucid rim just inside the limiting membrane and between it and the dense matrix (Maunsbach, 1966a). In addition to these structural features, histochemical tests for acid phosphatase are characteristic of lysosomes, as is their ability to accumulate exogenous material. In this last respect, they are unique among cytoplasmic organelles (de Duve, 1963).

Membrane Characteristics

The membrane of the lysosome, which forms the barrier between the cytoplasm and the arsenal of enzymes within, functions as the semipermeable membrane of an osmotic system. The simplest model of such a system would be the enzyme-containing bag first suggested by de Duve. This model does not imply that the contents are devoid of fine structure, but it does indicate that the hydrolases have freedom of movement when the barrier is broken (de Duve, 1963). The demonstration of the mobility of the enzymes by de Duve's laboratory and of the elution of the enzymes from lysosomal membranes by Tappel and his group (1963) suggested at that time that the enzymes were not closely bound in either the inner structure of the lysosome or in the lipoprotein of the membrane. However, present biochemical evidence suggests that some of the lysosomal enzymes are constituents of the membrane itself and, furthermore, that a portion of the soluble enzymes are bound to the membrane and possibly form a protective lining. Three lysosomal enzymes have been identified as constituent parts of the membrane: β-N-acetyl-glucosaminidase, a-glucosidase, and sialidase. Other enzymes have been shown to be bound to membranes under experimental conditions. Although lysosomes contain a variety of proteases, the enzymes that are part of or bound to membranes appear stable and quite resistant to the proteolytic enzymes (Tappel, 1969). The lysosomal membrane, therefore, must differ from that of other organelles since the membranes of mitochondria and endoplasmic reticulum are hydrolyzed within the confines of the lysosome.

Despite the content of highly active hydrolytic enzymes, autolysis does not usually occur in the cell, and this has been attributed to what de Duve calls *structure-linked latency* of the lysosomal hydrolases. In other words, the extralysosomal cytoplasm remains intact because any heterolytic digestive action of the lysosome takes place only after a substrate has come within the confines of the lysosomal membrane. It follows that a break in the membrane must precede any autolytic activity. It is the membrane shield or the *structure* which is responsible for and *linked* to the inactive presence or *latency* of the enzymes. The integrity of the membrane was thought to be secured by the fact that neither lipases nor phospholipases had been identified, but no longer can this be a comfort since it appears that lysosomes have a complete complement of hydrolytic enzymes for the breakdown of lipids (Tappel, 1969), along with the enzymes acting on proteins, glycogen, nucleic acids, and mucopolysaccharides.

De Duve (1963) suggested the membrane was responsible for the latency of the enzymes and that the lysosome may be comparable to a bag of fluid in which the enzymes are suspended or dissolved. Koenig (1962), however, suggested that the lysosomes may be solid complexes and that the latency depends on ionic binding of the enzymes to acidic glycolipids, which renders them inactive. This is the *matrix binding theory,* in which the lysosome is regarded as a membrane-limited polyanionic lipoprotein granule. According to this model (Koenig, 1969), the hydrolytic enzymes within the lysosome are in an inert state by electrostatic binding to the acidic groups of the lipoprotein matrix. The active sites of the hydrolases are unavailable to react with their substrates because of ionic linkage to the lysosomal matrix. The acidic lipoprotein acts as an inhibitor of lysosomal enzymes, and the membraneous envelope serves mainly to limit the freedom of the enzyme-lipoprotein complex. Studies with phospholipase C indicate that the phosphoryl groups of the lipoprotein phospholipids play an important role in the structural latency of the lysosomal enzymes. Fig. 14.3 shows how the phosphoryl groups probably serve as binding sites for the

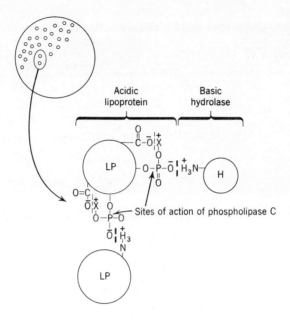

Fig. 14.3 Matrix binding theory of the lysosome. The basic groups of the phospholipid are represented as being internally neutralized through electrostatic interaction with adjacent carboxylic groups of the lipoprotein, leaving the negatively charged phosphoryl group free for binding the cationic hydrolases (or other lipoprotein macromolecules). (From H. Koenig, Lysosomes in the Nervous System, *Lysosomes in Biology and Pathology,* Vol. 2, J. T. Dingle and H. B. Fell, eds., Wiley-Interscience, N. Y., 1969, p. 142.)

acid hydrolases. The remaining phospholipid phosphate, which is less accessible to the action of the enzyme, according to Koenig (1969), seems to be essential for the maintenance of the structural integrity of the lysosomal particle.

Whether or not there is a fine structure to the interior of the lysosome is yet to be revealed. The disclosure of details of an internal structure may help to pinpoint the responsibility for latency. It may also indicate whether a nonenzymatic constituent of lysosomes that gives a histochemical reaction indicating the presence of mucopolysaccharide or glycolipid is a part of the membrane or, possibly, a part of the still undiscovered fine structure.

Membrane Stabilizers and Labilizers

The stability of the membrane defining the lysosome and holding its package of potentially powerful hydrolytic enzymes is of major importance in the normal physiology of the cell. Those agents which favor the maintenance of lysosomal membrane integrity have been termed *stabilizers*. In contrast, agents which disturb cellular pH, osmotic relations, chemical stability, or perhaps electrical charge of the membrane are all potentially disruptive and can promote the liberation of the contained enzymes into the cellular contents. Such agents are *labilizers* of the lysosomal membrane. An intact lysosomal membrane would be dependent upon the counterbalancing influences of membrane stabilizers over membrane labilizers. Just as the cell is dependent upon the nutrients coming in from its environment, so are the organelles dependent upon and affected by the nutrients available in the intracellular environment. It should come as no surprise that specific nutrients have been shown to exert either stabilizing or labilizing influences on the lysosomal membrane.

Vitamin A was reported to be an extremely effective labilizer of the lysosomal membrane. Several investigators including Dingle (1963) and Weissman and Thomas (1963) showed in *in vivo* and *in vitro* studies that vitamin A alcohol or acid acted directly on lysosomes releasing the confined enzymes. Tissues from hypervitaminotic A animals consistently released more enzymes than control tissues. It was suggested that a reaction occurs between the lipoprotein membrane of the lysosome and the vitamin in which the vitamin penetrates the membrane and causes expansion of the lipoprotein components, thus leading to instability of the membrane and the consequent release of enzymes. Fell (1965) suggested that spontaneous fractures observed as a result of excess dosage of vitamin A is due to the release of lysosomal enzymes from cartilage and bone cells into the extracellular environment. One could speculate that this capacity of vitamin A to labilize lysosomal membranes and release the confined enzymes is also a specific mechanism employed in normal bone growth, perhaps triggered by growth hormone or thyrotropin.

The labilizing effect attributed to vitamin A became confused when Roels et al. (1964) demonstrated that vitamin A deficiency in rats also led to a considerable degree of lability of liver lysosomes. However, administration of oral retinyl acetate restored lysosomal fragility to normal. No conclusion could be reached concerning whether the effect was a specific one because of vitamin A deficiency or to the general tissue degeneration accompanying the advanced deficiency state (Roels, 1969). Here was an instance where both a plethora and a deficiency of vitamin A had a labilizing effect on lysosomal membranes. Vitamin A has also been shown to be terato-genic in both deficiency and in excess, and Lloyd and Beck (1969) suggest that the effect of excess may be due to lysosomal rupture. They indicate that the teratogenicity of vitamin A deficiency could be due to action of vitamin A on biological membranes although the exact mechanism is not clear.

Other labilizers of the lysosomal membrane are ultraviolet light and ionizing radiation, both of which are extremely effective in disrupting the membrane and causing the enzymes to leak out into the surrounding area. The effect is due to the sensitivity of the membrane to damage by free radicals. Free radicals are produced when ionizing radiations hitting the cells are absorbed by the water in the cell, ionizing and decomposing the water. Hydroxyl and perhydroxyl radicals are formed as well as oxidizing compounds such as hydrogen peroxide and organic peroxides. These can be extremely toxic to tissue, leading to blistering and other more serious symptoms such as those observed in severe sunburn and X-ray burn. This effect of free peroxides can only be counteracted by the action of the iron-containing enzyme catalase, which can decompose hydrogen peroxide to water and oxygen. When free radical generation exceeds the capacity of the catalase reaction, the toxic effects become evident.

Vitamin E acts as a membrane stabilizer since its antioxidant properties prevent lipid peroxidation and the consequent generation of a free radical system (Tappel, 1972) leading to the disruption of the lysosomal membrane (see Chapter 9). However, there is contro-versy as to whether the antioxidant theory of vitamin E action is sufficient to explain its role in maintaining membrane stability. According to Green (1972), the role of vitamin E at membrane sites has yet to be clarified.

Some of the conflicting reports on the effects of vitamin E on lysosomal membrane stability apparently are due to the levels of the vitamin used. When small quantities were employed in *in vitro* work (Guha and Roels, 1965), there was stabilization of lysosomal membranes; but when large doses were employed (de Duve et al., 1962), labilization of the membrane occurred. Roels (1969) concludes that the *in vitro* effect of vitamin E on lysosomes greatly depends on the quantity: doses in the physiological range tend to stabilize the membrane, whereas large amounts tend to produce labilization.

When the interaction of vitamins A and E on lysosomes was studied in rat liver (Roels et al., 1965; Guha and Roels, 1965), it was concluded that vitamin A appeared to regulate the stability of lysosomal membranes and that its effect was dependent upon the level of a-tocopherol in the diet. In vitamin A-deficient rats, increasing amounts of a-tocopherol had an increasingly stabilizing effect on the lysosomal membrane.

An interaction was also observed between vitamin E and selenium (Brown and Pollack, 1972). Using low levels of selenium and vitamin E, a potentiating effect was observed; that is, the combination of the two nutrients produced stabilization of lysosomal membranes at levels that neither could do alone. However, if vitamin E and selenium were given in the same ratio but at 100 times the level, labilization of lysosomal membranes was observed.

Zinc markedly stabilizes lysosomal membranes and its effect appears to be at the surface of the membrane. Since cadmium and lead are also effective, although less so than zinc, the suggested action is one of interfering with oxidation of membrane components (Chvapil et al., 1972).

The lysosomal membrane depends for its successful functioning on controlled instability, that is, sufficient lability to permit it to function in endo- and exocytosis, secondary lysosome formation, and other kinds of membrane fusion (Lucy, 1972). The relationships between the stabilizers and labilizers of the membrane structure, therefore, must in some way participate in jointly establishing that control. How this occurs remains the lysosomes' secret.

ORIGIN, DEVELOPMENT, AND FATE OF LYSOSOMES

The *primary lysosome* is believed to develop in the cell through the combined activities of the endoplasmic reticulum and the Golgi

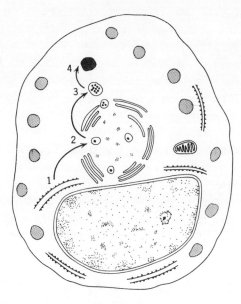

Fig. 14.4 Illustration of flow of tritiated lysine through the cytoplasm of rabbit myelocyte. 10 min after a pulse, label is found over the rough endoplasmic reticulum (1). By 30 min there is peak Golgi labeling (2). 180 min after a pulse, label over granules (3, 4) has risen and Golgi labeling has fallen. (From Z. A. Cohn and M. E. Fedorko, *Lysosomes in Biology and Pathology*, Vol. 1, J. T. Dingle and H. B. Fell, eds., Wiley-Interscience, N. Y., 1969, p. 50.)

complex. Lysosome formation has been studied in granular leucocytes of the rabbit since these cells permit ease of identification of primary lysosomes, that is, *storage granules*, whose enzymes participate in digestion after phagocytosis. Using tritiated lysine in both *in vivo* and *in vitro* studies, Fedorko and Hirsh (1966) followed its incorporation in the formation of the granules in the membrane-bound primary lysosome. Within 5 to 10 minutes after the pulse, the label was highest (71 percent) over the rough endoplasmic reticulum and cytoplasmic matrix, fell to 50 percent and was maintained at that level. Label over the Golgi complex was 11 percent at 10 minutes, increased to 37 percent by 30 minutes, and then fell back to 11 percent by 180 minutes. The label over the cytoplasmic granules rose steadily to 37 percent by 180 minutes. The flow of the labeled lysine is illustrated in Fig. 14.4. From this and other studies, it was concluded that the Golgi complex receives the newly formed protein from the endoplasmic reticulum and packages it in membrane-bound cytoplasmic granules.

The formation of *secondary lysosomes* was studied in cultured macrophages by time-lapse cinematography (Cohn and Benson, 1965). Pinocytotic vesicles were formed at the peripheral membrane and migrated toward the cell interior with some fusing to form larger vesicles or *heterophagosomes*. Close to the Golgi complex they became smaller and denser. The actual fusion of the pinocytotic vesicles and the vesicle containing the granules that budded off from the Golgi saccule (the primary lysosome) was observed by Hirsh et al. (1970) just prior to the increase in density and decrease in size. At this stage the test for acid phosphatase, the characteristic enzyme of lysosomes, was strongly positive. Since these contained both environmental molecules and newly synthesized hydrolases, they are identified as *secondary lysosomes*, or *heterolysosomes*. Had they evolved from a merger of intracellular material, an *autophagosome*, and lysosome, they would be *autolysosomes*. A form of heterolysosome is the *multivesicular body*, which results from the penetration of intact Golgi vesicles through heterophagosome membranes (Novikoff et al., 1964). These form physiological time bombs according to Beck and Lloyd (1969) since they are in a position to release hydrolytic enzymes at any time after penetration into the phagosome. It is generally assumed that the contents of the lysosome are emptied into the phagosome after lysosome-phagosome fusion (Koenig and Jibril, 1962) and that the fusion itself is due to *fusion compatability* between these membranes compared to an incompatability between the lysosome and other intact organelles. The membrane of the secondary lysosome that is thus formed is partly plasma membrane that originally surrounded the phagosome and partly lysosomal membrane (see Daems et al., 1969).

After the first fusion of a pinocytotic vesicle with the primary lysosome to form the secondary lysosome, additional fusions with vesicles can occur leading to successive acts of digestion and the piling up of residues (de Duve and Wattiaux, 1966). Eventually sufficient residue is accumulated in the lysosomes and they can no longer pick up materials ingested by the cell (Daems, 1969). De Duve and Wattiaux (1966) suggest that these filled secondary lysosomes develop into *telolysosomes*, which develop lipofuscin granules as

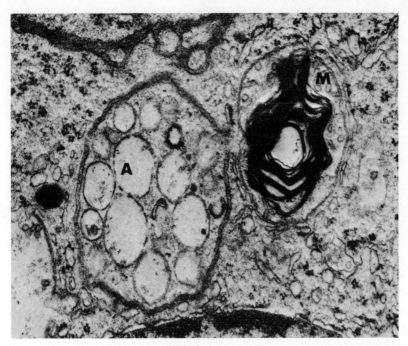

Fig. 14.5 Autophagic vacuole (A) and myelin figure (M) indicating degeneration of cellular organelles. Zona glomerulosa cell of the adrenal cortex of a pregnant rat fed a low sodium diet. Degenerative changes attributed to cellular exhaustion as a consequence of the inability of the cell to cope with the excessive demand for aldosterone secretion. Magnification 30,000. (Courtesy of Dr. Helen Smiciklas-Wright).

they age. According to Daems et al. (1969), telolysosomes are the secondary lysosomes that have reached their maximum loading capacity and no longer accumulate material nor renew their enzymes. Finally, a structure that is functionally and enzymatically inactive is formed that consists solely of digestive residues, the *residual body*. The residual bodies have an accumulation of electron-dense pigments, lipid droplets, myelin figures,[1] and amorphous masses (Fig. 14.5).

It has been suggested that the accumulated material in the residual bodies can leave the cell by defecation (Ericsson et al.,

[1]Degraded membrane fragments that appear as dense swirls in electron micrographs.

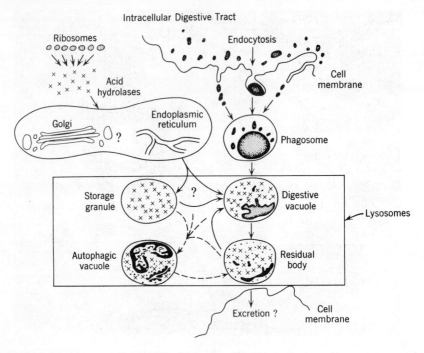

Fig. 14.6 Diagrammatic representation of the four functional forms covered by the lysosome concept and of their interrelationships. (From C. de Duve, "The Lysosome Concept" in *Ciba Foundation Symposium on Lysosomes,* A. V. S. de Rueck, and M. P. Cameron, eds., Little, Brown and Co., Boston, Mass., 1963 p. 20.)

1965) but the fact that pigment accumulation occurs in liver cells in jaundice (Novikoff et al., 1964) and that storage is progressive in pathological storage diseases suggests that a defecation mechanism, if it does exist, is not very efficient.

The discharge of some of the products of digestion by the lysosome into the cytoplasm of the cell certainly occurs in protists that depend on the lysosome as the source of digested materials for metabolism. It is assumed also that this occurs in cells of higher organisms without affecting the integrity of the lysosomal membrane; for example, the breakdown of colloid in thyroid cells leading to the release of thyroxin from thyroglobulin (Seljelid, 1967), and the release of iron from erythrocytes that have been engulfed by lysosomes (Daems, 1968). (Both of these examples will be discussed in a later section.)

With very slight modifications, de Duve's representation of the lysosomal forms and their interrelationships (Fig. 14.6) is still applicable. In fact, it clearly depicts the birth, life, and death of this organelle. For further detail on the formation and fate of lysosomes, see Dingle (1968) and Cohn and Fedorko (1969).

FUNCTION

The presence within a membrane-enclosed structure of a collection of acid hydrolases suggested to de Duve (1963) only one function, acid digestion. Since pinocytosis is a phenomenon that probably occurs in all cells, and since the pinocytotic invagination becomes the membrane-enclosed phagosome, de Duve postulated the merging of the enzyme-containing lysosome and the substrate-containing phagosome. This merger would enable the digestive process to occur entirely within the confines of an enclosing membrane. Residual materials could either be retained within the membrane-enclosed area in the cell or released from the cell by a process which could be called *exocytosis* or defecation (Fig. 14.6). Such a progressive digestive process could account for the diversity in appearance of the lysosomes and, in addition, make this characteristic understandable in terms of organelle function. Further, it could explain the mechanism involved in the phagocytic function of the specialized cells found in the blood, liver, spleen, and other tissues. Since few cell types in higher organisms are able to eliminate their digestive residues, de Duve (1963) suggested the possibility that accumulated residues in the cells may play an important part in the phenomenon of aging.

In the years following the description of lysosomes as discrete biological entities, they have been shown to be as much a part of the cell's dynamic state as the mitochondria and polysomes. The lysosome system is, in fact, crucial in the interactions between the cell and its environment. Lysosomal sensitivity to both the intra- and extracellular environment is either directly or indirectly involved in many physiological and pathological processes.

De Duve's (1969a) present concept of lysosomes describes five basic functions: (1) The simplest function of the lysosome is *storage* both of biosynthetic products within zymogen granules and other secretion granules in the primary lysosomes and of materials brought in by endocytosis. (2) Related to storage is the *exocytotic discharge* of stored materials. If the stored products were secretory materials, the process is called *secretion;* if the products had previously been taken in by endocytosis and are returned to the space from which they came, it is *regurgitation;* or, if they are released to another space, it is *transcellular transport.* (3) Another fundamental function results from the merger of the phagosome and a lysosome that results in the *digestion* of the material in the phagosome. (4) *Cellular autophagy* is still another function. It is a process whereby an autophagic vacuole fuses with a lysosome and enables the cell to rid itself of cytoplasmic fragments and damaged or worn out organelles. (5) The *release of storage material* either by defecation or exocytosis. The process may be excretory or secretory. Continued accumulation in storage without the mechanism of release leads to

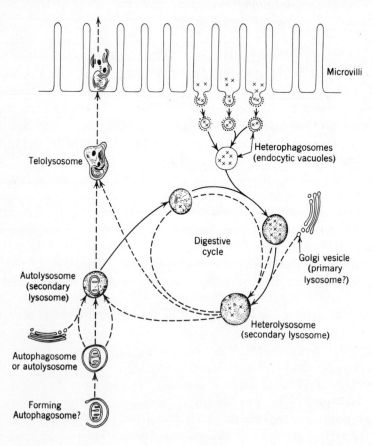

interference with normal cell function.

In the sections that follow, specific lysosomal activities will be discussed. In each case, one or more of the basic functions of this organelle system are involved.

Lysosomes and Kidney Function

Although lysosomal function has been studied in different sections of the nephron, the role in the proximal tubule is best known. Following careful differential centrifugation, several species of lysosomes that vary in fine structure have been identified in proximal tubule cells. It is assumed that different ultrastructural characteristics are associated with differences in function. Of particular interest is the evidence that cells of the proximal tubules have the ability to absorb proteins from the glomerular filtrate (Latta et al., 1967; Straus, 1967). This could be of importance in pathological conditions, but there is evidence that small amounts of protein, primarily albumin, are normally present in the filtrate of mammals (Dirks et al., 1964). This albumin is reabsorbed into the proximal tubule cell and catabolized there (Schultze and Heremans, 1966). The

---

Fig. 14.7 Diagram illustrating the probable relation between different components of the vacuolar apparatus in normal proximal tubule cells. The heterophagic pathways, which are shown in the right part of the diagram, begin with endocytic invaginations of the luminal cell membrane. The invaginations take up protein molecules (represented by crosses) from the tubule lumen, and pinch off as small heterophagosomes. The latter form large heterophagosomes, which transfer the protein to lysosomes for digestion. The heterolysosomes are used in many successive digestive events until eventually worn out and set aside as telolysosomes, which may be extruded from the cell. Acid hydrolases may continuously be fed into the heterolysosomes through Golgi vesicles representing primary lysosomes. The probable relation between the autophagic components of the vacuolar apparatus are shown in the lower left part of the diagram.

Unbroken arrows designate pathways that are proven or strongly suggested by experimental observations, and broken arrows indicate routes that are suggested by indirect evidence. Merging arrows symbolize fusion of structures. (From A. B. Maunsbach, *Lysosomes in Biology and Pathology*, Vol. 1, J. T. Dingle and H. B. Fell, eds., Wiley-Interscience, N. Y., 1969 p. 139.)

albumin first appears in the cells in endocytotic vacuoles that fuse with each other and then with lysosomes (Maunsbach, 1966a; 1966b). There is no evidence that the absorbed protein molecules are extruded from the cells. However, *in vitro* studies on purified lysosomes (Maunsbach, 1969) have indicated the presence of several albumin-degrading enzymes. He has proposed that the proximal tubule cell lysosomes function in protein catabolism (Fig. 14.7). In animals with experimental proteinuria, increased protein break-down was shown to occur in the kidney tubules (Katz et al., 1963; 1964). The suggestion is that under such conditions, or in human disorders in which proteinuria is heavy, the normal albumin absorption process is accelerated, and the lysosomes in the tubular cells are responsible for the increased protein catabolism.

There is evidence that all proteins are not handled as albumin and, indeed, that foreign proteins may become localized in particles that resemble lysosomes (Novikoff, 1963; Graham and Karnovsky, 1966). Allergic reactions initiated by antibodies to foreign protein and leading to lysosomal enzyme release have been impugned in various disorders including glomerulonephritis (Coombs and Fell, 1969).

Macrophages and Other Phagocytes

One of the principal functions of macrophages is the uptake of substances by endocytosis. Lymphoid macrophages, part of the reticulo-endothelial system, operate in the first line of defense for the removal of deleterious substances by sequestering them in their lysosomes. What happens to these substances subsequently depends on the lysosome. Those materials susceptible to lysosomal enzyme attack are digested; inert substances accumulate. The accumulations may be relatively harmless, as the dust collected in the lung cells; or painful, as the accumulations of uric acid crystals in gout; or seriously injurious, as the accumulation of asbestos and silica by lung macrophages (Allison, 1967). Whereas the accumulation of uric acid crystals appears to cause release of lysosomal enzymes and the subsequent inflammation and pain in the joints, silica and asbestos accumulated by macrophages in the lungs are far more damaging. These materials apparently react with the lysosomal membrane rendering it unstable and ultimately causing release of its hydrolytic enzymes. The silica or asbestos particles are released only to be reengulfed. This leads to further damage each time the cycle repeats and produces further necrosis and eventual fibrosis (Slater, 1969).

An active physiological process in which the macrophages participate is erythrophagocytosis (Daems, 1968), or the phagocytic action on the worn-out erythrocytes pulled into the spleen (Bowers, 1969). Whole erythrocytes have been observed inside lysosomes in electron micrographs of guinea pig macrophages in culture (North, 1966). Erythrocytes in various stages of digestion have been observed and the salvage of iron is important in the body's iron economy (see Chapter 16).

Another macrophage function that is part of a normal repair process involves white blood cells that migrate from the vascular system to the tissue involved. In wound healing, the lysosomes of the macrophages play an important role. The neutrophils, one of the group of granular leucocytes in the blood, phagocytose invading bacteria and subject them to lysosomal digestion. However, if no bacteria are there for the eating, the deprived neutrophil appears to succumb and, with the rupture of its cell membrane, it releases enzyme-containing granules into the wound site where they act on the cellular debris. Invasion of the wound by monocytes from the blood is next, and they complete the removal and digestion of tissue debris. This, too, is due to the activity of lysosomes (Ross, 1969). Only after this phagocytic activity can other cells move in for the synthesis of collagen, scar formation, and tissue synthesis in the process of healing.

Hormone Secretion and Regulation

The thyroid hormones, thyroxine and triiodothyronine, are synthesized in the thyroid gland linked to the protein, thyroglobulin. This is subsequently stored as colloid in the follicle of the gland. When the gland is stimulated to release the thyroid hormones, the thyroglobulin moves from the follicle back into the cell where the protein is hydrolyzed by the action of lysosomal enzymes before the hormones can be released.

Passage of thyroglobulin into the cell from the follicle occurs by endocytosis (Fig. 14.8). Pseudopods engulf large colloid droplets that are taken into the cell. They are found within five minutes

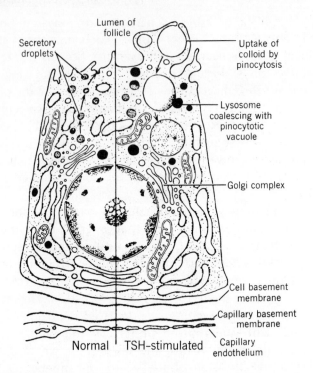

Fig. 14.8 Thyroid cell. Left: Normal pattern. Right: After marked TSH stimulation. The arrows on the left show the secretion of thyroglobin into colloid. On the right, pinocytosis of the colloid and merging of a pinocytotic vacuole with a lysosome are shown. The cell rests on a capillary with gaps (fenestrations) in the endothelial wall. (Modified from O. W. Fawcett, J. A. Long, and A. L. Jones, "The Ultrastructure of Endocrine Glands," *Recent Progr. Hormone Res.*, 25:315 1969.)

after stimulation with thyroid-stimulating hormone (TSH), and the number of droplets increases progressively (Shishiba et al., 1967). As the colloid droplets migrate toward the base of the cell they merge with dense granules, primary lysosomes, that migrate toward them carrying the necessary hydrolytic enzymes (Wetzel et al., 1965; Seljelid, 1967). The fusion appears to be rapid and hydrolysis of the thyroglobulin follows. Thyroxine and triiodothyronine are released to the blood. Probably mono- and diiodotyrosine are liberated in the cell, but they are deiodinated and the iodide reused (Greer and Grimm, 1968). Whether the thyroglobulin is hydrolyzed

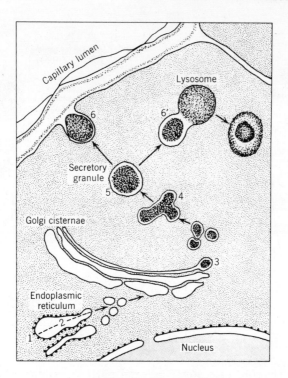

Fig. 14.9 Diagrammatic representation of the secretory process for lactogenic hormone in the anterior pituitary gland. The hormone is probably synthesized on ribosomes (1), segregated and transported by the rough endoplasmic reticulum (2), and concentrated into granules by the Golgi complex. Small granules arising within the Golgi cisterna (3) aggregate (4) to comprise the mature secretory granule (5). During active secretion, the latter fuse with the cell membrane (6) and are discharged into the perivascular spaces. (From M. G. Farquhar, *Lysosomes in Biology and Pathology*, Vol. 2, J. T. Dingle and H. B. Fell, eds., Wiley-Interscience, N. Y., 1969, p. 470.)

to amino acids or partially hydrolyzed to a "core" that is reused in synthesis is not known. For a detailed account of the secretion of thyroid hormones, see Wollman (1969).

The adrenal medulla synthesizes and stores the catecholamine hormones, epinephrine and norepinephrine, as chromaffin granules. Some of the cells in the medulla are specialized to secrete epinephrine and some, norepinephrine. (Synthesis of these hormones is discussed in Chapter 19.) The granules are formed in the Golgi

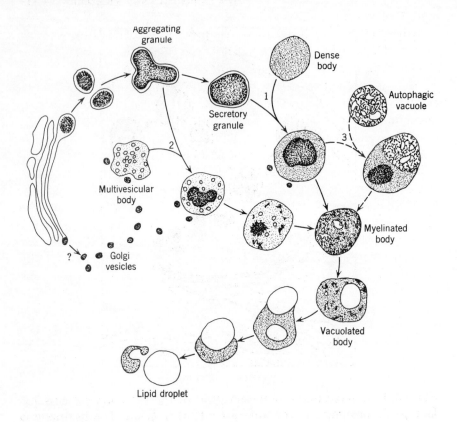

Fig. 14.10 Diagram to illustrate lysosomal digestion of stored lactogenic hormone in the anterior pituitary cell following suppression of secretion. Mature secretory granules are incorporated into dense bodies (arrow 1) and immature or aggregating granules into multivesicular bodies (arrow 2). Rough endoplasmic reticulum and ribosomes are sequestered in autophagic vacuoles which can merge with dense bodies (arrow 3). This last path is not obligatory but takes place primarily when there is pronounced cellular involution. In subsequent steps the material entering the lysosomal system through all three pathways is progressively degraded to yield a vacuolated dense body. The vacuole is shown successively protruding from, and eventually separating from the peripheral dense rim, leaving a free lipid droplet and a residual dense body. (From M. G. Farquhar, *Lysosomes in Biology and Pathology*, Vol. 2, J. T. Dingle and H. B. Fell, eds., Wiley-Interscience, N. Y., 1969, p. 471.)

region of the medullary cell (Holtzman, 1967) as are the enzyme constituents of the lysosomes. An interesting observation is that mature chromaffin granules are rich in lysolecithin, but neither lysolecithin nor the enzyme responsible for its formation from lecithin is present in early granules (Winkler et al., 1967). The enzyme responsible for the formation of 1-acyl lysolecithin is phospholipase A_2, which is found in the adrenal medulla only as a lysosomal enzyme. Smith and Winkler (1969) postulate that the phospholipase A_2, which is incorporated into the lysosomes in the Golgi region, may also be used at that locus to form the lysolecithin in the membranes that ultimately surround the chromaffin granules. (For discussion of the role of the Golgi in altering membrane enzyme content, see Chapter 12.)

If hormones are synthesized and stored as granules in the cells prior to secretion, some mechanism must exist to dispose of the accumulated secretory products. Farquhar (1969) reported on the role played by the lysosomes in degrading the undischarged granules. This was studied in the pituitary cell that secretes the lactogenic hormone. The normal sequence of events in Fig. 14.9 shows the synthesis of the hormone by the endoplasmic reticulum, passage through the Golgi complex, and release as the secretory granules. The granules coalesce and during active secretion they fuse with the cell membrane and leave the cell by exocytosis. However, when secretory activity is suppressed, the excess stored hormone does not fuse with the membrane but, instead, fuses with existing lysosomes in the cell (Fig. 14.10). This is followed by lysosomal digestion until only a lipid droplet and a residual body can be observed.

Bone Resorption

Osteoclasts, cells responsible for eroding cartilage in the shaft of the growing bone, preparatory to the deposition of bone salts, operate in association with acid phosphatase. Electron photomicrographs of osteoclasts show vacuoles in the cytoplasm and no conspicuous endoplasmic reticulum. Invaginations of the plasma membrane are associated with the cytoplasmic vacuoles and debris of the resorption (Scott and Pease, 1956).

The presence of lysosomes in bone cells has been clearly shown through biochemical studies. Nine acid hydrolases were found associated with the lysosomal fraction of bone homogenates (Vaes, 1965; Vaes and Jacques, 1965). Morphological studies, although less definitive, have indicated histochemically that several hydrolases appear in droplets that presumably are lysosomes (Hancox and Boothroyd, 1963). Furthermore, the presence of dense bodies similar to lysosomes were observed in the cytoplasm close to the ruffled border of osteoclasts (Scott, 1967) and chondroclasts (Schenk et al., 1967).

For bone resorption to occur, both collagen and mineral must be dissolved. It seems reasonable to assume that the mineral must be removed before enzymatic action on the remaining collagen can occur. The ruffled or striated border which osteoclasts show in electron micrographs is considered to be the edge of the bone that has been freed of mineral. Ham (1969, p. 411) suggests that an acid environment created by the osteoclast at the bone surface dissolves the mineral, and that lysosomal enzymes are liberated to the surface to digest the remaining collagen fibers. Although some investigators suggest that intracellular digestion by lysosomal enzymes occurs after the material is brought in by pinocytosis (Scott, 1967), Vaes

---

Fig. 14.11 A schematic view of the ultrastructural aspects of osteoclastic bone resorption showing the ruffled border of the osteoclast and the underlying sealed resorption zone at an approximate magnification of 20,000. Crystals of mineral (m) and demineralized collagen fibers (f) are free in the resorption zone (RZ) between the bone matrix (BM) and the osteoclast. Numerous channels (C) penetrate into the cytoplasm and are the sign of an extracellular digestion of the matrix. These elements are also seen more deeply in the cell in large pouches (P, pinosomes, phagosomes or digestive vacuoles) where their solubilization is completed. Between these vacuoles, numerous smaller vesicles (V) probably represent the primary lysosomes of the osteoclasts. They coalesce with the digestive pouches or vacuoles, or with the plasma membrane of the osteoclast (see arrow) and probably supply the lytic enzymes required to digest the pinocytosed material in these vacuoles as well as for the direct secretion of the lysosomal content in the extracellular resorption zone. A secretion of H^+ ions probably occurs at the same levels. SZ, sealing portion of the osteoclast; M, mitochondria; N, nuclei. (From G. Vaes, *Lysosomes in Biology and Pathology*, Vol. 1, J. T. Dingle and H. B. Fell, eds., Wiley-Interscience, N. Y., 1969, p. 227.)

(1968) proposes that the acid hydrolases of the lysosomes are excreted in bulk through exocytosis into the resorption zone and that an eroding action occurs on the organic components of the bone matrix (Fig. 14.11). This can proceed because of stimulation of the synthesis of lysosomal enzymes in the cells. Vaes (1969) postulates that acid excreted into the resorption zones as a result of aerobic glycolysis within the osteoclast permits solubilization of the mineral component of the matrix and favors the action of the acid hydrolases. Fragments of matrix released by this extracellular resorption are taken up into the osteoclasts by pinocytosis for further digestion intracellularly by lysosomal enzymes and H^+ ions. The observation that some of the large vacuoles at the ruffled surface are open to the extracellular resorbing zone suggests that there is continuous mixing of substrates and enzymes through endocytosis and exocytosis in which the pinocytotic vacuoles, the

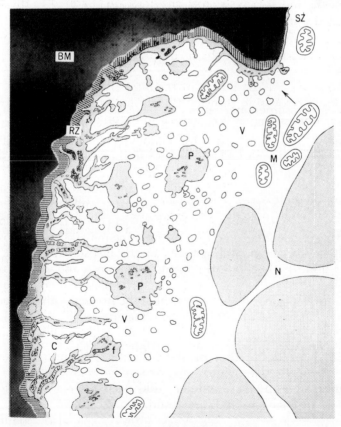

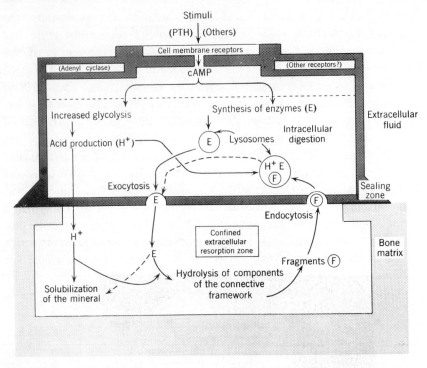

Fig. 14.12 Presumed mechanism of the osteoclastic bone resorption: a working hypothesis. Membrane receptors (adenylcyclase, ion transport systems, receptors for endocytosis, etc.), stimulated by parathyroid hormone (PTH), release intracytoplasmic messengers (cyclic AMP, ions, endocytosis vesicles, etc.) which, directly or indirectly, cause the various metabolic and cytological transformations leading ultimately to bone resorption: stimulation of glycolysis and of acid excretion; increased synthesis and exocytosis of lysosomal enzymes: extracellular digestion of the bone matrix; endocytosis and intracellular digestion of fragments in the lysosomal system. Some stimuli (dibutyryl cyclic AMP; possibly vitamin A and excess oxygen) may however directly penetrate through the plasma membrane of the cell into the cytoplasm, and exert there themselves, either directly or indirectly, alterations leading to the same end-result. (From G. Vaes, *Lysosomes in Biology and Pathology*, Vol. 1, J. T. Dingle and H. G. Fell, eds., Wiley-Interscience, N. Y., 1969, p. 244.)

lysosomes, and the extracellular fluid participate (Vaes, 1969). A suggested mechanism of bone resorption is shown in Fig. 14.12. For further discussion, see Vaes (1969); see also Chapter 17.

Since a lack of vitamin A has been shown to arrest bone growth, one might question whether this arrest is due to interference with the continuous destruction of cartilage and bone, which must take place as bones increase in length and shaft diameter. Is this effect of vitamin A deficiency due to an inability to labilize lysosomal membranes in the osteoclasts? Is the spontaneous fracturing that is a manifestation of vitamin A toxicity due to excessive labilization of the lysosomal membrane? These are interesting questions for nutritionists.

Cellular Autophagy

Not all materials destined for lysosomal digestion come from outside the cell. The formation of an autophagic vacuole in the cell may provide a neat procedure for the disposal of worn-out or damaged subcellular organelles as well as constituents of such organelles that are replaced at fairly constant rates. This "turnover" varies with the tissue, the organelle and the chemical constituent. The turnover of whole organelles—such as mitochondria—by autophagy and involving lysosomes is supported by evidence from electron microscopic studies (de Duve and Wattiaux, 1966). Autophagic activity under normal conditions rids the cell of worn-out organelles and pieces of cytoplasm without losing the constituent chemical components that can be reutilized by the cell. Since the half-life of liver mitochondria is approximately 10 days, and the half-life of the liver cell is about 150 days, the mitochondrial population of each liver cell is renewed about 15 times during the cell's lifetime (Ericsson, 1969). It has been estimated that 10^9 mitochondria per gram of liver tissue are destroyed per hour. What is true for mitochondria is probably true for other cellular components.

Cellular autophagy also plays a role in the disposal of whole organs that have outlived their usefulness. Examples are the regression of the tadpole tail in the metamorphosis of the frog (Weber, 1963; 1969) and regression of the Müllerian ducts in the male chick embryo (Sheib, 1963). In addition, normal involutionary changes occur in the mammary glands on cessation of lactation (Helminen and Ericsson, 1968), in skin keratinization (Farquhar and Palade, 1965), in thymus involution (Gad and Clark, 1968), and in bone due to the action of parathyroid hormone (see above and Chapter 17).

Another role for cellular autophagy is that of providing a survival mechanism in times of emergency. Through digestion of dispensable cellular contents, essential nutrients can be provided for high priority functions in the cell. Such an autolytic procedure during a period of starvation, when the cell decreases in volume, could be an important mechanism in the mobilization of proteins from liver cells for the return of amino acids to the blood for essential syntheses at other body sites (Swift and Hruban, 1964).

When cell injury occurs, augmented autophagy is a sequel and appears to be a mechanism that prevents spread of the insult to other parts of the cytoplasm.

Lysosomes and Disease

Storage Diseases.   Interference with a normal hydrolytic process within the cell may occur if the requisite lysosomal enzyme is missing or defective. Hers (1963) suggested that the inability to attack glycogen molecules, due to a lack of a-glucosidase in the complement of lysosomal enzymes, was the fundamental defect in the genetic disorder, Type II Glycogen Storage disease. This glycogenosis was the first disease to be clearly attributed to a missing lysosomal hydrolase. Electron microscopic examination of liver (Baudhuin et al., 1965) and other tissues (Hers and Van Hoof, 1969) indicated accumulation of glycogen in vacuoles surrounded by one membrane which were, in fact, enlarged lysosomes. Since there is also evidence of some glycogen in the cell outside the lysosome, such patients are not hypoglycemic since the glycogen dispersed in the cytoplasm can be mobilized for metabolism. The glycogen in the vacuole, however, is not available. The death of the patient results from muscle destruction due to disruption of the engorged lysosome followed by proteolytic destruction of the muscle (Hers and Van Hoof, 1969).

Other storage diseases in which genetic lysosomal enzyme defects have been implicated (see Hers and Van Hoof, 1969; Kint et al., 1973) result in excessive storage of mucopolysaccharides (Hurler syndrome), gangliosides (Tay-Sachs disease), glucocerebrosides (Gaucher disease), and sphingomyelin (Niemann-Pick disease).

Muscular Dystrophies and Vitamin E Deficiency.   The characteristic muscular dystrophy of vitamin E-deficient rabbits and chicks and of genetically dystrophic mice appears to be due to injury to the lysosomal membrane of muscle cells. Large quantities of at least four lysosomal enzymes have been detected in muscle cells from dystrophic animals (Tappel, 1963). For further discussion of lysosomal involvement in muscular dystrophies, see Weinstock and Iodice (1969).

The brain damage in vitamin E deficiency according to Kummerow (1964) occurs because the antioxidant effect of the vitamin is missing and the peroxides alter the structure of the cell membrane, perhaps deactivating specific enzyme systems. Since prompt administration of vitamin E will reverse such changes, and since vitamin E is a stabilizer of most intracellular membranes including that of the lysosome, it is tempting to think that the later irreversible brain damage that occurs is due not to the deactivating of enzymes but rather to the rupture of the lysosome, the release of enzymes, and the consequent digesting of surrounding intracellular material including some mitochondria and parts of the endoplasmic reticulum.

Rheumatoid Arthritis.   Suggestions have been offered concerning the role of lysosomes in rheumatoid arthritis (Weissmann, 1972). The primary reason for implicating lysosomes is that the local lesions of human disease can develop in laboratory animals injected with lysates of purified lysosomes. Histochemical and ultrastructural studies of synovial tissues of arthritic individuals have indicated abnormalities in lysosomes indicating that they may be more permeable to substrate (Hamermann, 1968). Weissmann (1972) proposes that macrophages crowd the inflamed synovial lining and that phagosomes still open at the external surface merge with lysosomes permitting "regurgitation during feeding." The lysosomal contents entering the synovial fluid and surrounding tissues lead to the local lesions.

It is also argued that arthritis may be associated with incomplete cellular autolysis, implying failure of lysosomal enzymes to perform their function of digesting dead cells and debris (Lack, 1969). Joint damage in rheumatoid arthritis involving both membrane and cartilage is mainly caused by lysosomal enzymes released from the cells of the synovial lining by infecting organisms. These organisms are normally phagocytosed by macrophages from the blood. If the scavenger mechanisms are defective possibly because of enzyme deficiencies, this would allow an abnormal persistence of debris.

This debris would subsequently be enveloped by fibrous tissue, a defense strategy employed by cells that isolate what cannot easily be digested. For further discussion, see Page Thomas (1969) and Lack (1969).

MICROBODIES OR PEROXISOMES

Another group of cell components, the *microbodies* or *peroxisomes*, share with lysosomes the characteristic single limiting membrane. However, microbodies differ from lysosomes in that they can be identified morphologically. They possess a moderately dense matrix that is finely granular and usually shows a denser core with a lattice structure varying in composition from one species to another (Baudhuin et al., 1965; Afzelius, 1965; Ericsson and Trump, 1966). Evidence that microbodies are different from lysosomes is based on the absence of acid phosphatase in microbodies (Miller and Palade, 1964); on the fact that they do not accumulate materials through pinocytosis (Shnitka, 1965); and on their characteristic enzymes that include catalase, urate oxidase, L-*a*-hydroxy acid oxidase, and D-amino acid oxidase (see de Duve and Baudhuin, 1966). They are usually found in close association with the smooth endoplasmic reticulum.

Little is understood of the biogenesis and turnover of rat liver peroxisomes, or of their relationships to each other within the cell (Poole, 1969). On the basis of the association of urate oxidase, xanthine dehydrogenase, and allantoinase with peroxisomes, Scott et al. (1969) concluded that they play a role in the degradation of purines. The suggestion has been made also that microbodies are important sites of hydrogen peroxide metabolism. However, de Duve and Baudhuin (1966) question their biological significance, particularly for man, because (1) urate oxidase is absent from many species, including man; (2) humans can survive with only trace amounts of catalase; (3) the function of D-amino acid oxidase in animals is questioned; and (4) the oxidation of L-*a*-hydroxy acids can proceed by several alternative routes.

De Duve (1969b) has speculated on the origin and evolution of peroxisomes and suggested that such thoughts might contribute to an understanding of their biological significance. The evolutionary survival of these organelles and their presence in large numbers in certain mammalian cells with high mitochondrial and gluconeogenetic activity have suggested that one common functional property of peroxisomes in various plants and microorganisms is gluconeogenesis. Another constant component of all peroxisomes and in remarkably high concentrations is catalase, suggesting that these microbodies may be vestiges of early respiratory mechanisms characteristic of primitive aerobes and that they appeared in response to hydrogen peroxide formation that arose either spontaneously or by catalysis. The possibility that this enzyme might be involved in some yet unsuspected role is also suggested. The D-amino acid oxidase and L-α-hydroxy acid oxidase are not vitally important, and de Duve (1969) suggests that if these enzymes perform the sole functions of microbodies in higher organisms, then microbodies decrease in importance as we go up the evolutionary scale. Perhaps, according to de Duve, the peroxisome is a dying organelle, at least in animals. For further details, see Hruban and Rechcigl (1969).

CONCLUSION

The lysosome functions as a digestive organ by making soluble and available the nutrients from phagocytosed particles; as a protective organ by engulfing and killing bacteria or foreign particles; as a site for mobilizing protein for the release of needed amino acids; as the assassin of worn-out cells; as a means of disposing of embarrassing appendages in the process of metamorphosis; and as an essential participant in processes such as bone growth. These are all normal physiological functions and, it is presumed, that precise and balanced mechanisms such as hormonal stimulation and nutrient supply would trigger the lysosomes into action at the proper time, thereby avoiding the untimely and disastrous activity of the hydrolytic enzymes.

Experimental evidence suggests that excess or deficit of certain nutrients may, by action on the lysosomal membrane, lead to widespread pathological manifestations. Such findings serve to emphasize that the effects of nutrient adequacy or potential toxicity must eventually be appraised at the cellular level.

The role of microbodies in animal cells, if indeed one exists, continues to be far from clear.

part four

specialized cells

Chapter 15   Hepatocytes
Chapter 16   Erythrocytes
Chapter 17   Bone Cells
Chapter 18   Muscle Cells
Chapter 19   Nerve Cells
Chapter 20   Adipose Cells

In a sense, all cells are specialized since the "typical cell" does not exist. The kind and degree of specialization of a cell or an organism is related to the life it leads, whether it is a free-living entity in a specific kind of environment or one of a myriad of highly specialized cells that function together as part of a unit, or organ, in a complex organism. The basic machinery with which the cell functions is present with modifications in practically all cells: nucleus, mitochondria, endoplasmic reticulum, plasma membrane. When a cell's capability to perform a specific function becomes enhanced through differentiation, it usually sacrifices the ability to carry out some other functions. However, certain metabolic processes essential to life continue: selective transport through the plasma membrane, synthesis of protein (although this, too, may be lost as in the mature erythrocyte that no longer has a nucleus), release of energy from cellular nutrients, and the trapping of this energy in ATP. Specialization often is accompanied by distinctive adjustments in nutrient needs, some of which are determined by morphological features and others by physiological characteristics.

When the fertilized ovum enters into a series of divisions they are, at first, quantitative; that is, there is an increase in number but not in kind. The resulting group of similar cells form the hollow ball or blastula stage in embryonic development which is followed by gastrulation and the formation of the germinal layers (see Grobstein, 1959). It is at this stage that differentiation begins and proceeds into the development of specialized tissues and organs. The tissues arising from the three germinal layers are both similar and diverse in their biochemical characteristics. From the one cell comes approximately 10^{14} cells that comprise a man, each identical insofar as its chromosomal endowment, or the coded information in its DNA, is concerned; yet they are different in that certain potentialities have been accentuated and others repressed or lost. For example, hemoglobin is synthesized only by the erythrocyte, insulin by the beta cell of the pancreas, hydrochloric acid by the parietal cell in the gastric mucosa. Extreme differences are also apparent in the way specialized structure is adapted to the specialized function: the long, insulated nerve fiber is irritable and has the capacity to conduct and transmit; the muscle, by virtue of the arrangement of its protein molecules, can adjust its length; the bone's affinity for calcareous matter and the arrangement of the mineral in spicules along the lines of force give the skeleton strength and rigidity. In each instance, a particular capability has been exploited and, as a result, the cell and its cytoplasmic proteins possess characteristics which differentiate it from other cells. It follows, then, that only a small fraction of the genes carried by any one cell are functional, that is, transmit their information by forming messenger RNA. The basic questions yet to be answered unequivocally: "What determines which of the genes in a particular cell are to be operative" or, "Which molecules of the DNA are to be transcribed into RNA?" were discussed in Chapter 10.

Despite the illusiveness of the mechanism, the process of specialization nonetheless occurs and is probably operative at the level of the gene. In a sense, the cells are what they synthesize. However, Grobstein (1964) clearly points out that in the multicellular organism the differentiations of individual cells are linked into a total pattern that "makes sense." It is therefore evident that intracellular controls operate to make the integrated whole.

Specialization and the consequent division of labor in a complex multicellular organism leads to a loss of independence. Each specialized cell becomes dependent upon other specialized cells for the performance of functions essential for the survival of the total organism. This interdependence is taken for granted when function proceeds undisturbed, but it becomes manifest, often strikingly, when there is interruption or interference with normal function. The total organism carries with it a great deal of insurance in the form of extra cells of all kinds. Rarely is the total number of like cells required for any specific function. However, when a sufficient number of cells specialized to perform unique functions can no longer operate, the effects will be spread throughout the functioning whole. The effects that we recognize we call disease.

Of all the cells in an organism the only ones that possess the ability to develop into any one of the specialized cells of the body are the *totipotent* germ cells such as the fertilized ovum. During development this totipotentiality is sequestered only in germ cells and not into the other cell types into which they differentiate.

Some cells are so highly specialized that soon after birth they lose all ability to reproduce. There is no way of replacing such cells when they have become worn out or destroyed. Such is the fate of nerve cells and, as a consequence, the total organism may be affected.

Some cells that are highly specialized and unable to reproduce have very short life spans due to wearing out or the sloughing off from surfaces. A steady population of such cells is maintained by cells that are called *stem cells* that have differentiated only so far as to become one of the family of cells. Steady reproduction of stem cells provides a supply of cells that can be stimulated to differentiate further to replace and maintain the cell population. Cell populations of this type that undergo continuous replacement from a pool of stem cells are the mucosal cells lining the gastrointestinal tract which last for only a few days, and the erythrocytes that have a span of about 120 days.

Some highly differentiated cells with long life spans that normally do not reproduce after full growth of the organ is attained can, under extraordinary circumstances, start to reproduce again. A description of such an event comes from Greek mythology: "Jupiter had him (Prometheus) chained to a rock on Mount Caucasus, where a vulture preyed on his liver, which was renewed as fast as devoured."[1] It seems unlikely that mere mortals can work quite that fast today, but the laboratory rat after two-thirds of its liver is removed can regenerate it fully within days through cell divisions of the remaining third. The liver which is indispensable is also resourceful. A protein factor in serum of rats found 12 hours after partial hepatectomy is capable of stimulating DNA synthesis specifically in livers (Morley and Kingdon, 1973). There is at present only a suggestion, but it appears to be released from the remaining portion of liver (Morley, 1974).

Cell specialization, however important in a multicellular society, carries with it the defects of its virtues.

[1]*Bullfinch's Mythology, The Age of Fable,* Chapter 2, p. 20, First Modern Library Edition, 1934.

chapter 15
hepatocytes

1. Structure
2. Specialized Functions
   a. Regulation of Blood Glucose Level
   b. Gluconeogenesis
   c. Acetoacetyl CoA and Ketone Body Formation
   d. Plasma Protein Synthesis
   e. Creatine Synthesis
   f. Urea Synthesis
   g. Plasma Lipid Synthesis
   h. Cholesterol Synthesis and Degradation
   i. Bile Acid Synthesis
   j. Bile Pigment Formation
3. Conclusion

The size of the liver and its prominence in the abdominal cavity was undoubtedly a factor in the importance that the ancient Babylonians ascribed to it. The liver was used in medical diagnosis, but interestingly, it was not the patient's liver but that of a sheep into whose nose the patient had breathed. The liver from the slaughtered sheep was compared to a clay liver which priests had carefully zoned into regions to indicate the nature of the disease. In a sense, the Babylonians could be considered prescient in the importance they placed upon liver function and appearance; but many centuries passed before the central role of the liver in the total metabolic scheme was recognized.

The structural plan of the liver is adapted to the diversity of hepatocyte function. Every cell is oriented so that the plasma membrane is adjacent on one side to the sinusoids that receive blood from both the portal and arterial circulation and on the other side to the bile canaliculi that form a communicating and collecting system for the bile synthesized by the liver cells. The cells thus form a narrow wall between the blood on one side and the bile on the other. The architectural plan of the liver showing a continuous mass of cells in plates of one cell thickness is shown in Fig. 15.1. These plates are usually curved, have many holes in them, and anastomose with each other. All of the spaces between the plates of hepatocytes are the blood sinusoids into which the individual hepatocytes deliver their synthetic products, except for the exocrine secretion, bile. Bile is delivered into the bile canaliculi, the spaces between the cells. The arrangement provides for close contact and exchange between the hepatocytes and both the blood and the exocrine ducts that carry the bile. In that way the hepatocytes can respond quickly to the demands of the total organism they serve.

Of the blood entering the liver, 65 to 75 percent comes via the portal vein and carries in it all of the nutrients absorbed into the blood from the small intestine; the remaining 25 to 35 percent is arterial blood that enters through the hepatic artery. The nutrients

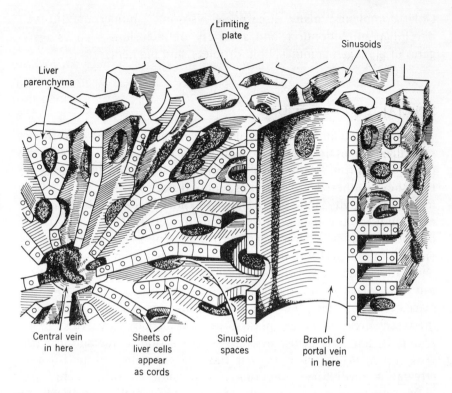

Central vein
in here

Sheets of
liver cells
appear
as cords

Sinusoid
spaces

Branch of
portal vein
in here

Fig. 15.1 Stereogram of a quadrant of a hepatic lobule. (Modified by Ham to the extent that labeling was added, from H. Elias, *Am. J. Anat.*, 85:379.)

absorbed into the lymph from the small intestine arrive at the liver cell with the arterial blood. The liver sinusoids, therefore, bring to the cells simultaneously arterial blood and all of the products of intestinal digestion. In a sense, the liver cells are transfer or nutrient redistribution centers that, under the influence of hormonal regulatory mechanisms, can store or metabolize nutrients and then transfer the metabolic products to the hepatic vein or the bile canaliculi.

STRUCTURE

The liver cell, or hepatocyte, displays no strikingly unique morphological characteristics. It contains a large nucleus, sometimes two nuclei, well developed rough and smooth endoplasmic reticulum,

Golgi complexes, many discernable lysosomes, numerous and well developed mitochondria, and a variety of inclusions such as aggregates of glycogen granules, lipid droplets, and pigment.

SPECIALIZED FUNCTIONS

The unspectacular appearance of the liver cell belies the diversity of specialization of its metabolic pathways. Most cells metabolize the major foodstuffs, synthesize ATP, and are self-sufficient in the sense that they synthesize the enzymes required both for their intracellular metabolic activity and for specialized export products. However, the magnitude of the liver's participation in such synthetic activities is probably its most characteristic attribute. The scope and variety of vital functions performed is variously estimated from 100 to perhaps over 500. Practically all the reactions of intermediary metabolism can take place in the liver, and some reactions occur in no other place. For example, the liver is primarily responsible for the synthesis of urea, creatine, plasma proteins, triacyl glycerols, phospholipids, and bile acids. Because of the scope of metabolic pathways open in the liver cell, it has the capability of performing integrated regulatory functions not possible in other cells, and upon which homeostasis depends in the complex multicellular organism as, for example, the fine regulation of the blood sugar concentration and the maintenance of plasma protein levels. The scope of liver synthetic function both in terms of products for export and enzymes for intrahepatocyte synthesis indicates that these cells have the capability of synthesizing unique types of RNA; that is, in these cells mechanisms must exist which permit the reading of more specific DNA regions of the genes than are read in other cells.

Regulation of Blood Glucose Level

The maintenance of the normal blood glucose concentration is a coordinated process in which the rate of glucose entry into the blood is balanced by its rate of withdrawal. The liver cell, responding to hormonal and various other influences during plethora, can withdraw glucose from the blood for the synthesis of glycogen for storage; or, in times of shortage, can supply glucose derived from its readily available stores of glycogen through glycogenolysis. Since liver glycogen capacity is rather limited, the hepatocyte is equipped to tap more extensive sources of ultimate glucose such as amino acids and fats, through gluconeogenesis.

In a postabsorptive state, blood glucose concentrations are maintained within the normal range of 80 to 100 mg/100 ml by the glycogenolysis and gluconeogenesis in the liver cell to counterbalance the glucose that is constantly withdrawn from the circulation for oxidative and synthetic activities of all of the cells of the complex organism. The efficiency and rapidity of regulation in the normal individual are such that, despite long periods of fasting, glucose concentrations in blood do not fall to hypoglycemic levels, nor do bouts of overeating lead to more than a transient rise. (Although the kidney cells in no way regulate plasma glucose concentration, they normally participate by preventing glucose excretion. See Chapter 7 for discussion of renal threshold.)

The antagonistic actions of insulin and glucagon on glycogenolysis, gluconeogenesis, and glycogenesis in the liver cell are part of the effective control on the level of blood glucose. The secretion of either one of these hormones is greatly enhanced by metabolites that cause a decrease of the other. For example, glucagon secretion is decreased and insulin secretion increased by the presence of glucose. The receptivity of the hepatocyte to hormonal stimulation is a characteristic of its plasma membrane. There is evidence that there are both glucagon and insulin receptors in the membrane that, when stimulated, initiate the metabolic response characteristic of each hormone.

Rodbell (1973) postulated that the glucagon-sensitive receptors in rat liver cell membranes are composed of regulatory and catalytic components (see Chapter 9). When glucagon binds to the regulatory receptor, the catalytic component converts ATP to cAMP and both glycogenolysis and gluconeogenesis are stimulated. Insulin inhibits the actions of glucagon on the liver cell (Mackrell and Sokal, 1969), and this is attributed to a reduction in the intracellular levels of cAMP. Whether the decrease in cellular cAMP levels produced by insulin is due to inhibition of the adenyl cyclase or to the activation of phosphodiesterase is not clear (Exton et al., 1971). Cuatrecasas (1973) has postulated several ways that the insulin action on the membrane receptor of the hepatocyte could produce a decrease in cAMP within the cell and promote entry of glucose into the cell followed by glycogenesis (see Chapter 9). The coordinate stimulation of glycogenolysis and inhibition of glycogenesis mediated by cAMP through protein kinase activation was presented in Chapter 11. The roles of glucagon in increasing cAMP in the cell appear to be clearly related to the activation of protein kinase and the cascade of events leading to glycogenolysis and inhibition of glycogenesis. The action of insulin associated with decreased cAMP according to Villar-Palasi et al. (1971) could be through the conversion of phosphorylase a into the inactive b form and, therefore, preventing glycogen breakdown.

In addition to the sensitivity to insulin and glucagon, the metabolsim of the hepatocyte may be responsive to the action of the glucocorticoids from the adrenal cortex. Although these hormones have usually been ascribed a role in gluconeogenesis, their impact on this liver function is becoming debatable and their influence on the regulation of blood sugar level questionable. It is clear that glucocorticoids influence peripheral tissues by promoting protein catabolism and thereby making available glucogenic substrates. However, the gluconeogenic role of these hormones on the liver cell has not been clarified. It is suggested that they exert a supportive action in gluconeogenesis only after the tissue level of cAMP is elevated through the action of glucagon. A possible role of the glucocorticoid activity in the liver may be one of promoting enzyme synthesis (Wicks et al., 1974). This would integrate the role in protein catabolism in peripheral tissue with the gluconeogenic role of glucagon in liver (Ensinck and Williams, 1972).

The liver cell, as is true of all other cells, is responsive to the availability of substrate. However, the liver cell's response appears to be of a broader nature in that its metabolic environment mirrors that of the total organism, and it functions in the homeostasis of that total metabolic environment to a far greater extent than other cells. Substrates arriving at the plasma membrane of the hepatocyte are accepted, metabolized, stored, or replenished according to the needs of the total organism. It seems reasonable to assume that coordination is effected through central nervous system control. Whether this control is mediated through the endocrine glands, or through the release of epinephrine or other neurotransmitters at nerve endings in hepatic tissue, or both, is not clear. Burr et al. (1971) suggests that such a single coordinating influence in the central nervous system is responsive to changes in the metabolic state. This influence is capable of initiating appropriately timed modifications in hormonal, hepatic, and peripheral tissue metabolic activities. Such a mechanism (Fig. 15.2) would implement the rapid adaptation to metabolic change essential for glucose homeostasis. Sutherland and Robison (1969) suggest that the adenyl cyclase-cAMP system in both hepatic and peripheral metabolism is the trigger point for blood glucose control at the level of the hepatocyte.

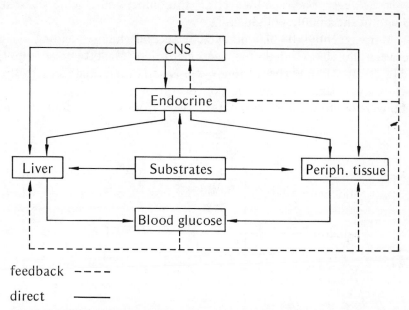

feedback   – – – –

direct   ———

Fig. 15.2 Model illustrating the concept of glucose homeostasis: direct effects are shown by continuous lines; feedback effects by dashed line. [From I. M. Burr, H. P. Taft, W. Stauffachen, and A. E. Renold, *Ann. N. Y. Acad. Sci.*, 185: 245 (1971).]

Gluconeogenesis

Gluconeogenesis is the synthesis of glucose and glycogen from several compounds: lactate, pyruvate, glycerol, and certain amino acids. The liver is the major site of gluconeogenesis but under certain circumstances, such as starvation, the kidney is equally as important as liver in this process. Gluconeogenesis is a primary source of providing glucose to body cells when carbohydrate intake is limited and body glycogen stores are depleted. This process further provides for the recycling of lactate (the Cori cycle) and glycerol when these compounds accumulate in muscle tissues, such as occurs following heavy exercise. When amino acids are degraded in normal metabolism or when excessive amounts are degraded, as occurs during starvation, a major pathway is the formation of glucose or glycogen. In prolonged starvation, the ammonia thus released, is significant in counteracting acidosis. Almost all amino acids are potentially glucogenic; however, only alanine, serine, threonine, and glycine give rise to significant amounts of glucose.

More recently the alanine cycle, a second glucose-yielding cycle between muscle and liver, has been identified (Mallette et al., 1969; Felig et al., 1970). The alanine cycle is somewhat analagous to the lactate cycle and involves the conversion of alanine to glucose and reconversion to alanine. Pyruvate derived from glucose oxidation in

ALANINE CYCLE

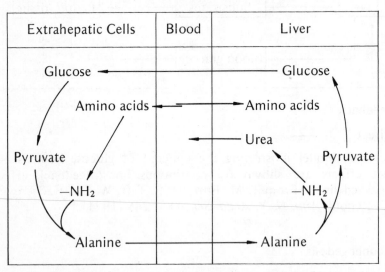

Fig. 15.3 Diagrammatic representation of the postulated role of alanine in the transfer of amino groups from extrahepatic tissues to the liver. [From L. E. Mallette, J. H. Exton, and C. R. Park, *J. Biol. Chem.*, 244: 5712 (1969).]

muscle is transaminated to form alanine, which is transported to the liver where its carbon skeleton is reconverted to glucose (Fig. 15.3). The cycle is important in gluconeogenesis as a source of glucose when exogenous supply is low and when metabolic demands for oxidizable substrate, as in exercise, are high. The cycle also is important in nitrogen metabolism since, in transferring amino groups from muscle to liver, alanine acts as a nontoxic alternative to ammonia.

For a detailed discussion of the alanine cycle see Felig and Wahren (1974).

Fig. 15.4 shows the pathways by which glucose and glycogen are formed from various other noncarbohydrate sources.

Acetoacetyl CoA and Ketone Body Formation

Normally fatty acid oxidation does not result in any significant accumulation of intermediary metabolites. However, under certain conditions, a normal intermediate, acetoacetyl CoA, is formed by reversal of the β-ketoacyl thiolase reaction resulting from condensation of two moles of acetyl CoA. Acetoacetyl CoA subsequently gives rise to free acetoacetic acid, β-hydroxybutyric acid, and acetone. These three compounds are referred to as *ketone bodies.*

In order to form free acetoacetate, acetoacetyl CoA must be converted in the liver to 3-hydroxy-3-methyl glutaryl CoA (HMG), an important intermediate in the biosynthesis of cholesterol. Cleavage of 3-hydroxy-3-methyl glutarate yields acetoacetic acid and acetyl CoA. These reactions are shown below.

$$\underset{\text{Acetoacetyl CoA}}{CH_3COCH_2COSCoA} + \underset{\text{Acetyl CoA}}{CH_3COSCoA} + H_2O \longrightarrow \underset{\substack{\text{3-Hydroxy-3-methyl}\\ \text{glutaryl CoA}}}{HOOCCH_2\overset{\overset{\displaystyle OH}{|}}{\underset{\underset{\displaystyle CH_3}{|}}{C}}CH_2COSCoA} + HSCoA$$

$$\text{3-Hydroxy-3-methylglutarylSCoA} \longrightarrow \text{acetoacetic acid} + \text{acetyl SCoA}$$

Acetoacetate, thus formed, may be reduced to form β-hydroxybutyrate in an easily reversible reaction or decarboxylated to form acetone.

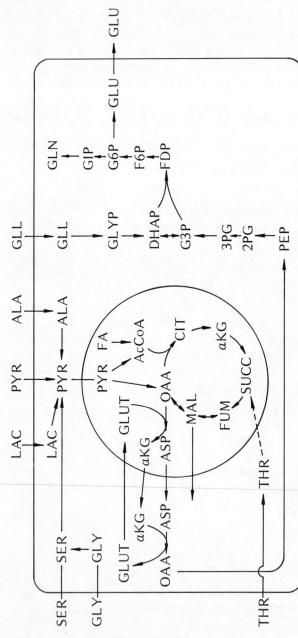

Fig. 15.4 Gluconeogenesis in the liver cell. Rectangle represents the plasma membrane; circle, a mitochondrion. Abbreviations are LAC, lactate; PYR, pyruvate; ALA, alanine; SER, serine; GLY, glycine; FA, fatty acid; AcCoA, acetyl CoA; CIT, citrate; α-KG, α-ketoglutarate; SUCC, succinate; FUM, fumarate; MAL, malate; OAA, oxalacetate; ASP, aspartate; GLUT, glutamate; THR, threonine; PEP, P-enol pyruvate; 2PG, 2-P-glycerate; 3PG, 3-P-glycerate; G3P, glyceraldehyde-3-P; DHAP, dihydroxyacetone-P; GLYP, glycerol-1-P; GLL, glycerol.; FDP, fructose-1, 6-di-P; F6P, fructose-6-P; G6P, glucose-6-P; G1P, glucose-1-P; GLU, glucose; GLN, glycogen. [From J. H. Exton, *Metabolism*, 21: 945 (1972).]

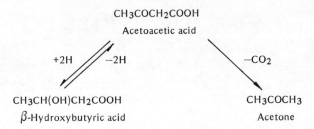

The reversible reaction between acetoacetate and β-hydroxybutyrate depends on the level of liver glycogen. When liver glycogen level is high, the reaction is chiefly in the direction of β-hydroxybutyrate formation; when liver glycogen is low, acetoacetate is the chief reaction product.

Liver mitochondria are incapable of oxidizing ketone bodies. Mitochondria of muscle cells and other extrahepatic cells, however, readily oxidize acetoacetate via the TCA cycle. In order to be oxidized, acetoacetic acid must be converted back to its CoA form. The conversion is accomplished by transfer of a CoA residue from succinyl CoA by the action of a specific thiophorase that apparently is present in muscle cells but not in liver. The acetoacetyl CoA, thus formed, may yield two molecules of acetyl CoA that are oxidized via the TCA cycle.

Fig. 15.5 illustrates the pathway of ketogenesis in the liver cell. Note that the fatty acyl CoA is converted to fatty acyl carnitine before it is transported into the liver cell mitochondrion. This is a necessary step in transport of acyl groups into and out of the mitochondrion since the mitochondrial membrane is impermeable to the fatty acyl CoA but permeable to the fatty acyl carnitine molecule. Two enzymes are involved. One, acetyl coenzyme A-carnitine acetyl transferase, catalyzes the acylation of carnitine with short chain fatty acids. The second enzyme, palmitoyl coenzyme A-carnitine palmitoyl transferase, catalyzes acetylation of long chain fatty acids.

Acetone may give rise to pyruvic acid by way of an initial conversion to propanediol and thus enters the TCA cycle by the glycolytic pathway. A second pathway for metabolism of acetone is through cleavage to form a two-carbon acetyl residue and a one-carbon formyl group.

Under certain conditions, such as markedly increased fat catabolism (as in the fasting state) and relatively decreased carbohydrate catabolism, acetoacetate is formed at a faster rate than it can be

PATHWAY OF KETOGENESIS

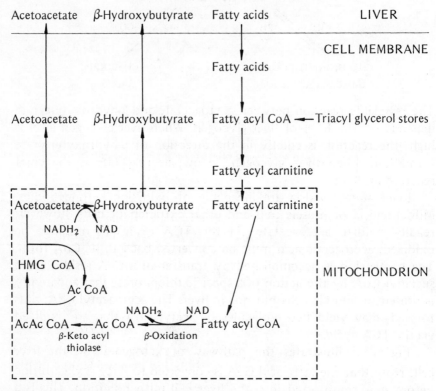

Fig. 15.5 Diagram of the pathways of ketogenesis from fatty acids in the liver. (From Best and Taylor's *Physiological Basis of Medical Practice,* J. B. Brobeck, ed., 9th ed., Williams and Wilkins Company, Baltimore, 1973, p. 7-140.)

oxidized. This leads to the accumulation of ketone bodies in blood (ketonemia). If the blood level exceeds the renal threshold for these compounds, ketone bodies also are excreted in large amounts in the urine (ketonuria). This condition is known as *ketosis.* The exact mechanism precipitating ketosis is not understood. It is clear, however, that under normal conditions ketone bodies are produced and oxidized and, moreover, under certain conditions ketone bodies may supply a major source of energy to the cell. Such a condition prevails in the fasting state. The brain, which normally utilizes glucose as its source of energy, shifts to a predominantly ketone body metab-

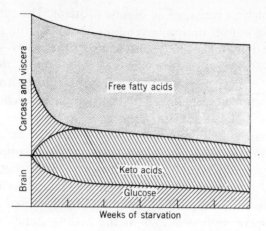

Fig. 15.6 Substrate oxidation in fasting man. Schematic representation of the transition from glucose to fatty acid utilization by the carcass and viscera and from glucose to ketoacids by the brain. (From G. F. Cahill, Jr. et al., *Adipose Tissue, Regulation and Metabolic Function*, B. Jeanrenaud and D. Hepp, eds., Acad. Press, N. Y., 1970, p. 181.

olism as fasting progresses (Fig. 15.6). Other tissues also use ketone bodies to a limited extent during fasting but rely chiefly on fatty acids as a source of energy. Thus, ketone bodies are a source of fuel for the body and function in the same way as glucose and fatty acids.

Plasma Protein Synthesis

The early work of Whipple and his associates (Madden and Whipple, 1940) suggested that the liver was the specific site for synthesis of plasma proteins. Only the synthesis of albumin and fibrinogen, however, is the exclusive function of liver cells. Roughly 80 percent of globulins (with the exception of gamma globulin) is synthesized in the liver (Miller and Bale, 1954). Gamma globulin, which contains most of the antibodies present in blood, is formed in extrahepatic cells, primarily in the spleen and to some extent in lymphoid tissue.

Albumin is by far the most abundant of the plasma proteins. Normally 150-250 mg albumin/kg body weight are synthesized daily in the adult human (see Rothschild et al., 1969). The turnover rate of albumin is high as is that of all plasma proteins. The synthesis and release of one albumin molecule requires about 30 minutes in man and in the rabbit (Peters, 1962), and some of the newly synthesized albumin probably stays within the cell for a short time. Peters (ibid.) has shown that the bulk of albumin is attached to the endoplasmic reticulum. About half as much is found in mitochondria, and traces appear in nuclei and lysosomes.

The synthesis of albumin is markedly lowered as a result of fasting or malnutrition. In children suffering from protein-calorie malnutrition, albumin synthesis was shown to range between 100-148 mg/kg/day as compared to 222-233 mg/kg/day in well nourished children (James and Hay, 1968). Studies with perfused livers from fasted rabbits have indicated that in the fasting state albumin synthesis was stimulated by tryptophan and, to a lesser extent, by isoleucine. No increase in synthesis occurred as a result of perfusion with methionine, lysine, leucine, valine, or threonine (Rothschild et al., 1969). Thus, albumin synthesis is determined not only by the available supply of amino acids but under some conditions may be responsive to specific amino acids.

Creatine Synthesis

The synthesis of creatine is a function of liver and of kidney cells. The amino acids—glycine, arginine, and methionine—each contribute a part of the molecule (Fig. 15.7). The synthesis begins with the reversible transfer of the guanidine moiety of arginine to glycine, a transamidination reaction catalyzed by the enzyme, transamidinase. The products of the reaction are guanidoacetic acid and ornithine. The final reaction is the methylation of guanidinoacetic acid to form creatine under the influence of the enzyme guanidinoacetate methyltransferase. The methyl group is donated by δ-adenosylmethionine, which is formed from methionine and ATP. As a result of the transmethylation, δ-adenosyl homocysteine and creatine are formed.

Creatine is converted to creatine phosphate or creatinine. In its phosphorylated form, creatine is the major source of high energy phosphate for the regeneration of ATP during muscle contraction (see Chapter 18). Creatinine is the major excretory product of creatine metabolism.

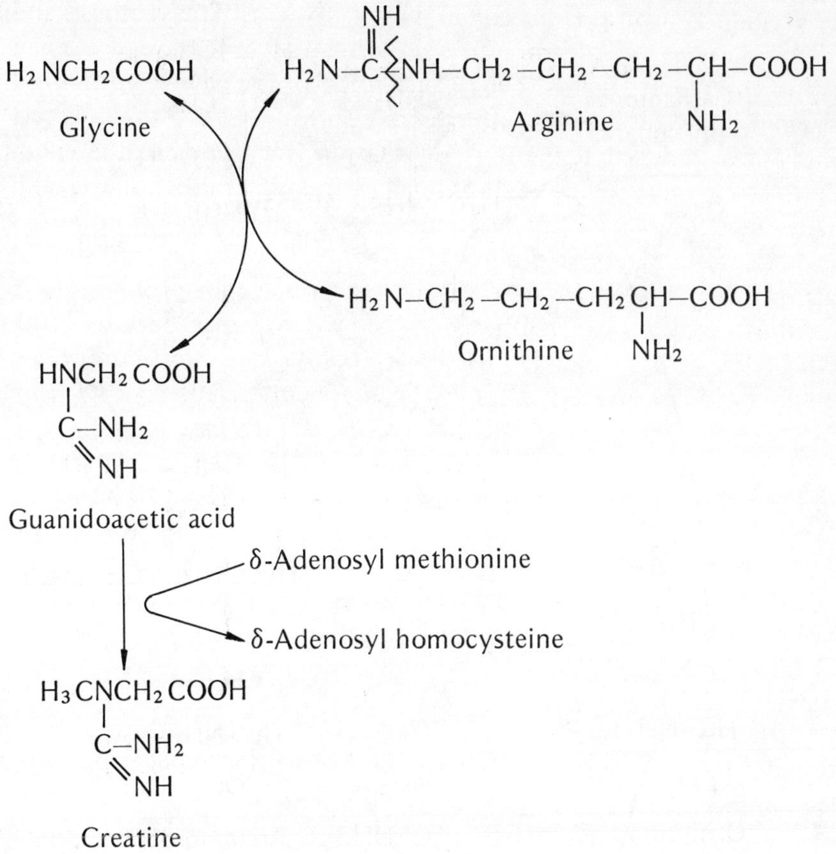

$$H_2NCH_2COOH$$

Glycine

$$\underset{\underset{NH_2}{|}}{H_2N-C\text{--}NH-CH_2-CH_2-CH_2-CH-COOH}$$

with NH double bond on the C.

Arginine

$$\underset{\underset{NH_2}{|}}{H_2N-CH_2-CH_2-CH_2 CH-COOH}$$

Ornithine

$$\underset{\underset{\underset{NH}{\diagdown\diagup}}{C-NH_2}}{HNCH_2COOH}$$

Guanidoacetic acid

δ-Adenosyl methionine

δ-Adenosyl homocysteine

$$\underset{\underset{\underset{NH}{\diagdown\diagup}}{C-NH_2}}{H_3CNCH_2COOH}$$

Creatine

Fig. 15.7 Creatine synthesis.

Urea Synthesis

A major and critical function of the liver is the synthesis of urea; this synthesis is the most significant pathway for disposal of ammonia arising from the deamination of amino acids and of amines, such as histamine or glutamine. Some ammonia synthesized from urea and other sources by intestinal bacteria is absorbed.

It will be recalled that all amino acids participate in transamination and thereby lose amino groups to form glutamic acid from α-ketoglutarate. Direct oxidative deamination, however, the final

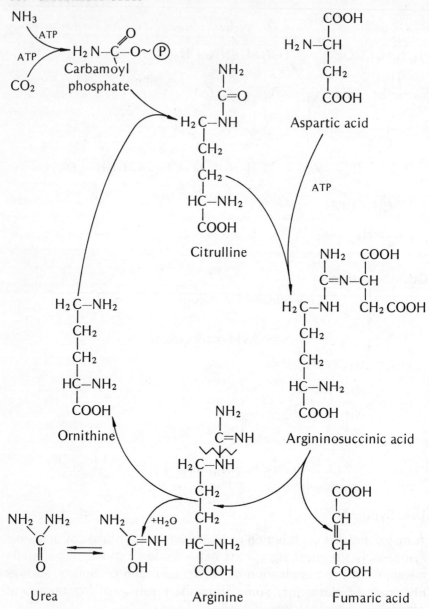

Fig. 15.8 Synthesis of urea.

pathway for disposal of amino acid nitrogen, is chiefly limited to deamination of glutamic acid in mammalian liver cells. Dehydrogenation of glutamate yields ammonia, a highly toxic compound, even in small quantities. The formation of urea, which can be tolerated in much higher concentrations, thus represents a detoxication mechanism in which the liver is the chief participant.

The mechanism of urea synthesis, first proposed by Krebs and Henseleit (1932), was based on *in vitro* experiments in which formation of urea in liver slices was observed to increase when either arginine, ornithine, or citrulline were added to the reaction medium. On the basis of these experiments coupled with results of earlier isolated studies reported in the literature, they proposed that formation of urea is a cyclic process accomplished through the breakdown and resynthesis of arginine. The scheme shown in Fig. 15.8 is only slightly different from the original Krebs-Henseleit proposal. They assumed that both atoms of urea nitrogen came from ammonia; now it is known that one nitrogen atom comes from ammonia and one from aspartic acid. The hydrolysis of arginine is the final step in the formation of urea; this reaction is catalyzed by the enzyme arginase. Borsook and Keighley (1933) established that urea synthesis, like most biosynthetic mechanisms, is an energy-requiring process. The ATP requirement for urea synthesis has been cited by Krebs (1964) as one factor contributing to the greater heat production following protein ingestion and will be discussed in a later section on the calorigenic effect of food (see Chapter 23).

Although urea formation is the chief means of disposing of ammonia, it is not the only mechanism. Ammonia also may be used in the synthesis of glutamine, the acid amide of glutamic acid, which then may give up its ammonia for synthesis of urea or other nitrogenous compounds, such as purines. Glutamine appears thus to serve as a temporary storage compound for ammonia until urea synthesis can proceed.

Plasma Lipid Synthesis

Whereas liver appears to be no more important than other tissues in the synthesis of fatty acids, it is the principal site of synthesis of the plasma triacyl glycerols and phospholipids and of their incorporation into lipoproteins that are fractions of the a- and β-globulins. The key compound for the formation of both the triacylglycerols and the phospholipids is phosphatidic acid. This compound can be synthesized in liver from either glycerol 3-phosphate or dihydroxyacetone phosphate.

The synthesis of phosphatidic acid via glycerol 3-phosphate occurs both in liver and adipose cells. The reaction shown below is preferential for the saturated and unsaturated C_{16} and C_{18} acyl CoA esters. Glycerol 3-phosphate is formed from the phosphorylation of free glycerol by glycerokinase and ATP, or by the reduction of dihydroxyacetone phosphate.

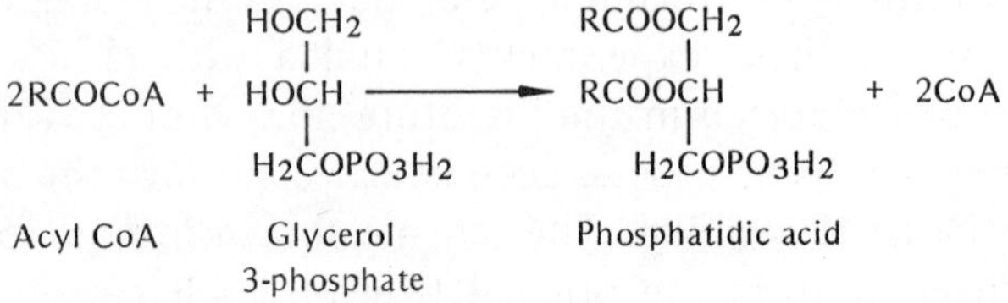

$$
\begin{array}{ccccc}
& & HOCH_2 & & RCOOCH_2 \\
& & | & & | \\
2RCOCoA & + & HOCH & \longrightarrow & RCOOCH & + & 2CoA \\
& & | & & | \\
& & H_2COPO_3H_2 & & H_2COPO_3H_2
\end{array}
$$

| Acyl CoA | Glycerol 3-phosphate | Phosphatidic acid |

Dihydroxyacetone phosphate can lead to the formation of phosphatidic acid, however, without being converted to glycerol 3-phosphate. The pathway is shown below.

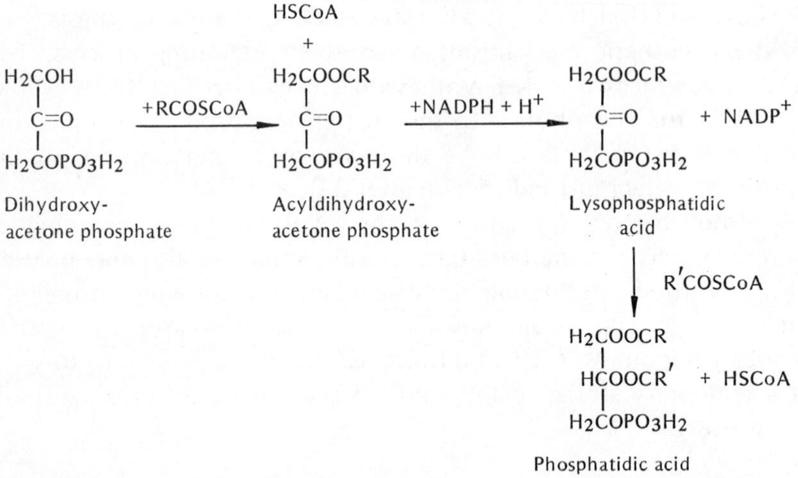

$$
\begin{array}{ccc}
& HSCoA & \\
& + & \\
H_2COH & H_2COOCR & H_2COOCR \\
| & | & | \\
C=O \xrightarrow{+RCOSCoA} C=O \xrightarrow{+NADPH + H^+} C=O + NADP^+ \\
| & | & | \\
H_2COPO_3H_2 & H_2COPO_3H_2 & H_2COPO_3H_2
\end{array}
$$

Dihydroxy-acetone phosphate   Acyldihydroxy-acetone phosphate   Lysophosphatidic acid

$$
\downarrow R'COSCoA
$$

$$
\begin{array}{c}
H_2COOCR \\
| \\
HCOOCR' \quad + \quad HSCoA \\
| \\
H_2COPO_3H_2
\end{array}
$$

Phosphatidic acid

The formation of acyldihydroxyacetone phosphate is catalyzed by a transacylase which is present in mitochondria and microsomes and which is specific for saturated fatty acids. The reduction of this compound to lysophosphatidic acid is catalyzed by a microsomal enzyme. The second acylation resulting in the formation of phosphatidic acid is accomplished also by a microsomal enzyme which is preferential for unsaturated fatty acyl CoA esters.

The synthesis of triacyl glycerols and phospholipids proceeds from phosphatidic acid which is hydrolyzed by a specific phosphatase to yield 1,2-diacylglycerol. Finally, as shown below, the diacylglycerol is fully acylated to yield a triacylglycerol or reacts with a cytidine diphosphate base (choline, serine, or ethanolamine) to form a phospholipid.

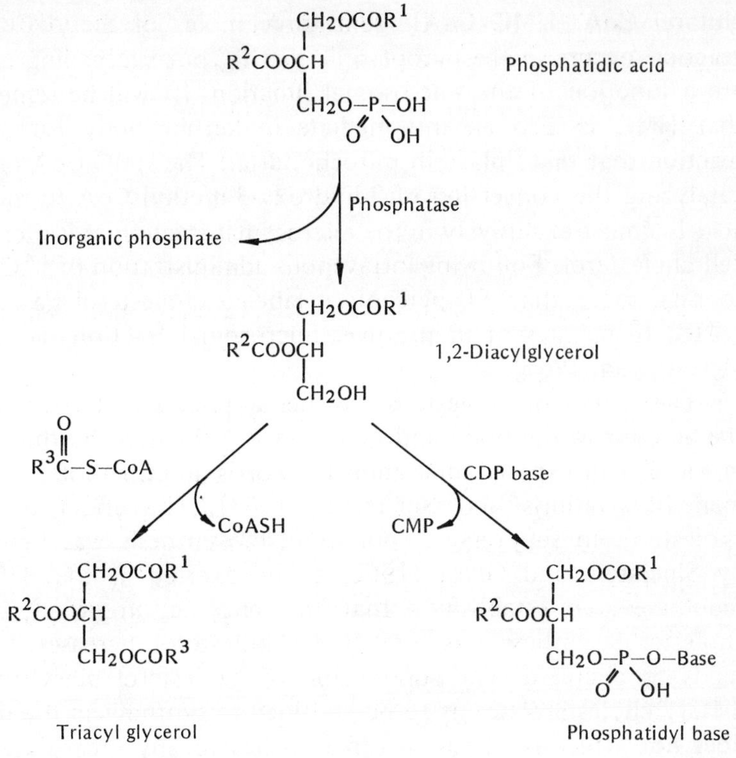

$$CH_2OCOR^1$$
$$R^2COOCH$$
$$CH_2O-P-OH$$
$$O \quad OH$$

Phosphatidic acid

Phosphatase

Inorganic phosphate

$$CH_2OCOR^1$$
$$R^2COOCH$$
$$CH_2OH$$

1,2-Diacylglycerol

$$R^3C-S-CoA$$

CoASH

CDP base

CMP

$$CH_2OCOR^1$$
$$R^2COOCH$$
$$CH_2OCOR^3$$

Triacyl glycerol

$$CH_2OCOR^1$$
$$R^2COOCH$$
$$CH_2O-P-O-Base$$
$$O \quad OH$$

Phosphatidyl base

The liver is also the site of plasma lipoprotein synthesis (with the exception of the chylomicrons which are synthesized in intestinal epithelium). The various fractions of lipoproteins function in the transport of triacylglycerols, phospholipids, and cholesterol esters (see Chapter 6).

Cholesterol Synthesis and Degradation

The liver and intestine are the principal organs of cholesterol synthesis, but synthesis also occurs in other tissues such as adrenals, skin, aorta, and reproductive organs. The liver, however, is the source of plasma cholesterol and is the major site for cholesterol catabolism.

All of the carbon atoms of cholesterol are derived from acetyl CoA. At least 26 steps are known to be involved in the biosynthesis of cholesterol; a gross outline of the major steps is shown in Fig. 15.9. The initial reaction is the formation of 3-hydroxy-3-methyl glutaryl CoA (HMG CoA) from three moles of acetyl CoA. This reaction occurs in the cytoplasmic matrix, but succeeding reactions are a function of the microsomal function. (It will be remembered that HMG is also an intermediate in ketone body formation, a reaction that takes place in mitochondria.) The HMG CoA reductase catalyzing the conversion of 3-hydroxy-3-methyl CoA to mevalonic acid is almost exclusively in the microsomal fraction as is most of the cell cholesterol. Following intravenous administration of ^{14}C acetate to rats, more than 90 percent of labeled cholesterol has been reported to be present in the liver microsomal fraction (Bucher and McGarrahan, 1956).

The extent of cholesterol synthesis appears to be regulated by the amount in the body and therefore is influenced by the quantity in the diet in experimental animals (Morris and Chaikoff, 1959) and man (Bhattathiris and Siperstein, 1963). The effect of dietary cholesterol in suppressing cholesterol biosynthesis was first shown by Siperstein and Guest (1960) to be exerted at the HMG CoA reductase step establishing that this enzyme, in effect, controls cholesterol synthesis. As total body cholesterol increases, synthesis tends to decrease. The suppression of cholesterol biosynthesis by dietary cholesterol seems to be confined to synthesis in the liver and does not affect synthesis in other tissues to any great extent. The effect of suppression of cholesterol biosynthesis on the overall economy of cholesterol metabolism varies with the amount absorbed. When high levels of the sterol are ingested the decrease in synthesis is not sufficient to prevent an increase in the total body pool of cholesterol.

Many other factors have been shown to influence cholesterol biosynthesis in experimental animals (Table 15.1). A high level of fat in the diet increases cholesterol synthesis whereas a low fat diet or fasting decrease cholesterol synthesis. Young animals and females, surprisingly, synthesize more cholesterol than older animals and males (see Bortz, 1973).

The regulation of blood cholesterol level depends not only on the rate of synthesis but also on the rate of degradation and excre-

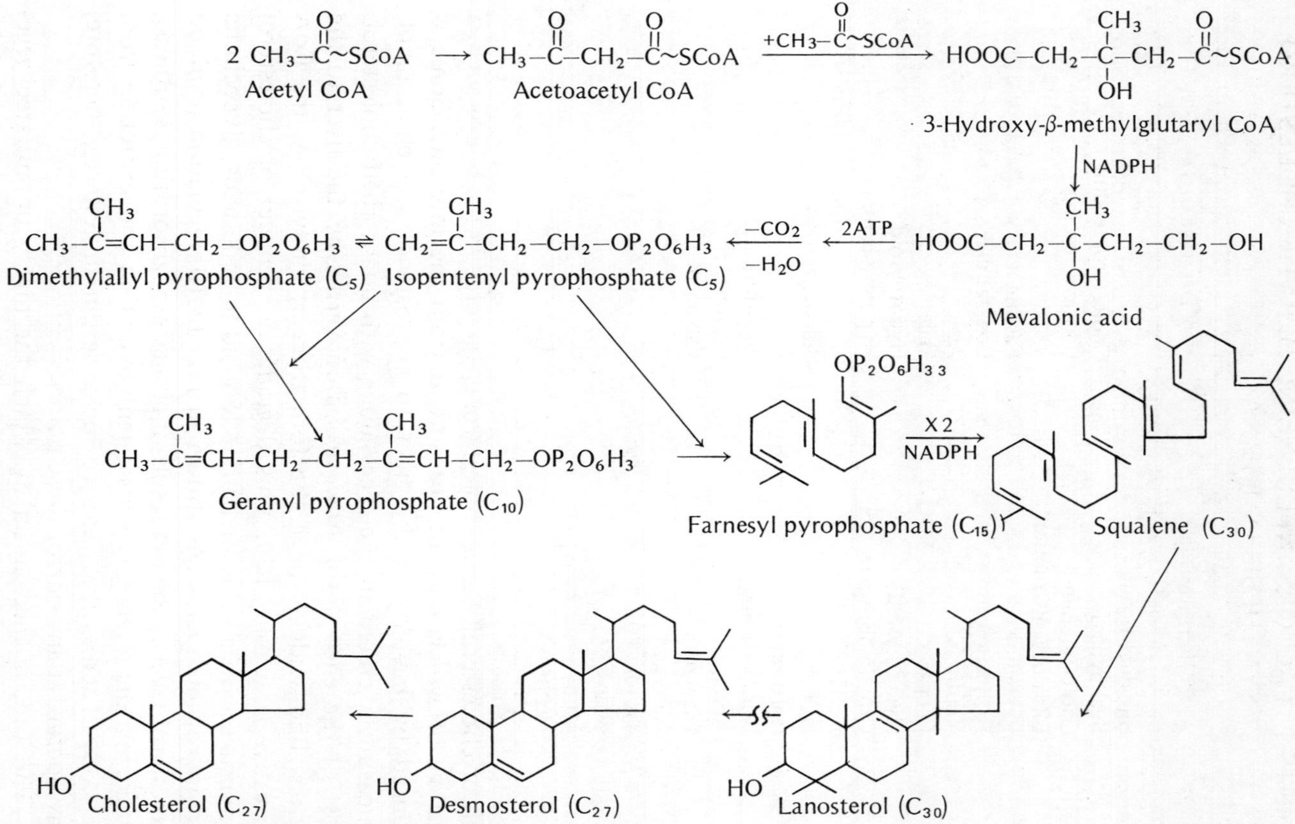

Fig. 15.9 Biosynthesis of cholesterol.

589

Table 15.1   FACTORS INFLUENCING HEPATIC CHOLESTEROL
SYNTHESIS IN THE RAT

Increase	Decrease
Bile duct fistula	
Ileal bypass	Cholesterol feeding
Cholestyramine	Bile acid feeding
Bile duct obstruction	
Refeeding	Fasting
Fat feeding	Low fat diet
Youth	Age
Female	Male
Hyperthyroid	Hypothyroid
Growth hormone	Hypophysectomy
ACTH	
DOCA	Adrenalectomy
Cortisone	
Noradrenaline	Nicotinic acid
Adrenalin	Clofibrate
Diabetes?	Estrogen
Glucagon	
Tiriton	
X-ray	
Stress	
Nephrosis	

tion of cholesterol. Some cholesterol is excreted in the bile as such, a portion of which may be reabsorbed from the intestine. Some is reduced by bacteria in the tract to coprostanol and cholestanol, which are excreted in the feces along with unabsorbed cholesterol. Most of the cholesterol, however, is converted by the liver to the various bile acids through the formation of cholyl CoA, the CoA derivative of cholic acid. This degradation product of cholesterol conjugates with glycine or taurine to yield the bile acids, glycocholic and taurocholic acids. As shown in Fig. 15.10, regulation of blood cholesterol level is the net result of cholesterol absorption, synthesis, uptake by the liver, and subsequent oxidation and excretion from the body. Factors that tend to lower serum cholesterol, therefore, may operate at any one of these points.

The precise mechanism by which the highly unsaturated vegetable oils act in lowering serum cholesterol level is uncertain. An

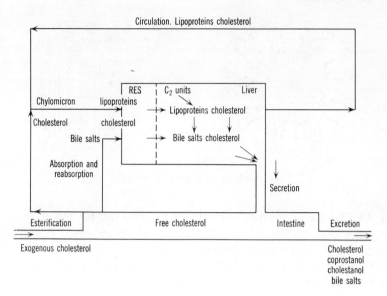

Fig. 15.10   Role of the liver in cholesterol metabolism. (From P. Favarger, "The Liver and Lipid Metabolism" in *The Liver*, Vol. I, Ch. Rouiller, ed., Acad. Press, N. Y., 1963, p. 587.)

inhibitory effect on synthesis does not seem likely, and experiments designed to show an effect on rate of cholesterol degradation are contradictory. Some years ago Okey and Lyman (1957) showed that unsaturated fatty acids increase liver uptake of cholesterol in rats. More recent indirect evidence with humans suggested a similar explanation (Grundy and Ahrens, 1970). The latter group found that neither a decrease in absorption of cholesterol nor an increase in excretion of bile acids occurred with the feeding of unsaturated fat suggesting that unsaturated fat caused a redistribution of cholesterol from plasma to tissue pools. Some workers, however, have reported an increase in bile acid excretion (Connor et al., 1969). A third explanation is unrelated to the unsaturation of vegetable oils but rather to their content of sitosterol and other plant sterols that decrease the absorption of cholesterol (Beveridge et al., 1964). Although a clear cut answer is not yet forthcoming because of the conflicting data reported in the literature, it seems possible that more than one factor may be operating.

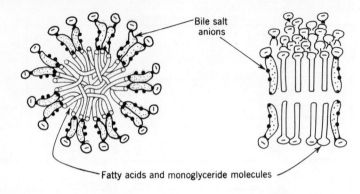

Fig. 15.11 Two proposed models for the bile salt-polar lipid micelle. The aggregate on the left is spherical; that on the right disc-shaped. (From A. F. Hofmann, *Medium Chain Triglycerides,* J. R. Senior, ed., Division of Graduate Medicine, Univeristy of Pennsylvania, 1968, p. 14.)

Bile Acid Synthesis

Bile acids, cholic and chenodeoxycholic acids, are the most important secretory products of the liver cell. These acids are conjugated with amino acids taurine or glycine and appear in the bile as the sodium or potassium salts. Bile acid synthesis is closely tied to the metabolism of cholesterol, its precursor. Through feedback control mechanisms, bile acids inhibit conversion of cholesterol to bile acids. The decrease in bile acids then leads to an increase in liver cholesterol which, in turn, is followed by a decrease in cholesterol synthesis. Beher et al. (1962) have described this as a double feedback mechanism.

Bile salts are of particular importance in the formation of micelles (Fig. 15.11) for the solubilization of lipid and lipid-soluble materials for absorption through the mucosal membrane of the small intestine (see Chapter 6).

Bile Pigment Formation

Another major constituent of bile is the pigment derived from heme breakdown. The chief bile pigment is bilirubin but small quantities of its oxidative derivative biliverdin are also present. Some bilirubin derived from nonhemoglobin heme proteins such as myoglobin, catalase, and cytochromes is degraded in the liver cell. The major portion of the bilirubin is derived from hemoglobin degradation. It is transported to the liver cell associated with serum albumin and conjugated there with glucuronic acid by the endoplasmic reticulum-associated enzyme, glucuronyl transferase, to form bilirubin glucuronide. Inhibition of action of this enzyme or its deficiency leads to hyperbilirubinemia manifested by jaundice. This condition has been found in breast-fed infants of mothers with an inherited defect in steroid metabolism, which leads to interference with glucuronyl transferase activity in the infant. Cases of nonhemolytic jaundice occurring in premature infants often are due to a deficiency of glucuronyl transferase, and in full term neonates may develop because of delayed development of the glucuronide conjugating system in the liver cell. The jaundice that appears in patients with liver disease is usually due to interference with the liver cell's ability to conjugate bilirubin which can be excreted only after conjugation.

CONCLUSION

The appearance of the hepatocyte does not proclaim its exploitation of some specific function as do the specialized cells in the chapters that follow. Its capabilities, nevertheless, are unique; its versatility awesome; its competence unquestioned; yet its design amazingly undistorted. It is, perhaps, the Leonardo of cells, with an innate genius for authoritative expression.

chapter 16

erythrocytes

1. A Cell Renewal System
2. Erythropoietin
   a. Characteristics and Origin
   b. Mechanism of Action
3. Maturation
4. Hemoglobin Synthesis
5. Iron Delivery
6. Globin Synthesis
7. Degradation
8. Conclusion

"Aren't these erythrocytes, as you call them, simply what are known as red blood cells?" he asked, stretching out beside Dr. Streets on the soft, velvety surface.

"Exactly so," was the answer. "In fact, erythros *means 'red' in Greek. The material which gives them that bright red color is known as hemoglobin and is a complicated chemical substance possessing great affinity for oxygen. When the blood stream passes through the lungs, these red blood cells absorb large amounts of oxygen and carry it along to various cell colonies in the body. In fact, although erythrocytes occupy less than fifty percent of the volume of the blood fluid, they can adsorb seventy-five times more oxygen than can possibly be dissolved in the plasma itself."*

"Must be a tricky substance," said Mr. Tompkins thoughtfully.

"So it is," agreed Dr. Streets. "And, as a matter of fact, biochemists have had to work hard to learn its exact composition."

George Gamow and Martynas Yčas,
Mr. Tompkins Inside Himself, 1967, p. 6

Blood is a connective tissue which differs from other types of connective tissue in that its intercellular substance is liquid. It constitutes a sizable mass, comprising one-eleventh to one-twelfth of body weight. Another distinctive feature of this tissue is the extremely rapid turnover of its cellular constituents. It has been estimated that 2.5 million erythrocytes, 20,000 white cells, and 5 million platelets are sent into the circulation *each second* (Bessis, 1961). Since the total number of cells in circulation remains fairly constant, one must assume that the number entering is balanced by an equal number of cells that are withdrawn from circulation. The successful execution of so relentless a task and one of such enormity is dependent upon precise cues, skillful coordination, and conservation of resources.

A CELL RENEWAL SYSTEM

The existence of a cell renewal system depends on the replacement of its relatively short-lived cells by proliferation and differentiation of less specialized precursor cells (Patt and Quastler, 1963). The three main lines of hematopoietic cells—erythroid, granulocytic, and thrombocytic—all arise in the bone marrow. They have certain characteristics in common: most of the cells in any one class are mature and highly differentiated; most of the mature cells have a relatively short life span of days or weeks; and all appear to be "end cells," that is, they cannot proliferate, and in the case òf the erythrocyte and platelet, this is carried to the extreme in that the mature cell even lacks a nucleus. In a cell renewal system such as that present in the epithelium of the intestinal villi, a progression in the renewal can be observed starting with cell generation in the crypt, to increasing maturity as the cell migrates up along the villus, to death in the lumen. In the blood, the mature cells circulate freely and independently with no obvious connections to their immediate ancestors that do not circulate.

It has long been debated as to whether there was one common ancestral cell from which all blood cells stemmed, a so-called pluripotential stem cell giving rise to several specialized lines of development; or whether each cell line has its own stem cell. As so often happens, both suggestions may turn out to be partially true. It appears that when cell lineages are traced back they seem to merge

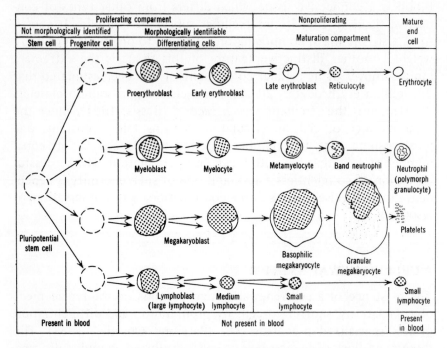

Fig. 16.1 Schematic diagram indicating the nomenclature, morphology and some properties of the various blood cells. (From D. Metcalf and M. A. S. Moore, *Haemopoietic Cells*, North-Holland Publishing Company, Amsterdam, 1971, p. 3.)

at the earliest stage. The *stem cell* has all options open to it. It can undergo a reversible transition from a state of rest to one of division (McCulloch, 1970), and it can serve as the target for control mechanisms to give rise to specific *precursor* or *progenitor cells* (Morse and Stohlman, 1966; Moore and Metcalf, 1970). Such progenitor cells are irreversibly *committed* to develop along a specific line leading to the mature cell at the end of that line (Fig. 16.1). It has been suggested that the bulk of the pluripotential stem cell compartment is in a steady state; that is, when cells are stimulated to differentiate, thereby decreasing the pluripotential stem cell compartment size, the remaining cells undergo mitosis and return the compartment to its original size (Stohlman, 1971). A negative feedback system is implied but no details are known of the feedback relationships between the pluripotential stem cells and the progenitor cell compartments.

The only external regulator of blood cell differentiation identified thus far is erythropoietin, which is responsible for stimulating the differentiation of the committed erythroid stem cell. Similar regulators have been postulated for the other stem lines. In the material that follows, only the line committed to erythropoiesis and responsive to erythropoietin will be discussed.

ERYTHROPOIETIN

The *erythropoiesis-stimulating factor (ESF), erythropoietin,* is a hormone that increases the total number and total volume of red blood cells in the circulation of normal animals. Its existence was postulated and effects attributed to it were demonstrated in 1906 by Carnot and Déflandre who called it *hématopoiétine* (see Fisher, 1968). Almost 50 years elapsed before there was verification of this original work. This was done by exposing one of a pair of parabiotic rats to air with lowered oxygen tension and its partner to normal air (Reissmann, 1950). The stimulation of erythropoiesis in both animals clearly indicated that an hormonal factor was involved. When Erslev (1953) injected an animal with plasma from an anemic animal and found that erythropoiesis was stimulated, the search began in earnest.

Characteristics and Origin

Erythropoietin is a glycoprotein containing sialic acid, galactose, mannose, glucose, and glucosamine. There are at least 17 or 18 amino acids in a single polypeptide chain. Its molecular weight has been established at 45,800 (Lowy, 1970; Keighley and Lowy, 1971; Goldwasser and Kung, 1971).

Plasma was used in the first demonstrations of the existence of erythropoietin. In order to determine its source, plasma erythropoietin was assayed after organ resections and a dramatic fall in erythropoietin levels was found after nephrectomy (Jacobson et al., 1957). Although this evidence strongly suggested that the kidney was the sole source of erythropoietin, it was soon found that some of the hormone could be produced even in the absence of the kidneys (Mirand et al., 1959). However, other sites of synthesis have not been identified. Then Kuratowska et al. (1964) reported that kidney was probably not the source of erythropoietin but of an enzymelike factor that was responsible for converting an erythropoietin precursor in the plasma to erythropoietin. They called this *renal erythropoietic factor (REF)* or *erythrogenin.* Contera and Gordon (1968) suggested that REF might be either an enzyme that acted on a plasma substrate to produce ESF or an ESF precursor that complexed with a plasma carrier to acquire erythropoiesis-stimulating activity. Kuratowska (1968) proposed that the kidney released the labile component, REF, that formed a relatively stable active complex with a-globulin in the plasma. This complex was postulated to be ESF, which circulated and acted on the blood-forming organs and was stored and catabolized in the liver. Since studies with labeled amino acids indicated increased protein synthesis in the liver induced by hypoxia, Katz et al. (1968) hypothesized that during the initial phases of hypoxia the kidney was stimulated to elaborate an activator or enzyme which converted a plasma substrate of liver origin into the active ESF. A model of the biogenesis of ESF proposed by Gordon and Zanjani (1970) is presented in Fig. 16.2, which depicts hypoxia as the fundamental

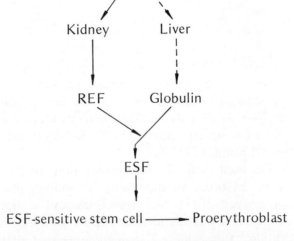

Fig. 16.2 Proposed scheme for renal-hepatic axis involvement in production of ESF. (From A. S. Gordon and E. D. Zanjani, *Regulation of Hematopoiesis,* A. S. Gordon, ed., Vol. I, Appleton-Century-Crofts, N. Y., 1970, p. 413.)

erythropoietic stimulus inducing the kidney to produce additional quantities of REF. They suggest that hypoxia also triggers production and release of additional quantities of the REF protein substrate by the liver. The REF and protein interact in either the kidney, the circulation, or both to produce ESF. The interaction according to these investigators may involve the splitting off of a portion of the protein substrate by the enzymatic action of REF. Such an action may be likened to that of the renin-angiotensin system (see Chapter 7).

The ability of cobalt to stimulate erythropoiesis is mediated through increased ESF production (Goldwasser et al., 1957), but the mechanism remained unclear until recently. Rogers et al. (1972) have shown that cobalt produces a rise in kidney cAMP, which activates REF and is followed by elevation of plasma ESF.

Mechanism of Action

The model of hematopoiesis (Fig. 16.3) suggested by Stohlman (1970a) shows the pluripotential stem cell giving rise to three lines of committed cells. The continuous accumulation of committed stem cells is prevented by the death of some that do not continue to differentiate. A feedback relationship appears to exist since depletion of the committed cell compartment leads to its replenishment from the pluripotential compartment. Although the pluripotential stem cell does not appear to be directly affected by ESF, both the committed stem cells and the differentiated compartment cells are ESF-sensitive.

The specific action of ESF on the committed stem cell appears to be initiation of hemoglobin synthesis. The suggested mechanism is at the nuclear level and perhaps involves derepressing a repressor and thereby permitting the transcription of mRNA for hemoglobin synthesis. In addition, ESF also appears to govern the rate of hemoglobin synthesis. A model (Fig. 16.4) of the kinetics of erythropoiesis suggests that the cytoplasmic concentration of hemoglobin constitutes a negative feedback and terminates RNA synthesis and cell division. Stohlman (1964) suggested that a critical level for hemoglobin concentration in the cell was perhaps about 20 percent. Since the interval between cell divisions appears fixed (Stohlman, 1970b), if nucleic acid synthesis is cut off when a critical level of hemoglobin is reached, then the rate of hemoglobin synthesis be-

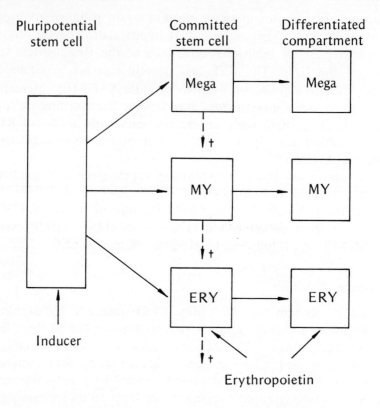

Pluripotential stem cell

Committed stem cell

Differentiated compartment

Fig. 16.3 Schematic model of hematopoiesis. Mega, megakaryocytic; MY, myelocytic; ERY, erythropoietic. Dashed line and cross indicate cell death. (From F. Stohlman, Jr., *Regulation of Hematopoiesis*, A. S. Gordon, ed., Vol. I, Appleton-Century-Crofts, N. Y., 1970, p. 317.

comes the factor determining the number of divisions between differentiation and the final cell division. It follows, therefore, that an accelerated rate of hemoglobin synthesis would cause fewer divisions to take place before the critical level was reached and the cells would be larger; whereas in iron deficiency, rate of hemoglobin synthesis would be decreased, and more divisions could take place before the critical concentration of hemoglobin was attained and microcytic cells would be formed. In the case of iron deficiency anemia, Conrad and Crosby (1962) have shown that microcytosis precedes hypochromia. Support for such a model was provided when the response to varying doses of iron in animals and humans with

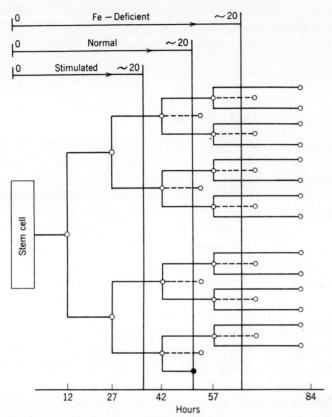

Hemoglobin concentration %

Fig. 16.4 Model of kinetics of erythropoiesis postulates that when hemoglobin concentration of ~20 percent is achieved, further nucleic acid synthesis and division cease. [From Stohlman et al., *Ann. N. Y. Acad. Sci.*, 149: 156 (1968).]

iron deficiency anemia were observed (Stohlman et al., 1963; Leventhal and Stohlman, 1966). When doses were high and iron was no longer rate-limiting, macrocytes were produced; but when doses of iron were low, although restoration to normal hemoglobin was attained, microcytes continued to be produced. If hypoxia is assumed to be the original stimulus to ESF production, then ESF action initiating and controlling the rate of hemoglobin synthesis would produce an increase in red blood cell mass and hemoglobin concentration in circulation. This would increase the oxygen-carrying power of the blood, relieve the hypoxia and act as a feedback mechanism in cutting off the stimulus to ESF production.

For the sake of clarity, the discussions of erythrocyte maturation and hemoglobin synthesis will be presented separately although, in fact, these two processes are inextricably linked and proceed simultaneously.

ERYTHROCYTE MATURATION

The progression of change in the committed stem cell under the influence of ESF leads to the chemical and structural specialization observed in the mature erythrocyte carrying its characteristic load of hemoglobin. The erythroid precursor cells start to proliferate and over a period of 4 to 7 days pass through several identifiable morphological stages, the first of which is the *proerythroblast*, also called *pronormoblast*. After 3 to 4 mitotic divisions, each primitive nucleated cell finally gives rise to 8 or 16 anucleate erythrocytes. The cells first appear in the circulation as *reticulocytes*, and after 1 to 2 days of further maturation become erythrocytes remarkably uniform in size, shape, and life span (See Hillman, 1970).

Although the normal sequence of differentiation, proliferation, and maturation is fairly steady under normal conditions, the time can be speeded up to 3 to 5 days with ESF stimulation. However, the time and maturation schedule is predicated on the presence of an adequate nutrient supply. Limitation of folic acid or vitamin B_{12} interferes with DNA replication and the number of cell divisions during maturation. This leads to fewer but larger and less mature cells, megaloblasts. Limitation of iron, by interfering with the attainment of the critical amount of hemoglobin to curtail cell division, leads to smaller or microcytic cells. With progression of an iron deficiency, synthesis of hemoglobin is further restricted, and the microcytic cells become hypochromic as well. In a cell renewal system of such magnitude any nutrient can interfere with cell proliferation when it becomes the limiting nutrient.

Tracing the earliest changes in development is complicated by the fact that the cells are not recognizably erythroid. Indeed, it has taken both morphological and biochemical sleuthing to discover which cells were destined to become mature erythrocytes. The earliest changes in the progression were presumed to be biochemical, and Krantz and Goldwasser (1965) were able to show that ESF added to an *in vitro* preparation of bone marrow cells produced an increase in RNA synthesis. Then, in an electron microscopic auto-radiographic study, Orlic et al. (1968) were able to identify ESF-sensitive stem cells by their almost immediate incorporation of ^{3}H-thymidine indicating DNA synthesis, and of ^{3}H-uridine indicating RNA synthesis. These cells had numerous ribosomes, sparse endoplasmic reticulum and mitochondria. Nucleoli were seen from 4 to 12 hours after activation, and these remained prominent in the maturation which followed. At 12 to 24 hours the cells developed into proerythroblasts, the earliest recognizable erythroid cell, and into erythroblasts at 48 to 72 hours of maturation, still showing a portion of the original tritium label. Originally in 1 to 4 cells, by 48 hours the radioactive material was diluted into 18 to 36 erythroblasts. The ^{3}H-uridine taken up at 5.5 hours after activation was still present 42 hours later suggesting its incorporation into a stable RNA fraction. Many reticulocytes emerged with the uridine label, and this was consistent with the knowledge that rRNA and mRNA for directing hemoglobin synthesis are stable and that synthesis of hemoglobin continues to occur after nuclear extrusion and reticulocyte maturation are completed. A schematic summary is presented in Fig. 16.5

From this and subsequent data, Orlic (1970) suggested that if ESF was, in fact, a derepressor of genes controlling the production of a specific erythroid substance (Krantz and Goldwasser, 1965), then its action was likely during the replication of DNA in cycling stem cells. Orlic (1970) also suggested, on the basis of ultrastructural observations, that the ribosomes were already present in the cyto-plasm of the stem cells and that the cells need only acquire specific mRNA molecules to begin undergoing erythroid changes. This, he suggested, was in accord with Krantz and Goldwasser's (1965) hypothesis that the primary regulating event in ESF-induced dif-ferentiation of stem cells was synthesis of mRNA coded for hemoglobin.

Well developed nucleoli are observed in the proerythroblasts, and these presumably are responsible for the synthesis of nearly all the erythroid-specifying RNA that is transcribed later during hemoglobin synthesis (Orlic, 1970). As the cells develop, there is nuclear condensation which continues until there are only a few small areas of chromatin material. How the nucleus is finally extruded is

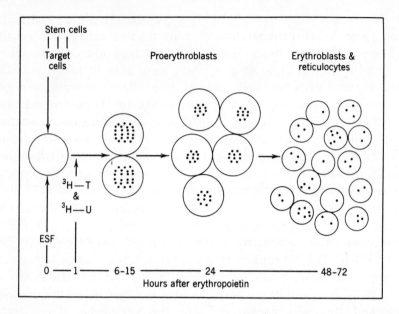

Fig. 16.5 The incorporation of ³H-nucleic acid precusors is represented by black dots (silver grains) over cells of the erythroid series. Both ³H-thymidine and ³H-uridine are incorporated within one hr after administration of erythropoietin, and ³H-uridine uptake continues at 1.5, 3.5, and 5.5 hours. After exposures (three months) erythroblast autoradiograms indicated greatly reduced numbers of silver grains per cell compared with the total found in proerythroblast autoradiograms exposed for shorter times (three to four weeks). This dilution of label appears to occur through cell division. [From D. Orlic et al., *Ann. N. Y. Acad. Sci.*, 149: 198 (1968).]

not well understood. It takes only about 10 minutes, as demonstrated by cinematography (Fig. 16.6), and the extruded nuclei are phagocytosed by macrophages in the marrow (Orlic, 1970). The cells never reach this stage in folic acid or vitamin B_{12} deficiency states.

The reticulocytes usually remain in the marrow for another 1 to 2 days during which time they synthesize additional hemoglobin. After penetrating the vascular lining cells, they enter the blood where, after another 1 to 2 days, they mature into biconcave discs devoid of all organelles but filled instead with hemoglobin. These cells are specialized to perform one major func-

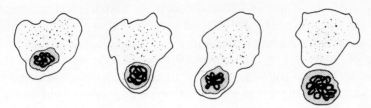

Fig. 16.6 Loss ·of nucleus from erythroblast taken from film sequence. (Redrawn from M. Bessis "The Blood Cells and Their Formation" in *The Cell,* Vol. V, J. Brachet and A. E. Mirsky, eds., Acad. Press, N. Y., 1961, p. 183.)

tion, that of transporting oxygen. The biconcavity increases the surface area and permits more rapid absorption and release of the gases. The loss of all organelles provides optimum space for hemoglobin and makes the cell more efficient per unit volume. The physical structure of the hemoglobin protein and the shape of the cells provide pliability and resiliency and keep them from being prematurely shattered during their frenzied trips through the turbulent vascular system. Defects in hemoglobin protein may be responsible for the excessive fragmentation of erythrocytes as, for example, in sickle cell anemia.

Despite the lack of standard organelle equipment, the mature erythrocyte is far from inert. It is a metabolizing cell that depends on glycolysis for its energy to maintain the high concentration of intracellular potassium and the functional state of reversible deoxygenation in hemoglobin. However, the major function of the erythrocyte requires no expenditure of energy. Both oxygen and carbon dioxide are transported through the plasma membrane by passive diffusion. The mature cell emerges from the bone marrow into the circulation with a supply of lipid, protein, lipoprotein, carbohydrate, ATP, and enzymes in addition to the extremely concentrated solution of hemoglobin, approximately 33 percent, which is just below the point of crystallization. Having lost its capacity for synthetic activity, its stockpile of nutrients and enzymes cannot be replenished. As the cells age, therefore, the complement of enzymes and available ATP decline, and electron-dense material called Heinz bodies which are thought to be aggregations of denatured hemoglobin accumulate. The cells that entered the circulation as trim, biconcave discs, full of energy become old and more spheroidal, worn out, and depleted. After about 120 days they are destroyed. The actual *coup de grace* is not known. It has been suggested that the Heinz bodies can be detected by phagocytes lurking in the spleen and that they pull the old cells out of circulation (Rifkind, 1965); or perhaps the cells merely fall by the wayside due to their senescence and the phagocytes act as the clean-up squad. Probably some cells are lost by fragmentation, hemolysis, or some combination of these.

For more detailed description of the development of erythrocytes, see Bloom and Fawcett (1968); Ham (1969); Metcalf and Moore (1971).

HEMOGLOBIN SYNTHESIS

A single red blood cell contains about 280 million molecules of hemoglobin, each of which has a molecular weight of 64,500. Hemoglobin contains 10,000 atoms, four of which are iron firmly chelated to protoporphyrin. In addition, there are four polypeptide chains arranged as two identical pairs that together contain a total of 574 amino acid units and constitute the globin portion of the hemoglobin molecule (Perutz, 1963; 1964). The protoporphyrin portion of the molecule is a key compound in many types of cells from different species and functions in photosynthesis (chlorophyll), oxygen transport (hemoglobin and myoglobin), and electron transport (cytochromes). The synthesis of protoporphyrin comes about through a series of reactions starting with the ubiquitous succinyl CoA and glycine which condense in the presence of pyridoxal phosphate, the enzyme δ-aminolevulinic acid synthetase (ALA-S) and possibly iron (Brown, 1958), to form δ-aminolevulinic acid (ALA) (Fig. 16.7). This reaction takes place in the mitochondria where succinyl CoA is readily available through the TCA cycle. The condensation of two molecules of ALA yields porphobilinogen and is catalyzed by ALA dehydrase which is located in the cytoplasm. ALA dehydrase depends on free sulfhydryl groups for its activity, as does the enzyme in the final formation of heme from iron and protoporphyrin. The inhibitory effect of lead at these two points in hemoglobin synthesis has been reported (Chisolm, 1971). The inhibition of ferrochelatase activity probably is responsible for the anemia of lead intoxication. Lamola and Yamane (1974) recently reported that in the anemias of both lead intoxication and severe

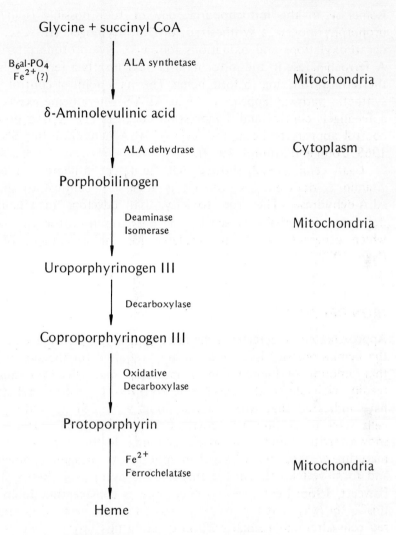

Fig. 16.7 Synthesis of heme.

iron deficiency, Zn^{2+} ions bind to the globin moieties and produce a fluorescent porphyrin. According to these investigators, this provides a simple and specific screening test for lead intoxication.

Recently, vitamin E deficiency, which has been associated with anemia in primates (Dinning and Day, 1957), was shown to produce a decrease in the activity of ALA dehydrase (Nair et al., 1972). From porphobilinogen, under the influence of a deaminase and an isomerase in the mitochondria, one of four possible isomers of uroporphyrinogen is synthesized, uroporphyrinogen III. A series of decarboxylations and oxidations follow to give protoporphyrin IX. A ferrochelatase in the mitochondria next inserts a ferrous ion into the tetrapyrrole ring to form heme. The main point of control in the synthetic pathway appears to be at ALA-S where heme exerts both a feedback control and a repression control. The second point of control appears to be at the level of ALA dehydrase (see Shemin, 1968; Conn and Stumpf, 1972).

Caasi et al. (1972) showed that the defect in heme synthesis in vitamin E deficiency in the rat is at a site identical to that of ALA-dehydrase. The iron toxicity that develops in vitamin E deficiency is perhaps caused by the decrease in protoporphyrin IX which otherwise would be available for the acceptance of iron (Nair, 1972).

IRON DELIVERY

Approximately 1 percent of the red cell mass is replaced each day by the hematopoietic tissue and the iron required for the synthesis of that amount of hemoglobin is about 25 mg. This iron must be readily available to the developing erythron. Ultrastructural studies have indicated that within a few hours after ESF-activation, stem cells start to accumulate ferritin (Orlic et al., 1965). Others have shown ferritin adhering to specialized areas in the glycocalyx of the maturing erythrocyte, which then appeared to invaginate, pinch off, and form vesicles that move through the cytoplasm (Bessis, 1961; Fawcett, 1966; Lentz, 1971). There now is considerable doubt that this is the way that the iron is presented to the mass of developing red cells although a small portion entering this way may be derived from catabolism of some erythrocytes in the marrow. Evidence that ferritin iron is the precursor of heme iron has been challenged. Primosigh and Thomas (1968) found that only a small and relatively fixed portion of iron that enters the cell is ferritin. The immature erythron appears to be able to obtain all the iron it requires for hemoglobin synthesis directly from the circulating iron-transferrin complex (Katz, 1970). Transferrin molecules bind at specific receptor sites on the surface of the immature red cells. The iron is transferred to the interior of the cell and the transferrin is released by the membrane. The site then receives another iron-transferrin complex and the process is repeated (Morgan et al., 1966). The entire process from the initial binding of iron by the cell surface receptors until its incorporation into hemoglobin requires only 6 to 8 minutes (Allen and Jandl, 1960). The iron transfer peaks at the earlier stages of maturation with less taken up by the reticulocyte and none by the mature cell. How this attraction between the cell membrane and transferrin operates is not known, but iron-transferrin has greater affinity for the receptor sites than apotransferrin indicating that the iron plays a part in the "fit." It may also be worthwhile recalling that transferrin is a glycoprotein, and this may endow it with a certain capacity for recognition of and affinity for the specific site on the membrane surface of the developing red cell.

It had long been recognized that copper was involved in some way in iron metabolism. The report of Osaki et al. (1966) established that the oxidase activity of ceruloplasmin, the copper-containing enzyme in the serum, is a controlling element in iron metabolism. In the absence of ceruloplasmin neither the rate of iron entry into the plasma nor its rate of oxidation are sufficient to meet the demands of the developing marrow or other tissues for iron. The presence of unsaturated transferrin (apotransferrin) in the serum is responsible for trapping the ferric ion and incorporating it into the transferring complex. The mechanism postulated for this action is shown in Fig. 16.8 (see also Fig. 5.1).

The release of ferric iron from ferritin apparently depends on a ferritin reductase system since iron must go through the ferrous state to be mobilized only to be reconverted to ferric iron for every step in iron metabolism including storage, transport, biosyntheses, and degradation. A system has been found in liver for the reductive release of iron from ferritin that requires NADH and FMN (Freiden, 1973).

The release of the transferrin iron for the formation of hemoglobin in the developing erythrocytes involves a ferrochelatase, an enzyme that has been found in vertebrate liver and erythrocytes (Frieden, 1973). Iron uptake, however, is not regulated solely by the rate of hemoglobin synthesis since developing cells remove iron from transferrin before hemoglobin synthesis starts. All erythroid cells can synthesize ferritin (Primosigh and Thomas, 1968), and this may occur when the iron is in excess of immediate needs. Myhre (1964) and Noyes et al. (1964) have shown that up to 90 per

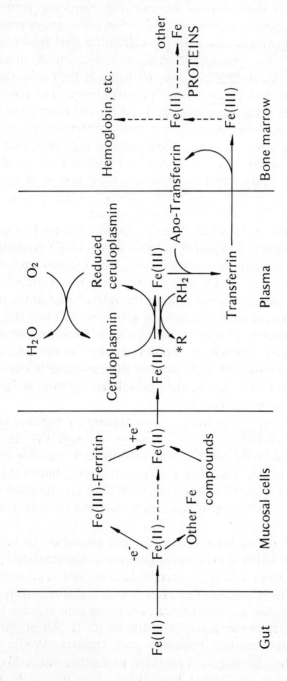

Fig. 16.8 Summary of some of the initial aspects of a prevailing theory of iron metabolism showing the possible role of ceruloplasmin promoting iron utilization. [From S. Osaki et al., *J. Biol. Chem.*, 241: 2746 (1966).]

*RH₂ : Ascorbate, R : Dehydroascorbate

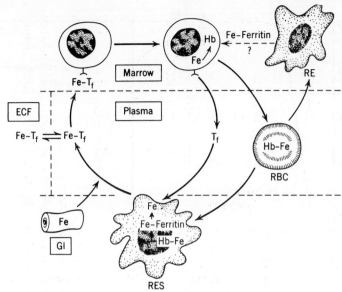

Fig. 16.9 Diagrammatic representation of cyclic mechanisms of iron delivery to bone marrow. Not illustrated is uptake of iron by other tissues of feedback of iron from the so-called labile pool, both of which may involve transferrin binding to membrane receptors. T_f, transferrin; RE, reticuloendothelial cells; RES, reticuloendothelial system; Hb, hemoglobin. [From J. H. Katz, *Ser. Haemat.*, 6: 15 (1965).]

cent of the iron entering the intact marrow is converted into heme within one hour. A diagrammatic representation of the mechanisms of iron delivery to developing red cells in the marrow is shown in Fig. 16.9. For a review of heme synthesis, see Finch (1968); Kaplan (1970).

GLOBIN SYNTHESIS

During development there is a change in the type of hemoglobin chains that are synthesized and this seems to be correlated with the source of the oxygen that the hemoglobin carries. The embryonic hemoglobin, Hb-Gower 1, the more common one, and Hb-Gower 2 circulate during the earliest stages of gestation when the source of oxygen is from maternal interstitial fluid. These chains are replaced by Hb-F by the tenth week of gestation when oxygen uptake is via

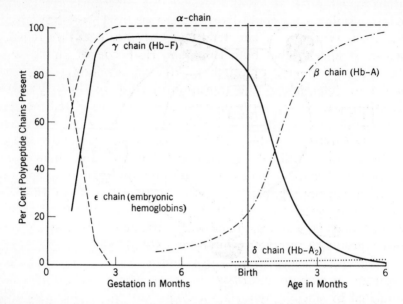

Fig. 16.10 The developmental changes in human hemoglobin chains. (From E. R. Huehns and G. H. Beaven, *The Biochemistry of Development,* P. Benson, ed., J. B. Lippincott, Philadelphia, 1971, p. 175.)

the placenta. From the newborn period onward, oxygen is obtained through the lungs, and Hb-F is replaced by Hb-A during the first six months of life (Fig. 16.10).

Studies on human embryonic hemoglobins are rather limited but Huehns et al. (1964) have shown that the ϵ chain is specific to the embryonic period and Hb-Gower 1 is probably made of four chains; Hb-Gower 2 has a structure of Hb-$a_2\epsilon_2$. The a and ϵ globin chains differ from one another by several amino acid substitutions. The a chains in both fetal and adult type Hb are identical; the non-a chains, γ chains in Hb-F and β chains in Hb-A, are alike in structure and consist of 146 amino acids, 39 of which are different.

The synthesis of each of the polypeptide chains is under separate genetic control, but there is little direct evidence of regulation of hemoglobin synthesis at the genetic level, and characterization of the DNA specifically responsible for the synthesis of globin has not yet been achieved (Bank et al., 1970). It has been suggested that DNA for particular globins might serve as templates for the synthesis of mRNA under different conditions; but the subcellular events that are responsible for the gradual, orderly change from γ chain synthesis to β chain synthesis in late fetal and early postnatal life remains unclear. It appears that both Hb-A and Hb-F coexist in the same cells during the period of switching. Preterm newborn infants were studied to determine if the transition of Hb-F to Hb-A synthesis was influenced by the birth process. The results indicated that the slow transition to Hb-A synthesis accelerates as the preterm infant approaches the thirty-eighth week of postconceptional age. At the postconceptional age corresponding to term, there is no statistical difference between the early preterm-born group and the full term newborn group. The rate of transition from Hb-F to Hb-A appears species-specific, and the switchover is related to the rate of biological maturation and is not affected in man by a precocious exposure to extrauterine life (Bard, 1973).

The persistence of Hb-F or its reappearance in adult life occurs in certain hemolytic disorders. In cases where erythropoiesis is stimulated by anemic hypoxia, Hb-F appears to provide a survival advantage to the erythrocyte containing it; in other cases, this explanation does not hold and no explanation can be offered for reversion to Hb-F (Bertles, 1970).

Comprehension of the logistics involved in the intricate coordination of globin chain synthesis and heme synthesis with the velocity of the maturation schedule of the mass-produced erythrocytes appears at once impossible and intriguing.

DEGRADATION OF ERYTHROCYTES

The 120-day life span of the erythrocytes is exceedingly long compared to that of some of the white blood cells, which may remain in the circulation for only 30 minutes, or the platelets that circulate for three to eight days. One can only be astounded at the magnitude and speed of the hematopoietic activity.

When the erythrocytes are withdrawn from the circulation they are taken up by the reticulum cells in the spleen, liver, and bone marrow and their digestion takes about 5 to 10 minutes (Bessis, 1961). Around the fragments of the phagocytosed red cell, granules of ferritin or larger masses of hemosiderin are visible in electron micrographs. Bessis (1961) suggests that the ferritin observed in the reticulum cells may come directly from phagocytosed red cells or may be the iron carried to the cell by transferrin and stored there as ferritin for use in the synthesis of hemoglobin in the developing cells. More likely, the ferritin iron is released to transferrin and circulated to the marrow for incorporation into the developing erythrocytes. Approximately 90 percent of the iron in new hemoglobin is obtained from such recycling. The appearance in the plasma of catabolized heme iron bound to transferrin is rapid (Garby and Noyes, 1959; Noyes et al., 1960). The protein of the hemoglobin molecule is also released, and these amino acids become part of the amino acid content of the cell. The porphyrin portion of the hemoglobin molecule is degraded by the reticuloendothelial cells of the liver, spleen, and bone marrow. The first step involves opening of the pyrrole ring to form biliverdin, the first of the bile pigments. This is readily reduced to bilirubin by bilirubin reductase (Singleton and Lasker, 1965). The bilirubin circulates in the plasma associated with albumin, and in the liver it conjugates with glucuronic acid catalyzed by glucuronyl transferase. The now water-soluble bilirubin is excreted with the bile into the intestinal lumen. In the colon, bilirubin is released from the glucuronide and undergoes progressive reduction by enzymes derived mostly from the anaerobic flora in the tract and eventually appears in the feces as stercobilin and urobilin (Watson, 1969; Lightner et al., 1969).

Recently a method utilizing measurement of labeled serum bilirubin for the determination of mean red blood cell life span has been reported which can be used clinically. The method also gives information about the capacity of the liver to clear the plasma of bilirubin and thus is useful in diagnosis of liver disease (Berk et al., 1970).

CONCLUSION

A cell renewal system of the magnitude required for the maintenance of the circulating erythrocytes, or one of even greater magnitude such as required for the mucosa of the gastrointestinal tract, can function only if the nutrients supplied to the generating tissues are adequate. Any limiting nutrient will affect the total system. The more fundamental the metabolic role of the nutrient in the cell renewal process, the more severe will be the effect. It becomes apparent why the effects of vitamin B_{12} and folic acid deficiencies are so dramatic in both the gastrointestinal tract and the blood. If the enzymes involved in nucleotide synthesis are blocked, cell division is blocked. If cell division is blocked, there can be no cell renewal.

chapter 17
bone cells

1. Bone as a Connective Tissue
2. Intercellular Substance
   a. Collagen Synthesis
   b. Mucopolysaccharide Synthesis
   c. Mineral Deposit
3. Bone Growth
4. Bone Loss
5. Calcium Homeostasis
   a. Parathyroid Hormone
   b. Thyrocalcitonin
   c. Vitamin D
   d. Interrelationships Among PTH, Thyrocalcitonin, and Vitamin D
6. Vitamin D Toxicity
7. Other Factors Affecting Bone Metabolism
8. Conclusion

"The mineral in the human skeleton is an integral part of a large calcium phosphate cycle which courses throughout the earth's biosphere....Over eons of time the extended leaching of...primary rocks by the earth's waters made calcium and phosphate (as well as other ions) available for mineralogical and/or biological redisposition throughout the world. Thus, the oceans, rivers, and lakes move calcium and phosphate through the earth just as the blood system in man moves these ions in solution to the desired locus of mineral formation."

A. S. Posner, "Bone Mineral on the Molecular Level,"
Fed. Proc., 32: 1933 (1973)

BONE AS A CONNECTIVE TISSUE

Bone, like blood, is a connective tissue, and the intercellular substance is its most distinguishing characteristic. Whereas in blood the intercellular substance is liquid and the tissue itself is composed almost entirely of cells, other connective tissues consist almost entirely of intercellular material and have relatively few cells. The differences between types of connective tissue are due to modifications of the intercellular material that consists of fibers and the amorphous ground substance in between. The fibers are the fibrous proteins, collagen and elastin; the ground substance in which they are embedded is primarily mucopolysaccharide. The interstitial or intercellular substance in bone is impregnated with mineral but, in the case of hyaline cartilage, it is a firm gel. However, bone is not calcified cartilage. Because of the character of the interstitial substance in cartilage, nutrients diffuse through it to the cells; but if calcification occurs, diffusion stops and the cells die. Calcification in bone develops differently. The bone cells are in spaces called lacunae and have access to nutrient supplies through cytoplasmic processes that extend into the canaliculi and, therefore, they are metabolizing cells (Fig. 17.1). These cells are so arranged that they are never more than a fraction of a millimeter from a capillary carrying the blood supply which flows through the bone at an estimated rate of 200 to 400 ml/min.

Bone and other connective tissue cells, like blood cells, develop from a pool of common stem cells that, under appropriate circumstances, can differentiate along different lines. In the material that follows, only those stem cells that differentiate into *osteogenic cells,* also called *preosteoblasts,* will be discussed. Osteogenic cells normally cover and line all bone surfaces, and they are the cells that eventually lead to the production of bone. They develop into *osteoblasts* that secrete organic intercellular substances around themselves and become *osteocytes.* The osteocyte has less cytoplasmic material since it no longer synthesizes and secretes protein and mucopolysaccharide. The calcification of the surrounding organic intercellular material that began when the cell was an osteoblast continues until the matrix is solidly impregnated with mineral.

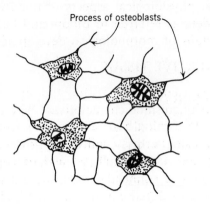

Process of osteoblasts

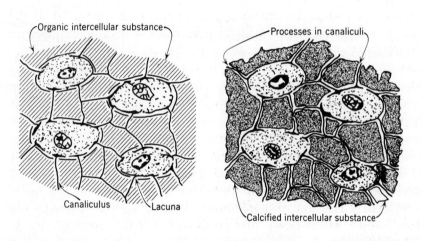

Organic intercellular substance

Processes in canaliculi

Canaliculus Lacuna

Calcified intercellular substance

Fig. 17.1 The osteoblasts secrete the organic intercellular substance of bone both around their cell bodies and around the cytoplasmic arms that extend from the cell bodies. The cytoplasmic arms serve as molds for tiny passageways called canaliculi which remain to provide communication between adjacent osteoblasts and the surface on which the bone is forming. When the osteoblasts are completely surrounded by the intercellular substance they have secreted, they are termed osteocytes. The organic intercellular substance then becomes impregnated with calcium salts. The canaliculi provide a means whereby materials can be transported between surfaces and the cells buried in the calcified intercellular substance. (From A. W. Ham, Histology, 5th ed., J. B. Lippincott Company, Philadelphia, Pa., 1965, p. 389).

618

The nutritional and physiological aspects of bone will be discussed below but the student is referred to Bloom and Fawcett (1968) or Ham (1974) for details of morphological development.

INTERCELLULAR SUBSTANCE

The osteoblasts of developing bone are similar to the fibroblasts of other connective tissues in their ability to synthesize and secrete intercellular substances such as collagen and mucopolysaccharides.

Collagen Synthesis

Collagen, a connective tissue protein, constitutes one-third of the total protein of the body and 57 percent of it is in bone. Collagen differs from most other proteins in that it is fibrous and it contains an unusual assortment of amino acids. One-third of its amino acid content is glycine, which occurs in every third position in the polypeptide chains. It is also rich in proline and lysine (Fig. 17.2). Collagen contains no tryptophan and no cysteine. A biochemical puzzle was revealed when it was reported that labeled hydroxy-proline was not incorporated into collagen and that free proline served as the source of both the proline and hydroxyproline in the molecule (Stetten and Schoenheimer, 1944; Stetten, 1949). Later it was shown that during collagen synthesis the polypeptide rich in proline and lysine was assembled and subsequently hydroxylated to hydroxyproline and hydroxylysine by the enzymes peptidyl proline hydroxylase and peptidyl lysine hydroxylase. Both enzymes are dependent upon molecular oxygen and not water as the source of the hydroxyl molecule (Fujimoto and Tamiya, 1962; Prockop et al., 1963). Other requirements are a-ketoglutarate as co-substrate (Hutton et al., 1967; Rhoads and Udenfriend, 1968), nonheme ferrous iron (Prockop and Juva, 1965; Prockop, 1971), and ascorbic acid (Stone and Meister, 1962). The nonheme iron in the enzyme is loosely bound (Pankalainen and Kivirikko, 1970) and activates the enzyme (Bhatnagar et al., 1972). Ascorbic acid had been considered a reducing agent in the reactions (Hutton et al., 1967), but recent evidence suggests that, in addition, it may be implicated in the conversion of the inactive precursor form of the enzyme to the

$-$ Gly $-$ Pro $-$ _Y_ $-$ Gly $-$ Pro $-$ Hypro $-$ Gly $-$ _X_ $-$ $-$ Gly $-$

(a)

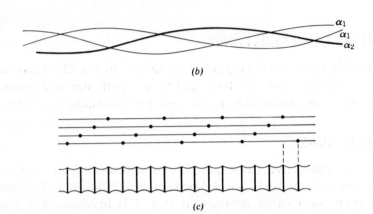

(b)

(c)

Fig. 17.2 (_a_) Typical amino acid sequence in collagen. _X_ and _Y_ are any amino acid other than Gly, Pro, Hypro, Lys, or Hylys. (_b_) Triple helix of tropocollagen showing two α_1-chains and one α_2-chain. (_c_) Staggered alignment of tropocollagen molecules accounting for the periodicity of the collagen fibril.

active enzyme (Stassen et al., 1973). These reactions appear to occur in the endoplasmic reticulum or in the cytoplasmic matrix.

It is assumed that immediately following hydroxylation, and while the chains are still on the polyribosomes, helix formation occurs. The alignment of the three individual chains into helix formation is thought to be aided by a number of extra amino acid sequences at the amino terminals of the procollagen chains. The removal of the amino-terminal extensions by procollagen peptidase (Bornstein et al., 1972) occurs subsequent to the attachment of the carbohydrate moiety, galactose or glucose, by the galactosyl or glucosyl transferases which are in the membranes of the Golgi complex (Weinstock and Leblond, 1974). The glycosylated procollagen in the secretory vacuoles from which the amino-terminal sequences have been removed is _tropocollagen_, which leaves the cell by exocytosis. Miller and Matukas (1974) suggest that the microtubule system in the cell plays a role in guiding the vacuoles to the membrane of the cell for secretion. A summary of the steps in biosynthesis is shown in Fig. 17.3.

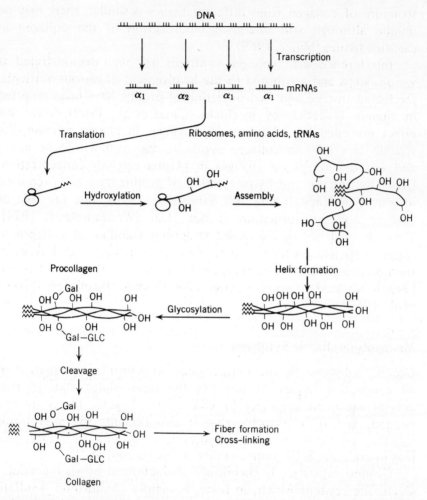

Fig. 17.3 Schematic diagram illustrating the steps involved in biosynthesis of the monomer collagen molecule. [From E. J. Miller and V. J. Matukas, *Fed. Proc.*, 33: 1197 (1974).]

Following extrusion from the cell, there is alignment of the monomers side to side and end to end in a staggered arrangement followed by cross-linking through interchain hydrogen bonds and through covalent bonds between the ranks of the monomers (see Fig. 17.2). Bone collagen is cross-linked rapidly and extensively, and it is suggested that this is a means of stabilizing the tissue prior to and during mineralization (Miller, 1969). Although primary structure of collagen from different tissues is similar, there may be unique although still unknown modification of the collagen in calcified tissues (Miller, 1969).

Interference with collagen synthesis has been demonstrated at various steps and attributed to the involvement of various nutrients. Decreased uptake and hydroxylation of proline have been reported in vitamin D deficiency in chicks (Canas et al., 1969). Since this effect preceded by 12 hours any changes in plasma calcium, the vitamin D effect on collagen synthesis was assumed to be direct and not dependent on changes in plasma calcium concentration. Decreased uptake and hydroxylation of proline have been reported in zinc deficiency (Lema and Sandstead, 1970), but the role of zinc in collagen formation is not clear (Westmoreland, 1971). There is evidence of decreased structural stability of collagen in copper deficiency which is attributed to decreased cross-linkage of the polypeptide chains (Carnes, 1971). Vitamin E deficiency has also been implicated in the defective cross-linking of collagen (Brown et al., 1967).

Mucopolysaccharide Synthesis

Ground substance is the extracellular, interfibrillar component of all connective tissues. It provides the intercellular material that acts as a cement substance in which the collagenic fibrils are embedded, and it is probable that it also cements the microfibrils together to form the fibrils. Synthesis of ground substance, like that of collagen, is the responsibility of the osteoblasts.

Ground substance is chemically characterized by its mucopolysaccharide content which, in bone, is mainly chondroitin 4-sulfate (chondroitin sulfate A), the polymer of glucuronic acid alternating with N-acetyl galactosamine in which the hydroxyl group on carbon 4 is sulfated (see Chapter 2). Synthesis of the mucopolysaccharide component of ground substance takes place in the well developed Golgi apparatus of the osteoblasts (see Ham, p. 394). The Golgi apparatus is also the site where sulfate is added to the carbohydrate (Neutra and Leblond, 1969). As the osteoblasts mature into osteocytes and become embedded in the mineralized matrix, synthetic activity is devoted mainly to maintenance of the bone matrix and is reflected morphologically by less prominent endoplasmic reticulum and Golgi apparatus.

The essentiality of manganese in mucopolysaccharide synthesis was revealed through study of the bone abnormalities in manganese-deficient chicks (Leach and Muenster, 1962; Leach, 1967). Manganese deficiency was found to interfere with the activity of the glycosyltransferase enzymes involved in chondroitin sulfate synthesis (Leach et al., 1969; Leach, 1971). Decreased sulfate uptake has been reported in zinc deficiency in rats (Lema and Sandstead, 1971) and chicks (Neilson and Ziporin, 1969). The poor control of calcification observed in these animals has been attributed to the decrease in sulfate groups in the matrix (Westmoreland, 1971). Alkaline phosphatases are zinc metalloenzymes and these, too, have been implicated in matrix formation (Miller et al., 1965).

Mineral Deposition

The process of calcification begins soon after the organic intercellular matrix is formed by transforming the ions in solution to the crystalline state in the calcifying tissue. By this time the osteoblasts have become osteocytes and lie in the lacunae. Crystal formation begins and progresses until the cell is completely surrounded by the hard bone mineral which is believed to be an hydroxyapatite, the basic formation of which is: $Ca_{10}(PO_4)_6(OH)_2$. The exact chemical composition is not accurately known because of a mixture of transition forms that are present as the bone matures and because of the various substitutions and exchanges of ions that occur in the crystal structure. It is well established that the mineral in bone is precipitated first as an amorphous material which is converted to a crystalline precipitate and then eventually to the final crystal (Eanes et al., 1967; Posner, 1973). In mature compact bone about 40 percent of the total mineral is present in the form of a non-apatite component, and the percentage is higher in young bone. The amorphous phase is lower in Ca/P and, with the addition of calcium as the bone matures, the ratio rises (Posner, 1967). The concept of bone maturation may be clearer if the young crystal is viewed with calcium ions missing at random throughout the crystal structure and maturation as a process of filling in the calcium. It is this process of maturation of the apatite that is disturbed in bones of vitamin D-deficient animals whose bones contain a higher amorphous content than do normal bones of the same age (Muller et al., 1966).

There are three zones in the crystal lattice: crystal interior, crystal surface, and hydration shell, all of which are involved in exchanges of ions. Ions at the interior have the slowest rate of turnover, and this is the site for the sequestration of strontium, radium, and lead for which bone has an affinity. These minerals replace calcium in the crystal lattice. Fluoride produces changes in the bone crystal by replacing the hydroxyl ion. This leads to growth and stabilization of the apatite crystal. Since larger crystals react more slowly than smaller ones, fluoride substitution produces more stable bone mineral (Posner, 1969). There is rapid turnover of ions at the crystal surface, and sodium, magnesium, citrate, and carbonate can be held by adsorption to the surface or by substitution on the surface. The hydration shell of the crystal allows diffusion of all the ions mentioned plus potassium and chloride. With age, the amount of water in bone decreases and the ions of bone salt are less accessible for exchange.

Bone crystals are ultramicroscopic in size and rodlike with a diameter averaging 50 Å. The surface area of the crystal is large in proportion to the mass; a single gram is reported to have a surface area in excess of 100 m^2. On this basis, McLean and Urist (1968) calculate that the total surface area of the bone crystals in the skeleton of a 70 kg man exceeds 100 acres, all of which is bathed by a few liters of bone fluid!

Normally one may view the ions on the surface of the crystals as being in equilibrium with those in the fluid bathing the bone. The entire system is a very dynamic one. However, bone fluid has been shown to differ markedly in composition from general extracellular fluids (Neuman, 1969). This is explained in terms of compartmentalization, presumably by a functional membrane that regulates the flow of cations. Rasmussen et al. (1970) strongly support the view that osteoblasts constitute an effective membrane separating the general extracellular fluids and the bone extracellular fluid. These cells control matrix synthesis and, in addition, regulate the exchange of ions between the general extracellular fluid and those of mineralizing bone collagen.

In addition to the physical process of ion exchange, there are hormonal factors involved in controlling deposition and release of mineral associated with bone metabolism and growth which will be discussed in a later section.

The canaliculi provide the means whereby nutrients and oxygen required by the cell can be transported from the bone surface, where the capillaries are situated, to the cell bodies embedded in the calcified intercellular substance. Such a system is obviously less proficient than one in which the plasma membrane of an individual cell lies in the aqueous nutrient medium. However, the proximity of the osteocytes to the capillary permits the system to operate efficiently.

BONE GROWTH

Most bones of the skeleton exist in embryonic life as cartilage models, and in development and growth the cartilage is gradually replaced by bone due to the activity of invading osteoblasts. The skeleton of a fetus becomes the skeleton of an adult through a series of coordinated processes in which new bone is formed on the preexisting outer bone surfaces and resorbed from the preexisting inner surfaces. These two processes of formation and resorption are balanced so that as new bone is added to the outside of a bone shaft during growth, bone is resorbed from the inner surface of the shaft to make the marrow cavity wider (Fig. 17.4). Resorption includes the processes necessary to put into solution the complicated structure of bone, and its component parts then can enter the circulation. The cells responsible for the resorption process are the *osteoclasts,* large cells often containing 15 to 20 nuclei. Osteo-clasts, like the other bone cells, arise from the stem cells that cover and line bone surfaces, but the multinuclear nature of these cells suggests that they may represent fused osteocytes and osteoblasts. It is not known what causes certain cells to develop into osteocytes whose function it is to build bone, and others from the same group of stem cells to become osteoclasts responsible for bone resorption. The manner in which the osteoclasts participate in bone resorption has not been clarified, but their direct involvement has been demon-strated by time-lapse motion pictures (Hancox and Boothroyd, 1961). According to McLean and Urist (1968) the organic and inorganic constituents of bone are resorbed at the same time. This requires that there be a continuous application to the inner resorbing surface of the bone of a solution that will depolymerize mucopolysaccharides, digest collagen, and hold calcium in solution. This could be accomplished by the combined action of an enzyme such as hyaluronidase, a protease, and a chelating agent all of which

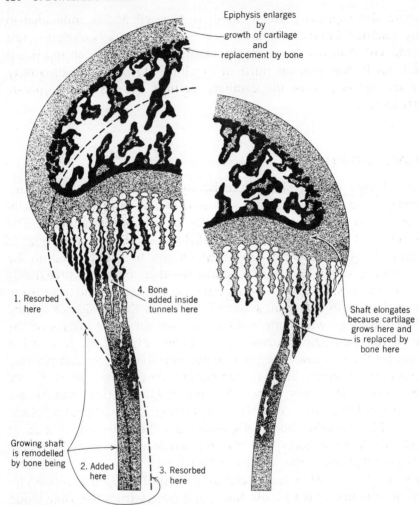

Epiphysis enlarges
by
growth of cartilage
and
replacement by bone

1. Resorbed
here

4. Bone
added inside
tunnels here

Shaft elongates
because cartilage
grows here and
is replaced by
bone here

Growing shaft
is remodelled
by bone being

2. Added
here

3. Resorbed
here

Fig. 17.4 Diagram showing surfaces on which bone is deposited and resorbed to account for the remodeling that takes place at the ends of growing long bones that have flared extremities. [From A. W. Ham, *J. Bone Joint Surg.*, 34-A:701 (1952).]

can function at the pH of body fluids. This forms the basis for a working hypothesis which is not in conflict with known facts but neither are there facts to support it (McLean and Urist, 1968). It will be recalled that involvement of lysosomes has been suggested (see Chapter 14), and there is evidence that lysosomes contain a collagenase, proteases, and organic acids that could help to solubilize bone. Ham (1969) questions the possibility of osteoclasts breaking down collagen when it is encased by mineral and suggests that first osteoclasts create an acid environment beside a bone surface that favors mineral removal. This, then, is followed by enzymatic digestion of the collagen fibrils that remain on the surface of the resorbing bone by lysosomal enzymes liberated by osteoclasts. Mueller et al. (1973) present evidence indicating that osteoclastic bone resorption in laying hens is associated with release of hydrogen ions. They have localized carbonic anhydrase in osteoclasts in physiologically significant quantities and suggest that it may play a major role in bone resorption (Gay and Mueller, 1974). A link for carbonic anhydrase into the web of agents implicated in the maintenance of calcium homeostasis has been provided by Waite (1972). He has shown that bone resorption in rats stimulated by parathyroid secretion is mediated through the activity of carbonic anhydrase which produces carbonic acid.

Although growth in size of bone ceases in the mature individual, bone tissue formation and destruction continue within the framework of the skeleton. The unit of structure of bone is the Haversian system or *osteon*. When fully formed, this is a thick-walled cylindrical branching structure with a narrow lumen carrying one or several capillaries or venules. The osteons are usually oriented along the long axis of a bone and the walls consist of concentric layers of *lamellae* containing large numbers of lacunae in which are found the osteocytes. The interconnections among the osteocytes, the canaliculi, and lumen of the osteon canal provide the circulatory system of the hard tissue and the means by which nutrients in the blood are transported to the bone cells (Fig. 17.5). For a more detailed discussion of bone structure, formation, and growth, see Ham (1969), McLean and Urist (1968).

When skeletal mass is increasing, bone formation predominates over resorption, whereas in old age resorption may predominate. In the normal adult, formation and resorption tend to balance each other. The overall balance between the formation of bone and its resorption is reflected in the difference between calcium intake and calcium excretion, provided the extraskeletal calcium content of the body does not change. Since the body does not normally tolerate large changes in the extraskeletal calcium, which accounts

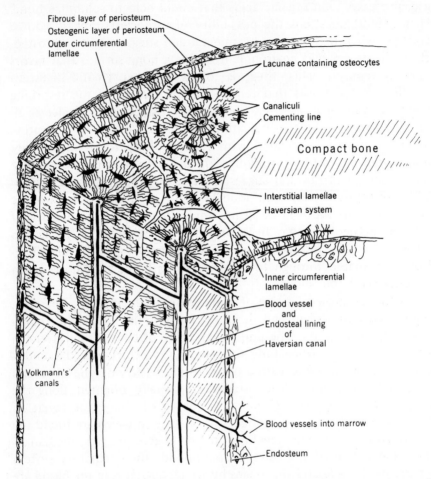

Fibrous layer of periosteum
Osteogenic layer of periosteum
Outer circumferential
lamellae

Lacunae containing osteocytes

Canaliculi
Cementing line

Compact bone

Interstitial lamellae
Haversian system

Inner circumferential
lamellae

Blood vessel
and
Endosteal lining
of
Haversian canal

Volkmann's
canals

Blood vessels into marrow

Endosteum

Fig. 17.5 A three-dimensional diagram showing the appearance of both a cross and a longitudinal section of the various components that enter into the structure of the cortex of the shaft of a long bone. (From A. W. Ham, *Histology*, 5th ed., J. B. Lippincott Company, Phila., Pa., 1965, p. 431.)

for approximately 1 percent of total body calcium, the calcium balance is usually positive when bone formation dominates, negative when resorption dominates, and equilibrium exists when formation and resorption balance. Calcium balance, then, is an indication *solely* of the relationship between the rates of formation and resorption of bone and in no way indicates the level of metabolic activity.

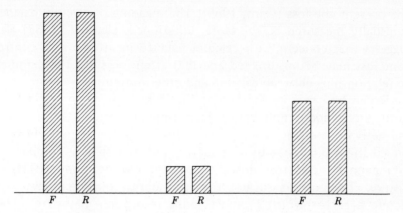

Fig. 17.6 A simple illustration of three levels of calcium balance. In each case bone formation (F) and resorption (R) proceed at equal rates and the calcium balance is zero; metabolic activity, however, is vastly different. (From G. C. H. Bauer, A. Carlsson, and B. Lindquist, "Metabolism and Homeostatic Function of Bone" in *Mineral Metabolism*, Vol. I, Part B, C. F. Comar and F. Bronner, eds., 1961, p. 617.)

The simple illustration from Bauer et al. (1961) in Fig. 17.6 clearly shows that bone formation and resorption may proceed at equal rates under conditions of widely different metabolic activity. In each instance calcium equilibrium is attained, but calcium balance, as nitrogen balance, can be attained at many different levels of intake (see Chapter 23).

BONE LOSS

Adult bone loss is a general phenomonon beginning at the fifth decade and progressing twice as fast in the female as in the male (Garn, 1967). Certain factors, such as small stature, hasten bone loss whereas less bone loss occurs in taller individuals. A larger skeletal mass attained by the fourth decade has been associated with slower evidence of bone loss in later life. At present, there is no satisfactory evidence to show that bone loss is due to low calcium intakes or that protection is afforded by high intakes. It is estimated that adult women lose approximately 30 mg of calcium per day or 900 mg per month, and intakes of even 1000 to 1500 mg/day do not prevent the loss (Garn, 1969). The meaning of calcium balance as usually measured is, therefore, questioned. Hegsted (1967) also suggests that concern with calcium balance in attempts to control bone loss may be misdirected and that attention should be centered on relationships between calcium and other nutrients.

Recently a soluble factor was found in supernatant fluid from cultures of blood lymphocytes which stimulates osteoclast formation and activity (Horton et al., 1972). This factor has tentatively been named the osteoclast-activating factor, and its activity is comparable to maximally effective doses of parathyroid hormone (PTH) in culture. The authors suggest that the ability of lymphocytes to secrete a factor which promotes bone resorption may play a role in the pathogenesis of bone loss near areas of chronic inflammation such as might occur in rheumatoid arthritis or periodontal disease.

The one most significant relationship discovered to date in preventing bone loss is fluoride consumption. Relatively high levels of fluoride intake have been associated with substantial reductions in osteoporosis in women (Bernstein et al., 1966). Gaster et al. (1967) have shown that fluoride increases bone crystallinity and decreases bone mobility. The mechanism of the fluoride action postulated by Rich (1969) is that fluoride which is absorbed is concentrated into bone crystals of newly formed bone at bone surfaces and along borders of osteocyte lacunae and canaliculi. The concentration of fluoride in extracellular fluid surrounding the osteocytes is low when bone is not being resorbed and high during bone resorption. High fluoride inhibits bone resorption because of its toxicity to the cells, and this inhibition leads to a compensatory increase in PTH just sufficient to maintain plasma calcium within normal range. There is evidence that fluoride stimulates osteoblastic differentiation within a few weeks of its administration (Reutter et al., 1969). Osteoblasts engaged in matrix production are less affected by fluoride in crystals at the surfaces of bone. Only when concentration of fluoride in extracellular fluid rises to a toxic level would osteoblastic function be altered. Therefore, bone formation proceeds and bone resorption is inhibited. For an extensive review of the role of fluoride in bone structure, see Gedalia and Zipkin (1973).

CALCIUM HOMEOSTASIS

Calcium in the blood and extracellular fluid is probably the best regulated ion in the body (Copp, 1960). About 65 percent of the calcium in normal plasma is present in the ionized form (Neuman and Neuman, 1958) and most of the remainder is protein bound. A third form—diffusable, nonionized calcium—is present only to the extent of 0.5 to 1 mg/100 ml. It is the ionized calcium concentration which controls and is controlled by the parathyroid secretion. This is the fraction involved in all aspects of calcium metabolism including muscle contraction (Imai and Takeda, 1967), nerve excitation (Koketsu and Miyamoto, 1961), and maintenance of the integrity of cell membranes (Streffer and Williamson, 1965). The constancy of blood calcium is maintained by absorption of calcium from the intestinal tract or that released by bone, counterbalanced by that deposited in the bone and excreted in the urine and feces. Maintenance of blood levels appears to depend on the integrated action of PTH, vitamin D, and thyrocalcitonin. The action of each of these will be discussed separately before an attempt is made to clarify their interrelationships.

Parathyroid Hormone

Parathyroid hormone (PTH) is a single chain polypeptide containing 84 amino acid residues and having a molecular weight of 8500. The complete amino acid sequence of bovine PTH was reported independently by two groups (Niall et al., 1970; Brewer and Ronan, 1970) and is shown in Fig. 17.7. A synthetic peptide consisting of the first 34 amino acids from the amino terminus in the naturally occurring hormone was shown to have biologic effects identical to those of the natural hormone (Potts et al., 1971).

The primary action of PTH has been debated for many years. Collip and his coworkers at Montreal suggested that the primary action of the hormone on the bone led to the release of calcium and phosphorus and this, in turn, led to the increased urinary excretion of these ions (Collip et al., 1934). The group at Harvard held that the primary action was on the kidney causing the increased excretion of phosphate which, by lowering of plasma phosphate, led to increased bone resorption (Albright and Reifenstein, 1948). The debate has continued with MacIntyre (1970) lending support to the primacy of bone action, and suggesting that the action occurred under the aegis of cAMP. The kidney as the principal target of PTH action received the support of Nordin and Peacock (1970) who suggested

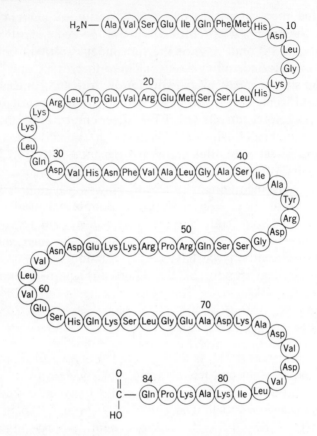

Fig. 17.7 Structure of parathyroid hormone: a linear polypeptide of 84 amino acids. The physiologic activities of the peptide on both skeletal and renal tissues are contained within the 34 amino acids counting from the amino terminal end of the molecule. (From H. A. Harper, *Review of Physiological Chemistry*, Lange Medical Publishers Los Altos, Cal., 1971, p. 423.)

the action led to tubular calcium reabsorption. Fourman and Royer (1968) and McLean and Urist (1968) diplomatically state that the bone and renal actions are independent effects of the same hormone directed toward elevating plasma calcium concentrations without a concomitant elevation of plasma phosphate. The action of PTH on kidney (Chase and Aurbach, 1968) and bone (Chase et al., 1969) have both been associated with the accumulation of cAMP. The investigations of this group (Aurbach and Chase, 1970; Aurbach et al., 1971) led them to suggest that the activation of adenyl cyclase constitutes the true primary action of PTH. In each of the target tissues the hormone binds to specific sites on the plasma membrane and then stimulates adenyl cyclase which is either an integral part of the binding site or next to it. The cAMP formed intracellularly activates specific processes within each tissue that account for the diverse physiological effects of PTH. The controversy that has existed from the early days of PTH research appears settled with cAMP as the arbiter, and both sides were right.

The activity of the parathyroid glands is directly related to the calcium ion concentration in the plasma to which it responds. The level of PTH secretion plays a decisive role in the homeostatic regulation of plasma calcium. By means of a system of negative feedback, the plasma calcium activates the regulatory mechanism: a shift toward hypocalcemia stimulates PTH secretion, which mobilizes calcium ions and elevates the plasma level; this, in turn, cuts off the stimulating effect. Such control regularly maintains the plasma level at approximately 10 mg/100 ml by stimulating osteoclastic activity and releasing calcium from stable bone mineral. This relatively slow action is responsible for the hour-to-hour and day-to-day adjustments, but the constancy of the plasma calcium level is maintained despite extremely rapid movement of calcium ions in and out of the blood. It has been estimated that one out of every four ions leaves the blood of adult man every minute, and in a young animal there may be a 100 percent exchange every minute (McLean and Budy, 1961). Rasmussen et al. (1970) suggest that the minute-to-minute plasma calcium regulation depends on the osteocytes that form functional units of bone and that are vitally concerned with calcium homeostasis. The osteocytes, according to these investigators, form a functional syncytium of membranes covering the bone surface and separate the general extracellular fluid and bone extracellular fluid. This concept is elaborated further by the presentation of a model (Fig. 17.8) that indicates regulation of calcium exchange through a membrane between a specialized compartment of the extracellular fluids (gastrointestinal fluids, bone extracellular fluid, and glomerular filtrate) and general extracellular fluids. In this view the osteoclasts are conceived as being primarily involved in skeletal homeostasis or bone remodeling, and only secondarily involved in mineral homeostasis. They become important in mineral homeostasis only in abnormal situations such as hyperparathyroidism.

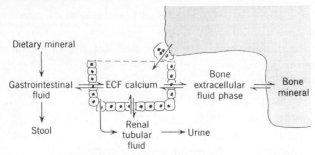

Fig. 17.8 Schematic representation of the regulation of blood and extracellular fluid calcium. Calcium homeostasis is achieved by regulating calcium exchange between the bulk extracellular fluids, and three specialized extracellular fluids (ECF): (1) gastrointestinal fluids, (2) renal tubular fluid, and (3) bone extracellular fluids. In addition osteoclastic reabsorption contributes directly to the bulk extracellular fluids. In the case of both intestine and kidney, an epithelial membrane separates the special compartment from the bulk ECF, but in the case of bone the membrane is a syncytium of mesenchymal cells consisting primarily of resting osteoblasts and osteocytes, and so the present scheme is a highly stylized representation of the situation of bone. [From Rasmussen et al., *Fed. Proc.*, 29: 1190 (1970).]

McLean and Urist (1968) have introduced the concept of a dual mechanism of control to account for the rapid calcium turnover in both directions between plasma and bone (Fig. 17.9). The slow acting part of the mechanism is mediated by the parathyroid glands and depends on their control of osteoclastic activity. When plasma calcium falls below 10 mg/100 ml, the parathyroids are stimulated and calcium is released from the stable hydroxyapatite crystals of bone. This is a feedback mechanism and, therefore, self-regulatory. If the parathyroid glands are removed, plasma calcium concentration falls to approximately 7 mg/100 ml but is then maintained at that level by the other part of the dual mechanism which is independent of the parathyroids. This part of the action is rapid and maintains an equilibrium between the labile or reactive bone mineral and the ions in the surrounding bone fluid. If calcium is removed from the blood, calcium ions are transferred from the surrounding bone fluid to the blood to restore the level. Calcium ions will then move from the labile bone mineral to the surrounding bone fluid to reestablish equilibrium. In contrast, addition of calcium to the blood leads to

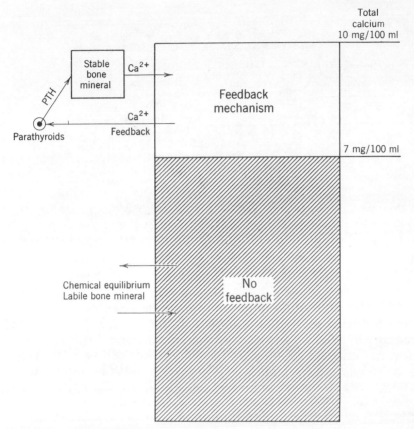

Fig. 17.9 Diagram to illustrate mechanism of exchange of calcium between blood plasma and bones. Chemical equilibrium with labile fraction of bone mineral is independent of parathyroid glands and is adequate to maintain plasma calcium level at 7 mg/100 ml. Parathyroid activity is under control of feedback from Ca^{2+} concentration in plasma and regulates release of calcium from stable hydroxyapatite crystals of bone mineral. This results in maintenance of plasma calcium at normal level of 10 mg/100 ml. (From McLean and Urist, *Bone: an Introduction to the Physiology of Skeletal Tissue*, University of Chicago Press, Chicago, 3rd ed., 1968, p. 143.)

transfer of calcium ions to the labile stores. The dual mechanism postulated by McLean and Urist effects calcium transfer by ion exchange from the labile fraction of bone and by bone resorption from the stable hydroxyapatite crystals of bone. For reviews of PTH action, see Potts et al. (1971); Aurbach et al. (1972).

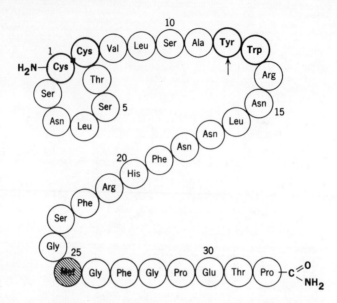

Fig. 17.10 Schematic representation of the covalent structure of porcine calcitonin. Residues important for biological activity are indicated in boldface and heavy circles. Methionine (shaded), residue 25, is not essential for biological activity. (From Potts, J. T., Jr., et al. in *Parathyroid Hormone and Thyrocalcitonin (Calcitonin)*, R. V. Talmage and L. F. Belanger, eds., Amsterdam: Excerpta Medica Foundation, 1968, p. 54.)

Thyrocalcitonin

A hypocalcemic factor released by the thyroid and parathyroid glands of dogs perfused with blood high in calcium was demonstrated by Copp et al. (1962). They postulated that the effect was due to a hormone released by the parathyroids that they named *calcitonin*. Others (Hirsch et al., 1963; Foster et al., 1964) attributed hypocalcemic activity to a hormone released by the thyroid gland and called it *thyrocalcitonin*. Although both names are used, the polypeptide hormone secreted by the C-cells of the mammalian thyroid is generally called thyrocalcitonin and that from the ultimobranchial glands of lower vertebrates is referred to as calcitonin.

The calcitonins of various species are polypeptides containing 32 amino acids. The complete amino acid sequence (Fig. 17.10) was determined independently by several groups (Potts et al., 1968;

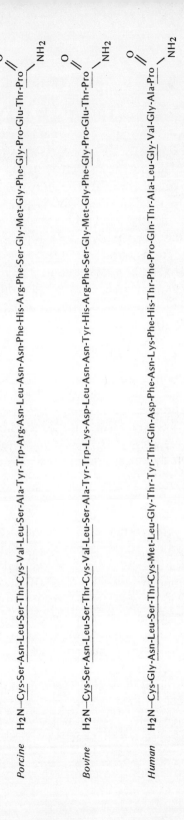

Fig. 17.11 Amino acid sequence of porcine, bovine, human, and salmon calcitonin. [From J. T. Potts, Jr., *Fed. Proc.,* 29: 1200 (1970).]

Neher et al., 1968; Bell et al., 1968). There is an homology in only a portion of the amino terminus among the calcitonins from different species (Fig. 17.11). Only 18 of the 32 amino acids in the human hormone correspond to the porcine hormone. However, in each instance the whole molecule appears to be necessary for biological activity. An unexpectedly high potency calcitonin has been found in the salmon (Guttmann et al., 1970). Despite having 16 of the amino acids different from the human hormone, it is particularly potent when assayed in comparison to other calcitonins. The potency of salmon calcitonin has been related to a longer half-life *in vivo* and resistance to degradation by plasma and tissue extracts (Habener et al., 1972; DeLuise et al., 1972). Marx et al. (1972), however, have presented additional evidence that salmon calcitonin has high affinity for specific tissue receptors in kidney and bone and that this is important in contributing to its potency.

Thyrocalcitonin acts as a physiological antagonist to parathyroid hormone. The concentration of thyrocalcitonin is directly proportional to plasma calcium concentration whereas PTH is inversely proportional. These relationships are shown in Fig. 17.12. The rates of secretion of these two hormones are controlled by plasma calcium in a direct feedback mechanism (Potts, 1970). The response of the thyroid gland to very small increments in plasma calcium by releasing thyrocalcitonin to the circulation protects against hypercalcemia. The rise in plasma calcium due to intestinal absorption is postulated to stimulate the release of thyrocalcitonin which, by inhibiting calcium resorption from bone, reduces the plasma calcium toward normal. This response to absorption would conserve calcium by diminishing calcium loss from the plasma through the urine and preventing resorption of skeletal calcium (Gray and Munson, 1969). Munson and Gray (1970) suggest that this is the physiological mechanism protecting against hypercalcemia during calcium absorption from the intestinal tract. The presence of calcium in the gastrointestinal tract was postulated to cause the secretion of a gastrointestinal hormone which, in turn, signals the thyroid gland to secrete thyrocalcitonin (Cooper et al., 1971). Using pentagastrin, a synthetic pentapeptide containing the biologically active portion of the hormone gastrin, a marked, rapid, and transitory increase in thyrocalcitonin secretion was observed in the pig (Cooper et al., 1971). It was suggested that gastrin or a related gastrointestinal

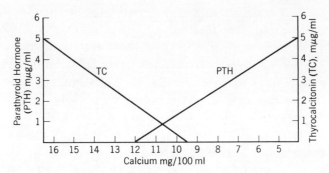

Fig. 17.12 Effects of changes in serum calcium on the concentration of parathyroid hormone and thyrocalcitonin in peripheral blood. The concentration of thyrocalcitonin is directly proportional to calcium concentration; the concentration of parathyroid hormone is inversely proportional to calcium concentration. [From Potts, J. T., Jr., *Ann. Intern. Med.*, 70: 1251 (1969).]

hormone, in concert with plasma calcium concentration, may be important in the physiological regulation of thyrocalcitonin secretion. There is circumstantial evidence that the secretion of thyrocalcitonin is increased by activation of adenyl cyclase in the C-cells (Care et al., 1971). How this activation might operate is not clear, but the suggestion is presented that cAMP can increase the permeability of cell membranes to calcium ions and thus increase the intracellular concentration of calcium. This might then cause a release of thyrocalcitonin stored as granules within the C-cells.

The thyrocalcitonin-produced hypocalcemia appears to result from the inhibition of bone resorption. It has been suggested that this action may be due to the action of cAMP in bone (Aurbach et al., 1971). Rasmussen et al. (1970) indicate their belief that the effect of thyrocalcitonin on bone cells is directly on cellular calcium exchange, either by decreasing the entry of calcium into the cell or by enhancing the rate of calcium efflux by increased activity of calcium-activated ATPase.

For reviews of thyrocalcitonin action, see Potts (1970), Potts et al. (1970).

Vitamin D

The effect of vitamin D on absorption of calcium from the small intestine is well established, and the postulated mechanism of action has been presented (see Chapter 6). Vitamin D also has a direct effect on the bone and, in the absence of vitamin D, bone resorption is impaired and plasma calcium levels fall (Rasmussen et al., 1963). It was found that vitamin D_3 did not stimulate bone resorption in culture but that 25-hydroxycholecalciferol (25(OH)D_3) was effective (Blunt et al., 1968). This led to the work that demonstrated kidney involvement in vitamin D_3 hydroxylation to 25(OH)D_3 and the greater activity following a second hydroxylation. The active metabolite of vitamin D_3 was identified as the dihydroxylated form synthesized in the kidney, 1,25-dihydroxycholecalciferol (1,25-(OH)$_2 D_3$); soon to be nudged aside by a second dihydroxy derivative also produced in the kidney, 24,25(OH)$_2 D_3$. It now appears that both dihydroxy forms share the responsibility for vitamin D_3 activity in bone, and the conditions that lead to the increased production of one lead to the decreased production of the other. According to work from DeLuca's laboratory (Holick et al., 1972) 1,25(OH)$_2$-D_3 is the predominant form produced by the kidney when plasma calcium is low; and 24,25(OH)$_2 D_3$ when plasma calcium is normal or high.

The role of inorganic phosphorus, long implicated in the functional relationship between vitamin D and calcium is now being elucidated. Data presented by Tanaka and DeLuca (1973) suggest that inorganic phosphorus regulates whether the second hydroxylation in the kidney is at the 1- or 24-position. They showed in work with rats that when the level of serum inorganic phosphorus is greater than 8 mg/100 ml the production of 24,25(OH)$_2 D_3$ is favored; when the level is less than 8 mg/100 ml, 1,25(OH)$_2 D_3$ is formed. Holick et al. (1972) had previously found that the 1,25-dihydroxy form predominated in hypocalcemia and the 24,25-dihydroxy form in normo- or hypercalcemia. Popovtzer et al. (1974) observed that 25 (OH)D_3 enhanced the tubular absorption of phosphorus in rats only in the presence of PTH. This PTH-dependent action, however, was unrelated to the formation of 1,25(OH)$_2 D_3$ since the latter failed to effect tubular reabsorption of phosphorus in parathyroidectomized rats. These reports are beginning to explain observations made half a century earlier, soon after the discovery of vitamin D, that both low calcium and high phosphorus diets contribute to the development of rickets.

The depressing effects of certain minerals on bone mineralization, for example cadmium, appears to be due to interference with the synthesis of $1,25(OH)_2D_3$ by the kidney (Feldman and Cousins, 1973).

In addition to the physiologic effect of vitamin D_3 on bone resorption, Canas et al. (1969) observed an increased incorporation of ^{3}H-proline into the ^{3}H-hydroxyproline fraction of rachitic chicks after vitamin D_3 treatment. Since the effect on proline incorporation preceded changes in serum calcium by 12 hours, these investigators concluded that vitamin D has a direct effect on collagen synthesis and that it is not secondary to changes in plasma calcium concentration. A related observation after vitamin D treatment to osteomalacic patients was increased urinary excretion of hydroxyproline which also was interpreted as an indication of a direct effect of vitamin D on collagen metabolism (Smith and Dick, 1968). Whether these findings are directly related to the monohydroxylated form of vitamin D_3, or to one or both of the dihydroxylated forms, is not known.

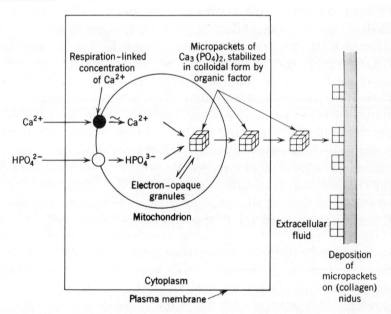

Fig. 17.13 Working hypothesis for the role of mitochondria in biological calcification. [From A. L. Lehninger, *Biochem. J.*, 119: 129 (1970).]

Additional evidence for an effect of vitamin D on bone growth is the pattern of intramitochondrial granules in chondrocytes. In normal rats a gradient of distribution was observed along the epiphyseal plate that is the area of active bone growth; whereas in vitamin D-deficient rats, the granules were mostly in the area of provisional calcification. The normal growth pattern was assumed when vitamin D was added to the diet (Matthews et al., 1970). Evidence supporting the concept that tiny packets of tricalcium phosphate collect in the mitochondria of bone cells before transference to the calcifying site (Fig. 17.13) has been summarized by Lehninger (1970). Granules containing calcium phosphate have been identified in bone cells by Hirschman and Nichols (1970). For a review of the regulation of vitamin D metabolism and function, see Wasserman and Corradino (1971); Omdahl and DeLuca (1973); Kodicek (1974).

Interrelationships among PTH, Thyrocalcitonin, and Vitamin D

The tight control on the plasma calcium and phosphate levels and, therefore, on the metabolism of bone cells, depends on the interaction of PTH, thyrocalcitonin, and vitamin D. The responsiveness of parathyroids and of the C-cells of the thyroid to the level of plasma calcium brings about a precise minute-to-minute regulation of plasma calcium concentration. This control depends on the ability of PTH to mobilize calcium from bone when plasma calcium falls below 10 mg/100 ml and on the inhibition of bone mobilization by thyrocalcitonin when plasma calcium rises above this level. The presence of vitamin D is required for the bone mobilization effect of PTH and, conversely, the presence of PTH is required for the physiologic action of vitamin D in bone mobilization. The amount of vitamin D required for PTH action is very small, and the effect of the two together appears to be synergistic in stimulating bone resorption, that is, the response to vitamin D_3 and PTH together is effective at levels at which neither of them could be effective alone. The reason becomes clear with the knowledge that PTH stimulates the activity of the kidney enzyme responsible for the conversion of $25(OH)D_3$ to $1,25(OH)_2 D_3$ (Rasmussen et al., 1972; Garabedian et al., 1972).

In contrast, the action of thyrocalcitonin does not require vitamin D_3, and thyrocalcitonin can reduce bone mobilization both in vitamin D deficiency and in PTH deficiency. Furthermore, thyrocalcitonin inhibits formation of $1,25(OH)_2 D_3$ in the kidney, and its secretion is stimulated by conditions for which PTH is not required—that is, hypercalcemia and hypophosphatemia—both of which favor the synthesis of $24,25(OH)_2 D_3$. Thyrocalcitonin can decrease bone mobilization induced by either vitamin D_3 or by PTH and, in addition, depress bone mobilization even when both these factors are absent.

In a vitamin D_3 deficiency, that part of the reduction in bone mobilization produced by thyrocalcitonin can be prevented by PTH (Morii and DeLuca, 1967); but when the vitamin is present, both PTH and thyrocalcitonin have their expected effects.

VITAMIN D TOXICITY

It has long been known that excessive vitamin D causes withdrawal of calcium from bone and a consequent hypercalcemia (Shelling, 1932). This effect appears to be an intensification of the normal physiologic action of the vitamin on bone (Lindquist, 1952) and is presumed to be responsible for the hypercalcemia and bone destruction in vitamin D intoxication (Carlsson and Lindquist, 1955). The therapeutic use of large doses of vitamin D in certain types of arthritis successfully removed calcium deposits but, unfortunately, led to deposition of calcium in soft tissues such as cardiac muscle.

Moderate overdose of vitamin D (1800 to 6300 I.U.) to infants was reported by Jeans and Stearns (1938) to have an adverse effect on linear bone growth. However, Fomon et al. (1966) report no effect on either bone growth or plasma calcium levels in infants receiving 400 or 1600 units of vitamin D when compared to breast-fed infants who received a 200 unit supplement.

OTHER FACTORS AFFECTING BONE METABOLISM

With all the synthetic activity accompanying growing bone, it becomes obvious that the growth pattern will be affected by any metabolic alterations that interfere with (1) cell multiplication, (2) the formation of intercellular substance, or (3) the mineralization of the organic matrix. The need for protein, calcium, and vitamin D has been repeatedly emphasized. Mineralization of bone, however, can take place only after a suitable matrix has been established.

Despite the fact that no disturbance exists in the mechanism of calcification, the abnormal matrix resulting from defective collagen in scorbutic animals is not normally calcifiable; the intercellular substance that does form, however, becomes heavily calcified. The retardation of ossification by the abnormal matrix is accompanied by the continuation of the resorptive process in bone with the result that the shaft of the growing bone becomes thin and porous, leading to spontaneous fractures. Piling up of calcified cartilage at the costochondral junctions is responsible for the so-called scorbutic rosary and pigeon chest. These lesions characteristic of ascorbic acid deficiency, but grossly similar to those of vitamin D deficiency, occur only in growing bone.

In a vitamin A deficiency the cartilage cells do not follow the normal pattern of growth, maturation, and degeneration and, as a result, bone formation ceases and abnormalities in shape appear. These effects are associated with diminished uptake of sulfur in the formation of chondroitin sulfate (Dziewiatkowski, 1954) and apparently are due to decreased activity of sulfate transferase (Carroll and Spencer, 1965) and ATP-sulfurylase (Subba Rao et al., 1963; Levi et al., 1968). Vitamin A does not appear to be an essential part of the sulfurylase enzyme but may be involved in its stabilization (Levi and Wolf, 1969). The neurological manifestations of vitamin A deficiency appear to be due to the failure of certain bony foramina to enlarge with the resultant pressure and subsequent degeneration of nerves (see McLean and Urist, 1968). The first evidence of the relationship between vitamin A and bone formation was reported by Mellanby, who also is known for his comprehensive description of the pathology of rickets (see Mellanby, 1950).

Dissolution of cartilage matrix occurs in hypervitaminosis A, and this leads to increased plasma levels of chondroitin sulfate and increased sulfur excretion (Thomas et al., 1960). The effect on bone growth due to increased osteoclastic activity, possibly mediated through the lysosomes, has been discussed (see Chapter 14). For a discussion of the postulated mechanism of action of excessive vitamin A on the lysosomal system of skeletal cells, see Fell (1970).

It should be evident that the effects of nutrients on bone are much more pronounced and more readily detected in the growing organism. In the adult, the amount of calcium in the skeleton is very large, and X-ray assessment of skeletal calcium content is generally insensitive to even a 30 percent loss in bone calcium (Lachmann, 1955). It is probably for this reason that adaptation can take place and that no clinical syndrome attributable solely to dietary calcium deficiency has been defined (Hegsted, 1967). With repeated stresses and drain on calcium stores coupled with consistently low dietary intakes of calcium and/or vitamin D, bone structure may be affected to the point where abnormality is clinically detectable. Such is probably the case in osteomalacia of pregnancy. A similar set of conditions has been suggested in the etiology of osteoporosis of old age, in which the stress is chronic, representing a small but steady drain on bone calcium as a result of low dietary intakes over the better part of a lifetime. However, the data are certainly controversial.

CONCLUSION

The bone cells are far from inert calcified vestiges organized to give shape and rigidity, as well as flexibility, to the mass of functioning cytoplasm that comprises the total organism. In fact, they are living, metabolizing cells. They are responsible for maintaining the calcium ion concentration of the blood and other extracellular fluids so that, as a result, intracellular concentrations of calcium are suitable for function of all body cells. The extracellular bank of bone calcium becomes available if the metabolizing bone cells provide the necessary conditions for withdrawal: carbonic anhydrase synthesis, lysosomal enzyme activity, and probably cAMP formation. Through sensitivity to hormonal signals received by the bone cells, the calcium homeostasis in the total organism is maintained.

chapter 18

muscle cells

1. Structural Organization
2. Structural Components
   a. Myosin
   b. Actin
   c. Actomyosin
   d. Tropomyosin and
      Other Proteins

3. Muscle Contraction
   a. Sliding Filaments
   b. Role of Calcium Ions
   c. Source of Energy
4. Conclusion

"Muscle, as a material of inquiry, offers great advantages. Its function is motion, one of the simplest and oldest signs of life which has always been looked upon by man as the criterion of life. Motion, owing to its mechanical character, can be observed with the naked eye and registered by relatively simple means. It is accompanied by very fast and intense chemical changes and changes in energy which can be measured with greater ease and accuracy than the relatively slow functions of parenchymatous organs. All this has made muscle the classical object of biological research and up to the present century the greater half of physiology was muscle physiology."

Albert Szent-Györgyi, *Nature of Life,* 1948, p. 9

The highly specialized muscle cell, or fiber, exploits the capacity of the cell to contract and produce movement. It does this by effectively transducing into mechanical work some of the ATP it synthesizes. The transduction is efficiently carried out because the structural organization of the fibers is closely integrated with the specialized function of unidirectional shortening or contraction

STRUCTURAL ORGANIZATION

The organization of striated muscle is somewhat like a box within a box. The muscle is an organ composed of many long cells or fibers which are composed of many longitudinally arrayed fibrils. The fibrils are composed of the myofilaments, myosin and actin (Fig. 18.1). Examination of the muscle fiber using a light microscope reveals its most characteristic feature, the cross striations of alternating light and dark bands. The striations are not part of the *sarcoplasm* (muscle cytoplasm) but are due to the close arrangement of myofibrils which are aligned in register with one another and give the impression that the bands cross the entire cell and are part of the fiber.

The dark bands are the anisotropic bands or *A bands;* the lighter bands, the isotropic or *I bands*. The dark appearance of the A bands is due to the thicker myosin filament; the lighter appearance of the I band, to the thinner actin filaments. In the middle portion of the A band is a less dense portion called the *H zone*. The myosin filament is continuous through the length of the A band. The I bands are bisected by a dark line, the *Z line*. The actin filaments begin at the Z line and are continuous through the I band extending into the A band and terminating at the H zone, the center of the A band. In good preparations, projections are visible from the thick myosin filaments. The portion of the muscle fiber between the two Z lines is the *sarcomere,* a complete unit that is repeated throughout the length of the fiber and is the contractile unit or mechanism which enables the muscle to perform its specialized function of unidirectional shortening or contraction. Fig. 18.2 illustrates the detail of one sarcomere.

In addition to the precise arrangement of fibrils and myofilaments, two other characteristics of muscle structure are visible through electron microscopy: vesicles and mitochondria. There are

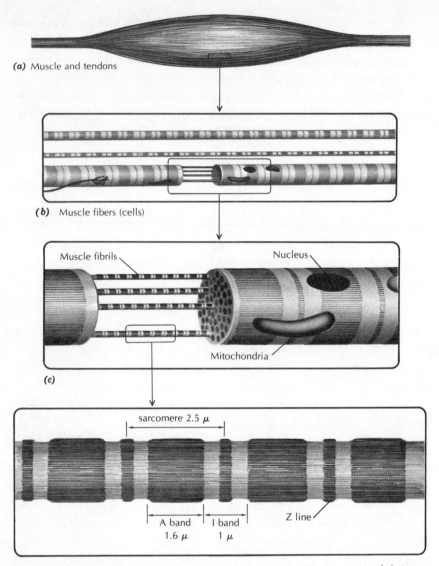

(a) Muscle and tendons

(b) Muscle fibers (cells)

Muscle fibrils

Nucleus

Mitochondria

(c)

sarcomere 2.5 μ

A band
1.6 μ

I band
1 μ

Z line

Fig. 18.1 The organization of striated muscle. The muscle (a) is an organ composed of numerous elongated cells or fibers (b). The fiber in turn is composed of numerous contractile elements or fibrils (c), which under the phase contrast microscope (d) can be seen to have a striated structure of repeating units (sarcomeres) composed of two types of bands—the A band and the I band. The latter is divided by a structure called the Z line. In the electron microscope the band structure can be seen in far greater detail. (From A. G. Loewy and P. Siekevitz, *Cell Structure and Function*, 2nd ed., Holt, Rinehart and Winston, Inc., N. Y., 1969 p. 402.)

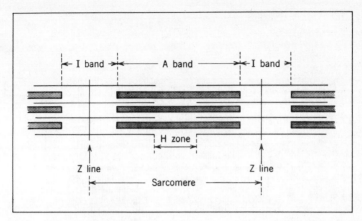

Fig. 18.2 Schematic diagram of morphology of striated muscle fibers. (From L. Mandelkern, *Contractile Proteins and Muscle,* K. Laki, ed., Marcel Dekker, Inc., N. Y. 1971, pp. 499.

two sets of vesicles which do not appear to connect with each other and are closely associated with the myofibrils: a system of transverse tubules called the *T-system,* and the *sarcoplasmic reticulum* (Fig. 18.3). The T-system appears to be invaginations of the cell membrane or *sarcolemma,* and this system of tubules comes close to every sarcomere of every myofibril. The sarcoplasmic reticulum is a series of interconnected transverse and longitudinal vesicles and is the muscle version of the endoplasmic reticulum. In most mammalian muscle, three circular profiles occur near the level of the junction of the A and I bands. The two lateral and larger vesicles are the terminal dilatations of the sarcoplasmic reticulum and the central vesicle is a section through the T-system. This group is called the *triad.*

Between the myofibrils and parallel to the muscle fiber are rows of elongated mitochondria. In muscles with a low rate of activity (Fig. 18.3*a*), relatively few mitochondria are in the area between the myofibrils and there are also few in the area at either end of the nucleus. The mitochondria have rather sparse cristae and a matrix of low density. In muscles with a high metabolic rate (Fig. 18.3*b*), the mitochondria are lined up in long chains between the myofibrils, and they are very abundant at either end of the nucleus. Each of the mitochondria has a complex arrangement of cristae and a dense matrix. Muscle cells with a high metabolic rate also have numerous lipid droplets close to the mitochondria and

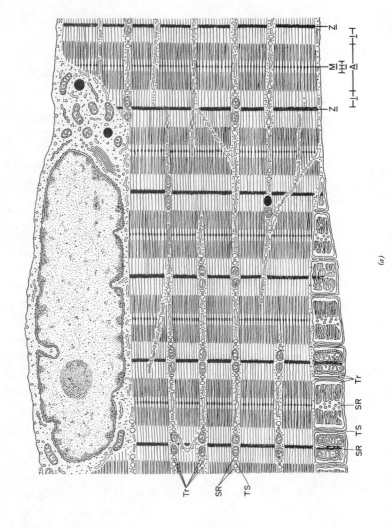

Fig. 18.3a Muscle with low metabolic activity. Tr, triad; SR, sacroplasmic reticulum; TS, tubular system. (From T. L. Lentz, *Cell Fine Structure*, W. B. Saunders Co., Phila. 1971.)

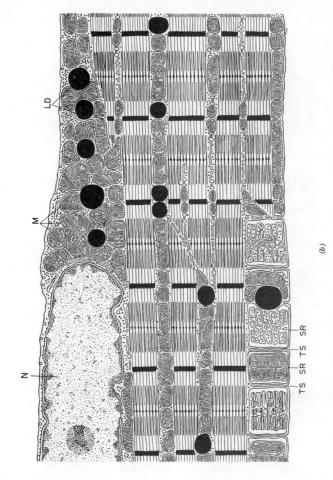

Fig. 18.3b Muscle with high metabolic activity. N, nucleus; M, mitochondria; LD, lipid droplets; TS, tubular system; SR, sarcoplasmic reticulum. (From T. L. Lentz, *Cell Fine Structure*, W. B. Saunders Co., Phila., 1971.)

(b)

often near the I band, whereas in muscles with a lower metabolic activity there are few lipid droplets but abundant glycogen granules.

The nuclei in striated muscle are elongated and at the periphery of the muscle fiber. The fibers are multinucleate, and there are usually one or two nucleoli. A small Golgi complex is usually near the end of the nucleus. There are few ribosomes and little visible sarcoplasmic matrix although it is present and does provide the

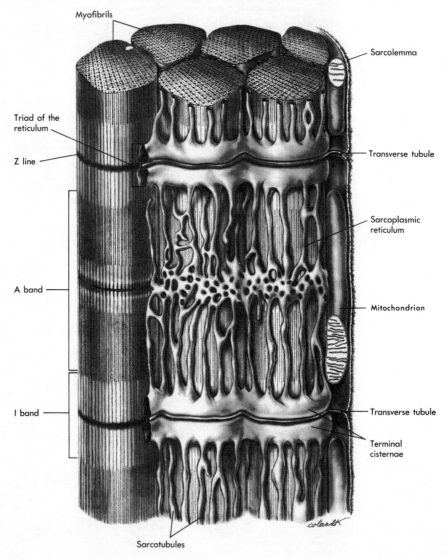

Myofibrils

Sarcolemma

Triad of the reticulum

Z line

Transverse tubule

A band

Sarcoplasmic reticulum

Mitochondrion

I band

Transverse tubule

Terminal cisternae

Sarcotubules

matrix in which the myofilaments are aligned. Its metabolic role is important to muscle function.

Cardiac muscle is striated in an identical manner, but there are several specific differences between it and skeletal muscle. The nucleus in cardiac muscle fibers is centrally located and surrounded by an area rich in mitochondria. The mitochondria between the myofibrils are large and numerous with many cristae, and they are associated with lipid droplets and large numbers of glycogen granules which are also between the myofilaments. Some differences are apparent also in the tubular systems. In skeletal muscle separate cellular units are not visible but in cardiac muscle cellular units are visibly connected with specialized arrangements of plasma membrane called *intercalated disks*. The disks do not extend across the width of the muscle fibers in a straight line but go across in a steplike manner. This arrangement is believed to provide sites of low electrical resistance to permit the spread of excitation throughout the cardiac muscle. The cardiac muscle is adapted structurally and metabolically for its sustained activity.

A three-dimensional representation of portions of several myofibrils puts into perspective all of the component structures of the muscle fiber (Fig. 18.4).

STRUCTURAL COMPONENTS

Skeletal muscle has been studied in greater detail than have either cardiac or smooth muscle. It is approximately 75 percent water

---

Fig. 18.4 Schematic representation of the distribution of the sarcoplasmic reticulum around the myofibrils of skeletal muscle. The longitudinal sarcotubules are confluent with transverse elements called the terminal cisternae. A slender transverse tubule (T tubule) extending inward from the sarcolemma is flanked by two terminal-cisternae to form the so-called triads of the reticulum. The location of these with respect to the cross banded pattern of the myofibrils varies from species to species. In frog muscle, depicted here, the triads are at the Z line. In mammalian muscle there are two to each sarcomere, located at the A-I junctions. (From W. Bloom and D. W. Fawcett, *A Textbook of Histology*, 9th ed., W. B. Saunders Company, Phila., p. 281.)

and 20 percent protein; the remaining 5 percent includes inorganic material, the so-called organic "extractives," and glycogen and its derivatives. Of the protein, 60 to 70 percent of the total quantity in muscle is structural protein, the protein of the fibrils; the remaining 30 to 40 percent is in the sarcoplasm. The water-soluble sarcoplasmic proteins, easily extractable with cold water, include all of the glycolytic enzymes and myoglobin. The enzyme-containing water extract is called *myogen*. The water-insoluble structural proteins are fibrous proteins and constitute almost 90 percent of the myofibril of which 54 percent is myosin, 20 to 25 percent actin, and 11 percent tropomyosin. The remaining 10 percent of the structural protein in the myofilaments is accounted for by troponin, α-actinin, and β-actinin.

Amino acid compositions of the various muscle proteins have been determined, but there is some question as to whether the analyzed preparations were uncontaminated.

Myosin

Myosin, the most abundant of muscle proteins, is the major component of the A band, It has a molecular weight of approximately 470,000 and is a long asymmetrical molecule with two identical, long polypeptide chains and two short ones. The long chains each contain about 1800 amino acids and are the longest known polypeptides. Each chain is an α-helix, and the two chains coil about each other in an α-helix. The two long chains form the tail of the molecule and part of the globular head that, in addition, contains the two small chains (Fig. 18.5). Myosin can be fragmented into two fractions: *light meromyosin,* the thin tail region, and *heavy meromyosin,* the more bulbous head region. It is the latter region that forms the side projections on the filaments and has ATPase activity and affinity for actin (Loewy et al., 1969). The light meromyosin has affinity for other myosin molecules and aligns them forming the backbone of the filaments. The structure of the myosin is closely integrated with its function.

Myosin is believed to be present as the magnesium salt, magnesium myosinate. It also binds sodium and potassium ions and practically all of the ATP present in muscle fibers is probably bound to myosin (Szent-Györgyi, 1958).

For further reading on myosin, see Laki (1971a).

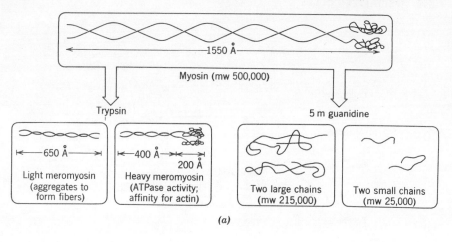

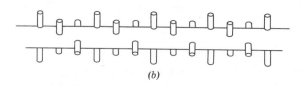

Fig. 18.5*a* Structure of myosin molecule. The molecule appears to be composed of two large chains and two small ones. The large chains form the long "tail" of the molecule. The "head" of the molecule is composed in part of the remainder of the large chains and in part of two small chains. The molecular weight of the chains can be measured by disaggregating the molecule and using the ultracentrifuge. (From A. G. Loewy and P. Siekevitz, *Cell Structure and Function,* 2nd ed., Holt, Rinehart and Winston, Inc. N. Y., 1969 p. 409.)

Fig. 18.5*b* Diagram of cross-bridge arrangement on thick myosin-containing filaments. [From H. E. Huxley, *Science,* 164: 1356 (1969).]

Actin

Actin appears to be a single polypeptide chain containing about 450 amino acids. Estimates of molecular weight range from approximately 45,000 to 70,000 (Laki, 1971b). Actin is present in two forms. In the absence of salts, it is in the form of globular *G-actin.* Each molecule binds one calcium ion and one ATP. Binding of ATP to G-actin leads to its polymerization and the formation of *F-actin*

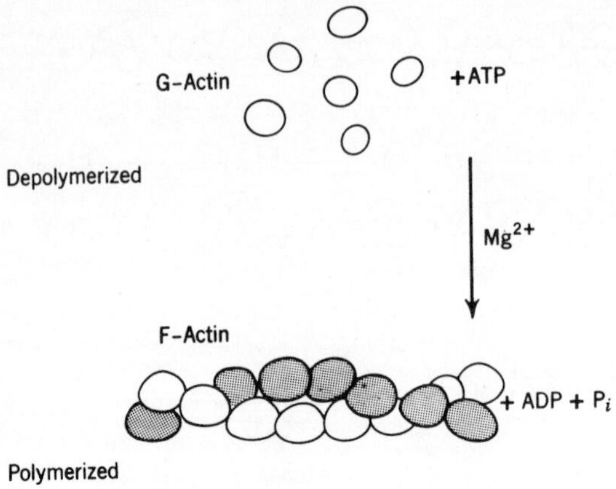

Fig. 18.6 Two forms of actin. Binding of ATP to G-actin leads to polymerization and the formation of F-actin.

(Fig. 18.6). F-actin is a supercoiled arrangement of two strands of G-actin (Huxley, 1963; Hanson and Lowy, 1963). For each molecule of G-actin added to the F-actin chain, one molecule of ATP is split. The ADP binds firmly to the actin and the phosphate is released. F-actin corresponds to the thin myofilaments seen in sections.

For some of the facts and some of the conjecture on actin, see Laki (1971b).

Actomyosin

When actin and myosin are mixed together *in vitro* they form actomyosin, which has high viscosity. This basic reaction was discovered by Szent-Györgyi many years ago (see Szent-Györgyi, 1947). This interaction is the foundation of muscle contraction. It is the heavy meromyosin fragment of the myosin molecule that combines with actin (Szent Kiralyi and Oplatka, 1969). The spatial arrangement of the actin and myosin is illustrated in Fig. 18.7

Actomyosin is not only a contractile protein, but it also functions as an enzyme that specifically hydrolyzes ATP and makes use of the energy of hydrolysis for muscle contraction. It is, therefore, responsible for the conversion of the chemical energy of ATP into the mechanical energy of contraction. Dissociation of actomyosin

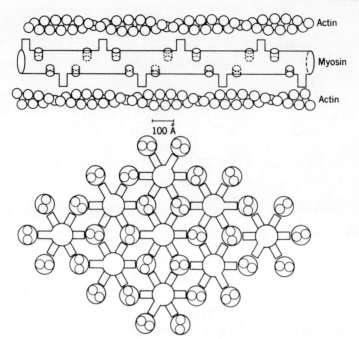

Fig. 18.7 Spatial arrangement of myosin and actin filaments in striated muscle. [From R. E. Davies, *Nature,* 199: 1068 (1963).]

accompanies the hydrolysis and, when hydrolysis is complete, actin and myosin reaggregate.

A paradox is apparent when the dissociation of actomyosin occurs in the presence of ATP and Mg^{2+} leading to a large and rapid decrease in viscosity *in vitro,* or a relaxed state. This reverts to rigor when there is no longer any ATP to hydrolyze, and actin and myosin reaggregate. How actomyosin requires the energy of ATP to maintain a relaxed state and also uses the energy of ATP to contract muscle is dependent upon whether Ca^{2+} ions are present. The role of Ca^{2+} ions becomes somewhat clearer with the understanding of the roles of some of the other muscle proteins.

Tropomyosin and Other Proteins

The tropomyosin fraction of muscle protein is small. Like light meromyosin it consists of two polypeptide chains twisted in an a-helix and coiled about each other. They are believed to be similar,

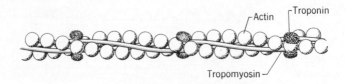

Fig. 18.8 Troponin-tropomyosin-F-actin complex is the relaxing protein. Troponin restrains the interaction of actin and myosin. Troponin restraint is released by Ca^{2+} ions leading to contraction. [From D. Ebashi, M. Endo, and I. Ohtsuki, *Quart. Rev. Biophys.,* 2: 351 (1969).]

if not identical, chains each having a molecular weight of about 70,000.

The tropomyosin which is usually referred to as tropomyosin A is found mostly in invertebrate muscle such as the hinge muscle in clams (Laki, 1971c), but tropomyosin B is in the filaments of the I band (Bodwell, 1971). It is associated with *troponin,* another minor protein with a major role, as part of the troponin-tropomyosin-F-actin complex (Fig. 18.8). This complex appears to be associated with the calcium regulatory functions in muscle.

Troponin is believed to be the calcium-receptive protein of muscle (Maruyama, 1971). It binds strongly to calcium, and this binding is not affected by the presence of either magnesium or ATP. How the calcium binding occurs is not yet known, but the presence of Ca^{2+} ions along with Mg^{2+} ions and ATP leads to muscle contraction. Ca^{2+} ions, therefore, by their presence convert the energy released by ATP into the energy of contraction. In the absence of Ca^{2+} ions, actomyosin requires ATP to maintain its relaxed state. Rigor sets in if muscle can no longer generate ATP.

MUSCLE CONTRACTION

What muscles do and their characteristic appearance have been known for centuries. How their structural characteristics are related to the function they perform is still, to a great extent, theoretical.

Sliding Filaments

The contractile material that forms the myofibrils consists of a long

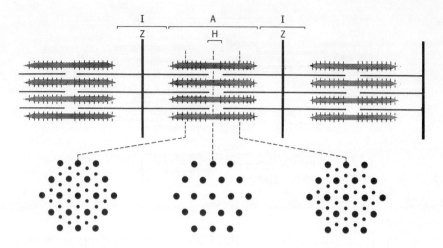

Fig. 18.9 Diagrammatic representation of the structure of striated muscle, showing overlapping arrays of actin- and myosin-containing filaments, the latter with projecting cross-bridges on them. For convenience of representation, the structure is drawn with considerable longitudinal foreshortening; with filament diameters and side-spacings as shown, the filament lengths should be about five times the lengths shown. [From H. E. Huxley, *Science,* 164: 1356 (1969).]

series of partially overlapping arrays of myosin and actin filaments which Huxley (1963) referred to as the *interdigitating filaments.* This is observed in the electron micrograph representation of striated muscle in Fig. 18.9. The change in muscle length (contraction) is postulated to occur without change in filament length and is due to the relation of the filaments to each other. Huxley's (1969) *sliding filament model* suggests that the change in muscle length occurs when the overlapping filaments slide past each other with the actin (I bands) being drawn further into the myosin filaments (A bands) as the muscle shortens. The I bands move out again as the muscle relaxes or lengthens (Fig. 18.10). The actual mechanism of the sliding action is still partly conjectural, but structural studies of the proteins involved are gradually supplying some of the missing clues.

According to Huxley (1969), the sliding of the filaments is accomplished by the formation of actomyosin. The globular part of the myosin molecule is the part that forms the visible cross-

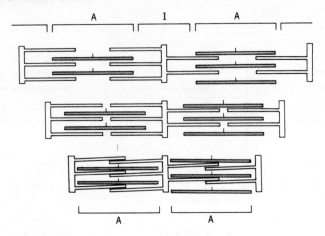

Fig. 18.10 Sliding filament model of muscle contraction. (From A. L. Lehninger, *Biochemistry*, Worth Publishers Inc., 1970 p. 586.)

bridge. The suggestion is that flexible joints in the myosin filament permit the globular head to interact with the actin filament. Huxley has suggested two alternate mechanisms for the linkage of the gobular head of myosin to actin, *i.e.*, the attachment of the thick and thin filaments (Fig. 18.11). In one, the tilting of the myosin head of the crossbridge would slide the actin filament along the myosin filament. In the other, a pair of subunits in the myosin head would tilt in opposite directions and produce the sliding movement of the actin along the myosin.

In a model suggesting how the head region of the myosin molecules form crossbridges, Murray and Weber (1974) suggest that the ATP becomes bound to a receptor site on the myosin head which causes the myosin-ATP to be converted into a "charged" intermediate form. The charged intermediate has great affinity for the actin molecule in the thin filament, and this binding is associated with the hydrolysis of the ATP and the release of energy. The energy release causes the crossbridge to swivel to a new angle pulling the thick filament along with respect to the thin filament thereby shortening the muscle. The detachment of the crossbridge occurs very rapidly when a new ATP binds to the actin-myosin complex causing it to revert to a low energy state. In a living cell, ATP is readily available for the recharging of the myosin head; but the absence of ATP accounts for the rigor mortis that develops in

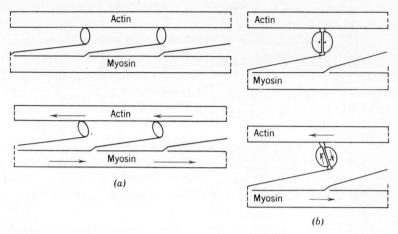

Fig. 18.11 Diagram illustrating possible mechanisms for producing relative sliding movement by tilting of cross-bridges. (*a*) If separation of filaments is maintained by electrostatic force-balance, tilting must give rise to movement of filaments past each other. (*b*) A small relative movement between two subunits of myosin could give rise to a large change in tilt, by the mechanism shown. [From H. E. Huxley, *Science*, 164: 1356 (1969).]

muscle after death. The low energy complexes, therefore, are called rigor complexes; the high energy state or the combination of actin with the charged ATP intermediates are the "active complexes" (Weber and Murray, 1973).

The characteristic feature of contraction in all models is the attachment of the globular head of the myosin to the actin followed by an active change in the angle of attachment thereby increasing the degree of filament overlap with contraction. This is associated with the hydrolysis of ATP. Calcium ions are essential for the actin, myosin, and ATP to function in muscle contraction.

Role of Calcium Ions

Regulation of muscle contraction depends on the presence of Ca^{2+} ions which are stored in sacs in the sarcoplasmic reticulum. The muscle fiber at rest is electrically polarized with the outside of the membrane positive with respect to the inside. Contraction is initiated when the nerve signal reaches the muscle cell, travels along the sarcolemma of the muscle fiber, and reaches the terminal dilatation of the triad. This induces a reversal of polarization and the release of Ca^{2+} ions from the reticulum sacs into the fluid surrounding the filaments. The Ca^{2+} ions, by binding to troponin, are directly responsible for activating the contractile mechanism. The restraint the troponin exerted as part of the troponin-tropomyosin-F-actin complex is released, permits the crossbridges to attach and contraction to occur (see Winegrad, 1968; Murray and Weber, 1974).

Calcium is quickly removed and returned to the storage vesicles in the membranes of the sarcoplasmic reticulum and the muscle relaxes. This is accomplished through the action of ATP in the operation of a calcium pump (Ebashi and Lipmann, 1962). A Ca^{2+}-activated ATPase localized in the outer surface of the sarcoplasmic reticulum is coupled to Ca^{2+} ion uptake (Hasselbach and Elfvin, 1967). Interference with the operation of the Ca^{2+} ion pump interferes with muscle relaxation, and the ATP-deprived muscle will go into a state of rigor. Both the initial release of the Ca^{2+} ions and the return to the storage sac is extremely rapid, usually requiring only a fraction of a second.

According to Maruyama (1971), "The most exciting prospect in the field of regulatory proteins is the elucidation of how the binding of calcium to troponin changes its conformation and how the changes are transmitted to F-actin through tropomyosin so as to permit the interaction between myosin and actin." Fortunately, we can continue to flex our muscles as we await the answer.

Source of Energy for Contraction

Glycolysis can provide the energy for muscle contraction and so can respiratory activity. The muscles of all vertebrates do both, but the amounts of ATP in muscle are extremely small compared to the chemical energy required to support muscle work. The immediate source of energy for muscle contraction is ATP. The ATPase in myosin is responsible for the hydrolysis of ATP to ADP and inorganic phosphate. However, analysis of ATP in muscle before and after single contractions shows no decrease in ATP nor any increase in ADP indicating another source of ATP (see Lehninger, 1970, p. 596). The high energy compound, creatine phosphate (phosphocreatine), is that source. The prompt resynthesis of ATP from ADP is achieved through the action of creatine kinase, which transfers a high energy phosphate from creatine phosphate to the ADP.

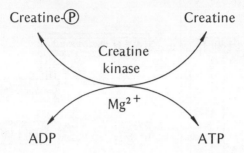

The creatine phosphate is regenerated by the transfer of high energy phosphate from ATP to creatine through aerobic metabolism using stored glucose for energy. The ATP and creatine phosphate are energy sources that can be used rapidly but the recharging of ATP by oxidative phosphorylation requires more time and occurs during the recovery period. At moderate rates of exercise a sufficient amount of ATP can be synthesized from stored glycogen. However, this cannot be maintained during rapid or prolonged strenuous exercise. Under such conditions, muscle contraction is carried on anaerobically, and large amounts of lactic acid accumulate leading to "muscle fatigue." Lactic acid disappears when fatigued muscle is exposed to oxygen, and the muscle's ability to contract is regained. After muscular exercise, any lactic acid that accumulates is reconverted into glycogen (see Chapter 11).

There are three phases in the operation of muscle in strenuous exercise. The first phase, involving prompt resynthesis of ATP through the action of creatine phosphate, lasts only a few seconds. The second phase is the arrival of oxygen through increased respiration for resynthesis of creatine phosphate. Only half the creatine phosphate is split during the peak period of activity and all of this can be resynthesized in a brief recovery period. The third energy contribution, glycolysis, comes about only after oxidation can no longer keep up with the need of muscle. The quantity of available glycogen depends on the nutritional state of the muscle. The payment of the oxygen debt after strenuous exercise is a slow process and may take more than an hour after the conclusion of the exercise. In studies designed to determine how energy for the most efficient muscular work can be provided, Margaria (1972) showed that short periods of strenuous muscle work interspersed with

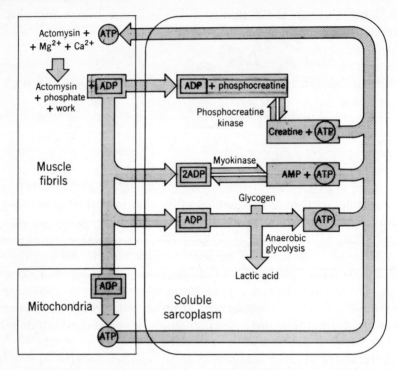

Fig. 18.12 Energy flow in muscle. The muscle is seen here as a mechanochemical transducer using energy from ATP to produce work. The ATP is generated locally by four separate systems: (1) by the mitochondria, (2) from phosphocreatine, (3) from ADP and myokinase, and (4) from the anaerobic glycolysis of glycogen to lactic acid. (Redrawn from Siekevitz, 1959.) (From A. G. Loewy and P. Siekevitz, *Cell Structure and Function,* 2nd ed., Holt, Rinehart and Winston, Inc., N. Y., 1969 p. 423.)

periods of rest could permit up to 30 times more work for the energy expended.

A picture of the energy flow in muscle is shown in Fig. 18.12. The muscle fiber operates as an energy converter of the chemical energy of ATP into mechanical work. The ATP is generated in the muscle through four separate systems: the mitochondria, from creatine phosphate, from ADP and myokinase, and from the anaerobic glycolysis of glycogen to lactic acid. The energy conversion is accomplished by exploiting certain cellular capabilities and certain potentialities of molecular structure. It is a beautiful example of the integration of structure and function which, when efficiently used, can become more efficient with use.

Man's skeletal muscle does not require the speed and efficiency of the hummingbird's wing, but his cardiac muscle must be equipped for non-stop activity. Metabolic adaptations in heart muscle and a high content of myoglobin permit the utilization of free fatty acids, ketones, and lactate as energy sources. Under basal conditions, 35 percent of the caloric needs of the heart are provided by carbohydrate, 60 percent by fat mostly as circulating free fatty acids, and the remainder by ketones and amino acids. As activity is increased, the nutrients used in the metabolic adaptations of heart muscle will depend, in part, on the nutritional status of the individual.

Goldberg (1972) reported that skeletal muscle catabolizes certain amino acids at a rapid rate and appears to be the major site in the body for the catabolism of leucine, isoleucine, and valine. Accompanying food deprivation, catabolism of leucine, isoleucine, and valine increased 3 to 5 times the rates in normal rats. The increased ability of muscle to catabolize branched chain amino acids in food-deprived rats coincides with the increased concentrations of these amino acids in the blood and with the reduced tendency to burn glucose. A similar situation with respect to these branched chain amino acids appears to prevail in physiological situations where muscle growth is decreased such as in diabetes or following hypophysectomy. Goldberg's (1972) studies have also indicated that six amino acids are preferentially catabolized by muscle: leucine, isoleucine, valine, alanine, aspartic acid, and glutamic acid; whereas other tissues catabolize the amino acids not degraded by muscle. Addition of other energy sources had little or no effect on this preferential catabolism by muscle. Whether the catabolism of certain amino acids by muscle plays a role in the control of muscle protein synthesis and degradation is not known.

CONCLUSION

Perhaps at times the explorations through these various specialized cells have seemed to probe rather deeply into the hows and whys but, as Szent-Györgyi (1948) has explained, "I cannot take the girl in my right arm and her smile in my left hand and study the two independently. Similarly, we cannot separate life from matter and what we can only study is matter and its reactions. But if we study this matter and its reactions, we study life itself." If we study nutrients and their reactions, we study living.

chapter 19

nerve cells

1. Neurons and Related Cells
2. Neuron Structure
   a. Perikaryon and Axon
   b. Myelin Sheath
3. Neuron Function
   a. Membrane Potential
   b. Propagation of the Nerve Impulse
      1. Local Circuit Theory
      2. Saltatory Conduction
      3. Synaptic Transmission
         a. The Synapse
         b. Synaptic Vesicles
         c. Receptor Sites
         d. Postsynaptic Potentials
         e. Mechanism of Action
4. Transmitter Substances
   a. The Catecholamines: Norepinephrine, Epinephrine, Dopamine
   b. Acetylcholine
   c. Gamma Aminobutyric Acid
   d. Serotonin
5. Conclusion

"The night before Easter Sunday of that year (1920) I awoke, turned on the light, and jotted down a few notes on a tiny slip of thin paper. Then I fell asleep again. It occurred to me at six o'clock in the morning that during the night I had written down something most important, but I was unable to decipher the scrawl. The next night, at three o'clock, the idea returned. It was the design of an experiment to determine whether or not the hypothesis of chemical transmission that I had uttered seventeen years ago was correct. I got up immediately, went to the laboratory, and performed a simple experiment on a frog heart according to the nocturnal design...its results became the foundation of the theory of chemical transmission of the nervous impulse."

Otto Loewi, "The Excitement of a Life in Science,"
Perspect. Biol. Med. 4:3-25 (1960)

The structure of the neuron creates certain logistical problems particularly in relation to nutrient supply. How does the center of synthetic activity located in the nucleus and other cell body organelles relate to the activity of the distant terminals? How do nutrients and metabolites enter and traverse the length of an axon, particularly one well insulated with a sheath of myelin? How are the nutrient needs and product requirements of the terminals monitored by the metabolic center in the cell body? These are only a few of the questions that are beginning to be asked and answered through the combined efforts of scientists from a variety of related and unrelated disciplines. In the sections to follow, certain aspects of specialized function peculiar to nerve cells, and significant to nutritionists, will be presented.

NEURONS AND RELATED CELLS

The *neurons* are the cells specialized to carry on the rapid communications required for coordinated function both within the organism and between the organism and its environment. The exploitation of two characteristics of protoplasm—irritability and conductivity—permit these cells to react to various stimuli in a fraction of a second and to transmit the excitation to another location. In addition, some nerve cells possess a secretory capability that enables integration of function through localized and selective effects.

During embryological development certain cells derived from neural epithelium do not develop as neurons but as cells that occupy space between neurons. These cells have been called *neuroglia* or *glial cells* from the suggestion that they were the neural glue that held the neuron population together (Bodian, 1967). The glial cells outnumber neurons by 10 to 1. They are generally divided into the macroglia and microglia. There are two types of macroglia cells: the *oligodendrocytes* and the *astrocytes*. In addition to macroglia and microglia, there are *ependymal cells* that line the cavities of the central nervous system much like an epithelial layer. These cells often have cilia and microvilli that extend into the ventricle lumens and spinal canal. Generally, the glial cells appear to act as the metabolic stabilizers of the neurons (Hyden, 1967); specifically, their functions are only beginning to be understood since early work centered on the neuron and the glial cells were considered merely supporting connective tissue.

The oligodendrocytes are the metabolic appendices of the neuron (Hyden, 1967) and both metabolic and functional collaboration exists between the two cell types. They may function in the provision of nutrients to the neurons they enclose. In the central nervous system these cells are thought to provide the myelin sheath much as the related Schwann cells do for the peripheral nerve fibers (see below). The astrocytes, interposed between capillaries and neurons, are believed to mediate ion transport and monitor the materials that pass into the neurons. In this way, they may function as part of the blood-brain barrier (Hyden, 1967).

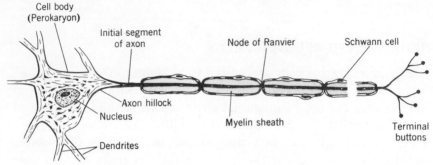

Fig. 19.1 Motor neuron with myelinated axon.

The microglia are smaller than the other glial cells. Their fine structure resembles that of macrophages, and they are believed to have a phagocytic function and to be active primarily in damaged nervous tissue.

Neuroglia that form myelin are sensitive to a variety of diseases involving the myelin sheath, the so-called demyelinating diseases, of which multiple sclerosis is one.

For detailed discussion of the fine structure of the glia cells, see Peters et al. (1970).

Each neuron and its immediate surrounding glia cells, mostly oligodendrocytes, form a biochemical and functional unit with a specificity that is the result of their relationship to other neurons in the nervous system (Peters et al., 1970). Most neurons are extremely elongated and bipolar so that one end normally receives information and the other pole transmits that information to other nerve cells or to muscle or gland cells. Information is received at points of contact on the *perikaryon* or *cell body* and on extensions from the cell body called *dendrites* (Fig. 19.1). The *axon,* or conducting portion of the nerve cell, arises from a cone-shaped region of the perikaryon called the *axon hillock.* The axon is a cylindrical structure that can vary in length from microns to meters, and it may have collateral branches along its course. It is capable of propagating an impulse at speeds up to 100 meters per second (Bodian, 1967). This is a rate of more than 3 miles per minute or 180 miles per hour! Axons surrounded by a single fold of a sheath cell are the unmyelinated fibers and are usually of extremely fine caliber. Axons enclosed in concentric wrappings of sheath cell membranes are myelinated axons. The *myelin sheath* is composed of layers of lipid and

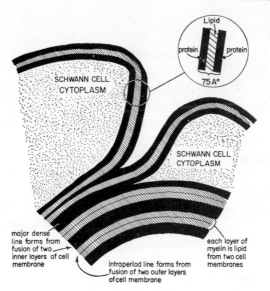

Inside circle: Lipid / protein / protein / 75 A°

SCHWANN CELL CYTOPLASM

SCHWANN CELL CYTOPLASM

major dense line forms from fusion of two inner layers of cell membrane

each layer of myelin is lipid from two cell membranes

intraperiod line forms from fusion of two outer layers of cell membrane

Fig. 19.2 Diagram illustrating the fine structure of cell membranes and how cell membranes of Schwann cells become myelin sheaths. (From A. W. Ham, *Histology*, 6th ed., J. B. Lippincott Company, Phila., 1969, p. 530.)

protein and is, in fact, a concentric lamellar specialization of the membrane of the Schwann cells (Fig. 19.2).

The myelin sheath is interrupted at regular intervals designated as the *nodes of Ranvier*. The distance from one node to another is proportional to the thickness of the fiber: the thicker the fiber, the longer its internodes. Each internode is formed by and surrounded by one Schwann cell.

The functional contact between neurons is the *synapse*, the site of transmission of impulses. Contact may occur between the axon and cell body, axo-somatic; between the axon terminals of one neuron and the dendrites of another, axo-dendritic; or more rarely, between axon and axon, axo-axonic. The term synapse includes the entire neurochemical mechanism and involves transmitter and receptor substances, synthetic and hydrolytic enzymes, and the membrane structures on each side of the contact. Details of the synapse will be presented in a later section. The cytoplasm of the two neurons is not continuous at a synapse; but the nerve impulse that has traveled down the axon of one neuron arrives at the terminals and sets off an impulse in the neuron with which it connects. This point of contact is dynamically polarized, that is, it transmits an impulse in one direction only. The number of synapses on a neuron varies from just a few to several hundred thousand.

The degree of differientation which enables the neuron to perform its highly specialized function occurs at the expense of other cellular capabilities. After embryonic and early postnatal life neurons are no longer capable of division and the number of neurons is not increased although changes in volume and in the complexity of the neuron processes and functional contacts can take place. The neuron is, in fact, one of the most active biosynthesizing cells in the body and such high rates of protein synthesis are often incompatible with cell division (Bodian, 1967). The high rate of protein synthesis and turnover is probably related to the continuous passage of protein from the perikaryon down the axon to the nerve endings for use there or for export. For a discussion of brain cell development during pre- and postnatal life, see Chapter 21.

It is estimated that there 14-30 billion nerve cells in man and, since no cell renewal takes place, the loss of each brain cell is a loss of capital. The contemplation of such downhill development is enough to make anyone nervous.

NEURON STRUCTURE

In common with all other cells, the surface of neurons is covered with a plasma membrane. However, there is both structural diversity and chemical heterogeniety among membranes in general and even among the membranes of nerve cells (see Johnston and Roots, 1972). Neuronal plasma membranes and those of glial cells and subcellular organelles differ from the myelin sheath structurally and in composition. The study of the morphology and biochemistry of all membranes, and especially nerve membranes, is a relatively new field of investigation and on its development rests our understanding of the specialized functions of the diverse membranes in the cells of the nervous system.

Perikaryon and Axon

The perikaryon is usually angular or polygonal with slight concavity

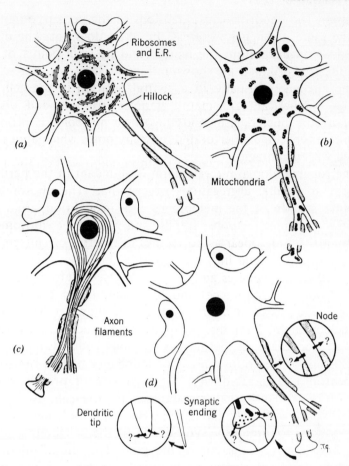

Fig. 19.3 Distribution of organelles within the neuron. (*a*) Ribosomes and endoplasmic reticulum (ER). (*b*) Mitochondria. (*c*) Axon filaments. (*d*) Possible points of egress of constituents synthesized in the cell center and translocated peripherad. (From F. O. Schmitt, "Molecular Neurobiology in the Context of the Neurosciences," *The Neurosciences*, G. C. Quarton, T. Meinechuk, and F. O. Schmitt, eds., Rockefeller University Press, N. Y., 1967, p. 211.)

of the surface between the points at which its dendrites and axon arise. Both size and shape of the cell body varies with different kinds of neurons. The cytoplasmic matrix, *neuroplasm*, is filled with organelles that appear to be in concentric formation around the nucleus. The neuroplasm that extends into the axon is called the *axoplasm.* The dendrites are extensions of the perikaryon and contain the same organelles; whereas the axon does not. The distribution of organelles within the neuron and possible points of egress of synthesized products are shown in Fig. 19.3.

The nucleus is usually in a central position in the cell and is large and spherical. Chromatin granules are fine and dispersed evenly in the nucleoplasm and the single nucleolus is prominent. The nuclear envelope is perforated by many pores which appear to be covered with diaphragms.

The rough endoplasmic reticulum is abundant in the perikaryon arranged as parallel aggregations of cisternae. The ribosomes stud the outer surface of the membranes and, in addition, are arranged on the membranes in loops, spirals, and rows. Free ribosomes also are abundant and appear as polysomes in rosettes or clusters in the neuroplasm and extend into the dendrites; however, they are absent where the axon originates and in the axon itself. Before examination by electron microscopy, chromophilic material in the perikaryon was designated as *Nissl bodies* which were shown to be principally ribonucleoprotein. Examination of the fine structure indicated that the Nissl bodies are, in fact, arrays of rough endoplasmic reticulum and clusters of free ribosomes. The abundance of free ribosomes in the neuron is associated with the high rate of protein synthesis required to replenish that metabolized by the cell. According to the axonal flow theory (Weiss and Hiscoe, 1948), new protein is more or less continuously synthesized in the cell body and flows from there down to the end of the axon. The rate of migration of labeled protein was shown to be approximately 1.5 mm per day (Droz and Leblond, 1963).

The Golgi complex is well developed and often arranged as an arc halfway between the nuclear envelope and the perikaryon membrane; but sometimes the Golgi complex completely encircles the nucleus. It consists of short stacks of flat cisternae with clusters of small vesicles nearby. Areas of the Golgi are connected with smooth endoplasmic reticulum which, in turn, are connected with cisternae of rough endoplasmic reticulum, but there are no sharp divisions in the sequence.

Mitochondria are small and numerous and are scattered throughout the perikaryon and down through the axon to its endings where they appear to be particularly numerous (Fig. 19.3*b*). They have few cristae and these sometimes run parallel to the long axis of the organelle. Neuron mitochondria have been shown to contain DNA (Lehninger, 1967) and may be involved in protein synthesis.

Neurotubules were first observed by De Robertis and Franchi (1953) in extruded axoplasm from myelinated nerves. They course through the perikaryon, into the dendrites, and down the axon running parallel to the long axis. They are unbranched, uniform in size, and straight, running without interruption from the cell body to the terminal synapses. They appear to be formed of 13 parallel filaments arranged to form the tubes and closely resemble the microtubules in cilia and flagella (Stephens, 1968). Neurotubules can be considered the microtubules of nerve cells. They consist of a single well-defined protein, *tubulin*, which is a globular protein, contains the nucleotide guanosine-5'-diphosphate and can be resolved into two slightly different subunits each with a molecular weight of about 55,000 (Bray, 1974).

Neurotubules appear to function as mechanical support and in transport down the axon to nerve endings of transmitter substances synthesized in the perikaryon (Smith et al., 1970). It has been suggested also that they function in the continual transport through the axon of protein synthesized in the cell (Droz and LeBlond, 1963). Dense cores in the neurotubules observed in electron micrographs are thought to be products in transit. Methods now available for isolating and preserving neurotubules should permit both ultrastructural and biochemical analysis and further insight into function (Bray, 1974).

Neurofilaments are the distinctive filaments of nerve cells and are chemically and structurally distinct from neurotubules. Bray (1974) suggests that these filaments may be unique to neurons. They are present in all parts of the cytoplasm of the cell body and also run down the axon (Fig. 19.3c). The number seen in cross section in an axon varies with the diameter of the axon. Neurofilaments are uniform in size, 80 to 100 Å in diameter, remarkably straight and run in parallel arrays without interruption from cell body to the terminal synapses. Neurofilament protein extruded from squid axon for study reveals that the acidic protein is formed of globular subunits which aggregate into helical filaments.

The functional role of the neurofilaments is not known. Wiseniewski et al. (1968) suggest that neurotubules and neurofil-

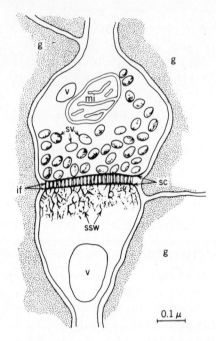

Fig. 19.4 A common form of synapse in the mammalian brain. The axonal (presynaptic) side above; the dendritic (postsynaptic) side below, g, glia; if, intersynaptic filaments; mi, mitochondria; sc, synaptic cleft; ssw, subsynaptic web; sv, synaptic vesicles; v, vesiculate body. (From E. D. P. DeRobertis, W. W. Nowinski, and F. A. Saez, *Cell Biology*, 5th ed., W. B. Saunders Company, Phila., 1970, p. 514.)

aments are interconvertible. Peters and Vaughn (1967) suggest that neurotubules form first and that neurofilaments are formed from the tubules. According to Bray (1974), however, neurofilaments function in conjunction with neurotubules in axoplasmic flow of materials from their site of synthesis in the body of the cell to the cell periphery.

Other but less definite fibrillar structures are the *microfilaments* which are thin, randomly dispersed structures which occur in parallel bundles close to the membrane surface or as a loose meshwork of filaments in actively moving regions of cells in culture (Bray, 1974). There is some evidence that these microfilaments resemble actin, but they have never been isolated or purified.

The *axon terminals* at the synapse are swollen to form different shapes called end-bulbs, end-feet or boutons, cups, and so forth. Each of these swollen terminals contains many mitochondria and numerous tiny vesicles, *synaptic vesicles,* which aggregate close to the terminal membrane. The membrane itself appears to be somewhat thicker as does the opposing membrane of the postsynaptic surface. Between the two membranes is the *synaptic cleft,* a separation approximately 200 Å in width (Fig. 19.4). The manner in which these structures function in the transmission of nerve impulses will be discussed in a later section.

Myelin Sheath

The myelin sheath became the model for ultrastructural investigation of membranes after its layered structure was first suggested by Schmitt and his coworkers (1935) and then verified by electron microscopy (Fernández-Moran, 1950; 1952). Perhaps this was because (1) it was the only membrane that could be obtained with any degree of purity and integrity and (2) it was so accessible. The formation of this interesting structure was shown to be the result of the spiral wrapping of the Schwann cell membrane around the axon (Geren and Schmitt, 1954) which produces a concentric tightly packed membrane of uniform thickness. In the formation of the myelin sheath, the axon lies in a trough formed by the cytoplasm of the Schwann cell which surrounds the axon. The cell rotates around the axon and produces the myelin spiral. According to Robertson (1955) the Schwann cells along an axon operate individually rather than in concert since the direction of the spiral is not consistent. A diagram illustrating how the Schwann cell membranes come together and fuse to form the spiral is shown in Fig. 19.5. For detailed molecular models based on X-ray diffraction and high resolution electron microscopy, see Vandenheuvel (1963), Fernández-Moran (1967), Kirschner and Casper (1972), and Worthington (1972).

Periodic interruptions occur in the myelin sheath that are designated the nodes of Ranvier. These nodes occur where two adjacent Schwann cells meet one another. Although no myelin is present at these areas of contact, there are villi and projections of the two Schwann cells that interdigitate (Fig. 19.6). As the myelin approaches the node, the lamellae of the membrane separate from

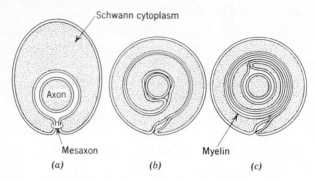

Fig. 19.5 Diagram of the development of nerve myelin. (*a*) Axon enveloped by a relatively large Schwann cell. (*b*) Intermediate stage. (*c*) Later stage showing formation of a few layers of compact myelin. [Adapted from J. D. Robertson, *Prog. Biophys.*, 10: 344, (1960).]

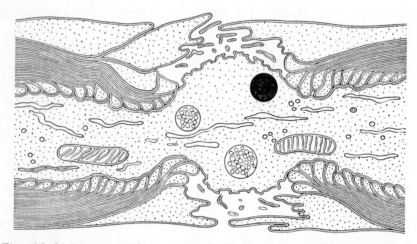

Fig. 19.6 Diagram of a node of Ranvier showing myelin sheath formed by two adjacent Schwann cells with unmyelinated gap between. Organelles are represented in axoplasm. [Redrawn from J. D. Robertson, *Prog. Biophys.*, 10: 344, (1960).]

the compact myelin, and each splits into its component plasma membranes which are continuous with a membrane from the adjacent layer. The interruptions in the myelin sheath at the nodes play a role in the speed of nerve conduction and will be discussed under function.

Myelin contains lipids, proteins, polysaccharides, salts, and water. Its unusual degree of metabolic inertness was demonstrated in early studies. Brain cholesterol of adult rats given deuterium did not become labeled whereas considerable amounts of deuterium were taken up by brain cholesterol in young rats (Waelsch et al., 1940; 1941). This suggested that the adult brain does not synthesize cholesterol. Studies indicated that the other major lipids in myelin—cerebroside, cephalins, and sphingomyelin—also underwent little metabolic turnover (Davison et al., 1959; Davison and Dobbing, 1960). It was concluded, therefore, that myelin was one of the more permanent tissues in the body although the reasons for the inertness were not clear.

The lipid composition of myelin in human brains from ages 10 months to 55 years was studied by O'Brien (1965). No differences in total lipid content of myelin were found related to age. Lipid constituted between 78 and 81 percent of the dry weight, the highest lipid content for any tissue of the body with the exception of adipose tissue. There was more than twice as much cholesterol as any of the other lipids in myelin. Only 1 in 17 fatty acids was polyunsaturated, and 1 in 5 fatty acids had a chain longer than 18 carbon atoms. The stability of myelin is attributed to both the small proportion of lipids containing polyunsaturated fatty acids and the presence of very long chain fatty acids (O'Brien, 1965). Data on erythrocyte membranes had provided evidence that an increase in the proportion of lipids containing unsaturated fatty acids led to a less stable membrane (Kogl et al., 1960). Myelin has been shown to have a low proportion of polyunsaturated fatty acids and, therefore, should be expected to have greater stability. (For a discussion of the relation of chain saturation to lipid packing, see Chapter 9).

Sphingolipids containing fatty acids with chain lengths of 19 to 26 carbon atoms are proportionately 10 times greater in myelin than in any other membrane analyzed. In certain genetic disorders, for example, Niemann-Pick disease, there is a seven- to tenfold deficiency of sphingolipids containing these long chain fatty acids (O'Brien, 1964). Similar deficiencies in sphingolipids containing long chain fatty acids have been reported for multiple sclerosis (Gerstl et al., 1963). O'Brien (1965) concluded that deficiency of long chain sphingolipid molecules results in either cessation of

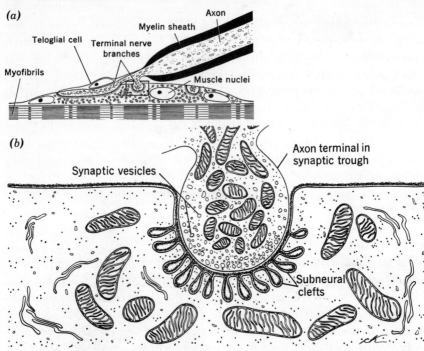

(a)

Axon

Myelin sheath

Teloglial cell   Terminal nerve
branches

Myofibrils

Muscle nuclei

(b)

Axon terminal in
synaptic trough

Synaptic vesicles

Subneural
clefts

Fig. 19.7 Diagram of a motor end plate for neuromuscular transmission in striated muscle. (a) Based on appearance under light microscope. (b) Based on an electron micrograph of an area comparable to rectangle on (a). (From W. Bloom and D. W. Fawcett, *A Textbook of Histology*, 9th ed., W. B. Saunders Company, Phila., 1968, p. 287.)

myelin formation or production of unstable myelin. Since myelin formed in the baby is "chemically mature," O'Brien (1965) suggested that myelination begins only when a specific chemical composition is reached; that is, when saturated glycerophosphatides and long chain sphingolipids are present in high proportions.

NEURON FUNCTION

The primary function of a neuron is to receive information in the form of an impulse and to carry that information along its axon to its terminals. These two facets of nerve function, *excitation* and *conduction*, depend on electrical activity. Excitation refers to the series of events that lead to a change in membrane potential when the impulse is received; and conduction to the propagation of that change in potential away from the point of excitation. Once started, conduction is a self-propagating process and depends on expenditure of energy by the nerve cell. Neurons function in sequence and in parallel, activity from one being transmitted to another (Grundfest, 1967). Neurons also transmit information to effectors such as secretory cells and muscle fibers and the message may be excitatory or inhibitory. A diagram of a motor end plate for transmission from nerve to striated muscle is shown in Fig. 19.7.

Membrane Potential

The specialized function of the neuron depends on the exploitation of a characteristic of the plasma membrane: the maintenance of a difference in composition between the intra- and extracellular fluids thereby establishing an electrical potential across the membrane; in other words, nerve cells are electrogenic. A *resting membrane potential* is present in all cells, with the interior of the cell negative to the exterior; but the magnitude of the potential varies with the type of cell. In most polarized cells, the resting membrane potential is kept within narrow limits; however, in nerve (and muscle) cells a decrease in membrane potential changes the characteristics of the membrane and permits a sudden increase in permeability to Na^+ ions. It is this unique difference that permits the generation of self-propagating impulses described below.

The neuron, like all other cells, maintains a higher concentration of K^+ ions in its intracellular fluid than is present in the extracellular environment. Extracellular fluid has a higher concentration of Na^+ ions. The plasma membrane of the neuron forms the boundary between these two fluids. In the resting condition, the plasma membrane is highly permeable to K^+ ions but only slightly permeable to Na^+ ions (Fig. 19.8*a*). As a result of this and its gradient, K^+ ions tend to leak out of the axon at a fairly high rate. This results in an excess of negative charges inside the cell due to the negative charges of the macromolecular proteins. The differential concentrations of the Na^+ ions and K^+ ions are maintained by the metabolic activity of the neuron involving the sodium pump and the electrical

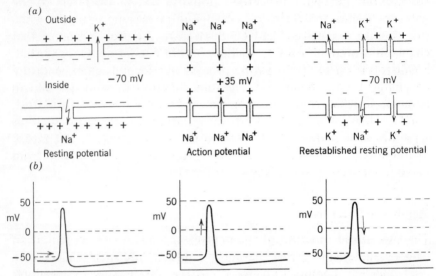

Fig. 19.8   (a) Movement of sodium and potassium ions during action potential. In resting condition, membrane is highly permeable to K^+ but only slightly to Na^+. Na^+ ions are pumped out and the leaked K^+ ions pumped back in. When stimulated, membrane becomes very permeable to Na^+ ions leading to depolarization and to peak of action potential. Reversal in polarity occurs when membrane again becomes essentially impermeable to Na^+ ions and more permeable to K^+ ions. (b) Action potential spike showing rapid reversal in polarity from -70 mV to $+35$ mV and back again.

gradient across the membrane (see Chapter 9). Na^+ ions which leak into the neuron are pumped back out, and the K^+ ions which diffuse out are pumped back in. As a result, there is a concentration of K^+ ions within the cell at least 10 times higher than outside, and a concentration of Na^+ ions that is 10 times lower. The interior of the cell is about -70 mV in relation to the extracellular fluid. This is the *resting potential* of the nerve cell.

When the nerve is stimulated, an alteration of the membrane's permeability to ions occurs. The membrane becomes very permeable to Na^+ ions that enter at a rate faster than they can be pumped out and depolarization is initiated. Immediately following the movement of Na^+ ions into the cell, K^+ ions diffuse out. After an initial decrease of 15 mV, the *firing level*, the rate of depolarization increases and the membrane potential drops to zero. This depolarization lasts for only a few milliseconds and reaches a peak at about +35 mV.

The increased voltage difference from the resting potential to this peak is the *action potential.* A sudden reversal occurs, and the potential falls rapidly at first toward the resting level, becoming slower after repolarization is about two-thirds complete. The rapid reversal in polarity from -70 mV to +35 mV and back again is called the *spike* (Fig. 19.8*b*). This reversal is brought about when the "Na$^+$ gate" closes and the membrane once again becomes essentially impermeable to Na$^+$ ions and more permeable to K$^+$ ions, thus permitting repolarization and reestablishment of the resting potential.

The action potential has two characteristics that are important in nerve stimulation. (1) After reaching a certain threshold of activation, regardless of the intensity of the stimulation, the height of the spike remains the same. This is referred to as an *all-or-none* response, which occurs at the point where and the moment when the impulse arises. (2) The impulse is *nondecremental,* that is, the amplitude of the spike remains the same as it is propagated along the course of the fiber. This characteristic is particularly important for conduction of impulses over long distances.

Propagation of the Nerve Impulse

The architecture of the neuron is particularly well adapted to its function of transmitting information over relatively long distances. The propagation of the nerve impulse depends upon the elongated conductile portion, the axon, that both separates and connects the areas of information reception and output. The characteristics of the axon enable it to generate signals that can be propagated rapidly along the cell with as little distortion as possible despite its length. This is achieved by the interaction of the intracellular fluid of the axon, the extracellular fluid surrounding the axon, and the membrane that separates these two compartments (Baker, 1966). The electrical system established is capable of generating spikes that can propagate themselves along the conductile membrane to the end of the axon. The manner in which this occurs intracellularly differs between myelinated and unmyelinated nerves. The *local circuit theory* describes conduction in unmyelinated nerves. Conduction in myelinated nerves is referred to as *saltatory conduction.* Intercellular conduction, or the transfer of information from one neuron to the others or to effector cells, is referred to as *synaptic*

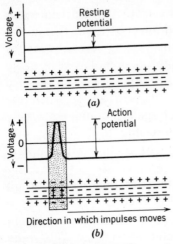
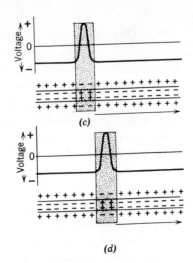

Fig. 19.9 Conduction of nerve impulse in nonmyelinated nerve. The curves represent electrical changes, and the cylinders represent an axon and the electrical charges inside and outside its membrane. (a) In a resting nerve cell (one that is not conducting an impulse) the inside of the cell is negative to the outside. Thus a voltage difference exists which is referred to as the resting potential (electrical potential = voltage). (b) When the axon is stimulated, the inside becomes positive or depolarizes at the point of stimulation. This increased voltage difference is called the action potential. Although the excited region quickly recovers its original negativity or repolarizes the impulse does not disappear. (c) Instead it moves forward along the axon. At the same time that the original excited region repolarizes, the region in front of it depolarizes. (d) These events are repeated down the length of the axon, which in this way conducts an impulse. (From J. D. Ebert, A. G. Loewy, R. S. Miller, and H. A. Schneiderman, *Biology*, Holt, Rinehart and Winston, Inc., N. Y., 1973, p. 406.)

transmission. Each of these will be discussed separately.

Local Circuit Theory. When a receptor is stimulated, a nerve impulse, or spike, is induced. This is an all-or-none response and is propagated along the axon without decrement. Each spike is followed by a short period of complete refractoriness during which it cannot react to another stimulus. This ensures that each spike is separated from the next. This type of propagation is restricted almost exclusively to axons and operates in the following manner: the point of stimulation becomes depolarized, or positive on the inside and negative on the outside. The next adjacent region still has a normal resting potential, and this causes a current to flow from the stimulated or depolarized area to the adjacent polarized area causing it to become depolarized. The area toward which the current flows is referred to as a sink. The area from which the current flowed is returned to its normal state of polarization. Repetition of this series of events causes the impulse to be propagated: each depolarized area setting up a flow of current that depolarizes the adjacent area and the action potential thereby travels along the membrane as a chain reaction (Fig. 19.9). The wave of depolarization is followed by such a rapid wave of repolarization that only a very short section of the axon is depolarized at one time.

The energy required for the specialized activity of the neuron involves the operation of the sodium pump which depends on the generation of a supply of ATP. It is suggested that the active ion transport involved in impulse propagation may be the major energy-consuming process of the neuron, and it has been correlated with the presence of a Na^+- and K^+-stimulated ATPase in the membrane. There is reason to believe that an electrogenic sodium pump is present in nerve cells; that is, a pump that generates a potential because the Na^+ ions pumped out are not balanced by K^+ ions coming in (see Kerkut and York, 1971). It is suggested that an electrogenic pump might provide a mechanism for metabolism to control the critical level of the membrane potential of the cell. However, both the electrogenic and the coupled Na^+-K^+ pumps have identical properties, and it is suggested that the efflux of Na^+ ions may occur through both mechanisms. There is still much to be learned about how important a role, if any, an electrogenic pump may have in the activity and control of the neuron. However, whether the pump is electrogenic or a coupled Na^+-K^+ pump, the energy required to drive it appears to be generated by the mitochondria present in the axoplasm and released by the ATPase in the membrane.

Saltatory Conduction. A pattern of current flow similar to that described by the Local Circuit Theory occurs in myelinated axons but, since the myelin sheath is a relatively effective insulator, little current can flow through it. Instead, the depolarization of the myelinated axon leaps from one node of Ranvier to the next. This is called saltatory conduction (after the Latin, *salta,* a leap or jump). The internodes act as passive conductors and the depolarization leaps from

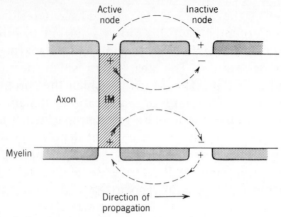

Fig. 19.10 Saltatory conduction. Local current flow around an impulse in a myelinated nerve. IM = Impulse. [From W. F. Ganong, *Review of Medical Physiology*, Lange Medical Publications, Los Altos, Ca., 1971, p. 25.)

node to node (Fig. 19.10). At each node the action potential is boosted to the same height by the ionic mechanism. The amount of Na^+ ions and K^+ ions that are exchanged is much reduced, and much less work is required for saltatory propagation. Since the myelin sheath improves the efficiency of the axon, the rate of conduction is 50 times faster in myelinated than in nonmyelinated axons. Furthermore, the thicker the myelin and the longer the internodes, the faster the conduction of the action potential.

Synaptic Transmission. Synaptic transmission involves the transfer of the information or impulse carried by a neuron to either another neuron or to effector sites. In most instances the transfer must be accomplished across a gap between membranes, the *synaptic cleft,* and this is accomplished through the aegis of a chemical waiting to be released for the performance of this particular mission, the *transmitter substance.*

The Synapse. The term *synapse* was coined by Sherrington in 1897 from the Greek meaning "to fasten together," and was meant to designate a site where the axon terminal of one neuron made functional contact with another neuron. The term has been expanded to include not only the axon to dendrite contact but also functional contacts between neurons and effector cells such as muscle and gland cells. The synapse then becomes the most important structure of the nerve cell, one that enables it to perform its primary function, the transmission of impulses. However, the synapse is not a site of cytoplasmic contact. It is an interface at which two neurons or neurons and effector cells are functionally related (see Fig. 19.4).

The *presynaptic membrane* is the plasma membrane of the axon; the *postsynaptic membrane* is the plasma membrane of the dendrite cell body, axon, or effector site of an adjoining cell. A salient functional characteristic of the synapse is that it is polarized. Electrical activity is transmitted across the synaptic cleft only from the presynaptic to the postsynaptic membrane. The transmission is mediated by means of a chemical released from the presynaptic ending. Such a synapse is referred to as a chemical synapse.

Through synaptic transmission the integrative function of the nervous system operates, permitting the action potential of an axon to exert its influence across the synaptic cleft. This is effected by the release of specific neurotransmitter substances at the nerve terminal which, in turn, affect the excitability of the postsynaptic membrane.

Synaptic Vesicles. Neurotransmitters accumulate in synaptic vesicles clustered against the presynaptic membrane (Hubbard and Kwanbunbumpen, 1968; Jones and Kwanbunbumpen, 1968). There is considerable evidence that the neurotransmitter in some vesicles is acetylcholine (Whittaker and Sheridan, 1965) and, in others, may be serotonin (5-hydroxytryptamine, 5-HT), γ-aminobutyric acid, and three catecholamines: epinephrine, norepinephrine, and dopamine (Rude et al., 1969; Tranzer et al., 1969). The vesicles containing the various transmitter substances are found within the presynaptic bouton at the axon ending along with numerous mitochondria. The mitochondria may be concerned with the need to provide energy for the energy-consuming processes involved in the synthesis of transmitter substances, the formation of the vesicles, and the storage of the neurotransmitters.

Synaptic vesicles are a constant and specific component of practically all synapses (Palay, 1967). De Robertis and Bennett (1954) showed, by use of the electron microscope, that vesicles are related to the secretion of the acetylcholine demonstrated at nerve endings by Fatt and Katz (1952). Later work has shown that the synaptic vesicles are the basic structural unit for the storage and quantal release of transmitter substance.

Receptor Sites. The involvement and release of transmitter substance presupposes that there are receptor sites on the post-synaptic membrane. De Robertis (1971) has shown that the receptor sites are proteolipid in character and undergo conformational changes when the transmitter binds to the receptor on the outer surface of the membrane. This produces the conformational change that permits translocation of ions through the membrane during synaptic transmission. There is evidence also that the isolated receptor sites show group specificity for various bivalent amines.

Postsynaptic Potentials. When the action potential reaches the presynaptic membrane, instead of crossing the membrane, it causes the release of discrete units of constant size, or quanta, of trans-mitter substance from the synaptic vesicles (Fatt and Katz, 1952). The release of the soluble constituents of the granules from the vesicles appears to be by a process of reverse pinocytosis also called exocytosis (Axelrod, 1974). The neurotransmitter crosses the gap in a few microseconds and attaches to specific receptor sites on the postsynaptic membrane. In the case of *excitatory synapses,* the attachment of the transmitter to the receptor sites causes fine channels in the membrane to open permitting Na^+ ions and K^+ ions to flow through the membrane. This produces an intense ionic flux that depolarizes the membrane. When a critical level of about -60 mV is reached the neuron discharges an impulse, the *excitatory post-synaptic potential* (EPSP). This may last for only a millisecond and by then the transmitter has either diffused out into surrounding areas or has become degraded by enzymes. For example, the enzyme acetylcholinesterase is known to destroy the neurotransmitter acetyl-choline, which is released from some synaptic vesicles (De Robertis, 1967).

Structurally the *inhibitory synapse* appears very similar to the excitatory one when examined with an electron microscope, but its stimulation produces an inhibitory effect by driving the internal voltage of a nerve cell in a negative direction. If the resting potential of the cell is -70 mV, and inhibitory impulses drive it down to -75 or -80 mV, the result is an increase in membrane potential and depres-sion of neuronal excitatory impulses. The transient increase in membrane potential is the *inhibitory postsynaptic potential* (IPSP).

The action of both inhibitory and excitatory synapses is due to changing the permeability of the synaptic membrane to the flow of ions. In the case of inhibitory synapses, Eccles (1965) has shown that it is the outward flow of K^+ ions through the membrane that

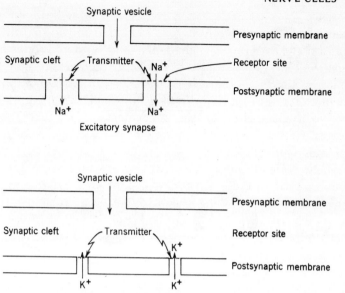

Fig. 19.11 Diagram showing excitatory transmission with inward flow of Na$^+$ ions and inhibitory transmission with outward flow of K$^+$ ions.

increases the negative potential within the cell. It appears that hydrated ions, to which the membrane is permeable under the influence of inhibitory transmitter substances, are smaller than the hydrated ions to which the membrane is impermeable. The hydrated Na$^+$ ion is larger than the hydrated K$^+$ ion. The difference between excitatory and inhibitory synaptic transmission is that the membrane is freely permeable to Na$^+$ ions in excitatory transmission and blocks their passage in inhibitory synaptic transmission. It appears likely that the channels through which the ions flow are selectively opened by transmitter substance; the excitatory neurotransmitter opening the larger channels to permit flow of Na$^+$ ions, and the inhibitory neurotransmittor opening the smaller channels to permit flow of K$^+$ ions (Fig. 19.11).

Mechanism of Action. The molecular mechanism responsible for the release of transmitter substance has not yet been clarified, but most of the relevant information suggests a role for Ca^{2+} ions in enabling transmitter release (Radouco-Thomas, 1971). Suggested mechanisms include triggering the migration of vesicles toward the membrane for transmitter release (Kopin, 1966); activation of

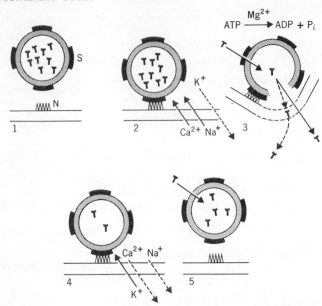

Fig. 19.12 Schematic diagram to explain release of transmitter material as a result of interaction between neurin (N) associated with synaptic membranes and stenin (S) associated with vesicle membranes. Stage 1, synaptic vesicle close to the presynaptic membrane. Stage 2, synaptic vesicle in intimate contact with the presynaptic membrane and the influx of Ca^{2+} in response to stimulation. Stage 3, the Ca^{2+} triggers interaction between neurin and stenin. Conformational changes in the membranes result in opening of the membranes. Transmitter (T) is released into the synaptic cleft or replaces transmitter in the membrane. Stage 4, the action is terminated by efflux of Ca^{2+}. Stage 5, the vesicle separates from the membrane. [From S. Berl, S. Puszkin, and W. J. Nicklas, *Science*, 179:441 (1973).]

release sites (Costa, 1968); and binding of the ions to a receptor complex and then in some manner providing a pore for the release of a quantal package of transmitter (Dodge and Rahaminoff, 1967). At myoneural junctions the amount of transmitter released varies directly with the Ca^{2+} ion concentration and inversely with the Mg^{2+} ion concentration at the terminal membrane.

An actomyosin-like protein, *neurostenin*, has been isolated from mammalian brain (Puszkin et al., 1968). It is comprised of a neuro-

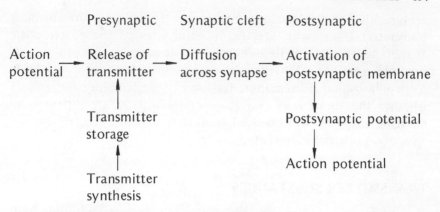

Fig. 19.13 Outline of processes involved in storage and release of chemical transmitter. (From *Best and Taylor's Physiological Basis of Medical Practice*, 9th ed., J. R. Brobeck, ed., Williams and Wilkins Company, Baltimore, 1973, p. 1-58.)

tubular protein, *neurin*, which has actin-like properties (Puszkin and Berl, 1970), and *stenin*, which has myosin-like properties. Berl et al. (1973) postulate that these proteins may be the means by which transmitter release takes place. Drawing an analogy to actomyosin, these investigators suggest that neurin may be associated with the membrane and stenin with the vesicles. Like actomyosin, neurostenin is a Mg^{2+}- and Ca^{2+}-activated ATPase. A model of transmitter substance release involving neurostenin at synaptic junctions is shown in Fig. 19.12. Synaptic vesicles in contact with the presynaptic membrane come under the influence of Ca^{2+} ions either released from binding sites in the membrane or entering the synaptic ending following depolarization that follows electrical stimulation. The Ca^{2+} ions trigger interaction between neurin and stenin, which is associated with conformational change in the membranes. Transmitter is then released into the synaptic cleft. The action is terminated by the efflux of Ca^{2+} ions, and the vesicle then separates from the membrane. This model suggests that transmitter release is similar to many other secretory processes in its dependence upon Ca^{2+} ions.

The chemical theory of synaptic transmission as enunciated by De Robertis (1971) suggests that a chemical substance acts to amplify the electrical signal and that this occurs between the presynaptic and postsynaptic membranes. In addition, the chemical transmitter reacts with specific receptor sites on the postsynaptic membrane which leads to a change in ionic permeability of the postsynaptic membrane. Whether the change in ionic permeability leads to depolarization or hyperpolarization of the membrane determines whether the stimulus is excitatory or inhibitory. An outline summarizing the processes involved leading to synaptic transmission of an action potential is presented in Fig. 19.13.

TRANSMITTER SUBSTANCES

The transmitter substances are relatively simple compounds and, except for acetylcholine, are derived from simple amino acid precursors: the three catecholamines, norepinephrine, epinephrine, and dopamine from tyrosine; γ-aminobutyric acid from glutamic acid; and serotonin from tryptophan. The precursors of acetylcholine are equally ubiquitous, choline and acetyl CoA. It is generally accepted that these are the neurotransmitters released from nerve endings. Amino acids proposed as transmitters are glycine, glutamic and aspartic acids, and proline (Snyder et al., 1973). It is also accepted that transmitter substance is synthesized within the neuron, packaged and stored in vesicles, and released through the presynaptic membrane into the synaptic cleft where it exercises its function as a transmitter and then is either metabolized or removed from the site. It appears quite clear that the cells from which the transmitters are released are responsible for their synthesis. Snyder et al. (1973) propose that the nerve terminals that utilize certain amino acids as transmitters have high affinity selective transport systems for the accumulation of those particular amino acids.

The Catecholamines: Norepinephrine, Epinephrine, and Dopamine

The synthesis of catecholamines was at first assumed to take place in the cell body, and von Euler (1958) suggested that the storage granules were transported down the axon to the endings by axoplasmic flow. There is evidence also (Dahlström and Häggendahl, 1966) that synthesis occurs all along the axon and that storage particles are filled with transmitter both during passage and in the axon terminals. The process leading to catecholamine formation according to Axelrod (1974) starts with synthesis of the four required enzymes

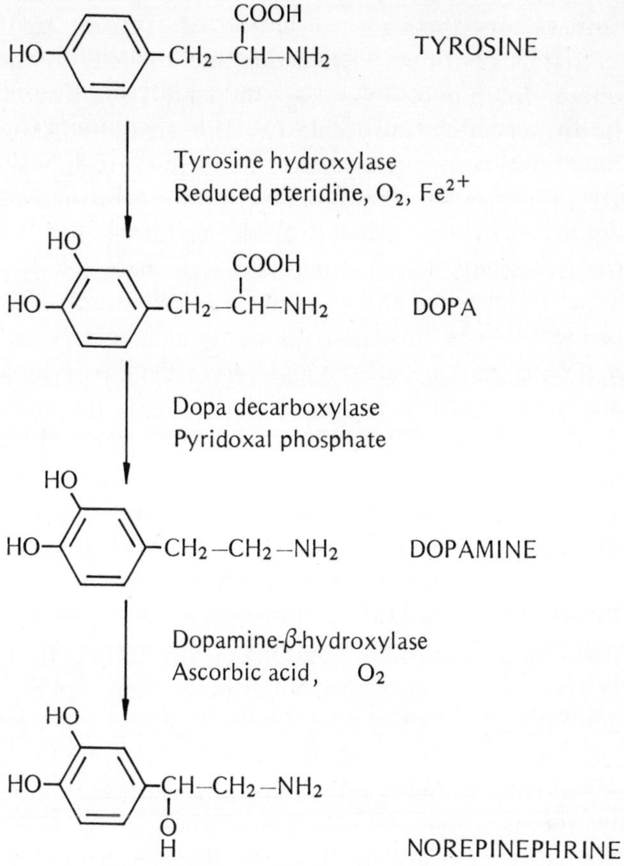

Fig. 19.14 The enzymatic steps in the synthesis of norepinephrine from tyrosine. [From N. Weiner, *Ann. Rev. Pharmacol.*, 10: 273 (1970).]

in the cell body and their passage down the axon to the nerve endings where the catecholamine synthesis takes place. Dopamine-β-hydroxylase is packaged in the vesicles along with norepinephrine and is released with it. This appears to be important in relation to a number of disorders which will be mentioned in a subsequent section.

The pathway for synthesis of all three catecholamines was established by Udenfriend's laboratory (Nagatsu, 1964). Synthesis proceeds through tyrosine to norepinephrine in three enzymatically catalyzed sequential steps (Fig. 19.14). The hydroxylation of tyrosine to dopa is the first and the rate-limiting step in norepinephrine synthesis and occurs through the action of tyrosine hydroxylase, an enzyme that is confined to neurons and to cells in the adrenal medulla where norepinephrine is synthesized (Udenfriend, 1966). Tyrosine hydroxylase can also catalyze the prior hydroxylation of phenylalanine to tyrosine (Nagatsu et al., 1964). It appears to be a soluble enzyme present in the axoplasm of the neuron (Wurzberger and Musacchio, 1971). A reduced pteridine factor and oxygen are required for its activity (Brenneman and Kaufman, 1964), and iron is an essential cofactor for the enzyme action (Petrack et al., 1968).

Decarboxylation of dopa to dopamine is catalyzed by the L-aromatic amino acid decarboxylase, dopa decarboxylase (Lovenberg et al., 1962), which is relatively nonspecific and requires pyridoxal phosphate for activity (Sourkes, 1966; 1972). This enzyme has been located in the cytosol.

The last step in synthesis requires the action of dopamine-β-hydroxylase to catalyze the formation of norepinephrine from dopamine. This is a copper-containing enzyme synthesized only in neurons and adrenal medulla (Kaufman, 1966). The reaction requires oxygen, ascorbic acid, and fumarate. The ascorbic acid serves as a reducing agent for the Cu^{2+} ions and acts as a co-substrate. Fumarate apparently speeds up the reoxidation of the Cu^{2+} ions. Catalase is also necessary to destroy peroxides formed by the auto-oxidation of ascorbate and dopamine (Axelrod, 1972). This reaction takes place in the vesicle where the product is stored (Geffen and Livett, 1971). Dopamine-β-hydroxylase has been located both in cell bodies and at the terminals (Mollinoff et al., 1970). At the terminal, it is present both in the membrane of the granule and in the soluble contents of the vesicle (Viveros et al., 1968).

Dopamine, a precursor of norepinephrine, has also been located in abundance in certain nerve terminals. In patients with Parkinson's disease there is depletion of dopamine in brain ganglia apparently due to low activity of dopamine-β-hydroxylase. Therapeutic administration of L-dopa produces an increase in enzyme activity (Lieberman et al., 1972), and eases the symptoms of the disease. This apparent paradox is due to decreased decarboxylation of L-dopa peripherally, which apparently makes more dopa available for entry into the brain where it may be decarboxylated to dopamine (Dairman et al., 1972).

Lower than normal dopamine-β-hydroxylase activity has also been noted in the brains of schizophrenic patients and, in addition, both tryptophan and methionine administration have been found to exacerbate the symptoms of this disorder. One clue appears to be related to the relative quantities of the N-methylated and O-methylated products that are produced by the amine-methylating enzymes in the brain which use 5-methyltetrahydrofolic acid as the methyl donor (Snyder et al., 1974).

Axelrod (1974) has found that the concentration of dopamine-β-hydroxylase released into the blood was low in a variety of other disease states including Down's syndrome, a neurological disease involving muscle spasticity (torsion dystonia), a cancer of nervous tissue (neuroblastoma), and in certain forms of hypertension. These findings suggest to him that functional abnormalities in the autonomic nervous system are associated with low levels of dopamine-β-hydroxylase in the blood.

The conversion of norepinephrine to epinephrine occurs almost exclusively in the adrenal medulla (Axelrod, 1972) and is catalyzed by the enzyme phenylethanolamine-N-methyl-transferase (PNMT). This enzyme is the only one unique to epinephrine production. The methyl group for the methylation was found to come from methionine. For discussion of epinephrine synthesis and secretion, see Fuller (1973).

Both norepinephrine and epinephrine are in constant flux, continuously being released, metabolized, synthesized, and reaccumulated; yet the level in the tissues is maintained remarkably constant (Axelrod, 1971). Biosynthesis is under precise control. One factor affecting rate of synthesis was shown to be its release from synaptic vesicles (Weiner and Alousi, 1967); another, the rapid feedback inhibition which appears to control tyrosine hydroxylase activity (Sedvall and Kopin, 1967). The suggestion is that concentration of free neuronal norepinephrine is reduced following transmitter release, and this cuts off the feedback inhibition thus stimulating the activity of tyrosine hydroxylase (Weiner et al., 1972). The activity and amounts of tyrosine hydroxylase, dopamine-β-hydroxylase, and PNMT transferase appear to be regulated physiologically. The activity of the enzymes may be influenced by endogenous inhibitors. The amount of the enzymes is subject to neuronal and hormonal influences such as glucocorticoids from the adrenal cortex (Fuller, 1973).

The storage of catecholamines is in the form of granules in

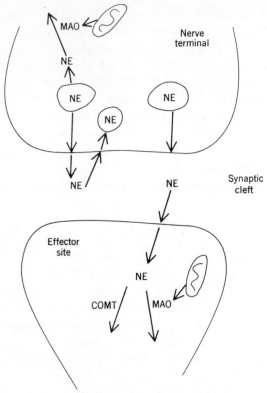

Fig. 19.15 Schematic drawing of fate of norepinephrine (NE) released from nerve terminal into synaptic cleft. NE binds to effector site to elicit response. Its activity is terminated either through action of catecholamine-*O*-methyl-transferase (COMT) or monoamine oxidase (MAO), which is released by mitochondrion. A major mechanism for terminating activity is reuptake and storage by the nerve terminal.

synaptic vesicles at nerve endings and also in the adrenal medulla. The granules also contain ATP in the ratio of one mole of ATP to four moles of the catecholamine; a specific protein with a molecular weight of about 40,000; and Mg^{2+} ions (Potter, 1966). The storage vesicles for norepinephrine have been observed by electron microscopy as dense-core vesicles at the nerve endings. Only the bound amines in the vesicles and not those in the soluble fraction are released by stimulation of the nerve (Kopin, 1967).

The release of the catecholamine from the synaptic vesicle involves the presence of Ca^{2+} ions and takes place along with the

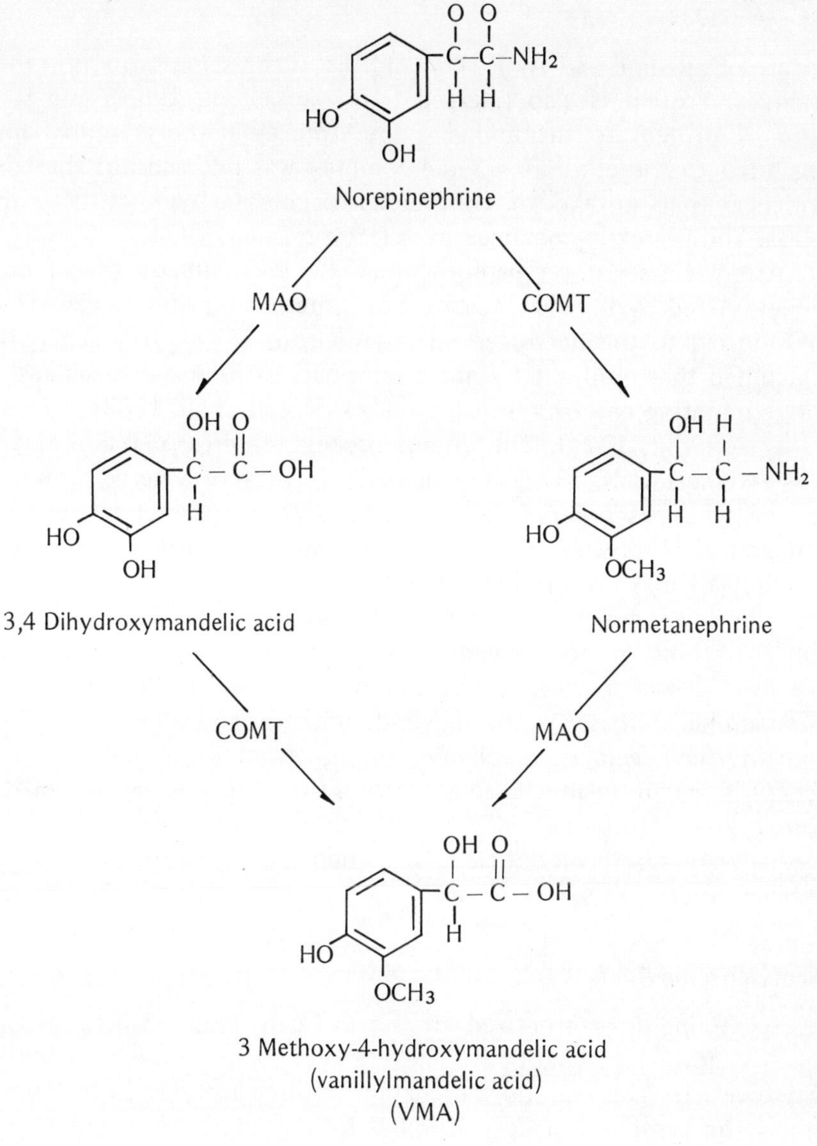

Norepinephrine

MAO

COMT

3,4 Dihydroxymandelic acid

Normetanephrine

COMT

MAO

3 Methoxy-4-hydroxymandelic acid
(vanillylmandelic acid)
(VMA)

MAO = monoamine oxidase; COMT = catechol-O-methyl transferase

Fig. 19.16 Pathways of norepinephrine metabolism. (From I. J. Kopin, "The Adrenergic Synapse," *The Neurosciences*, G. C. Quarton, T. Melnechuk, and F. O. Schmitt, eds., Rockefeller University Press, N. Y., 1967, p. 431.)

release of adenine and AMP. The AMP is in the same ratio as in the granules. Protein is also released (Kirshner et al., 1966), and the ratio of protein to the amine is the same as in the granule. This suggested that the whole granule complex was released but there is evidence that uptake of transmitter occurs concomitantly with release and is greatly enhanced by ATP (von Euler, 1971).

After release, norepinephrine may be taken up by the blood, O-methylated by the enzyme catechol-O-methyl-transferase (COMT), or returned to the nerve terminals (Axelrod, 1971). It is generally concluded that reuptake by nerve terminals is the major mechanism for terminating neurotransmitter action (Rosell et al., 1963; Iversen, 1967; Axelrod, 1974). The uptake process requires ATP and Mg^{2+} ions (Weiner et al., 1972). A schematic drawing of a nerve terminal that synthesizes norepinephrine, releases it, reaccumulates, or inactivates it, is shown in Fig. 19.15. The pathways for norepinephrine metabolism are shown in Fig. 19.16.

Riboflavin deficiency has been associated with decreased tissue concentrations of norepinephrine and epinephrine, particularly in the liver. This has been attributed to decreased hepatic levels of monoamine oxidase in riboflavin-deficient rats (Sourkes, 1972), and interference in catecholamine uptake from the blood for conversion to vanillylmandelic acid. Sourkes (ibid.) has shown that MAO contains covalently bound FAD and that activity can be restored gradually in riboflavin-deficient rats when the vitamin is added to a deficient diet.

Acetylcholine

Acetylcholine is synthesized in nerve fibers and retained in an inactive form in synaptic vesicles (Ritchie and Goldberg, 1970). These vesicles also contain the enzyme choline acetylase, which promotes the synthesis of acetylcholine from choline and acetyl CoA. For optimal activity, this enzyme requires Mg^{2+}, K^+, and Ca^{2+} ions. Ca^{2+} ions are required for the release of acetylcholine from the vesicles into the synaptic cleft. The receptor site has not been identified, but it is presumed to be a membrane protein which enables a permeability change to take place when activated by the acetylcholine.

Synthesis and release of acetylcholine appear to be closely regulated. In studies of acetylcholine release from ganglia, Birks and

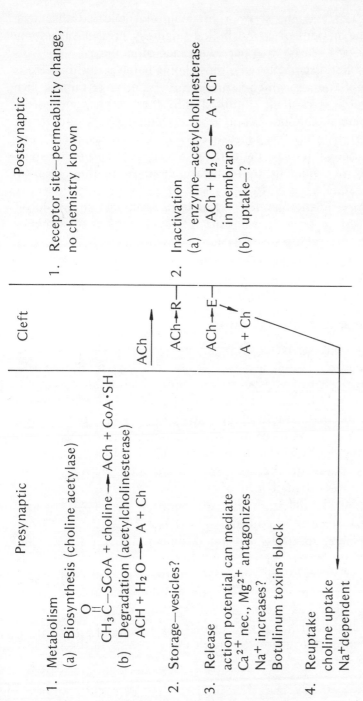

Fig. 19.17 Synaptic chemistry of acetylcholine. (From E. A. Kravitz, "Acetylcholine, Aminobutyric Acid and Glutamic Acid: Physiological and Chemical Studies Related to Their Roles as Neurotransmitter Agents," *The Neurosciences*, G. C. Quarton, T. Melnechuk, and F. O. Schmitt, eds., Rockefeller University Press, N. Y., 1967, p. 439).

MacIntosh (1961) could show a total amount released that was five times the amount of acetylcholine originally present suggesting that synthesis and release kept pace with each other.

Acetylcholine is hydrolyzed almost immediately after its release by acetylcholinesterase, which is present at the nerve terminals. The released choline is partially returned into the presynaptic neuron terminal where it can be reused for acetylcholine synthesis (MacIntosh, 1959). The uptake depends on Na^+ ions (Birks, 1963) and appears as though it may be part of an active transport system utilizing the Na^+ gradient to transport choline into the cell. The fate of the acetate is not clear.

A reduction in the number of functional acetylcholine receptor sites is thought to be responsible for the symptoms of myasthenia gravis, a neuromuscular disorder (Fambrough et al., 1973).

A summary of the synaptic chemistry of acetylcholine is presented in Fig. 19.17.

Gamma Aminobutyric Acid (GABA)

Gamma aminobutyric acid and the enzyme that synthesizes it (glutamate decarboxylase) are exclusively localized in the central nervous system (Wingo and Awapara, 1950). The pathway may be viewed as a shunt around the oxidative decarboxylation of a-ketoglutarate to succinate via succinyl-S-CoA (Fig. 19.18). It has been estimated that up to 40 percent of the metabolism of a-ketoglutarate is through this pathway (McKhann et al., 1960). Since transamination restores glutamate that has been decarboxylated there is no net change in the glutamate level of the cell.

Although some investigators have reported that GABA exists in the central nervous system and that it can be synthesized from succinic semialdehyde (Bessman and Fishbein, 1963, Fishbein and Bessman, 1964), these reports have not been confirmed.

Many gaps exist in our knowledge of the action of GABA as a transmitter substance and, in fact, its physiological role in mammalian central nervous system is still speculative (Kravitz, 1967). However, if it indeed has a role in mammals it may be that of an inhibitory transmitter, a function it clearly performs in the nervous system of the lobster.

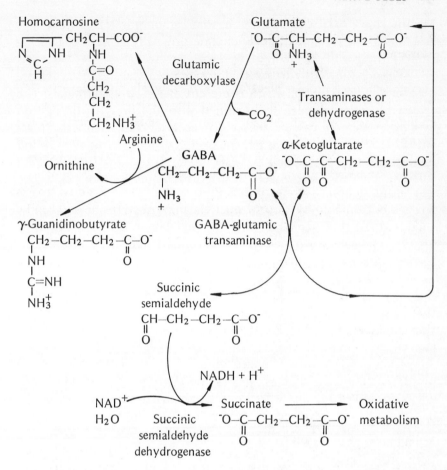

Fig. 19.18 Sequence of reactions for the synthesis and destruction of GABA. (From E. A. Kravitz, "Acetylcholine, Aminobutyric Acid and Glutamic Acid: Physiological and Chemical Studies Related to Their Roles as Neurotransmitter Agents," *The Neurosciences,* G. C. Quarton, T. Melnechuk, and F. O. Schmitt, eds., Rockefeller University Press, N. Y., 1967, p. 441.)

Serotonin

Serotonin, 5-hydroxytryptamine (5-HT), has been associated with nerve terminals especially in the brain. Its function, in a manner similar to acetylcholine in lower animals, led to the belief that 5-HT functions as a transmitter substance in mammals (Page, 1969). Subsequently, the storage of 5-HT coexisting with storage of nor-epinephrine was demonstrated in large granular vesicles in pineal nerve terminals through electron microscopy (Jaim-Etcheverry and Zieher, 1971). Selective depletion of the vesicles at pineal nerve endings was produced by an inhibitor of 5-HT synthesis at the hydroxylation step (Koe and Weissman, 1966). Through electron microscopic autoradiography, Bloom and Costa (1971) have shown certain synapses in the brain that are specific 5-HT synapses.

The oxidation of tryptophan to the hydroxy derivative is analagous to the conversion of phenylalanine to tyrosine and can be catalyzed by the same enzyme, phenylalanine hydroxylase (Fig. 19.19). The subsequent decarboxylation of 5-hydroxytryptophan is carried out by 5-hydroxytryptophan decarboxylase (Clark et al., 1954) to yield 5-hydroxytryptamine, or serotonin. The latter reaction can also be catalyzed by aromatic L-amino acid decarboxylase that also catalyzes the decarboxylation of dopa to dopamine (Lovenberg et al., 1962). Pyridoxine depletion affects the decarboxylase enzymes more than the transaminases (Scriver and Hutchinson, 1963). The personality changes reported in subjects placed on a pyridoxine-deficient diet as well as the abnormal electroencephalograms observed could well be related to interference with the decarboxylation involved in production of the catecholamines, serotonin, and GABA (Sauberlich et al., 1970).

The synthesis of serotonin, like the synthesis of the catecholamines, occurs in the tissues where it is found. In the case of serotonin, the major loci are the brain and gastrointestinal tract.

Further metabolism of serotonin is by way of oxidative deamination to form 5-hydroxyindoleacetic acid (5-HIAA) (Fig. 19.20) and this reaction is catalyzed by a monoamine oxidase (MAO). The urinary excretion of 5-HIAA amounts to 2-8 mg per day.

Several investigators have reported diurnal peaks of serotonin concentration (Dixit and Buckley, 1967; Sheving et al., 1968). There is evidence to suggest that this variation is related to diurnal fluctuations of plasma and brain tryptophan concentration. The functional meaning of the changes in concentration of serotonin are not clear (Bloom and Costa, 1971), but a recent report provides for interesting speculation especially for nutritionists. Fernstrom

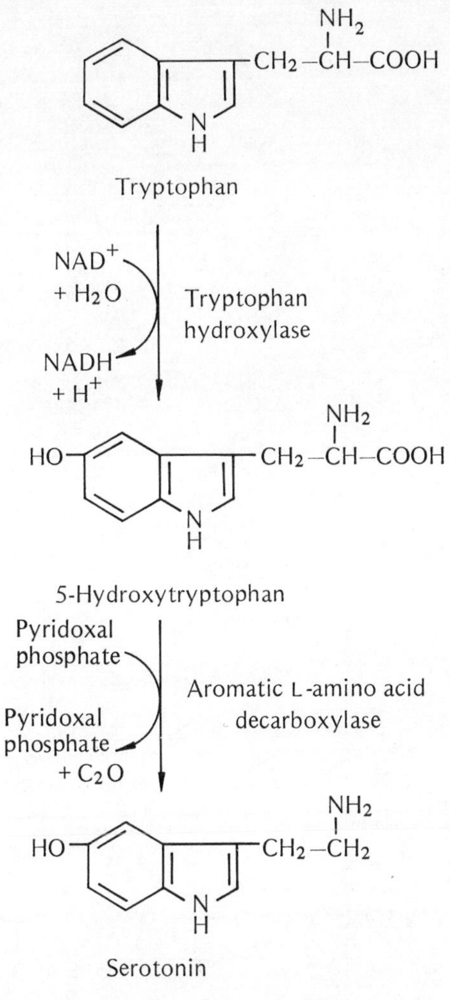

Fig. 19.19 Biosynthesis of serotonin.

and Wurtman (1974) have found that following the ingestion of a meal high in carbohydrate there is an increase in the rate at which the brain synthesizes the neurotransmitter serotonin. This response occurs in rats within an hour after eating and is preceded by a change in the concentration of amino acids in the plasma. The concentration of most amino acids decreases, but the concentration of tryptophan increases in the plasma, and there is a

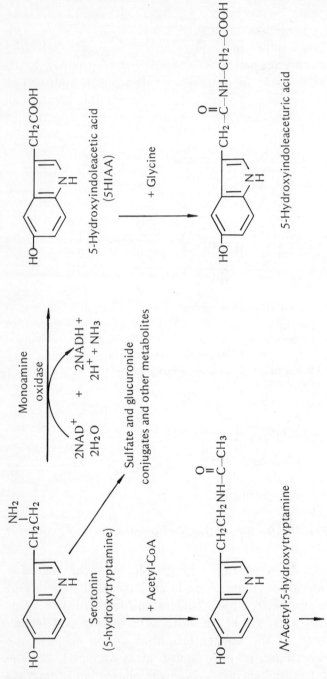

Fig. 19.20 Catabolism of serotonin. In oxidative deaminations catalyzed by monoamine oxidase, an aldehyde is formed first and then oxidized to the corresponding acid. Some of the aldehyde is also reduced to the corresponding alcohol. The heavy arrow indicates the major metabolic pathway. (From W. F. Ganong, *Review of Medical Physiology*, Lange Medical Publications, Los Altos, Ca., 1971, p. 182.)

proportional increase in the uptake by the brain. The rate of serotonin synthesis also increases in the serotonergic neurons. This increase in the availability of tryptophan for serotonin synthesis takes on added interest when it is realized that tryptophan is the least abundant amino acid in protein, and tryptophan hydroxylase is a low affinity enzyme. Therefore, only when the tryptophan concentration is higher than normal can the enzyme function at the maximum rate. When the available tryptophan was increased by injection, the brain tryptophan and brain serotonin increased, and the diurnal variations in plasma were paralleled by changes in brain serotonin.

Since insulin lowers the amino acid concentration of plasma, plasma tryptophan levels were determined following insulin injection. Contrary to expectation, plasma tryptophan, and brain tryptophan and serotonin, were increased. Never before had there been evidence of neurotransmitter synthesis in the brain being increased by a hormone.

Further work indicated that plasma tryptophan was increased by protein intake but that neither brain tryptophan nor serotonin were elevated. It soon became apparent that brain tryptophan and serotonin were more a reflection of the ratio of tryptophan to other neutral amino acids than of the plasma level of tryptophan alone. A high protein diet would elevate all amino acids and thereby lower the ratio of tryptophan to other amino acids; but a high carbohydrate diet would, through stimulation of insulin secretion, increase the ratio. It then became apparent that the reason plasma tryptophan did not decrease following insulin administration was that it, like fatty acids, was carried by plasma albumin and, under usual circumstances, it competed with the other neutral amino acids for the transport system into the brain. Insulin not only released fatty acids from the albumin carrier and pulled them from the plasma, it also pulled amino acids from the plasma; that is, all the amino acids with exception of tryptophan that immediately became attached to the albumin that the fatty acids had freed. As a result, tryptophan content of the plasma remained high, and the tryptophan was protected from the action of insulin. Fernstrom and Wurtman (*loc. cit.*) postulate that the sensitivity of brain serotonin concentration to dietary change suggests that the serotoninergic neurons release more serotonin into synapses with a high carbohydrate diet, thereby transmitting specific signals through the neurons and conveying the message of "carbohydrate-richness" to other parts of the brain or to neuroendocrine mechanisms, to bring about some metabolic consequence. It has also been suggested that brain serotonin level in rats can influence both motor activity and food consumption.

The possibilities for speculation are enticing: Lát (1967) has shown that associative and discriminatory types of learning are closely correlated with "nonspecific excitability level" or "tonus" of the central nervous system. He also showed that rats with an inherited high excitability level self-selected a high carbohydrate diet. If such rats were fed a high protein diet their excitability levels decreased. Similarly, rats with a low excitability level self-selected high protein diets and their excitability levels increased when fed high carbohydrate. Could it be that such dietary responses are related to plasma-borne messages to the brain which are translated into behavior by neurotransmitters? An interesting thought.

CONCLUSION

Understanding of the mechanisms involved in nerve cell function and the roles played by electrolytes in conduction and transmission of nerve impulses should make it apparent that any disturbance in the maintenance of electrolyte concentrations in the intra- and intercellular environment could interfere with function. Since the single neuron is ineffective unless its message can be passed along to other neurons or to effector cells, the synthesis of transmitter substances becomes a key factor in the coordination attained by the nerve cells. These simple transmitter chemicals which, except for acetylcholine, are derived from amino acids or are amino acids themselves, may be closely associated with nutrient intake or dependent upon specific nutrients for their synthesis. The well-known associations of electrolytes such as Ca^{2+}, Mg^{2+}, and Na^+ to nerve function, and of vitamins such as thiamine, pyridoxine, nicotinic acid, ascorbic acid, and vitamin B_{12}, make abundantly clear that an intimate relationship exists between those nutrients and nerve function. The prominence of nerve function derangement in disorders of amino acid metabolism can be understood both in relationship to the high rate of protein synthesis in the neuron and the need for substrate for the synthesis of transmitter substance. This definitely becomes a case of matter over mind.

chapter 20

adipose cells

1. **White Fat Cell**
   a. Structure
   b. Function
      1. Lipogenesis
         a. Fatty Acid Transport
         b. Glucose Transport
         c. Fatty Acid Synthesis
         d. Triacyl glycerol Synthesis
      2. Lipolysis
         a. Fatty Acid Acceptors
         b. Fate of Liberated Glycerol

2. **Brown Fat Cell**
   a. Structure
   b. Function
3. **Conclusion**

"If one attempts to summarize the results of the isotope work on fats, one is compelled to conclude that the normal animal's body fats, despite their qualitative and quantitative constancy, are in a state of rapid flux. It can readily be understood why the classical methods of metabolism, which were mainly limited to the measurement of changes in amount or relative composition, failed to detect this dynamic state."

Rudolf Schoenheimer, *The Dynamic State of Body Constituents,*
1949, p. 23-24

Fat cells are normally present in loose connective tissue either singly or in small groups. When large numbers of these cells are organized, the resulting lobules constitute adipose tissue. The specialized capability of fat cells is the storage of a fuel reserve, which may vary in extent from an approximate 40-day reserve in the average person to one sufficient for a year or more in some obese individuals. At first, fat cells were thought to be placid repositories of excess fuel which, when organized into subcutaneous layers, served as insulating material to prevent loss of body heat. Another recognized function of adipose tissue was its ability to cushion and support abdominal organs. However, the highly specialized role of fat cells in the homeostasis of the organism was established by Schoenheimer and Rittenberg (1935), who demonstrated that even when the quantity of depot fat remained constant, it was continually being degraded and synthesized.

In most mammals there are two distinct types of fat cells which differ considerably in size, number, distribution, and metabolic activity. The bulk of the fat cells are the *white adipose cells* organized as adipose tissue in the subcutaneous layers, the mesenteries and omentum, the retroperitoneal regions, and as isolated fat cells in loose connective tissue. *Brown adipose cells* are much less abundant and occur only in restricted areas. Although present in man and other primates to a limited extent, brown adipose cells are abundant in hibernating animals and their specialized role will be discussed in a later section. Unless otherwise indicated, the material that follows refers to white or ordinary adipose cells.

WHITE FAT CELL

Structure

The number, dimensions, and composition of fat cells varies with individuals, with subcutaneous site sampled, and with nutritional state. The fat cell number in human subjects calculated by dividing the total body fat by the average fat cell content ranges from approximately 21 to 43 x 10^9 (Salans et al., 1971). It is generally believed that the number of adipose cells reaches a maximum during adolescence or early adult life and tends to remain fixed after that (Hirsch and Knittle, 1970). However, it is granted that years of excessive calorie intake in adult man could lead to hyperplasia as well as hypertrophy of existing cells (Salans et al., 1971). Bray and Gallagher (1970) reported a marked increase in cell number in an adult who became obese after the development of a hypothalamic tumor.

Overfeeding in infancy results in an increase in the number of fat cells. This appears to play an important role in adult obesity since there are more cells available waiting to be filled (Knittle and Hirsch, 1967). Moderate overfeeding of an adult leads only to larger cells, with no increase in number (Hirsch et al., 1966; Björstein and Sjöström, 1971). A difference in fat cell size and in the appearance of the cells in the adipose tissue in a 2-day old and an 8-week old rat is pictured in Fig. 20.1.

The prominent and distinguishing feature of the fat cell is the large central lipid droplet that dwarfs and dislocates the other cellular contents. The lipid, surrounded by a thin rim of cytoplasm, appears homogeneously opaque in electron micrographs (Fig. 20.2). The nucleus, distorted to a crescent shape, lies between the lipid and the plasma membrane. In histological preparations the lipid is

2 days   8 weeks

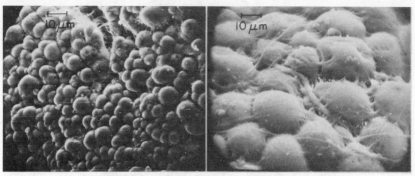

Fig. 20.1 Adipose tissue taken from a 2-day old and an 8-week old rat showing difference in size of fat cell. Scanning electron micrograph of epididymal adipose tissue. Magnification 1000. (Courtesy of Dr. Jerry Regunburg.)

dissolved out, and the fat cell in cross section often looks like a signet ring. All the cell organelles are distributed in the rim of cytoplasm between the lipid and the plasma membrane. The mitochondria tend to be spherical and contain a dense matrix. The cristae extend across the entire organelle. In addition, there is a small Golgi complex, a few short cisternae of rough endoplasmic reticulum, and some free ribosomes. The plasma membrane often has pinocytotic invaginations.

Whether or not the conspicuous lipid droplet is surrounded by a membrane is not clear. Fawcett (1966) suggests that since the lipid accumulates in the cytoplasmic matrix and not within the organelles, it is not membrane-bound. The dense interface between the lipid and the cytoplasm that appears in some preparations does not have any of the characteristics of typical lipoprotein membranes. To call it a membrane can only be a misinterpretation (Fawcett, 1966). Even though electron micrographs do not reveal a typical membrane surrounding the lipid in the adipose cell, during cell fractionation the cell lipases are extracted with the lipid. It is assumed that a close structural relationship must exist between the lipid and the lipases. Galton (1971) doubts that the enzymes "lie naked" at the interface and suggests that the presence of a membrane would provide for both the stabilization and attachment of the

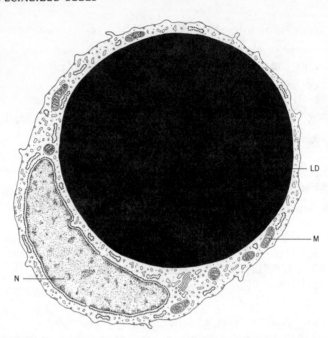

Fig. 20.2 White Adipose cell. N, nucleus; M, mitochondrion; Ld, lipid droplet. (From T. L. Lentz, *Cell Fine Structure*, W. B. Saunders Co., Phila., 1971.)

enzymes. Despite the ready-made function waiting to be assigned, no membrane has as yet been identified.

Function

The constant turnover of the lipid content of the fat cell requires the controlled transport of glucose and fatty acids into the cell where they are converted to triacyl glycerol during lipogenesis, and the transport of fatty acids and glycerol out of the cell after they have been released during lipolysis.

Lipogenesis. The liver is recognized as the primary site of fatty acid synthesis in man (Shrago et al., 1966) and in pigeons (Goodridge and Ball, 1966). Even in the rat whose fat cells have a much higher capability for fatty acid synthesis, the major portion of fat that is eventually stored in adipose tissue cells is derived from hepatic synthesis (Markscheid and Shaffir, 1965;

Zurier et al., 1967; Hollenberg, 1967). The liver exports fatty acids to the circulation as lipoproteins. In addition to the fatty acids synthesized in the liver from acetyl CoA, fatty acids are taken up from the circulating free fatty acids, incorporated into triacyl glycerols in the liver and exported to the plasma. Another source of plasma triacyl glycerols are those arriving via the lymphatic system after intestinal absorption and incorporation into chylomicra and lipoproteins (see Chapter 6).

Fatty Acid Transport. Neither lipoproteins nor chylomicra can leave the plasma by penetrating the endothelial wall of the capillaries. The enzyme *lipoprotein lipase,* also known as the *clearing factor* or *clearing factor lipase,* has been found in human adipose tissue (Marshall, 1965). It probably is bound to the endothelial surfaces of the capillaries supplying the tissue (Patten and Hollenberg, 1967; Ho et al., 1967). It liberates the triacyl glycerol from the molecules (Harlan et al., 1967) and may also be involved in the uptake of the triacyl glycerol and fatty acids by the tissue (Nestel et al., 1969). Also present in loose connective tissue, and particularly numerous along the small blood vessel walls, are the *mast cells* which are distinguished in stained preparations by large quantities of dense granules. These granules contain two substances: histamine and the sulfated mucopolysaccharide, heparin. Heparin, secreted by the mast cell into the intercellular substance of loose connective tissue, participates in the action of lipoprotein lipase (Patten and Hollenberg, 1967). The mechanism of its participation is not clear. It apparently causes lipoprotein lipase to be released and increases its binding to its substrate. It may activate the enzyme, stimulate its production, act in tandem with it, or furnish a part of the active enzyme molecule. In any case, heparin is essential for the effect of lipoprotein lipase in "clearing" the plasma; that is, dissipating the chylomicra which give plasma a milky appearance.

Much of the free fatty acid penetrates the endothelium and then associates with the membrane of the fat cell (Vaughan et al., 1964; Knittle and Hirsch, 1965; Donabedian and Karmen, 1967). The mechanism controlling subsequent passage of the free fatty acids through the plasma membrane has not been clarified. It is assumed to be an active process (Shapiro et al., 1957; Galton et al., 1971), and could be similar to fatty acid transport through mitochondrial membranes. The free fatty acid remaining in the plasma and the glycerol released are circulated back to the liver or to other tissues.

Lipoprotein lipase activity is integrated into the total metabolic scheme. It has high activity in the fed state when lipogenesis is required, and low activity during fasting or starvation when fat must be mobilized from fat cells (Hollenberg, 1959). An inverse correlation has been observed in man between the activity of lipoprotein lipase activity of adipose tissue and the levels of serum triacyl glycerols (Persson et al., 1966). Insulin, which promotes lipogenesis, appears to increase the activity of lipoprotein lipase, but whether this is a primary or secondary function of insulin is not clear (Avruch et al., 1972).

Glucose Transport. Insulin is of particular importance in the transport of glucose into the fat cell (Renold, 1965). In addition to the insulin requirement, the process is an active one that is Na^+-dependent (Letarte and Renold, 1969; Morgan and Neely, 1972). The mechanism by which insulin facilitates glucose entry is the subject of intensive study.

Cuatrecasas (1973a) has demonstrated that insulin receptors are located on the outer surface of the fat cell membrane and that approximately 10,000 molecules of insulin can be bound per fat cell (Cuatrecasas, 1971a). The binding of insulin to the membrane is a saturable, time- and temperature-dependent reaction. The binding is highly specific for insulin, the binding of proinsulin being 20 times less (Cuatrecasas, 1971b). The binding molecule on the membrane appears to be glycoprotein in nature (Cuatrecasas and Tell, 1973b) and is restricted to the external surface of the membrane (Bennett and Cuatrecasas, 1973).

The mechanism by which insulin acts to permit the entry of glucose into the fat cell is not clear. Since insulin promotes lipid synthesis and cAMP promotes lipid breakdown, it has been suggested that the action of insulin involves the inhibition of adenyl cyclase activity thereby decreasing the concentration of cAMP in adipose cells (Butcher et al., 1968). It has been suggested also that insulin may directly modulate cAMP activity (Illiano and Cuatrecasas, 1972) or that it might modify adenyl cyclase activity by producing a change in the conformation of the membrane (Cuatrecasas, 1973). However, a decrease in response to insulin such as observed during starvation is not accompanied by an observable defect in the receptor site (Bennett and Cuatrecasas, 1972).

The presence of cGMP as well as cAMP in all living tissues suggested to Goldberg et al. (1973) that bidirectional cellular processes may be controlled by the interaction of these two nucleotides. These investigators have shown that insulin is associated with rapid increase in the intracellular concentrations of cGMP in systems where it promotes responses opposite to those produced by cAMP. The fat cell qualifies as such a system since insulin promotes lipogenesis and is associated with low cAMP, whereas lipolysis is associated with an increase in cAMP. Whether cGMP is indeed involved in the action exerted by insulin on the fat cell membrane leading to the entry of glucose into the cell remains speculative but intriguing.

Still another hypothesis to explain insulin action on the fat cell suggests that the insulin molecule combines with the plasma membrane at a site near the glucose carrier. An alteration in membrane structure takes place, and this, in turn, enhances the carrier activity (Galton, 1971).

For further discussion of the mechanism of insulin action at the fat cell membrane, see Avruch et al. (1972).

The responsiveness of the fat cell to insulin was reported to be related to the size of the cell: the larger the mean cell size, the less responsive it was to insulin (Salans et al., 1968). Adipose cells of obese individuals which are larger and filled with lipid displayed a diminished response to insulin, but after weight loss and reduction of adipose cell size, the response to insulin returned to normal. One explanation offered was that the overfilled cell might have distorted membrane receptor sites (Jungas, 1966) which returned to normal after weight loss. However, some investigators were unable to find differences in the sensitivity to insulin in adipose cells from obese and nonobese individuals (Davidson, 1972), and others (Bray, 1969) suggested that the state of nutrition as well as cell size affected insulin-stimulated glucose metabolism in the fat cell. In a recent report, Salans et al. (1974) suggest the disparity in results attributed to insulin in human adipose tissue reflects the composition of the diet ingested prior to tissue sampling as well as cell size; and that the dietary and morphologic effect could be dissociated. Adipose cells examined under conditions of similar nutrition and growth showed no difference in insulin response according to size.

Upon entry into the adipose cell glucose may proceed through the glycolytic pathway to the cleavage of fructose-1,6-diphosphate to the trioses, dihydroxyacetone phosphate, and phosphoglycer-

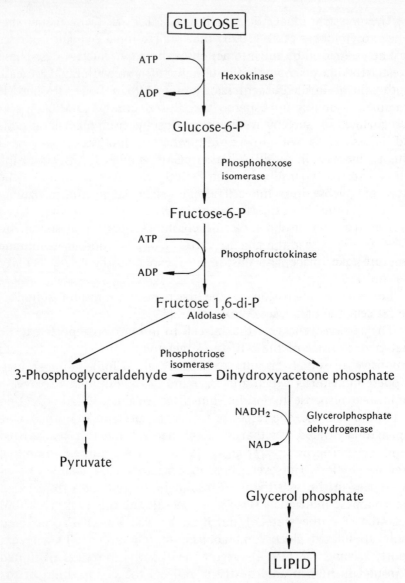

Fig. 20.3 Glycolytic sequence leading to the formation of glycerol phosphate.

aldehyde. Oxidative breakdown of dihydroxyacetone phosphate can continue, or it can be reduced to glycerol phosphate. The reaction is catalyzed by an NAD-linked glycerol phosphate dehydrogenase and provides the link between glycolysis and lipogenesis (Fig. 20.3).

The glycerol phosphate is a major acceptor for long chain fatty acids in the synthesis of neutral lipid.

Fatty Acid Synthesis. The conversion of glucose into lipid occurs readily. In mouse adipose cells, 90 percent of ^{14}C-glucose appears in glyceride fatty acids (Jansen et al., 1966a; 1966b). In human fat cells, only 16 percent or less is found in the fatty acid moiety and 80 percent in the glyceride-glycerol. Human adipose tissue does not appear to be an important site for synthesis of fatty acids based on ^{14}C recovery (Bjorntorp et al., 1968) and on studies of key enzyme levels (Shrago et al., 1966). However, data supporting fatty acid synthesis in human adipose cells have been presented by Jacob (1963) and by Goldrick et al. (1969).

The enzymes involved in fatty acid synthesis in the fat cell show an adaptive response to changes in diet and in hormonal balance. These changes are referred to as long-term changes and take two to four days to come into effect (Lowenstein, 1972). These responses in the fat cell have been ascribed to the rate of glucose utilization, which is controlled by insulin. However, there is no evidence that insulin exerts a direct effect on the enzyme levels for fatty acid synthesis.

If the fatty acids are not synthesized in the human fat cell, they are transported there by lipoprotein triacyl glycerols and phospholipids after hepatic synthesis. For further details of fatty acid synthesis, see Chapter 13.

Triacyl glycerol Synthesis. Glucose can be used by adipose tissue to form the entire triacyl glycerol molecule (Farvarger, 1965). Long chain fatty acids synthesized in the fat cell from glucose or transported there following hepatic synthesis react with L-α-glycerophosphate leading to the formation of diacylglycerols and then triacylglycerols (see Chapter 13). The metabolic sequence shown in Fig. 20.4 has been demonstrated in mitochondria from rat adipose tissue (Shapiro et al., 1960; Steinberg and Vaughan, 1961; Roncari and Hollenberg, 1967). The importance of this pathway to lipid synthesis in human adipose cells is not established.

Lipolysis. The hydrolysis of fat prior to its release from the fat cell is a tightly controlled series of reactions—so tightly controlled in some individuals that one wonders if it occurs at all. All of the steps in the pathway leading from stored lipid in the fat cell to fatty acids and glycerol available for transport are separate from the pathways leading to lipogenesis. This separation of power increases

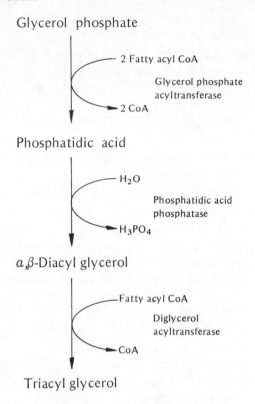

Glycerol phosphate

2 Fatty acyl CoA

Glycerol phosphate
acyltransferase

2 CoA

Phosphatidic acid

H_2O

Phosphatidic acid
phosphatase

H_3PO_4

a,β-Diacyl glycerol

Fatty acyl CoA

Diglycerol
acyltransferase

CoA

Triacyl glycerol

Fig. 20.4   Steps in the synthesis of triacyl glycerol.

the complexity of metabolic activity in the fat cell but also provides for finer control.

Since a specific function of the fat cell is to store fuel in periods of plenty and to release it during periods of deprivation, it is particularly important that the reactions leading to storage and release of fat be integrated with the needs of the total organism. *Hormone-sensitive lipase*, the enzyme that catalyzes triacyl glycerol hydrolysis in adipose tissue (Vaughan et al., 1964), is much more active in fat cells of fasted than of fed animals (Hollenberg, 1965). Increased activity of the enzyme occurs also after brief exposure of fat cells to epinephrine, norepinephrine, glucagon, ACTH, and several other hormones (Vaughan, 1966; Butcher and Sutherland, 1967). Activity of the enzyme is decreased after fat cells are exposed to insulin or prostaglandin E_1 (Butcher and Baird, 1968; Manganiello et al., 1971). Since hormone-sensitive lipase is the rate-determining

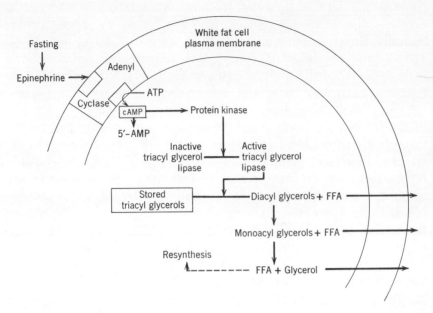

Fig. 20.5 Model of lipolysis in white fat cell. Adipose cell of rat responds to glucagon and ACTH; human adipose cell does not. Level of cAMP is the major controlling factor in lipolysis.

enzyme in lipolysis, its activity controls the overall rate of lipolysis (Hollett and Auditore, 1967).

Changes in hormone-sensitive lipase activity induced by hormones are associated with changes in the intracellular content of cAMP (Manganiello et al., 1971). The model shown in Fig. 20.5 incorporates the second messenger concept of cAMP action (Sutherland, 1972), the theory of allosteric regulation suggested by Monod et al. (1965), and the concept of enzymatic interconversion as postulated by Segal (1973) or by Rodbell (1973). The hormone that initiates lipolysis binds to the regulatory site of adenyl cyclase on the outer surface of the plasma membrane of the fat cell. An allosteric effect exposes the catalytic component on the inner surface of the membrane, which converts ATP to cAMP in the cell. The activation of protein kinase is effected by binding of cAMP, which causes dissociation of a receptor unit-catalytic unit complex thereby liberating the free catalytic unit (see Chapter 11). The protein kinase then transforms the inactive hormone-sensitive triacyl glycerol lipase to the active form. It is this hormone that controls the rate of lipolysis. Hormone stimulation of lipolysis in human adipose tissue appears to be effected by a mechanism basically similar to that in rat adipose tissue (Khoo et al., 1974). The di- and monoacyl glycerol lipase activities are not correlated with the level of the hormone (Vaughan, 1967), but their activities follow sequentially after the rate-controlling lipase is activated.

Fatty Acid Acceptors. The fatty acids released by hydrolysis in the fat cell are made water-soluble for transport by the plasma through the formation of an albumin-FFA complex. Lipolysis in the fat cell, therefore, is influenced by the plasma albumin available for the removal of the fatty acids from the cell. Increase in the amount of albumin available for transport is effected not by increasing albumin synthesis but simply by the expedient of increasing the blood flow to the adipose tissue. This has been shown to occur when fat mobilization is increased by norepinephrine, glucagon, or fasting in man (Nielson et al., 1968) and in rats (Mayerle and Havel, 1969). Although the concentration of fatty acids in the plasma is low, a significant amount can be transported to other tissues because of its rapid turnover. For discussion of the importance of fatty acids in the total fuel economy, see Chapter 23.

Fate of Liberated Glycerol. For want of an enzyme glycerol is lost. Lost, that is, as far as the metabolic machinery of the fat cell is concerned. Almost all of the glycerol liberated by hydrolysis of triacyl glycerol diffuses into the plasma because the fat cell lacks glycerokinase thereby preventing the re-use of the glycerol in the esterification of acyl CoA. Glycerokinase has recently been found in rat adipose tissue (Robinson and Newsholme, 1967), but its activity does not appear to have any significance. The glycerol liberated by hydrolysis is carried by the plasma to tissues, such as the liver and kidney, that can provide the enzyme required for its phosphorylation.

BROWN FAT CELL

Brown fat, a specialized form of adipose tissue, is much less widely distributed than white fat. However, at birth brown fat is usually more abundant than the common white variety. It is found in newborn animals and in adult cold-adapted animals where it forms what

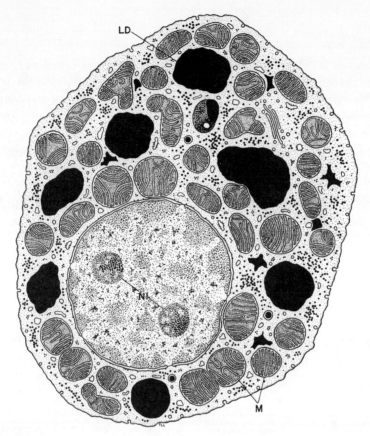

Fig. 20.6 Brown adipose cell. LD, lipid droplet; M, mitochondron; NI, nucleoli. (From T. L. Lentz, *Cell Fine Structure*, W. B. Saunders Co., Phila., 1971.)

is sometimes called the hibernating gland. Brown fat develops during embryonic life in certain specific sites: the interscapular region, back of the neck, and the axillae in rodents and humans; also, in humans, around the neck, kidneys, adrenals and in the abdomen (Dawkins and Hull, 1965; Aherne and Hull, 1966; Dyer, 1968). No new areas develop after birth except in animals subjected to prolonged cold (Smith and Horwitz, 1969). Although the fat content in brown adipose tissue usually decreases with age, some masses are present even in old individuals. Total depletion of brown fat has been reported for both children and adults dying of cold exposure.

Structure

Brown fat cells are not only smaller than the white cells but contain more cytoplasm in relation to the lipid, and the lipid is in many smaller droplets (Fig. 20.6). The nucleus, usually with two nucleoli, is not generally in a central position but it does not have a distorted shape. There are many large mitochondria with abundant cristae and relatively dense matrices. However, the subunits usually observed on the inner membrane of the cristae have not been demonstrated. This finding suggests that oxidative phosphorylation, a key function of mitochondria, probably does not take place. According to Afzelius (1966) this is consistent with the thermogenic function of the tissue (see below). There are few cisternae of either smooth or rough endoplasmic reticulum. Some free ribosomes and glycogen granules can be observed in the cytoplasm as well as a small Golgi apparatus. Pinocytotic vesicles appear at frequent intervals in the plasma membrane (Napolitano, 1965). A rich blood supply comes to brown adipose tissue and is in part responsible for its color. Color is due also to the high content of iron-containing cytochromes in the mitochondrial membranes.

Function

The functions of brown fat in newborn mammals and adult hibernating animals remained a mystery until the early 1960s. Smith (1961) observed the high heat-producing potential of brown fat and suggested that production of heat was its specific function. The high concentrations of cytochromes in the numerous mitochondria and the ample quantities of fat for substrate suggested a high capacity for oxidative metabolism. It was soon found that the oxygen consumption of these cells when expressed on a lipid-free dry weight basis was higher than that of any other body cells (Joel, 1965). In a series of experiments on newborn rabbits, Dawkins and Hull (1965) clearly demonstrated that brown fat cells are the main site of heat production in response to cold. The rich blood supply in the tissue rapidly removes the heat to other parts of the body, thereby protecting the bare-skinned newborn rabbit. The explanation of how exposure to cold in most mammalian neonates including humans leads to increased heat production without shivering becomes apparent. Pigs and calves, having no brown fat, must shiver for extra heat production (Hull, 1966), as do all other mammals when their brown fat storage is gradually replaced by white fat, since white fat plays no part in nonshivering thermogenesis. A clear demonstration of the specialization of brown fat cells for this purpose was presented by Hull and Segall (1966), who showed that the cells of brown fat became depleted when newborn rabbits were exposed to cold for 48 hours but there was little change in the white fat cells. In contrast, starving newborn rabbits in a warm environment depleted white fat cells, but the brown fat cells were unchanged. Hittleman et al. (1969) also demonstrated that the stimulus to lipolysis in brown fat of rabbits was cold; in white fat, lack of calories.

Both the structure and function of brown fat in animals and humans appears similar. Silverman et al. (1964) reported that skin temperature was maintained best at the interscapular region in infants exposed to cold. Cold exposure was also related to increased plasma glycerol levels indicating lipolysis (Dawkins and Scopes, 1965).

There is a considerable body of evidence indicating that the oxidative metabolism of brown fat is mediated by norepinephrine (Hull and Segall, 1965a; Schiff et al., 1966). This apparently occurs through local secretion at sympathetic nerve endings (Hull and Segall, 1965b) since the response to cold is very rapid. Furthermore, electrical stimulation leads to heat production and cutting the sympathetic nerves supplying the tissue abolishes this response. When brown fat is removed from newborn rabbits the oxygen consumption following injection of norepinephrine is greatly reduced (Hull and Segall, 1965b).

The metabolic specialization of the brown fat cell is its capacity to shift to oxidation of fatty acids for the production of heat. The shift is initiated by temperature receptors in the skin which stimulate the temperature regulating center in the brain. Impulses are relayed through the sympathetic nerves to brown fat tissue leading to norepinephrine release at the nerve endings. A suggested model of the sequence that follows is presented in Fig. 20.7. Norepinephrine at the brown fat cell membrane interacts with adenyl cyclase and stimulates the production of cAMP. The ensuing events leading to

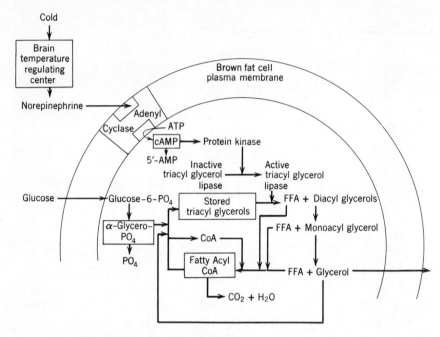

Fig. 20.7 Model of lipolysis in brown fat cell.

triacyl glycerol hydrolysis are probably similar to those postulated for the white fat cell: cAMP binds to the receptor unit-catalytic unit complex and liberates the free catalytic unit which activates the protein kinase. The protein kinase converts the hormone-sensitive lipase to the active state leading to hydrolysis of stored triacyl glycerol into glycerol and FFA. However, the presence of glycerokinase in the brown fat cell (Treble and Ball, 1963) permits re-utilization of some of the free glycerol. The increased concentration of FFA has been shown by Prusiner et al. (1968) to uncouple oxidation and phosphorylation in brown fat cells. Myant (1971) suggests that reversible uncoupling of mitochondria, combined with the increased supply of oxidizable substrate, may be the explanation for the increased oxygen consumption in brown fat cells of cold-stressed newborn animals. There is evidence also that coupling of oxidative phosphorylation can be restored to brown fat tissue by the removal of endogenously produced fatty acids (Bulychev et al., 1972). This finding is of particular interest when considered along with a report on the presence of a fatty acid binding protein (FABP) in the cytosol in many tissues including adipose tissue (Ockner et al., 1972). The FABP appears to be a regulator of cellular fatty acid concentration. These two lines of evidence point to the possibility that the FABP, through control of the concentration of the liberated fatty acids in the brown fat cells, can shift mitochondrial metabolism so that oxidation and phosphorylation become uncoupled and thermogenesis is possible.

Although in most species born with brown fat the tissue is converted to white fat by adulthood, in some animals it is retained and can increase; for example, in laboratory rats kept in a cold environment. The blood supply from the brown adipose tissue conducts the heat produced to warm the body without shivering much as the water pipes in a hot water home heating system provide a similar service. In animals that hibernate, a large quantity of brown fat remains throughout life. The importance of the brown fat is not so much in providing comfort during the long sleep but rather in providing the source of heat for awakening and emergence from the hibernating state. The stimulus for increased heat production in brown fat is the release of the norepinephrine at nerve endings as the animal begins to arouse. This initiates the lipolytic reesterification cycle that produces the heat carried by the blood to warm the rest of the body. The heat generated by brown fat in a bat arousing from hibernation has been visually demonstrated by thermography. A scan of the temperature-dependent intensity of infrared radiation from the body surface was registered on a photographic plate. A sharply delineated hot area corresponded to the location of the interscapular fat (Hayward and Ball, 1966). Skin temperature measurements between the shoulder blades of newborn babies have indicated the presence of brown fat which has been identified morphologically as well (Dyer, 1968; Mrosovsky and Rowlatt, 1968).

CONCLUSION

In the white adipose tissue cell there is a continual cycle of hydrolysis of triacyl glycerols to glycerol and fatty acids followed by triacyl glycerol resynthesis. The a-glycerophosphate for resynthesis is derived from glycolysis in the cell. Some of the fatty acids released are reincorporated into triacyl glycerol; some are synthesized in the cell; and some are derived from the triacyl glycerols of the lipo-proteins and chylomicra delivered by the plasma. Free fatty acids are continually released into the plasma where a small quantity circulates free and the rest are picked up by albumin. The quantity of free fatty acids released by the fat cell and circulated to supply fuel needs is determined by the relative rates of lipolysis and lipo-genesis which are under hormonal control and closely integrated into the total body need for endogenous lipid as an energy source.

The continual cycle of hydrolysis in the brown fat cell differs from that in the white fat cell in that the major portion of fatty acids are not released to the circulation for an energy source but are oxidized by the mitochondria of the brown fat cell for the purpose of producing heat. Triggered by the stimulus of cold, the cutaneous nerve endings elicit the series of events leading to non-shivering thermogenesis in neonates. Although the original stimulus to norepinephrine release may differ in arousal from hibernation, the mechanisms of thermogenesis appear to be the same.

part five

the complex organism

Chapter 21   Cellular Growth
Chapter 22   Body Composition
Chapter 23   Determination of Nutrient Needs: Energy, Protein,
              Minerals
Chapter 24   Determination of Nutrient Needs: Vitamins
Chapter 25   Dietary Standards
Chapter 26   Nutrition Surveys

"Man is, first of all, a nutritive process. He consists of a cease-less motion of chemical substances. One can compare him to the flame of a candle, or to the fountains playing in the gardens of Versailles. Those beings, made of burning gases or of water, are both permanent and transitory. Their existence depends on a stream of gas or of liquid. Like ourselves, they change according to the quality and the quantity of the substances which animate them. As a large river coming from the external world and returning to it, matter perpetu-ally flows through all the cells of the body. During its passing, it yields to tissues the energy they need, and also the chemicals which build the temporary and fragile structures of our organs and humors. The corporeal substratum of all human activities originates from the inanimate world and, sooner or later, goes back to it. Our organism is made from the same elements as lifeless things. Therefore, we should not be surprised, as some modern physiologists still are,

727

to find at work within our own self the usual laws of physics and of chemistry as they exist in the cosmic world. Since we are parts of the material universe, the absence of those laws is unthinkable."

Alexis Carrel, *Man the Unknown*, 1935, p. 88

chapter 21
cellular growth

1. The Stages of Development
2. Determination of Cell Number and Size
3. Phases of Cell Growth
4. Cell Growth of Specific Tissues
   a. Placenta
   b. Brain
   c. Muscle
5. Malnutrition and Growth Retardation
6. Cellular Basis for Permanent Growth Retardation
7. Malnutrition and Cellular Growth of Specific Tissues
   a. Placenta
   b. Brain
   c. Muscle
8. Malnutrition, Mental Development, and Behavior
9. Conclusion

"I wish you wouldn't squeeze so," said the Dormouse, who was sitting next to her. *"I can hardly breathe."*

"I can't help it," said Alice very meekly: *"I'm growing."*

"You've no right to grow here,*"* said the Dormouse.

"Don't talk nonsense," said Alice more boldly; *"you know you're growing too."*

"Yes, but I grow at a reasonable pace," said the Dormouse; *"not in that ridiculous fashion."* And he got up very sulkily and crossed over to the other side of the court.

Lewis Carroll, *Alice's Adventures in Wonderland*

To paraphrase the Dormouse, "growth does not occur in a ridiculous fashion." Growth of the total organism is a series of highly regulated processes that begins with the fertilization of the ovum and terminates with maturity; maturity being defined as the attainment of the body size, conformation and physiological capabilities characteristic of the species, and of the hereditary material with which the organism is endowed. Growth is represented by an increase in size and weight, the acquisition of active protoplasmic mass, and the accumulation of adipose tissue.

The changes in body composition accompanying normal growth will be discussed in the following chapter. This chapter will deal with the phenomenon of growth at the cellular level and the effect of nutrition upon the course of cellular growth.

THE STAGES OF DEVELOPMENT

The life span of all living organisms can be divided into two discrete phases: prenatal life that culminates with birth and postnatal life that ends with death. Each of these periods is further divided into several periods each of which is characterized by discrete morphological, physiological, and biochemical features. The rate of change and the timing of these events differ among various species, but the pattern is common to all.

The stages of development from conception to maturity in the human are described in Table 21.1. The human differs from most mammalian species in one major respect: the relative length of the periods of childhood and adolescence. No other animal can boast of enjoying so long a period between birth and maturity. Indeed, a period comparable to adolescence in the human is virtually non-existent in other species. Brody (1945) observed that growth curves of many animals are superimposed on each other when growth is expressed in terms of weight as a percentage of mature weight (Fig. 21.1). The curve for the human, however, shows a long slow period of growth unmatched by any other species and one that does not conform to the pattern of other mammals until mid-adolescence.

Different species are born at different levels of maturity as determined by body composition and physiological function. Birth is not a mark of equal development. However, certain physiological

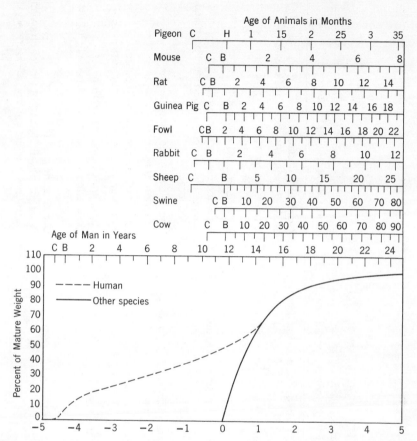

Fig. 21.1 Weight-growth equivalence of farm animals, laboratory animals, and man. (From S. Brody, *Bioenergetics and Growth*, Reinhold Pub. Co., N.Y., 1945, p. 492.)

events tend to occur sequentially in many species. There are exceptions, of course, and the time intervals vary, but for the most part mammalian species tend to grow and develop in a recognizable pattern. Extrapolations then can be made from one species to another if they are made with care; consideration must be given to the variation in time at which a specific event occurs. The latter point is especially important in extrapolating from one species to another in terms of cellular growth and the effects of malnutrition during critical periods of growth. The critical period varies from one

Table 21.1 AGE PERIODS OF LIFE BEFORE MATURITY

Name of Period	Ages Represented (approximate)	Some Characterizing Features
Embryonic	First trimester of prenatal life	Rapid differentiation Establishment of systems and organs
Early fetal	Second trimester of prenatal life	Accelerated growth Elaboration of structures Early functional activities
Late fetal	Third trimester of prenatal life	Rapid increase in body mass Completion of preparation for postnatal experience
Parturient	Period of labor and delivery	Risk of trauma and anoxia Cessation of placental function
Neonatal and early infancy	First month of postnatal life	Postnatal adjustments in circulation Initiation of respiration and other functions
Middle infancy	1 month to 1 year	Rapid growth and maturation Maturation of functions, especially of nervous system
Late infancy	1 to 2 years	Decelerating growth Progress in walking and other voluntary motor activities and in control of excretory functions

Childhood Preschool	2 to 6 years	Slow growth Increased physical activity Further coordination of functions and motor mechanisms Rapid learning
School	Girls: 6 to 10 years Boys: 6 to 12 years	Steady growth Developing skills and intellectual processes
Adolescent Prepubertal (late school or early adolescent)	Girls: 10 to 12 years Boys: 12 to 14 years	Accelerating growth Rapid weight gain Early adolescent endocrine and sex organ changes
Pubertal (adolescence proper)	Girls: 12 to 14 years Boys: 14 to 16 years	Secondary sex character maturation Maximum postnatal growth increase
Postpubertal	Girls: 14 to 18 years Boys: 16 to 20 years	Decelerating and terminal growth Rapid muscle growth and increased skills Rapid growth and maturing functions of sex organs Need for self-reliance and independence

From P. S. Timiras, *Developmental Physiology and Aging*, The MacMillan Co., N. Y., 1972, p. 4.

733

species to another. For a specific organ or tissue, it may be prenatal in one species and postnatal in another.

DETERMINATION OF CELL NUMBER AND SIZE

The number of cells can be determined from the amount of DNA present in an organ or tissue. With the exception of liver cells, most body cells contain a single diploid nucleus. Since cellular DNA is located almost entirely in the nucleus, and since the amount of DNA is constant within the diploid nucleus (Mirsky and Ris, 1949), the number of nuclei (i.e., the number of cells) may be determined by dividing total organ DNA by the amount of DNA known to be present in the cell. For the rat this amount has been shown to be 6.2 micromicrograms (Enesco and Leblond, 1962). The number of cells may be calculated from the following formula:

$$\text{Number of nuclei (millions)} = \frac{\text{total organ DNA (mg)} \times 10^3}{6.2}$$

The size of the cell thus may be calculated by dividing organ weight by the number of cells as shown below.

$$\text{Weight/nucleus (ng)} = \frac{\text{total organ weight (gm)} \times 10^3}{\text{number of nuclei (millions)}}$$

This formula may be used also to calculate protein, RNA, or any other cell constituent by dividing the total organ content of the substance by the number of nuclei.

These calculations are valid only for cells containing a diploid nucleus. The parenchymal cells of liver, however, are polyploid and, in addition, contain different quantities of DNA. Measurement of DNA in liver, therefore, does not give an accurate assessment of cell number. Total DNA, however, is closely associated with total liver mass (Campbell and Kosterlitz, 1950).

PHASES OF CELL GROWTH

Using the techniques described above, Enesco and Leblond (1962) and Winick and Nobel (1965) studied cell growth in the prenatal and

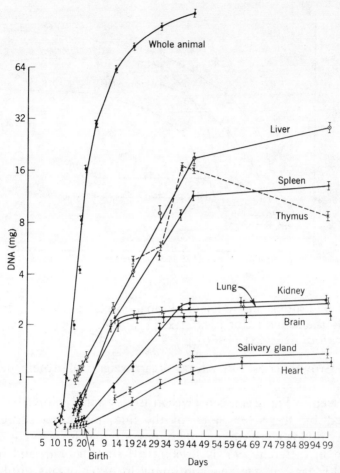

Fig. 21.2 DNA (mg) during normal growth in the rat. Points represent mean values for at least ten animals or organs. I represents range. [From M. Winick and A. Noble, *Develop. Biol.*, 12: 451 (1965).]

postnatal rat. Growth was shown to occur in three stages. Initially, growth proceeds by cell division alone as indicated by increasing amounts of DNA. Then growth proceeds by simultaneous cell division and cell enlargement as indicated by increase in weight or protein per nucleus. Finally, cell division ceases and growth occurs only by cell enlargement, that is, DNA content of the organ remains relatively constant but weight or protein content continue to in-

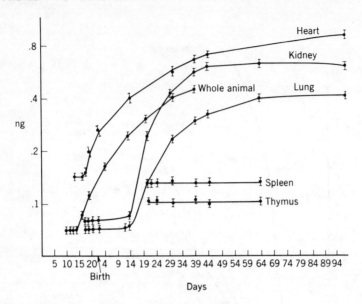

Fig. 21.3 Protein per nucleus during normal growth in the rat. Symbols the same as for Fig. 21.2. [From M. Winick and A. Noble, *Develop. Biol.*, 12: 451 (1966).]

crease. Growth ends when total organ weight or protein becomes constant.

As seen in Fig. 21.2, cell division is very rapid in prenatal life as indicated by the steep slope of the lines indicating tissue DNA content. Following birth, cell division continues for varying periods of time in different organs leveling off first in brain and lung at about 13 days of age and continuing in other organs until about 44 to 65 days of age. When ^{14}C-thymidine incorporation into DNA was used as a measure of DNA synthesis it was found that by 20 days synthesis in the brain had ceased and was markedly decreased in the lung. By 44 days synthesis ceased in kidney, spleen, and thymus whereas it was continued in heart, salivary gland, and skeletal muscle at a minimal rate. It is interesting that total DNA decreased in thymus after the thirty-ninth day, an indication of the loss of cells associated with atrophy of the gland.

The total protein content of organs, like organ weight, increases until maturity (Fig. 21.3). During early prenatal life cellular protein and DNA increase proportionately indicating that growth is due to cell division alone. In the late prenatal period and thereafter, protein

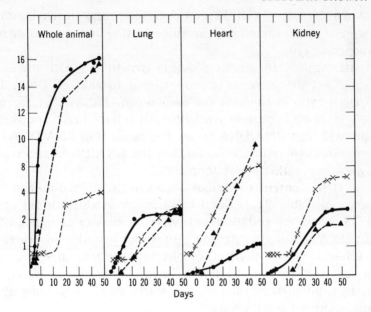

Fig. 21.4 Comparison between DNA content, total protein content, and protein per nucleus in various organs during normal growth of the rat. ●--● DNA (mg); ▲---▲ total protein (mg x 10^{-2}); X---X protein per nucleus. [From M. Winick and A. Noble, *Develop. Biol.*, 12: 451 (1966).]

increases more rapidly than DNA because cell growth is largely due to increase in cell size. When protein synthesis and degradation come into equilibrium, growth ceases. This situation is reflected in the change from a positive nitrogen balance as seen in growing animals and nitrogen equilibrium as observed in the adult.

Protein content per nucleus remains static in spleen and thymus indicating that growth in these organs occurs chiefly by cell proliferation.

A comparison of DNA, total protein, and protein per nucleus is shown in Fig. 21.4 for the whole animal body, and for lung, heart, and kidney, and emphasizes the differences in patterns of growth for various organs. It will be noted that the increase in number of cells is very rapid in early life and gradually tapers off as protein increases. Enesco and Leblond (1962) estimate that the number of cells for the whole rat body increases from 52 x 10^6 cells at 10 days before birth to 3000 x 10^6 at birth and then to 67,000 x 10^6 at 95 days of age. When the rate of cell division decreases, total protein continues to increase at the same rate, thereby resulting in a marked increase in protein per cell.

Total organ RNA increases during growth and, with the exception of liver, the increase is proportional to that of DNA. Thus RNA/DNA ratio is constant for each organ. Tissues that are most actively involved in protein synthesis such as liver, heart, and skeletal muscle have high RNA/DNA ratios. The patterns of RNA/DNA ratio and protein/DNA ratio are similar, but the RNA/DNA ratio reaches its highest level earlier in development.

The DNA content of various organs in the normal human fetus is shown in Table 21.2. Total cell number increases in all organs from 13 weeks of gestation until term. Cell size as indicated by weight/DNA remains unchanged throughout gestation in heart, kidney, spleen, thyroid, thymus, esophagus, stomach, large and small intestines, and tongue. In brain, lungs, liver, adrenal gland, and diaphragm, an increase in cell size starts slowly beginning at the seventh month of gestation.

CELL GROWTH OF SPECIFIC TISSUES

Placenta

Growth of the placenta follows the same three-stage pattern described for other tissues (Winick and Noble, 1966). In the rat placental DNA increases until the seventeenth day of gestation, that is, four days before term. Placental weight, protein, and RNA increase until day 19 (Fig. 21.5). Until day 16, cell number increases with no increase in cell size as indicated by proportional increases in DNA and protein. From day 16 through 18 hyperplasia and hypertrophy occur simultaneously; thereafter, placental cell growth is by hypertrophy alone.

Human placenta follows the same pattern of growth. Cell division ceases at about 34 to 36 weeks of pregnancy; weight, protein, and RNA increase until near term (Winick et al., 1967). RNA/DNA ratio of human placenta, however, is only half that of the rat. The reason for this difference is not known.

Table 21.2 DNA CONTENT OF VARIOUS ORGANS IN NORMAL HUMAN FETUSES (MILLIGRAMS)

Weeks of gestation	13	17	23	25	27	31	33	34	49	40
Fetal weight (gm)	31.7	163	320	580	610	1080	1525	1720	3300	4040
Brain	25	85	134	251	240	285	385	–	620	685
Heart	0.51	2.8	8.1	15.4	17.3	18.2	38.6	40.2	54.7	55.6
Liver	16.5	50	53.9	97.3	105.1	175	203	247	328	329
Kidney	0.72	6.8	–	38.7	59.6	–	73	79	107	128
Spleen	0.41	1.2	2.5	7.7	9.8	15.3	–	64.4	84.6	90.9
Thyroid	0.02	0.10	–	0.84	0.97	2.7	–	4.5	5.8	6.9
Adrenal	0.24	0.71	1.31	1.87	2.14	5.84	6.97	8.04	10.2	12.6
Right lung	3.0	23.6	50.9	64	–	66.4	68.5	–	148.7	166.8
Left lung	2.5	18.7	37.5	41.8	–	55.6	59.4	–	126	132
Thymus	0.39	3.99	10.96	21.8	26.5	47.3	105.4	160.6	249	303
Esophagus	0.17	0.60	0.64	0.78	0.80	1.38	3.69	4.21	6.1	6.9
Stomach	0.53	2.3	3.6	5.0	5.7	6.8	22.3	26.8	32.7	40.7
Small intestine	3.8	6.1	16.2	26.3	32.8	48.7	157	179	512	529
Large intestine	0.37	2.97	5.8	10.0	11.2	26.3	47.2	525	129.6	137.2
Diaphragm	0.38	2.1	5.2	6.8	7.2	18.7	24.7	31.7	385	45.3
Tongue	0.39	1.21	2.4	3.5	3.7	4.9	–	–	–	–

From M. Winick et al., *Nutrition and Development*, Wiley, N. Y., 1972, p. 88.

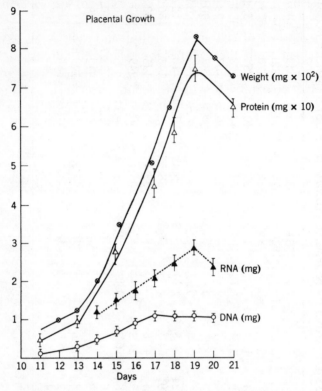

Fig. 21.5 Total weight, protein, DNA, and RNA during development of rat placenta. Each point represents the average of at least 15 separate determinations. The bars on the figure represent the range. [From M. Winick and A. Noble, *Nature*, 212: 34 (1966).]

Brain

Different regions of the brain exhibit different patterns of growth (Fish and Winick, 1969). In the rat, cell division in the cerebellum ceases at 17 days postnatally, in cerebral cortex at 21 days, and in brain stem as early as 14 days. There is a well defined increase in DNA in the hippocampus between the fourteenth and seventeenth days, which is probably due to migration of neurons into this area. Total protein content of cerebellum is not reached until nearly 100 days of age. Net protein synthesis decreases in cerebrum, and cerebral cells decrease in size with aging. In contrast, the protein/DNA ratio increases in brain stem cells due not only to an increase in cell size but also to myelination and extension of neuronal processes from other brain regions into the brain stem.

Less is known of cell growth in human brain. Analysis of brain tissue obtained from therapeutic abortions and autopsy of healthy infants who died from accidents suggest that DNA synthesis is nearly linear prenatally, begins to decline after birth, and reaches a maximum at 8 to 12 months of age (Winick, 1970). In more detailed

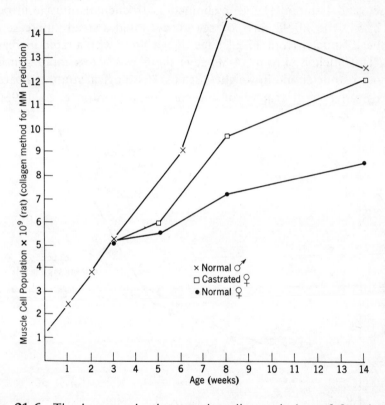

Fig. 21.6 The increase in the muscle cell population of female rats is compared with that of the male. Note the lesser number of muscle cells in the female. Castrated female rats show muscle cell growth resembling more that of the male. The value for the number of muscle nuclei for males at 8 weeks equals 15.09 ± 1.38 and at 14 weeks the value is 12.52 ± 1.56 (p < 0.02). At 22 weeks the value is 12.30 ± 1.33. Possibly the peak for the muscle nuclei at 8 weeks is due to enhanced mitoses. (From D. B. Cheek, ed., *Human Growth*, Lea and Febiger, Phila., 1968, p. 311.)

studies, Dobbing and Sands (1970) described two peaks of DNA synthesis in human brain, one occurring at about 26 weeks of gestation and the second around the time of birth. These peaks were interpreted as a reflection of the peak rates of neuronal division and of glial division respectively.

Muscle

Enesco and Leblond (1962) examined gastrocnemius muscle in rats at 17, 34, and 80-95 days of age. They noted a steady increase in number of nuclei from 17-34 days of age along with a rapid increase in weight/nucleus. From 34-56 days there was a less rapid gain in number of nuclei and in weight/nucleus. Histological study indicated a progressive hypertrophy of muscle fibers. Gordon et al. (1966)

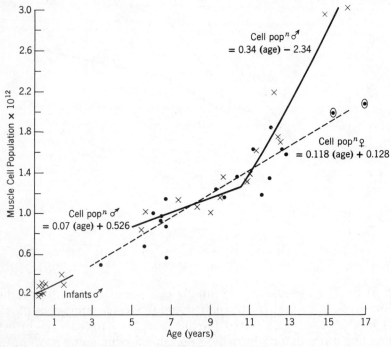

Fig. 21.7 Muscle cell population against age is shown for male infants, for boys, and for girls. Note the sex difference and the breaking line relationship (or quadratic relationship) for boys. The intersection of the 2 lines for boys occurs at 10½ years. The points with a circle represent sexually mature girls. (From D. B. Cheek, ed., *Human Growth*, Lea and Febiger, Phila., 1968, p. 340.)

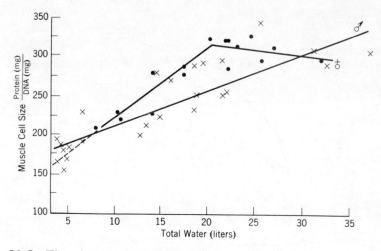

Fig. 21.8 The changes in muscle cell size with growth are shown for male infants, boys, and girls. Note that the increase in cell size for girls outstrips that for boys but eventually boys overtake girls and finally have bigger muscle cells. (From D. B. Cheek, ed., *Human Growth*, Lea and Febiger, Phila., 1968, p. 345.)

reported that hyperplasia of muscle fiber nuclei ceases at about 90 days of age in the rat, but hypertrophy of muscle fibers continues to approximately 140 days.

Cheek et al. (1968) also have reported on changes in muscle cell population from analysis of DNA in the noncollagen protein in carcass (eviscerated animal minus skin) for male and female rats up to 14 weeks of age. As shown in Fig. 21.6, male rats contain considerably more muscle cells than females. Following castration, however, muscle cell number in females approaches that of males.

Sex differences in muscle cell number and size in humans have been observed. In boys, the increase in muscle cell number from two months to 16 years of age is fourteen-fold (Cheek, 1968). There is a marked increase in muscle cell number at 10.5 years of age so that when number of cells is plotted against age there is a steep slope from age 10.5 to age 16 (Fig. 21.7). On the other hand, muscle cell number increases linearly for girls and after age 11 is well below the levels reported for males.

Cheek (1968) also has compared cell size as determined by protein/DNA ratio with body size (indicated by total body water) in boys and girls (Fig. 21.8). Muscle cell size tends to increase

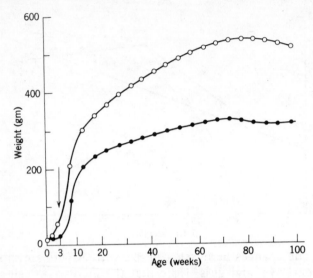

Fig. 21.9 Body weight of rats suckled in small (○) and large (●) litters. Arrow shows weaning. [From R. A. McCance and E. M. Widdowson, *Proc. Roy. Soc. B*, 156: 326 (1962).]

linearly in boys. In girls, muscle cell size is higher than that for boys throughout childhood and early adolescence. Thereafter muscle cell size increases in males and surpasses that of girls.

MALNUTRITION AND GROWTH RETARDATION

Early studies suggested that malnutrition in young animals and children can result in permanent growth retardation and that the likelihood of permanent damage is greater the earlier the period of malnutrition (Dunn et al., 1947). Systematic studies of the effects of malnutrition at various periods in the life of rats were carried out by McCance and Widdowson (see Widdowson, 1964; McCance and Widdowson, 1974). Malnutrition was produced in rats during the suckling period (the first three weeks of life) by increasing the size of the litter suckled by one dam to 17-20 young. These young were unable to obtain enough milk from the lactating female and therefore grew poorly. Other rats were suckled in small groups of 3 rats; these animals grew rapidly and were moderately overnourished. At weaning, all animals were given unlimited

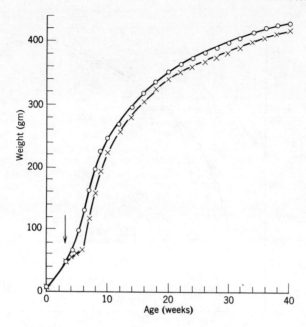

Fig. 21.10 The effect of undernutrition from the 3rd to the 6th week of life on the growth in weight of rats suckled in small groups. ○, Unlimited food after weaning; x, unlimited food after the 6th week. Arrow shows weaning. [From E. M. Widdowson and R. A. McCance, *Proc. Roy. Soc. B,* 158: 329 (1963).]

access to food. The undernourished rats grew rapidly for a few weeks, then weight gain slackened and at 100 weeks of age they were considerably smaller than the initially well nourished rats (Fig. 21.9).

When well nourished rats were restricted in food intake from the third to sixth week and then allowed to refeed, they also grew rapidly at the outset of refeeding but never attained the full body size of rats well nourished for the entire period (Fig. 21.10). However, final body weight was much greater than that of animals subjected to malnutrition during the first three weeks of life.

When food restriction occurred as late as the ninth to twelfth week of life no permanent effect on growth resulted (Fig. 21.11). Animals rapidly attained normal weight and even slightly surpassed their continually well nourished counterparts.

These studies clearly demonstrate that malnutrition in very

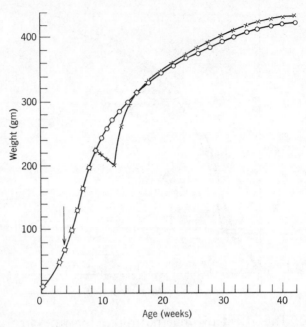

Fig. 21.11 The effect of undernutrition from the 9th to the 12th week on the growth in weight of rats suckled in small groups. ○, Unlimited food after weaning; x, unlimited food except from the 9th to the 12th week. Arrow shows weaning. [From E. M. Widdowson and R. A. McCance, *Proc. Roy. Soc. B*, 158: 329 (1963).]

early life in the rat results in permanent growth stunting and further, that beyond a certain period of life, transient malnutrition has no long-term effect on growth.

CELLULAR BASIS FOR PERMANENT GROWTH RETARDATION

In a classic study, Winick and Noble (1966) tested a hypothesis to establish the cellular basis for permanent growth retardation in animals subjected to malnutrition in early life. They reasoned that if malnutrition occurred during the period of cell division, permanent damage would result; but if malnutrition occurred when cell size only was affected then the animal likely would recover. Since the timing of periods of cellular growth of different organs was known to be different it was expected that the critical period would vary from organ to organ.

In order to test this hypothesis, three groups of animals were subjected to food deprivation during one of three periods: birth to 21 days of age, 21 to 42 days, and 65 to 82 days. Following the period of food restriction, animals were allowed access to unlimited food until they reached 133 days of age when the experiment was terminated. Analyses for DNA, RNA, and protein were made on organs from groups of animals at the end of the restriction period and at the end of the recovery period. *Ad libitum* fed animals of the same age served as controls. Weight and DNA content of some organs following food restriction are shown in Table 21.3 and the same data following refeeding are shown in Table 21.4. In general, RNA and protein content of the animal body and organs followed the pattern for weight.

Food restriction resulted in reduced weight, total protein, and RNA in all animals regardless of the timing of the period of malnutrition. DNA, however, was lowered only in those organs in which cell division was occurring at the time of food deprivation. When food intake was restricted from birth to 21 days of age (when cell division is most rapid in all organs), animals failed to recover body or organ size because of the permanent decrease in cell number. In animals who were restricted from 21 to 42 days of age, all organs were permanently reduced in cell number and size except brain and lung (cell division had ceased in these organs prior to the period of food deprivation). In animals 65 to 82 days of age at the time of food restriction, cell number was reduced only in the lymphoid organs (thymus and spleen) although cell size was reduced to varying degrees in all organs as indicated by decreased organ weight without reduction in DNA content. At the end of refeeding, recovery was complete for all organs except thymus.

With this simple but elegant study Winick and Noble (1966) defined the events occurring at the cellular level which clarified the significance of timing of nutritional insult on later development of the animal. Cell division is time dependent. Thus, reduction in cell number as a result of malnutrition results in permanent stunting of growth.

Table 21.3 WEIGHT AND DNA CONTENT OF ANIMAL AND ORGANS AFTER FOOD RESTRICTION

	Period of Restriction								
	Birth-21 days		21-42 days		65-82 days				
	Weight gm	DNA mg	Weight gm	DNA mg	Weight gm	DNA mg			
Whole animal: control	59	97.8	119	—	267	—			
restricted	29	42.2	62	—	188	—			
Brain: control	1.49	2.18	1.59	2.94	1.80	3.28			
restricted	1.23	1.48	1.40	2.81	1.67	3.39			
Lung: control	0.39	1.96	1.11	3.17	1.50	3.56			
restricted	0.14	1.06	0.64	3.48	1.16	3.61			
Heart: control	0.36	0.622	0.65	0.798	1.01	1.39			
restricted	0.19	0.377	0.55	0.698	0.75	1.33			
Thymus: control	0.33	2.74	0.38	10.3	0.75	1.06			
restricted	0.07	0.99	0.15	2.85	0.43	0.76			
Spleen: control	0.29	2.30	0.48	5.29	0.77	10.62			
restricted	0.06	0.76	0.17	2.07	0.30	2.67			

Adapted from M. Winick and A. Noble, *J. Nutr.*, 89: 300 (1966).

Table 21.4 WEIGHT AND DNA CONTENT OF ANIMAL AND ORGANS AFTER REFEEDING

| | Period of Restriction | | | | | | | | | | |
| | Birth-21 days | | | | 21-42 days | | | | 65-82 days | | |
	Weight gm	DNA mg			Weight gm	DNA mg			Weight gm	DNA mg
Whole animal: control	376	—			382	—			374	—
restricted	297	—			314	—			379	—
Brain: control	1.88	3.10			1.92	2.97			1.87	3.02
restricted	1.60	2.42			1.88	2.92			1.91	3.13
Lung: control	2.21	3.34			2.19	3.28			2.16	3.18
restricted	1.87	1.82			2.20	3.20			2.10	3.22
Heart: control	1.42	1.43			1.31	1.40			1.28	1.47
restricted	0.94	1.12			1.01	1.09			1.34	1.45
Thymus: control	0.72	1.47			0.65	1.30			0.65	1.32
restricted	0.40	0.82			0.29	0.96			0.33	1.07
Spleen: control	0.56	0.68			0.60	10.58			0.58	10.06
restricted	0.37	6.94			0.48	7.63			0.59	9.94

Adapted from M. Winick and A. Noble, *J. Nutr.*, 89: 300 (1966).

MALNUTRITION AND CELLULAR GROWTH OF SPECIFIC TISSUES

Placenta

Malnutrition during gestation markedly reduces placental weight (Winick, 1969; Zamenhof et al., 1971) essentially because of a decrease in cell number. Cell size remains normal. Winick (1969) reported that rats fed a severely deficient protein diet (5 percent casein) from day 5 of gestation had small placentas containing reduced amounts of DNA and protein but elevated levels of RNA (Table 21.5). As a result RNA/DNA ratio is about twice that for

Table 21.5   EFFECT OF MATERNAL MALNUTRITION ON RAT PLACENTA

Parameter	Mg/placenta	
	Control	Experimental
Weight	0.405	0.320
Protein	23.0	21.7
RNA	1.00	1.80
DNA	1.06	0.82
RNA/DNA	0.99	2.10
Protein/DNA	27.0	28.2

From M. Winick, *Diagnosis and Treatment of Fetal Disorders*, K. Adamsons, ed., Springer-Verlag, N. Y., 1969.

normal placental tissue. The significance of this finding is not known. High RNA/DNA ratios are found in tissues requiring protein synthesis. The increase in RNA/DNA may represent an attempt by the organ to promote protein synthesis by a compensatory increase in RNA synthesis per cell.

Reduction in cell number in placental tissue apparently also occurs in human malnutrition. Examination of placentas from a population in which malnutrition was common indicated a reduction in cell number as compared with placentas obtained from well nourished women (Winick et al., 1972). Incidence of low birth weight infants was also high in this malnourished population and may reflect intrauterine growth retardation resulting from maternal malnutrition.

Brain

More attention has been given to the effect of malnutrition on cell growth in brain than in any other body tissue. The studies of Winick and Noble (1966) indicated that brain weight and cell number were decreased when rats were subjected to malnutrition during the first 3 weeks of life and that these changes could not be reversed by subsequent adequate feeding. Malnutrition later in life produced a reduction in cell size only, which was readily reversed in the nutritionally rehabilitated animal. This work was rapidly confirmed and extended by a number of investigators. Guthrie and Brown (1968) subjected rats to malnutrition for 3, 5, 7, and 9 weeks after birth. Depression of brain weight and DNA was no greater in the nutritionally rehabilitated rats that had been malnourished for 5 to 9 weeks than for those that had been malnourished for only 3 weeks. These data indicate that malnutrition beyond the critical period in postnatal brain development is of no further detriment to the animal.

Decrease in brain cell number as a result of malnutrition in postnatal life is due almost entirely to reduction in cells of the cerebellum. According to Chase et al. (1968), cells of the cerebrum are not affected. When fetal growth retardation occurs as a result of maternal dietary restriction, the number of cells of the cerebral region also is reduced although not nearly to the extent of those of cerebellar (Fig. 21.12). Other areas of the brain also are markedly affected. Malnutrition during either prenatal or postnatal life results in a reduction of brain cells to about 85 percent of normal. The combined effects of nutritional insult in both prenatal and postnatal life result in a reduction of cell number to 40 percent of normal brain (Winick, 1980).

Malnutrition during the first 3 weeks of life also has been shown to interfere with the synthesis of lipids in rat brain. This results in substantially reduced quantities of cholesterol (Dobbing, 1964), cerebroside (Culley and Mertz, 1965), and slightly reduced amounts of phospholipid (Culley and Mertz, ibid). It has been found that the incorporation of sulfatide into myelin of rat brain is re-

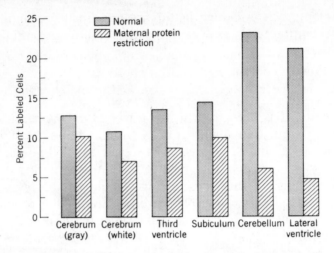

Fig. 21.12 Effect of maternal protein restriction on regional DNA content of fetal brain. [From M. Winick, *Fed. Proc.*, 29: 1510 (1970).]

duced both *in vivo* and *in vitro* and that the activity of galacto-cerebroside sulfokinase, the enzyme catalyzing the incorporation of sulfatide, also is reduced (Chase et al., 1967). Myelination is retarded when malnutrition occurs early in life (Fishman et al., 1971), but is relatively unaffected in the later phase of myelination even under the condition of severe undernutrition (Fishman et al., 1972).

In children, malnutrition during the first year of life results in a reduction in the number of brain cells. Brain tissue of children who died of malnutrition before age one was found to contain fewer cells than normal. Children who died of protein-calorie malnutrition at an older age and who presumably were reasonably well nourished during the first year of life had brains of normal cell number but somewhat lower in cell size (Winick, 1970). Thus the protein/DNA ratio was reduced. These data are similar to observations in rats and confirm that, in the human, malnutrition during the first year of life interferes with cell division. Malnutrition beyond one year interferes with cell size only. In the latter case, recovery should have been possible had the children lived.

Muscle

Muscle tissue is markedly affected by malnutrition during both prenatal and postnatal life. Widdowson (1970) has reported that the quadriceps muscle of guinea pigs born of poorly nourished mothers weighed about half as much as muscle from young of well nourished mothers. Protein content was reduced about half; DNA was reduced by about one-quarter. Muscle fiber size was normal, but the number of muscle fibers was markedly reduced.

Food restriction in the postnatal rat was reported to result in proportionate decreases in DNA and protein in gastrocnemius muscle so that cell number was reduced but cell size remained essentially normal (Winick and Noble, 1966). In rats above the age of 65 days, only cell size was affected and complete recovery from the effects of malnutrition were attained when the animals were allowed an adequate diet. Similarly, Graystone and Cheek (1969) found muscle cell size to be normal or large in young rats fed a diet restricted in calories but adequate in protein and other nutrients. However, cell division was decreased as was total muscle mass.

In contrast, marked reductions in muscle cell size occurred in infants suffering from malnutrition during the first year of life (Cheek and Hill, 1970). After rehabilitation, the number of muscle nuclei increased to normal for the body size of the child, but cells did not attain normal size. Cheek and Hill (ibid) suggest that these differences are due to differences in the type of food restriction imposed. In protein-calorie restriction small muscle fibers are found, but with low calorie intake (as in their animal studies) muscle size is normal or increased. In protein-calorie malnutrition small cell size is associated with reduced circulating levels of insulin, whereas in caloric restriction normal to large cell size is associated with high levels of pituitary growth hormone. Cheek and Hill (ibid.) theorize that protein intake through its influence on insulin secretion affects muscle cell size while calorie intake influences growth hormone and affects cell number. This interesting hypothesis suggests that the nature of the nutritional insult as well as the timing of the insult may affect the cellular response to malnutrition in early life.

MALNUTRITION, MENTAL DEVELOPMENT, AND BEHAVIOR

Few recent developments in the area of nutritional science have attracted as much public attention as the possible effect of early malnutrition on later mental development and behavior. The observation that children suffering from protein-calorie malnutrition were apathetic, listless, and unresponsive to environmental stimuli suggested that there may have been an impairment in learning behavior that persisted during and following nutritional rehabilitation. Detailed observations on children who had recovered from protein-calorie malnutrition suggested that there was some impairment in learning ability as compared with other children living in the same social environment (Cravioto and Robles, 1965; Cravioto et al., 1966). It was not clear, however, if the apparent retardation was a reflection of lowered intelligence or a retardation in the development of learning behavior as a result of loss of learning time. Cravioto et al. (1966) suggested that malnutrition could act in two ways: one deriving from a direct interference with the development of the central nervous system (as indicated from studies with experimental animals), and a second from a series of indirect effects including interference with learning during a critical period of development and changes in motivation and personality. Learning progresses in stages. By failing to respond to learning stimulation during the period of malnutrition, the child would become less able to benefit from later experiences. As a result he would fail to learn because there was no foundation for the next developmental stage.

Most of the early animal experiments were designed to test the hypothesis that early malnutrition produced irreversible damage to the central nervous system which would be reflected in "animal intelligence" and that could be measured by problem solving tests. As an example, Barnes et al. (1966) used a Y-shaped water maze to evaluate the learning of visual discrimination. Rats were forced to swim from the base of the Y to the point of choice; one direction led to a platform and the other to a dead end from which there was no escape from the water. Learning consisted of making the correct choice to the platform after several trials and, in addition, relearning when the position of the platform was reversed. The performance on the position-reversal test was poorest in young rats that had been suckled in large litters and fed on a low (4 percent) protein diet for eight weeks following weaning.

Subsequent studies in a number of laboratories tended to show that the *behavioral* responses of previously malnourished animals were perhaps more significant than scores on tests of "learning" (Barnes, 1967; Levitsky and Barnes, 1970). Studies of animal behavior have shown a lack of exploratory behavior as evidenced by limited activity when given free access to an "open field" (Frankova and Barnes, 1968a; Guthrie, 1968; Hsueh et al., 1971; Simonson et al., 1971), increased excitability and heightened emotional activity (Frankova and Barnes, 1968b; Guthrie, 1968; Simonson et al., 1971). The most characteristic change in adult behavior according to Levitsky and Barnes (1970) is in emotional responsiveness.

Early social or environmental isolation have been shown to result in an increase in emotional responsiveness in the adult rat whereas various forms of environmental stimulation (such as daily handling) have been shown to decrease emotionality. Levitsky and Barnes (1972) therefore studied the interactions between early malnutrition and environmental conditions on various aspects of adult behavior. Environmental stimulation was provided by handling the rats for 3 minutes once a day and providing a one-hour "play" period 5 days a week with 5 other animals in a box containing toys. The results of the experiment indicated that the behavioral effects of early malnutrition were completely eliminated by environmental stimulation early in life although these animals were severely retarded in body weight (and presumably in brain weight and brain cell number). Thus, it would seem that the structural and biochemical deficits of brain resulting from early malnutrition cannot account entirely for learning and behavioral problems in later life.

The protective effect of early stimulation is not well understood but possibly could be due to a true physiological effect on brain tissue. Bennett et al. (1969) have demonstrated that brain weight of malnourished rats allowed access to toys and other environmental stimuli were comparable to those of normal controls. The effect of stimulation also could be entirely behavioral in nature. Thus, as Cravioto et al. (1966) suggested earlier, the effect of malnutrition on development as reflected in intellectual performance may be due to the behavioral responses resulting from malnutrition. Monckeberg et al. (1972) also have stressed the significance of the interaction of malnutrition and environment on mental development in the human.

In a recent experiment Lát et al. (1973) attempted to correlate behavioral responses of rats to biochemical response. They used exploratory behavior as a measure of excitability and incorporation of ^{14}C-leucine into brain protein as the biochemical response. The rats were fed a standard laboratory stock diet and were divided into 3 groups on the basis of their exploratory behavior. These workers found a strong positive correlation between excitability and specific activity of various regions of the brain. These results cannot be applied directly to malnourished animals since all animals in this study were well fed, and the range of excitability may have been similar to what one might expect to find in a "normal" human population. This intriguing approach, however, suggests possibilities for further study on the effects of malnutrition on behavior.

It is clear from animal studies that malnutrition in early life is associated both with defects in development of the central nervous system and with impaired behavioral response. Observations on malnourished children (Cravioto and Robles, 1965; Cravioto et al., 1966; Winick, 1970; Hertzig, 1972) suggest that similar effects occur in the human. Although extrapolations from animal studies to humans must be made with caution as Dobbing (1972) has warned, the beneficial effects of environmental stimulation upon subsequent behavioral development of malnourished animals may apply to the malnourished human as well. Thus, diet and environment appear to interact in the complex series of events that lead to normal behavioral response and intellectual performance. The effect of malnutrition upon mental development obviously is much more complicated than the early animal studies seemed to imply.

CONCLUSION

Cellular growth is a carefully regulated process that proceeds in three stages: hyperplasia, hyperplasia with simultaneous hypertrophy, and hypertrophy alone. Hyperplasia represents the critical stage in development and occurs in different organs for varying periods of time. Malnutrition during the period of cell division results in permanent growth retardation. Malnutrition at any time following the period of cell division results in reduction of cell size from which the system can recover with adequate feeding.

The three phases of cell growth underlie all the complex changes that occur in the growing animal and in its development into a mature adult. The long term consequences of malnutrition depend on the phase of cell growth that is interrupted.

chapter 22
body composition

1. **Methods**
   a. Chemical Analysis
   b. Nutritional Anthropo-
      metry
   c. Skinfold Thickness
   d. Body Density
   e. Simultaneous Multiple
      Isotope Dilution
   f. ^{40}K Analysis

2. **Compositional Changes During the Life Cycle**
   a. Human Fetal Develop-
      ment
   b. Maternal Weight Gain
      1. Distribution
      2. Composition
   c. Nutrient Requirements
      During Pregnancy
   d. Compositional Changes
      Between Birth and
      Maturity
   e. Compositional Changes
      with Weight Change
      1. Obesity
      2. Physical Activity
3. **Summary**

Primitive man believed that by consuming the flesh of an animal he would acquire the characteristics of that animal: that eating the lion's heart would make a person brave, but a jackal's heart would make him timid; the deer's flesh would make him swift, but the bear's, clumsy. One might interpret such statements as evidence that man, from earliest times, has suspected that the food he ate became part of his substance and contributed specific characteristics. Such interpretation, perhaps, attributes unwarranted prescience to our forebears, but, despite the mask of Greek mythology, drinking the water in which a steel sword rusted could lead to the acquisition of strength if the individual happened to be anemic, and such practices and rites could indeed influence the composition of the body.

The Arabic scientist, Al-Biruni, who lived in the first half of the eleventh century stated in his *Book of Drugs:* "...the body in equilibrium has the power to transform nutriment into its own substance by complete digestion and by assimilation, thus replacing what part of the diet has been lost by disassimilation. That is the reason why the body must act on food before it can derive any benefit from it." (See Taton, 1963.) And in *Hamlet* Shakespeare said, "A man may fish with the worm that hath eat of a king, and eat of the fish that hath fed of that worm." A vivid illustration of the cycle of Nature and the continuity of matter; yet this predates by 200 years Lavoisier's experimental establishment of the Law of Conservation of Mass! Indeed, we could idly speculate about elements in our body constituents that at one time might have contributed to Pepys' dyspepsia or Solomon's sagacity.

What started as magic and progressed through myth and into the arena of science has come within the purview of the physical anthropologist, the physicist, the radiologist, the physician, as well as the various "sects" in human biology. Perhaps of greatest concern to the nutritionist are the compositional changes associated with the entire life cycle from the developing embryo to the extremes of aging. If we can assume that compositional changes determine nutrient needs, then knowledge of changing body composition constitutes the *matériel* for nutritionists.

Except for a few isolated studies, all the reported work investigating human body composition has appeared within the last 35 years and was inaugurated by the first of a series of papers from

Behnke's laboratory (1941-42). Although the literature has become extensive and the methodology expanded, it is easy to agree with Brozek (1961), who suggests "that the field is in the state of late adolescence rather than full-blown maturity."

METHODS

The interest centered upon the estimation of the chemical composition of the human body during the last few decades has led to the development of nondisruptive methods, some of which give some insight into the dynamic state of metabolism. Final tests of their validity would be a comparison with data from chemical analysis. The purpose of this section is not to delve deeply into the specifics of each method but to understand the rationale behind them and the parameters they measure.

Chemical Analysis

Ways of estimating chemical composition of the human appear at first to be both obvious and impossible: Obvious because the gross chemical composition of most biological materials can be determined by analytical laboratory procedures; impossible because chemical dissection of humans today is frowned upon just slightly less than anatomical dissection was in Leonardo da Vinci's day. However, despite mores and the tedious unpleasantness of the work, several nineteenth-century investigators reported on chemical analyses of human cadavers (see McCance and Widdowson, 1951). Not until the middle of the twentieth century were the results of detailed

Table 22.1 PERCENTAGE OF WATER AND FAT IN FIVE ADULT BODIES

Subject	2	3	4	5	7
Age	46	60	48	25	42
Weight as percentage of standard	84	110	95	100	70
Percentage of fat in body	19.4	27.0	4.3	14.9	23.6
Percentage of water in body	55.1	51.4	70.8	61.8	56.0

From E. M. Widdowson, "Chemical Analysis of the Body," *Human Body Composition*, J. Brozek, ed., Pergamon Press, Oxford, 1965, p. 35.

chemical analyses of adults published in the United States by Mitchell et al. (1945) and by Forbes et al. (1953; 1956) and in England by Widdowson and her co-workers (1951). A compilation by Widdowson (1965) of the data from these original studies which utilized dissimilar laboratory techniques revealed that the most variable body constituent was fat and this, of course, was no real surprise (Table 22.1). However, when calculations were made on the basis of fat-free tissue, the largest constituent, water, was shown to be remarkably consistent, as were the electrolytes associated with body water (Table 22.2). The greatest range in these studies was

Table 22.2 COMPOSITION OF THE FAT-FREE BODY TISSUE OF FIVE ADULTS

Subject	2	3	4	5	7	Mean
Water, %	69.4	70.4	73.0	72.5	73.2	71.7
Total N, gm/kg	37.5	38.1	33.0	31.1	31.0	34
Na, mEq/kg	82.6	78.2	—	92	97	80[a]
K, mEq/kg	66.5	66.6	—	71.5	73	69
Cl, mEq/kg	43.9	55.5	—	—	—	50
Ca, gm/kg	24.0	21.5	20.7	21.3	24.8	22.4
P, gm/kg	11.6	11.3	11.1	14.0	12.9	12.0
Mg, gm/kg	—	0.49	0.47	0.48	0.43	0.47
Fe, mg/kg	—	—	—	87.5	60.0	74
Cu, mg/kg	—	—	—	1.6	1.8	1.7
Zn, mg/kg	—	—	—	33.3	22.0	28
B, mg/kg	0.30	0.36	0.45	—	—	0.37
Co, mg/kg	0.022	0.024	0.018	—	—	0.021

From E. M. Widdowson, "Chemical Analysis of the Body," *Human Body Composition*, J. Brozek, ed., Pergamon Press, Oxford, 1965, p. 37.
[a]Mean of subjects 2 and 3 only.

apparent in the quantities of iron reflecting obvious differences in intakes coupled with limited capacity of the body to excrete this mineral. The data are expressed on a fat-free basis in order to compensate for the most variable component, the adipose or neutral fat stores. Essential lipid, which is part of every cell, is not included in the fat-free body. The differences among *fat-free body, lean body mass,* and *body cell mass* will become apparent.

The disadvantages of direct analysis, both apparent and real, coupled with the importance of studying living organisms, led to the exploration of various indirect approaches to the problem of body composition.

Nutritional Anthropometry

Even to the unpracticed eye, body measurements are a fair indication of the stores of fat, and thus of relative body composition. Certainly body weight has been used (and misused) as such a measure and can often give a fair indication of the magnitude of adipose stores in an individual. However, if body measurements are to be used for assessing human nutriture, it is apparent that selection and standardization of measurements are essential. A Committee on Nutritional Anthropometry established by the Food and Nutrition Board of the National Research Council employed the combined talents of physical anthropologists and nutritionists. The report of the Committee (Brozek, 1956) lists the minimum number of measurements that would indicate skeletal build and the thickness of subcutaneous fat: height, weight, and skinfold thickness.

Although height-weight relationships are the most readily attained parameters for comparison and are simple to use, they are neither definitive nor instructive by themselves. Gross departures from norms become evident but probably would be so by just visual appraisal. One danger inherent in the use of such tables is the attempt to evaluate population groups of unlike genetic and nutritional backgrounds with norms for the United States. However, comparison within groups can be informative (Mitchell, 1963).

Attempts at relating anthropometric measurements to age of children in some parts of the world is difficult when birth dates cannot be verified, and Jelliffe (1969) has stressed the need for measurements that are independent of age. So-called age-independent measurements are based on the ratio of a nutritionally labile tissue such as muscle mass or subcutaneous fat to a measurement likely to be less affected by acute short-term malnutrition such as height, head circumference, or the length of a single bone. A suggested measurement of weight for height has the disadvantage of possibly masking a general growth failure with a body weight that is relatively proportional to height (Downs, 1964). Jelliffe and Jelliffe (1971) suggest that in areas where malnutrition is prevalent in childhood, anthropometric tests of nutritional status may have to take into consideration the age incidence of malnutrition in that

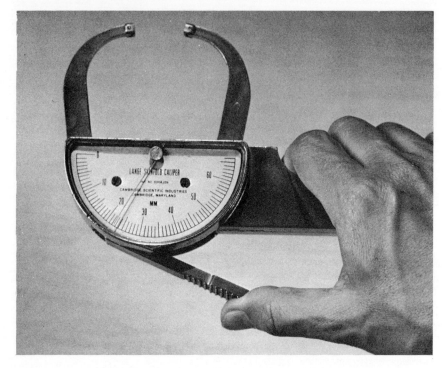

Fig. 22.1   A standard skinfold caliper.

locale. They suggest the development of composite anthropometric indices including weight, height or possibly arm length, midarm muscle, and fat measurements that might be used to indicate mass, linear growth, and protein and calorie reserves, respectively.

The ease and rapidity of obtaining anthropometric measurements with tape measure and calipers make them extremely attractive for estimating body fat, body muscle, and the weight of the lean body mass. Behnke (1963) presents the formulas used and the data obtained on groups of individuals to support the value of specific body measurements in screening procedures.

Skinfold Thickness

Since the subcutaneous adipose tissue constitutes approximately 50 percent of the adipose tissue stores, skinfold measurements can serve a useful purpose in judging the total body fat of individuals. In addition, they are simple, rapid, easily interpreted, and can be used in the clinic or in the field. Keys and Brozek (1953) have

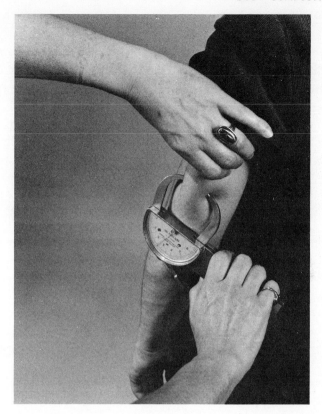

Fig. 22.2 Skinfold caliper measuring a relatively thick triceps skinfold in a young woman.

reviewed the literature on skinfold measurements with respect to standardization, sites, and consistency of measurements. Data on young American soldiers were included in the report of the 1956 conference (Newman, 1956; Pascale et al., 1956). At subsequent conferences, data were presented on middle-aged men (Brozek et al., 1963), older women (Young et al., 1963a; Wessel et al., 1963), adolescent boys and girls in different cultures (Young, 1965), and trained and untrained athletes (Pařízková, 1965).

Standardization of skinfold measurements involves both site of measurement and the pressure exerted by the calipers on the double fold. Specially designed calipers (Fig. 22.1) exert a pressure of 10 gm/mm^2 on a contact surface of 20-40 mm^2. A trained technician using standard calipers on the triceps (Fig. 22.2) or subscapular skinfold can obtain a rapid estimation of total body fatness. Several investigators using only the triceps, which is easiest to measure, have obtained extensive data which permit determination of the normal variation in the American population (Brozek et al., 1963; Seltzer and Mayer, 1965; Seltzer et al., 1965).

A report published by the Department of Health, Education and Welfare (1973a) presents data on the distribution of skinfold measurements, at three anatomical sites, on children aged 6 through 11 years in the United States. Data on over 7000 children are discussed as related to age, sex, race, and geographic regions. This report is the second in 25 to be published on body dimensions and composition. A report on height and weight of youths 12 through 17 (DHEW, 1973b) presents an analysis of the adolescent growth spurt.

Garn et al. (1971) have studied the relative values of subscapular and triceps fat fold measurements made under actual field conditions. They found that correlations of the two measurements were high and that the subscapular fold systematically had higher correlations with weight than the triceps fat fold. They were able to demonstrate also that summing the two fat fold measurements did not offer any advantage. Based on their analysis of the data from the Michigan phase of the Ten-State Nutrition Survey, they concluded that fat fold measurements effectively provide indications of fatness under field conditions in a mass scale nutrition survey.

The triceps fat fold measurement can be used to ascertain the arm muscle circumference through the use of a nomogram. The arm muscle circumference is read where a line joining the fat fold measurement and the arm circumference crosses. Figures are given also for determining the equivalent muscle area, arm area, and fat area (Gurney and Jelliffe, 1973).

A high correlation has been shown between pinch-caliper and X-ray measurements of skin and subcutaneous fat (Garn, 1956) and, since the fat-plus-skin thickness at the midaxillary line at the level of the lowest rib can be measured on full-size or miniature chest plates, Garn (1957) suggests that mass radiography as used in tuberculosis detection could be extended to the assessment of obesity. Young et al. (1963b) reported good correlation between skinfold thickness and X-ray measurements of fat-pad thickness made at lower thorax and suprailiac locations in young women. Theoretically, the skinfold measurements should be twice the X-ray measurement since the calipers measure a double thickness; however, a correction has to be made for compression even though standard calipers are used, and Young et al. (1963b) point out that compression varies with location.

Body Density

Early studies by Behnke et al. (1942) and Welham and Behnke (1942) on Navy personnel, some of whom were overweight according to height-weight standards but obviously not overfat, led to the use of body density for estimating the variable quantity of body fat. From this emerged the concept of *lean body mass*, which they defined as the whole body minus nonessential or excess lipids. The lean body mass was conceived as relatively constant in gross chemical composition with fat acting as a diluent (Behnke, 1941-1942). The concept was quantitatively expressed by Pace and Rathbun (1945) on the basis of an average water content of 73.2 percent of the lean body mass. On this basis, they developed the equation:

$$\% \text{ body fat } = 100 - \frac{\% \text{ body water}}{0.732}$$

This concept of lean body mass differs from the fat-free body in that essential structural lipids are included. Behnke's group first estimated essential lipids as constituting 10 percent of the total mass, but later this was revised to 2 percent. Although the concept is different, the actual discrepancy between the fat-free body and the lean body mass that contains 2 percent essential lipid is negligible.

The rationale of Behnke's group for using body density as an estimate of body composition was based on the concept of a relatively constant lean body mass coupled with a variable fat mass. Since the density of fat is less than that of other body components, as the percentage of body fat increases, the body density decreases. In practice, specific gravity is substituted for density and calculated as weight divided by volume:

$$\text{Sp. gr. } = \frac{W}{V}$$

The essential measurement, body volume, may be obtained by employing Archimedes' principle of water displacement. Body

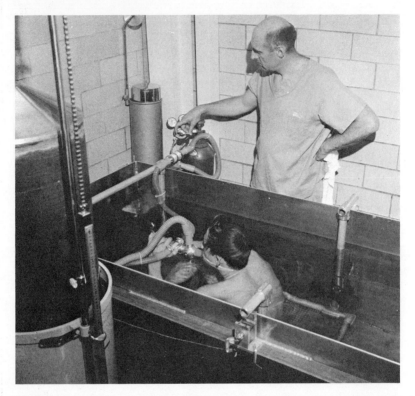

Fig. 22.3 Subject in position for obtaining underwater weight which is measured using a suspended metal mesh cot. The outputs from four transducers placed at each corner of the cot frame are balanced and integrated into one voltage that is recorded on a strip chart. The subject bends forward so that his head goes underwater and his weight is recorded. He exhales as he submerges and continues to exhale until he reaches voluntary end-expiration. At this point his breathing circuit is switched to a small demand spirometer and he breathes pure oxygen for seven minutes. The volume of air in his lungs at the time the subject is weighed is determined by the quantity of nitrogen he expires in seven minutes (nitrogen wash-out method for determining the residual volume of the lungs). (Courtesy of Dr. E. R. Buskirk, The Pennsylvania State University.)

volume therefore is calculated by subtracting the weight under water from the weight in air:

$$V = \text{wt in air} - \text{wt under water}$$

Several methods have been devised for obtaining weight under water, one of which is shown in Fig. 22.3. Corrections must be made for residual air in the lungs.

On the basis of chemical analyses and specific gravity determinations on shaved, eviscerated guinea pigs, Rathbun and Pace (1945) derived an equation for the conversion of specific gravity to percent body fat. The values presented in Table 22.3 are based on the

Table 22.3   CONVERSION OF VALUES FOR BODY SPECIFIC GRAVITY OF MAN TO FAT CONTENT ON BASIS OF EQUATION, PERCENT FAT = 100 [5.548/ (SPECIFIC GRAVITY) MINUS 5.044]

Body Sp. Gr.	Percent Fat of Body Weight	Body Sp. Gr.	Percent Fat of Body Weight
1.002	49.3	1.052	23.0
1.004	48.2	1.054	22.0
1.006	47.1	1.056	21.0
1.008	46.0	1.058	20.0
1.010	44.9	1.060	19.0
1.012	43.8	1.062	18.0
1.014	42.7	1.064	17.0
1.016	41.7	1.066	16.1
1.018	40.6	1.068	15.1
1.020	39.5	1.070	14.1
1.022	38.5	1.072	13.1
1.024	37.4	1.074	12.2
1.026	36.3	1.076	11.2
1.028	35.3	1.078	10.3
1.030	34.2	1.080	9.3
1.032	33.2	1.082	8.4
1.034	32.2	1.084	7.4
1.036	31.1	1.086	6.5
1.038	30.1	1.088	5.5
1.040	29.1	1.090	4.6
1.042	28.0	1.092	3.7
1.044	27.0	1.094	2.7
1.046	26.0	1.096	1.8
1.048	25.0	1.098	0.9
1.050	24.0	1.100	0.0

From E. N. Rathbun and N. Pace, *J. Biol. Chem.*, 158: 667 (1945).

following equation, which was corrected for the density of human fat:

$$\% \text{ body fat} = 100 \left(\frac{5.548}{\text{sp. gr.}} - 5.004 \right)$$

Using this formula and the formula by which percent body fat is derived (shown previously), Pace and Rathbun (1945) derived the equation to predict from specific gravity both the fat content and water content of the whole body.

$$\% \text{ body water} = 100 \left(4.24 - \frac{4.061}{\text{sp. gr.}} \right)$$

Since the estimation of specific gravity involves the use of expensive equipment and an extremely cooperative subject, it cannot be used in the clinic to estimate body fatness. Equations for predicting specific gravity from skinfold thickness measurements of men have been presented by Brozek and Keys (1951), and Young et al. (1962) have presented a formula for predicting specific gravity of young women from one skinfold measurement and the percentage of "standard weight." The predicted specific gravity can then be converted to percent fat using the Rathbun-Pace formula. Based on such calculations, Young et al. (1962) presented data on the Cornell reference young woman of normal weight (Table 22.4).

Table 22.4   CORNELL REFERENCE YOUNG WOMAN

	Percent	Percent
Fat	29	0[a]
Water	52	73
Cell solids	14	20
Bone mineral	5	7

From C. M. Young et al., *J. Amer. Diet. Ass.*, 40: 102 (1962).
[a]Calculated on fat-free basis.

The difficulties and restrictions encountered in measuring body density by hydrometry led to the development of methods for measuring body volume by helium displacement (Siri, 1953; Fomon et al., 1963) and by air displacement (Falkner, 1963; Gnaedinger et al., 1963), each of which obviates the necessity for correcting for residual air in the lungs. However, each of these methods and the chambers they require for use are of value as research tools but do not provide any quick and easy means for determining body volume.

Simultaneous Multiple Isotope Dilution

Dilution techniques freed the investigator from the limitations imposed by either chemical analysis of a cadaver or the indirect and somewhat imprecise methods of anthropometry and densitometry for estimation of body composition *in vivo*. The more illusive compartmentalization of body components could now be studied. Dilution methodology is based on the concept that certain substances distribute themselves evenly within a specific body water compartment and that the dilution of a known amount of substance introduced into an unknown volume permits calculation of that unknown volume. Antipyrine distributes itself evenly throughout the total body water and therefore can be used for the determination of total body water. Thiocyanate and inulin distribute themselves within the extracellular fluid but do not penetrate the plasma membrane. The use of simultaneous measurement of total body water and extracellular water permits the calculation of intracellular water by difference.

The most detailed and extensive compilation of data employing the multiple isotope dilution method comes from the laboratories of Moore and his associates at Harvard and the Peter Bent Brigham Hospital in Boston. Table 22.5 indicates the direct measurements that were made employing the multiple isotope dilution technique and those that could then be derived. From this listing, it is readily apparent that research in body composition has attained a certain degree of sophistication. For the methods, both biochemical and statistical, and the detailed data from clinical studies, the reader is referred to the published monograph (Moore et al., 1963). Only a few of the pertinent concepts will be discussed here.

Since total body water (TBW) can be determined directly, the formula of Pace and Rathbun (1945) can be employed to calculate the percent of body fat, and from that the simple calculations for total body fat (TBF), total body solids (TBS), and fat-free solids (FFS):

Table 22.5 COMPOSITIONAL RATIOS AND DERIVATIONS

Ratio or Derivation	Abbreviation	Dimensions	Normal Range[a]
Total body fat	TBF	kg or % B.Wt.[b]	12-20 % B.Wt.
Total body solids	TBS	kg or % B.Wt.	40-60 % B.Wt.
Fat-free solids	FFS	kg or % B.Wt.	25-40 % B.Wt.
Intracellular water	ICW	L. or % B.Wt.	30-40 % B.Wt.
Residual sodium	Res Na	mEq or % Na_e	8-15 % Na_e
Average intracellular potassium concentration	Av. ICK conc.	mEq/liter	140-160 mEq/liter
Ratio of whole body hematocrit to large vessel hematocrit	WBH/LVH	%/%	0.85-0.91
Ratio of total exchangeable sodium to total exchangeable potassium	Na_e/K_e	mEq/mEq	0.85-1.00
Ratio of sum of total exchangeable sodium plus total exchangeable potassium to body weight	Na_e+K_e/B.Wt.	mEq/kg	70-90 mEq/kg
Concentration of total exchangeable cation (sodium plus potassium) in total body water	Na_e+K_e/TBW	mEq/liter	150-160 mEq/liter
Body cell mass	BCM	kg or % B.Wt.	35-45 % B.Wt.
Ratio of intracellular water to total body water; relative predominance of the cell	ICW/TBW	liter/liter x 100	50-55 %
Ratio of red cell volume to total exchangeable potassium	RV/K_e	ml/mEq	0.50-0.55 ml/mEq
Ratio of total exchangeable potassium to dry body weight	K_e/DBW	mEq/kg	90-110 mEq/kg
Ratio of total exchangeable potassium to fat-free solids	K_e/FFS	mEq/kg	200-250 mEq/kg
Ratio of red cell volume to plasma volume	RV/PV	ml/ml	0.70-0.80
Ratio of plasma volume to total exchangeable sodium	PV/Na_e	ml/mEq	0.95-1.10 ml/mEq
Dry fat-free, marrow-free whole bone (matrix plus mineral)	B	kg or % B.Wt.	6-8 % B.Wt. (10.3 % FFB)
Ratio of total exchangeable potassium to resting 24-hour creatinine excretion	K_e/creatinine	mEq/mg	1.75-2.25 mEq/mg

From F. D. Moore et al., *The Body Cell Mass and Its Supporting Environment*, W. B. Saunders Co., Philadelphia, Pa., 1963, p. 20.

[a]Broad range only.

[b]The term "B.Wt." is used for body weight throughout.

$$(1) \ \% \text{ fat} = 100 \ - \ \frac{\% \text{ water}}{0.732}$$

$$(2) \ \text{TBF (kg)} = \% \text{ fat} \ \times \ \frac{\text{B.Wt. (kg)}}{100}$$

$$(3) \ \text{TBS (kg)} = \text{B.Wt. (kg)} \ - \ \text{TBW}$$

$$(4) \ \text{FFS} = \text{TBS} \ - \ \text{TBF}$$

A nomogram illustrating the relationship between the water phase and the fat-free solid phase of the body is shown in Fig. 22.4. The theoretical aspects of the relationship between body water and fat-free solids permit evaluation of both normal and abnormal conditions of hydration on the basis that water content of fat-free tissue normally ranges from 69-74 percent.

From the direct determination of total exchangeable potassium (K_e) by isotope dilution using ^{42}K another important concept has evolved, that of *body cell mass*. The body cell mass as defined by Moore et al. (1963) is the "chemically homogeneous mass of tissue in the body that contains all the cellular elements concerned with respiration, physical and chemical work, and mitotic activity." It is comprised of all the cells of the body capable of converting or using the chemical energy of food. It does not include the fluids bathing the cells nor any solids outside the cell membrane. The body cell mass is the composite of oxygen-requiring, carbon dioxide-producing, glucose-metabolizing cells of the body and constitutes from 35 to 45 percent of the body weight in the normal adult male and from 30 to 40 percent in the adult female. The body cell mass differs from both the *fat-free body* of chemical analysis and the concept of *lean body mass* set forth by Behnke. Each of the latter designations is heterogeneous both in its chemistry and energy exchange and includes not only the metabolizing cells but also skeletal and cartilaginous material, collagen and other noncellular, nonfat portions which are not actively metabolizing nor even constant in mass.

All cells in the normal body contain potassium at a concentration of approximately 150 mEq/kg cell water (Moore and Boyden, 1963). Potassium is not present to any extent in the extracellular compartment. Thus the total amount of potassium in the body is a linear function of the body cell mass:

$$\text{BCM (gm)} = K_e \times 8.33$$

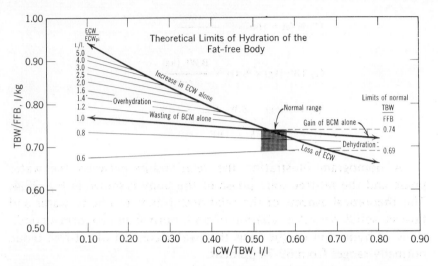

Fig. 22.4 Theoretical limits of hydration of the fat-free body. The hydration coefficient of the fat-free body (the ratio TBW/FFB shown on the vertical coordinates) in the normal adult is usually assumed to be 0.732. It is variously estimated by dissection in animals and in man as varying from 0.67 to 0.74. These limits of normal (TBW/FFB) are shown to the right, as well as in the shaded area identified as "normal range" and coordinated with an ICW/TBW ratio (horizontal coordinates of 0.51 to 0.58). This ratio, ICW/TBW, indicates the relative predominance of the cell mass in the aqueous phase of body composition.

One other ratio is needed to express relative hydration. This is the ratio of the observed extracellular water to the extracellular water before illness. ECW/ECW$_{pi}$, shown as an added coordinate to the left.

If the body wastes by a loss of body cell mass alone, the average hydration of the fat-free body increases slightly because the average water content of the body cell mass is lower than that of the extracellular fluid within which this wasting occurs.

If body composition changes by an increase in extracellular water alone, then average hydration of the fat-free body increases sharply, and this describes the upper limit of body hydration.

The overhydration commonly observed in a wide variety of pathologic states lies somewhere between these two limits. Its exact position can be estimated by the ratio of extracellular water as observed to that predicted from regression relations, before illness.

Given the observed ICW/TBW ratio and the calculated ratio

where K_e is the total exchangeable potassium in mEq and 8.33 is the coefficient applied to yield the wet weight of the body cell mass in grams. Moore and Boyden (1963) point out that the coefficient is not precise but lies somewhere between 7.0 and 10.0. Thus the measurement of exchangeable potassium can be converted into body cell mass in grams.

The body cell mass is comprised essentially of two large groups of tissues: muscle, both skeletal and smooth; and parenchyma (heart, brain, liver, kidneys, diaphragm, and endocrine glands). These two moieties differ in that the muscle functions intermittently, resting between contractions, whereas the parenchymal cells are unceasingly involved in the oxidative and synthetic processes basic to all cell life. In terms of total body energy expenditure, the muscle is concerned primarily with "activity" (including gastrointestinal activity) and the parenchyma with the basal metabolic rate. Since the muscle mass may vary widely among individuals or even in the same person depending upon use and state of health, a partition of the K_e into these two components can provide important information. Creatinine excretion is a linear function of the skeletal muscle mass and remains relatively constant in the normal individual. Determination of creatinine excretion permits the calculation of the K_e/creatinine ratio:

$$\text{Muscle mass} = \frac{K_e}{\text{creatinine}}$$

The K_e/creatinine ratio reported for normal subjects in the Moore monograph ranged around 2.0 mEq/mg. Distortions in the ratio are indicative of changes in the relationship between the creatinine-producing and the noncreatinine-producing moieties comprising the body cell mass. As the athlete builds up skeletal muscle, the ratio

---

Fig. 22.4 (Continued)
ECW/ECW$_{pi}$, this diagram can be used as a nomogram to read off the TBW/FFB ratio. From this, in turn, body fat may be calculated with greater accuracy than that resulting from the use of a fixed coefficient such as 0.732.

The much rarer dehydration states are described by similar limits and are shown to the right of the normal range. (From Moore et al., *The Body Cell Mass and Its Supporting Environment*, W. B. Saunders Co., Phila., 1963, p. 16.)

falls; however, in wasting disease, the ratio rises.

Creatinine excretion alone can be used as a predictor of the mass of muscle tissue since a highly significant linear relationship exists between creatinine excretion during growth and muscle mass. A factor of 20 was derived by Cheek (1969, p. 191) indicating 1 gm of urinary creatinine per day as equivalent to 20 kg of muscle mass, and he presented equations to show that this factor could be used with a high degree of confidence.

Since the body cell mass is the energy-exchanging, work-producing moiety of body tissue, we should expect to find a relationship with total energy expenditure. Kinney et al. (1963) studied a group of hospitalized patients and found that a strong correlation did indeed exist between total energy expenditure and body cell mass. Allen et al. (1969), using ^{40}K (see below), also reported a linear relationship in healthy young male subjects. These findings are support for Rubner's early concept of the relationship of body heat production to the active tissue mass and illustrate how advances in methodology may eventually (in this case one-half century later) provide data to substantiate a logical but unverifiable concept.

The techniques involved in simultaneous multiple isotope dilution call for skilled personnel, expensive equipment, cooperative subjects, and time. The vast amount of statistically analyzed data on both normal subjects and hospital patients presented in the monograph by Moore and his associates (1963) has probed into the details, provided interpretation, and extracted concepts concerning normal body composition. In addition to providing data in depth through the direct and derived measurements in this elegant series of integrated studies, it also has provided a means for detecting and interpreting compositional shifts in pathological conditions.

^{40}K Analysis

Isotopic dilution using ^{42}K involves the intravenous injection of the radioisotope into the subject, a waiting time for equilibration, and the subsequent withdrawal of samples for analysis of dilution, whereas measuring the naturally occurring ^{40}K involves only counting the gamma rays emitted from the body. Since ^{40}K comprises 0.012 percent of naturally occurring potassium, the quantity in the body can be measured by a low level scintillation counter and, from the count, the total body potassium can be calculated.

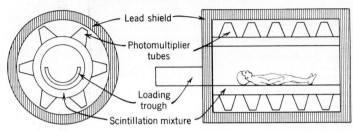

Schematic drawing of whole body counter

Lead shield

Photomultiplier tubes

Loading trough

Scintillation mixture

Fig. 22.5 Schematic representation of 4-pi whole body liquid scintillation counter. (From R. C. Reba, F. C. Leitnaker, and K. T. Woodward in D. B. Cheek, ed., *Human Growth,* Lea and Febiger, Phila., 1968, p. 675.)

A schematic representation of a whole body scintillation counter is shown in Fig. 22.5. The counter is 6 feet in length with an inner diameter of 20 inches for the subject. The motor-driven canvas sling on which the subject lies is moved into the well of the counter which is surrounded by a layer of liquid scintillator solution about 6 inches in thickness. The scintillator converts the photon energies of the gamma rays into light impulses or scintillations which are detected, amplified, and counted. For additional details, see Reba et al. (1969). The rapid procedure (3-30 minutes depending upon the instrument) is without risk or discomfort to the subject. These advantages tend to offset the high cost and complexity of the instrument. The results obtained are highly reproducible permitting comparisons between laboratories. Data showing the relationship of total body potassium to body weight from different laboratories is shown in Fig. 22.6.

Methods for the measurement of total potassium content of the human by means of ^{40}K were first reported by Anderson and Langham (1959). In 1590 individuals ranging in age from one to 79 years, sex differences and age trends were observed in the ratio of muscle mass to the other body constituents which contain little or no potassium. The use of whole body ^{40}K counting for the estimation of body fat was conceived by Forbes et al. (1961), who reported on 50 subjects, both males and females, ranging in age from 7 to 44 years. From the ^{40}K count, total body potassium was calculated, based on a potassium content of 68.1 mEq/kg:

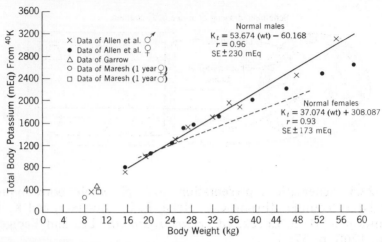

Fig. 22.6 Relationship of total body potassium to body weight. Values obtained from the literature relating total K to weights outside the range of those reported in the present study are added. The solid lines are the calculated regression relationships obtained in the present study. A sex difference becomes apparent after body weight exceeds 21 kg. (From R. C. Reba, F. C. Leitnaker, and K. T. Woodward in D. B. Cheek, ed., *Human Growth,* Lea and Febiger, Phila., 1968, p. 679.)

$$\text{LBW (kg)} = \frac{\text{measured total K (mEq)}}{68.1}$$

Fat content was then calculated as the difference between total body weight and lean body weight. The authors were able to show good correlations with skinfold thickness and weight/height ratio indices of fatness.

In subsequent studies, Forbes and Hursh (1963) and Barter and Forbes (1963) indicate their awareness of the variation in potassium content of individual body tissues and of how contributions from bone and viscera could lead to error in the calculation of lean body mass. Therefore, Forbes (1972) included correction figures for both the influence of adiposity and for the calibration of their instrument in estimating LBM by ^{40}K counting. These data were compared with estimates obtained from body density and total body water measurements. The data derived through these three methods are comparable when height differences are taken into account and when only narrow age groupings are compared, indicating that a

Table 22.6   PERCENTAGE COMPOSITION OF MAN ON A FAT-FREE BASIS

Age	Investigator	No. of Individuals	Water (percent)	Nitrogen (percent)	Ash (percent)
		Fetus			
35 days	Fehling[a]	1	97.54	0.39	0.001
2.5 months	Michel[b]	1	93.82	0.69	
3 months	Fehling[a]	2	91.84	0.81	1.005
3-4 months	Michel[b]	1	89.95	1.1	1.73
4 months	Fehling[a]	2	92.46	0.92	1.23
4.5 months	Fehling[a]	5	90.38	1.11	1.62
5 months	Fehling[a]	3	87.43	1.26	2.40
5 months	Michel[b]	1	87.81	1.32	1.95
5 months	Michel[b]	1	86.73	1.39	2.49
6 months	Michel[b]	1	85.03	1.64	2.51
6 months	Fehling[a]	4	86.00	1.78	2.72
7 months	Fehling[a]	1	84.97	1.71	2.89
7 months	Michel[b]	1	84.74	1.56	2.49
Full term	Fehling[a]	1	81.52	2.08	2.81
		Extrauterine			
Newborn	Camerer and Söldner[c]	6	81.87	2.13	3.08
Newborn	Klose[d]	1	80.2	2.32	3.52
3 months	Sommerfeld	1	80.73	2.61	3.14
4 months	Steinitz and Weigert[e]	1	77.75	2.97	3.94
33 yr	Moleschott[f]	1	69.33	3.3	9.44?

From C. R. Moulton, *J. Biol. Chem.*, 57: 79 (1923).

[a] H. Fehling, *Arch. Gynäk.*, 1877, xi, 523.

[b] C. Michel, *Compt. rend. Soc. biol.*, 1899, li, 422.

[c] W. Camerer, *Z. Biol.*, 1900, xxxix, 173; xl, 529; 1902, xliii, 1. Söldner, *Z. Biol.*, 1903, xliv, 61.

[d] E. Klose, *Jahrb. Kinderh.*, 1900, xxx, 253.

[e] F. Steinitz and R. Weigert, *Beitr. chem. Physiol. u. Path.*, 1905, vi, 206.

[f] J. Moleschott, *Physiologie der Nahrungsmittel*, Giessen, 2nd edition, 1859, 224.

properly calibrated whole body counter can provide valid estimates of LBM.

COMPOSITIONAL CHANGES DURING THE LIFE CYCLE

Pioneer studies of the effects of age and species on body composition were carried out over a century ago by von Bezold (1857), who reported that every individual animal possessed a normal water, organic matter, and salt content that was typical of its species and age and that was approximately constant in higher vertebrates. The classic analytical studies of Moulton (1923) on the changes during development of several different mammalian species, which he compared to data he assembled for man, led to his concept of *chemical maturity*. Moulton defined chemical maturity as the point at which the concentration of water, proteins, and salts becomes comparatively constant in the fat-free body. He showed that there was a rapid decrease in the water content of fat-free mammalian tissue and an increase in protein and ash content from conception to the time of chemical maturity, when the change became suddenly less and a practically constant concentration was reached. The data he assembled for man are shown in Table 22.6. There is a striking inverse relationship of water to both nitrogen and ash (Fig. 22.7). Comparable data on cattle are shown in Fig. 22.8. Curves for swine, guinea pigs, dogs, cats, rabbits, rats, and mice show similar slopes.

Moulton related the variation in mammalian composition at birth to relative maturity: animals born with a high water content were less mature, and those with a relatively low water content more mature. He also related chemical development to the degree of physical development at birth: animals with relatively great development, such as guinea pigs and cattle, quickly get on their feet at birth and are well developed physically, whereas rats and mice, which are very immature at birth, have the highest water content and the greater part of their chemical development occurs after birth. Man, the pig, the dog, and the cat are in an intermediate group.

Decades later confirmation of Moulton's suggestion relating chemical development to physiological development was presented by Widdowson and Dickerson (1964). Table 22.7 presents data on the chemical composition of newborn for eight mammalian species. The guinea pig contains the highest concentration of nitrogen, calcium, magnesium, and phosphorus, making it the most highly developed chemically. It is also the most highly developed functionally. In contrast, rats, rabbits, and mice are least developed both chemically and functionally.

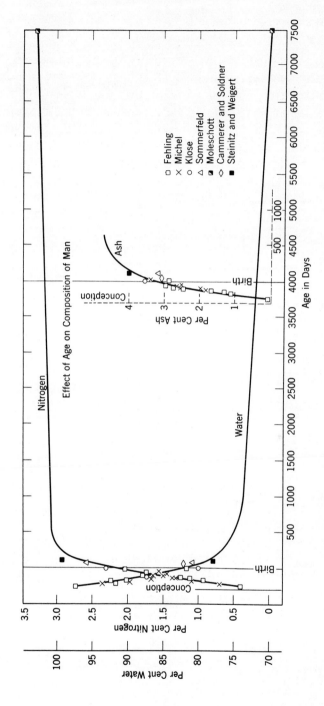

Fig. 22.7 Effect of age on the composition of man. [From C. R. Moulton, *J. Biol. Chem.*, 57:79 (1923).]

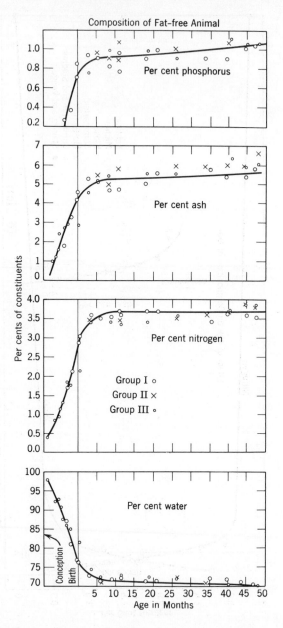

Fig. 22.8 Effect of age on the composition of cattle. Data of Moulton and coworkers. [From C. R. Moulton, *J. Biol. Chem.*, 57:79 (1923).]

Table 22.7 CHEMICAL COMPOSITION OF NEWBORN MAMMALS

Constituent	Man	Pig	Dog	Cat	Rabbit	Guinea Pig	Rat	Mouse
Body weight (gm)	3560	1260	328	118	54	80	5.9	1.6
Composition[a]								
Water (gm)	82.3	82.0	84.5	82.2	86.5	77.5	86.2	85.0
Total N (gm)	2.3	1.8	2.1	2.4	1.8	2.9	1.6	2.1
Ca (gm)	1.0	1.0	0.5	0.7	0.5	1.2	0.3	0.3
P (gm)	0.6	0.6	0.4	0.4	0.4	0.8	0.4	0.3
Mg (gm)	0.03	0.03	0.02	0.03	0.02	0.05	0.03	0.03
Fe (mg)	9.4	2.9	—	5.5	13.5	6.7	5.9	6.7
Cu (mg)	0.5	0.3	—	0.3	0.4	0.7	0.4	0.7
Zn (mg)	1.9	1.0	—	2.9	2.3	3.5	2.4	4.6

From E. M. Widdowson and J. W. T. Dickerson, "Chemical Composition of the Body," *Mineral Metabolism*, Vol. II, Part A, C. L. Comar and F. Bronner, eds., Acad. Press, N. Y., 1964, p. 40.

[a]Data expressed per 100 gm fat-free body tissue.

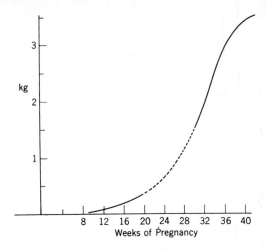

Fig. 22.9 The average curve of fetal growth. The curve up to 20 weeks is based on unpublished data of Dr. T. Lind; from 32 weeks to term on data of Thomson et al. 1968. The intermediate dotted line has been fitted arbitrarily. (From F. E. Hytten and I. Leitch, *The Physiology of Human Pregnancy*, 2nd ed., Blackwell Scientific Publications, Oxford, 1971, p. 292.)

Human Fetal Development

Investigation of the human fetus presents problems not encountered in animal studies, and establishing criteria for normality of the fetus in an interrupted pregnancy may be difficult. Despite the vastness of the problem and the enormity of the difficulties encountered, Hytten and Leitch (1971) have amassed and presented data on chemical changes during fetal development and the associated changes in the human maternal organism from their own studies at Aberdeen and from selected sources in the literature. Fig. 22.9 presents the weight gain of the human fetus during the gestation period. As the fetus grows and develops, total body water, which is the largest contributor to weight, falls from approximately 92 percent to 70 or 72 percent at term. This change is accompanied by an increase in protein and, particularly during the last two months of gestation, by an increase in fat content. The relative amounts of nitrogen, fat, and water in the developing fetus are shown in Fig. 22.10. Deposition of protein far exceeds that of fat until the last

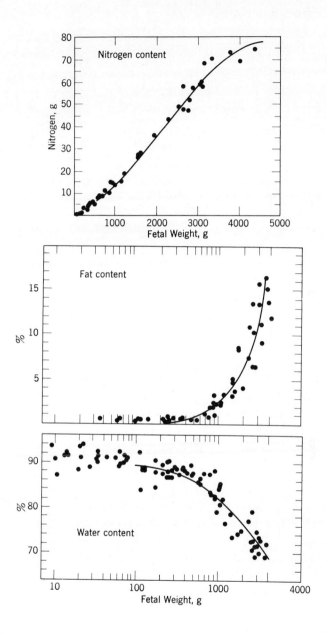

Fig. 22.10 Nitrogen, fat, and water content of human fetus. (From F. E. Hytten and I. Leitch, *The Physiology of Human Pregnancy*, 2nd ed., Blackwell Scientific Publications, Oxford, 1971, pp. 371, 373.)

2 months of gestation when relatively large amounts of fat are accumulated. The premature human infant whose body weight may be half that of a full term baby may have only 10 percent of the fat; this, in itself, is enough to explain the scrawny appearance of prematures and the need to protect them against body heat loss.

The concentration of calcium in the fetus increases progressively from under 2 gm/kg for the smallest fetuses to over 8 gm/kg at term, or approximately 28 gm. Sodium content also rises progressively to 6-7 gm at term and, when calculated on the basis of concentration per 100 gm of fat-free tissue, it remains almost constant at 230-240 mg during fetal development. About 30 percent of the sodium in the skeleton is nonexchangeable and therefore not measured by dilution techniques. Potassium rises to about 6 gm at term and on the basis of 100 gm of fat-free tissue the values increase from approximately 165 mg in the smallest fetuses to about 205 mg at term. The potassium is primarily in the intracellular water and hence is related to cell mass. Great variation is observed in the iron content of fetuses and the analyses of Widdowson and Spray (see Hytten and Leitch, 1971, p. 376) show a range of from 200 mg in smaller to approximately 375 mg in full term fetuses.

Body composition changes in 41 fetuses of malnourished Indian mothers were reported to be more closely related to body weight than to gestational age (Apte and Lyengar, 1972). Although the calcium, phosphorus, and magnesium contents of the body per unit of fat-free weight increased progressively with gestational age, the values were considerably lower than those reported in the literature. Body iron was almost 30 percent lower than reported values. This study emphasizes that the chemical composition of nutrient stores in the developing fetus can be considerably influenced by the state of maternal nutrition.

Susceptibility to modification of body composition in the premature infant may be comparable to that of the fetus. Kagan et al. (1972) found that even minor changes in the diet during the first month affected the body composition of prematures. The differences in body composition, which were apparent in total body water and the distribution of body water into the intra- and extracellular compartments, were influenced primarily by the amount of the electrolytes in the milks offered and the ratio of electrolytes, particularly potassium, to protein. The data presented make it clear that the metabolism of the young premature infant is modified by the composition of the diet offered to him.

The fetus is but one of three products of conception, albeit the most important with respect to size and consequence. The comparative increments during development of protein, fat, and calcium in fetus, placenta, and amniotic fluid are shown in Table 22.8. There are insufficient data on iron, but it is estimated that the fetus and placenta together contain approximately 450 mg.

Table 22.8 PROTEIN, FAT, AND CALCIUM IN THE PRODUCTS OF CONCEPTION

	Weeks of Pregnancy			
	10	20	30	40
		Protein		
Fetus	0.3	27	160	440
Placenta	2	16	60	100
Amniotic fluid	0.08	0.5	2	3
Total	2	44	222	543
		Fat		
Fetus	2	2	80	440
Placenta		1	3	4
Amniotic fluid		0.1	0.4	0.5
Total	2	3	83	445
		Calcium		
Fetus	Negligible	1.5	10	28
Placenta	Negligible	0.05	0.13	0.65
Amniotic fluid	Negligible	Negligible	Negligible	Negligible
Total	Negligible	1.5	10	29

From F. E. Hytten and I. Leitch, *The Physiology of Human Pregnancy*, 2nd ed., Blackwell Scientific Publications, Oxford, 1971, p. 382-383.

Maternal Weight Gain

Distribution. In addition to the nutrients incorporated into the products of conception, significant additions occur in the maternal body. However, in order to evaluate the composition of the weight gain, it is important to know whether any interference with

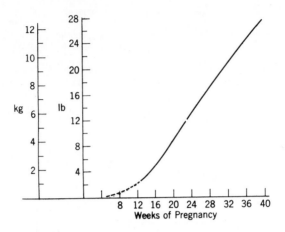

Fig. 22.11 Mean weight gain in pregnancy of 2868 normotensive primigravidae (Thomson and Billewicz, 1957). (From F. E. Hytten and I. Leitch, *The Physiology of Human Pregnancy,* 2nd ed., Blackwell Scientific Publications, Oxford, 1971, p. 280.)

the normal physiological adjustment was imposed through dietary restriction. Regulation of weight gain during pregnancy has long been the subject of debate and, until relatively recently, many obstetricians have tried to manipulate weight gain. Fortunately this practice is falling into disrepute, and evidence is accumulating that restriction of weight gain during pregnancy may significantly affect the incidence of prematurity, low birth weight, and the attendant mortality and morbidity (Singer et al., 1968). Weight gain in a healthy young woman who eats to appetite during pregnancy is estimated to be approximately 27.5 lb (12.5 kg) at term. The estimated weight gain at 10 weeks is 1.5 lb (0.65 kg); at 20 weeks, 9 lb (4 kg); at 30 weeks, 19 lb (8.5 kg); with the remainder during the last 10 weeks of pregnancy (Fig. 22.11). The distribution of this weight gain among the products of conception during the course of pregnancy and the more difficult estimations of the weight of the uterus, breasts, and blood volume, each of which add considerably to the total, is summarized in Table 22.9. In this analysis of weight gain there is approximately 3.5 kg which is not accounted for and assumed to be fat (Hytten and Leitch, 1971, p. 357). An estimated weight gain of up to 25 lb was recommended by the Committee on Maternal Nutrition (1970).

Table 22.9 ANALYSIS OF WIEGHT GAIN

Tissues and Fluids Accounted For and Total Weight Gained	Increase in Weight Up to:			
	10 weeks	20 weeks	30 weeks	40 weeks
	(gm)	(gm)	(gm)	(gm)
Fetus	5	300	1500	3400
Placenta	20	170	430	650
Amniotic fluid	30	350	750	800
Uterus	140	320	600	970
Mammary gland	45	180	360	405
Blood	100	600	1300	1250
Extracellular extravascular fluid				
1. No edema or leg edema	0	30	80	1680
2. Generalized edema	0	500	1526	4897
Total				
1. No edema or leg edema	340	1950	5020	9155
2. Generalized edema	340	2420	6466	12372
Total weight gained				
1. No edema or leg edema	650	4000	8500	12500
2. Generalized edema	650	4500	10000	14500
Weight not accounted for				
1. No edema or leg edema	310	2050	3480	3345
2. Generalized edema	310	2080	3534	2128

From F. E. Hytten and I. Leitch, *The Physiology of Human Pregnancy*, 2nd ed., Blackwell Scientific Publications, Oxford, 1971, p. 356.

Composition. Measurement of changes in body composition during pregnancy are a summation of the changes in the maternal tissue and the products of conception. Estimates of body composition rely primarily on measurements of body water employing the usual dilution and tracer techniques and/or body density. From these measurements body fat and lean body mass can be calculated according to the formulas presented previously. However, the validity must be questioned for pregnancy since the constant proportions of water to lean body mass cannot be fixed at 73 percent as for the nonpregnant. Some of the nonfat weight added during pregnancy has a water content of 90 percent. Whether or not the ratio between protein and mineral of the lean mass is unchanged during pregnancy

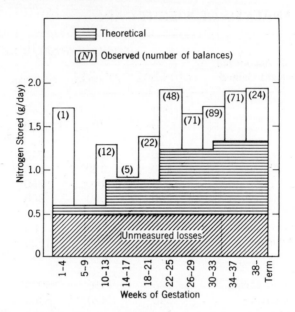

Fig. 22.12 Observed nitrogen retention of women during gestation. The theoretical values are from Hytten and Leitch. (From D. H. Calloway, *Nutrition and Fetal Development,* Vol. 2, p. 79, M. Winick, ed., Wiley, N. Y., 1974.)

will determine whether body fat can be estimated using both body water and body density measurements. There have been few studies in which these methods have been applied during pregnancy (Mc-Cartney et al., 1959).

Lean body mass was determined by whole body ^{40}K counting in pregnant teenagers (King et al., 1973) at the beginning and end of a 100-day study period. The increase in potassium deposition amounted to twice the estimate of Hytten and Leitch and was supported by nitrogen retention data from the same subjects, which also were twice the accepted estimates of daily deposition during the third trimester of pregnancy. The observed nitrogen retentions of women during pregnancy compared to the theoretical gain according to Hytten and Leitch is shown in Fig. 22.12. The interesting and important point brought out by King et al. (1973) is that the retention appears to be similar during the three trimesters and is considerably greater than the theoretical gain. This study emphasizes that women stored more nitrogen on higher intakes and this was accumulated as maternal lean body mass.

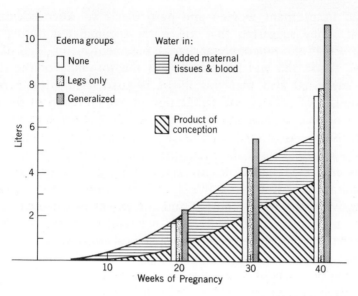

Fig. 22.13 The measured gain in body water during pregnancy in three edema groups compared to the calculated water accumulation in the product of conception and added maternal blood and tissues. (From F. E. Hytten and Leitch, *The Physiology of Human Pregnancy*, 2nd ed., Blackwell Scientific Publications, Oxford, 1971, p. 349.)

Estimations of total body water have been the subject of major interest to obstetricians because of their concern with the development of edema. This concern has probably led to widespread but fortunately, in most cases, mild iatrogenic disorders brought about by the use of diuretic agents. The change in body water observed during the course of pregnancy (Fig. 22.13) indicates that at term there is an excess of approximately 2.5 liters of water over what can be accounted for in the maternal tissue and the products of conception. In some cases this excess was observable as edema although in most cases the edema was clinically slight. This water has been a source of worry to obstetricians who assumed it to be indicative of some derangement in metabolism when, instead, it appears to be of physiological rather than pathological significance.

If there is an accumulation of approximately 2.5 liters of water and, in most cases, this is not visible as edema, the question of where the water is located becomes intriguing. Hytten and Leitch (1971, p. 353) point to a neglected paper (Fekete, 1964) that reported increased uptake of water in the connective tissue which was marked in pregnant women and particularly so when edema was present. They suggested that the water accumulated during pregnancy was in the mucopolysaccharide basement membranes of connective tissue and was associated with the softening of the tissue. They suggested also that this might be associated with increased diffusibility of solutes and facilitation of the nutrition of the cells. Such a normal accumulation of fluid is called physiological edema and is usually associated with better reproductive performance and fewer low birth weight and premature infants. The presence of such edema and the changes in the skin during pregnancy have been corroborated by Robertson (1971). Clarification of the changes in connective tissue water content and the extent of these changes in normal pregnancy could resolve the question of whether the edema of pregnancy is indeed a normal physiological adjustment.

That part of the maternal weight gain that cannot be accounted for in the products of conception or maternal tissue is assumed to be fat (Hytten and Leitch, 1971, p. 357) and amounts to approximately 3.5 kg. Calloway (1974) questions whether some of this unaccounted weight gain should not instead be attributed to increase in lean body mass accumulated when the nitrogen and energy intakes during pregnancy are sufficiently high. In an animal model (Naismith, 1971), fat stored during pregnancy was used as a source of energy during lactation. Carcass analyses in lactating rats on days 2 and 16 postpartum showed that, when the protein intake was high (25 percent), 70 percent of the fat stored during pregnancy was lost during lactation with no loss of body protein; whereas, on low protein intakes (11 percent), 10 percent of body protein in addition to the calories from fat were used for the synthesis of a reduced volume of milk. Such a study supports the suggestion that stored fat during pregnancy may indeed be a source of energy for lactation and serve to protect lean body mass.

Nutritional Requirements During Pregnancy

Meeting both fetal and maternal requirements and hence setting up nutrient allowances for pregnancy has, for the most part, been based on the suggested allowances for the nonpregnant woman with the superimposed additional requirements for pregnancy. Such an additive approximation of need has been questioned by Beaton

(1961), who points out that physiological and nutritional adaptations occur that permit pregnancy to proceed if the minimal nutrient requirements are met. When the minima are not met, harm results to the mother or fetus; above the minimal levels, the pregnant woman can adapt to wide ranges of intakes. This also appears to be evident in the data presented by Thomson (1958, 1959a, 1959b) and by Oldham and Sheft (1951).

Metabolic alterations promoting the retention of essential nutrients probably are dependent on adjustments in hormonal regulation. Animal studies suggest that growth hormone acts to decrease protein catabolism during pregnancy, thereby promoting retention (Beaton et al., 1955; Beaton, 1957). The increased demand for oxygen, by stimulation of erythropoietin secretion, and the consequent stimulation of hematopoiesis lead to increased oxygen-carrying power in the form of more erythrocytes carrying hemoglobin. Increased hemoglobin synthesis coupled with the higher plasma transferrin levels that are present during pregnancy undoubtedly are associated with increased iron absorption. The need for sodium to maintain the increased body water compartments is accomplished by stimulation of aldosterone secretion, which promotes sodium reabsorption by the kidney tubules. Physiological adaptation in pregnant rats to levels of sodium intake adequate for nonpregnant animals is observed in the histological evidence of increased renin secretion which, in turn, triggers increased secretion of aldosterone (Pike et al., 1966). As long as the required increase in hormone production can be maintained, the requisite increase in retention will occur. A fundamental question arises about the degree of stress to which the pregnant body should be subjected in order to meet its nutritional requirements and to maintain body composition. From studies of rats on restricted sodium intake, physiological adjustment leading to increased stimulation of aldosterone secretion takes place to the point of disruption in the fine structure of aldosterone-secreting cells (Smiciklas et al., 1971a; 1971b) and in loss of aldosterone-secreting capacity (Khokhar and Pike, 1973). Maternal weight gain was reduced, the young were smaller and lighter, and there were significant reductions in tissue sodium and plasma volume. What starts as a physiological adjustment can be extended until it attains pathological proportions.

The bases for recommended allowances set up by various national and supranational organizations vary (see Chapter 25). The ranges

Table 22.10 DAILY RECOMMENDED ALLOWANCES FOR NONPREGNANT AND PREGNANT WOMEN DOING LIGHT WORK

	United Nations		U.S.A.		United Kingdom	
	Nonpregnant	Pregnant	Nonpregnant	Pregnant	Nonpregnant	Pregnant
Weight, kg	55		58		55	
Weight gain, kg		10 ± 2		11		12.5
Energy, kcal	2200	2485	2000	2300	2200	2400
Protein, gm	29	38	46	76	55	60
Calcium, gm	0.4-0.5	1.0-1.2	0.8	1.2	0.5	1.2
Iron , mg	14-28	14-28[a]	18	18	12	15
Vitamin A, IU	2500	2500	4000	5000	2500	2500
Vitamin D, IU	100	400	None	400	100	400
Thiamin, mg	0.9	1.0	1.0	1.3	0.9	1.0
Riboflavin, mg	1.3	1.4	1.2	1.5	1.3	1.6
Nicotinic acid, mg equiv.	15.2	16.5	13	15	15	18

				N.R.C. 1974		D.H.S.S. 1969	
Vitamin B6, mg	—	—		2.0	2.5	—	—
Folate, µg	200	400		400	800	—	—
Vitamin B12, µg	2.0	3.0		3.0	4.0	—	—
Ascorbic acid, mg	30	50		45	60	30	60

Sources

Energy:
  FAO 1973
Protein:
  FAO/WHO 1965
Calcium:
  FAO/WHO 1962
Iron:
  FAO/WHO 1970
Vitamins:
  FAO/WHO 1967
  FAO/WHO 1970

[a] Assuming previous iron intake has been satisfactory.
Lower level is the recommendation where over 25 percent of calories are from animals foods.
Upper level is the recommendation where under 10 percent of calories are from animal foods.

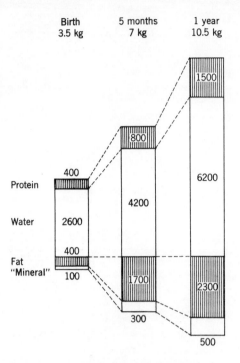

Fig. 22.14 Body composition in a normal newborn infant and at 5 and 12 months of age. [From B. Friis-Hansen, *Ped.,* 47: 264 (1971).]

suggested for various nutrients for pregnancy are shown in Table 22.10.

Compositional Changes between Birth and Maturity

Only one study giving chemical analysis of a child has appeared in the literature (see Widdowson and Dickson, 1964), and it is presented in Table 22.11 along with data on a full term baby and an adult. Although it had been suggested that some dehydration may have taken place before death, the water, nitrogen, and potassium contents appear to have attained a composition similar to that of the adult. Values lower than the adult for calcium, phosphorus, and magnesium indicate that the bones were not chemically mature. Copper and zinc concentrations were not yet at the adult level and the low iron was apparently indicative of anemia. Fig. 22.14 shows

Table 22.11 COMPOSITION OF THE WHOLE BODY OF A 4½ YEAR OLD BOY COMPARED WITH THAT OF A FULL TERM BABY AND AN ADULT

	Full Term Baby	Boy 4½ Years	Adult
Body weight (kg)	3.5	14.0	65
Composition[a]			
Water (gm)	823	695	720
Total N (gm)	22.6	38.2	34.0
Na (mEq)	82	—	80
K (mEq)	53	65	69
Cl (mEq)	55	—	50
Ca (gm)	9.6	21.1	22.4
P (gm)	5.6	10.5	12.0
Mg (gm)	0.26	0.36	0.47
Fe (mg)	93.9	64.2	74
Cu (mg)	4.7	3.3	1.7
Zn (mg)	19.2	22.3	28

From E. M. Widdowson and J. W. T. Dickerson, "Chemical Composition of the Body." In *Mineral Metabolism*, C. L. Comar and F. Bronner, eds., Vol. II, Part A, Acad. Press, N. Y., 1964, p. 17.

[a]Results expressed per kilogram of fat-free body tissue.

how the composition of the newborn changes when the body weight doubles at 5 months and triples at one year.

Garn et al. (1956) studied a group of 300 clinically healthy infants from 1 to 12 months of age to determine whether subcutaneous fat was indicative of nutritive status and concluded that it was not. They noted that the amount of subcutaneous fat increased rapidly in all infants from 1 to 6 months of age but that thereafter some gained and others lost fat and group differences disappeared. No relationship appeared to exist between the amount of fat deposited during the first 6 months and the subsequent rate of growth.

Fig. 22.15 shows the continuous increase observed in triceps fat fold measurements in males and females from age 1 to 80. Fat fold measurements in females is unchanged until the sharp prepubertal gain, which is followed by an equally sharp increase during the adolescent stage. A short plateau lasting until approximately age 22 is followed by the adult gain with peak fatness occurring at about

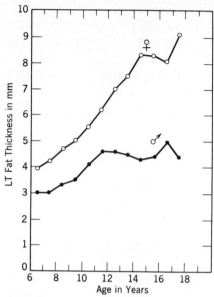

Fig. 22.15 Continuous increase in lower thoracic (LT) fat in girls and parallel increase in boys, terminating at 11.5 years. By 14.5 years the adult female/male fat ratio of 180 per cent has been attained. [From S. M. Garn and J. A. Haskell, *Science,* 129:1615 (1959).]

age 45. Fat loss then occurs into old age. The picture for males differs sharply from females after age 3, when there is a preschool loss that is not regained until the prepubertal gain between ages 8 and 13. This is followed by another loss during the adolescent stage reaching a trough about age 18. Adult gain in triceps fat fold measurement peaks about age 50 followed by the drop associated with increased age.

A study measuring total body water throughout the life span using deuterium dilution (Edelman et al., 1952) included a group of 11 children with an average age of 4.5 years. The mean total body water was 58.9 percent of body weight, a figure not too different from the Widdowson data, which calculated to 53.8 percent and which the authors indicated might have been abnormally low. A summary of total body water as a function of age in normal children clearly indicated the reduction in percentage of body water from birth to nine years of age (Table 22.12). A sex differential becomes

Table 22.12 SUMMARY OF TOTAL BODY WATER DATA AS A FUNCTION OF AGE IN NORMAL CHILDREN

No. Subjects	Age, Range	Weight, kg	Surface Area, m^2	Total Body Water, liters		Total Body Water, % B.Wt.		Total Body Water, liters/m^2	
				Mean	Range	Mean	Range	Mean	Range
6	2-28 (days)	3.16	0.198	2.42	1.67-3.17	76.7	71.8-83.0	12.1	9.8-13.8
9	1-9 (months)	6.94	0.328	4.27	3.08-6.15	62.6	53.0-70.9	12.9	11.3-14.6
11	1-9 (years)	16.6	0.650	9.77	5.90-16.2	58.9	55.2-62.8	14.2	13.1-16.7

Adapted from I. S. Edelman et al., *Surg. Gynec. Obstet.*, 95: 1 (1952).

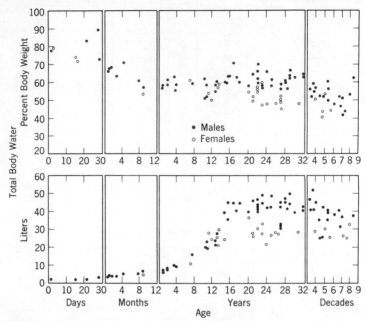

Fig. 22.16 Total body water as a function of age. In the upper section, the body water is plotted as percentage of body weight (i.e., relative water volume). In the lower section the body water is plotted in liters (i.e., absolute water volume). [From Edelman et al., *Surg. Gynec. Obstet.*, 95:1 (1952).]

apparent in the 10 to 16 age group, and the female has a lower percentage of body water associated with added increments of body fat. Fig. 22.16 which shows the absolute and relative amounts of body water as a function of age illustrates this clearly. Similar and confirming data for total body water measured in 86 subjects ranging in age from 1 day to 15 years were obtained by Friis-Hansen (1961). Thirty-seven of these subjects received a thiosulfate injection simultaneously with the deuterium, thereby permitting estimation of both total body water and extracellular fluid volume, and calculation of intracellular fluid volume (Table 22.13).

In an attempt to determine whether a correlation exists between subcutaneous fat and total body fat in healthy children in the age groups 9-12 and 13-16, Pařízková (1961) determined body density and skinfold thickness in 123 boys and 118 girls. In both age groups and sexes high correlations were observed, suggesting that the rela-

Table 22.13 MEAN VALUES OF TOTAL BODY WATER, EXTRA-CELLULAR WATER, AND INTRACELLULAR WATER[a] (PERCENT OF BODY WEIGHT)

Age of Subjects	TBW	ECW	ICW
0-1 day	78.4	44.5	33.9
1-30 days	74.0	39.7	31.8
1-3 months	72.3	32.2	43.3
3-6 months	70.1	30.1	42.1
6-12 months	60.4	27.4	35.2
1-2 years	58.7	25.6	33.6
2-3 years	63.5	26.7	38.3
3-5 years	62.2	21.4	(45.7)
5-10 years	61.5	22.0	(42.3)
10-15 years	57.3	18.7	(46.7)

From B. Friis-Hansen, *Ped.*, 28: 169 (1961).

[a]TBW minus ECW is not in all cases equal to ICW because both determinations were not carried out in all subjects within each group. The figures in parentheses are based on only one or two measurements and are less significant.

tionship of the density and percentage of fat in children is similar to that found in adults. Nomograms were constructed for each sex in each age group for determining body density and hence percentage fat from two skinfold measurements.

Hunt and Giles (1956) have suggested that in addition to consideration of chemical maturity as defined by Moulton, *mature hydration*, although more limited, might be useful. Mature hydration, according to their definition, is the minimal, or mature, percentage of water in the fat-free body. Hunt and Heald (1963) in a study of 55 adolescent boys found extreme variability in the hydration of the fat-free body early in adolescence. They suggest that perhaps mature hydration occurs temporarily before adolescence but that this is followed by fattening and accumulation of enough body water to make the fat-free body as hydrated as the newborn. Later the body becomes more lean, its composition more stable, and by 18 years body composition is that of mature males.

Forbes and Hursh (1963), on the basis of ^{40}K measurements and calculation of lean body mass, found that the weight of the lean body rises rapidly in males during the midportion of the second decade, reaching a maximum by the nineteenth year, after which

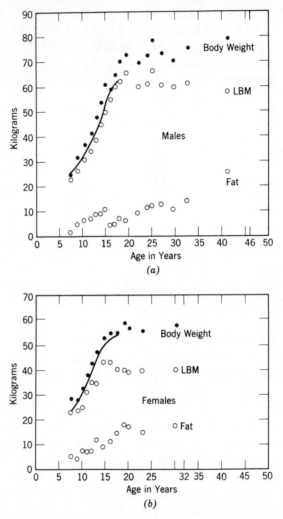

Fig. 22.17 Plot of average body weight, lean body mass (LBM), and fat for males (a) and females (b). The solid lines represent the fiftieth percentile for body weight for normal children. [From G. B. Forbes and J. B. Hursh, *Ann. N. Y. Acad. Sci.*, 110:255 (1963).]

there is a slow fall. They also reported an increase in fat during the early "teen" years, but at a much slower rate (Fig. 22.17). An abrupt fall in fat at age 16 is followed by a slow sustained rise during middle age. It is the concomitant rapid increase in lean body mass and decrease in fat to which they attribute the "muscular"

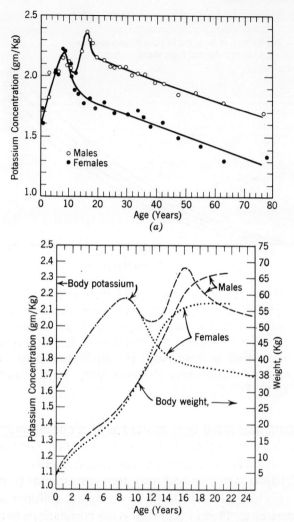

Fig. 22.18 (*a*) Average body potassium concentrations of males and females as a function of chronologic age (grams per kilogram of gross body weight). (*b*) Change in male and female potassium concentrations in relation to growth (as indicated by weight gain). [From E. C. Anderson and W. H. Langham, *Science*, 130:713 (1959).]

appearance of the male in late adolescence. The rise in lean body mass in females is less rapid than in males and the maximum, two-thirds that of the male, is reached at about 15 years of age. The increase in total fat is greater in females during the early years and the

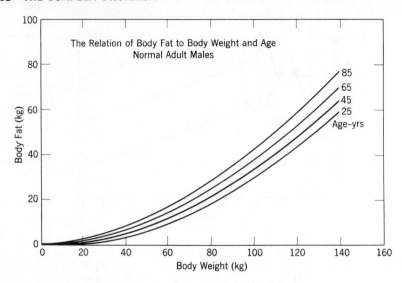

Fig. 22.19 Body fat and body weight in relation to age in normal adult males of various age groups. This plot can also be used as a nomogram entered with body weight and age. Note that with progressing increase of weight the fraction of fat increases even in a population identified as "normal," (From Moore et al., *The Body Cell Mass and its Supporting Environment*, W. B. Saunders Co., Phila., 1963, p. 162.)

curve is an uninterrupted one. Plotted as ^{40}K concentrations related to age, the peak occurs at about age 9 and then falls; however, a second peak in body potassium concentration occurs in males at age 16 (Fig. 22.18). It is this second peak that corresponds to the one described by Forbes and Hursh. In a study of children and young adults, Forbes et al. (1961) reported good correlations between ^{40}K measurements and both skinfold thickness and height-weight ratios, and between ^{40}K and both circumferential measurements and total fat (Barter and Forbes, 1963).

Attainment of maturity does not imply cessation of change, and alterations in relative and absolute body composition do, indeed, continue in adult life. These changes, however, proceed at a slower rate as the individual ages and are observable, often without benefit of the investigator's tools, as increases in body fat in males (Fig.

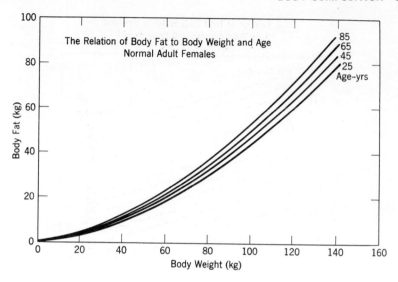

Fig. 22.20 The relation of body fat and body weight to age in normal adult females of various age groups. This figure is drawn as is Fig. 22.19 for use in predicting the degree of obesity in normal adult female subjects. Both here and in the previous figure the standard hydration coefficient for the fat-free body (0.732) is used. (From Moore et al., *The Body Cell Mass and Its Supporting Environment,* W. B. Saunders Co., Phila., 1963, p. 163.)

22.19) and females (Fig. 22.20). Increases in age are associated also with decreases in both body water (Fig. 22.21) and body cell mass. Table 22.14 shows clearly the concomitant and related changes in the three parameters with age at a constant body weight. The sex difference in adult body composition is readily apparent. Comparable data have been obtained by densitometry (Behnke et al., 1942; Brozek, 1952; Young et al., 1963), skinfold measurements (Brozek, 1952; Brozek et al., 1963), creatinine excretion (Norris et al., 1963), exchangeable potassium (Moore et al., 1963; Olesen, 1965), ^{40}K measurements (Forbes and Hursh, 1963; Anderson and Langham, 1959: Meneeley et al., 1963), and total body water measurements (Edelman et al., 1952; Siri, 1956; Friis-Hansen, 1965). For an extensive review of the *in vivo* quantification of human fat, muscle, and bone, see Malina (1969).

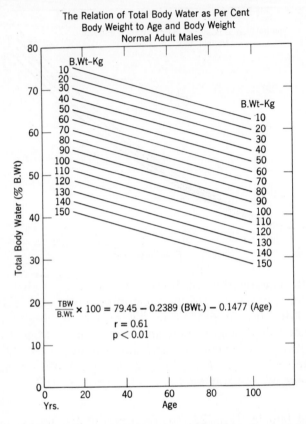

The Relation of Total Body Water as Per Cent
Body Weight to Age and Body Weight
Normal Adult Males

Fig. 22.21 Total body water (as per cent of body weight) related to age and body weight in normal adult males of all ages. This chart can be used as a nomogram. It is entered with the person's age; progressing vertically upward to the observed body weight. The vertical coordinate is then crossed to the predicted total body water, indicated not in liters, but in per cent of body weight. The parabolic expression upon which this nomogram is based is shown at the bottom. (From Moore et al., *The Body Cell Mass and Its Supporting Environment*, W. B. Saunders Co., Phila., 1963, p. 159.)

Compositional Changes with Weight Change

Since the major components of body weight are water, fat, and body cell mass, changes in weight can be reflections of alterations in any one of these fractions. Excessive hydration, which is observed

Table 22.14 NORMAL VALUES FOR FAT, TOTAL BODY WATER, AND BODY CELL MASS RELATED TO BODY WEIGHT AND AGE

Wgt. (kg)	Fat (kg)				Total Body Water (liters)				Body Cell Mass[a] (kg)			
	Age				Age				Age			
	25	45	65	85	25	45	65	85	25	45	65	85
Adult Males												
60	9.6	12.0	14.5	17.0	36.9	35.1	33.3	31.5	27.3	24.6	22.1	19.8
80	18.1	21.3	24.5	27.8	45.3	43.0	40.6	38.2	33.5	30.1	27.0	24.0
100	29.1	33.2	37.2	41.3	51.9	48.9	46.0	43.0	38.3	34.3	30.6	27.1
120	42.8	47.6	52.5	57.3	56.5	53.0	49.4	45.9	41.8	37.3	32.9	28.9
140	59.1	64.7	70.3	76.1	59.2	55.1	51.0	46.8	45.7	38.7	33.9	29.4
Adult Females												
60	17.9	19.8	21.8	23.5	30.8	29.4	28.0	26.7	21.2	19.6	18.3	16.8
80	29.5	32.0	34.6	37.1	37.0	35.1	33.2	31.4	25.6	23.4	21.7	19.8
100	44.0	47.1	50.3	53.4	41.0	38.7	36.4	34.1	28.2	25.7	23.8	21.4
120	61.3	65.1	68.9	72.6	43.0	40.2	37.4	34.7	29.6	26.8	24.5	21.8
140	81.4	85.8	90.3	94.6	42.9	39.7	36.4	33.2	29.6	26.4	23.8	20.9

Data from F. D. Moore et al., *The Body Cell Mass and Its Supporting Environment*, W. B. Saunders Co., Philadelphia, Pa., 1963, p. 167, 168.
[a]Calculated as $K_e \times 8.33$.

in a variety of pathological conditions, may be due to increase of extracellular water or wasting of body cell mass or both (see Fig. 22.4). Dehydration, which occurs more rarely, results from the reverse situation: loss of extracellular water or gain in body cell mass. These abnormal conditions are not relevant in this context. Changes in the relative proportions of fat comprising body weight may attain pathological status, but such conditions may be viewed as the extremes in the continuum from emaciation to obesity. Increases in body cell mass are the result of intensive physical activity and are observed in trained athletes.

Obesity. The effects of plethora rather than paucity of body fat is of major concern in the United States, where the combination of an abundant food supply and energy-conserving devices has made obesity a major public health problem. However, in many countries of the world where food shortages and famines are endemic, accumulation of excess body fat, though no less a health problem to the individual, may be an economic status symbol.

Body weight gain in the adult indicates an increase in both the absolute and relative amounts of body fat, but in spite of rather widespread misconception, the body weight gain is not due to fat alone: it includes water, body cell mass, and cell solids. The predicted body composition for an obese young man and young woman shows the composition of the weight increment over a "reference" man or woman (Table 22.15). Although the largest fraction of the increased weight is due to fat, a substantial proportion is due to the increase in water, body cell mass, and cell solids. Similar findings on "obesity tissue" were obtained by densitometric (Brozek et al., 1963) and by multiple isotope dilution techniques (Moore et al., 1963).

Pařízková (1972) has reported that obese children are sometimes taller and have a larger lean body mass than normal children of the same age. Skeletal development may also be greater than in normal weight children and bicristal (pelvic) width greater in obese boys but not girls (Table 22.16). The distribution of fat was described as similar to that in an old woman with the usual sexual difference in fat distribution not apparent (Fig. 22.22).

Body weight loss in the obese individual is not just loss of excess body fat but also includes loss of body water and body cell mass. A partitioning of the "obesity tissue" lost by obese young men (Brozek et al., 1963) indicates that fat constituted 64 percent; extracellular water, 4 percent; and cell residue, 32 percent. Some of the confusion that crops up in the literature concerning the composition of weight loss stems from the partition of body weight into two components: body fat and lean body weight. In this context, lean body weight includes body cell mass plus skeletal and supporting structures. As body weight decreases, the proportional weight of the skeletal and supporting tissues to total weight increases, thereby masking any decrease in body cell mass which accompanies weight loss. In addition, an increase in muscle mass during weight reduction due to

Table 22.15 a. COMPOSITION OF "EXCESS TISSUE" IN A 25 YEAR OLD, NORMAL MALE OF 100 KG BODY WEIGHT (A NORMAL 25 YEAR OLD MALE, OF 70 KG BODY WEIGHT, IS USED AS A "REFERENCE MAN")

Compartments	Predicted Normal Body Composition		"Excess Tissue" Absolute	Relative
	70 kg	100 kg	+ 30.0 kg	100%
Fat	13.7 kg	29.1 kg	+ 15.4 kg	51%
Extracellular water	17.2 l.	21.8 l.	+ 4.6 l.	15%
Body cell mass	30.6 kg	38.3 kg	+ 7.7 kg	26%
Remainder	8.5 kg	10.8 kg	+ 2.3 kg	8%

b. COMPOSITION OF "EXCESS TISSUE" IN A 25 YEAR OLD, NORMAL FEMALE OF 90 KG BODY WEIGHT (A NORMAL 25 YEAR OLD FEMALE, OF 60 KG BODY WEIGHT, IS USED AS A "REFERENCE WOMAN")

Compartments	Predicted Normal Body Composition		"Excess Tissue" Absolute	Relative
	60 kg	90 kg	+ 30.0 kg	100%
Fat	17.9 kg	36.6 kg	+ 18.7 kg	63%
Extracellular water	14.2 l.	18.2 l.	+ 4.0 l.	13%
Body cell mass	21.2 kg	26.7 kg	+ 5.5 kg	18%
Remainder	6.7 kg	8.5 kg	+ 1.8 kg	6%

From K. H. Olesen, "Body Composition in Normal Adults," *Human Body Composition,* J. Brozek, ed., Pergamon Press, Oxford, 1965, p. 185.

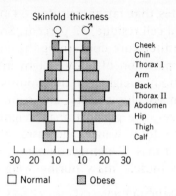

Fig. 22.22 Differences in skinfold thickness at different sites in normal and obese boys and girls. (From J. Pařizková, *Physical Activity — Human Growth and Development*, G. L. Rarick, ed., Acad. Press, N. Y., 1973, p. 114.)

physical activity obscures a decrease in body cell mass. Just such an erroneous interpretation of observed constancy in lean body weight appears in the data of Christian et al. (1963), who ascribe weight loss in obese individuals to loss of excess body fat only. In a study of weight loss in adolescent girls in which estimates of body composition were made by skinfold thickness, anthropometric measurements, and underwater determinations of specific gravity, Goldman et al. (1963) found two subjects in whom weight loss appeared to be 90-100 percent fat, and two who exceeded 100 percent! These subjects had been exercising and had undoubtedly added to their muscle mass, and the authors point to this to account for the illusion that the estimated fat loss was so high a proportion of the total weight loss.

In a study of obese young men weight loss, fat loss, and percent weight loss as fat (evaluated through density, anthropometric and skinfold measurements) appeared to be inversely related to the level of carbohydrate in isocaloric, isoprotein diets; but there were no differences in nitrogen, sodium, or potassium balances (Young et al., 1971). The level of carbohydrate that appeared to be most suitable for long term use was slightly over 100 gm. Why the weight loss and fat loss was greater on that level of carbohydrate was not clear. If due to changes in total body water, the

Table 22.16 MEAN VALUES OF ANTHROPOMETRIC MEASURES AND BODY COMPOSITION IN NORMAL AND OBESE BOYS AND GIRLS (13-14 YEARS)

	Height (cm)	Weight (kg)	Fat (%)	LBM (kg)	Bicristal Breadth (cm)	Chest Circum. (cm)	Arm (cm)	Femor. Cond. Breadth (cm)
Boys								
Normal	161.8	50.4	12.5	43.9	22.8	78.6	23.1	9.6
Obese	161.2	68.9	29.5	48.6	27.7	88.3	27.0	10.1
Girls								
Normal	156.9	50.4	18.1	40.7	26.8	79.2	24.3	8.6
Obese	157.5	88.9	31.9	46.7	27.4	95.1	29.6	10.0

From J. Pařízková, *Nutritional Aspects of Physical Performance*, J. F. De Wijn and R. A. Binkhorst, eds., Nutricia Ltd., Zoetermeer, The Netherlands, 1972, p. 148.

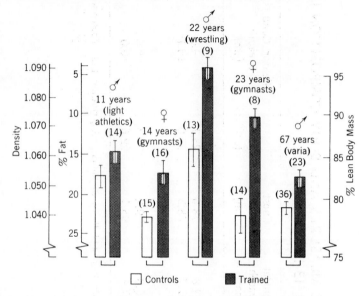

Fig. 22.23 Differences between trained and untrained control subjects of different ages in body density, fat, and lean body mass proportions. (From J. Pařizková, *Physical Activity — Human Growth and Development*, G. L. Rarick, ed., Acad. Press, N. Y., 1973, p. 100.)

techniques used in the study were not sufficiently precise to measure them.

The effect of weight reduction on body composition was studied in rats by direct chemical analysis after a 41-day total fast, and after a 41-day fast accompanied by exercise (Babirak et al., 1974). The percentage of weight loss was similar in both groups although the rate was greatly accelerated in the exercised animals. At the end of the experimental period there were no significant differences in body composition in the fasted animals with and without exercise.

Physical Activity. If comparison is made between physically active and inactive individuals of the same age, height, and weight, the physically active always have a higher body density, indicating a greater proportion of lean body mass. Pařizková (1963, 1965) has shown this for both sexes at all age levels (Fig. 22.23). In a study of gymnasts training for Olympic competition, Pařizková (1963) observed that body weight did not change during the first stage of training but that both the amount of subcutaneous and total body

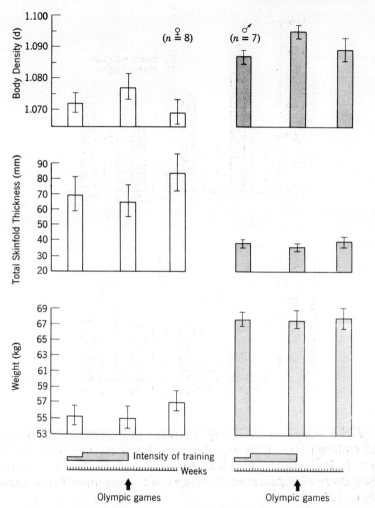

Fig. 22.24 Body density, skinfold thickness, and weight changes in gymnasts during the following Olympic training. [From J. Pařizková, *Ann. N. Y. Acad. Sci.*, 110:661 (1963).]

fat fell significantly with a concurrent development of lean body mass. After interruption of training, changes occurred in the opposite direction (Fig. 22.24). There was no difference in the response of male and female athletes. The effects of physical activity were also observed in obese children who were subjected to the combined effects of a reduction diet and intense physical training (Pařizková, 1965). At the end of a 6 to 7 week period all the children lost

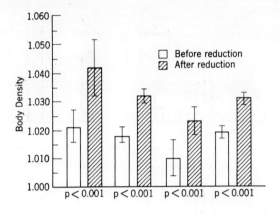

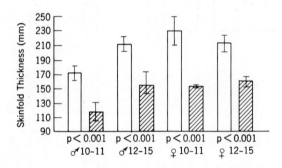

Fig. 22.25 Changes in body density and skinfold thickness in obese children after program of physical activity in a summer camp. (From J. Pařizková, "Physical Activity and Body Composition," *Human Body Composition*, J. Brozek, ed., Pergamon Press, Oxford, 1965, p. 166.)

weight and showed a reduction in skinfold thickness and an increase in body density (Fig. 22.25). Similar results have been reported from other laboratories (Goldman et al., 1963) for adolescent girls and boys. In a study involving obese high school boys Christakis et al. (1966) reported that planned physical activity increased body weight loss and was accompanied by a reduction in skinfold thickness. Indeed, the effect of physical activity on body composition, observed as "overweightness" but obviously not "overfatness" in Navy personnel and in professional football players (Behnke et al., 1942;

Welham and Behnke, 1942), served as the catalyst for studies on body composition.

SUMMARY

Under the thicknesses of their skinfolds, all men are surprisingly alike; and for women, beauty may not be skin, but skinfold deep, the depth varying with the fashion of the times. Today's fashion, for health rather than cosmetic reasons, is leanness for both men and women since excess fat has been implicated in the etiology of many of the diseases of middle age, and actuarial tables hold dire warnings for the obese. Estimation of body composition by various analytical laboratory methods has helped to establish norms and is invaluable to the physician and surgeon in patient management. Normative data permit evaluation and calibration of simpler methods that become the tools of the investigator of large population groups or of the practitioner in office or clinic. Since it is not only what we eat, but how much and what the body does with it, that makes us what we are, the nutritionist is an integral part of the team in prophylaxis and therapeutics.

Claude Bernard said, "Every time that a new and reliable means of experimental analysis makes its appearance, we invariably see science make progress in the questions to which this means of analysis can be applied." How clearly this has been demonstrated in the investigation of body composition.

chapter 23

determination of nutrient needs: energy, protein, minerals

1. Definition of Requirements
2. Summary of Methods for Determining Nutrient Needs
3. Balance Studies
   a. Interpretation of Balance Studies
   b. Uses and Limitations of the Balance Technique

4. Energy Requirement
   a. Principles of Calorimetry
   b. Total Energy Expenditure: Heat Loss Plus External Work Performed
   c. Factors Contributing to the Total Energy Requirement
      1. Basal Metabolism
      2. Factors Affecting Basal Metabolism
      3. Calorigenic Effect of Food
      4. Activity
   d. Calorimetry
      1. Direct Calorimetry
      2. Indirect Calorimetry
         a. Calculation of Heat Production from R. Q.
         b. Calculation of Heat Production from Oxygen Consumption Alone
   e. Energy Balance
   f. Energy Value of Foods

5. **Protein Requirement**
   a. Factors Affecting Nitrogen Balance
      1. Physiological State and Body Protein Reserves
      2. Energy Intake
      3. Essential Amino Acid and Total Nitrogen Intake
      4. Plasma Amino Acids
      5. Amino Acid Imbalance
      6. Amino Acid Toxicities and Antagonisms
   b. Evaluation of Protein Quality
      1. Amino Acid Score
      2. Protein Efficiency Ratio
      3. Biological Value
      4. Nitrogen Balance Index
      5. Net Protein Utilization
      6. Net Dietary Protein Calories Percent
      7. Slope-Ratio Assay

6. **Calcium Requirement**
7. **Iron Requirement**
8. **Summary**

Methods for assessment of nutrient needs are based on the fundamental concepts of nutrition already discussed: ingestion of food, digestion, absorption, transportation to the cells, metabolism in cells, storage, and finally excretion from the body (including expired gases, urine, feces, and sweat). Quantitatively, nutrient requirements depend upon the additive needs of the individual cells, which vary according to physiological demands imposed by the life cycle: growth, reproduction, lactation. The amounts supplied by the diet, however, must be sufficient to cover the net cellular requirements plus both unabsorbed nutrients and endogenous losses. In other words, the gross dietary requirement is the sum of cellular needs plus overall body losses.

It is at this point that we integrate the physiological and biochemical aspects of nutrition with the "nutritional aspects of nutrition." The additional responsibility of the nutritionist is to determine nutrient requirements and how they can be met.

The assessment of nutritional requirements, like so many complex subjects, is easier to discuss than to accomplish. At best, experiments designed to determine nutrient needs can provide only estimations of actual requirements. Biological systems are complex and highly variable and, in this respect, human beings are notorious. Genetic background, previous diet, environment, stress, and other factors influence to varying degrees the response to diet. Many of these factors can be controlled in carefully conducted experiments with laboratory animals of relatively short life span. Every human being, however, represents a multitude of uncontrollable variables even when maintained under the most rigid conditions.

A second complicating factor is that studies with humans rarely can be carried out for long periods of time partly because of expense of operation, but more often because few subjects will remain cooperative for more than several weeks at a time. The regimentation of eating prescribed kinds and amounts of foods and of collecting excreta require a fair degree of motivation even for a short period. The few studies that have been conducted over a period of months, however, suggest that long-term effects of diet may be quite different from effects observed in the usual periods of 6 to 8 weeks.

In spite of the difficulties inherent in human metabolic research, however, a large body of data has accumulated to form a working basis for evaluating the nutrient needs of man.

DEFINITION OF REQUIREMENTS

The term requirement has been loosely used and often misused. *Minimum requirement* has referred to the least amount of a nutrient that will prevent clinical symptoms of deficiency or support a well defined biochemical response such as maintenance of nitrogen equilibrium in the adult, normal hemoglobin levels, or a specified level of a metabolite in blood or urine. As will be seen later, these are very different criteria and do not necessarily measure the same state of nutrition. Therefore quantitative estimations of minimum requirement should *always* be expressed in terms of the criterion used for evaluation.

A question remains regarding *what* criterion should be used to evaluate minimum requirement. Is the minimum the lowest level that will prevent deficiency symptoms, or is it some undefined point in cellular adaptation to diminishing nutrient supply? Adaptation is a normal process in maintaining cell function, but when the adaptive shift becomes the fixed metabolic pathway, abnormalities ensue. It would seem that the true minimum requirement lies somewhere between the initial shift to alternative metabolic pathways and the final expression of adaptive failure and, in a complex organism, will vary among cells according to their metabolic rates and requirements. Simply stated, the problem is that there is at present no definitive criterion for determining the point in the continuum at which adaptive mechanisms are no longer normal. The inability to define precisely minimum requirement is a valid reason for the margin of safety used in developing dietary standards. The margin of safety is, in a sense, a cushion against ignorance.

SUMMARY OF METHODS FOR DETERMINING NUTRIENT NEEDS

Early attempts to determine the nutrient needs of animals were based on studies of body composition on the logical assumption that substances present in the body are primarily those necessary for life. The mere presence of substances in tissues does not establish a dietary requirement; many substances are synthesized in cells from dietary components or are simply carried in the food or water as contaminants. However, the proportions of nutrients comprising the animal body suggest grossly the relative amounts needed or retained in the body and thus very early provided clues to the nutrient needs of man.

Survey studies of nutrient intake also provide reasonable estimates of human nutrient needs. Dietary intake of a group of healthy persons, for example, compared with nutrient intake of a population group in which nutritional disease is endemic, yields data that distinguish roughly between nutrient intakes that are compatible with health and those that lead to disease. Similarly, many estimates of the energy needs of children are based on actual energy intakes of normally growing children. The British Medical Association's standard for ascorbic acid also is based on the results of dietary surveys which indicated that intakes of 30 mg were compatible with apparent health in the majority of the population of Great Britain (1950). Dietary surveys, however, cannot provide *precise* estimates of nutrient requirements; quantitative estimations of nutrient needs demand the refinement of controlled experiments.

One of the earliest recorded controlled dietary studies was the classical experiment on scurvy patients performed by James Lind about 1747 (from Todhunter, 1962). To 12 seamen with scurvy, Lind gave a basic diet and to 2 he gave daily supplements including cider, elixir of ferric sulphate, vinegar, sea water, citrus fruit, and an obscure medical treatment of the period. The result of Lind's rather crude experiment is nutrition history. The important characteristics of Lind's experiment are first, the control of dietary intake and second, the measurement of change in clinical condition as a result of dietary change alone.

Similarly, the determination of quantitative human requirements demands that dietary intake be precisely controlled in order to correlate nutrient intake with organism response. In other words, a specific response is measured against a known intake. The kinds of studies applicable to determination of human requirements are grouped arbitrarily below and will be discussed here and in Chapter 24.

1. Balance studies.
   (a) Energy balance.
   (b) Chemical balance.
2. Biochemical measurements of nutrient, nutrient metabolites or related functional and structural components.
   (a) Urinary excretions.
   (b) Blood levels.
3. Clinical evaluation and performance tests.

Other techniques such as those involving isotope tracers or tissue biopsy are essentially variations of 1 and 2. The basis of metabolic experiments is depicted in Fig. 23.1; factors most commonly measured are indicated by bold type.

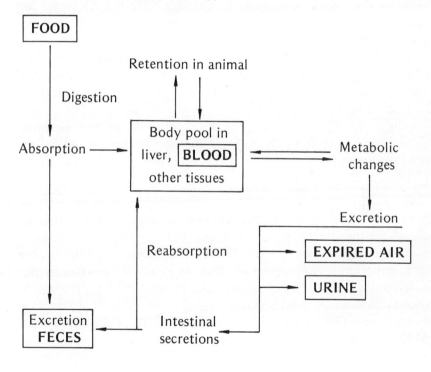

Fig. 23.1 Summary of nutrient metabolism. (After P. L. Altman and D. S. Dittmer, eds., *Biology Data Book. Fed. Amer. Soc. Exp. Biol.*, Washington, D. C., 1964, p. 192.)

BALANCE STUDIES

Balance studies are based on the principle of the conservation of energy and matter. In terms of body metabolism, as shown in Fig. 23.1, the balance method is simply a comparison of nutrient intake and output (loss from the body) and thus is a measurement of body gain or loss. The technique is applicable only when a stable component is under study or when end products of metabolism are clearly recognized. For example, heat is the end product of energy metabolism and all forms of energy may be expressed as heat. Therefore the balance experiment may be used in studies of energy exchange. Protein balance is determined by measurement of its metabolically stable component, nitrogen. Mineral elements are stable substances and therefore lend themselves to the balance technique.

On the other hand, vitamins are not biologically stable substances; the end products of vitamin metabolism are numerous and many are as yet unidentified. Vitamins synthesized by bacteria of the gastrointestinal tract further complicate the picture. The balance technique therefore is not generally applicable to the vitamins.

In its simplest form the balance method is represented by the following equation:

$$\text{Balance} = \text{Intake} - \text{Excretion products}$$

Excretion products are usually defined as substances excreted by way of the intestinal tract and kidneys, but in certain instances, for example energy balance, excretion via the lungs and skin is even more important. Although excretion by way of sweat need not be determined in studies of protein and mineral balance, the significance of these losses must be taken into account in the *interpretation* of data (see Consolazio et al., 1963a, 1963b; Calloway et al., 1971).

Interpretation of Balance Studies

The terminology used in interpretation of balance studies tends to be confusing: positive balance, negative balance, and equilibrium. A positive balance is expressed mathematically by a dietary intake greater than excretion products and indicates that the body is gain-

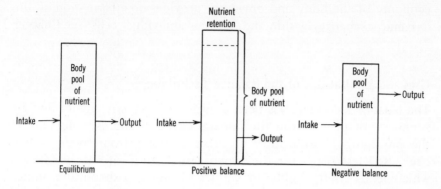

Fig. 23.2 Relationship between nutrient intake and output in balance experiments.

ing in the nutrient under study. Positive balance is the normal response to growth or gain in body substance and therefore is expected during childhood, adolescence, late pregnancy, and repletion following dietary restriction or loss of body substance as a result of surgery, injury from burns, or other trauma.

Conversely, negative balance means that excretion of a nutrient is greater than the intake and indicates that dietary intake is too low to replace nutrients lost from the body or to prevent destruction of body tissue. Loss of body weight, for example, is usually indicative of a negative energy balance.

Equilibrium represents the steady state, when intake and excretion are essentially equal. The normal adult maintained on an adequate diet, therefore, should be in a state of equilibrium with respect to energy, nitrogen, and the mineral elements assuming first that he is maintaining his weight, and second, that the quantity of nutrient in the body remains relatively constant. The adult is, in a sense, in a dynamic steady state.

The theoretical relationship between nutrient intake and output in balance studies is shown in Fig. 23.2. The use of the terms positive balance and negative balance is unfortunate; one does not readily conceive of balance under conditions of obvious imbalance. The terms are widely accepted, however, and must be clearly understood. Returning to the balance equation and Fig. 23.2 it should be clear that, on constant dietary intake, as the body gains in a nutrient, it must excrete less; when the body loses nutrient, it excretes more. Balance, then, must be interpreted as referring to the overall economy of the body and obviously provides no information on the dynamic exchanges within and between individual cells (see Chapter 7).

Uses and Limitations of the Balance Technique

The balance technique has been used widely as a criterion of dietary adequacy of protein and the mineral elements and as a measure of the physiological utilization of these nutrients from foods. It has been used less often for the experimental study of energy balance which lends itself readily to studies of energy expenditure alone.

In the normal adult, nitrogen and mineral equilibrium may be obtained at any level above the minimum requirement. Therefore reliable data on requirements may be obtained by measuring balance at various levels of dietary intake and calculating the intake at equilibrium by regression.

Balance studies, however, reflect previous dietary intake (Hegsted et al., 1952; Kelley and Ohlson, 1954; Allison, 1957). In addition, the animal body adapts to different levels of intake, although the time required for adaptation varies among nutrients. Adaptation to varying levels of protein occurs within days (Allison, 1957), whereas adaptation to changes in calcium intake may require several months (Malm, 1958). With the proper attention given to the effect of previous intake and the power of adaptation, the balance technique is a useful and valuable tool for the study of nutrient requirements.

ENERGY REQUIREMENT

From an experimental standpoint, the determination of energy requirement does not necessarily involve the balance of energy intake against output. Methods for determination of energy needs are based primarily on energy expenditure alone and include the direct measurement of heat loss from the body or calculation of heat production from gaseous exchange (oxygen consumed and carbon dioxide expired). The various instruments used in determining energy exchange have been described by Swift and French (1954) and Consolazio and Johnson (1971). The following discussion will stress the principles underlying calorimetric methods and scant attention will be given to details of operation.

Principles of Calorimetry

In studies of animal energy exchange, the use of the kilocalorie, a heat unit, must be considered a convenience rather than a primary concern. Interest in the origin of animal heat sparked the early work in calorimetry, and body heat loss has long been known to result from oxidation processes within the cell. The *primary* biological advantage, however, is not the production of heat to warm the body but the transformation of the energy bound in foodstuffs into a form of energy that can be used by the animal for internal and external work. Heat produced as an end result of cellular oxidation is beneficial to the animal in maintaining body temperature, but it is of no value as a source of external or internal work. (An exception is the brown adipose tissue that functions solely as a source of body heat.) Heat is a byproduct of metabolism. In other words, heat is a fringe benefit of animal oxidations; ATP is the net income that maintains life (see Chapter 13).

The animal's source of useful energy is the chemical energy supplied by food. Other forms of energy, such as solar energy utilized by the green plant for syntheses, are useless to animals in driving cellular reactions. Lying on a sunny beach, for example, can produce a beautiful suntan, but it is the picnic lunch that you bring along that sustains you.

Obviously, if an animal does not eat, the body's need for energy must be supplied by its own substance. Glycogen from liver and muscle, fatty acids from adipose tissues, or even structural protein all serve as substrate for cellular oxidation equally as well as the carbohydrate, fat, and protein from ham sandwiches and deviled eggs.

The oxidation of foodstuffs provides chemical energy for cellular reactions. As energy is transformed from one form to another (as occurs in the metabolism of foodstuffs in the cell), the capacity of the total energy to perform work decreases. The transformation of chemical energy (as in food) to mechanical energy (work) is never complete (see Fig. 23.3). When the large molecules of carbohydrates, fats, and proteins are broken down into progressively smaller fragments by the enzymes of intermediary metabolism, the change is from a highly organized to a disorganized state. The step-by-step process, however, insures the capture of about 40 percent of the

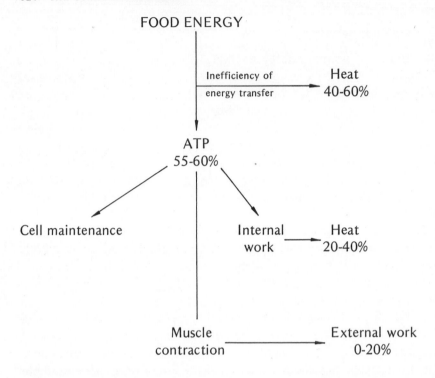

Fig. 23.3 Summary of animal energy expenditure and heat loss. (Adapted from A. C. Brown and G. Brengelmann, "Energy Metabolism," *Physiology and Biophysics*, T. C. Ruch and H. D. Patton, eds., Saunders, Phila., 1965, p. 1034.)

energy in the useful form of ATP. The rest is lost as heat (see Chapter 13). On the other hand, when molecules are disrupted violently, as in the oxygen-charged atmosphere of a bomb calorimeter, the state of disorganization is such that all of the potential energy of the food is manifested as heat.

When ATP is utilized for cellular synthetic reactions and in work performance, still more energy is wasted. Lehninger (1965) has estimated that the total energy required for synthesis of phosphatidyl choline is about 17 kcal/mole of the complete molecule. The synthesis of 1 mole of phosphatidyl choline is accomplished, however, at the expense of 8 moles of ATP or a total of about 56 kcal (8 x 7 kcal). The efficiency of synthesis therefore is only about 34 percent.

The synthesis of a complex protein is even more expensive in terms of ATP utilization. Each peptide bond with a free energy of about 5 kcal requires an investment of at least 3 high energy phosphate bonds yielding a biosynthetic efficiency of roughly 25 percent.

Muscle contraction also is a fairly expensive process. The overall ability of the animal body to convert potential energy of food to mechanical work amounts to only 20 to 25 percent of the total available energy. In comparison with man-made machines, however, the efficiency of the animal body is very good.

Total Energy Expenditure: Heat Loss Plus External Work

All of the energy transformed within the animal body may be accounted for as heat eliminated from the body and as work done by the animal on the environment. In the resting animal (that is, when no external work is being performed), essentially all of the energy transformed within the body is dissipated as heat. This state is referred to as the *resting metabolism*. Heat loss thus includes both the heat produced from inefficient transfer of the energy of oxidation and final degradation of internal work into heat. For example, the work of the heart and lungs is converted into heat by the friction of blood in the capillaries and the movement of air in and out of the body.

When external work is performed, energy expenditure is equivalent to the heat produced *plus* the work done. All forms of work, however, are not easily measured. Lifting a known weight to a known height or riding a stationary bicycle to which an ergometer is attached are forms of work that may be calculated easily as heat energy. The heat equivalent of work energy is 1 kcal to 427 kilogram meters of work where kilogram meters = weight x distance.

If, conceivably, a gymnasium-size calorimeter could be constructed and an individual allowed (or forced) to perform all his usual activities within, the total amount of heat measured should be quite close to the individual's actual energy expenditure. In certain instances, such as lifting an object, a small amount of energy would reside in the object lifted; in other instances, such as freely riding a bicycle, heat is produced by friction of the wheels. Heat produced during the latter activity therefore emanates from the object, not from the individual.

In any case, the direct measurement of heat loss is expensive and complicated in operation and is rarely used now in practical human calorimetry. Lavoisier's work suggested that oxygen consumption and heat production were closely correlated in the resting animal. Atwater and Rosa (1899) proved conclusively that the *total* energy expenditure is related quantitatively to oxygen consumption. The calculation of energy expenditure in kcal from oxygen consumption is known as *indirect calorimetry*. This method is simple and relatively inexpensive in operation and offers the added advantage of measuring the total energy expenditure, that is, resting metabolism plus work performed. For these reasons, indirect calorimetry has generally replaced measurement of heat loss as a method for determining energy expenditure in man.

Factors Contributing to the Total Energy Requirement

Total metabolism and therefore total energy expenditure ultimately are determined by the internal and external work of the body and are, in effect, a result of mitochondrial activity in cells in which respiratory rate may differ widely. In the rat, for example, kidney tissue respires at a very high rate; liver, heart, brain, and diaphragm are less active than kidney but also respire at high rates. In comparison, skin, skeleton, ligaments, and blood respire at relatively low rates (Field et al., 1939).

Total energy expenditure can be viewed most conveniently as an overall expression of varying degrees of tissue (or mitochondrial) activity necessary for the internal and external work of the body. Moreover, internal and external work are inseparable when external work is performed, because it is obvious that any form of activity (or external work) affects the internal work of the body.

The determination of energy needs, therefore, requires a separation of the total energy expenditure into physiological entities that can be defined and measured. The most significant factors that affect the total energy requirements of an individual are:

1. Basal metabolism.
2. Calorigenic effect of food (specific dynamic action or specific dynamic effect).
3. Activity.

Basal Metabolism. The energy expenditure during basal metabolism has been aptly called "the cost of living" and is loosely comparable to the minimum requirement for the nutrients. It refers to the metabolic activity required to maintain life: respiration, heart beat, maintenance of body temperature, and other essential functions.

Many factors influence the internal work of the body even when at rest, for example, physiological state, environmental temperature, food intake, and such subtleties as degree of muscle tension. In order to minimize influences that would raise metabolic activity and invalidate baseline comparison among individuals, the degree of cellular metabolism or basal metabolic rate (BMR) must be determined under closely controlled and standardized conditions. The BMR therefore is determined when an individual is in the post-absorptive state (at least 12 hours after eating) and is lying down, completely relaxed in a room of comfortable temperature.

Numerous determinations of basal metabolic rate have been made on humans and other species.[1] It is clear that metabolic rate varies with body size. For many years, however, there has been considerable discussion and disagreement in attempts to establish a constant relationship between metabolic rate and a unit of body size that would apply to large and small animals alike.

In clinical practice it is customary to express BMR in relation to surface area, that is, kcal per hour per square meter (m^2) of body surface ($kcal/hr/m^2$). This relationship is based on the assumption that heat loss and therefore BMR are proportional to surface area. Many formulas for calculation of body surface from weight and height have been proposed; the formula of DuBois and DuBois (1916) is one that appears to be well accepted:

$$A = W^{0.425} \times H^{0.725} \times 71.84$$

where A is surface area in m^2; W is weight in kg, and H is height in cm. Simple, easy-to-use clinical tables as shown in Table 23.1 have been substituted for the formula for most practical work.

[1] See Sargent (1961, 1962) for evaluation of basal metabolic data on infants and children in the United States.

Table 23.1 THE MAYO FOUNDATION NORMAL STANDARDS CALORIES PER SQUARE METER PER HOUR

Males		Females	
Age at Last Birthday	Mean	Age at Last Birthday	Mean
6	53.00	6	50.62
7	52.45	6½	50.23
8	51.78	7	49.12
8½	51.20	7½	47.84
9	50.54	8	47.00
9½	49.42	8½	46.50
10	48.50	9-10	45.90
10½	47.71	11	45.26
11	47.18	11½	44.80
12	46.75	12	44.28
13-15	46.35	12½	43.58
16	45.72	13	42.90
16½	45.30	13½	42.10
17	44.80	14	41.45
17½	44.03	14½	40.74
18	43.25	15	40.10
18½	42.70	15½	39.40
19	42.32	16	38.85
19½	42.00	16½	38.30
20-21	41.43	17	37.82
22-23	40.82	17½	37.40
24-27	40.24	18-19	36.74
28-29	39.81	20-24	36.18
30-34	39.34	25-44	35.70
35-39	38.68	45-49	34.94
40-44	38.00	50-54	33.96
45-49	37.37	55-59	33.18
50-54	36.73	60-64	32.61
55-59	36.10	65-69	32.30
60-64	35.48	a	
65-69	34.80		

[a]Obtained by extrapolation.

From a comparison of data on metabolic rate of several mammalian species, however, Kleiber concluded that although metabolic rate is not proportional to body weight *per se*, there is a linear rela-

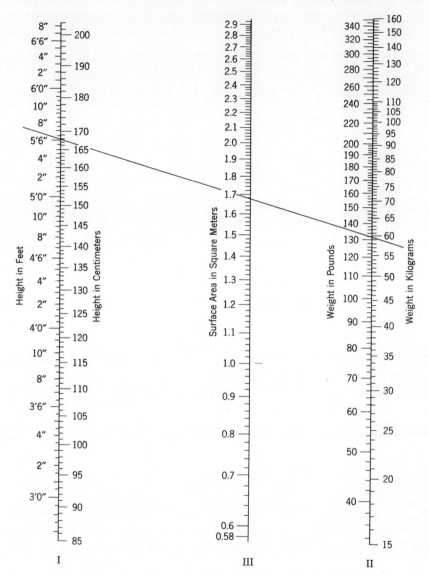

Fig. 23.4 Nomogram for calculating surface area.

tionship between metabolic rate and the three-fourth power of body weight (see Kleiber, 1947). Moreover, this relationship is more precise than that of BMR and surface area and thus is applicable to all species. Originally proposed in 1932, the concept of metabolic body size defined as body weight in kg$^{3/4}$ was officially accepted at the Conference on Energy Metabolism in Tyrone, Scotland, in 1964. As a general rule covering all species, metabolic rate may be computed in kcal per day as 70 x $W^{3/4}$. More precise formulas for predicting metabolic rate of humans are:

For men: $M = 71.2 \times W^{3/4}[1 + 0.004(30 - a) + 0.010(s - 43.4)]$
For women: $M = 65.8 \times W^{3/4}[1 + 0.004(30 - a) + 0.018(s - 42.1)]$

where M = metabolic rate in kcal per day
        W = body weight in kg
        a = age in years (formula is based on assumption of a decrease of about 0.4 percent of the metabolic rate for each year above age 30)
        s = specific stature in cm/$W^{1/3}$ (assuming each additional cm per kg$^{1/3}$ in specific stature produces an average increase of 1 percent of the metabolic rate of men and 1.8 percent of the metabolic rate of women)

Table 23.2   METABOLIC BODY SIZE, $W^{3/4}$ FOR BODY WEIGHTS FROM 1 TO 100 KG

W, kg	$W^{3/4}$ kg$^{3/4}$	W, kg	$W^{3/4}$ kg$^{3/4}$	W, kg	$W^{3/4}$ kg$^{3/4}$	W, kg	$W^{3/4}$ kg$^{3/4}$	W, kg	$W^{3/4}$ kg$^{3/4}$
1	1.00	21	9.8	41	16.2	61	21.8	81	27.0
2	1.68	22	10.2	42	16.5	62	22.1	82	27.2
3	2.28	23	10.5	43	16.8	63	22.4	83	27.5
4	2.83	24	10.8	44	17.1	64	22.6	84	27.7
5	3.34	25	11.2	45	17.4	65	22.9	85	28.0
6	3.83	26	11.5	46	17.7	66	23.2	86	28.2
7	4.30	27	11.8	47	18.0	67	23.4	87	28.5
8	4.75	28	12.2	48	18.2	68	23.7	88	28.7
9	5.19	29	12.5	49	18.5	69	23.9	89	29.0
10	5.62	30	12.8	50	18.8	70	24.2	90	29.2
11	6.04	31	13.1	51	19.1	71	24.4	91	29.4
12	6.44	32	13.5	52	19.4	72	24.7	92	29.7
13	6.84	33	13.8	53	19.6	73	25.0	93	29.9
14	7.24	34	14.1	54	19.9	74	25.2	94	30.2
15	7.62	35	14.4	55	20.2	75	25.5	95	30.4
16	8.00	36	14.7	56	20.5	76	25.8	96	30.7
17	8.38	37	15.0	57	20.8	77	26.0	97	30.9
18	8.75	38	15.3	58	21.0	78	26.2	98	31.1
19	9.10	39	15.6	59	21.3	79	26.5	99	31.4
20	9.46	40	15.9	60	21.6	80	26.7	100	31.6

A comparison of metabolic rate of the human calculated either from surface area or the three-fourth power of body weight yields comparable results. For example, daily basal energy expenditure for a 132 lb (60 kg) woman, 5 ft 6 in (167 cm) tall, 45 years old, then may be calculated from a surface area of 1.68 m² (Fig. 23.4). At 34.9 kcal/m²/hr, the total expenditure would be approximately 1409 kcal (1.68 x 34.9 x 24). Using the Kleiber formula, metabolic rate is calculated as 1416 kcal (1417 − 0.94 + 0.03). It should be noted, however, that despite close agreement within species, $W^{3/4}$ yields data applicable to all mammalian species and therefore is to be preferred for research in comparative animal calorimetry. Table 23.2 provides $W^{3/4}$ for body weights ranging from 1 to 100 kg.

Factors Affecting Basal Metabolism. The effect of age on basal metabolic rate is shown in Fig. 23.5. BMR is highest per square meter during the first one and one-half to two years of life, decreases in early childhood, and increases slightly at puberty; thereafter BMR declines steadily. The reason for these age differences is not well understood. It is clear, however, that BMR is highest during periods of rapid growth and undoubtedly is associated with the increased biosynthetic activity of growth.

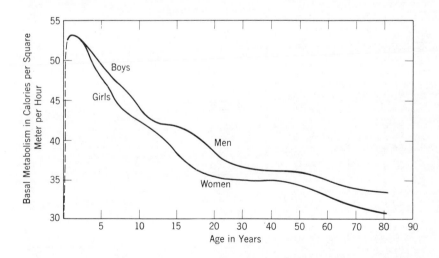

Fig. 23.5 Effect of age on basal metabolism. (From H. H. Mitchell, *Comparative Nutrition of Man and Domestic Animals*, Vol. I, Acad. Press, N. Y., 1962, p. 43.)

Table 23.3 BASAL METABOLIC RATES ACCORDING TO WEIGHT AND SEX

Body Weight (kg)	Kcal per 24 Hours		MJ per 24 Hours	
	Males	Females	Males	Females
3.0	150	136	0.6	0.6
4.0	210	205	0.9	0.8
5.0	270	274	1.1	1.1
6.0	330	336	1.4	1.4
7.0	390	395	1.6	1.6
8.0	445	448	1.9	1.9
9.0	495	496	2.1	2.1
10.0	545	541	2.3	2.3
11.0	590	582	2.5	2.4
12.0	625	620	2.5	2.6
13.0	665	655	2.8	2.7
14.0	700	687	2.9	2.9
15.0	725	718	3.0	3.0
16.0	750	747	3.1	3.1
17.0	780	775	3.3	3.2
18.0	810	802	3.4	3.3
19.0	840	827	3.5	3.5
20.0	870	852	3.6	3.6
22.0	910	898	3.8	3.8
24.0	980	942	4.1	3.9
26.0	1070	984	4.5	4.1
28.0	1100	1025	4.6	4.3
30.0	1140	1063	4.8	4.4
32.0	1190	1101	5.0	4.6
34.0	1230	1137	5.1	4.8
36.0	1270	1173	5.3	4.9
38.0	1305	1207	5.5	5.0
40.0	1340	1241	5.6	5.2
42.0	1370	1274	5.7	5.3
44.0	1400	1306	5.9	5.5
46.0	1430	1338	6.0	5.6
48.0	1460	1369	6.1	5.7
50.0	1485	1399	6.2	5.8
52.0	1505	1429	6.3	6.0
54.0	1555	1458	6.5	6.1
56.0	1580	1487	6.6	6.2
58.0	1600	1516	6.7	6.3
60.0	1630	1544	6.8	6.5
62.0	1660	1572	6.9	6.6
64.0	1690	1599	7.1	6.7

Table 23.3   Continued

66.0	1725	1626	7.2	6.8
68.0	1765	1653	7.4	6.9
70.0	1785	1679	7.5	7.0
72.0	1815	1705	7.6	7.1
74.0	1845	1731	7.7	7.2
76.0	1870	1756	7.8	7.3
78.0	1900	1781	7.9	7.4
80.0	–	1805	–	7.5
82.0	–	1830	–	7.7
84.0	2000	1855	8.4	7.8

From FAO/WHO, "Energy Requirements and Protein Requirements," *WHO Tech. Rep. Ser.*, No. 522 (1973), pp. 107-108.

The sex difference noted throughout the life span often is attributed to differences in body composition between males and females. The female body generally contains more fat than the male and therefore a lower lean body mass or active protoplasmic tissue (Behnke, 1953). According to Kleiber (1961) and Mitchell (1962), the effect of the sex hormones on BMR may be more direct than their effect on body composition. Estimated basal metabolic rates for males and females over a wide range of body weight are shown in Table 23.3.

Basal heat production is increased in late pregnancy (Sandiford and Wheeler, 1924; Enright, 1935). Leitch (1957) has attributed the increase to fetal growth and growth of maternal tissues such as mammary and uterine tissues. According to Kleiber (1961), however, the increase in BMR of pregnant rats is due mainly to increased metabolic rate of maternal tissues other than those directly involved in the reproductive process. The reason for increased BMR during pregnancy is therefore uncertain.

Racial differences apparently do not affect basal metabolic rate and the effect of environmental temperature is uncertain. Although some reports indicate that individuals living in tropical climates tend to have a basal metabolic rate lower than those living in temperate or cold climates, Consolazio et al. (1961) have reported no effect of excessively hot climates on the basal metabolism.[2]

[2]BMR is measured under highly standardized conditions so that, in fact, the BMR is a measure of inherent tissue metabolic rates. Resting metabolism assumes only that the

Certain pathological conditions, such as hyperthyroidism and fever, increase basal metabolism. In fever, the increase is about 7 percent for each degree (F) rise in body temperature or 13 percent for each degree (C). Both fasting and chronic undernutrition decrease the BMR to about an equal degree. Early studies by Benedict (1915) on a professional faster indicated a decrease in BMR of about 25 percent on the twentieth day of fasting; thereafter BMR remained relatively stable. Keys' studies (Keys et al., 1950), during World War II, on men maintained on low calorie rations indicated a reduction of about 20 percent. The decrease in BMR as a result of undernutrition is interpreted as an adaptive mechanism of the body that conserves energy by operating at a lower level of metabolic activity; probably some of the decrease is due also to a decrease in weight and a subsequent decrease in surface area of the body.

Many attempts have been made to show that BMR is higher for athletes than nonathletes due presumably to a greater mass of active protoplasmic tissue (see Mitchell, 1962). Slight increases have been shown in the trained athlete but differences between athletes and nonathletes generally appear to be negligible.

Calorigenic Effect of Food. Determination of the basal metabolic rate requires that the subject be in the postabsorptive state, that is, without food for at least 12 hours prior to the test. The reason for withholding food is that following ingestion of food, heat production increases above the resting state. This effect was first recognized by Rubner in 1902 and was called the *specific dynamic effect* of food. The effect of food on heat production was clearly demonstrated, however, in Lavoisier's experiments (see Chapter 1). When foodstuffs were fed individually, the increase in heat production following ingestion of protein was observed to be considerably greater than that following carbohydrate and fat. In an ordinary mixed diet consisting of all foodstuffs, however, the calorigenic effect amounts to about 6 percent of the energy value

---

individual is at rest, that is, not performing work; environmental factors are not controlled. Consequently, temperature effects are reflected in resting metabolism. The effect of environmental temperature on the resting metabolism was first shown by Lavoisier (see Chapter 1). An increase in metabolism occurs at either extreme of the temperature scale; in cold, the increase is accomplished by shivering: muscular contractions that result in an increase in heat production both from the inefficient transfer of the high energy of ATP and the friction of contracting muscle fibers. In severe heat, additional energy is paradoxically required to maintain body temperature; that is, the process of maintaining temperature homeostasis requires extra energy.

of the dietary intake (Benedict and Carpenter, 1918). The proportions of carbohydrate, fat, and protein in the diet do not significantly influence the calorigenic effect. The use of high protein diets in weight reduction in the belief that the calorigenic effect will be increased is without scientific basis. High protein and low protein diets produce similar effects (Bradfield and Jourdan, 1973).

In passing, it might be noted that the extra heat production following ingestion of food is known also as the *specific dynamic action* (SDA) of food. We prefer the term *calorigenic effect* as a more suitable description of this confusing phenomenon.

The cause of extra heat production following ingestion of food, and particularly protein, has plagued nutritionists for many years. Numerous theories have been proposed but there is no general agreement yet. The early belief that the work of digestion caused the increase in heat production was easily disproved since even when nutrient substances were injected (thus bypassing the intestinal tract), the calorigenic effect was observed.

The calorigenic effect, then, was assumed to be related to the fate of foodstuffs after absorption. Voit proposed that when foods are ingested and transported to the cells the cellular mechanism is temporarily overwhelmed by a flood of metabolizable nutrients that, in some indefinable way, speed up the metabolic rate. The greater calorigenic effect observed for protein was attributed by Lusk (1931) to the more complicated series of reactions required for the metabolism of amino acids, that is, deamination.

Probably the most definitive early reports on this difficult and confusing subject are those of Wilhelmj et al. (1928) and Borsook and Winegarden (1931), which extended earlier work of Terroine and Bonnet (1926). The latter authors attributed the high heat increment of protein to the quantity of amino nitrogen ingested and, more specifically, to the amount of amino nitrogen deaminated, that is, urinary nitrogen. Wilhelmj et al. (1928) expressed the relationship between the calorigenic effect and ingested protein in terms of calories per millimole of deaminated amino acid (calculated from urinary nitrogen), and Borsook and Winegarden (1931) reported a positive correlation between metabolic rate and urinary nitrogen.

Passmore and Ritchie (1957) have suggested that the calorigenic effect of food is a two-fold process. They observed an increase in heat production in subjects within five minutes after a test meal.

This finding suggests that the work of the digestive tract does indeed contribute in part to the total rise in heat production. The cellular mechanism contributing to extra heat production following the ingestion of foodstuffs remains speculative.

The most likely theory to date was proposed by Krebs (1964), who related the calorigenic effect of food to the energy requirement for synthesis of ATP. Calculating ATP yield from oxidation of triglyceride (tristearin) and carbohydrate (glucose residue from starch), he estimated that 18.1 kcal and 17.4 kcal are required to obtain 1 mole ATP when fat and carbohydrate, respectively, are oxidized, assuming complete oxidation of these foodstuffs. ATP synthesized from protein oxidation was calculated from the gross yield of ATP from each of the amino acids present in an individual protein. Calculation of ATP yield was corrected for two factors: (1) ATP required for urea synthesis and (2) incomplete oxidation of amino acids. (Much of the dietary glycine, for example, is used in the synthesis of creatine, porphyrin, or purines; some cystine and cysteine are used for synthesis of taurocholic acid; and tryptophan and, to some extent, all amino acid carbon skeletons may be incompletely oxidized.) Assuming that about 12 percent of amino acid carbon was not oxidized, and that 2 moles ATP are utilized for disposal of each gram atom of amino acid nitrogen in urea synthesis, Krebs calculated that when a protein such as ovalbumin is oxidized, at least 21.2 kcal are required to yield 1 mole ATP. Calorigenic effect was then calculated as the percentage increase in energy requirement for ATP synthesis from protein as compared with that from carbohydrate and fat, and amounted to approximately 20 percent for most proteins, varying by one or two percent according to amino acid content of the protein source.[1] Calorigenic effect thus represents the additional calories necessary for ATP formation when protein rather than carbohydrate or fat serves as oxidative substrate.

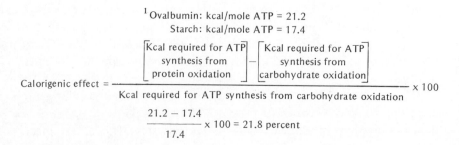

[1] Ovalbumin: kcal/mole ATP = 21.2
Starch: kcal/mole ATP = 17.4

$$\text{Calorigenic effect} = \frac{\left[\begin{array}{c}\text{Kcal required for ATP}\\ \text{synthesis from}\\ \text{protein oxidation}\end{array}\right] - \left[\begin{array}{c}\text{Kcal required for ATP}\\ \text{synthesis from}\\ \text{carbohydrate oxidation}\end{array}\right]}{\text{Kcal required for ATP synthesis from carbohydrate oxidation}} \times 100$$

$$\frac{21.2 - 17.4}{17.4} \times 100 = 21.8 \text{ percent}$$

Krebs' calculations, which are based on cellular energy transformations, represent a new approach to the problem of the calorigenic effect of food. Grisolia and Kennedy (1966) have criticized Krebs' calculations as being incomplete since no correction is made for ATP utilized in protein or other syntheses requiring nitrogen (purines, amino sugars, etc.). These authors do not question the basic reasoning underlying the calculation, but rather the validity of any such calculation. Doubtless, the problem of the calorigenic effect of food will continue to be debated, and whether experimental evidence *can* be obtained that will precisely explain its metabolic basis is a moot question. The fact remains, however, that the extra heat production following ingestion of food represents a wastage of metabolizable energy and therefore is considered in establishing dietary energy requirement. In other words, the total energy intake must allow for an increase above the estimated energy expenditure. A 6 percent increase for persons consuming an ordinary varied diet is generally accepted as satisfactory.

Activity.   Activity is the most variable factor affecting the total energy requirement. It is the external work of the body but, clearly, external work must involve a speeding up of the internal work and therefore an increase in the metabolic rate. Moreover, as described by Benedict and Cathcart (1913) from studies of muscular work, there are essentially two components of external activity: metabolism especially involved in production of work and extraneous motion incidental to the performance of work. It is the extraneous motion that often determines the difference in energy expenditure between two individuals performing the same task.

Activity requirements also vary with body size. Obviously, more energy is required to move a large body than a small body. Energy cost of activities involving whole body movement varies too with the intensity of activity. For example, both the speed of walking and body weight influence the energy required in walking (Table 23.4).

Energy costs for various activities have been studied extensively. A large amount of the published data has been compiled by Passmore and Durnin (1955). Some average data on energy expenditure for various activities are shown in Table 23.5. These figures are not representative of the cost of activity alone; they include the basal expenditure as well, and therefore they represent the total energy expenditure when activity is performed.

Table 23.4 RELATIONSHIP BETWEEN ENERGY EXPENDITURE (KCAL/MIN OR KJ/MIN) AND SPEED OF WALKING(MPH) AND GROSS BODY WEIGHT (LB)

	Weight (lb)							
	100		120		140		180	
Speed (mph)	kcal/min	kJ/min	kcal/min	kJ/min	kcal/min	kJ/min	kcal/min	kJ/min
2.0	2.2	9.2	2.6	10.9	2.9	12.1	3.5	14.6
2.5	2.7	11.3	3.1	13.0	3.5	14.6	4.2	17.6
3.0	3.1	13.0	3.6	15.1	4.0	16.7	4.8	20.1
3.5	3.6	15.1	4.2	17.6	4.6	19.2	5.4	22.6
4.0	4.1	17.2	4.7	19.7	5.2	21.8	6.4	26.8

Adapted from R. Passmore and J. V. G. A. Durnin, *Physiol. Rev.,* 35: 801 (1955).

Table 23.5 AVERAGE ENERGY EXPENDITURE FOR VARIOUS ACTIVITIES[a]

Activity	kcal/minute	kJ/minute
Lying at ease	1.4-1.5	5.9-6.3
Sitting at ease	1.6	6.7
Sitting, writing	1.9-2.2	8.0-9.2
Sitting, playing cards	2.1-2.4	8.8-10.0
Sitting, playing woodwind instrument	2.0	8.4
Sitting, playing piano	2.5	10.5
Sitting, playing violin	2.7	11.3
Sitting, playing organ	3.2-3.5	13.4-14.6
Sitting, playing drums	4.0-4.2	16.7-17.6
Standing at ease	1.7-1.9	7.1-8.0
Cycling (5.5 mph)	4.5	18.8
Cycling (9.4 mph)	7.0	29.3
Cycling (13.1 mph)	11.1	46.4
Dancing, foxtrot	5.2	21.8
Dancing, rumba	7.0	29.3
Volleyball	3.5	14.7
Archery	5.2	21.8
Tennis	7.1	29.7
Football	8.9	37.2
Swimming, breaststroke (30 yd/min)	7.5	31.4
Swimming, breaststroke (40 yd/min)	10.0	42.0

Adapted from R. Passmore and J. V. G. A. Durnin, *Physiol. Rev.*, 35: 801 (1955).
[a]Weight range 60-75 kg.

The total energy requirement for activity may be estimated and expressed as percent above basal expenditure; however, this is rarely done in describing the energy cost of individual activities.

Calorimetry

Early workers in calorimetry knew little of the details of energy transformations in the animal body. Indeed, the means by which animals utilize food and produce heat are not essential to an understanding of gross calorimetry and, in contrast to many other areas of nutrition investigation, much of the basic work in calorimetry was accomplished by 1920. Consolazio and Johnson (1971) have reviewed some of the more recent work.

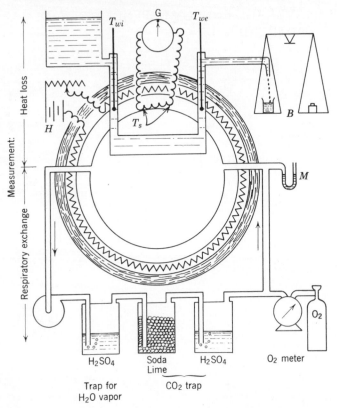

Fig. 23.6 Schematic diagram showing principle of Atwater-Rosa respiration calorimeter. The subject is surrounded by two concentric walls. The outer wall is kept at the same temperature T_s as in the inner wall by means of a heat source H and controlling galvanometer G. The heat produced by the subject is carried away by water that flows into the chamber at the temperature T_{wi} and leaves the chamber at the temperature T_{we}. The rate of flow is measured by the balance B. Maintenance of constant pressure is monitored by means of the manometer M. [From M. Kleiber, *Calorimetric Measurements in Biophysical Research Methods*, F. M. Uber, ed., Wiley-Interscience, N. Y. (1950).]

There have been refinements in instrumentation in recent years. Basically, however, all methods of calorimetry are based on two broad principles: the measurement of heat lost from the body (direct calorimetry) or the calculation of heat production from gaseous exchange (indirect calorimetry).

Table 23.6 HEAT LOSS FROM ADULT MEN IN THE RESTING AND ACTIVE STATE

Subject	Number of Days on Experiment	Average Kcal per Day				Total
		By Radiation and Conduction	In Urine and Feces	In Water Vaporized	Heat Equivalent of External Work	
H. F. (resting)	3	1471	8	425	—	1904
A. L. (resting)	2	2157	22	510	—	2689
A. L. (at work)	3	2391	13	1958	459	4821

From F. G. Benedict and T. M. Carpenter, "The Metabolism and Energy Transformations of Healthy Men During Rest," Carnegie Inst., Wash., 1910.

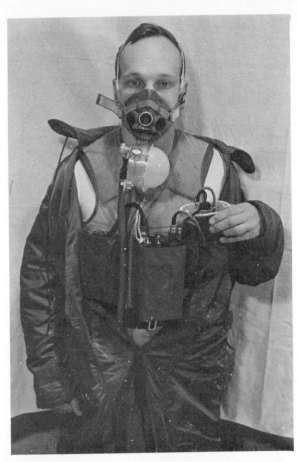

Fig. 23.7 Integrating motor pneumotachograph (IMP). The IMP is a portable battery-operated unit designed to measure total ventilation and oxygen consumption in man under field conditions. It was designed by Wolff (1955, 1958) and is shown as modified for use under arctic conditions by Rogers et al. (1963). The flowmeter is the plastic unit attached to the face mask. Movements of the flowmeter diaphragm generate small electrical signals proportional to the extent and duration of the diaphragm displacement during expiration. These signals are amplified and drive an integrating motor which turns a counter (odometer) in the unit carried in the center pocket of the vest shown. The odometer reading, multiplied by a previously obtained calibration factor, yields the total volume of expired air.

At the same time, a pump, located in the same unit as the odometer, pulls 0.5 ml samples of mixed expired air from the flowmeter after every liter or so of expiration and stores them in a neoprene

Direct Calorimetry. The direct measurement of heat loss is theoretically simple but, in practice, is cumbersome and expensive. Total energy output includes sensible heat given off from the body, the latent heat of vaporized water from lungs and skin, and the heat of combustion of urine and feces.

The calorimeter is an insulated double-walled adiabatic chamber (Fig. 23.6); that is, the temperature of the two walls must be kept equal so that heat cannot flow in either direction and thus escape from the calorimeter. Heat eliminated from the subject is removed by water flowing in coils of pipe within the chamber walls. Heat loss is calculated from the difference in temperature and amount of water flowing in and out of the pipes. Heat removed by vaporization of water is calculated by measuring moisture of air leaving the calorimeter (carbon dioxide is usually absorbed in soda lime and water in sulfuric acid). For each gram of water vaporized, 0.580 kcal are required at 30°C, the temperature of the skin. In addition, corrections must be made for changes in body temperature and for any food or drink introduced into the chamber.

The data in Table 23.6 were taken in part from experiments on adult men published by Benedict and Carpenter in 1910 and indicate the magnitude of heat eliminated from the body by various avenues. Note that losses in urine and feces are minor and that a major loss in either the resting state or while performing work is by radiation and conduction from the body. Note also the differences in water vaporization between the resting and active states.

Indirect Calorimetry. Indirect calorimetry refers to calculation of heat production from measurement of gaseous exchange: oxygen consumed and carbon dioxide expired or both. The respiration

---

Fig. 23.7 Continued
bag container carried in a plexiglass container in the pocket to the subject's left. Samples collected over a period of an hour or more are representative of the mixed expired air, and, then, appropriate gas analysis, together with the integrated ventilated volume measurement, permits calculation of the oxygen consumption and carbon dioxide production. (The loss of carbon dioxide by diffusion out of the neoprene bag can be prevented by first filling the space between the outside of the bag and the inside walls of the plexiglass container container with expired air.) The pocket on the subject's right carries the battery pack. (Courtesy of Dr. Terence A. Rogers.)

calorimeter, a chamber somewhat similar to that used in direct calorimetry, was the first instrument to be used for the measurement of respiratory exchange. More recently, mobile lightweight and more versatile instruments have been devised; these instruments consist of masks with attachments that can be strapped to the subject for collection of gas and permit easy movement of the subject in performing various activities (see Fig. 23.7).

The heat equivalent of respiratory exchange is not only calculated from oxygen consumed and carbon dioxide expired but also is dependent upon the ratio of the moles of carbon dioxide produced to the moles of oxygen consumed, or the *respiratory quotient* (R.Q.):

$$\text{R.Q.} = \frac{\text{moles } CO_2}{\text{moles } O_2}$$

The R.Q. varies when carbohydrate, fat, and protein are oxidized because of differences in composition of the foodstuffs that determine the amount of oxygen required for complete oxidation and, consequently, the volume of carbon dioxide that is given off. For carbohydrate the R.Q. is 1.0 since in combustion of carbohydrate the amount of molecular oxygen required for oxidation is equal to the carbon dioxide produced. The oxidation of glucose, for example, is shown below:

$$C_6H_{12}O_6 + 6\,O_2 \longrightarrow 6\,CO_2 + 6\,H_2O$$

Fats require more oxygen than carbohydrates for combustion because the fat molecule contains a low ratio of oxygen to carbon and hydrogen. Thus for a fat such as tristearin, the R.Q. may be represented as:

$$2\,C_{57}H_{110}O_6 + 163\,O_2 \longrightarrow 114\,CO_2 + 110\,H_2O$$

$$\frac{CO_2}{O_2} = \frac{114}{163} = 0.70$$

Calculation of the R.Q. for protein is more complicated than that for fat or carbohydrate because protein is not completely oxidized and both carbon and oxygen are excreted in the urine chiefly as urea. When adjustment is made for urinary excretion, the ratio of carbon dioxide produced to oxygen consumed is approximately 1:1.2 and thus is equivalent to an R.Q. of 0.80.

The R.Q.s for individual carbohydrates, fats, and proteins differ slightly, but the average figures of 1.0, 0.7, and 0.8 respectively are accepted as representative of the foodstuffs. The R.Q. for an ordinary mixed dietary consisting of the three foodstuffs is approximately 0.85. Obviously, it is impossible to make assumptions about the relative amounts of foodstuffs undergoing oxidation except at extremes of the R.Q. range. For example, if the R. Q. is nearly 1.0, one may safely assume that the foodstuff is largely carbohydrate. Similarly, an R.Q. of about 0.7 indicates a predominantly fatty acid metabolism. At intermediate levels of R.Q., no safe assumption can be made.

Since the nature of the foodstuff consumed in cellular respiratory processes determines both oxygen consumption and carbon dioxide formation (that is, the R.Q.), the caloric equivalent for a given volume of oxygen or carbon dioxide also will vary with the R.Q. Caloric equivalents of oxygen and carbon dioxide for R.Q. values between 0.7 and 1.0 are shown in Table 23.7. It is apparent from the table that when fat is oxidized heat production represented by 1 liter of oxygen consumed is only 0.3 kcal less than when carbohydrate is oxidized, a difference of about 6 percent. The variation in caloric equivalent for carbon dioxide, however, is on the order of 30 percent. These figures apply only to mixtures of carbohydrate and fat and therefore represent what is referred to as the nonprotein R.Q.

For work requiring great accuracy the extent of protein oxidation may be calculated from urinary nitrogen, and the nonprotein R.Q. then may be estimated. In practice, the error incurred by ignoring protein metabolism is relatively small and, particularly in short term studies, no correction is made for the effect of protein metabolism on R.Q. Calculation of heat production is made as if only fat and carbohydrate were oxidized.

Calculation of Heat Production from R.Q. Calculation of heat production from gaseous exchange is relatively easy. Oxygen consumed and carbon dioxide produced over a known period of time are corrected to standard conditions (760 mm mercury, dry, 0°C). The R.Q. is calculated and the appropriate caloric equivalent is used to determine the total heat production. For example, consider the following hypothetical data:

Vol. O_2 consumed (standard conditions) = 14.4 liter per hour

Table 23.7 CALORIC VALUES FOR OXYGEN AND CARBON DIOXIDE FOR NONPROTEIN R.Q.

Nonprotein Respiratory Quotient	Caloric Value of 1 Liter of O_2	Caloric Value of 1 Liter of CO_2	Percentage of Total O_2 Consumed by Fat	Percentage of Total Heat Produced by Fat
0.707	4.686	6.629	100.0	100.0
0.71	4.690	6.606	99.0	98.5
0.72	4.702	6.531	95.6	95.2
0.73	4.714	6.458	92.2	91.6
0.74	4.727	6.388	88.7	88.0
0.75	4.739	6.319	85.3	84.4
0.76	4.751	6.253	81.9	80.8
0.77	4.764	6.187	78.5	77.2
0.78	4.776	6.123	75.1	73.7
0.79	4.788	6.062	71.7	70.1
0.80	4.801	6.001	68.3	66.6
0.81	4.813	5.942	64.8	63.1
0.82	4.825	5.884	61.4	59.7
0.83	4.838	5.829	58.0	56.2
0.84	4.850	5.774	54.6	52.8
0.85	4.862	5.721	51.2	49.3
0.86	4.875	5.669	47.8	45.9
0.87	4.887	5.617	44.4	42.5
0.88	4.899	5.568	41.0	39.2
0.89	4.911	5.519	37.5	35.8
0.90	4.924	5.471	34.1	32.5
0.91	4.936	5.424	30.7	29.2
0.92	4.948	5.378	27.3	25.9
0.93	4.961	5.333	23.9	22.6
0.94	4.973	5.290	20.5	19.3
0.95	4.985	5.247	17.1	16.0
0.96	4.998	5.205	13.7	12.8
0.97	5.010	5.165	10.2	9.51
0.98	5.022	5.124	6.83	6.37
0.99	5.035	5.085	3.41	3.18
1.00	5.047	5.047	0	0

After N. Zuntz and H. Schumberg, with modifications by G. Lusk, E. P. Cathcart, and D. P. Cuthbertson, *J. Physiol. (London)*, 72: 349 (1931).

Vol. CO_2 produced (standard conditions) = 12.0 liter per hour

$$R.Q. = \frac{12.0}{14.4} = 0.83$$

From Table 23.7, the caloric equivalent for an R.Q. of 0.83 is 4.383 for 1 liter of O_2 and 5.829 for 1 liter of CO_2.

Heat production = 14.4 x 4.838 = 69.7 kcal per hour

or = 12.0 x 5.829 = 69.9 kcal per hour

The agreement in caloric values obtained by calculation from either oxygen consumption or carbon dioxide production is quite good. However, because variation in caloric equivalents is less for oxygen than carbon dioxide over the full range of R.Q. values, measurement of oxygen consumption is preferred for most experimental work.

Calculation of Heat Production from Oxygen Consumption Alone. When only oxygen consumption is determined, an *average* caloric equivalent of 4.83 may be used to calculate total heat production. The average caloric equivalent of 1 liter of oxygen yields final computations that vary little from those obtained by first determining R.Q., since the entire range of caloric equivalents of oxygen varies by only 6 percent. The accuracy of an average computation is heightened by the fact that rarely in practice does one encounter an R.Q. at either extreme of the range. For the most part, human beings oxidize a mixture of foodstuffs that yield R.Q. values near the middle of the range.

For example, if only oxygen consumption had been determined in the illustration cited above, heat production calculated from an average caloric equivalent of 4.83 is 69.6 kcal/hour (4.83 x 14.4) compared with 69.7 kcal/hour calculated from R.Q. Therefore, for many forms of work this simplified method is quite acceptable.

Energy Balance

Data from calorimetric studies as just described are the basis for the establishment of energy requirements for *groups* of people (see Chapter 25). These data also provide reasonable guides for the prediction of energy requirements of individuals; however, as in all determinations of nutrient requirements, studies of energy expenditure are less accurately applied to individuals than to groups. For example, differences in body size significantly affect the energy cost of the basal metabolism and activities involving whole body movement. Caloric adjustments for body size are relatively accurate for estimation of basal energy expenditure but are apt to be less accurate when applied to expenditure for activity.

Other factors also contribute to the variance among individuals. Efficiency in the performance of tasks is an obvious factor. Anyone who has seen a seasoned performer and a novice working side by side is aware of the difference. However, as Tepperman (1962) has pointed out, differences in muscle tone alone could account for the variations in energy need between two individuals apparently similar in body build and activity pattern. Relaxation of muscles during restful sleep may reduce the BMR by as much as 10 percent. Conceivably, and indeed very likely, the act of sitting quietly could require much more energy for the "high-tone" individual than for the "low-tone" individual.

One method of estimating energy expenditure requires the subject to keep an accurate record of daily activities over a period of time, usually about one week. The data shown in Table 23.8, for example, illustrate the compilation of a weekly activity record and calculation of energy expenditure for a relatively inactive man employed as a clerk (Passmore and Durnin, 1955). A similar approach was used by Widdowson et al. (1954) to estimate the energy expenditure of a group of cadets in active training. Data on energy costs for many occupational activities were compiled in the review of Passmore and Durnin (1955). On the basis of these and similar data, occupations have been classified arbitrarily as "sedentary," "light activity," and so forth. Although no system of arbitrary classification is infallible, most certainly this kind of estimation is valuable in planning group feeding programs and in roughly evaluating individual energy needs.

In this connection, it is worth mentioning that energy expenditure for certain individual activities may tend to be overestimated. Pollack et al. (1958) cite football and tennis as activities requiring a large energy expenditure when the body is in motion, but which, in fact, require only intermittent motion. In such cases, energy expended over the total period of play must be calculated separately for the periods of active play (to which figures of energy expenditure

Table 23.8 ENERGY OUTPUT AND INTAKE OF A CLERK OVER ONE WEEK (AGE 29; HT, 66 IN.; WT, 66 KG)

Activity	Total Time Spent Hr	Min	Kcal/Min	KJ/Min	Kcal for Activity	MJ for Activity	Total Kcal	Total MJ
In bed	54	4	1.13	4.73	3670	15.4		
Daytime dozing	1	43	1.37	5.73	140	0.59	3810	16.0
Recreational and off work								
Light sedentary activities	31	14	1.48	6.19	2810	11.8		
Washing, shaving, dressing	3	18	3.0	12.6	590	2.47		
Playing with child		30	3.2	13.4	100	0.42		
Light domestic work	7	14	3.0	12.6	1300	5.44		
Walking	8	35	6.6	27.6	3400	14.2		
Gardening	2	48	4.8	20.1	810	3.40		
Standing activities	6	45	1.56	6.52	630	2.64		
Watching football	2	10	2.0	8.37	260	1.09		
Total recreational and off work							9800	41.0
Working								
Sitting activities	22	22	1.65	6.90	2210	9.25		
Standing activities	25	57	1.90	7.95	2960	12.4		
Walking	1	22	6.6	27.6	540	22.6		
Total working							5710	24.0
Grand total							19,320	80.8
Daily average							2760	11.5
Food intake (daily average determined by diet survey)							2620	11.0

Adapted from R. Passmore and J. V. G. A. Durnin, *Physiol. Rev.*, 35: 801 (1955).

apply) *and* for periods of relative inactivity which require no greater energy expenditure of the player than that of the spectator standing on the sidelines.

The maintenance of energy balance is so obvious that it barely merits explanation. Positive balance is indicated by an energy intake greater than expenditure and leads to weight gain which, in the adult, is largely evidenced by sagging jowls and a thickening waistline, or worse. Negative balance is synonymous with weight loss and indicates that fewer calories are taken in than are expended. The ideal for the adult, of course, is equilibrium, when energy intake and energy expenditure are nicely balanced.

Many persons are able to maintain a favorable balance of energy with little effort; appetite, thus food intake, is geared to energy expenditure. The work of Edholm et al. (1955) indicates that energy expenditure tends to regulate food intake but that the effect is delayed. This conclusion was based on the observation that caloric intake of their subjects reflected the energy expenditure of two days earlier. Clearly, the balance of energy is not a day-to-day phenomenon but is governed over a period of time. The increasing rate of obesity in the United States and other affluent countries, however, is generally accepted to be the result of reduced energy output rather than a marked increase in food intake.

ENERGY VALUE OF FOODS

The energy value of foods usually is expressed in nutrition in terms of the kilocalorie and traditionally designated the large Calorie. The trend, however, is slowly moving away from the use of the term Calorie toward the more accurate practice of calling the kilocalorie by its own name.

Since Lavoisier's classic experiments on the origin of animal heat, it has been known that foods burned outside the body produce the same amount of heat as foods oxidized by the slow processes of intermediary metabolism. If, then, foods are burned and heat produced is measured, the quantity of heat expressed in kilocalories represents the *gross energy value* or *heat of combustion* of the food. The instrument used to determine heat of combustion is known to all students of nutrition as the bomb calorimeter (Fig. 23.8), that,

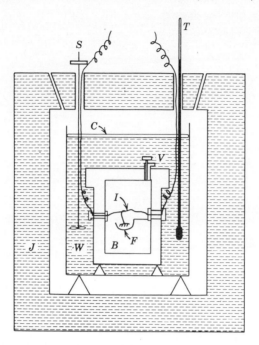

Fig. 23.8 Cross section of a bomb calorimeter. J = water jacket; W = weighed amount water; S = stirrer; T = thermometer; F = platinum sample dish; B = bomb chamber; I = ignition wire. (From chapter by Kleiber in Uber's *Biophysical Research Methods*, Wiley-Interscience, N. Y., 1950, p. 194.)

in effect, consists of a bomb or small chamber immersed in a container of water. The bomb is filled with oxygen and the food contained therein is ignited by means of an electric spark. As the food burns, heat produced leads to a rise in temperature of the surrounding fluid. Thus heat production can be accurately measured. An early designed bomb calorimeter was described by Atwater and Snell (1903). Present models, though more sleek, are technically similar to instruments used 60-odd years ago.

The heats of combustion for individual carbohydrates, proteins, and fats differ somewhat. The gross energy yield of sucrose, for example, was determined by Atwater to be 3.96 kcal/gm, whereas starch yielded 4.23 kcal/gm. Energy yield of butterfat was found to be 9.21 kcal/gm and that of lard, 9.48 kcal/gm (Atwater and Bryant, 1899). For practical use, individual figures were averaged to apply to the major foodstuffs as groups. These average (and familiar) figures are shown below:

Foodstuff	Gross Energy Value kcal/gm
Carbohydrate	4.15
Fat	9.4
Protein	5.65

The gross energy value of foodstuffs, however, does not represent the energy actually available to body cells, since no potentially oxidizable substrate can be considered available until it is presented to the cell for oxidation. None of the foodstuffs is completely absorbed; some potential energy, therefore, never enters the body and is excreted in the feces. Digestibility of the major foodstuffs, however, is high; on the average 97 percent of ingested carbohydrates, 95 percent of fats, and 92 percent of proteins are absorbed from the intestinal lumen.

In addition, although carbohydrates and fats are oxidized completely to carbon dioxide and water in the processes of cellular metabolism as in the calorimeter, the cell is less efficient in oxidizing protein than is the calorimeter. In biological systems, urea, uric acid, creatinine, and other nitrogenous compounds derived from protein are excreted in the urine. Determination of both the heat of combustion and nitrogen content of urine indicates that approximately 7.9 kcal/gm of urine nitrogen is equivalent to 1.25 kcal/gm of protein (7.9/6.25). This energy represents metabolic loss and must be subtracted from the "digestible" energy of protein.

When heat of combustion is corrected for losses in digestion and for unmetabolized urinary substances, energy value of foods is designated *available energy* or *physiological fuel value.* Available energy of the major foodstuffs is shown in Fig. 23.9. The terms digestible energy and metabolizable energy are more accurately designated *apparent digestible energy* and *apparent metabolizable energy.* Fecal matter always contains some bacterial debris and materials of metabolic or body origin, sloughed off mucosal cells, and secretions. These substances contribute to energy value of feces and, therefore, digestibility figures must represent apparent rather than true digestibility of individual foods.

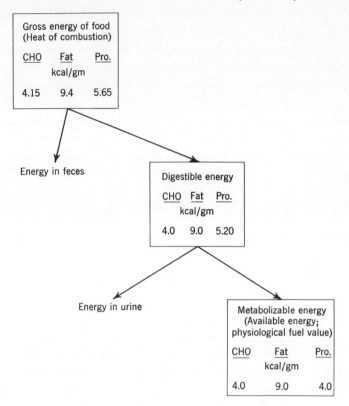

Fig. 23.9 Energy value of food.

Both malic and citric acid occur in varying amounts in some fruits and vegetables. These acids are absorbed and thus contribute to the tricarboxylic acid pool to yield energy. On the average, these organic acids yield approximately 2.45 kcal/gm of acid; 2.47 kcal/gm for citric acid and 2.42 kcal/gm for malic (FAO, 1947).

The contribution of organic acids to total energy value is fairly low for some vegetables and fruits. For example, cabbage, carrots, Brussels sprouts, head lettuce, and pineapple contain only 2-4 percent of organic acids as compared to total available carbohydrate. Higher amounts occur in prunes, plums, oranges, cranberries, and grapefruit. Lemon juice, however, contains a substantial amount of acids, 62.5 percent of total carbohydrate. Current food tables include organic acids as a part of total available energy.

Traditionally, tables of food composition have included data on energy, proximate composition, and the minerals and vitamins for which the National Research Council has made recommended dietary allowances, with the exception of vitamin D. Data for phosphorus content of foods also is included. The trend toward more detailed identification of nutrients present in foods is evident in the last revision of *Handbook 8* (Watt and Merrill, 1963) that, in addition to usual data, now includes figures on sodium and potassium of foods and limited tables on fatty acids, cholesterol, and magnesium. The tables compiled by Widdowson and McCance (1960) include limited figures for copper, sulfur, and chloride as well. As new commercially processed foods become available the task of keeping food composition data up to date becomes tremendous.

PROTEIN REQUIREMENT

Although it is convenient to speak of the protein requirement of man, because protein is the source of nitrogen in the human diet, the true requirement is not for protein as such, but rather for specific amounts and proportions of the essential amino acids and of nonessential amino acid nitrogen. The amino acids must adequately provide for cellular synthesis of both proteins and nonprotein nitrogenous compounds. The latter requirement may be met by simple nitrogen-containing compounds such as diammonium citrate or urea (Rose et al., 1949) as well as by the naturally occurring or synthetic amino acids.

The dependence of nutrient needs upon physiological state was discussed in Chapter 22, and little need be added here. Obviously, both growth and body size must affect nitrogen requirements, and, as shown in Fig. 23.10, both factors also affect the nature of the requirement. Thus the need for nitrogen shifts from a high-growth, low-maintenance requirement in early infancy to a high-maintenance, low-growth requirement in adulthood. The growth requirement of the adult (adult growth), defined by Mitchell (1949) as syntheses necessary for growth of hair and nails and replacement of epidermal cells, obviously is only a fraction of the maintenance requirement of the adult body.

Maintenance requirement can be estimated from nitrogen losses from the body when subjects are maintained on a diet free, or nearly free of nitrogen. These losses include endogenous urinary loss, metabolic fecal loss, and losses in sweat and from sloughing of

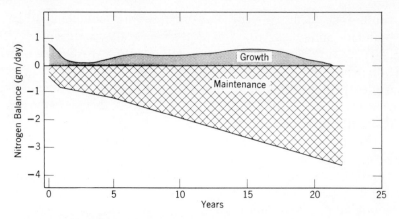

Fig. 23.10 Minimum nitrogen for maintenance and growth. [From J. B. Allison, 5th Int. Cong. on Nutrition (1960).]

dermal tissues. Recently other miscellaneous sources of loss have been quantitatively defined (Calloway et al., 1971).

The endogenous urinary nitrogen was shown by Smuts (1935) to be proportional to the basal metabolism (and therefore to body surface area and weight) and to be of the order of 2 mg N/basal kcal. This figure was confirmed in a number of mammalian species and was assumed to be applicable to man. Bricker et al. (1945) estimated that the true endogenous urinary losses were even lower. Subsequent studies with human subjects including those of Young and Scrimshaw (1966) and Calloway and Margen (1971) indicate that these losses amount to somewhere between 1.3 and 1.7 mg N/basal kcal (see FAO/WHO, 1973).

The metabolic fecal nitrogen (estimated at 0.7 to 1.1 gm/day) and losses through the skin (about 300 mg/day) are added to the endogenous urinary loss to obtain total nitrogen losses as a means of estimating the *maintenance* requirement for the adult. The total losses so determined are reckoned to be about 3.7 gm/day (FAO/ WHO, 1973; Food and Nutrition Board, 1974). Minimum protein requirement for maintenance then may be estimated as 23 gm protein/day (3.7 x 6.25) or 0.33 gm/kg for a 70 kg adult man.

The determination of body losses (and acquisition) of a nutrient as described above is one means of estimating protein and mineral requirements and is known as the factorial method. Theoretically, the provision of the equivalent of body losses should allow for adult maintenance. This concept, however, assumes complete utilization of dietary intake, a situation that does not occur even when the highest quality protein is fed (see Holmes, 1965; FAO/WHO, 1973). Thus, when this method is used, as in the determination of recommended protein intakes for population groups, corrections must be made to account for the discrepancy between calculated losses and dietary utilization (see Chapter 25).

The technique most generally accepted for the evaluation of human amino acid and nitrogen requirements is the nitrogen balance technique. Interpretation of nitrogen balance data is based on the premise that equilibrium in the adult is attained when the supplies of essential amino acids and total nitrogen are adequate for replacement of endogenous losses that occur through the kidney, intestinal secretions, sweat, and desquamation of epithelial cells and for synthesis of such tissues as hair and nails. Theoretically the balance of nitrogen is expressed as:

$$B = I - (U + F + S)$$

where B is nitrogen balance, I is nitrogen intake, U is urinary nitrogen, F is fecal nitrogen, and S is loss of nitrogen through the skin. The last factor most often is overlooked in the interpretation of nitrogen balance data, and the failure to take these skin losses into account has been cited by Mitchell (1949) as a source of error in nitrogen balance studies that may lead to underestimation of nitrogen requirement. Accordingly, Mitchell (ibid.) suggested a small retention of approximately 0.77 gm/m^2 as adequate to cover *adult growth.* In addition, he estimated losses in sweat to be on the average 0.36 gm nitrogen per day under minimal sweating conditions with markedly increased losses during periods of heavy sweating (Mitchell et al., 1949; Consolazio et al., 1963a). These figures are within the general range of more recent studies (Holmes, 1965; Calloway et al., 1971).

Wallace (1959) suggested that errors in nitrogen balance experiments arise through the manipulations involved in feeding and in collecting excreta and that these errors are more likely to lead to overestimation rather than underestimation of nitrogen requirements. A small quantity of the food intake is apt to be lost in feeding, and a small portion of the excreta invariably cannot be recovered. (These "unavoidable" losses have been estimated by

Calloway et al. (1971) to be of the order of 115 mg N/day.)

Clearly, there are other limitations to balance methodology. The balance of nitrogen intake against output is the sum of total body gains and losses. It is possible therefore, in a state of nitrogen equilibrium and possibly nitrogen retention, for some body tissues to be in positive balance while others are losing nitrogen. Such a state is implied by a study reported by Nasset (1954) in which hemoglobin levels fell in rats fed a low histidine ration, although nitrogen balance was satisfactory. Evidence suggests further that some cells may not be capable of synthesizing *all* of the nonessential amino acids and thus may require an extracellular source (Piez, 1958). Shifting of amino acids within the total metabolic pool and possible deprivation of individual cells cannot be ascertained by the gross evaluation of the nitrogen balance technique; this factor is probably the most significant of the limitations to balance methodology.

Factors Affecting Nitrogen Balance

Nitrogen balance, thus the interpretation of nitrogen balance data, represents the interaction of several factors. The most important of these are physiological state, body protein reserves, caloric value of the diet, and the essential amino acids and nonessential amino acid nitrogen provided by the diet.

Physiological State and Body Protein Reserves. Strong positive balances are characteristic of the growing child or the woman in late pregnancy when growth of fetal tissue is most rapid (see Calloway, 1974). Adults depleted of labile protein respond to nitrogen feeding in the same way, that is nitrogen retention and positive balance (Whipple, 1948). Furthermore, the extent of positive balance will reflect quantitatively the extent of protein depletion, and as protein reserves are replenished, the subject approaches equilibrium (see Allison, 1957).

Even when there is no marked depletion of body protein, nitrogen balance initially will reflect the previous intake. An initial negative balance in a subject placed on an experimental diet thus clearly indicates that previous dietary intake of nitrogen was higher than that of the experimental regimen, but it does not necessarily indicate that the experimental diet is inadequate. In the human, adjustment to changes in dietary protein occurs within a few days, as indicated by a relatively constant excretion of urinary nitrogen. Under this condition, data from balance studies over as few as three or four days following adjustment appear to be as valid as studies over longer periods of time (Bricker et al., 1949a). The length of the adjustment period, however, often varies from one study to another. Forbes (1973) has suggested that the period of time required for adjustment is likely longer than generally allowed and cites this possibility as a source of error in metabolic balance studies.

Energy Intake. The effect of energy intake on nitrogen balance has been widely studied (Benditt et al., 1948; Rosenthal and Allison, 1951; Oldham and Sheft, 1951; see Calloway, 1974). If dietary energy is reduced below a critical level then energy rather than nitrogen becomes the limiting factor in nitrogen balance. Adequate energy intake as evidenced by maintenance of body weight is essential to prevent loss of tissue protein. When energy intake is low, increased excretion of nitrogen in the urine reflects the inadequacy of energy rather than a lack of dietary nitrogen.

Essential Amino Acid and Total Nitrogen Intake. Assuming that energy and nutrient intakes are adequate, nitrogen balance is dependent primarily upon: (1) the amounts and proportions of essential amino acids provided by the diet and (2) the total nitrogen intake. The minimum protein requirement therefore is a variable estimate which is affected both by the level of essential amino acids and of nonessential amino acid nitrogen in the diet. The interrelationship between amino acid composition of the diet and total nitrogen intake, for example, was illustrated in early · studies by Sherman (1920), who showed that replacement of 10 percent of the protein content of a cereal diet by milk resulted in a decrease by almost 10 gm in the estimated protein requirement to maintain nitrogen equilibrium.

Data from studies by Bricker (1945) which are shown in Table 23.9 further illustrate the effect of amino acid composition, expressed here as biological value, upon total protein requirement. (For discussion of biological value, see next section.)

Because the protein requirement is a variable estimate depending upon the composition of protein fed, the ultimate problem in protein nutrition is the requirement for the essential amino acids and, further, the determination of minimum levels of nonessential amino acid nitrogen required at minimum intakes of the essential amino

Table 23.9   EFFECT OF PROTEIN QUALITY ON PROTEIN REQUIREMENT

Source of Protein	Biological Value	Protein Required for Equilibrium	Protein Required for Adult Growth
		gm protein/day	gm protein/day
Milk	74	22.4	33.9
White flour	41	38.7	58.6
Soy flour	65	23.4	36.7
Soy-white flour	55	27.4	42.8

From M. Bricker et al., *J. Nutr.*, 30: 269 (1945).

acids. Studies on amino acid requirements necessitate the use of partially purified diets in which synthetic amino acids are incorporated. When any one of the essential amino acids is excluded from the diet, subjects immediately go into negative nitrogen balance. The missing amino acid is then fed at graded levels until the criterion of adequacy is reached.

For a comprehensive review of studies related to protein requirements see Irwin and Hegsted (1971).

Amino acid requirements have been reported for infants (Holt et al., 1960) and for children (Nakagawa et al., 1964). Requirements of adult humans are based primarily on studies by Rose et al. (1955), Swendseid et al. (1956a, 1956b), and Leverton (1959). Adult requirements and the amino acid content of self-selected diets in this country are shown in Table 23.10. Requirements reported for men are, in general, larger than those obtained from studies with women; this finding may be due in part to the larger body size of men. However, differences in interpretation of minimum requirement from the studies on men and women suggest a more reasonable explanation for the higher levels reported for men. Rose defined minimum requirement as the smallest amount of an amino acid that would support a distinctly positive nitrogen balance and selected the value obtained from the subject with the highest requirement in the group studied as the proper figure to report. On the other hand, both Leverton and Swendseid defined minimum requirement as the amount of the amino acid that would keep a subject in nitrogen equilibrium or in a state in which the difference between

Table 23.10   MINIMUM REQUIREMENTS OF ADULTS FOR ESSENTIAL AMINO ACIDS AND AMINO ACID CONTENT OF SELF-SELECTED DIETS IN THE UNITED STATES

	Amino Acid Requirements		Amino Acids in Self-Selected Diets		
Amino Acid	Women[a]	Men[b]	Futrell[c]	Mertz[d]	Wharton[e]
	gm/day	gm/day	gm/day	gm/day	gm/day
Isoleucine	0.45	0.70	2.49-5.73	0.7-4.5	2.8-3.1
Leucine	0.62	1.10	3.28-7.35	1.3-7.8	4.4-4.9
Lysine	0.50	0.80	1.7-8.6	1.3-5.6	3.5-4.0
Methionine Cystine	0.55	1.10	0.90-2.54	0.7-2.7	0.9-1.0
Phenylalanine Tyrosine	1.12	1.10	1.98-4.88	0.9-3.77	2.5-2.7
Threonine	0.31	0.50	1.68-3.44	0.9-3.8	2.6-2.9
Tryptophan	0.16	0.25	0.5-1.28	—	0.4-0.5
Valine	0.65	0.80	2.85-5.39	0.8-4.9	3.1-3.4

[a] Leverton, *Protein and Amino Acid Nutrition* (1959).
[b] Rose, *J. Biol. Chem.*, 217: 997 (1955).
[c] Futrell et al., *J. Nutr.*, 46: 299 (1952)
[d] Mertz et al., *J. Nutr.*, 46: 313 (1952).
[e] Wharton et al., *J. Amer. Diet. Ass.*, 29: 573 (1953).

intake and output is no more than ±5 percent. Results reported from these two studies are similar. The essential amino acid content of self-selected diets in this country (Table 23.10) are in general well above the minimum requirements.

A recent study (Kopple and Swendseid, 1973) indicates that histidine may be an essential amino acid for the human adult. Subjects maintained on 40 gm of protein were in negative balance after 25 days on a diet deficient in histidine. When histidine was added subjects went into positive balance and remained so for at least 25 days. These results are particularly interesting because histidine has been thought previously to be nonessential for the human adult. In addition, the experimental period in this study was longer than often used in nitrogen balance studies and may account for the results obtained. Finally, the results of this study suggest that a reevaluation of short term studies might be in order.

Studies on amino acid requirements of young women on low nitrogen intakes suggested to Fisher et al. (1965, 1971) that essential amino acid requirements vary according to the level of nitrogen in the diet. As shown in Table 23.11, essential amino acid levels

Table 23.11   ESSENTIAL AMINO ACID REQUIREMENTS OF YOUNG WOMEN

	Requirements			
	Leverton and Swendseid[a]		Fisher[b]	
Essential Amino Acid	Mg Amino Acid/Day	Mg N/Day	Mg Amino Acid/day	Mg N/Day
Lysine	500	96	50	10
Tryptophan	160	22	50	7
Phenylalanine + tyrosine	1120	57	400	34
Threonine	310	36	200	24
Methionine + cystine	550	33	150	14
Leucine	620	66	150	16
Isoleucine	450	48	100	11
Valine	650	78	200	24
	3710	436	1300	140

Adapted from H. Fisher, *J. Agric. Food Chem.*, 22: 174 (1974).
[a]Diet contains approximately 9 gm nitrogen.
[b]Diet contains approximately 5 gm nitrogen.

necessary to maintain young women in nitrogen equilibrium on a diet containing 5 gm of nitrogen were found to be considerably lower than those reported for young women fed approximately 9 gm of nitrogen. These data raise interesting questions concerning requirements for essential amino acids and protein particularly in view of the projected world shortage of protein.

The importance of nonessential amino acid nitrogen and other forms of nitrogen (nonspecific nitrogen) on the adequacy of dietary protein and on essential amino acid requirements has more recently been appreciated (see Kies, 1974). Snyderman et al. (1962) found that when milk protein was reduced until weight gain and nitrogen retention in infants were adversely affected, both weight gain and nitrogen retention could be restored to normal by administration of nonessential nitrogen in the form of glycine or urea, that is, a nonessential amino acid or a nonprotein source of nitrogen. Scrimshaw et al. (1966) studied the effect of varying levels of egg protein diluted to a constant nitrogen intake with glycine and diammonium citrate. According to their results, the minimum ratio of grams of essential amino acids per gram of total nitrogen (E/T_N) for diets approximating the amino acid pattern in whole egg apparently lies between 1.85 and 2.16; at this level, essential amino acids account for 21 to 25 percent of the total dietary nitrogen. These findings suggest that the relative proportions of essential and nonessential amino acids in the diet are more important than has been supposed.

Plasma Amino Acids. The levels of plasma amino acids and in particular the ratio of essential to nonessential amino acids has been used as a means of evaluating response to low protein or low essential amino acid diets. Swendseid et al. (1963) reported that essential amino acids in plasma were decreased in subjects maintained on a low protein diet, whereas the amount of nonessential amino acids was not affected. Whitehead and Dean (1964), among others, have utilized the ratio of plasma nonessential to essential amino acids as a means of evaluating response to treatment of children suffering from protein-calorie malnutrition. In protein-calorie malnutrition the ratio is high (usually above 2) and gradually decreases as the clinical condition of the child improves under dietary treatment. The decreased ratio is due primarily to an increase in essential amino acid levels; nonessential amino acids remain unchanged. Similar changes in plasma amino acid levels were reported by Scrimshaw et al. (1966) when experimental subjects were fed diets containing decreasing levels of egg protein.

More recently, the level of amino acids in plasma has emerged as a means for determining dietary amino acid requirements. Studies in rats (McLaughlan and Illman, 1967) and pigs (Mitchell et al., 1968) indicated that the limiting amino acid accumulated in plasma only when the dietary requirement had been exceeded. Results obtained by this method were in good agreement with those obtained from the growth method in young animals. In adult human males, Young et al. (1971) found the tryptophan requirement to be 3 mg/kg of body weight using the plasma tryptophan level as criterion as compared with 2 to 2.6 mg/kg of body weight by the nitrogen balance technique. Because skin and sweat losses were not taken into consideration in determining nitrogen balance, it is likely that the values obtained by the two methods are closer than the figures imply. This method has been found to be satisfactory for determining the requirement for valine (Young et al., 1972) and threonine (Tontisirin et al., 1974). The plasma response to threonine, however, was not as pronounced as was observed for tryptophan.

The determination of plasma amino acid levels is considerably more convenient (to investigators and experimental subjects) than the nitrogen balance technique. It may be that the plasma amino acid method also is more accurate.

Evaluation of Protein Quality

The quality of a protein is dependent upon its amino acid composition. Biological evaluation is the preferred method for determination of protein quality since it is the ability of a protein to support growth and maintenance, that is, cellular synthesis, that determines its ultimate value. Methods for evaluation of protein quality are therefore based on the retention of nitrogen in the body. Some methods, for example those utilizing nitrogen balance or growth as criteria of nitrogen retention, can be applied to studies with human subjects. The large majority of reports in the literature, however, are of studies performed with experimental animals and that sometimes utilize techniques, such as carcass analysis, that obviously are not suitable for studies with humans.

Amino Acid Score (Chemical Score). A simple nonbiological device for estimating protein quality is called the amino acid score or chemical score. This method involves a comparison of the amino acid composition of a test food with that of a high quality protein such as egg or milk or, as is now preferred, to an amino acid reference pattern (FAO/WHO, 1973) shown in Table 23.12. The score is calculated from the following equation:

$$\text{Amino acid score} = \frac{\text{mg of amino acid in 1 gm of test protein}}{\text{mg of amino acid in 1 gm of reference pattern}} \times 100$$

The lowest score for any of the essential amino acids designates the "limiting amino acid" and gives a rough estimate of the protein quality of the food. In practice, only scores for lysine, methionine + cystine, and tryptophan need be calculated since one of these amino

Table 23.12 PROVISIONAL AMINO ACID SCORING PATTERN

Amino Acid	Suggested Level	
	Mg per Gm Protein	Mg per Gm Nitrogen
Isoleucine	40	250
Leucine	70	440
Lysine	55	340
Methionine + cystine	35	220
Phenylalanine + tyrosine	60	380
Threonine	40	250
Tryptophan	10	60
Valine	50	310
Total	360	2250

From FAO/WHO Energy requirements and protein requirements, *WHO Tech. Rep. Ser.* No. 522 (1973), p. 63.

acids is usually limiting in most common foods. Although a rather crude instrument for evaluating protein quality, the amino acid score often agrees well with the results of biological evaluation.

Protein Efficiency Ratio (PER). Protein efficiency ratio is a measure of weight gain of a growing animal divided by protein intake:

$$PER = \frac{\text{weight gain (gm)}}{\text{protein intake (gm)}}$$

The PER was used as early as 1917 by Osborne and Mendel in their studies establishing differences in protein quality (Osborne et al., 1919). It has most often been applied to studies on laboratory rats, but it is also applicable to studies with human infants. It is the simplest method for evaluating protein quality since it requires only an accurate measure of dietary intake and weight gain. However, the method requires strict adherence to certain conditions: the calorie intake must be adequate and the protein must be fed at an adequate but not excessive level since at high levels of dietary protein, weight gain does not increase proportionately with protein intake.

The greatest source of error in the PER method lies in the use of weight gain *per se* as sole criterion of protein value. Weight gain cannot be assumed to represent proportional gain in body protein under all conditions. Methods that precisely define protein retention therefore are likely to yield more consistently accurate results. In terms of speed of operation and expense, however, the PER method is advantageous.

Biological Value (BV). Biological value is a measure of nitrogen retained for growth or maintenance and is expressed as nitrogen retained divided by nitrogen absorbed (Mitchell, 1923). It is determined by nitrogen balance and is applicable to humans as well as laboratory animals. In a quantitative sense, BV may be expressed more explicitly as:

$$BV = \frac{I - (F - F_0) - (U - U_0)}{I - (F - F_0)}$$

where I is nitrogen intake, U is urinary nitrogen, F is fecal nitrogen and U_0 and F_0 are urinary and fecal nitrogen excreted when subjects are maintained on a nitrogen-free or nearly nitrogen-free diet. BV calculated from this equation accounts for metabolic (or endogenous) nitrogen losses. If the correction is not made, that is, if U_0 and F_0 are not in the equation, BV obtained is designated *apparent biological value.* The practice of ignoring metabolic nitrogen is not uncommon, so many values for BV represent apparent biological value of protein.

Nitrogen Balance Index. Nitrogen balance index is essentially the same as biological value (Allison, 1955). It may be determined from the slope of the line when nitrogen balance is plotted against absorbed nitrogen. More simply, nitrogen balance index may be calculated from the following equation:

$$\text{Nitrogen balance index} = \frac{B - B_0}{A}$$

where B is nitrogen balance; B_0 is nitrogen balance when nitrogen intake is zero; and A is absorbed nitrogen. Since B_0 represents metabolic nitrogen, the nitrogen balance index is a measure of dietary nitrogen retained. This method is not used as often as are some other measures of protein quality.

Net Protein Utilization (NPU). Quantitatively, NPU is represented by a simple formula: N retained/N intake. The NPU thus is equivalent to biological value x digestibility and is a measure both of the digestibility of food protein and the biological value of the amino acid mixture absorbed from food.

NPU represents the proportion of *food* nitrogen retained, whereas both BV and nitrogen balance index represent the proportion of *absorbed* nitrogen retained. NPU therefore is related directly to dietary intake of nitrogen. Nitrogen retention may be measured by nitrogen balance studies (Bender and Miller, 1953) or by direct analysis of the animal body (Miller and Bender, 1955). The latter method is preferred. In any case, the method requires two groups of experimental animals equivalent in weight and age. One group is fed the test protein and the other is fed a protein-free diet. At the end of the feeding period, carcasses are analyzed for water from which nitrogen content can be calculated (see Chapter 22). The formula for calculating NPU is as follows:

$$NPU = \frac{\text{Body N of test group} - \text{body N of nonprotein group} + \text{N consumed by nonprotein group}}{\text{N consumed by test group}}$$

Other terms may be used to define NPU. NPU standardized (NPU_{st}) refers to determinations of NPU when proteins are fed at minimum requirement or below. NPU operative (NPU_{op}) refers to NPU determined under any other conditions.

The net dietary protein value (NDpV) is a variation of NPU proposed by Platt and Miller (1959) and is determined by multiplying dietary protein concentration by NPU obtained. NDpV may be written with the percentage level of dietary protein as subscript to define more clearly the calculated value. For example, when protein is fed at an 8 percent level of the diet, NDpV may be written NPU_8.

Net Dietary Protein Calories Percent (NDpCal %). NDpCal % relates protein quality to energy intake (Platt et al., 1961). This method appears to be especially useful in evaluation of human diets in which the relation of protein to total calories may vary markedly. Thus dietary protein is expressed as percent of total calories rather than as percent of total weight.

Quantitatively, NDpCal % is obtained by the following formula:

$$NDpCal \% = \frac{\text{protein calories}}{\text{total caloric intake}} \times 100 \times NPU_{op}$$

According to calculated values from protein of highest quality, either

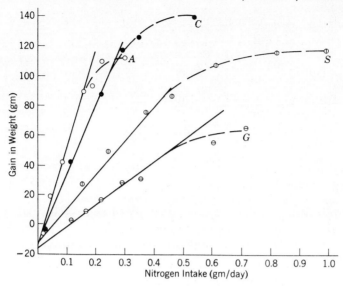

Fig. 23.11 Relationship between weight gain and nitrogen intake. Broken lines drawn by inspection. Solid lines are the regression lines calculated through the points that appear to be in the linear range. *A* = albumin; *C* = casein; *S* = soy protein; *G* = gluten. [From D. M. Hegsted and Y. Chang, *J. Nutr.*, 85: 159 (1965).]

whole egg or human milk, a diet that provides less than 5 percent of calories in the form of available protein will not meet protein needs of the human adult. For children, at least 8 percent is required (see FAO, Protein Requirements, 1965).

Slope-Ratio Assay.   The slope-ratio assay has been used to determine protein quality in growing rats (Hegsted and Chang, 1965; 1965a) and has been applied to adult rats (Said and Hegsted, 1969). The method is essentially an application of standard bioassay procedure and involves feeding proteins at varying levels of intake including a protein-free diet. Growth is used as measure of response to dietary protein. Weight gain or loss is plotted against nitrogen intake, and the data fitted to regression lines. The value of the protein is proportional to the slope of the regression line relating dose and response. Relative potency of the test protein is determined by comparison of its slope with that of a high quality standard protein such as albumin or lactalbumin, which is assigned a potency of 100 (see Fig. 23.11 and Table 23.13).

Table   23.13   RELATIVE   POTENCY   OF   PROTEINS   BY   THE SLOPE-RATIO ASSAY[a]

Protein	Slope	Relative Potency
Albumin	656	100
Casein	460	70.0
Soy protein	221	33.7
Gluten	143	21.8

From D. M. Hegsted and Y. Chang, *J. Nutr.*, 85: 159 (1965).
[a] Regression lines shown in Fig. 23.11.

In adult animals, maintenance of body nitrogen (calculated from body water) is the criterion of response to dietary nitrogen. Protein evaluations obtained with adult animals do not always agree with those obtained with growing animals since the relative amino acid requirements for growth and maintenance are different.

CALCIUM REQUIREMENTS

The greatest loss of dietary calcium occurs through the feces rather than urine and represents calcium that is not absorbed from the intestinal lumen and that secreted into the lumen in intestinal juices. Calcium absorption varies from roughly 15 percent to 35 percent or more. Outhouse et al. (1941) reported an average absorption of 24 percent for seven adults maintained on intakes ranging from 231 to 575 mg/day. A similar average absorption, 21 percent, was reported by Bricker et al. (1949b) for adult subjects on diets containing 206 to 752 mg calcium. Steggerda and Mitchell (1946) estimated average absorption to be about 30 percent.

Absorption of calcium and ability to maintain equilibrium on low calcium intakes varies with the previous intake of the experimental subject and the length of the experimental period. For example, Hegsted et al. (1952) found that 9 of 10 men required less than 400 mg to maintain calcium equilibrium; the subjects were inmates in a Peruvian prison and presumably had consumed a diet low in calcium for many years. Similarly, Malm (1958) in a study of men in Oslo found the calcium requirement for equilibrium to be less than 500 mg for 21 of 26 subjects. Subjects maintained for several months on approximately 450 mg/day after consuming about 950 mg for several months absorbed about 45 percent of the intake, compared with 25 percent on the higher intake. With the increase in percentage absorption, however, the total amount of calcium absorbed was approximately the same for both levels of intake.

It is significant that some subjects in the Malm study never adjusted to low intakes of calcium over a period of several months. Other studies also indicate that in addition to the problem of adaptation to calcium intake, individual variation in calcium balance is great. In a study of 12 young college women consuming self-chosen diets containing 1000 to 1050 mg calcium, which presumably represented customary intake, McKay et al. (1942) reported balances ranging from -394 to +250 mg. Meyer et al. (1955) reported balances ranging from -242 to +288 for 8 young college women on controlled intakes of 725 mg calcium. The wide range of calcium intakes reported to maintain equilibrium is evident from reviews of the literature summarized by Sherman (1920), Mitchell and Curzon (1939), and Leitch and Aitken (1959).

It would seem that calcium balance data from studies with children would be simpler to interpret since the need for calcium to support normal skeletal development is obviously high and should result in calcium retention. However, retention of dietary calcium varies considerably in children without demonstrable differences in either growth response or skeletal development. The infant fed cow's milk formula, for example, retains about 50 percent more calcium than the breast fed infant but shows no advantage for having done so. Leitch and Aitken (1959) estimated retention of calcium necessary for skeletal growth to be between 75 and 150 mg/day between the first and tenth years of life and about 400 mg/day during the maximal pubertal growth spurt; these retentions could be effected with intakes ranging from 600 mg to 1000 mg or more.

Recent evidence indicates that calcium retention is markedly affected by the level of protein in the diet (Johnson et al., 1970; Walker and Linkswiler, 1972; Anand and Linkswiler, 1974). This effect is observed even when the source of nitrogen is pure L-amino acids (Margen et al., 1974). In the studies by Linkswiler and associates, adult males maintained on a low protein diet (47 gm) retained calcium when the diet contained as little as 500 mg of calcium whereas those fed 97 gm of protein retained calcium only

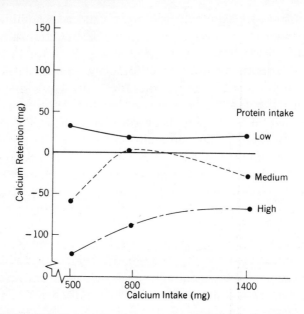

Fig. 23.12 Calcium retention at three levels of calcium and three levels of protein intake; ——— = low protein; ---- = medium protein and —·—·— = high protein. [From H. M. Linkswiler, *Trans. N. Y. Acad. Sci.* (Series II), 36: 333 (1974).]

when dietary calcium was 800 mg or more (Fig. 23.12). On a diet containing 142 gm of protein only 3 out of 15 subjects retained calcium on levels of 1400 mg of calcium; none were in balance at lower levels of calcium intake. Calcium absorption was increased somewhat at higher protein intakes, but this advantage was offset by markedly increased excretion of calcium in the urine. The reason for these findings is not clear. Linkswiler (1974) cites an hypothesis proposed by Wachman and Bernstein (1968) that dissolution of bone is greater in individuals who consume a diet high in acid ash (such as a high protein diet). Certainly the urinary excretion of calcium observed in these studies was of a magnitude that would indicate significant losses from bone. One wonders, however, if the acid-forming property of the diet is perhaps a too simplistic answer to this problem.

The influence of dietary protein on calcium retention could account, in part, for variations in estimated requirement from various studies. The problem of calcium requirements, however, is complicated by the lack of clinical evidence of calcium deficiency.

There is no conclusive evidence that low calcium intakes significantly reduce growth rate or result in altered structure or composition of bone (Walker, 1954; Walker and Arvidsson, 1954; A.M.A. Council of Foods and Nutrition, 1963). In adults, low calcium intakes have been implicated in the etiology of senile osteoporosis (Whedon, 1959; Nordin, 1961, 1962). Other investigators (Garn et al., 1967; Newton-John and Morgan, 1967) view osteoporosis as a physiological consequence of aging. It seems likely that neither view is entirely accurate. Ellis et al. (1972) reported the incidence of osteoporosis to be higher among omnivores than among vegetarians. The recent finding that high protein diets reduce calcium retention could possibly account for the low incidence of osteoporosis among vegetarians and the variable reports on the relation of calcium intake to osteoporotic disease. This, of course, is only speculation.

Coulston and Lutwak (1972) have presented evidence suggesting that dietary calcium deficiency results in periodontal disease. This finding is interesting and, if confirmed, will provide the first evidence of calcium deficiency in man.

Until more precise measurements are devised for determining calcium requirements, and until the significance and limitation of physiological adaptation are fully evaluated, the problem of calcium requirements will continue to be debated as it is presently, on the basis of point of view rather than upon meaningful experimental evidence.

IRON REQUIREMENTS

As discussed in Chapter 6, iron is poorly absorbed from the intestinal lumen, but once absorbed very little is excreted via the kidneys. The inability of the intestinal mucosa to absorb more than 10 to 20 percent of the total dietary intake places the dietary requirement for iron far above the actual metabolic requirement. However, the ability of the body to conserve iron tenaciously by reusing iron from hemoglobin degradation results in a much lower dietary requirement than could be possible if iron so released were excreted in the urine. Urinary loss of iron is almost negligible (Dubach et al., 1955).

The amount of iron lost in sweat is variable and ill-defined and includes iron in sloughed off epithelial cells (Mitchell and Edman, 1962). Fecal loss includes iron contained in desquamated intestinal mucosal cells and minute amounts in intestinal secretions as well as the dietary iron that never enters the mucosal cell. The former are true losses from the body but obviously are difficult to differentiate from unabsorbed iron by the usual balance technique. Radioisotope studies indicate that the total body turnover of iron including losses through the gastrointestinal and urinary tracts, and skin amount to approximately 14 μg/kg of body weight per day (Finch, 1959; Green et al., 1968). This loss amounts to a physiological requirement of about 0.9 mg/day for a 69 kg man and 0.8 mg/day for a nonmenstruating woman weighing 55 kg.

In women of child-bearing age, further losses occur in the menses. Menstrual blood losses vary considerably. In a study on a small group of women, Frenchman and Johnston (1949) reported losses to amount to from 0.8 to 2.6 mg/day when averaged for a monthly period. In a study with a larger number of women, Hallberg et al. (1966) found menstrual losses to be less than 1.4 mg/day for all but 10 percent of normal women and less than 2.0 mg/day for all but 5 percent.

In pregnant women additional iron is required for expansion of the red cell mass, for deposition in the fetus and placenta, and to cover the blood loss at delivery. These needs are compensated in part by the cessation of menstruation. In an early study by Coons (1932) an average positive balance of 3.2 mg was observed in 9 pregnant women who were consuming on the average 14.7 mg of iron daily. These data were later confirmed by radioisotope studies (Hahn et al., 1951) and shown to be caused by increased absorption in late pregnancy as well as conservation of iron normally lost through the menses. Further confirmation of the increased absorptive capacity during pregnancy has been provided by the studies of Apte and Lyengar (1969). Hahn et al. (1951) also reported percentage uptakes similar to the positive balance reported by Coons in 1932 when pregnant women were given a single dose of radioactive iron in amounts ranging from 1.8 to 9.0 mg. At 18 mg intakes, however, percentage uptake decreased. The latter finding is not unexpected as it is well known that therapeutic doses of iron are absorbed less efficiently than physiological doses. Despite relatively poor absorption, however, the absolute amount of iron absorbed from a therapeutic dose would be higher than that from a lower intake (Smith and Pannacciulli, 1958).

The chemical balance method measures the overall retention or loss of iron from the body and has been useful in determining absorption from various foods (Schlaphoff and Johnston, 1949). The use of radioactive isotopes of iron, however, has all but replaced the older technique in studies of iron metabolism. Radioisotope studies permit more definitive studies of the fate of dietary iron; yet it is surprising that the chemical balance technique and radioisotope technique have yielded similar estimates of the average dietary requirement for iron. For example, Leverton and Marsh (1942) in early balance studies found an average of 15.9 mg of iron to be necessary for equilibrium in young women; 12.9 mg was adequate for 87 percent of their subjects. This figure is not markedly different than that obtained from estimated losses of iron from the body and radioisotope studies on availability of iron (Layrisse et al., 1968; Cook et al., 1972; see Chapter 6).

In practical terms, the dietary requirement for iron depends largely on the ability to absorb iron, which depends on the character of the diet. The establishment of a recommendation for a population group, therefore, will be influenced by usual diets consumed (see Chapter 25). Because of wide individual variability, dietary allowances must be established with the view of reducing the risk of deficiency in vulnerable groups (see Beaton, 1972).

SUMMARY

Many of the techniques for determining nutrient requirements have not changed for many years. The limitations of these methods are now more readily recognized and, indeed, new interpretations have on occasion been applied to old data. As new and more refined techniques emerge, knowledge of human requirements will be refined both in terms of the individual nutrient and the effect of nutrient interrelationships upon dietary requirements. These data are necessary to establish rational allowances for normal population groups and may be critical in planning dietaries for therapeutic purposes.

chapter 24

determination of nutrient needs: vitamins

1. Clinical Evaluation
2. Urinary Excretion
3. Blood Level
4. Urinary Excretion and Blood Level Following a Test Dose

5. Enzyme Activity and Other Related Tests
6. Conclusion

Methods for determination of vitamin requirements are of necessity different from those applicable to energy, protein, and minerals. Techniques for determining vitamin needs also have changed more over the years than those for the other nutrients and continue to change. Yet many of the classic studies conducted 30 years ago remain valid and indeed form the basis for the recommended dietary allowances and other standards. Confirmation of early data by new techniques, however, has increased confidence in our knowledge of human vitamin requirements and removed some of the "guess work" from the margin of safety allowed in most dietary standards. Perhaps more important, new techniques have permitted the early and accurate detection of vitamin deficiency states.

The vitamins are different chemically, and they behave differently in the metabolism of living organisms. Consequently no single method for the assessment of vitamin requirements is equally satisfactory for all vitamins. In general, techniques that have been used to evaluate response to controlled dietary intake may be grouped into 5 categories:

1. Clinical evaluation.
2. Urinary excretion.
3. Blood level.
4. Urinary excretion and blood level following a test dose of vitamin.
5. Enzyme activity and/or other biochemical or histochemical tests related to vitamin function.

In addition to differences in response among the vitamins, these techniques do not necessarily yield comparable data for any one vitamin, because, in effect, they measure different states of vitamin nutriture. Assuming that a well-nourished, healthy person is placed on a diet deficient in a single vitamin, the sequence of the developing deficiency is:

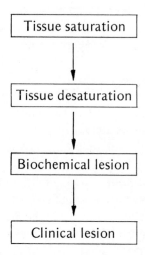

Theoretically, the five general methods for assessment of vitamin requirements should correlate with each level of vitamin status represented in the diagram; life would be simpler for the experimental nutritionist if this were so. In practice, as will be seen later, there is considerable variability and overlapping. In other words, some techniques for assessing vitamin requirements are more sensitive measurements for some vitamins than for others.

Tissue saturation applies to an optimal state of nutrition when a significant increase in tissue concentration of vitamin cannot be accomplished by an increase in dietary intake. The term is meaningful when applied to the water-soluble vitamins, but has little significance in relation to the fat-soluble vitamins. Water-soluble vitamins are excreted in the urine and do not accumulate in the body to any great degree. Although the upper limit varies, for example, 100 mg or less for thiamin and 4 to 5 gm for ascorbic acid, there is general agreement that beyond a certain point further loading of the body with water-soluble vitamins enriches the urine but not the body. Under this condition, the tissues are said to be saturated.

On the other hand, fat-soluble vitamins are not readily excreted in the urine and apparently can be stored to an unlimited degree in certain tissues. Since there is no apparent upper limit of accretion for these vitamins, there is no reasonable level that could be described as tissue saturation. Depletion of the body through inadequate intake of fat-soluble vitamins therefore is a long term process; the length of time required for depletion depends primarily upon the extent of tissue stores. Determination of dietary requirements for the fat-soluble vitamins thus is considerably more difficult than for the water-soluble vitamins and is limited to methods 1, 3, and 5 listed above. In addition, blood levels of fat-soluble vitamins are more difficult to interpret; a high level may merely represent mobilization from tissue stores as a result of transient inadequate dietary intake. Low levels may not be reached for months on an apparently low dietary level of vitamin when tissue stores initially are high.

Statements of minimum requirements therefore require definition of the criterion used for evaluation. The minimum requirement to prevent deficiency disease often is well below the requirement to support blood levels and/or urinary excretion. If we theorize that tissue saturation represents what is often called an optimal state of nutrition, the pathway leading to frank clinical lesions requires first that the tissues become depleted of their vitamin supply. As depletion proceeds, aberrations in cellular function result since vitamins are required chiefly as coenzymes for the biochemical reactions of cell metabolism. The appearance of clinical lesions is the final manifestation of diminishing cellular supply of a needed nutrient but does not imply that all cells are uniformly depleted. The real challenge to the experimental nutritionist is to ascertain the *order of cellular depletion*, for herein may lie the answer to the truly puzzling question, "What is minimum requirement?"

The nutritive state between tissue saturation and appearance of deficiency symptoms is an ambiguous area and is perhaps the most difficult state to evaluate. Clearly, a rather wide range of dietary intakes will support apparent health, yet they will not allow for tissue saturation. Measurement of urinary excretion and blood levels of vitamins or related metabolites in subjects maintained on varying vitamin intakes are attempts to evaluate better this gray area of nutrition. The so-called fitness tests also have occasionally been used to determine the ability of human subjects to function properly as a *total organism;* these include such criteria as endurance, reflex action, and psychological response.

CLINICAL EVALUATION

The chief significance of clinical evaluation is to establish the clinical course of vitamin deficiency in subjects maintained on carefully controlled vitamin intakes and thus to determine dietary levels that will prevent physical deterioration. Such studies properly should be carried on over a period of several months, since intakes that appear adequate for a short period may result in deficiency symptoms over longer periods of time as tissue supplies of vitamin are gradually depleted. Especially significant is the identification of early symptoms of deficiency that appear before the onset of the frank disease syndrome. These early physical or mental changes correlated with analyses of blood or urine provide the basis for biochemical evaluation of nutritional status.

Table 24.1 indicates some symptoms that have been observed in vitamin deficiency states. Known minimum dietary levels that will prevent clinical symptoms are also listed. In the case of vitamin B_6 and vitamin E where requirement depends on intake of protein and PUFA respectively, the minimum listed is that obtained at low levels of the interrelated nutrient.

Table 24.1 SOME CLINICAL EVIDENCES OF DEFICIENCY OF CERTAIN VITAMINS

Vitamin	Symptoms	References
Thiamin (below 0.2-0.3 mg/1000 kcal)	Anorexia Nausea with vomiting Constipation Calf muscle tenderness Weakness Irritability Depression Lowered blood pressure	Williams et al. (1942) Elsom et al. (1942) Najjar and Holt (1943) Foltz (1944) Brozek (1957) Horwitt et al. (1948)
Riboflavin (below 0.6 mg/day)	Cheilosis Angular stomatitis Seborrheic dermatitis (particularly nasolabial)	Horwitt et al. (1948) Hills et al. (1951)
Nicotinic acid (below 4.4 mg/1000 kcal)	Dermatitis Glossitis Stomatitis Diarrhea Proctitis and vaginitis Mental depression, anxiety	Goldsmith (1956)
Ascorbic acid (below 10 mg/day)	Hyperkeratotic papules Petechiae Perifolliculosis Swollen, spongy gums Poor wound healing Fatigue Coiled hair Muscular aches Swollen joints Edema	Crandon et al. (1940) Peters et al. (1948) Hodges et al. (1971)
Vitamin B_6 (below 1.25 mg/day)	Seborrheic dermatitis Glossitis, stomatitis, cheilosis Depression Confusion Abnormal electro-encephalogram Convulsions	Mueller and Vilter (1950) Coursin (1954) Baker et al. (1964)

Table 24.1 Continued

Folacin (below 50 μg/day)	Weakness, tiredness Dyspnea Sore tongue Irritability and forget-fullness Diarrhea Headache Palpitation	Herbert (1968)
Vitamin B$_{12}$ (below 0.5 μg/day)	Weakness, tiredness Sore tongue Paresthesia Constipation Headache Palpitation Macrocytic anemia Neurological damage	Herbert (1968)
Vitamin A (below 23-40 IU/kg)	Poor dark adaptation White papules Abnormal electro-retinogram Acne Follicular hyperkeratosis Abnormalities of balance, taste, and smell	Booher et al. (1939) Hume and Krebs (1949) Hodges and Kolder (1971)
Vitamin E (below 3 mg/day)	Edema (infants) Anemia Increased erythrocyte hemolysis	Ritchie et al. (1968) Horwitt et al. (1963)

Some of the reported symptoms are highly subjective, particularly those associated with thiamin deficiency. Apprehension, anxiety, and other mental changes are difficult to evaluate. Brozek (1957) used the Minnesota Multiphasic Personality Test for the evaluation of psychological changes in his subjects, but he was not certain that the changes observed were due entirely to effects of the deficiency or to possible negative response to the experimental regimen. Daum et al. (1949) found work output as measured by both performance on a stationary bicycle and a standardized measure of reflex action to be more sensitive determinants of thiamin status than the appearance of symptoms, which in early thiamin deficiency are almost always of a subjective nature. Keys et al. (1943) used several tests of "fitness" for the evaluation of response to varying levels of thiamin.

More recently Kinsman and Hood (1971) have reported behavioral changes in experimental ascorbic acid deficiency as determined by a battery of personality and psychomotor tests including the Minnesota Multiphasic Personality Test. Subjects deprived of ascorbic acid scored high in the areas of hypochondriasis, depression, and hysteria, the so-called "neurotic triad." The results are similar to those reported in thiamin deficiency and in semistarvation (Keys et al., 1950). Because high and low levels of the vitamin were fed at different times within the study period and psychological changes were noted only during periods of low ascorbic acid intake, these workers were able to eliminate reaction to the monotony of the experimental diet as a contributing factor. In the ascorbic acid-deficient subjects personality changes preceded impaired function in tests of physical fitness; the latter appeared to be due to muscular and joint pains resulting from lack of the vitamin.

For some vitamins, the minimum requirement has been determined from the amount of the vitamin necessary to cure deficiency symptoms. Such is the case for folacin and vitamin B_{12}. A minimum of 50 μg/day of crystalline pteroylglutamic acid has been shown to bring about a complete remission of hematologic symptoms in patients with uncomplicated folacin deficiency (Herbert, 1968). Similarly as little as 0.1 μg/day of vitamin B_{12} given intramuscularly to patients with pernicious anemia produced a reticulocyte and red cell response and a gradual return of serum vitamin B_{12} levels to normal. At least 0.5 μg/day, however, was required for complete remission of hematologic and neurologic symptoms (Herbert, 1968).

Curative doses of retinol for symptoms of vitamin A deficiency also have been reported (Hodges and Kolder, 1971) and are of especial interest because so little work has been done on the requirement for vitamin A. As can be seen in Table 24.2, the curative dose varies considerably according to the deficiency symptom, from as little as 75 μg of retinol for correcting impaired dark adaptation to 600 μg for curing cutaneous lesions including follicular hyperkeratosis and acne. Extrapolating on the basis of pure retinol these levels are equivalent to 250 to 1998 IU. In terms of human dietaries con-

Table 24.2 APPROXIMATE DAILY DOSE OF RETINOL OR BETA-CAROTENE REQUIRED TO CORRECT CLINICAL DEFECTS

	Clinical Defect	Dose in Micrograms	
I	Impaired dark adaptation	<75	Retinol
		≥ 150	Beta-carotene
II	Abnormal ERG	≥ 150	Retinol
		≥ 300	Beta-carotene
III	Abnormalities of balance,	≥ 300	Retinol
	taste, smell	≥ 600	Beta-carotene
IV	Cutaneous lesions	≥ 600	Retinol
	Follicular hyperkeratosis	≥ 1200	Beta-carotene
	Acne		

From R. E. Hodges and H. Kolder in Summary of proceedings, Workshop on biochemical and clinical criteria for determining human vitamin A nutriture, Food and Nutrition Board, National Academy of Sciences, Washington, D.C., (1971), pp. 10-16.

taining both preformed vitamin A and carotene, the amounts are approximately 375 to 3000 IU. See Chapter 25 for further discussion of retinol equivalents and IU.

URINARY EXCRETION

Whereas clinical evaluation provides an estimate of minimum requirements to prevent deficiency symptoms, biochemical lesions clearly must precede physical manifestation of deficiency. Measurement of urinary excretion of vitamins is a commonly used method for determination of vitamin status. Carefully controlled studies in which dietary intake was correlated with urinary excretion and appearance or absence of deficiency symptoms have formed the basis for evaluation of dietary intakes compatible with a "desirable" state of nutrition.

Urinary excretion levels may be interpreted as rough estimates of cellular function. Theoretically, as intake decreases excretion in the urine decreases; therefore at high levels of intake, increasingly larger amounts of vitamin should be excreted in the urine. Both the absolute amount of vitamin excreted in the urine and the percentage of the intake excreted increase as the dietary intakes increase. For most water-soluble vitamins the relationship between intake and excretion is fairly linear over certain ranges of intake. For example, the data in Table 24.3, taken from a report by Horwitt et al. (1950), demonstrate the effect of varying levels of riboflavin intake on excretion of the vitamin.

Table 24.3   EFFECT OF RIBOFLAVIN INTAKE ON URINARY EXCRETION

No. of Subjects	Riboflavin Intake (mg)	Riboflavin Excretion in 24 Hours	
		Amount (μg)	Percent of Intake (%)
15	0.55	37	6.7
11	0.75	73	9.7
12	0.85	76	8.9
28	1.1	97	8.8
39	1.6	434	26.5
12	2.15	714	33.2
13	2.55	849	33.3
13	3.55	1714	48.3

From M. K. Horwitt et al., *J. Nutr.*, 41: 247 (1950).

Symptoms of ariboflavinosis, angular stomatitis, and seborrheic-type dermal lesions appeared in subjects maintained on 0.55 mg riboflavin/day before the fourth month of experiment, but only one of the subjects receiving 0.75 and 0.85 mg/day for as long as two years showed any outward signs of deficiency. Since riboflavin excretion increased markedly when intake was 1.6 mg as compared to 1.1 mg, these investigators concluded that tissue saturation could be reached at some point between 1.1 and 1.6 mg/day.

It would be fallacious to assume that urinary excretions of all water-soluble vitamins correlate in the same manner with dietary intake or reflect dietary changes within comparable periods of time. However, certain similarities exist. Thiamin excretion also correlates with dietary intake between intakes of 0.5 and 2.0 mg/day but does not correlate well at extremely low intakes (Oldham et al., 1946; Mickelsen et al., 1947). Excretions of about 100 μg thiamin/

day have been reported to be compatible with adequate nutrition (Williams et al., 1942; Hathaway and Strom, 1946), but lower levels of excretion, between 50 and 100 μg, also have been judged adequate when correlated with other tests (Keys et al., 1945; Meyer et al., 1955).

According to studies of Ziporin et al. (1965), thiamin excretion approaches zero after three weeks on a diet containing less than 0.2 mg thiamin/1000 kcal, but thiamin metabolites, pyrimidine and thiazole, remain at high levels. These workers propose that the level of metabolite output represents a measure of the rate at which body stores of thiamin are being depleted. On the basis of this assumption, minimum requirement is estimated as the amount that would replace the vitamin used for metabolic needs. Minimum requirement as estimated on this basis amounted to 0.27 to 0.33 mg/1000 kcal.

Nicotinic acid metabolism is measured by the presence of its metabolites, N'-methylnicotinamide or the 2- and 6-pyridone of N'-methylnicotinamide, in urine. Evaluation of nicotinic acid intake

Table 24.4 THE 4-PYRIDOXIC ACID EXCRETION AS AFFECTED BY LEVEL OF VITAMIN B_6 INTAKE AND PROTEIN INTAKE

No. of Days on Specified Vitamin B_6 Intake	Vitamin B_6 Intake (mg/day)	4-Pyridoxic Acid Excretion (mg/day)
	Low Protein Diet	
6	1.66	1.01 ± 0.32[a]
2	0.16	0.67 ± 0.30
5	0.16	0.18 ± 0.18
20	0.16	0.11 ± 0.08
40	0.16	0.05 ± 0.08
7	0.76	0.12 ± 0.05
	High Protein Diet	
8	1.66	0.88 ± 0.11
2	0.16	0.46 ± 0.04
5	0.16	0.25 ± 0.13
17	0.16	0.25 ± 0.02
13	0.76	0.25 ± 0.02
2	50.16	26.20 ± 3.42

[a] S.D.

From J. Kelsay et al., *J. Nutr.*, 94, 490 (1968).

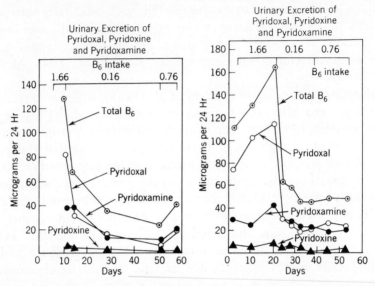

Fig. 24.1   Effect of the level of intake of vitamin B₆ on the urinary excretion of pyridoxal, pyridoxamine and pyridoxine by subjects fed a 54 gm protein diet and a 150 gm protein diet. [From J. Kelsay et al., *J. Nutr.*, 94: 490 (1968).]

must take into account the tryptophan content of the diet. Horwitt et al. (1956) and Goldsmith et al. (1961) used excretion of nicotinic acid metabolites as the basis for experiments designed to determine the extent of tryptophan conversion to nicotinic acid in the human (see Chapter 3).

Adjustment of urinary excretion of ascorbic acid to changes in dietary intake occurs fairly rapidly, within 10 to 15 days (Dodds et al., 1950). On intakes of between 50 and 60 mg reduced ascorbic acid, subjects excrete an average of 11 mg (ibid.), but may excrete half this amount. Moderate to high levels of ascorbic acid intake reflect dietary intake closely (Ritchey, 1965). However, when dietary intake is below 10 mg, urinary excretions approach zero long before clinical evidence of ascorbic acid deficiency becomes apparent (Crandon, 1940).

The three forms of vitamin B₆ and of the metabolite, 4-pyridoxic acid, also decrease rapidly in response to a low vitamin B₆ diet (Table 24.4; Fig. 24.1). Other tests to be described in a later section appear to be more significant in describing changes in vitamin B₆ nutrition (Baker et al., 1964; Cinnamon and Beaton, 1970).

In general, urinary excretion is a useful although imprecise tool for evaluation of response to dietary intake of many water-soluble vitamins. At low intakes, other tests appear to provide more definitive criteria.

BLOOD LEVELS

Tissue levels of vitamins are good indicators of the state of nutrition. When laboratory animals are studied, autopsies may be performed on them and various organs may be removed for analysis of tissues or subcellular particles to determine the amount and distribution of vitamins within the body. The human subject obviously is not a suitable candidate for such studies. Except for recent work on liver, skin, muscle, and adipose tissue obtained by biopsy, tissue analyses of humans are generally restricted to the most accessible tissue: blood.

Both the liquid (plasma or serum) and cell fractions of blood have been analyzed. Correlation with dietary intake depends not only upon the distribution pattern peculiar to the vitamin but also upon the sensitivity of analytical procedures used for determination of vitamin level. In general, blood cells contain larger amounts of vitamins than plasma, since it is within the cell that metabolic reactions that require vitamins take place. Vitamins contained in plasma, however, tend to represent nutrient available to *all* body cells, and some of these vitamins are more sensitively related to dietary intake than the content of blood cells. In other instances, the reverse is true.

Measurement of plasma levels of thiamin and riboflavin have not been used frequently in experimental studies. An adaptation of the fluorometric method for thiamin was shown to roughly correlate with dietary intake, but there was considerable overlapping at different dietary levels (Burch et al., 1950; Dube et al., 1952). Measurement of riboflavin in red cells was shown to reflect dietary intake rather accurately (Bessey et al., 1956). The microbiological methods described by Baker and Frank (1968) likely are the most accurate methods presently available for plasma thiamin and ribo-flavin and are used in clinical and nutrition survey studies.

Blood levels of ascorbic acid are closely related to dietary intake. At comparable levels of intake blood levels of the vitamin are

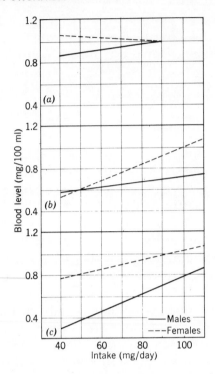

Fig. 24.2 Regressions of ascorbic acid blood levels with ascorbic acid intake, males and females, (a) 4 to 12 years of age; (b) 13 to 20 years; and (c) 20 years and over. [From M. L. Dodds, *J. Amer. Diet. Ass.,* 54: 32 (1969).]

higher among females than males. Dodds (1969) has compiled published data on ascorbic acid blood levels of 2130 males and 2865 females of different ages who were maintained on known intakes of the vitamin. Below the age of puberty no difference was found between blood values for males and females (Fig. 24.2). Above the age of puberty, however, females maintain blood levels well above those of males. The sex difference is most apparent in adults above the age of 20. These data were interpreted as evidence of hormonal regulation of ascorbic acid metabolism. The implications of this finding in terms of ascorbic acid requirements is not clear.

In studies of ascorbic acid deficiency, Hodges et al. (1971) reported plasma ascorbic acid levels to fall rapidly during the first month and then to be maintained at low but measurable levels as symptoms of scurvy developed. In contrast, urinary excretion of the

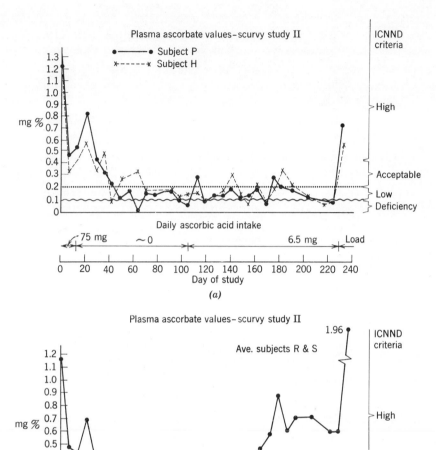

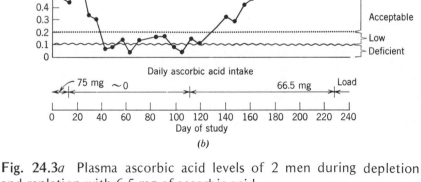

Fig. 24.3*a* Plasma ascorbic acid levels of 2 men during depletion and repletion with 6.5 mg of ascorbic acid.

Fig. 24.3*b* Average plasma ascorbic acid levels of 2 men during depletion and repletion with 66.5 mg of ascorbic acid. [From R. E. Hodges et al., *Amer. J. Clin. Nutr.*, 24: 432 (1971).]

vitamin was essentially nil after one month. As little as 6.5 mg of ascorbic acid was sufficient to relieve clinical symptoms of deficiency with no effect on ascorbic acid blood levels (Fig. 24.3a). Subjects given 66.5 mg of ascorbic acid, however, responded with an immediate increase in plasma levels and prompt remission of clinical symptoms (Fig. 24.3b).

Hodges and his associates further noted that, in the presence of frank scurvy, plasma levels often were as high as 0.2 mg/100 ml. This finding is of particular interest since this level is above the range which was classified as a "low" level (0.1 to 0.19 mg/100 mg) of serum ascorbic acid in the National Nutrition Survey (see Chapter 26).

Measurement of blood vitamin A levels is of little value as an experimental tool. Individuals in a good state of vitamin A nutrition can tolerate a vitamin A-deficient diet for one to nearly two years without showing a significant decrease in the vitamin A of serum (Hume and Krebs, 1949; Hodges and Kolder, 1971). Circulating levels of this vitamin tend to be maintained as long as liver stores are available. When liver stores are depleted, blood levels fall precipitously. There is, however, considerable individual variation between serum levels of retinol and the time that symptoms appear. The data for three subjects in the study by Hodges and Kolder (1971) are shown in Table 24.5. Although a failure of dark adaptation has been thought to be an early symptom of vitamin A deficiency it was a relatively late symptom in these subjects. One subject showed symptoms of follicular hyperkeratosis and impaired dark adaptation with only a small reduction in serum retinol. These results, obtained under highly controlled conditions, clearly demonstrate the almost terrifying reality of biological variation.

No experiments on vitamin A deficiency with children have been attempted. It is well known that children respond to low dietary intakes more quickly than adults, perhaps within a few months. The relative vulnerability presumably is due to the demands of growth and possibly to smaller liver stores than adults. Underwood (1970) has shown, however, that the concentration of vitamin A is higher in livers of children than adults. The total liver storage is most likely less than adults due to smaller liver size.

Levels of carotene in serum reflect changes in dietary intake of the provitamin (Moore, 1957), but they are of little value in determining the state of nutrition with respect to vitamin A. Attempts to determine minimum vitamin A requirement by measurement of

Table 24.5 SERUM RETINOL LEVELS AT TIME OF ONSET OF CLINICAL SIGNS AND SYMPTOMS

Subject	Time on Deficient Diet (days)	Clinical Signs and Symptoms	Serum Retinol Micrograms per 100 ml
1	260	White papules, anterior and shoulders	22
	321	Impaired dark adaptation	11
	449	Follicular hyperkeratosis, thighs and back	11
3	185	White papules, chest, back, and shoulders	25
	282	Follicular hyperkeratosis	25
	414	Severe acne	14
	420	Impaired dark adaptation	12
8	372	Follicular hyperkeratosis, thighs	35
	621	Impaired dark adaptation	27

From R. E. Hodges and H. Kolder in Summary of proceedings, Workshop on biochemical and clinical criteria for determining human vitamin A nutriture, Food and Nutrition Board, National Academy of Sciences, Washington, D. C., (1971), pp. 10-16.

blood levels admittedly have been discouraging.

Tocopherol blood levels also respond slowly when subjects are fed a diet deficient in the vitamin. Following depletion, however, a steady high level in plasma is reached after only one month of tocopherol feeding (Horwitt et al., 1956). Other tests, such as erythrocyte hemolysis (see following section), are thought to be more meaningful in evaluating dietary intakes of this vitamin.

URINARY EXCRETION AND BLOOD LEVELS FOLLOWING A TEST DOSE OF VITAMIN

The degree of tissue saturation can be estimated by feeding a fairly large dose of the vitamin to subjects and measuring excretion over a specific period of time, usually four hours. Such tests, sometimes called *load tests*, have been used in numerous experimental studies, and appear to be helpful in the interpretation of 24-hour excretion data.

The term *test dose return* refers to the percentage of the test dose excreted in urine samples collected during the period immediately following administration of the vitamin. Interpretation of the test dose return is based on the assumption that subjects in a state of saturation will excrete a large proportion of the administered vitamin within a relatively short period. As percentage return decreases, it is apparent that body tissues are avidly retaining the needed nutrient.

The response of blood levels to a test dose of vitamin also may be used as a means for evaluating tissue levels. A combination of the two measurements, urinary excretion and various blood levels, often may provide more easily interpreted data than either alone. For example, Wang et al. (1962) observed no difference in plasma total ascorbic acid level following a test dose of erythorbic acid (an inactive isomer of the vitamin) and of L-ascorbic acid, although urinary excretion of total ascorbic acid was markedly increased in subjects fed the isomer. A later report from the same laboratory (Rivers et al., 1963) indicated that although erythorbic acid could be detected in plasma and thus contribute to the total ascorbic acid measured, white cell level did not increase. Therefore the larger excretion following ingestion of the isomer was due to its rejection by the cell membrane transport system, thus providing a possible explanation for the failure of erythorbic acid to substitute metabolically for the active vitamin.

A strict comparison of studies reported in the literature is difficult because of differences in the amount of vitamin administered and the method of administration (orally or parenterally). Methods of test dose administration and evaluation of data have been reviewed by Unglaub and Goldsmith (1954). Basically the methodology remains unchanged.

ENZYME ACTIVITY AND OTHER RELATED TESTS

One of the long term objectives of nutrition research has been to uncover sensitive tests to evaluate human response to diet. It is clearly not enough to know that a certain level of nutrient will prevent clinical deficiency; what we need to know is the level that will support normal cellular metabolism, since it seems likely that clinical lesions result only when cellular adaptive mechanisms no longer are able to cope with a diminishing supply of nutrient.

Such tests are based on known metabolic functions of the vitamins and effectively combine knowledge of cellular biochemical reactions with response of the whole organism. For example, it has been known for many years that the oxidative decarboxylation of pyruvate is dependent upon an adequate supply of thiamin and that in a state of severe thiamin deficiency, pyruvate and lactate tend to accumulate in the blood. Blood pyruvate levels, however, are not directly related to the degree of thiamin deficiency and show little or no elevation in the mild deficiency state. In an attempt to develop a test which would more nearly define the aberration in cell metabolism, Horwitt and Kreisler (1949) combined glucose administration and mild exercise as a *metabolic load.* As a result of their tests a formula was developed for carbohydrate metabolism index:

$$CMI = \frac{L - G/10 + 15P - G/10}{2}$$

where CMI is carbohydrate metabolism index, L is blood lactate, P is blood pyruvate, and G is glucose blood level. Carbohydrate metabolism indices above 15 were correlated with subsequent development of thiamin deficiency and indicated an inability to efficiently oxidize available glucose in the presence of obvious extra energy requirement (exercise). This test has not been used extensively, but it is significant as one of the earliest tests designed to examine cellular function as a measure of nutritional adequacy.

A more recent test believed to be very sensitive to early thiamin deficiency is based on the requirement for TPP in the transketolase reaction of the pentose phosphate shunt (Brin, 1962). This enzyme system appears to be highly responsive to dietary thiamin intake. When rats are placed on a thiamin-deficient diet, for example, the enzyme activity decreases even before growth rate is affected. In humans transketolase activity is measured in red cell hemolysates. Depression of transketolase activity is assumed to indicate thiamin deficiency. *In vitro* stimulation of the system by addition of TPP provides conclusive evidence of thiamin deficiency.

The levels of riboflavin and niacin coenzymes in blood have been studied and have been shown to be imprecise measures of vitamin nutriture. Flavin mononucleotide levels of plasma were found to decrease in subjects maintained on a deficient diet, but the relationship between coenzyme level and dietary intake was highly variable (Bessey et al., 1956). Flavin adenine dinucleotide is very little affected by variations in riboflavin intake. The measurement of the activity of the enzyme glutathione reductase, however, appears to reflect riboflavin status accurately (Tillotson and Baker, 1972). The niacin coenzyme NAD has been determined for whole blood, serum, and red blood cells of well nourished adults (Burch et al., 1955), but the coenzyme is not a sensitive measurement at low intakes of nicotinic acid (Goldsmith, 1959). Apparently these coenzymes are maintained in blood even with extreme dietary deprivation and may not be reduced significantly even when clinical lesions are present.

Several metabolic tests related to vitamin B_6 have been evaluated. The excretion of xanthurenic acid is greatly increased following a load test of tryptophan when the diet does not contain pyridoxine, and this appears to be a highly sensitive test of vitamin B_6 deprivation (Baker et al., 1964). The test is based on the requirement for pyridoxal phosphate in the conversion of the tryptophan metabolite 3-hydroxykynurenine to 3-hydroxyanthranilic acid. In the absence of pyridoxine, 3-hydroxykynurenine is converted to xanthurenic acid (see Chapter 3). Administration of the vitamin, however, returns xanthurenic acid excretion to normal within 24 hours (Cinnamon and Beaton, 1970). This finding suggests that although xanthurenic acid excretion is a valid test for vitamin B_6 deprivation under controlled conditions, there may be little validity in results obtained randomly (as in a clinical or survey situation). A small dose of the vitamin prior to testing could conceivably obscure a long term deficiency of the vitamin.

The activities of serum transaminases also have been evaluated in terms of vitamin B_6 nutriture. It is generally agreed that serum glutamic-pyruvate transaminase (GPT) is more closely related to dietary intake than serum glutamic-oxaloacetic transaminase (GOT) (Babcock et al., 1960; Brin et al., 1960; Cinnamon and Beaton, 1970). In vitamin B_6-depleted subjects serum transaminases return to normal only after 3 to 4 weeks of vitamin B_6 feeding (Cinnamon and Beaton, 1970). Raica and Sauberlich (1964) suggested that the *in vitro* stimulation of serum GOT activity with pyridoxal phosphate would provide a more definitive answer to the question of vitamin B_6 involvement in decreased serum GOT activity. This procedure would satisfy at least in part the criticism by Baysal et al. (1966) that serum transaminases range so widely in normal individuals that these analyses cannot be used as an indication of vitamin B_6 nutriture.

The erythrocyte hemolysis test is a test for vitamin E deficiency and is based on the effect of the vitamin in stabilization of cell membranes. The test measures the *in vitro* resistance of the erythrocyte membrane to hemolysis by hydrogen peroxide. As shown in Table 24.6, dietary supplementation of subjects depleted of vitamin E resulted in increased plasma tocopherol levels within one month, but hemolysis of red blood cells did not decrease significantly until after 9 months. This test rather than tocopherol plasma levels

Table 24.6 EFFECT OF SUPPLEMENTATION OF DEPLETED SUBJECT WITH TOCOPHEROL (15 MG/DAY)

Months	Plasma Tocopherol (mg/100 ml)	Hemolysis (%)
0	0.48	61
1	0.95	46
3	0.70	52
8	0.85	40
9	0.90	12
10	0.95	10

From M. K. Horwitt et al., *Amer. J. Clin. Nutr.*, 8: 408 (1960).

was the basis for the determination of vitamin E requirement in relation to polyunsaturated fatty acid content of the diet (Horwitt et al., 1960).

CONCLUSION

Most of the studies on which human requirements and dietary standards of the major vitamins are based were done during a 20-year period, roughly between 1940 and 1960. More highly refined tests are needed not only for establishing definitive criteria for the determination of human requirements but also for the accurate diagnosis of nutritional lesions that are amenable to dietary treatment. In addition, such tests are needed to identify cellular metabolic aberrations resulting from genetic, infectious, and degenerative diseases and of the drugs used in treatment.

As stated by Goldsmith (1959):

"Nutritional diagnosis implies evaluation of the biochemical milieu within and outside of the cells, as well as detection of abnormalities of function and structure of the organs and tissues of the body. Recent studies of the role of mitochondria and other cellular units in oxidative metabolism link cytology and biochemistry closely together and may lead to better correlation between pathologic anatomical changes and biochemical abnormalities of body tissues and fluids."

New approaches to the problems of cellular metabolic disturbances will continue to be initiated primarily through studies with experimental animals followed by carefully conducted observations on humans. The measurement of enzyme activity and other functional tests appear to be superior to measurement of the vitamin itself as techniques for the determination of vitamin requirements. Nutrition research, therefore, is focusing more and more on identification of primary biochemical lesions that relate cellular function to human health. More of these lesions will become apparent as vitamin participation in cellular structure and function is better understood.

chapter 25
dietary standards

1. Uses of Dietary Standards
2. Requirements and Allowances
3. Recommended Dietary Allowances
   a. Energy
   b. Protein
   c. Calcium and Phosphorus
   d. Iron
   e. Magnesium, Zinc, and Iodine
   f. Ascorbic Acid
   g. Thiamin, Riboflavin, and Niacin
   h. Vitamin B_6
   i. Folacin and Vitamin B_{12}
   j. Vitamin A
   k. Vitamin D
   l. Vitamin E.
   m. Other Nutrients
4. Canadian and British Standards
5. FAO/WHO Standards
   a. Energy
   b. Protein
   c. Calcium
   d. Iron
   e. Vitamins
6. Other Dietary Standards
7. Summary

Dietary standards are derived from compilations of experimental studies designed to determine the nutrient requirements of the human. Quantitatively, standards are not *requirements* but, rather, are estimations of reasonable levels of nutrient intakes that should support normal function in most people. Thus they are intended as a basis for planning and evaluating diets of *groups* of people. Standards tend to vary slightly among countries primarily because populations and environmental conditions vary and because the interpretation of adequate levels of dietary intake also vary. Theoretically, standards are considered valid only for the group for which they are formulated. The rather widespread practice of using dietary standards as a basis for the evaluation of *individual* dietaries is not without value but is clearly dependent upon the user's understanding of the philosophical and scientific rationale for the standards and the recognition that individuals vary as widely in nutrient needs as they do in other physiological responses.

The first organized attempt at developing a dietary standard came as a result of food shortages during World War I when it became necessary for the United States government to devise a rational basis for shipments of food from this country to its allies in Europe. With the limited knowledge at that time of nutrition in general and of human nutrient needs in particular, recommendations could be made only for energy and, with reservations, for protein. In 1933, the British Medical Association proposed a limited set of standards, and in the same year the United States Department of Agriculture (Stiebeling, 1933) made more extensive proposals including recommendations for energy value, protein, calcium, iron, phosphorus, vitamin A, and ascorbic acid. Both sets of proposals were based primarily upon results of dietary surveys from which could be calculated average nutrient intakes of presumably healthy population groups. In the mid-1930s, the vitamin era was at its peak but very few data had accumulated on the metabolic needs of the human.

The greatest impetus to the development of dietary standards (and consequently to the encouragement of laboratory research directed toward the establishment of human nutrient requirements) came as a result of the work of the League of Nations Technical Commission on Nutrition (Burnet and Aykroyd, 1935). The Commission focused international attention on the significance of diet in preventive medicine and as a means of improving the public health. Dietary standards were proposed for energy and protein expressed as an average requirement on the basis of age, sex, and activity. In retrospect, however, the proposal of standards was a minor accomplishment of the Commission. Rather, as a result of the Commission's efforts, a number of the League member governments formed nutrition councils geared specifically to the improvement of health through nutrition, and it was the lack of experimental data available to the councils that helped to stimulate research on human nutrient requirements.

A more detailed discussion on the development of dietary standards can be found in the review by Leitch (1942); the subject also has been reviewed briefly by Young (1964).

USES OF DIETARY STANDARDS

If it is recognized that dietary standards represent, in effect, value judgments based on the kinds of experimental data described in Chapters 23 and 24 and subject to the limitations of human metabolic studies, it should be clear that the applications of standards must be broad in scope. Dietary standards thus are most useful for dietary planning and for evaluating diets consumed by population groups. They serve as a basis for regulating the food supply, for example, for governmental recommendations regarding agricultural practices and the extent of food exports and imports.

In evaluating the results of dietary surveys, standards serve as the yardstick by which the nutrient intake of a population group may be judged. Such evaluations are valid when applied to groups of people but can be misleading if applied to individuals. It is in this way that standards are most often misused. Numbers tend to give an illusion of exactness and accuracy which may lead to errors in judgment when used indiscriminately. These errors are likely to be magnified in the evaluation of individual dietaries. However, with recognition of the limitations of the standard and of survey methodology (see Chapter 26), useful information may be obtained.

A last and highly practical use of the dietary standard is in the development of *food plans* that, loosely described, are a translation of human nutrient needs into foods or food groups that may be used conveniently by nonprofessionals in planning diets. Quantitative expressions of nutrients (in terms of milligrams, grams, etc.) have meaning for the nutritionist or dietitian, but they are of little value to the layman. Nearly all countries have developed some type of food plan based on the dietary standards adopted and the food habits and food supply of the population. The *Basic Four* used in nutrition education in this country is an example of a food plan constructed to meet nutrient needs, with the exception of calories, and is specifically adapted to common dietary practices of the American population. It is not applicable, however, to other cultures in which food habits and thus food sources of nutrients are likely to differ markedly from those of this country.

REQUIREMENTS AND ALLOWANCES

Dietary standards are not dietary requirements. The term *minimum requirement* as defined in Chapter 23 represents basic physiological need and is compatible with the smallest amount of a nutrient that will prevent deficiency symptoms or support a well-defined physiological or biochemical response. The term *average requirement* is often used to denote the amount of a nutrient that will support health in most persons of a given population group and implies that the true requirement for individuals may be either above or below the average for the group. The two terms are ambiguous; the meanings tend to overlap and thus are confusing. Both, however, refer to quantitative estimates that are based upon data of uncertain precision obtained from a limited number of subjects. The perfect tool for determining human requirements has not yet been devised, nor has the perfect criterion of physiological response yet been ascertained. Even if such perfection could be attained, the results would be accurate only for the individual tested at the particular time tested. An average requirement based on a broad sample still would be subject to the errors inherent in any average.

It is for this reason that the term *requirements* is usually avoided in dietary standards. *Allowances* is a more accurate description and implies the addition of an amount above the estimated requirement to cover both the variation among individuals and the lack of precision inherent in the estimated requirement. This additional amount is a safety factor referred to as a *margin of safety* or *allowance for safety*. The differences among dietary standards are largely due to the amount of the safety factor added, an amount determined by the philosophical goals of those who help to set the standard.

RECOMMENDED DIETARY ALLOWANCES

The dietary standards used in this country are the Recommended Dietary Allowances (RDA) which were developed by the Food and Nutrition Board of the National Research Council, National Academy of Sciences. Every student of nutrition should be familiar with the RDA and with the basis for their formulation.

The first allowances were published in 1943 as the result of nearly two years of deliberation and study of the available literature (see Roberts, 1958). In presenting the first set of allowances, the following points were emphasized:

1. "That they were recommended allowances, not standards (i.e., requirements). They were goals, not necessarily absolute requirements.

2. "That they were based on the best knowledge available at the time they were formulated.

3. "That they were subject to change as soon as more evidence became available."

Consequently, the RDA were revised in 1945, again in 1948, and every five years since (1953, 1958, 1963, 1968, 1974). The latest revision is shown in Table 25.1 and includes recommendations for one additional nutrient. The allowances are described as "the levels of intake of essential nutrients considered, in the judgment of the Food and Nutrition Board on the basis of available scientific knowledge, to be adequate to meet the known nutritional needs of practically all healthy persons."

The recommendations of the Food and Nutrition Board are discussed in detail in the report on the 1973 RDA (Food and Nutri-

Table 25.1 FOOD AND NUTRITION BOARD, NATIONAL ACADEMY OF SCIENCES–NATIONAL RESEARCH COUNCIL RECOMMENDED DAILY DIETARY ALLOWANCES,[a]

Designed for the maintenance of good nutrition of practically all healthy people in the U.S.A.

	Age (yrs)	Weight (kg)	Weight (lbs)	Height (cm)	Height (in)	Energy (kcal)[b]	Protein (gm)	Fat-Soluble Vitamins				Water-Soluble Vitamins							Minerals					
								Vitamin A Activity (RE)[c]	Vitamin A Activity (IU)	Vitamin D (IU)	Vitamin E Activity[e] (IU)	Ascorbic Acid (mg)	Folacin[f] (µg)	Niacin[g] (mg)	Riboflavin (mg)	Thiamin (mg)	Vitamin B6 (mg)	Vitamin B12 (µg)	Calcium (mg)	Phosphorus (mg)	Iodine (µg)	Iron (mg)	Magnesium (mg)	Zinc (mg)
Infants	0-.5	6	14	60	24	kg×117	kg×2.2	420[d]	1,400	400	4	35	50	5	0.4	0.3	0.3	0.3	360	240	35	10	60	3
	.5-1	9	20	71	28	kg×108	kg×2.0	400	2,000	400	5	35	50	8	0.6	0.5	0.4	0.3	540	400	45	15	70	5
Children	1-3	13	28	86	34	1,300	23	400	2,000	400	7	40	100	9	0.8	0.7	0.6	1.0	800	800	60	15	150	10
	4-6	20	44	110	44	1,800	30	500	2,500	400	9	40	200	12	1.1	0.9	0.9	1.5	800	800	80	10	200	10
	7-10	30	66	135	54	2,400	36	700	3,300	400	10	40	300	16	1.2	1.2	1.2	2.0	800	800	110	10	250	10
Males	11-14	44	97	158	63	2,800	44	1,000	5,000	400	12	45	400	18	1.5	1.4	1.6	3.0	1,200	1,200	130	18	350	15
	15-18	61	134	172	69	3,000	54	1,000	5,000	400	15	45	400	20	1.8	1.5	2.0	3.0	1,200	1,200	150	18	400	15
	19-22	67	147	172	69	3,000	54	1,000	5,000	400	15	45	400	20	1.8	1.5	2.0	3.0	800	800	140	10	350	15
	23-50	70	154	172	69	2,700	56	1,000	5,000		15	45	400	18	1.6	1.4	2.0	3.0	800	800	130	10	350	15
	51+	70	154	172	69	2,400	56	1,000	5,000		15	45	400	16	1.5	1.2	2.0	3.0	800	800	110	10	350	15

Females	11-14	44	97	155	62	2,400	800	4,000	400	12	45	400	16	1.3	1.2	1.6	3.0	1,200	1,200	115	18	300	15
	15-18	54	119	162	65	2,100	800	4,000	400	12	45	400	14	1.4	1.1	2.0	3.0	1,200	1,200	115	18	300	15
	19-22	58	128	162	65	2,100	800	4,000	400	12	45	400	14	1.4	1.1	2.0	3.0	800	800	100	18	300	15
	23-50	58	128	162	65	2,000	800	4,000		12	45	400	13	1.2	1.0	2.0	3.0	800	800	100	18	300	15
	51+	58	128	162	65	1,800	800	4,000		12	45	400	12	1.1	1.0	2.0	3.0	800	800	80	10	300	15
Pregnant		+30				+300	1,000	5,000	400	15	60	800	+2	+0.3	+0.3	2.5	4.0	1,200	1,200	125	18[h]	450	20
Lactating		+20				+500	1,200	6,000	400	15	80	600	+4	+0.5	+0.3	2.5	4.0	1,200	1,200	150	18	450	25

[a]The allowances are intended to provide for individual variations among most normal persons as they live in the United States under usual environmental stresses. Diets should be based on a variety of common foods in order to provide other nutrients for which human requirements have been less well defined.

[b]Kilojoules (kJ) = 4.2 × kcal.

[c]Retinol equivalents.

[d]Assumed to be all as retinol in milk during the first six months of life. All subsequent intakes are assumed to be half as retinol and half as β-carotene when calculated from international units. As retinol equivalents, three-fourths are as retinol and one-fourth as β-carotene.

[e]Total vitamin E activity, estimated to be 80 percent as α-tocopherol and 20 percent other tocopherols.

[f]The folacin allowances refer to dietary sources as determined by *Lactobacillus casei* assay. Pure forms of folacin may be effective in doses less than one-fourth of the recommended dietary allowance.

[g]Although allowances are expressed as niacin, it is recognized that on the average 1 mg of niacin is derived from each 60 mg of dietary tryptophan.

[h]This increased requirement cannot be met by ordinary diets; therefore, the use of supplemental iron is recommended.

901

tion Board, 1974) and a general background of the basis for the new recommendations is reviewed by Harper (1974). Only a few pertinent explanations and comments will be made in the sections that follow.

Energy

Energy allowances probably have less applicability to the individual than those of any other nutrient. The allowances are set for different age groups for which an *average* height and weight is assumed. Therefore, individual energy needs that vary with body height and weight as well as age can only roughly be surmised from the recommendations since normal people exist in many different sizes and shapes. More important than body size, however, is individual activity. The energy allowance is set at the lowest value that appears to be compatible with good health. Even so, it is recognized that some persons will need less because of the sedentary activity pattern characteristic of a large number of Americans. For these persons, an increase in energy expenditure rather than a significant decrease in energy intake is recommended. Reasons for this view as listed in the 1973 RDA (Food and Nutrition Board, 1974) follow. ". . . (1) Many of the essential nutrients, particularly the minerals, are distributed widely and in low concentration in foods, especially in the low-cost staple commodities. It is therefore difficult to assure nutritional adequacy of diets that are low in energy content (less than 1800 − 2000 kcal) unless fats, sugar, and alcohol are more rigidly restricted than is customary in most American households. (2) Evidence from human population groups and experimental studies in animals indicates that energy intake is usually not regulated adequately to maintain balance at very low levels of work output, with the result that sedentary individuals become obese (Mayer et al., 1956). (3) There is evidence that a sedentary life contributes to degenerative arterial disease, as well as to obesity and its many complications, notably diabetes mellitus (WHO, 1969)."

A decrease in recommended energy allowance with increasing age is consistent with the known decrease in basal metabolic rate that occurs with aging and with a possible decrease in physical activity. Desirable weights for height suggested for adults remain constant for all adults over 25 years of age (Table 25.2). Accordingly, recommended energy intakes for persons over 50 years of age are 90 percent of those for younger adults. If the individual remains active, the necessary reduction in energy intake is less.

Energy needs of children vary even more widely than those of adults, primarily because activity patterns differ markedly among individual children. Individual adjustments, therefore, are necessary. The allowances can only be considered as approximate and are useful primarily for planning food service for groups.

Little adjustment is believed to be necessary for climate in this country. Individuals are usually well protected from cold, and with increased use of air conditioning, many are equally well protected from extreme heat. A small increase (2.5 percent) is suggested to cover energy expended in carrying heavy clothing. No adjustment is necessary for persons living in climates between 20 and 30°C or for inactive persons living in warmer climates. Consolazio et al. (1961) have presented evidence suggesting that at temperatures above 30°C persons engaged in hard work expend extra energy in maintaining temperature homeostasis due to increases in both metabolic rate and body temperature. A small *increase* in energy intake therefore may be necessary; the recommendation is for an increase of 0.5 percent for every degree rise in temperature between 30 and 40°C.

A modest increment of 300 kcal is recommended during the latter half of pregnancy because of limited physical activity associated

Table 25.2 DESIRABLE WEIGHT FOR HEIGHT.

Height[a] (in)	Weight[a] in Pounds	
	Men	Women
60		109±9
62		115±9
64	133±11	122±10
66	142±12	129±10
68	151±14	136±10
70	159±14	144±11
72	167±15	152±12
74	175±15	

From Food and Nutrition Board NRC *Recommended Dietary Allowances*, 1974. Modified from Table 80, Hathaway and Ford, 1960, Heights and weights of adults in the U. S., Home Economics Research Report No. 10, ARS, USDA.
[a]Heights and weights are "without shoes and other clothing." To convert inches to centimeters, multiply by 2.54. To convert pounds to kilograms, multiply by 0.454.

with labor-saving devices, general pattern of living, and possible decrease in activity due to body bulk in late pregnancy. For most women this increase should assure a desirable weight gain of about 20 to 25 lb (Committee on Maternal Nutrition, 1970). An increase of 500 kcal/day is recommended for milk production during lactation and is based on the assumption that approximately 850 ml of milk are produced daily with a caloric yield of 120 kcal/100 ml with an efficiency of 80 percent. The latter figure is in contrast to the previous assumption of 60 percent efficiency, which is clearly too low (Thomson et al., 1970). About one-third of the energy cost of lactation is assumed to be provided by maternal fat stores accumulated during pregnancy (See Chapter 22).

Protein

Recommended daily allowance for protein for adults is 0.8 gm/kg desirable weight. The recommendation assumes 70 percent efficiency in utilization of dietary protein and amounts to 56 gm/day for men and 46 gm/day for women of reference body size. These figures are roughly 10 gm lower than the RDA for 1968. The reduction in the recommendations for protein has been criticized as being incompatible with sound nutritional planning (Calloway, 1974) primarily on the basis that high protein foods provide many other nutrients, including vitamin B_6 and some of the trace elements, the needs of which may be difficult to meet with the current recommendations for protein and energy. The probability of widespread deficiencies of these nutrients occurring among the general population seems remote since habitually Americans consume higher intakes of protein than are presently recommended. However, in institutions in which emphasis is given to reducing operating costs, reduction in dietary protein (the most expensive food item) in adherence to the lower recommendation could result in inadequate intakes of other nutrients unless very careful attention is given to the nutrient content of other components of the diet. It should be emphasized that the controversy concerning the recommendation for protein is not directed to protein intake per se. There is no question but that the allowance is more than adequate to cover the requirement to maintain adults in nitrogen equilibrium as well as to allow for inefficiency of nitrogen utilization and individual variation. The question, instead, applies to the consequences of reducing protein intake in view of the present intake of sugar, fats, and alcohol as major energy (but low nutrient) components of the American diet and the inadequacy of present knowledge on the role and availability of trace minerals in the human diet.

Protein allowances for infants and children are based on growth rates and changes in body composition (see Chapter 22). For infants, the quantity of milk which will result in satisfactory growth provides about 2 to 2.4 gm protein/kg body weight decreasing to about 1.5 gm/kg by the sixth month. For children after infancy, protein recommendations are also based on growth rates and the assumption that the efficiency of protein utilization is similar to that for maintenance in the adult.

Nitrogen balance studies indicate that the efficiency of protein utilization during pregnancy is lower than has been assumed. For this reason and because of suggestions of improved reproductive performance with generous protein intakes (Committee on Maternal Nutrition, 1970, 1973), an increment of 30 gm of protein is recommended during the latter half of pregnancy. The protein intake during lactation is based on a protein yield in milk of 10 to 15 gm/day assuming the efficiency of utilization of dietary protein to be the same as for maintenance of nitrogen equilibrium.

Calcium and Phosphorus

The recommendation for calcium has always been controversial and has remained at 800 mg for many years. The recommendation has been based partially on balance data and partially on calculations from estimated endogenous losses and absorption of calcium. The allowance of 800 mg assumes absorption of approximately 40 percent of ingested calcium (320 mg) and further assumes that this amount is required to replace the daily endogenous loss of approximately 124 mg in feces, 175 mg in urine, and 20 mg in sweat. Results from balance studies indicate that most adults are likely to maintain calcium equilibrium on the 800 mg intake; others, however, adjust to and maintain equilibrium on intakes of 200-400 mg or less.

The present recommendation represents a reluctance to lower the recommendation in the absence of any more reliable data on the calcium requirement of man. As stated by Harper (1974), "Discussions of calcium allowances, like those of ascorbic acid, are likely to generate more heat than light." The relationship of protein intake to calcium retention (see Chapter 23) is a possible justification for maintaining the calcium level at 800 mg since high protein intakes (which Americans consume) tend to increase dietary calcium requirement. However, with the reduction in the recommendation for protein, the calcium allowance of 800 mg appears in theory to be inconsistent.

Calcium allowances for infants are set at the higher level available from cow's milk formulas and are intended specifically for the artificially-fed infant. The breast-fed infant obtains less calcium from his mother's milk despite somewhat better absorption. Although it hardly seems reasonable to set the allowance at a level higher than that available from breast milk, in the absence of data indicating that at *comparable* calcium intakes artificial feeding and breast feeding are equally satisfactory, the higher calcium recommendation is made to insure adequate intakes from cow's milk formulas. The RDA for calcium thus applies only to infants fed formulas.

The calcium allowance for children 1 to 10 years of age also is set at 800 mg, which appears to be compatible with the relatively slow, steady growth of children in this age range. For the preadolescent child and the rapidly growing adolescent a higher intake of 1200 mg is recommended. This amount is in the range at which maximum retention of calcium occurs in children.

A recommendation of 1200 mg/day is also made for pregnancy and lactation on the basis that 200 to 300 mg calcium is deposited in the fetus during the last 2 to 3 months of pregnancy, and a similar amount is present in milk secreted during lactation.

The allowance for phosphorus is the same as that for calcium for all age groups except for the young infant. A calcium:phosphorus ratio of 1.5:1 appears to be more suitable for the infant. (Cow's milk contains a ratio of 1.2:1 whereas human milk contains a ratio of 2:1 calcium to phosphorus.)

Iron

The recommendation for iron is based partly on absorption and balance studies and partly on the demonstrated prevalance of iron deficiency anemia among infants and very young children, and among women of childbearing age. The recommendations of 10 to 15 mg for infants and young children and 18 mg for females above 11 years of age cannot be supplied by usual diets and require that the diet be supplemented. The typical American diet contains about 6 mg of iron/1000 kcal; thus an adult woman could reasonably have an intake of roughly 12 mg/day. Infants on an all milk diet would have access to negligible amounts of iron without supplementation.

Supplements of 30 to 60 mg iron are recommended during pregnancy although there is evidence that lower amounts are effective in preventing lowering of iron stores in pregnant women (Committee on Maternal Nutrition, 1970).

Magnesium, Zinc, and Iodine

For the first time the table of recommended allowances has included zinc. Although rough estimations have been made previously for this nutrient improvements in methodology permitting the accurate analysis of food and body tissues have accelerated the accumulation of data.

The recommendations for magnesium for adults are based on balance studies on adult men and are compatible with amounts of magnesium found in usual American diets. The allowance for zinc is about one-third higher than the 8 to 10 mg/day required for equilibrium in the adult male (Food and Nutrition Board, 1970) and is at the upper limit of amounts analyzed in usual dietaries (Sandstead et al., 1967). Allowances for infants for magnesium and zinc are based on the content of these elements in human and cow's milk. Allowances for children and adolescents are regarded as reasonable estimates.

The recommendations for iodine are similar to those proposed in 1968. The apparent differences are due to changes in age-group categories.

Ascorbic Acid

The recommended allowance for ascorbic acid was lowered to 55 to 60 mg for adults in 1968 and is now lowered to 45 mg. This level is based on recent experiments with adult males indicating that an intake of 45 mg/day will maintain an adequate body pool of 1500 mg of the vitamin (Baker et al., 1971). About 10 mg ascorbic acid will prevent scurvy. About 30 mg will maintain relatively low blood levels and is sufficient to replace the amount of ascorbic acid metabolized daily.

Doses of 1 gm or more of ascorbic acid have been reported to prevent the common cold (Pauling, 1970) or to lessen symptoms of a cold (Anderson et al., 1972). These suggestions are of interest. However, a possible pharmacologic action of the vitamin should not be equated with the RDA (see Alfin-Slater, 1974). The pharmacologic effects of ascorbic acid certainly deserve further research particularly in view of some of the undesirable side effects produced by massive doses of the vitamin (Rhead and Schauzer, 1971; see Chapter 3).

The requirement for ascorbic acid in infants and young children is not well defined. The RDA for the infant is based on the ascorbic acid content of human milk; for older children, 40 mg is recommended. Increases in ascorbic acid of 15 and 35 mg are recommended during pregnancy and lactation respectively. These levels are not based on experimental evidence but are presumed to be adequate.

Thiamin, Riboflavin, and Niacin

Recommended intakes of thiamin, riboflavin, and niacin are based on experimental studies, as described in Chapter 24; all are expressed in terms of mg/1000 kcal of dietary intake. The recommended allowance for thiamin remains at 0.5 mg/1000 kcal. This level has been based primarily on a study indicating that normal red cell transketolase activity is maintained in subjects receiving more than 0.5 mg thiamin/1000 kcal (Haro et al., 1966). For older people who apparently utilize thiamin less efficiently than younger adults (Horwitt et al., 1948; Oldham, 1962) an intake of at least 1 mg a day is recommended even if their caloric intake is less than 2000 kcal. An increase of 0.1 mg/100 kcal is recommended during the last trimester of pregnancy. An increase in total thiamin during lactation is compatible with the increased energy intake of this period.

Riboflavin allowances are calculated on the basis of 0.6 mg/1000 kcal. The conclusion that riboflavin need is closely related to energy expenditure was derived from a review of the literature (Bro-Rasmussen, 1958) and is based largely on the participation of flavoproteins in cellular respiration. Horwitt (1966) questioned the validity of relating riboflavin allowances to energy intake and cited experimental evidence indicating that riboflavin need, like protein requirement, does not increase with increased energy expenditure. Expression of riboflavin allowance in terms of energy intake, therefore, is a convenience and must apply only to persons of moderate activity. There is no evidence that riboflavin requirement is increased as energy needs are increased. An additional 0.3 mg is recommended for pregnancy and 0.5 mg during lactation.

Allowances for niacin are expressed as mg niacin rather than as niacin equivalents, a term that includes preformed niacin and that formed from tryptophan (60 mg tryptophan = 1 mg niacin). The allowance for adults is 6.6 mg/1000 kcal but not less than 13 mg when caloric intakes are below 2000 kcal. In estimating the amount of niacin available from foods, however, it is suggested that the contribution of tryptophan to niacin should be considered. In essence then, the recommendation is exactly the same as when the term niacin equivalents was used. Very little is known about the niacin requirements of infants and children. The allowance for infants is based on the niacin and tryptophan content of human milk. Reasonable estimates are made for older children. An increase during pregnancy and lactation is based on the increased energy needs and amounts to an increment of 2 mg and 4 mg respectively.

Vitamin B_6

Recommendations for vitamin B_6 were first made in the 1968 revision of the RDA; the allowance was set at 2.0 mg/day for adults and remains unchanged. This level of the vitamin should cover the requirements over a wide range of protein intake (Baker et al., 1964). Using xanthurenic acid excretion following a tryptophan load test as criterion, it was found that optimum intake of vitamin B_6 on a low protein (30 gm) diet was 1.25-1.5 mg/day, whereas on a high protein (100 gm) diet 1.75-2 gm vitamin B_6 was necessary.

The requirements of children and adolescents have received little experimental study. The allowance for infants is based on the vitamin B_6 content of human and cow's milk and on studies by Bessey et al., (1957) on the excretion of xanthurenic acid by normal babies. At least 0.3 mg was required by infants to prevent excretion of abnormal tryptophan metabolites following a load test.

Very little is known about the needs for vitamin B$_6$ during pregnancy and lactation. An increment of 0.5 mg is assumed to be adequate.

Folacin and Vitamin B$_{12}$

Recommendations for folacin and vitamin B$_{12}$ also were first made in the 1968 revision of the RDA. The adult allowance of 400 μg for folacin remains the same. The level is possibly high. Approximately 50 μg of crystalline folic acid has been shown to be adequate to prevent symptoms of folacin deficiency (Herbert, 1968); levels of 100-200 μg/day, however, are necessary to return serum levels to normal in persons with folacin deficiency. The RDA was set at 400 μg on the basis that 25 percent of folic acid activity in an ordinary mixed diet will be absorbed and allows for the variance in the absorptive availability of the folate conjugates in foods.

As is the case for many nutrients, allowances for infants are based on the folacin content of human and cow's milk. Allowances for children are reasonable estimates. The requirement for folacin is increased with use of oral conceptives; and that for pregnant women has been shown to be markedly increased over the nonpregnant state (Alperin, 1966). The extent of the increase can only be surmised. For this reason, the allowance for women during pregnancy is set at twice that for the nonpregnant adult. An increment of 200 μg is judged to be sufficient for the lactating woman.

The allowance for vitamin B$_{12}$, however, was believed to be considerably overestimated in the first attempt at setting the standard. (Historically, first standards have tended to be high; with meager information available, the higher figure has usually been taken as the safer.) As a result the allowance was reduced from 5 μg for adults to 3 μg. The adult requirement has been shown to range tenfold from 0.1 μg to 1 μg/day when reticulocyte response in pernicious anemia patients was used as criterion (Herbert, 1968). Studies of turnover of vitamin B$_{12}$ in deficient patients indicated that daily losses of the vitamin ranged from 0.25-1.05 μg/day (FAO/WHO, 1970). Assuming that approximately 50 percent of vitamin B$_{12}$ in food is absorbed, the RDA was set at 3 μg/day for adults and adolescents. In the absence of data on the requirements for infants, young children, and pregnant and lactating women, reasonable estimates were proposed on much the same basis as was done for other nutrients for which there was no clear evidence.

Vitamin A

In the present revision of the RDA, the allowance for vitamin A activity is expressed in terms of retinol equivalents (RE) as well as the more familiar International Units (IU). One IU of vitamin A activity is equivalent to 0.3 µg of retinol (or 0.344 µg of retinyl acetate), and 0.6 µg of β-carotene. The vitamin A value of foods, expressed as retinol equivalents can be calculated from the following equivalencies:

$$
\begin{aligned}
1 \text{ retinol equivalent} &= 1 \text{ µg retinol} \\
&= 6 \text{ µg β-carotene} \\
&= 12 \text{ µg other provitamin A carotenoids} \\
&= 3.33 \text{ IU vitamin activity from retinol} \\
&= 10 \text{ IU vitamin A activity from β-carotene}
\end{aligned}
$$

To calculate retinol equivalents the following formula should be used:

1. If retinol and β-carotene are given in µg

$$\text{µg retinol} + \frac{\text{µg β-carotene}}{6} = \text{RE}$$

2. If both are given in IU

$$\frac{\text{IU retinol}}{3.33} + \frac{\text{IU β-carotene}}{10} = \text{RE}$$

3. If β-carotene and other provitamin A carotenoids are given in µg

$$\frac{\text{µg β-carotene}}{6} + \frac{\text{µg other carotenoids}}{12} = \text{RE}$$

Previously the recommended dietary allowance for the adult was estimated to be comprised of 2500 IU as retinol and 2500 IU as provitamin A. Expressed as retinol equivalents, the amounts are 750 µg of retinol and 250 retinol equivalents as β-carotene, a total of

1000 RE. A conversion factor of 5, therefore, is used to convert the RDA in RE to IU.

Experiments designed to determine the requirement for vitamin A have been reviewed by Rodriguez and Irwin (1972). From the available data the RDA for vitamin A has been based primarily on the classic study of Hume and Krebs (1949) and the more recent study by Hodges and Kolder (1971). The conclusions from both studies are in general agreement and indicate that a minimum of 500-600 μg of retinol is required to maintain adequate blood levels of the vitamin and to prevent all deficiency symptoms.

The allowance for adult men was set at the same level as previous recommendations, 1000 RE (5000 IU). Because of the smaller body size of women the recommendation was changed to 800 RE (4000 IU). The allowance for infants is based on the vitamin A activity of human milk; allowances for infants and children were extrapolated from those for infants and adults considering body size and arbitrary amounts to meet the needs of growth.

See Chapter 4 for discussion of vitamin A toxicity.

Vitamin D

Recommendations for vitamin D remain unchanged and are uniformly set at 400 IU for growth, pregnancy, and lactation. Relatively little new data are available on human requirements of vitamin D. It seems well established, however, that 400 IU will promote maximum calcium absorption and is well below toxicity levels (see Chapter 4).

Vitamin D intakes are usually expressed as IU. However, designation is sometimes made by weight of the vitamin. The conversion can be made on the basis that 100 IU of vitamin D are equivalent to 2.5 μg of cholecalciferol.

Vitamin E

A recommended allowance for vitamin E was first established in the 1968 revision of the RDA and was based on experimental studies in man (Horwitt et al., 1963) and on available data on the vitamin E content of customary diets. The latter figure has been found to be an overestimation (Bunnell et al., 1965; Bieri and Evarts, 1973), and this finding is a primary reason for the recent changes in the RDA for vitamin E. Because there is no clinical or biochemical evidence to indicate that vitamin E intake from customary diets is inadequate, the RDA have been revised downward from 30 to 15 mg for the adult male and 25 to 12 mg for the adult female. It should be noted that these figures refer to total vitamin E activity estimated to be 80 percent as α-tocopherol and 20 percent other tocopherols.

Recommendations for infants are based on the tocopherol content of human milk; other recommendations are given as reasonable estimates.

The requirement for vitamin E is known to be related to the PUFA content of the diet and of body tissues. Vitamin E, however, is associated with the PUFA content of foods (i.e., vegetable oils) so that the vitamin E intake increases along with the PUFA intake. Accordingly, the allowance for vitamin E can vary considerably from the tabulated figure. Unless PUFA intakes are extremely high the amount of vitamin E carried along with PUFA in foods should be adequate (Bieri, 1974).

Other Nutrients

Certain of the nutrients known to be essential to man are not included in the table of recommended allowances either because there is insufficient evidence on which to base a recommendation or because adequate amounts presumably will be provided by customary American diets. Information on these nutrients is summarized in Table 25.3.

CANADIAN AND BRITISH DIETARY STANDARDS

Both the dietary standards formulated by the Canadian Council on Nutrition (1964; Supplement, 1968; 1974) and the Department of Health and Social Security of the United Kingdom (1969) are somewhat different from the RDA in quantitative recommendations (Tables 25.4 and 25.5). The purposes of the standards are very similar (see Campbell, 1974), and clearly the differences in nutrient standards are the result of differences in philosophy concerning the means to presumably the same end. The RDA are "to be adequate to meet the known nutrition needs of practically all healthy persons." The

Table 25.3. ESTIMATED NEEDS FOR OTHER NUTRIENTS (RDA)

Nutrient	Estimated Requirement	Comment
Carbohydrate	No basis for recommendation.	Some carbohydrate in the diet is needed to avoid ketosis and loss of cations, especially sodium. 50-100 mg/day will offset undesirable effects of high fat diets. Complex carbohydrate is recommended.
Fat	No specific recommendation for fat. Essential fatty acid requirement 1-2% of total calories	Recommend that fat intake not exceed 35% of total calories because of relationship of high fat diets to heart disease.
Water	1 ml/kcal of food is reasonable allowance for adults; 1.5 ml/kg for infants; includes water of solid foods and metabolic water.	Higher intakes necessary when sweat losses are high.
Sodium	Unknown	Usual intake of adults 6-18 gm sodium/day. Extra amounts needed when water given to replace sweat losses.
Potassium	Adults need about 2.5 gm/day.	Customary diets appear adequate.
Copper	2 mg/day required for balance in adults; 1.2-1.3 mg promote retention in preadolescent girls.	Customary diets provide 2 mg/day.

Nutrient	Requirement	Remarks
Fluorine	Unknown	1 ppm in drinking water is effective in reducing incidence of dental caries.
Cobalt	Unknown	Appears to function in man only as a component of vitamin B_{12}.
Manganese	Unknown	No deficiency shown in man suggesting that customary intakes of 2.5-7 mg/day meet requirement.
Selenium	Unknown	0.1 μg/gm in diet prevents deficiency in animals; approximately the same amount is present in customary diets.
Molybdenum	Unknown	No deficiency shown in man. Estimated intakes of 45-500 μg/day probably meet requirement.
Choline	Unknown. Requirement depends on amount synthesized by the body and the content of methionine and other methyl donors available.	Customary diets provide 400-900 mg/day.
Pantothenic acid	5-10 mg probably adequate for adults; upper level suggested for pregnant and lactating women.	Diets contain 5-20 mg/day.
Biotin	Unknown. Some biotin provided by intestinal microorganisms.	Customary diets contain 100-300 μg/day.
Vitamin K	Unknown. Some vitamin K provided by intestinal microorganisms.	Customary diets appear adequate.

Table 25.4 RECOMMENDED DAILY NUTRIENT INTAKES—REVISED 1974 COMMITTEE FOR REVISION OF THE CANADIAN DIETARY STANDARD, BUREAU OF NUTRITIONAL SCIENCES, HEALTH AND WELFARE CANADA.

Age (years)	Sex	Weight (kg)	Height (cm)	Energy[a] (kcal)	Protein (gm)	Water-Soluble Vitamins							Fat-Soluble Vitamins			Minerals					
						Thiamin (mg)	Niacin[e] (mg)	Ribo-flavin (mg)	Vit. B6[f] (mg)	Folate[g] (µg)	Vit. B12 (µg)	Ascorbic Acid (mg)	Vit. A (µg RE)[i]	Vit. D (µg cholecalciferol)[j]	Vit. E (mg α-tocopherol)	Ca (mg)	P (mg)	Mg (mg)	I (µg)	Fe (mg)	Zn (mg)
0-6 mo.	Both	6	–	kgx117	kgx2.2 (2.0)[d]	0.3	5	0.4	0.3	40	0.3	20[h]	400	10	3	500[1]	250[1]	50[1]	35[1]	7[1]	4[1]
7-11 mo.	Both	9	–	kgx108	kgx1.4	0.5	6	0.6	0.4	60	0.3	20	400	10	3	500	400	50	50	7	5
1-3	Both	13	90	1400	22	0.7	9	0.8	0.8	100	0.9	20	400	10	4	500	500	75	70	8	5
4-6	Both	19	110	1800	27	0.9	12	1.1	1.3	100	1.5	20	500	5	5	500	500	100	90	9	6
7-9	M	27	129	2200	33	1.1	14	1.3	1.6	100	1.5	30	700	2.5[k]	6	700	700	150	110	10	7
7-9	F	27	128	2000	33	1.0	13	1.2	1.4	100	1.5	30	700	2.5[k]	6	700	700	150	100	10	7
10-12	M	36	144	2500	41	1.2	17	1.5	1.8	100	3.0	30	800	2.5[k]	7	900	900	175	130	11	8
10-12	F	38	145	2300	40	1.1	15	1.4	1.5	100	3.0	30	800	2.5[k]	7	1000	1000	200	120	11	9
13-15	M	51	162	2800	52	1.4	19	1.7	2.0	200	3.0	30	1000	2.5[k]	9	1200	1200	250	140	13	10
13-15	F	49	159	2200	43	1.1	15	1.4	1.5	200	3.0	30	800	2.5[k]	7	800	800	250	110	14	10
16-18	M	64	172	3200	54	1.6	21	2.0	2.0	200	3.0	30	1000	2.5[k]	10	1000	1000	300	160	14	12
16-18	F	54	161	2100	43	1.1	14	1.3	1.5	200	3.0	30	800	2.5[k]	6	700	700	250	110	14	11

19-35	M	70	176	3000	56	1.5	20	1.8	2.0	200	3.0	30	1000	2.5[k]	9	800	800	300	150	10	10
	F	56	161	2100	41	1.1	14	1.3	1.5	200	3.0	30	800	2.5[k]	6	700	700	250	110	14	9
36-50	M	70	176	2700	56	1.4	18	1.7	2.0	200	3.0	30	1000	2.5[k]	8	800	800	300	140	10	10
	F	56	161	1900	41	1.0	13	1.2	1.5	200	3.0	30	800	2.5[k]	6	700	700	250	100	14	9
51+	M	70	176	2300[b]	56	1.4	18	1.7	2.0	200	3.0	30	1000	2.5[k]	8	800	800	300	140	10	10
	F	56	161	1800[b]	41	1.0	13	1.2	1.5	200	3.0	30	800	2.5[k]	6	700	700	250	100	9	9
Pregnant				+300[c]	+20	+0.2	+2	+0.3	+0.5	+50	+1.0	+20	+100	+2.5[k]	+1	+500	+500	+25	+15	+1[m]	+3
Lactating				+500	+24	+0.4	+7	+0.6	+0.6	+50	+0.5	+30	+400	+2.5[k]	+2	+500	+500	+75	+25	+1[m]	+7

[a] Recommendations assume characteristic activity pattern for each age group.

[b] Recommended energy allowance for age 66+ years reduced to 2000 for men and 1500 for women.

[c] Increased energy allowance recommended during second and third trimesters. An increase of 100 kcal per day is recommended during first trimester.

[d] Recommended protein allowance of 2.2 gm/kg body weight for infants age 0-2 mo. and 2.0 gm/kg body weight for those age 3-5 mo. Protein recommendation for infants, 0-11 mo., assumes consumption of breast milk or protein of equivalent quality.

[e] Approximately 1 mg of niacin is derived from each 60 mg of dietary tryptophan.

[f] Recommendations are based on the estimated average daily protein intake of Canadians.

[g] Recommendation given in terms of free folate.

[h] Considerably higher levels may be prudent for infants during the first week of life to guard against neonatal tyrosinemia.

[i] One μg retinol equivalent (1 μg RE) corresponds to a biological activity in humans equal to 1 μg retinol (3.33 IU) and 6 μg β-carotene (10 IU).

[j] One μg cholecalciferol is equivalent to 40 IU vitamin D activity.

[k] Most older children and adults receive enough vitamin D from irradiation but 2.5 μg daily is recommended. This recommended allowance increases to 5.0 μg daily for pregnant and lactating women and for those who are confined indoors or otherwise deprived of sunlight for extended periods.

[l] The intake of breast-fed infants may be less than the recommendation but is considered to be adequate.

[m] A recommended total intake of 15 mg daily during pregnancy and lactation assumes the presence of adequate stores of iron. If stores are suspected of being inadequate, additional iron as a supplement is recommended.

Table 25.5 RECOMMENDED DAILY INTAKES OF ENERGY AND NUTRIENTS FOR THE UK

Age Range[a]	Occupational Category	Body Weight[c] (kg)	Energy[d] (kcal)	(MJ)[e]	Protein[f] (gm)	Thiamin[g] (mg)	Riboflavin (mg)	Nicotinic Acid (mgeq)[h]	Ascorbic Acid (mg)	Vitamin A (μgRE)[i]	Vitamin D (μg)[j]	Calcium (mg)	Iron (mg)
Boys and Girls													
0 to 1 year[b]		7.3	800	3.3	20	0.3	0.4	5	15	450	10	600[l]	6[i]
1 to 2 years		11.4	1200	5.0	30	0.5	0.6	7	20	300	10	500	7
2 to 3 years		13.5	1400	5.9	35	0.6	0.7	8	20	300	10	500	7
3 to 5 years		16.5	1600	6.7	40	0.6	0.8	9	20	300	10	500	8
5 to 7 years		20.5	1800	7.5	45	0.7	0.9	10	20	300	2.5	500	8
7 to 9 years		25.1	2100	8.8	53	0.8	1.0	11	20	400	2.5	500	10
Boys													
9 to 12 years		31.9	2500	10.5	63	1.0	1.2	14	25	575	2.5	700	13
12 to 15 years		45.5	2800	11.7	70	1.1	1.4	16	25	725	2.5	700	14
15 to 18 years		61.0	3000	12.6	75	1.2	1.7	19	30	750	2.5	600	15
Girls													
9 to 12 years		33.0	2300	9.6	58	0.9	1.2	13	25	575	2.5	700	13
12 to 15 years		48.6	2300	9.6	58	0.9	1.4	16	25	725	2.5	700	14
15 to 18 years		56.1	2300	9.6	58	0.9	1.4	16	30	750	2.3	600	15
Men													
18 to 35 years	Sedentary	65	2700	11.3	68	1.1	1.7	18	30	750	2.5	500	10
	Mod. active		3000	12.6	75	1.2	1.7	18	30	750	2.5	500	10
	Very active		3600	15.1	90	1.4	1.7	18	30	750	2.5	500	10
35 to 65 years	Sedentary	65	2600	10.9	65	1.0	1.7	18	30	750	2.5	500	10
	Mod. active		2900	12.1	73	1.2	1.7	18	30	750	2.5	500	10
	Very active		3600	15.1	90	1.4	1.7	18	30	750	2.5	500	10
65 to 75 years	Assuming a	63	2350	9.8	59	0.9	1.7	18	30	750	2.5	500	10
75 and over	sedentary life	63	2100	8.8	53	0.8	1.7	18	30	750	2.5	500	10

		Body weight (kg)	Energy (kcal)	Energy (MJ)	Protein (g)	Thiamin (mg)	Riboflavin (mg)	Nicotinic acid (mg equiv.)	Vitamin A (μg retinol equiv.)	Vitamin D (μg)	Calcium (mg)	Iron (mg)
Women												
18 to 55 years	Most occupations very active	55	2200	9.2	55	0.9	1.3	15	30	750	2.5	500	12
	Assuming a sedentary life		2500	10.5	63	1.0	1.3	15	30	750	2.5	500	12
55 to 75 years		53	2050	8.6	51	0.8	1.3	15	30	750	2.5	500	10
75 and over		53	1900	8.0	48	0.7	1.3	15	30	750	2.5	500	10
Pregnancy, 2nd & 3rd trimester			2400	10.0	60	1.0	1.6	18	60	750	10[k]	1200[m]	15
Lactation			2700	11.3	68	1.1	1.8	21	60	1200	10	1200	15

From Department of Health and Social Security, *Recommended Intakes of Nutrients for the United Kingdom*, Her Majesty's Stationery Office, London (1969), p. 4.

a The ages are from one birthday to another: 9 to 12 is from the 9th up to, but not including, the 12th birthday. The figures in the table in general refer to the midpoint of the ranges, though those for the range 18 up to 35 refer to the age 25 years, and for the range 18 to 55, to 35 years of age.

b Average figures relating to the first year of life.

c The body weights of children and adolescents are averages and relate to London in 1965. (Taken from Tanner, Whitehouse & Takaishi, 1966; Tables IV A and IV B, 50th centile.) The body weights of adults do not represent average values; they are those of the FAO (1957) reference man and woman, with a nominal reduction for the elderly.

d Average requirements relating to groups of individuals.

e Megajoules (10^6 joules). Calculated from the relation 1 kilocalorie = 4.186 kilojoules, and rounded to 1 decimal place.

f Recommended intakes calculated as providing 10 percent of energy requirements.

g The figures, calculated from energy requirements and the recommended intake of thiamin of 0.4 mg/1000 kcal, relate to groups of individuals.

h Figures given in mg equivalents. 1 nicotinic acid equivalent = 1 mg available nicotinic acid or 60 mg tryptophan.

i Figures given in retinol equivalents. 1 retinol equivalent = 1 μg retinol or 6 μg β-carotene or 12 μg other biologically active carotenoids.

j Figures given in μg cholecalciferol. No dietary source may be necessary for those adequately exposed to sunlight, but the requirement for the housebound may be greater than that recommended.

k For all three trimesters.

l These figures apply to infants who are not breast fed. Infants who are entirely breast fed receive smaller quantities; these are adequate since absorption from breast milk is higher.

m For the third trimester only.

Canadian standards are proposed "as adequate for the maintenance of health among the majority of Canadians." The British standards are defined "as the amounts sufficient or more than sufficient for the nutritional needs for practically all healthy persons in a population." Yet there are major differences in the recommendations for calcium, iron, and ascorbic acid and minor differences for other nutrients. The Canadian and British standards are more similar to each other than either is to those of the United States.

FAO/WHO STANDARDS

The Food and Agriculture Organization (FAO) and World Health Organization (WHO) of the United Nations have established standards for energy, protein, calcium, iron, and several vitamins. These standards are intended for international use and, therefore, for many varied population groups. The standards, with the exception of those for protein and energy, are defined as "recommended intakes," that is, "amounts considered sufficient for the maintenance of health in nearly all people" (FAO/WHO, 1970). The committee responsible for developing protein standards preferred the expression "safe level of intake," which is defined as "the amount of protein considered necessary to meet the physiological needs and maintain the health of nearly all persons in a specified group" (FAO/WHO, 1973). It seems that "safe level of intake" and "recommended intake" are similar in concept and for practical purposes may be considered as different terms for essentially the same standard.

In a somewhat different vein, characteristic of most dietary standards, *energy requirement* is defined as "the energy intake that is considered adequate to meet the energy needs of the average healthy person in a specified category." Thus, some persons will need less and others more than the average requirement.

Energy

Energy requirements represent average requirements and are based on the FAO-originated reference man and woman (FAO, 1957). The reference man and woman as presently described by FAO/WHO are between the ages of 20 and 39 years, moderately active, and weigh 65 kg and 55 kg, respectively.

Table 25.6 ACTIVITY LEVELS AS DEFINED BY FAO/WHO

Light activity

Men: Office workers, most professional men (such as lawyers, doctors, accountants, teachers, architects, etc.), shop workers, unemployed men

Women: Office workers, housewives in houses with mechanical household appliances, teachers, and most other professional women

Moderately active

Men: Most men in light industry, students, building workers (excluding heavy labourers), many farm workers, soldiers not on active service, fishermen

Women: Light industry, housewives without mechanical household appliances, students, department store workers

Very active

Men: Some agricultural workers, unskilled labourers, forestry workers, army recruits and soldiers on active service, mine workers, steel workers

Women: Some farm workers (especially peasant agriculture), dancers, athletes

Exceptionally active

Men: Lumberjacks, blacksmiths, rickshaw-pullers

Women: Construction workers

From FAO/WHO, "Energy and Protein Requirements," *WHO Tech. Rep. Ser.*, No. 522 (1973), p. 25.

The chief factors considered in developing energy requirements were body size and activity. Table 25.6 indicates activity level as defined by FAO/WHO. Average energy requirements as adjusted for activity and body weight are shown in Table 25.7. Finally, energy requirements for all age groups and for the moderately active man and woman are shown in Table 25.8.

Table 25.7 THE EFFECTS OF BODY WEIGHT AND OCCUPATION ON ENERGY REQUIREMENTS

MEN

Body Weight (kg)	Light Activity (kcal)	(MJ)	Moderately Active (kcal)	(MJ)	Very Active (kcal)	(MJ)	Exceptionally Active (kcal)	(MJ)
50	2 100	8.8	2 300	9.6	2 700	11.3	3 100	13.0
55	2 310	9.7	2 530	10.6	2 970	12.4	3 410	14.3
60	2 520	10.5	2 760	11.5	3 240	13.6	3 720	15.6
65	2 700	11.3	3 000	12.5	3 500	14.6	4 000	16.7
70	2 940	12.3	3 220	13.5	3 780	15.8	4 340	18.2
75	3 150	13.2	3 450	14.4	4 050	16.9	4 650	19.5
80	3 360	14.1	3 680	15.4	4 320	18.1	4 960	20.8

WOMEN

Body Weight (kg)	Light Activity (kcal)	(MJ)	Moderately Active (kcal)	(MJ)	Very Active (kcal)	(MJ)	Exceptionally Active (kcal)	(MJ)
40	1 440	6.0	1 600	6.7	1 880	7.9	2 200	9.2
45	1 620	6.8	1 800	7.5	2 120	8.9	2 480	10.4
50	1 800	7.5	2 000	8.4	2 350	9.8	2 750	11.5
55	2 000	8.4	2 200	9.2	2 600	10.9	3 000	12.6
60	2 160	9.0	2 400	10.0	2 820	11.8	3 300	13.8
65	2 340	9.8	2 600	10.9	3 055	12.8	3 575	15.0
70	2 520	10.5	2 800	11.7	3 290	13.8	3 850	16.1

From FAO/WHO, "Energy and Protein Requirements," *WHO Tech. Rep. Ser.*, No. 522 (1973), p. 31.

Protein

As a basis for determining the safe level of intake of protein, egg or milk protein was used as the reference high quality protein. Average requirements for nitrogen were determined by the factorial method that first requires determination of the obligatory losses of nitrogen when a protein-free diet is eaten and, second, the amounts of nitrogen

Table 25.8 ENERGY REQUIREMENTS OF CHILDREN AND ADOLESCENTS BY AGE PERIODS

Age (years)	Body Weight (kg)	Energy per kg per Day		Energy per Person per Day	
		(kcal)	(kJ)	(kcal)	(MJ)
Children					
<1	7.3	112	470	820	3.4
1-3	13.4	101	424	1 360	5.7
4-6	20.2	91	382	1 830	7.6
7-9	28.1	78	326	2 190	9.2
Male adolescents					
10-12	36.9	71	297	2 600	10.9
13-15	51.3	57	238	2 900	12.1
16-19	62.9	49	205	3 070	12.8
Female adolescents					
10-12	38.0	62	259	2 350	9.8
13-15	49.9	50	209	2 490	10.4
16-19	54.4	43	179	2 310	9.7
Adult man (moderately active)	65.0	46	192	3 000	12.6
Adult woman (moderately active)	55.0	40	167	2 200	9.2

From FAO/WHO, "Energy and Protein Requirements," *WHO Tech. Rep. Ser.*, No. 522 (1973), p. 35.

accrued during growth or pregnancy or secreted in milk during lactation. Values so obtained were increased by 30 percent because balance studies have indicated that even high quality protein such as egg or milk is not utilized at 100 percent efficiency. Thus, the amount equivalent to nitrogen losses and growth needs must be increased in order to maintain nitrogen equilibrium in adults and retention in children.

Table 25.9 SAFE LEVELS OF INTAKE OF EGG OR MILK PROTEIN

Age	A Total Nitrogen Requirements—Obligatory Losses and Growth (mg nitrogen per kg per day)		B Adjusted Nitrogen Requirements—Increased by 30% in Accordance with Balance and Growth Data (mg nitrogen per kg per day)		C Safe Level of Intake (adjusted requirements + 30% to allow for individual variability) (mg nitrogen per kg per day)		D (gm protein per kg per day)	
(Months)								
< 3					384[a]		2.40[a]	
3-6					96[a]		1.85[a]	
6-9	154		200		260		1.62	
9-11	136		177		230		1.44	
(Years)								
1	120		156		203		1.27	
2	112		146		190		1.19	
3	106		138		179		1.12	
4	100		130		169		1.06	
5	96		125		162		1.01	
6	92		120		156		0.98	
7	88		114		148		0.92	
8	83		108		140		0.87	
9	80		104		135		0.85	
	M	F	M	F	M	F	M	F
10	78	77	101	100	132	130	0.82	0.81
11	77	72	100	94	130	122	0.81	0.76
12	74	70	96	91	125	118	0.78	0.74
13	73	64	95	83	123	108	0.77	0.68
14	68	59	88	77	115	100	0.72	0.62
15	63	56	82	73	107	95	0.67	0.59
16	61	55	79	71	103	93	0.64	0.58
17	58	54	75	70	98	91	0.61	0.57
Adult	54	49	70	64	91	83	0.57	0.52

From FAO/WHO, "Energy and Protein Requirements," *WHO Tech. Rep. Ser.*, No. 522 (1973), p. 70.

[a]Based on observed intakes (mean + 2 standard deviations) of healthy infants.

Table 25.10 SAFE LEVEL OF PROTEIN IN TERMS OF DIETS OF PROTEIN QUALITIES OF 60%, 70%, AND 80% RELATIVE TO MILK OR EGGS

Age Group	Body Weight (kg)	Safe Level of Protein Intake		Adjusted Level for Proteins of Different Quality (gm per person per day)		
		(gm protein per kg per day)	(gm protein per person per day)	Score[a] 80	Score 70	Score 60
Infants						
6-11 months	9.0	1.53	14	17	20	23
Children						
1-3 years	13.4	1.19	16	20	23	27
4-6 years	20.2	1.01	20	26	29	34
7-9 years	28.1	0.88	25	31	35	41
Male adolescents						
10-12 years	36.9	0.81	30	37	43	50
13-15 years	51.3	0.72	37	46	53	62
16-19 years	62.9	0.60	38	47	54	63
Female adolescents						
10-12 years	38.0	0.76	29	36	41	48
13-15 years	49.9	0.63	31	39	45	52
16-19 years	54.4	0.55	30	37	43	50
Adult man	65.0	0.57	37	46[b]	53[b]	62[b]
Adult woman	55.0	0.52	29	36[b]	41[b]	48[b]
Pregnant woman, latter half of pregnancy			Add 9	Add 11	Add 13	Add 15
Lactating woman, first 6 months			Add 17	Add 21	Add 24	Add 28

From FAO/WHO, "Energy and Protein Requirements," *WHO Tech. Rep. Ser.*, No. 522 (1973), p. 74.

[a]Scores are estimates of the quality of the protein usually consumed relative to that of egg or milk. The safe level of protein intake is adjusted by multiplying it by 100 divided by the score of the food protein. For example, 100/60 = 1.67, and for a child of 1-4 years the safe level of protein intake would be 16 x 1.67, or 27 gm of protein having a relative quality of 60.

[b]The correction may overestimate adult protein requirements.

For any average value, some individuals will require more and some less. In order to correct for individual variation, a value of 30 percent above the average was taken to cover the needs of the majority of the population. This figure is twice the coefficient of variation of 15 percent for the protein requirements for maintenance and growth. Nitrogen requirement as determined by obligatory nitrogen losses, adjusted nitrogen requirement, and safe levels of egg or milk protein are shown in Table 25.9. For infants below 6 months of age, no figure is listed for obligatory nitrogen losses. The requirement for the very young infant was based on average intakes of breast milk.

Because neither all foods nor mixed diets approach the quality of egg or milk protein, a further correction for safe level of protein may be necessary. Table 25.10 lists the total protein intake calculated when protein score is 80, 70, or 60 (see Chapter 23). Thus, as the quality of dietary protein decreases, the amount of protein needed to provide a safe level of intake increases.

Calcium

Calcium needs are defined by FAO/WHO in terms of dietary intakes known to be compatible with health and attainable in many areas of the world. Recommended levels are considerably lower than those of the RDA but are similar to those of Canada, the United Kingdom and many other countries (Table 25.11).

Table 25.11 PRACTICAL ALLOWANCES FOR CALCIUM (FAO)

Age	Practical Allowance
	mg/day
0-12 months[a]	500-600
1-9 years	400-500
10-15 years	600-700
16-19 years	500-600
Adult	400-500

Adapted from FAO/WHO, "Calcium Requirements," WHO Tech. Rep. Ser. 230, (1962).
[a]Artificially fed only.

Allowances of 1000-1200 mg are recommended for pregnant and lactating women.

Iron

Recommended intakes for iron were based on physiological losses from the body and increments in body iron during growth. These intakes are intended to maintain iron stores of 500 mg or more in healthy adults. The recommendations were derived from estimates of the highest amounts of iron that would be absorbed from three types of diets varying in proportions of foods of animal origin (Table 25.12). As the proportion of animal protein increases, absorption of iron increases, thus necessitating a lower level of dietary iron. Recommended daily intakes for age-group categories are shown in Table 25.13. Iron needs of pregnant and lactating women with adequate body iron stores of about 500 mg are presumed to be similar to those of nonpregnant, nonlactating women of childbearing age. For women with no iron stores, however, the absorbed iron requirement during the second half of pregnancy could be as high as 6.6 mg to cover basal loss as well as increase in red cell mass and losses to fetus and placenta. This amounts to 33-66 mg of dietary iron, depending upon the percent of intake absorbed, and would require supplementation.

Table 25.12   ABSORPTION OF IRON FROM DIETS CONTAINING
DIFFERENT PROPORTIONS OF FOODS OF
ANIMAL ORIGIN

Type of Diet	Assumed Upper Limit of Iron Absorption by Normal Individuals (percent)
Less than 10% of calories from foods of animal origin	10
10-25% of calories from foods of animal origin	15
More than 25% of calories from foods of animal origin	20

From FAO/WHO, "Requirements of Ascorbic Acid, Vitamin D, Vitamin B_{12}, Folate, and Iron," *FAO Nutr. Mtg. Rep.*, Rep. Ser. No. 47, (1970), p. 50.

Table 25.13 RECOMMENDED DAILY INTAKES OF IRON

		Absorbed Iron Required (mg)	Recommended Intake According to Type of Diet Proportion of Animal Foods		
			Below 10% of Calories	10-25% of Calories	Over 25% of Calories
Infants	0-4 months	0.5	[a]	[a]	[a]
	5-12 months	1.0	10	7	5
Children	1-12 years	1.0	10	7	5
Boys	13-16 years	1.8	18	12	9
Girls	13-16 years	2.4	24	18	12
Menstruating women[b]		2.8	28	19	14
Men		0.9	9	6	5
Pregnancy		see text			
Lactation					

Adapted from FAO/WHO, "Requirements of Ascorbic Acid, Vitamin D, Vitamin B_{12}, Folate, and Iron," *FAO Nutr. Mtg. Rep.*, Ser. No. 47, (1970), p. 54.

[a]Breast-feeding is assumed to be adequate.
[b]For non-menstruating women the recommended intakes are the same as for men.

Table 25.14 RECOMMENDED INTAKES FOR VITAMINS (FAO/WHO)

	Ascorbic[a] Acid (mg)	Vitamin D[a] (IU)	Vitamin B_{12}[a] (µg)	"Free"[a] Folate (µg)	Vitamin A[b] (µg retinol)
0-6 months	c	400	0.3	40	a
7-12 months	20	400	0.3	60	300
1-6 years	20	400	0.9-1.5	100	250-300
7-12 years	20	100	1.5-2.0	100	400-575
13 years and over	30	100	2.0	200	725-750
Pregnancy	30[d]	400	3.0	400	750
Lactation	30[d]	400	2.5	300	750

[a] Figures taken from FAO/WHO, "Requirements of Ascorbic Acid, Vitamin D, Vitamin B_{12}, Folate, and Iron (1970).
[b] Figures taken from FAO/WHO, "Requirements of Vitamin A, Thiamin, Riboflavin, and Niacin" (1967).
[c] These intakes are best met by breast-feeding from a well-nourished mother.
[d] Figures taken from FAD, "Handbook of Human Nutritional Requirements" (1974).

Vitamins

Recommended intakes for ascorbic acid, vitamin D, vitamin B_{12}, "free" folate, and vitamin A are shown in Table 25.14. Because individual vitamin intakes were not always given for the same age categories (see FAO/WHO 1967, 1970), an arbitrary regrouping has been made and some vitamin levels, therefore, are expressed in ranges. Folacin is listed as "free" folate, which does not take into account variances in capacity to absorb folate conjugates in foods (as do the RDA).

Thiamin, riboflavin, and niacin intakes are expressed in terms of caloric intake and are 0.4 mg, 0.55 mg, and 6.6 niacin equivalents respectively per 1000 kcal. Total intakes, therefore, are determined by energy intakes for all age categories (including pregnancy and lactation).[1]

OTHER DIETARY STANDARDS

Dietary standards have been established by many other countries including Australia, Norway, Holland, South Africa, Philippines, Japan, Central America and Panama, Columbia, Guatemala, USSR, and India. It is not practical to include all of the existing standards here. Table 25.15 includes protein and energy standards for women for eight countries for purposes of comparison. A thorough examination of the four standards presented should emphasize the limitations of present knowledge concerning human nutrient requirements and the divergence of opinion as to the interpretation of experimental data and how these data should be applied in improving the nutrition of population groups.

SUMMARY

Dietary standards are necessary and useful tools and are a means through which the science of nutrition can be applied for the im-

---

[1] Addendum, in press. For a compilation of FAO/WHO recommended daily nutrient intakes, see Food and Agriculture Organization of the United Nations, "Handbook on Nutritional Requirements," FAO, Rome, 1974, 66 pp.

Table 25.15 PROTEIN AND ENERGY ALLOWANCES FOR WOMEN IN VARIOUS COUNTRIES

Country	Body Weight (kg)	Protein[a] (gm/day)					Energy (kcal/day)	
		Non-pregnant (per kg)	Added for Pregnancy[b]	Total	Non-pregnant (per kg)	Added for Pregnancy[b]	Total
Australia, 1965	58	1.00	8	66	36	150	2250
Canada, 1974[c]	56	0.73	20	61	38	300	2400
Colombia, 1955	55	1.09	12	72	36	200	2200
Guatemala, 1969	55	1.18	10	75	36	200	2200
India, 1968	45	1.00	10	55	49	300	2500
Philippines, 1970	49	1.12	10	65	39	400	2300
United Kingdom, 1969	55	1.00	5	60	40	200	2400
United States, 1974[c]	58	0.8	30	76	36	300	2300

From D. H. Calloway, *Nutrition and Fetal Development*, Vol. 2, M. Winick, ed., Wiley, N.Y., 1974, pp. 79.

[a]Includes correction for assumed 60 to 70% net protein utilization.
[b]Standard allowance irrespective of body weight.
[c]Canadian and United States Allowances recalculated for 1974 revisions.

provement of human health. Standards serve as guides in planning dietaries, in evaluating food consumption of population groups, and in devising rational plans for maintaining an adequate food supply. They are never static but are assessed periodically and revised as new data become available. Standards differ among nations and reflect, in part, the needs of the population group for which they are intended and, in part, the philosophy of those who establish the standards.

chapter 26

nutrition surveys

1. Contributory Information
   a. Agricultural Data. Food
      Balance Sheets
   b. Vital and Health Statistics
2. Dietary Surveys
   a. Household Food
      Consumption
      1. Food Account
      2. Food List
      3. Food Record
      4. Weighed Household
         Consumption
      5. Summary
   b. Individual Food
      Consumption
      1. Estimation by Recall
      2. Food Record
      3. Weighed Intake
      4. Diet History
      5. Summary
   c. Calculation and Interpre-
      tation of Dietary Intake
   d. Summary
3. Biochemical Evaluation of
   Nutritional Status
4. Clinical Evaluation of
   Nutritional Status
5. Correlation of Dietary,
   Biochemical, and Clinical Data

"Well in our country," said Alice, still panting a little, "you'd generally get to somewhere else—if you ran very fast for a long time as we've been doing."

"A slow sort of country!" said the Queen. "Now here, you see, it takes all the running you can do, to keep in the same place. If you want to get somewhere else, you must run at least twice as fast as that!"

Lewis Carroll, *Through the Looking-Glass*

A nutrition survey is similar to any other community survey in that its goal is to define a population in terms of specific factors. It is epidemiological in nature and, in this respect, it is designed to identify the extent and distribution of malnutrition. The survey is the chief but not the only means of providing information necessary for the planning of realistic nutrition programs consistent with the needs and habits of a community and for evaluating the effect of nutrition programs already existing within a community. There are other less direct means for obtaining a fair concept of the nutritional status of population groups, but the survey as usually conducted has the advantage of providing the kind of quantitative data necessary to convince legislators (and the public) to support and encourage direct action programs for the benefit of the public health.

The classic methods for the determination of nutritional status yield three kinds of evaluative data: (1) dietary, (2) biochemical, and (3) clinical. The three methods measure different states of nutriture and therefore do not necessarily correlate with each other. It is generally agreed that the dietary surveys evaluate current food intake, biochemical data reflect recent nutritional status, and clinical examinations evaluate long-term nutritional history. Any one or combination of the three methods may be used in survey studies, but there is no question that interpretation of results becomes more difficult as the number of evaluative criteria increase. Perhaps surveys, more than any other kind of nutritional studies, help to remind investigators of the limitations of the procedures presently available for the evaluation of human nutritional status and of the variability inherent within the human race. In spite of the limitations, however, useful data can be obtained that *grossly* define the nutritional status of *groups* of people.

CONTRIBUTORY INFORMATION

Certain kinds of accessory information provide indications of nutritional status and should be investigated prior to or at the same time as a population survey. These factors have been elegantly summarized in a WHO publication (1963a) and are shown in Table 26.1. The table is self-explanatory and only two of the factors will be commented on here. Clearly, an investigator working in unfamiliar territory should become as familiar as possible with all factors that could influence nutrition and food habits if he is to logically plan a nutrition survey within a community. Such information often may be obtained through the study of agricultural and health records as well as any available literature describing the cultural and sociological aspects of the community.

Agricultural Data. Food Balance Sheets.

The FAO has developed food balance sheets for many countries that relate agricultural production and import and export data to arrive at a presumptive figure grossly approximating the amount of food available to a population. Similarly, the astute nutritionist or medical worker can learn much of the general nutritional status of a population by studying available agricultural records. Such data can be valuable in roughly estimating the presence or absence of widespread malnutrition, but they obviously provide no information on the distribution of available food within the different segments of the population.

Vital and Health Statistics

Mortality and morbidity ratios are affected by many factors including environmental conditions of sanitation and the extent of immunization and medical care; infants are especially vulnerable to environ-

Table 26.1 INFORMATION NEEDED FOR ASSESSMENT OF NUTRITIONAL STATUS

Sources of Information	Nature of Information Obtained	Nutritional Implications
1. Agricultural data Food balance sheets	Gross estimates of agricultural production Agricultural methods Soil fertility Predominance of cash crops Overproduction of staples Food imports and exports	Approximate availability of of food supplies to a population
2. Socioeconomic data Information on marketing, distribution, and storage	Purchasing power Distribution and storage of foodstuffs	Unequal distribution of available foods between the socioeconomic groups in the community and within the family
3. Food consumption patterns Cultural-anthropological data	Lack of knowledge, erroneous beliefs, prejudices, and indifference	
4. Dietary surveys	Food consumption	Low, excessive, or unbalanced nutrient intake
5. Special studies on foods	Biological value of diets Presence of interfering factors (e.g., goitrogens) Effects of food processing	Special problems related to nutrient utilization
6. Vital and health statistics	Morbidity and mortality data	Extent of risk to community Identification of high-risk groups
7. Anthropometric studies	Physical development	Effect of nutrition on physical development
8. Clinical nutritional surveys	Physical signs	Deviation from health due to malnutrition
9. Biochemical studies	Levels of nutrients, metabolites, and other components of body tissues and fluids	Nutrient supplies in the body Impairment of biochemical function
10. Additional medical information	Prevalent disease patterns, including infections and infestations	Interrelationships of state of nutrition and disease

From WHO Report of Expert Committee on Medical Assessment of Nutritional Status, *Tech. Rpt. Series No. 258* (1963a).

mental stresses and neglect. There is evidence suggesting that the high mortality rate observed among children 1 to 4 years of age in many areas of the world is the result of malnutrition as well as infectious disease. Scrimshaw and Behar (1958) reported that deaths that had been attributed to diarrhea or parasitic infection among children under 5 years of age in a Central American community were, in fact, caused by or associated with malnutrition. It is generally accepted that the mortality rate in the preschool age range of 1 to 4 years may serve as a rough index of malnutrition in a community (Wills and Waterlow, 1958).

The occurrence of high mortality rates in a community therefore suggests that for each child who dies in early life, many others live who are being handicapped by incipient malnutrition (see Chapter 21). Unfortunately, accurate health and vital statistics are not available in all countries, and even when statistics are available, the investigator can estimate only that a nutritional problem exists. The identification of the problem requires more definitive evaluation.

DIETARY SURVEYS

Just as the first organized attempts to develop dietary standards came as a result of the work of the League of Nations Technical Commission on Nutrition, so did the first organized efforts to evaluate the nutritional status of population groups. Bigwood's *Guiding Principles for Studies on the Nutrition of Populations* (1939) is a classic in the area of nutrition surveys, and although many of the details of procedure and methodology have been extended, improved, or replaced, the basic approach and philosophy are essentially the same today as they were nearly 40 years ago.

Dietary surveys may be planned to determine food consumption of families or of individuals. Family food consumption or household consumption, as it is more appropriately called, is an estimate of the total amount of food consumed by an entire household for a fixed period of time, usually one week. The most commonly used methods are the food account, food list, and food record.

Household Food Consumption

Food Account. The food account is a record of all food purchased or produced for family consumption over a period of several weeks. The length of time depends on the complexity of the diet since no record is made of food already in the household or of that remaining at the end of the study period. When the diet is relatively monotonous or few food supplies are routinely stored in the home, a period of two weeks is often satisfactory since under these conditions food purchases tend to represent food consumed within a brief period of time. A family that relies upon a well-stocked freezer to provide a large portion of the weekly food intake is not well suited to this type of study. For this reason, the method is almost never used in the United States and has been used chiefly in areas where the diet is less complex than that of the average American family.

Food List. The food list is essentially a recall method. The homemaker is asked to estimate the quantity of food consumed by the entire household during the previous week by weight, retail unit, or household measure. The method requires a well-trained interviewer who can help the homemaker recall by daily menu or purchases all food consumed by the household. The food list is advantageous in that only one visit to the household is necessary; because it requires little time and effort on the part of the homemaker, cooperation usually is good.

The food list method is used for many of the food consumption surveys conducted by the United States Department of Agriculture and most often is the basis for the per capita food consumption data published by the Department. Accuracy of the food list is judged to be satisfactory for this purpose; errors tend to be due to omission of food items or incorrect estimation of amounts of food consumed.

Food Record. This method involves a weighed inventory of foods at the beginning and close of the study period, usually one week, together with a day-by-day record by weight of food brought into the home during the week. Records of plate and kitchen wastes are sometimes, but not always, included. The method is time consuming and therefore more expensive than the food list. At least two visits to the home are required of the interviewer and considerably more time is demanded of the homemaker. Accuracy of the method is relatively high although it is generally believed that the food list is an equally satisfactory and much less expensive means for obtaining household food consumption data.

Weighed Household Consumption. In some cases it is both feasible and advisable to obtain household food consumption by daily weighing of food prepared and served in the home. This method usually requires that an investigator be present in the home at the time that food is prepared. The method has the advantage of providing more precise information than can be obtained by recall or record. It is perhaps the best approach to use in rural or small village situations where much food is obtained from home gardens or local barter and where retail measures or weights are uncertain. However, the method requires a greater investment in time and personnel than other techniques and is seldom used unless it is certain that data of comparable validity cannot be obtained by other means.

Summary.   Surveys of household food consumption are designed to yield essentially two kinds of data: economic consumption, that is, the monetary value of food entering the home or food available for consumption; and/or physiological consumption, food actually eaten by the family. In any case, certain kinds of accessory information must be obtained, such as the number of individuals usually fed from the family food supply, the number of meals eaten away from home, and the number of guests entertained during the study period. The accuracy of the calculation of per capita intake depends on these factors as well as on the composition of the family unit. Formulas taking into consideration family composition by age and the number of meals eaten in and out of the home have been proposed (Francois, 1970; Cresta, 1970).

If wastes from purchased and prepared foods are ignored, food consumption data represent economic but not physiological consumption. For this reason, economic food consumption, such as the per capita food supply data, tends to be higher than physiological consumption (See Call, 1965). In either case, data on family food consumption yield no information on the distribution of food within the family.

Details of these methods may be found in several publications (Norris, 1949; NRC, 1949; Reh, 1962; FAO, 1964).

Individual Food Consumption

Evaluation of individual nutritional status leading to identification of vulnerable groups within a population group requires study of food actually consumed by a given individual. Four methods are commonly used to determine individual food consumption: estimation by recall, food record, dietary history, and weighed intake.

Estimation by Recall. Recall of food intake is almost always for a 24-hour period only, and for this reason it is generally designated the 24-hour recall. The subject is asked to recall all food consumed during the previous day and to estimate quantities in ordinary measures or servings. In order to increase accuracy of quantities of food consumed, the subject may be provided with measuring cups or other devices to aid in estimation. Information obtained by this method obviously is not necessarily representative of usual intake of an individual. The method, therefore, is most useful when relatively large numbers of subjects are involved and provides a qualitative rather than a quantitative description of group dietary patterns. As a rough evaluation of food habits, however, the 24-hour recall can serve as a basis for educational programs or gross evaluation of dietary intake of large groups. It is not valid as an accurate measure of food intake of *one* individual. When large numbers of subjects are involved, the method is considered to be indicative of the dietary pattern characteristic of the group. Because of ease of obtaining data, the 24-hour recall has gained in usage.

Food Record. This method requires that the subject keep a record of food eaten for varying lengths of time, usually 3 to 7 days. Quantities of food are estimated in common household measures; occasionally the subject may be asked to measure his food intake. Accuracy of the method depends largely on the diligence and integrity of the subject and, when food is not measured, on his ability to estimate quantities of food. The method appears to be a fairly accurate estimate of food consumption *over a specific period of time.*

Weighed Intake. A very accurate record of food consumption may be obtained by having a subject or a trained person weigh all food consumed during a given period of time. This method of obtaining food consumption data is obviously expensive and time consuming and consequently is rarely used in nutrition surveys. In spite of the accuracy of data obtained on quantities of food consumed, the method is limited in other ways. Because of the tediousness of the procedure, subjects are prone to try to find shortcuts and thus to change from their usual eating patterns.

The weighed food intake, however, is standard procedure in a laboratory-controlled metabolic study and, although a few surveys have involved weighed data, this method most often is limited to research studies. Under these circumstances, it is the researcher rather than the subject who bears the burden of tedium.

Diet History. The diet history is designed to discover the *usual* food intake pattern over a relatively long period of time and is most often obtained by interview. A series of food records kept at intervals over a period of months or years yields data comparable to the diet history but obviously is a more expensive procedure both in terms of time and personnel. The diet history is often used for studies of food habits or in clinics or hospital dietetics. Burke (1947), however, devised a method for calculation of diet histories and for their use as research tools.

The research dietary history has the disadvantage of requiring highly skilled interviewers in order to obtain useful data. Quantitative significance of the data, however, has been questioned, and in unskilled hands, the history may yield erroneous information (Maynard, 1950). When properly conducted, it has an advantage over other methods in that it relates food intake over a relatively long period of time. The method measures frequency of intake of a large number of foods or groups of foods and thus smooths out seasonal variations in food intake.

As originally devised by Burke, the diet history method is rather time consuming. A modification of the history applicable to epidemiological studies involving thousands of subjects has been described by Stefanick and Trulson (1962). The method requires less time than the diet history and is regarded as a qualitative estimation of frequency of food intake. Mann et al. (1962) have described a similar modification of the Burke dietary history in which the procedure was restricted to a selection of nutrients pertinent to the problem under study. The diet history and modifications of the history technique appear to be especially useful in epidemiological studies, in which interest is directed toward the usual food pattern over a period of several years.

Summary. Since all known methods for obtaining dietary data have certain advantages as well as limitations, the choice of method should depend on the population sample to be surveyed and the specific use for which the data are intended. Flores (1962), for example, has pointed out some differences in collection of dietary information in nonmodernized societies as compared to modernized communities. For further discussion of the advantages and disadvantages of methods for obtaining individual food consumption see Young et al. (1952), Chalmers et al. (1952), Trulson and McCann (1959), Adelson (1960), Cellier and Hankin, (1963), Pekkarinen (1970), Balogh et al. (1971), and Marr (1971).

In addition to the choice of method, the investigator must decide how the collected data will be handled. He may need to know only the general pattern of food intake or he may need to know the range of nutrient intake for a population and the specific food groups from which nutrients are obtained. In certain epidemiological studies, the pattern of eating throughout the day may be as important as total nutrient intake. Furthermore, the consumption of food in commercial establishments and the use of highly processed convenience foods in the home have increased. It will, most likely, become important to assess the contribution of food consumed from these sources and their effect upon total nutrient intake.

Calculation and Interpretation of Dietary Intake

The laborious computation of nutrient intake from food records is familiar to every student of nutrition. Calculation of dietaries, however, has been greatly simplified by the use of computers. Tullis et al. (1965), Hankins et al. (1965), and Moe et al. (1970) have discussed computer calculations for a number of purposes; surveys, hospital and clinic records, institution dietaries, and so forth. All foods listed in *Handbook 8* are provided with code numbers for use in computer calculations, and methods for coding and preparing coded data for analysis are described in a publication of the United States Department of Agriculture (Davenport, 1964).

When the diet is complex and consists of many mixed food dishes, accurate calculation is difficult and depends on having a detailed description of the dish and, if possible, the recipe used by the homemaker in preparation. Merrill et al. (1966) have described methods for calculating mixed dishes from home-prepared foods; methods also are described by the ICNND (1963).

Several short methods for the calculation of dietary intake have been described (Leichsenring and Wilson, 1951; Clark and Cofer, 1962). Foods similar in nutritive content are grouped together, and average values are used to calculate nutritive content of foods included in each group. Results obtained by these shortened procedures tend to agree rather well with the more detailed dietary calculations when large samples are involved. A short procedure described by Mann et al. (1962) was designed for the Framingham epidemiological study relating environmental and other factors to incidence of heart disease. This was aimed at identifying dietary intake as high, medium, or low in regard to specific nutrients. The accuracy of the procedure appeared to be high since even after a lapse of two years, dietary intake obtained from a second dietary history almost always fell into the same general category (Dawber et al., 1962). This type of procedure appears to have special merit for epidemiological studies in which interest is centered both upon specific dietary components and the relation of diet over a long period of time to a specific health problem. The gross identification of dietary intake as high, medium, or low appears to be a reasonable approach to interpretation of data from nutritional status studies as well. Even the most precise mathematical manipulations cannot remove the sources of error inherent both in the methods for collecting data and in the food tables from which these data are calculated; therefore the use of numerical values in describing food intakes often implies a degree of accuracy that does not actually exist.

The limitations of tables of food composition in evaluating dietary intakes have been subject to both discussion and investigation (Toscani, 1948; Mayer, 1960; Eagles et al., 1966). In addition to the wide variation in nutrient content of foods in the raw state due to differences in cultivation, harvesting, and storage, there is a paucity of data on commercially prepared and processed foods and on nutrient losses during preparation and cooking. Clearly, however, tremendous variation exists in methods of food preparation in the home, and this is particularly true in the case of mixed dishes. For these reasons, differences between calculated values and values obtained by laboratory analyses of meals and individual mixed dishes may be considerable and thus confirm the suspicion that calculated values may not represent the actual nutrient value of food consumed.

In a study of nutritive values of weighed school lunches, calculated data compared well with analytical values for energy, protein, fat, and calcium; however, values for thiamin and ascorbic acid were higher and for riboflavin lower than those obtained by chemical analysis (Meyer et al., 1951). The close agreement for the more stable nutrients likely was influenced by the extent of detailed

Table 26.2 GUIDE TO INTERPRETATION OF NUTRIENT INTAKE DATA

Kcal Standards		Protein Standards	
Age	Kcal/Kg Body Weight	Age	Gm Protein/Kg Body Weight
0-1 month	120	0-11 months	2.2
2-5 months	110		
6-11 months	100	12-23 months	1.9
12-23 months	90		
24-47 months	86	24-47 months	1.7
48-71 months	82		
6-7 years	82	48-71 months	1.5
8-9 years	82		
10-12 years		6-9 years	1.3
Male	68	10-16 years	1.2
Female	64		
13-16 years		17-19 years	1.1
Male	60		
Female	48	20 years and over	1.0

For 2nd and 3rd trimesters of pregnancy, increase basic standard 20 gm.
For lactating, increase basic standard 25 gm.

Kcal Standards (cont.)		Calcium Standards	
17-19 years		Age	Mg/Day
Male	44	0-11 months	550
Female	35		
20-29 years		12-71 months	450
Male	40		
Female	35	6-9 years	450
30-39 years			
Male	38	10-12 years	650
Female	33		
40-49 years		13-16 years	650
Male	37		
Female	31	17-19 years	550
50-59 years			
Male	36	Adults	400
Female	30		
60-69 years			
Male	34		
Female	29		
>70 years			
Male	34		
Female	29		

For 2nd and 3rd trimesters of pregnancy, increase basic standard 200 kcal.
For lactating, increase basic standard 1000 kcal.

For 3rd trimester of pregnancy, increase standard 400 mg.
For lactating, increase standard 500 mg.

Table 26.2   (continued)

Vitamin B Standards

Age	Thiamin	Riboflavin	Niacin
For all age groups including adults	0.4 mg/ 1000 kcal	0.55 mg/ 1000 kcal	6.6 mg/ 1000 kcal

Iron Standards

Age	Mg/Day
0-11 months	10
12-47 months	15
48-71 months	10
6-9 years	10
10-12 years	
Male	10
Female	18
13-19 years	
Male	18
Female	18
20 years and over	
Male	10
Female (to 55)	18
Female (55 on)	10

Vitamin A Standards

Age	International Units
0-1 month	1,500
2-5 months	1,500
6-11 months	1,500
12-23 months	2,000
24-47 months	2,000
48-71 months	2,000
6-7 years	2,500
8-9 years	2,500
10-12 years	2,500
>12 years	3,500

For lactating, increase standard 1000 IU.

Vitamin C Standards (ascorbic acid)

All age groups	30 mg/day

From U.S. Department of Health, Education and Welfare, Publication No. (HSM) 72-8133 (N.D.)

information obtainable under institutional methods of preparation. Harris (1962) found that analyzed values for a number of nutrients of foods prepared in the home were 5-30 percent lower than values calculated from food tables. Whiting and Leverton (1960) reported close agreement between calculated and analyzed values for protein, but fat content was overestimated in nearly 50 percent of cases studied. Undoubtedly, the variation reported depends upon the nature of the diet as well as the tables used for calculation and the analytical methods employed. Buzina et al. (1971) reported analyzed values for riboflavin 50-80 percent higher than calculated values when meals were analyzed by a chemical method but close agreement when a microbiological method was used. For thiamin, analyzed and calculated values agreed most closely when computed data were based on results of analyses of local foods rather than upon averages from food tables.

A guide for the evaluation of dietary intakes was developed for use in a nutrition survey of ten states by the Nutrition Section of the U. S. Department of Health, Education and Welfare (referred to as the Ten State Nutrition Survey). These data are shown in Table 26.2. (The Nutrition Section now is administered under the Center for Disease Control, HEW. Formerly, it was known as the Inter-departmental Committee on Nutrition for National Defense and was affiliated with the Office of International Research.) This survey is one of the most comprehensive thus far attempted in this country. The standards for evaluation of dietary data were developed by an ad hoc committee and are based on the Recommended Dietary Allowances (1968) and FAO/WHO standards (See Chapter 25). The standards developed for energy, protein, and iron are approximately the same as the RDA although energy and protein are expressed in terms of body weight for all age groups. Calcium, vitamin A, and ascorbic acid standards are lower than the RDA and are similar to the FAO/WHO standards. which were considered to be more realistic for evaluation of dietary data. Thiamin, riboflavin, and niacin are expressed in relation to energy intake as are those of FAO/WHO; absolute values, however, are similar to those of the RDA. Standards for pregnancy and lactation were adapted from the RDA.

Summary

Proper interpretation of dietary data requires a sound knowledge of dietary requirements and an appreciation of the errors inherent in the methods for collecting and analyzing the data. One cannot depreciate the value of survey data as an *indication* of nutritional status, but there is little virtue in assigning to such data an accuracy that cannot possibly pertain. The human being is a highly variable creature, and the human living in an uncontrolled community setting is even more variable. There are many pitfalls in the study of population groups, and they should be recognized. For a compilation of nutritional status and dietary evaluation studies conducted in the United States between 1957 and 1967, see Kelsay (1969).

BIOCHEMICAL EVALUATION OF NUTRITIONAL STATUS

Data accumulated on human response to diet under controlled conditions, that is, metabolic studies, have been used to establish standards for evaluation of the nutritional status of population groups. Biochemical tests for appraisal of nutritional status, however, have usually been selected on the basis of simplicity of the analytical procedure. Sensitivity of the method has, perhaps, too often been of secondary concern. When the study sample is large and the objective of the study is to identify nutritional problems of possible public health significance, emphasis is on the group rather than the individual. Under these circumstances, the approach is to select the most practical method that will yield useful data.

Methods applicable to the biochemical appraisal of nutritional status have been reviewed by Lowry (1952), Pearson (1962), Sauberlich et al. (1973) among others. Analytical procedures are described in the ICNND manual (1963) and in a compilation by Consolazio (1951). Micromethods that require only a few drops of blood obtained by fingerprick have been described by Lowry and Bessey (1945); they are suitable for the study of some nutrients. Highly sensitive microbiological methods also have been described (Baker and Frank, 1968) and have been applied in survey studies (Baker et al., 1967; Christakis et al., 1968). Various modifications and new methodologies also have been recently described, including a modified thiochrome procedure for determination of urinary thiamin (Leveille, 1972), enzymatic measurement of riboflavin status (Sauberlich et al., 1971; Tillotson and Baker, 1971), and an evaluation of several methods for measuring pyridoxine status in the human (Sauberlich et al., 1972a).

Just as biochemical analyses are limited primarily to blood and excreta in human metabolic studies, so are analyses for surveys limited to blood and urine. Collection of urine samples obviously presents more problems than blood. A 24-hour sample rarely can be obtained and investigators are fortunate if they can obtain a timed sample over a period of 4 or 6 hours. Most often a single voided sample is analyzed and may be a fasting sample collected in the morning before any food is eaten, or a random sample, taken at any time during the day. Excretion data from single samples are expressed in relation to creatinine content of the same sample on the assumption that creatinine excretion is relatively constant and thus can serve as a basis for equating excretion data from different individuals. This method is generally accepted for practical purposes but is acknowledged to be limited by vagaries of creatinine and nutrient excretions (Edwards et al., 1969; Pollack, 1970). Hair has been proposed as a possible tissue for analysis for zinc (Klevay, 1970a) and copper (Klevay, 1970b). The value of such tests for nutrition surveys has not yet been adequately tested.

The techniques most commonly used in surveys are measurements of thiamin, riboflavin, and N'-methylnicotinamide in urine; and hemoglobin, vitamin A, carotene, and ascorbic acid in blood (see ICNND, 1963). With the exception of carotene, the validity of these tests appears to be relatively high in terms of identifying nutritional problems within a population. Data on serum carotene apparently are traditionally collected but rarely yield useful information. Iodine in urine was also determined in the National Nutrition Survey in order to correlate these data with clinical evidence of goiter in the American population.

Serum proteins are often determined although it is generally conceded that these data are less definitive than some other measurements. The determination of essential and nonessential amino acid ratio in plasma (Swendseid, 1963; McLaughlan, 1963; Whitehead and Dean, 1964; Arroyave, 1970) and urea nitrogen/creatinine ratio in urine (Arroyave, 1962) appear to be useful tools for evaluation of protein nutritional status. Measurement of the prealbumin fraction of plasma proteins (Ingenbleek, 1972) and examination of hair roots (Bradfield, 1972) are more recent additions to proposed procedures for assessment of protein-calorie malnutrition. Microtechniques for the automated analysis of serum total protein and albumin, urinary urea, creatinine, and hydroxyproline have been described for use in developing countries (Coward et al., 1971). The sensitivity of the hydroxyproline/creatinine index in urine as proposed by Whitehead (1967) as well as the examination of buccal smears (Squires, 1965) remain questionable.

Guides for interpretation of data on urinary excretion of riboflavin, thiamin, N'-methylnicotinamide, and iodine, and for blood hematocrit, hemoglobin, iron transferrin saturation, serum proteins, serum vitamin A, carotene, ascorbic acid, and folic acid are shown in Table 26.3 (see O'Neal et al., 1970). The rationale behind these standards has been discussed by Plough and Bridgeforth (1960), Pearson (1962, 1967) and Wilson et al. (1964). It is interesting that the interpretation of biochemical measurements has changed little in the last 30 years (see Bessey and Lowry, 1945; NRC, 1949). Special problems in the biochemical assessment of nutritional status during pregnancy evolved from the Vanderbilt study of pregnant women (Darby et al., 1948; Dawson et al., 1969), and it is clear that standards for pregnant and nonpregnant women differ. More data are needed on the biochemical evaluation of nutritional status of young children.

CLINICAL EVALUATION OF NUTRITIONAL STATUS

The physical examination of subjects was the earliest means of evaluating nutritional status since knowledge of the nutrients evolved from the observation of deficiency symptoms. Clinical evaluation, however, is by far the most subjective area in the determination of nutritional status, and for this reason it is recommended that all clinical evaluations be conducted by one physician trained in recognition of deficiency symptoms. When the number of subjects is so large that more than one examining physician is needed, best results are obtained if physicians are trained in a group. In spite of all precautions, however, physicians are people, and people are prone to subjectivity, so clinical data must be scrutinized carefully with the human error in mind.

Whereas the dietary survey is indicative of current food intake and biochemical analysis of relatively recent food intake, the clinical examination is more apt to reflect the result of long-term nutritional status. Scars of early skin lesions and mild skeletal deformities, for example, provide evidence of earlier deprivation even when present diet appears adequate. Clinical lesions, moreover, may be influenced by other factors, such as intestinal parasites or infection, which influence absorption and metabolism of nutrients independent of

Table 26.3 GUIDELINES FOR CLASSIFICATION AND INTER-
PRETATION OF GROUP BLOOD AND URINE DATA
COLLECTED AS PART OF THE TEN STATE NUTRI-
TION SURVEY

| | Classification Category | | |
| | Less than Acceptable | | |
Determination	Deficient	Low	Acceptable[a]
Hemoglobin, gm/100 ml			
6-23 months	< 9.0	9.0-9.9	≧10.0
2-5 yr	<10	10.0-10.9	≧11.0
6-12 yr	<10	10.0-11.4	≧11.5
13-16 yr, male	<12	12.0-12.9	≧13.0
13-16 yr, female	<10	10.0-11.4	≧11.5
>16 yr, male	<12	12.0-13.9	≧14.0
>16 yr, female	<10	10.0-11.9	≧12.0
Pregnant, 2nd trimester	< 9.5	9.5-10.9	≧11.0
Pregnant, 3rd trimester	< 9.0	9.0-10.4	≧10.5
Hematocrit, %			
6-23 months	<28	28-30	≧31
2-5 yr	<30	30-33	≧34
6-12 yr	<30	30-35	≧36
13-16 yr, male	<37	37-39	≧40
13-16 yr, female	<31	31-35	≧36
>16 yr, male	<37	37-43	≧44
>16 yr, female	<31	31-37	≧38
Pregnant, 2nd trimester	<30	30-34	≧35
Pregnant, 3rd trimester	<30	30-32	≧33
Hemoglobin conc. MCHC g/100 ml RBC			
All ages	—	30	≧30
Serum iron, µg/100 ml			
0-5 months		—	—
6-23 months		< 30	≧30
2-5 yr		< 40	≧40
6-12 yr		< 50	≧50
>12 yr, male		< 60	≧60
>12 yr, female		< 40	≧40
Transferrin saturation, %			
0-5 months		—	—
6-23 months		< 15	≧15
2-12 yr		< 20	≧20
>12 yr, male		< 20	≧20
>12 yr, female		< 15	≧15

Table 26.3 (continued)

Determination	Classification Category		Acceptable[a]
	Less than Acceptable		
	Deficient	Low	
Red cell folacin, ng/ml			
All ages	<140	140-159	≧160-650
Serum Folacin, ng/ml	3.0	3.0-5.9	≧ 6.0
Serum protein, gm/100 ml			
0-11 months		<5.0	≧ 5.0
1-5 yr		<5.5	≧ 5.5
6-17 yr		<6.0	≧ 6.0
Adult	<6.0	6.0-6.4	≧ 6.5
Pregnant, 2nd and 3rd trimester	<5.5	5.5-5.9	≧ 6.0
Serum albumin, gm/100 ml			
0-11 months		< 2.5	≧ 2.5
1-5 yr		< 3.0	≧ 3.0
6-17 yr		< 3.5	≧ 3.5
Adult	<2.8	2.8-3.4	≧ 3.5
Pregnant, 1st trimester	<3.0	3.0-3.9	≧ 4.0
Pregnant, 2nd and 3rd trimester	<3.0	3.0-3.4	≧ 3.5
Serum vitamin C, mg/100 ml			
0-11 months	—	—	—
>1 yr	<0.1	0.1-0.19	≧ 0.2
Plasma carotene, μg/100 ml			
0-5 months		<10	≧ 10
6-11 months		<30	≧ 30
1-17 yr		<40	≧ 40
Adult	<20[b]	20-39	≧ 40
Pregnant, 2nd trimester		30-79	≧ 80
Pregnant, 3rd trimester		40-79	≧ 80
Plasma vitamin A, μg/100 ml			
0-5 months	<10	10-19	≧ 20
0.5-17 yr	<20	20-29	≧ 30
Adult	<10	10-19	≧ 20
Urinary thiamine, μg/g creatinine			
1-3 yr	<120	120-175	≧176
4-6 yr	< 85	85-120	≧121
7-9 yr	< 70	70-180	≧181
10-12 yr	< 60	60-180	≧181
13-15 yr	< 50	50-150	≧151
Adult	< 27	27-65	≧ 66
Pregnant, 2nd trimester	< 23	23-54	≧ 55
Pregnant, 3rd trimester	< 21	21-49	≧ 50

Table 26.3 (continued)

	Classification Category		
	Less than Acceptable		
	Deficient	Low	Acceptable[a]
Urinary riboflavin, μg/gm creatinine			
1-3 yr	<150	150-499	≥ 500
4-6 yr	<100	100-299	≥ 300
7-9 yr	< 85	85-269	≥ 270
10-15 yr	< 70	70-199	≥ 200
Adult	< 27	27-79	≥ 80
Pregnant, 2nd trimester	< 39	39-119	≥ 120
Pregnant, 3rd trimester	< 30	30-89	≥ 90
Urinary iodine, μg/gm creatinine	< 25	25-49	≥ 50

From O'Neal et al., *Pediat. Res.*, 4:103 (1970).

[a]Excessively high levels may indicate abnormal clinical status or toxicity.

[b]May indicate unusual diet or malabsorption.

dietary intake. A carefully taken medical history may help reveal significant factors contributing to nutritional status.

Symptoms and signs have been classified by WHO (1963a) and are shown in Table 26.4. Those listed as of value in nutrition surveys are similar to clinical signs observed in most general nutrition surveys. It should be obvious that frank clinical lesions are easily recognized and evaluated. In the clinical examination as in all aspects of evaluating nutritional status, it is the marginal cases that are so difficult to define. Standard guides for interpretation of clinical signs of nutritional inadequacy have been proposed by ICNND (1963). Excellent discussions of the clinical examination as a means of determining nutritional status are given by the NRC (1949) and by Goldsmith (1959).

Growth, as represented by height and weight for age, is believed to be one of the most definitive indications of nutritional status of young children. On the basis of data collected on children 6 to 11 years of age, Ferro-Luzzi (1966) suggests that these simple anthropometric measurements in addition to clinical examination provide more information at low cost than other more extensive and expensive methods of survey. When the age of the child is not accurately known, as is often the case in some primitive societies, weight/height

Table 26.4 CLASSIFIED LIST OF SIGNS USED IN NUTRITION SURVEYS

Area of Examination	Group 1: Signs Known to be of Value in Nutrition Surveys	Group 2: Signs That Need Further Investigation	Group 3: Some Signs Not Related to Nutrition
1. Hair	Lack of lustre Thinness and sparseness Dyspigmentation of proximal part of hair Flag sign Easy pluckability		Alopecia Artificial discoloration
2. Face	Diffuse depigmentation Naso-labial dyssebacea Moon-face	Malar and supraorbital pigmentation	Acne vulgaris Acne rosacea Chloasma
3. Eyes	Xerosis conjunctivae Xerophthalmia (including keratomalacia) Bitot's spots Angular palpebritis	Conjunctival infection Circumcorneal infection Circumcorneal and scleral pigmentation Corneal vascularization Corneal opacities and scars	Follicular conjunctivitis Blepharitis Pingueculae Pterygium Pannus
4. Lips	Angular stomatitis Angular scars Cheilosis	Chronic depigmentation of lower lip	Chapping from exposure to harsh climates
5. Tongue	Edema Scarlet and raw tongue Magenta tongue Atrophic papillae	Hyperemic and hypertrophic papillae Fissures Geographic tongue Pigmented tongue	Aphthous ulcer Leucoplakia
6. Teeth	Mottled enamel	Caries Attrition Enamel hypoplasia Enamel erosion	Malocclusion
7. Gums	Spongy, bleeding gums	Recession of gum	Pyorrhea
8. Glands	Thyroid enlargement Parotid enlargement	Gynecomastia	Allergic or inflammatory enlargement of thyroid or parotid

953

Table 26.4 (continued)

Area of Examination	Group 1: Signs Known to be of Value in Nutrition Surveys	Group 2: Signs That Need Further Investigation	Group 3: Some Signs Not Related to Nutrition
9. Skin	Xerosis Follicular hyperkeratosis, types 1 and 2 Petechiae Ecchymoses Pellagrous dermatosis Flaky paint dermatosis Scrotal and vulval dermatosis	Mosaic dermatosis Intertriginous lesions Thickening and pigmentation of pressure points	Folliculosis Ichthyosis Acneiform eruptions Miliaria Epidermophytoses Sunburn Onchocercal dermatosis
10. Nails	Koilonychia	Brittle, ridged nails	
11. Subcutaneous tissue	Edema Amount of fat		
12. Muscular and skeletal systems	Intramuscular or subperiosteal hematomas Craniotabes Frontal and parietal bossing Epiphyseal enlargement (tender or painless) Beading of ribs Knock-knees or bow-legs Diffuse or local skeletal deformities	Winged scapula Deformities of thorax	Funnel chest Kyphoscoliosis
13. Internal systems:			
(a) Gastrointestinal	Hepatomegaly Ascites		Splenomegaly
(b) Nervous	Psychomotor change Mental confusion Sensory loss Motor weakness Loss of position sense Loss of vibratory sense Loss of ankle and knee jerks Calf tenderness	Condition of ocular fundus	
(c) Cardiovascular	Cardiac and peripheral vascular dysfunction Pulse rate	Blood pressure	

From WHO Report of Expert Committee on Medical Assessment of Nutritional Status, *Tech. Rpt. Series No. 258* (1963a).

ratio for very young children may be a useful criterion of nutritional status. Dugdale (1971) has shown that the weight/height ratio for children one to five years of age is independent of age but correlates with nutritional status. In older children, however, normal weight for height has been observed in children well below norms for their ages (Downs, 1965). These children apparently suffered from malnutrition in early life which led to continued growth retardation; that is, although weight was proportional to height, both were similar to that observed in children of younger age.

The Stuart-Meredith standards based on measurements of children in Boston in the early 1940s and of Iowa City children and adolescents in the 1930s (see Nelson, 1946) are frequently used as standards for the evaluation of height/weight data in surveys throughout the world. Despite the obvious objection of applying height/weight standards compiled nearly 40 years ago to the present population and to various racial groups, children of various racial backgrounds who come from homes of high economic status tend to fall within the standards (Bohdal and Simmons, 1969). This finding suggests that nutritional status may be a more significant factor in promoting growth than genetic makeup per se, but the controversy of nutrition versus genetics is far from solved. For example, the Ten State Nutrition Survey indicated differences in anthropometric measurements of American black and white adolescents, which suggested that separate standards for evaluation might be appropriate. Clearly, additional data are needed on the effect of nutrition, genetic potential for growth, and environment upon the growth of children before the controversy can be resolved.

Standards for children ages six and one-half to 10 years of age have been compiled from more recent health survey data collected between 1962 and 1965 (U.S. Department of Health, Education and Welfare, 1971). These data possibly reflect more accurately the growth of normal children in the general population today and may be more representative of the widely varied gene pool in this country.

CORRELATION OF DIETARY, BIOCHEMICAL, AND CLINICAL DATA

The degree of correlation that can be expected among dietary, biochemical, and clinical data is limited. In general, dietary and biochemical data for most nutrients correlate to a greater extent than either criterion correlates with clinical examination. One might expect that serum ascorbic acid should reflect dietary intake fairly well and results of surveys tend to bear this out. Clinical evidence of ascorbic acid deficiency, such as spongy or bleeding gums, also tends to correlate rather well with a low intake of the vitamin and low or negligible levels in serum.

Urinary excretion of thiamin, riboflavin, and N'-methylnicotinamide roughly parallels dietary intake, but data generally do not agree well enough to predict either parameter from a measurement of the other. In the case of vitamin A, however, little correlation can be expected, except in extreme long-term deprivation, and little correlation is generally obtained.

The investigator of population nutritional status always runs the risk of gathering data that cannot be adequately explained. Because the survey is limited both by current methodology and by the variability of population groups, interpretation of survey data should be made with recognition of the limitations of the procedures. Clearly, however, there is a need for improved methodology for assessing nutritional status of population groups and for standardization of methods of evaluating data obtained. Surveys as presently conducted are valuable in grossly defining nutritional status; whereas they rarely resolve problems of a nutritional nature, they often raise questions that can be answered in the more precisely controlled environment of the research laboratory.

bibliography

Abdul-Nour, B. and G. C. Webster. Biological activity of reconstituted ribosomes. *Exper. Cell Res.* 20:226-227 (1960).

Abels, J. and R. F. Schilling. Protection of intrinsic factor by vitamin B_{12}. *J. Lab. Clin. Med.* 64:375-384 (1964).

Abels, J., J. J. M. Vegter, M. G. Woldring, J. H. Jans, and H. O. Nieweg. The physiologic mechanism of vitamin B_{12} absorption. *Acta Med. Scand.* 165:105-113 (1959).

Abraham, E. P. Experiments relating to the constitution of alloxazine-adenine-dinucleotide. *Biochem. J.* 33:543-548 (1939).

Adelson, J. W. and S. S. Rothman. Selective pancreatic enzyme secretion due to a new peptide called chymodenin. *Science* 183:1087-1089 (1974).

Adelson, S. Some problems in collecting dietary data from individuals. *J. Amer. Diet. Ass.* 36:453-461 (1960).

Adibi, A. A. and S. J. Gray. Intestinal absorption of essential amino acids in man. *Gastroenterol.* 52:837-845 (1967).

Afzelius, B. A. The ultrastructure of the nuclear membrane of the sea urchin oocyte as studied with the electron microscope. *Exper. Cell Res.* 8:147-158 (1955).

Afzelius, B. A. The occurrence and structure of microbodies. A comparative study. *J. Cell Biol.* 26:835-843 (1965).

Aggeler, P. M., S. G. White, M. B. Glendening, E. W. Page, T. B. Leake, and G. Bates. Plasma thromboplastin component (PTC) deficiency: A new disease resembling hemophilia. *Proc. Soc. Exp. Biol. Med.* 79:692-694 (1952).

Aherne, W. and D. Hull. Brown adipose tissue and heat production in the newborn infant. *J. Pathol. Bacteriol.* 91:223-234 (1966).

Ahrens, H. and W. Korytnyk. Pyridoxine chemistry. XXI. Thin-layer chromatography and thin-layer electrophoresis of compounds in the vitamin B_6 group. *Anal. Biochem.* 30:413-420 (1969).

Aikawa, J. K. *The Role of Magnesium in Biologic Processes.* Charles C. Thomas, Springfield, Ill. (1963).

Alam, S. Q. Inositols IX. Biochemical systems. In *The Vitamins*, Vol. III, pp. 380-394, W. H. Sebrell, Jr. and R. S. Harris, Eds., Academic Press, N.Y. (1971).

Albright, F. and E. C. Reifenstein. *The Parathyroid Glands and Metabolic Bone Disease; Selected Studies.* Williams & Wilkins, Baltimore, Md. (1948).

Alfin-Slater, R. B. Fats, essential fatty acids, and ascorbic acid. *J. Amer. Diet. Ass.* 64:168-170 (1974).

Allen, D. W. and J. H. Jandl. Kinetics of intracellular iron in rabbit reticulocytes. *Blood* 15:71-81 (1960).

Allen, E. H., E. Glassman, E. Cordes, and R. S. Schweet. Incorporation of amino acids into ribonucleic acid. II. Amino acid transfer ribonucleic acid. *J. Biol. Chem.* 235:1068-1074 (1960).

Allen, T. M., E. C. Anderson, and W. H. Langham. Total body potassium and gross body composition. *J. Gerontol.* 15:348-357 (1960).

Allfrey, V. G. Biosynthetic reactions in the cell nucleus. In *Aspects of Protein Biosynthesis*, Part A, pp. 247-365, C. B. Anfinsen, Jr., Ed., Academic Press, N. Y. (1970).

Allfrey, V. G., V. C. Littau, and A. E. Mirsky. On the role of histones in regulating ribonucleic acid synthesis in the cell nucleus. *Proc. Natl. Acad. Sci.* 49:414-421 (1963).

Allgood, J. W. and E. B. Brown. The relationship between duodenal mucosal iron concentration and iron absorption in human subjects. *Scandinav. J. Haematol.* 4:217-229 (1967).

Allison, A. Lysosomes and disease. *Sci. Amer.* 217(5):62-72 (1967).

Allison, J. B. Biological evaluation of protein. *Physiol. Rev.* 35:664-700 (1955).

Allison, J. B. Interpretation of nitrogen balance data. *Fed. Proc.* 10:676-683 (1957).

Allison, J. B., R. W. Wannemacher, Jr., and W. L. Banks, Jr. Influence of dietary proteins on protein biosynthesis in various tissues. *Fed. Proc.* 22:1126-1130 (1963).

Alperin, J. B., H. T. Hutchinson, and W. C. Levin. Studies of folic acid requirements in megaloblastic anemia of pregnancy. *Arch. Intern. Med.* 117:681-688 (1966).

Altman, P. L. and D. S. Dittmer, Eds., *Biology Data Book*. Fed. of Amer. Soc. for Exp. Biol., Washington, D. C. (1964).

Alvarado, F. Transport of sugars and amino acids in the intestine: Evidence for a common carrier. *Science* 151:1010-1013 (1966).

Alvarado, F. and R. K. Crane. Phlorizin as a competitive inhibitor of the active transport of sugars by hamster small intestine, *in vitro. Biochim. Biophys. Acta* 56:170-172 (1962).

A. M. A. Council on Foods and Nutrition. Symposium on human calcium requirements. *J.A.M.A.* 185:588-593 (1963).

American Academy of Pediatrics Committee on Nutrition. The prophylactic requirement and the toxicity of vitamin D. *Pediat.* 31:512-513 (1963).

American Academy of Pediatrics Committee on Nutrition. Vitamin D intake and the hypercalcemic syndrome. *Pediat.* 35:1022-1023 (1965).

Ames, S. R. Bioassay of vitamin A compounds. *Fed. Proc.* 24:917-923 (1965).

Ames, S. R. Factors affecting absorption, transport and storage of vitamin A. *Amer. J. Clin. Nutr.* 22:934-935 (1969).

Ames, S. R. The joule—unit of energy. *J. Amer. Diet. Ass.* 57:415-416 (1971).

Ames, S. R. Tocopherols IV. Estimation in foods and food supplements. In *The Vitamins*, Vol. V, pp. 225-233, Sebrell, W. H., Jr., and R. S. Harris, Eds., Academic Press, N.Y. (1972).

Anderson, B. B., C. E. Fulford-Jones, J. A. Child, M. E. J. Beard, and C. J. T. Bateman. Conversion of vitamin B_6 compounds to active forms in the red blood cell. *J. Clin. Invest.* 50:1901-1909 (1971).

Anderson, E. C. and W. H. Langham. Average potassium concentration of the human body as a function of age. *Science* 130:713-714 (1959).

Anderson, T. W., D. B. W. Reid, and G. H. Beaton. Vitamin C and the common cold: a double-blind trial. *Can. Med. Assoc. J.* 107:503-508 (1972).

Andersson, B. Thirst—and brain control of water balance. *Amer. Sci.* 59:408-415 (1971).

Andersson, B., M. F. Dallman, and K. Olsson. Observations on central control of drinking and of the release of antidiuretic hormone (ADH). *Life Sci.* 8:425-432 (1969).

Andersson, B., L. Eriksson, and R. Oltner, Further evidence for angiotensin-sodium interaction in central control of fluid balance. *Life Sci.* Part I, 9:1091-1096 (1970).

Andersson, B., K. Olsson, and R. G. Warner. Dissimilarities between the central control of thirst and the release of antidiuretic hormone (ADH). *Acta Physiol. Scand.* 71:57-64 (1967).

Andersson, B. and O. Westbye. Synergistic action of sodium and angiotension on brain mechanisms controlling fluid balance. *Life Sci.* Part I, 9:601-608 (1970).

Andersson, S. Gastric and duodenal mechanisms inhibiting gastric secretion of acid. In *Handbook of Physiology*, Section 6: Alimentary Canal, Vol. II, pp. 865-877, C. F. Code, Ed., American Physiological Society, Washington, D.C. (1967).

Andersson, S. Secretion of gastrointestinal hormones. *Ann. Rev. Physiol.* 35:431-452 (1973).

Andre, J. and V. Marinozzi, Presence dans les mitochondries de particules ressemblant aux ribosomes. *J. Microscopie* 4:615-626 (1965).

Angier, R. B., J. H. Boothe, B. L. Hutchings, J. H. Mowat, J. Semb, E. L. R. Stokstad, Y. SubbaRow, C. W. Waller, D. B. Consulich, M. J. Fahrenback, M. E. Hultquist, E. Kuh, E. H. Northey, D. R. Seeger, J. P. Sickels, and J. M. Smith, Jr. The structure and synthesis of the liver L. casei factor. *Science* 103:667-669 (1946).

Anning, S. T., J. Dawson, D. E. Dolby, and J. T. Ingram. The toxic effects of calciferol. *Quart. J. Med.* 17:203-228 (1948).

Apte, S. V. and L. Lyengar. Absorption of dietary iron in pregnancy. *Amer. J. Clin. Nutr.* 23:73-77 (1969).

Apte, S. V. and L. Lyengar. Composition of the human foetus. *Brit. J. Nutr.* 27:305-312 (1972).

Arens, J. F. and D. A. van Dorp. Synthesis of some compounds possessing vitamin A activity. *Nature* 157:190-191 (1946).

Arora, R. B. and C. N. Mathur. Relationship between structure and anti-coagulant activity of coumorin derivatives. *Brit. J. Pharmacol.* 20:29-35 (1963).

Arroyave, G. The estimation of relative nutrient intake and nutritional status by biochemical methods: Proteins. *Amer. J. Clin. Nutr.* 11:447-461 (1962).

Arroyave, G. Comparative sensitivity of specific amino acid ratios versus "essential to nonessential" amino acid ratio. *Amer. J. Clin. Nutr.* 23:703-706 (1970).

Arroyave, G., F. Viteri, M. Béhar, and N. S. Scrimshaw. Impairment of intestinal absorption of vitamin A palmitate in severe protein malnutrition (Kwashiorkor). *Amer. J. Clin. Nutr.* 7:185-190 (1959).

Arroyave, G., D. Wilson, J. Méndez, M. Béhar, and N. S. Scrimshaw. Serum and liver vitamin A and lipids in children with severe protein malnutrition. *Amer. J. Clin. Nutr.* 9:180-185 (1961).

Asatoor, A. M., B. W. Lacey, D. R. London, and M. D. Milne. Amino acid metabolism in cystinuria. *Clin. Sci.* 23:285-304 (1962).

Ashworth, C. T. and J. M. Johnston. The intestinal absorption of fatty acid: A biochemical and electron microscope study. *J. Lipid Res.* 4:454-460 (1963).

Ashworth, C. T., V. A. Stembridge, and E. Sanders. Lipid absorption, transport and hepatic assimilation studied with electron microscopy. *Amer. J. Physiol.* 198:1326-1328 (1960).

Association of Official Agricultural Chemists. *Official Methods of Analysis.* Collegiate Press, George Banta Co., Inc., Menasha, Wisc. (1960).

Association of Vitamin Chemists, Inc. *Methods of Vitamin Assay*, 3rd Ed., Wiley-Interscience, N. Y. (1966).

Ast, D. B., D. J. Smith, B. Wachs, and K. T. Cantwell. Newburgh-Kingston caries fluorine study. XIV. Combined clinical and roentgenographic dental findings after ten years of fluoride experience. *J. Amer. Dent. Ass.* 52:290-325 (1956).

Astaldi, G., G. Meardi, and T. Libino. The iron content of jejunal mucosa obtained by Crosby's biopsy in hemochromatosis and hemosiderosis. *Blood* 28:70-82 (1966).

Atwater, W. O. and A. P. Bryant. The availability and fuel value of food materials. *Storrs Agr. Ext. Sta. Ann. Rept.,* 1899, pp. 73-110.

Atwater, W. O. and E. B. Rosa. Description of new respiration calorimeter and experiments on the conservation of energy in the human body. *U. S. Dept. Agr. Off. Exp. Sta. Bull.* 63 (1899).

Atwater, W. O. and J. F. Snell. Description of a bomb calorimeter and method of its use. *J. Amer. Chem. Soc.* 25:659-699 (1903).

Auerbach, C. The chemical production of mutations. *Science* 158:1141-1147 (1967).

Aurbach, G. D. and L. R. Chase. Cyclic 3', 5'-adenylic acid in bone and the mechanism of action of parathyroid hormone. *Fed. Proc.* 29:1179-1182 (1970).

Aurbach, G. D., H. T. Keutman, H. D. Niall, G. W. Tregear, J. L. H. O'Riordan, R. Marcus, S. J. Marx and J. T. Potts, Jr. Structure, synthesis and mecahnism of action of parathyroid hormone. *Rec. Progr. Horm. Res.* 28 353-398 (1972).

Aurbach, G. D., R. Marcus, J. Heersche, and S. Marx. Hormones and other factors regulating calcium metabolism. *Ann. N. Y. Acad. Sci.* 185:386-394 (1971).

Avioli, L. V. Current concepts of vitamin D_3 metabolism in man. In *The Fat-Soluble Vitamins*, pp. 159-172, H. F. DeLuca and J. W. Suttie, Eds., The University of Wisconsin Press, Madison (1970).

Avruch, J., J. R. Carter, and D. B. Martin. The effect of insulin on the metabolism of adipose tissue. In *Handbook of Physiology*, Section 7, Vol. I, pp. 545-562, R. O. Greep and E. B. Astwood, Eds., American Physiological Society, Washington, D. C. (1972).

Axelrod, J. Noradrenaline: Rate and control of its biosynthesis. *Science* 173:598-606 (1971).

Axelrod, J. Dopamine-β-hydroxylase: Regulation of its synthesis and release from nerve terminals. *Pharmacol. Rev.* 24:233-243 (1972).

Axelrod, J. Neurotransmitters. *Sci. Amer.* 230(6):58-71 (1974).

Babcock, M. J., M. Brush, and E. Sostman. Evaluation of vitamin B_6 nutrition. *J. Nutr.* 70:369-376 (1960).

Babirak, S. P., R. T. Dowell, and L. B. Oscai. Total fasting and total fasting plus exercise: Effects on body composition of the rat. *J. Nutr.* 104:452-457 (1974).

Bai, P., M. Bennion, and C. J. Gubler. Biochemical factors involved in the anorexia of thiamin deficiency in rats. *J. Nutr.* 101:731-738 (1971).

Baker, E. M., J. E. Canham, W. T. Nunes, H. E. Sauberlich, and M. E. McDowell. Vitamin B_6 requirement for adult men. *Amer. J. Clin. Nutr.* 15:59-66 (1964).

Baker, E. M. III, D. C. Hammer, S. C. March, B. M. Tolbert, and J. E. Canham. Ascorbate sulfate: a urinary metabolite of ascorbic acid in man. *Science* 173:826-827 (1971a).

Baker, E. M., R. E. Hodges, J. Hood, H. E. Sauberlich, S. March, and J. E. Canham. Metabolism of ^{14}C- and ^3H-labeled L-ascorbic acid in human scurvy. *Amer. J. Clin. Nutr.* 24:444-454 (1971b).

Baker, E. M., J. C. Saari, and B. M. Talbert. Ascorbic acid metabolism in man. *Amer. J. Clin. Nutr.* 19:371-378 (1966).

Baker, H. and O. Frank. *Clinical Vitaminology.* Wiley-Interscience, N.Y. (1968).

Baker, H., O. Frank, S. Feingold, G. Christakis, and H. Ziffer. Vitamins, total cholesterol, and triglycerides in 642 New York City school children. *Amer. J. Clin. Nutr.* 20:850-857 (1967).

Baker, H., O. Frank, J. J. Fennelly, and C. M. Leevy. A method for assaying thiamine status in man and animals. *Amer. J. Clin. Nutr.* 14:197-201 (1964).

Baker, H., O. Frank, V. B. Matovitch, I. Pasher, S. Aaronson, S. H. Hutner, and H. Sobotka. A new assay method for biotin in blood, serum, urine, and tissues. *Anal. Biochem.* 3:31-39 (1962).

Baker, H. and H. Sobotka. Microbiological assay methods for vitamins. In *Advances in Clinical Chemistry*, pp. 173-235. H. Sobotka and C. P. Stewart, Eds., Academic Press, N.Y. (1962).

Baker, H., H. Ziffer, I. Pasher, and H. Sobotka. A comparison of maternal and foetal folic acid and vitamin B_{12} at parturition. *Brit. Med. J.* 1:978-979 (1958).

Baker, P. E. The nerve axon. *Sci. Amer.* 214(3):74-82 (1966).

Balaghi, M. and W. N. Pearson. Metabolism of physiological doses of thiazole-2-^{14}C-labeled thiamine by the rat. *J. Nutr.* 89:265-270 (1966).

Balazs, E. A. *Chemistry and Molecular Biology of the Intercellular Matrix.* Vol. 2, Glycosaminoglycans and Proteoglycans. Academic Press, N.Y. (1970).

Balcerzak, S. P. and N. J. Greenberger. Iron content of isolated intestinal epithelial cells in relation to iron absorption. *Nature* 220:270-271 (1968).

Balogh, M., H. A. Kahn, and J. H. Medalie. Random repeat 24-hour dietary recalls. *Amer. J. Clin. Nutr.* 24:304-310 (1971).

Bank, A., R. A. Rifkind, and P. A. Marks. Regulation of globin synthesis. In *Regulation of Hematopoiesis*, Vol. I, pp. 701-729, A. S. Gordon, Ed., Appleton-Century-Crofts, N.Y. (1970).

Barakat, M. Z., S. K. Shehab, N. Darwish, and A. El-Zoheiry. New titrimetric method for the determination of vitamin C. *Anal. Biochem.* 53:245-251 (1973).

Bard, H. Postnatal fetal and adult hemoglobin synthesis in early preterm newborn infants. *J. Clin. Invest.* 52:1789-1795 (1973).

Barer, R., S. Joseph, and G. A. Meek. The origin of the nuclear membrane. *Exper. Cell Res.* 18:179-182 (1959).

Barker, H. A., H. Weissbach, and R. D. Smyth. A coenzyme containing pseudovitamin B_{12}. *Proc. Natl. Acad. Sci.* 44:1093-1097 (1958).

Barnard, T. and B. A. Afzelius. The matrix granules of mitochondria: A review. *Sub-Cell. Biochem.* 1:375-389 (1972).

Barnes, M. J. Ascorbic acid and the biosynthesis of collagen and elastin. *Bibl. Nutr. Dieta.* 13:86-98 (1969).

Barnes, R. H. Experimental animal approaches to the study of early malnutrition and mental development. *Fed. Proc.* 26:144-147 (1967).

Barnes, R. H., S. R. Cunnold, R. R. Zimmermen, H. Simmons, R. B. McLeod, and L. Krook. Influence of nutritional deprivations in early life on learning behavior of rats as measured by performance in a water maze. *J. Nutr.* 89:399-410 (1966).

Barnes, R. H., G. Fiala, and E. Kwong. Decreased growth rate resulting from prevention of coprophagy. *Fed. Proc.* 22:125-128 (1963).

Barnett, W. E. and D. H. Brown. Mitochondrial transfer ribonucleic acids. *Proc. Natl. Acad. Sci.* 57:452-458 (1967).

Barnett, W. E., D. H. Brown, and J. Epler. Mitochondrial-specific amino-acyl-RNA synthetases. *Proc. Natl. Acad. Sci.* 57:1775-1781 (1967).

Barnett, W. E. and J. L. Epler. Fractionation and specificities of two aspartyl-ribonucleic acid and two phenylalanyl-ribonucleic acid synthetases. *Proc. Natl. Acad. Sci.* 55:184-189 (1966).

Barondes, S. H. and M. W. Nirenberg. Fate of a synthetic polynucleotide directing cell-free protein synthesis. II. Association with ribosomes. *Science* 138:813-817 (1962).

Barrnett, R. J. and J. Rostgaard. Absorption of particulate lipid by intestinal microvilli. *Ann. N. Y. Acad. Sci.* 131:13-23 (1965).

Barter, J. and G. B. Forbes. Correlation of potassium-40 data with anthropometric measurements. *Ann. N. Y. Acad. Sci.* 110:264-270 (1963).

Barton, P. G. Lipoproteins of blood coagulation. In *Structural and Functional Aspects of Lipoproteins.* E. Tria and A. M. Scanu, Eds., Academic Press, N.Y. (1969).

Baudhuin, P., H. Beaufay, and C. DeDuve. Combined biochemical and morphological study of particulate fractions from rat liver. *J. Cell Biol.* 26:219-243 (1965).

Bauer, G. C. H., A. Carlsson, and B. Lindquist. Metabolism and homeostatic function of bone. In *Mineral Metabolism*, Vol. I, Part B., pp. 609-676, C. F. Comar and F. Bronner, Eds., Academic Press, N.Y. (1961).

Baugh, C. M. and C. L. Krumdieck. Naturally occurring folates. *Ann. N. Y. Acad. Sci.* 186:7-28 (1971).

Baugh, C. M., C. L. Krumdieck, H. J. Baker, and C. E. Butterworth. Studies on the absorption and metabolism of folic acid. I. Folate absorption in the dog after exposure of isolated intestinal segments to synthetic pteroylpolyglutamates of various chain lengths. *J. Clin. Invest.* 50:2009-2021 (1971).

Baugh, C. M., J. H. Malone, and C. E. Butterworth, Jr. Human biotin deficiency. A case history of biotin deficiency induced by raw egg consumption in a cirrhotic patient. *Amer. J. Clin. Nutr.* 21:173-182 (1968).

Baxter, J. H. Origins and characteristics of endogenous lipid in thoracic duct lymph in rat. *J. Lipid Res.* 7:158-166 (1966).

Baxter, R. Origin and continuity of mitochondria. In *Origin and Continuity of Cell Organelles*, pp. 46-64, J. Reinert and H. Ursprung, Eds., Springer-Verlag, N.Y. (1971).

Bayless, T. M. and N. S. Rosensweig. A racial difference in incidence of lactase deficiency. *J.A.M.A.* 197:968-972 (1966).

Baysal, A., B. A. Johnson, and H. Linkswiler. Vitamin B_6 depletion in man: blood vitamin B_6, plasma pyridoxal-phosphate, serum cholesterol, serum transaminases and urinary vitamin B_6 and pyridoxic acid. *J. Nutr.* 89:19-23 (1966).

Beams, H. W. and R. G. Kessel. The Golgi apparatus: Structure and function. *Internatl. Rev. Cytol.* 23:209-276 (1968).

Bean, W. B. and R. E. Hodges. Pantothenic acid deficiency induced in human subjects. *Proc. Soc. Exp. Biol. Med.* 86:693-698 (1954).

Beaton, G. H. Urea formation in the pregnant rat. *Arch. Biochem. Biophys.* 67:1-9 (1957).

Beaton, G. H. Nutritional and physiological adaptations in pregnancy. *Fed. Proc.* 20, Part III, Suppl. No. 7, pp. 196-201 (1961).

Beaton, G. H. and N. A. Fernandez. The use of nutritional requirements and allowances. In *Proceedings, Western Hemisphere Nutrition Congress* II, pp. 356-363, Futura Pub. Co., Inc., Mount Kisco, N.Y. (1972).

Beaton, G. H., M. H. Ryu, and E. W. McHenry. Studies on the role of growth hormone in pregnancy. *Endocrinology* 57:748-754 (1955).

Beattie, D. S. The synthesis of mitochondrial proteins. *Sub-Cell. Biochem.* 1:1-23 (1971).

Beck, F. and J. B. Lloyd. Histochemistry and electron microscopy of lysosomes. In *Lysosomes in Biology and Pathology*, Vol. 2, pp. 567-599, J. T. Dingle and H. B. Fell, Eds., *Frontiers of Biology*, Vol. 14A, Wiley, N.Y. (1969).

Beck, W. S. Deoxyribonucleotide synthesis and the role of vitamin B_{12} in erythropoiesis. *Vitamins Hormones.* 26:413-442 (1968).

Bédard, Y. C., P. H. Pinkerton, and G. T. Simon. Radioautographic observations on iron absorption by the normal mouse duodenum. *Blood* 38:232-245 (1971).

Beermann, W. and U. Clever. Chromosome puffs. *Sci. Amer.* 210(4):50-58 (1964).

Béhar, M., F. Viteri, R. Bressani, G. Arroyave, R. L. Squibb, and N. S. Scrimshaw. Principles of treatment and prevention of severe protein malnutrition in children (Kwashiorkor). *Ann. N. Y. Acad. Sci.* 69:954-968 (1959).

Beher, W. T., G. D. Baker, and W. L. Anthony. Feedback control of cholesterol biosynthesis in the mouse. *Proc. Soc. Exper. Biol. Med.* 109:863-868, (1962).

Behnke, A. R. Fat content and composition of the body. *Harvey Lect.* 37:198-226 (1941-42).

Behnke, A. R. The relation of lean body weight to metabolism and some consequent systematizations. *Ann. N.Y. Acad. Sci.* 56:1095-1142 (1953).

Behnke, A. R. Anthropometric evaluation of body composition throughout life. *Ann. N. Y. Acad. Sci.* 110:450-464 (1963).

Behnke, A. R., B. G. Feen, and W. C. Welham. The specific gravity of healthy men. *J.A.M.A.* 118:495-498 (1942).

Beiler, J. M., J. N. Moss, and G. J. Martin. Formation of a competitive antagonist of vitamin B_{12} by oxidation. *Science* 114:122-123 (1951).

Bell, P. H., W. F. Barg, Jr., D. F. Colucci, M. C. Davies, C. Dziobkowski, M. E. Englert, E. Heyder, R. Paul, and E. H. Snedeker. Purification and structure of porcine calcitonin-1. *J. Amer. Chem. Soc.* 90:2704-2706 (1968).

Bell, R. R., H. H. Draper, and J. G. Bergan. Sucrose, lactose, and glucose tolerance in northern Alaskan Eskimos. *Amer. J. Clin. Nutr.* 26:1185-1190 (1973).

Bemis, J. A., G. M. Bryant, J. C. Arcos, and M. I. Argus. Swelling and contraction of mitochondrial particles: A reexamination of the existence of a contractile protein extractable with 0.6 M-potassium chloride. *J. Molec. Biol.* 33:299-307 (1968).

Bender, A. E. and D. S. Miller. A new brief method of estimating net protein value. *Biochem. J.* 53:vii (1953).

Benditt, E. P., E. M. Humphreys, R. W. Wissler, C. H. Steffee, L. E. Frazier, and P. R. Cannon. The dynamics of protein metabolism. I. The interrelationship between protein and caloric intakes and their influence upon the utilization of ingested protein for tissue synthesis by the adult protein-depleted rat. *J. Lab. Clin. Med.* 33:257-268 (1948a).

Benedict, F. G. and T. M. Carpenter. The metabolism and energy transformations of healthy men during rest. Carnegie Institute of Washington Pub. No. 126 (1910).

Benedict, F. G. and E. P. Cathcart. *Muscular Work*. (A metabolic study with special reference to the efficiency of the human body as a machine). Carnegie Institute of Washington Pub. No. 187 (1913).

Benjamin, H. R., H. H. Gordon, and E. Marples. Calcium and phosphorus requirements of premature infants. *Amer. J. Dis. Child.* 65:412-425 (1943).

Bennett, E. L., M. R. Rosenzweig, and M. C. Diamond. Rat brain: effects of environment enrichment on wet and dry weights. *Science* 163:825-826 (1969).

Bennett, G. Migration of glycoprotein from Golgi apparatus to cell coat in the columnar cells of the duodenal epithelium. *J. Cell Biol.* 45:668-673 (1970).

Bennett, G. and C. P. Leblond. Formation of cell coat material for the whole surface of columnar cells in the rat small intestine, as visualized by radioautography with L-fucose-^{3}H. *J. Cell Biol.* 46:409-416 (1970).

Bennett, G. V. and P. Cuatrecasas. Insulin receptor of fat cells in insulin-resistant metabolic states. *Science* 176:805-806 (1972).

Bennett, M. V. L. Function of electrotonic junctions in embryonic and adult tissues. *Fed. Proc.* 32:65-75 (1973).

Bennett, V. and P. Cuatrecasas. Preparation of inverted plasma membrane vesicles from isolated adipocytes. *Biochim. Biophys. Acta* 311:362-380 (1973).

Benson, A. A. On the orientation of lipids in chloroplast and cell membranes. *J. Amer. Oil Chem. Soc.* 43:265-270 (1966).

Benzonana, G., B. Entressangles, G. Marchis-Mouren, L. Pasero, L. Sarda, and P. Desnuelle. Further studies on pig pancreatic lipase. In *Metabolism and Physiological Significance of Lipids*, pp. 141-154, R. M. C. Dawson and D. N. Rhodes, Eds., Wiley, N.Y. (1964).

Berendes, H. D. Factors involved in the expression of gene activity in polytene chromosomes. *Chromosoma* 24:418-437 (1968).

Berg, P. and E. J. Ofengand. An enzymatic mechanism for linking amino acids to RNA. *Proc. Natl. Acad. Sci.* 44:78-86 (1958).

Berger, E. Y. Intestinal absorption and excretion. In *Mineral Metabolism*, Vol. I, Part A, pp. 249-286, C. L. Comar and F. Bronner, Eds., Academic Press, N.Y. (1960).

Bergström, S., Prostaglandins: members of a new hormonal system. *Science* 157:382-391 (1967).

Bergström, S., H. Danielsson, and B. Samuelsson. The enzymatic formation of prostaglandin E_2 from arachidonic acid. Prostaglandins and related factors 32. *Biochim. Biophys. Acta* 90:207-210 (1964).

Bergström, S., R. Ryhage, B. Samuelsson, and J. Sjövall. The structure of prostaglandin E, F_1, and F_2. *Acta Chem. Scand.* 16:501-502 (1962).

Bergström, S. and B. Samuelsson. Prostaglandins. *Ann. Rev. Biochem.* 34:101-108 (1965).

Berk, P. D., R. B. Howe, J. R. Bloomer, and N. I. Berlin. The life span of the red cell as determined with labeled bilirubin. In *Formation and Destruction of Blood Cells*, pp. 91-107, T. J. Greenwalt and G. A. Jamieson, Eds., J. B. Lippincott, Philadelphia (1970).

Berl, S., S. Puszkin, and W. J. Nicklas. Actomyosin-like protein in brain. *Science* 179:441-446 (1973).

Berlin, J. D. The localization of acid mucopolysaccharides in the Golgi complex of intestinal goblet cells. *J. Cell Biol.* 32:760-766 (1967).

Bernard, R. A. and B. P. Halpern. Taste changes in vitamin A deficiency. *J. Gen. Physiol.* 52:444-464 (1968).

Bernhard, W. and N. Granboulan. Electron microscopy of the nucleolus in vertebrate cells. In *The Nucleus*, vol. 3, pp. 81-149, *Ultrastructure in Biological Systems*, A. J. Dalton and C. Haguenau, eds., Academic Press, N. Y., (1968).

Bernstein, D. S., N. Sadowsky, D. M. Hegsted, C. D. Guri, and F. J. Stare. Prevalence of osteoporosis in high- and low-fluoride areas in North Dakota. *J.A.M.A.* 198:499-504 (1966).

Bernstein, L. H., S. Gutstein, S. Weiner, and G. Efron. The absorption and malabsorption of folic acid and its polyglutamates. *Amer. J. Med.* 48:570-579 (1970).

Berry, H. K. Hereditary disorders of amino acid metabolism associated with mental deficiency. *Ann. N. Y. Acad. Sci.* 66-73 (1969).

Bertles, J. F. The occurrence and significance of fetal hemoglobins. In *Regulation of Hematopoiesis*, Vol. I, pp. 731-765, A. S. Gordon, Ed. Appleton-Century-Crofts, N. Y. (1970).

Bessey, O. A., D. J. Adam, and A. E. Hansen. Intake of vitamin B_6 and infantile convulsions: a first approximation of requirements of pyridoxine in infants. *Pediat.* 20:33-44 (1957).

Bessey, O. A., M. K. Horwitt, and R. H. Love. Dietary deprivation of riboflavin and blood riboflavin levels in man. *J. Nutr.* 58:367-383 (1956).

Bessis, M. The blood cells and their formation. In *The Cell*, Vol. V, pp. 163-217, J. Brachet and A. E. Mirsky, Eds., Academic Press, N. Y. (1961).

Bessman, S. P. and W. N. Fishbein. Gamma-hydroxybutyrate, a normal brain metabolite. *Nature* 200:1207-1208 (1963).

Best, C. H. and M. E. Huntsman. The effects of the components of lecithine upon deposition of fat in the liver. *J. Physiol.* (London) 75:405-412 (1932).

Beveridge, J. M. R., H. L. Haust, and W. F. Connell. Magnitude of the hypocholesterolemic effect of dietary sitosterol in man. *J. Nutr.* 83:119-122 (1964).

von Bezold, A. Untersuchungen uber die Vertheilung von Wasser, organischer Materie und anorganischen Verbindungen im Thierreiche. *Z. wissensch. Zool.*, viii, 487 (1857).

Bhatnagar, R. S., S. S. R. Rapaka, T. Z. Liu, and S. M. Wolfe. Hydralazine-induced disturbances in collagen biosynthesis. *Biochem. Biophys. Acta* 271:125-132 (1972).

Bhattacharyya, M. H. and H. F. Deluca. The regulation of rat liver calciferol-25-hydroxylase. *J. Biol. Chem.* 218:2969-2973 (1973).

Bhattathiry, E. P. M. and M. D. Siperstein. Feedback control of cholesterol synthesis in man. *J. Clin. Invest.* 42:1613-1618 (1963).

Bidder, F. and C. Schmidt. *Die Verdauungssaefte und der Stoffwechsel.* Reyher, Mitau (1852).

Biehl, J. P. and R. W. Vilter. Effects of isoniazid on pyridoxine metabolism. *J.A.M.A.* 156:1549-1552 (1954).

Bieri, J. G. Biological activity and metabolism of *N*-substituted tocopheramines: Implications on vitamin E function. In *The Fat-Soluble Vitamins*, pp. 307-316, H. F. DeLuca and J. W. Suttie, Eds., The University of Wisconsin Press, Madison (1970).

Bieri, J. G. Fat-soluble vitamins in the eighth revision of the recommended dietary allowances. *J. Amer. Diet. Ass.* 64:171-174 (1974).

Bieri, J. G. and R. P. Evarts. Tocopherols and fatty acids in American diets. The recommended allowance for vitamin E. *J. Amer. Diet. Ass.* 62:147-151 (1973).

Bieri, J. G., E. G. McDaniel, and W. E. Rogers, Jr. Survival of germfree rats without vitamin A. *Science* 163:574-575 (1969).

Biggs, R., A. S. Douglas, R. G. MacFarlane, J. V. Dacie, W. R. Pitney, C. Merskey, and J. R. O'Brien. Christmas disease. A condition previously mistaken for haemophilia. *Brit. Med. J.* ii:1378-1382 (1952).

Bigwood, E. J. Guiding principles for studies on the nutrition of populations. League of Nations Health Organization, Geneva, March, 1939.

Bihler, I. and R. K. Crane. Studies on the mechanism of intestinal absorption of sugars. V. The influence of several cations and anions on the active transport of sugars, *in vitro*, by various preparations of hamster small intestine. *Biochim. Biophys. Acta* 59:78-93 (1962).

Binder, H. J., D. C. Herting, V. Hurst, S. C. Finch, and H. M. Spiro. Tocopherol deficiency in man. *New Eng. J. Med.* 273:1289-1297 (1965).

Bird, O. D., E. L. Wittle, R. Q. Thompson, and V. M. McGlohon. Pantothenic acid-antagonists. *Amer. J. Clin. Nutr.* 3:298-304 (1955).

Birks, R. I. The role of sodium ions in the metabolism of acetylcholine. *Canad. J. Biochem. Physiol.* 41:2573-2597 (1963).

Birks, R. and F. C. MacIntosh. Acetylcholine metabolism of a sympathetic ganglion. *Canad. J. Biochem. Physiol.* 39:787-827 (1961).

Birnstiel, M. L., M. I. H. Chipchase, and W. G. Flamm. On the chemistry and organization of nucleolar proteins. *Biochim. Biophys. Acta* 87:111-122 (1964).

Bischoff, T. L. W. and C. Voit. Die gestze der ernahrung des fleischfressers. Winter, Leipzig (1860).

Bito, L. Z. Blood-brain barrier: Evidence for active cation transport between blood and the extracellular fluid of brain. *Science* 165:81-83 (1969).

Bizzi, A., E. Veneroni, S. Garattini, L. Puglisi, and R. Paoletti. Hypersensitivity to lipid mobilizing agents in essential fatty acid (EFA) deficient rats. *Eur. J. Pharmacol.* 2:48-52 (1967).

Björn-Rasmussen, E., L. Hallberg, and R. B. Walker. Food iron absorption in man. I. Isotopic exchange between food iron and inorganic iron salt added to food: studies on maize, wheat, and eggs. *Amer. J. Clin. Nutr.* 25:317-323 (1972).

Björnstein, I. and L. Sjöström. Number and size of adipose tissue fat cells in relation to metabolism in human obesity. *Metabolism* 20:703-715 (1971).

Björntorp, P., T. Schersten, and A. Gottfries. Effects of glucose infusions on adipose tissue lipogenesis in man. *Acta med. Scand.* 183:565-571 (1968).

Blair, J. A. Isolation of *iso*xanthopterin from human urine. *Biochem. J.* 68:385-387 (1958).

Blair, P. V., T. A. Oda, D. E. Green, and H. Fernandez-Moran. Studies on the electron transfer system. IV. Isolation of the units of electron transfer. *Biochemistry* 2:756-764 (1963).

Bland, J. H. *Clinical Metabolism of Body Water and Electrolytes*. W. B. Saunders Company, Philadelphia (1963).

Blankenhorn, D. H., J. Hirsh, and E. H. Ahrens, Jr. Transintestinal intubation: Technique for measurement of gut length and physiological sampling at known loci. *Proc. Soc. Exp. Biol. Med.* 88:356-362 (1955).

Blomstrand, R. and E. H. Ahrens, Jr. Absorption of fats studied in a patient with chyluria. *J. Biol. Chem.* 233:327-330 (1958).

Blomstrand, R. and L. Forsgren. Intestinal absorption and esterification of vitamin D_3-1,2-^{3}H in man. *Acta Chem. Scand.* 21:1662-1663 (1967).

Bloom, F. E. and E. Costa. The effects of drugs on serotonergic nerve terminals. *Adv. Cytopharmacol.* 1:379-395 (1971).

Bloom, W. and D. W. Fawcett, *A Textbook of Histology*, 9th Ed., W. B. Saunders Company, Philadelphia (1968).

Blunt, J. W., Y. Tanaka, and H. F. DeLuca. 25-hydroxycholecalciferol. A biologically active metabolite of vitamin D_3. *Biochemistry* 8:671-675 (1969).

Boass, A. and T. H. Wilson. Intestinal absorption of intrinsic factor and B_{12}-intrinsic factor complex. *Amer. J. Physiol.* 207:27-32 (1964).

Bodian, D. Neurons, circuits, and neuroglia. In *The Neurosciences,* pp. 6-24, G. C. Quarton, T. Melnechuk, and F. O. Schmitt, Eds., Rockefeller University Press, N. Y. (1967).

Bodwell, C. E. Tropomyosin B. In *Contractile Proteins and Muscle.* pp. 155-177, K. Laki, Ed., Marcel Dekker, Inc., N. Y. (1971).

Boguth, W. Aspects of the action of vitamin E. Vitamins Hormones 27:1-15 (1967).

Bohdal, M. and W. K. Simmons. A comparison of the nutritional indices in healthy African, Asian and European children. *Bull. World Health Organiz.* 40:166-174 (1969).

Bolin, T. D. The effect of diet on lactase activity in the rat. *Gastroenterol.* 60:432-437 (1971).

Booher, L. E., E. C. Callison and E. M. Hewston. An experimental determination of the minimum vitamin A requirements of normal adults. *J. Nutr.* 17:317-331 (1939).

Booth, C. C. Effect of location along the small intestine on absorption of nutrients. In *Handbook of Physiology,* Section 6: Alimentary Canal, Vol. III, pp. 1513-1527, C. F. Code, Ed., American Physiological Society, Washington, D. C. (1968).

Booth, C. C. and M. C. Brain. The absorption of tritium-labelled pyridoxine hydrochloride in the rat. *J. Physiol.* 164:282-294 (1962).

Booth, C. C. and D. L. Mollin. The site of absorption of vitamin B_{12} in man. *Lancet* 1:18-21 (1959).

Börgstrom, B. Digestion and absorption of fat. *Gastroenterol.* 43:216-219 (1962).

Börgstrom, B. Fat digestion and absorption. In *Intestinal Absorption,* Biomembranes, Vol. 4B, pp. 555-620, D. H. Smyth, Ed., Plenum Press, London (1974).

Borle, A. B. Calcium metabolism at the cellular level. *Fed. Proc.* 32:1944-1950 (1973).

Bornstein, P., H. P. Ehrlich, and A. W. Wyke. Procollagen: conversion of the precursor to collagen by a neutral protease. *Science* 175:544-546 (1972).

Borsook, H. and G. Keighley. The energy of urea synthesis. I and II. *Proc. Nat. Acad. Sci.* 19:626-631; 720-725 (1933).

Borsook, H. and H. M. Winegarden. The work of the kidney in the production of urine. *Proc. Nat. Acad. Sci.* 17:13-28 (1931).

Bortz, W. M. On the control of cholesterol synthesis. *Metabolism* 22:1507-1523 (1973).

Bovina, C., B. Tolomelli, C. Rovinetti. Effect of estradiol on folate coenzymes in the rat. *Int. J. Vit. Res.* 41:453-456 (1971).

Bowen, R. H. The Golgi apparatus—its structure and functional significance. *Anat. Rec.* 32:151-193 (1926).

Bowers, W. E. Lysosomes in lymphoid tissues: spleen, thymus, and lymph nodes. In *Lysosomes in Biology and Pathology,* Vol. I, pp. 167-191, J. T. Dingle and H. B. Fell, Eds., *Frontiers of Biology,* Vol. 14A, Wiley-Interscience, N.Y. (1969).

Boyd, W. C. Applications of biochemistry to problems of variation and heredity. *Ann. N. Y. Acad. Sci.* 134:858-863 (1966).

Boyle, I. T., R. W. Gray, and H. F. DeLuca. Regulation by calcium of *in vivo* synthesis of 1,25-dihydroxycholecalciferol and 21,25-dihydroxycholecalciferol. *Proc. Nat. Acad. Sci.* 68:2131-2134 (1971).

Bradfield, R. B. A rapid tissue technique for the field assessment of protein-calorie malnutrition. *Amer. J. Clin. Nutr.* 25:720-729 (1972).

Bradfield, R. B. and M. H. Jourdan. Relative importance of specific dynamic action in weight-reduction diets. *Lancet* (Sept. 22):640-643 (1973).

Brain, M. C. and C. C. Booth. The absorption of tritium-labelled pyridoxine HCl in control subjects and in patients with intestinal malabsorption. *Gut* 5:241-247 (1964).

Brandt, P. W. and A. R. Freeman. Plasma membrane: substructural changes correlated with electrical resistance and pinocytosis. *Science* 155:582-585 (1967).

Branton, D. and D. W. Deamer. *Membrane Structure,* Springer-Verlag, Wien-N. Y. (1972).

Bray, D. The fibrillar proteins of nerve cells. *Endeavor* 33:131-136 (1974).

Bray, G. A. Effect of diet and triiodothyronine on the activity of sn-glycerol-3-phosphate dehydrogenase and on the metabolism of glucose and pyruvate by adipose tissue of obese patients. *J. Clin. Invest.* 48:1413-1422 (1969).

Bray, G. A. and T. F. Gallagher, Jr. Regulatory obesity in man. *Clin. Res.* 18:537A (1970).

Breeze, B. B. and A. B. McCoord. Vitamin A absorption in celiac disease. *J. Pediat.* 15:183-196 (1939).

Brenneman, A. R. and S. Kaufman. The role of tetrahydropteridines in the enzymatic conversion of tyrosine to 3,4-dihydroxyphenyl alanine. *Biochem. Biophys. Res. Commun.* 17:177-183 (1964).

Bretscher, M. S. Membrane structure: Some general principles. *Science* 181:622-629 (1973).

Bricker, M., H. H. Mitchell, and G. M. Kinsman. The protein requirements of adult human subjects in terms of the protein contained in individual foods and food combinations. *J. Nutr.* 30:269-283 (1945).

Bricker, M., R. E. Shively, J. M. Smith, H. H. Mitchell, and T. S. Hamilton. The protein requirements of college women on high cereal diets with observations on the adequacy of short balance periods. *J. Nutr.* 37:163-183 (1949a).

Bricker, M. L., J. M. Smith, T. S. Hamilton, and H. H. Mitchell. The effect of cocoa upon calcium utilization and requirements, nitrogen retention and fecal composition. *J. Nutr.* 39:455-461 (1949b).

Brin, M. Erythrocyte transketolase in early thiamine deficiency. *Ann. N. Y. Acad. Sci.* 98:528-541 (1962).

Brin, M. The antithiamine effects of amprolium in rats on tissue transketolase activity. *Toxicol. Appl. Pharmacol.* 6:454-458 (1964).

Brin, M. A simplified Toepfer-Lehmann assay for the three vitamin B_6 vitamers. In *Methods in Enzymology,* XVIII, Part A, pp. 519-523 D. B. McCormick and L. D. Wright, Eds., Academic Press, N. Y. (1970).

Brin, M., M. Tai, A. S. Ostashever, and H. Kalinsky. The relative effects of pyridoxine deficiency on two plasma transaminases in the growing and in the adult rat. *J. Nutr.* 71:416-420 (1960).

Brindley, D. N. The intracellular phase of fat absorption. In *Intestinal Absorption,* Bio-membranes, Vol. 4B, pp. 621-671, D. H. Smyth, Ed., Plenum Press (1974).

Brinkhous, K. M. Plasma prothrombin; Vitamin K. *Medicine* 19:329-416 (1940).

Britton, G. and T. W. Goodwin. Biosynthesis of carotenoids. In *Methods in Enzymology,* Vol. XVIII, Part C, pp. 654-706, D. B. McCormick and L. D. Wright, Eds., Academic Press, N. Y. (1971).

Brobeck, J. R., Ed. *Best and Taylor's Physiological Basis of Medical Practice,* 9th ed., Williams and Wilkins Company, Baltimore, (1973).

Brody, S. *Bioenergetics and Growth.* Reinhold Pub. Co., N. Y. (1945).

Bronner, F. Dynamics and function of calcium. In *Mineral Metabolism,* Vol. II, Part A, pp. 341-444, C. L. Comar and F. Bronner, Eds., Academic Press, N. Y. (1964).

Bronner, F. and R. S. Harris. Absorption and metabolism of calcium in human beings, studied with calcium[45]. *Ann. N. Y. Acad. Sci.* 64:314-325 (1956).

Broquist, H. P., E. L. R. Stokstad, and T. H. Jukes. Biochemical studies with the "Citrovorum factor." *J. Lab. Clin. Med.* 38:95-100 (1951).

Bro-Rasmussen, F. The riboflavin requirement of animals and man and associated metabolic relations. Part II. Relation of requirement to the metabolism of protein and energy. *Nutr. Abstr. Rev.* 28:369-386 (1958).

Brown, E. G. Evidence for the involvement of ferrous iron in the biosynthesis of δ-aminolaevulinic acid by chicken erythrocyte preparations. *Nature* (London) 182:313-315 (1958).

Brown, F. and J. F. Danielli. The cell surface and cell physiology. In *Cytology and Cell Physiology*, pp. 239-310, G. H. Bourne, Ed., Academic Press, N. Y. (1964).

Brown, J. H. and S. H. Pollack. Stabilization of hepatic lysosomes of rats by vitamin E and selenium *in vivo* as indicated by thermal labilization of isolated lysosomes. *J. Nutr.* 102:1413-1419 (1972).

Brown, R. G., E. M. Button, and J. T. Smith. Effect of vitamin E deficiency on collagen metabolism in the rat's skin. *J. Nutr.* 91:99-106 (1967).

Brown, R. R. Normal and pathological conditions which may alter the human requirement for vitamin B_6. *Agric. Food Chem.* 20:498-505 (1972).

Brown, R. R., D. P. Rose, J. M. Price, and H. Wolf. Tryptophan metabolism as affected by anovulatory agents. *Ann. N. Y. Acad Sci.* 166:44-56 (1969).

Brozek, J. Changes of body composition in man during maturity and their nutritional implications. *Fed. Proc.* 11:784-793 (1952).

Brozek, J., Ed., *Body Measurements and Human Nutrition*. National Research Council Committee on Nutritional Anthropometry. Wayne University Press, Detroit (1956).

Brozek, J. (with technical assistance of H. Guetzkow). Psychologic effects of thiamine restriction and deprivation in normal young men. *Amer. J. Clin. Nutr.* 5:109-120 (1957).

Brozek, J. Body composition. *Science* 134:920-930 (1961).

Brozek, J. and A. Keys. Evaluation of leanness-fatness in man: Norms and interrelationships. *Brit. J. Nutr.* 5:194-206 (1951).

Brozek, J., J. K. Kihlberg, H. L. Taylor, and A. Keys. Skinfold distributions in middle-aged American men: a contribution to norms of leanness-fatness. *Ann. N. Y. Acad. Sci.* 110:492-502 (1963).

Brutlag, D. and A. Kornberg. Enzymatic synthesis of deoxyribonucleic acid. XXXVI. A proofreading function for the $3'{\to}5'$ exonuclease activity in deoxyribonucleic acid polymerases. *J. Biol. Chem.* 247:241-248 (1972).

Bucher, N. L. R. and K. McGarrahan. The biosynthesis of cholesterol from acetate-1-C[14] by cellular fractions of rat liver. *J. Biol. Chem.* 222:1-15 (1956).

Buell, G. C. and R. Reiser. Glyceride-glycerol precursors in the intestinal mucosa. *J. Biol. Chem.* 234:217-219 (1959).

Bulychev, A., R. Kramar, Z. Drahata, and O. Lindberg. Role of a specific endogenous fatty acid fraction in the coupling-uncoupling mechanism of oxidative phosphorylation of brown adipose tissue. *Exper. Cell Res.* 72:169-187 (1972).

Bunnell, R. H., J. Keating, A. Quaresimo, and G. K. Parman. Alpha-tocopherol content of foods. *Amer. J. Clin. Nutr.* 17:1-10 (1965).

Burch, H. B., T. Salcedo, Jr., E. O. Carrasco, C. Ll. Intengan, and A. B. Caldwell. Nutrition survey and tests in Bataan, Philippines. *J. Nutr.* 42:9-30 (1950).

Burch, H. B., C. A. Storvick, R. L. Bicknell, H. C. Kung, L. G. Alejo, W. A. Everhart, O. H. Lowry, C. G. King, and O. Bessey. Metabolic studies of precursors of pyridine nucleotides. *J. Biol. Chem.* 212:897-907 (1955).

Burchenal, J. H. Folic acid antagonists. *Amer. J. Clin. Nutr.* 3:311-320 (1955).

Burk, R. F., Jr., W. N. Pearson, R. P. Wood II, and F. Viteri. Blood-selenium levels and *in vitro* red blood cell uptake of ^{75}Se in kwashiorkor. *Amer. J. Clin. Nutr.* 20:723-733 (1967).

Burke, B. The dietary history as a tool in research. *J. Amer. Diet. Ass.* 23:1044-1046 (1947).

Burnet, E. and W. D. Aykroyd. Nutrition and public health. *League of Nations Quarterly Bulletin IV*, No. 2 (1935).

Burr, G. O. and M. M. Burr. A new deficiency disease produced by the rigid exclusion of fat from the diet. *J. Biol. Chem.* 82:345-367 (1929).

Burr, I. M., H. P. Taft, W. Stauffacher, and A. E. Renold. On the role of cyclic AMP in insulin release: II. Dynamic aspects and relations to adrenergic receptors in the perifused pancreas of adult rats. *Ann. N. Y. Acad. Sci.* 185:245-262 (1971).

Butcher, R. A., C. E. Baird, and E. W. Sutherland. Effects of lipolytic and antilipolytic substances on adenosine 3',5'-monophosphate levels in isolated fat cells. *J. Biol. Chem.* 243:1705-1712 (1968).

Butcher, R. W. and E. W. Sutherland. The effects of the catecholamines, adrenergic blocking agents, prostaglandins E_1, and insulin on cyclic AMP levels in the rat epididymal fat pad *in vitro*. *Ann. N. Y. Acad. Sci.* 139:849-859 (1967).

Butcher, R. W. and C. E. Baird. Effects of prostaglandins on adenosine 3',5'-monophosphate levels in fat and other tissues. *J. Biol. Chem.* 243:1713-1717 (1968).

Butterworth, C. E., Jr., C. M. Baugh, and C. L. Krumdieck. A study of folate absorption and metabolism in man utilizing carbon-14-labeled polyglutamates synthesized by the solid phase method. *J. Clin. Invest.* 48:1131-1142 (1969).

Buzina, R., A. Brodarec, M. Jusic, N. Milanovic, K. Bernhard, G. Brubacher, S. Christeller, and J. P. Vuilleumier. The assessment of dietary vitamin intake of 24 Istrian farmers: I. Laboratory analysis versus food tables. *Internat. J. Vit. Nutr. Res.* 41:129-140 (1971).

Caasi, P. I., J. W. Hauswirth, and P. P. Nair. Biosynthesis of heme in vitamin E deficiency. *Ann. N. Y. Acad. Sci.* 203:93-102 (1972).

Caddell, J. L. Magnesium deficiency in protein-calorie malnutrition: a follow-up study. *Ann. N. Y. Acad. Sci.* 162:874-890 (1969).

Cahill, G. F., Jr., E. B. Marliss, and T. T. Aoke. Fat and nitrogen metabolism in fasting man. In *Adipose Tissue, Regulation and Metabolic Function*, B. Jeanrenaud and D. Hepp, Eds., pp. 181-185, Academic Press, N. Y. (1970).

Call, D. L. An examination of caloric availability and consumption in the United States, 1909-1963. *Amer. J. Clin. Nutr.* 16:374-379 (1965).

Callender, S. T. Iron absorption. In *Intestinal Absorption*, Biomembranes, Vol. 4B, pp. 761-791, D. H. Smyth, Ed., Plenum Press, London (1974).

Callender, S. T., B. J. Mallett, and M. D. Smith. Absorption of hemoglobin iron. *Brit. J. Haematol.* 3:186-192 (1957).

Callender, S. T., S. R. Marney, and G. T. Warner. Eggs and iron absorption. *Brit. J. Haematol.* 19:657-665 (1970).

Callender, S. T. and G. T. Warner. Iron absorption from bread. *Amer. J. Clin. Nutr.* 21:1170-1174 (1968).

Callow, R. R., E. Kodicek, and G. A. Thompson. Metabolism of tritiated vitamin D. *Proc. Roy. Soc.* (Biol.) 164:1-20 (1966).

Calloway, D. H. Nitrogen balance during pregnancy. In *Nutrition and Fetal Development*, Vol. 2, M. Winick, Ed., pp. 79-94, Wiley, N. Y. (1974).

Calloway, D. H. Recommended dietary allowances for protein and energy, 1973. *J. Amer. Diet. Ass.* 64:157-162 (1974).

Calloway, D. H. and S. Margen. Variation in endogenous nitrogen excretion and dietary nitrogen utilization as determinants of human protein requirement. *J. Nutr.* 101:205-216 (1971).

Calloway, D. H., A. C. F. Odell, and S. Margen. Sweat and miscellaneous nitrogen losses in human balance studies. *J. Nutr.* 101:775-786 (1971).

Campbell, H. A. and K. P. Link. Studies on the hemorrhagic sweet clover disease. IV. The isolation and crystallization of the hemorrhagic agent. *J. Biol. Chem.* 138:21-33 (1941).

Campbell, J. A. Approaches in revising dietary standards. *J. Amer. Diet. Ass.* 64:175-178 (1974).

Campbell, R. M. and H. W. Kosterlitz. The effects of growth and sex in the composition of the liver cells in the rat. *J. Endocr.* 6:308-318 (1950).

Canadian Council on Nutrition. Dietary standard for Canada. *Canadian Bulletin on Nutrition.* 6:1-76 (1964); Supplement (1968); Supplement (1974).

Canadian Pediatric Society. The use and abuse of vitamin A. *Canad. Med. J.* 104:521-522 (1971).

Canas, F., J. S. Brand, W. F. Neuman, and A. R. Terepka. Some effects of vitamin D_3 on collagen synthesis in rachitic chick cortical bone. *Amer. J. Physiol.* 216:1092-1096 (1969).

Cannigia, A., C. Gennari, L. Cesari, and S. Romano. Intestinal absorption of ^{45}Ca in adult and old human subjects. *Gerontologia* 10:193-198 (1964).

Capaldi, R. A. A dynamic model of cell membranes. *Sci. Amer.* 230(3):26-34 (1974).

Carafoli, E. and C. S. Rossi. Calcium transport in mitochondria. *Adv. Cytopharmacol.* 1:209-227 (1971).

Carafoli, E., P. Gazzotti, F. D. Vasington, G. L. Sottocasa, G. Sandri, E. Panfil, and B. deBernard. Soluble Ca^{2+} binding factors isolated from mitochondria. In *Biochemistry and Biophysics of Mitochondrial Membranes*, pp. 623-640, G. F. Azzone, E. Carafoli, A. L. Lehninger, E. Quagliariello, and N. Siliprandi, Eds., Academic Press, N. Y. (1972).

Carafoli, E., P. Patriarca, and C. S. Rossi. A comparative study of the role of mitochondria and the sarcoplasmic reticulum in the uptake and release of Ca^{++} by the rat diaphragm. *J. Cell. Physiol.* 74:17-30 (1969).

Cardell, R. R., S. Badenhausen, and K. R. Porter. Fine structure of rat intestinal cells during fat absorption. *J. Cell Biol.* 27:120A-121A (1965).

Care, A. D., R. F. L. Bates, and H. J. Gitelman. Evidence for a role of cyclic AMP in the release of calcitonin. *Ann. N. Y. Acad. Sci.* 185:317-326 (1971).

Carlisle, E. M. Silicon as an essential element. *Fed. Proc.* 33:1758-1766 (1974).

Carlsson, A. and B. Lindquist. Comparison of intestinal and skeletal effects of vitamin D in relation to dosage. *Acta Physiol. Scand.* 35:53-55 (1955).

Carnes, W. H. Role of copper in connective tissue metabolism.*Fed. Proc.* 30:995-1000(1971).

Caro, L. G. and G. E. Palade. Protein synthesis, storage and discharge in the pancreatic exocrine cell. An autoradiographic study. *J. Cell Biol.* 20:473-495 (1964).

Carr, F. H. and E. A. Price. Colour reactions attributed to vitamin A. *Biochem. J.* 20:497-501 (1926).

Carroll, J. and B. Spencer. Vitamin A and sulphotransferases in foetal rat liver. *Biochem. J.* 96:79P (1965).

Carter, H. E., P. Johnson, and E. J. Weber. Glycolipids. *Ann. Rev. Biochem.* 34:109-142 (1965).

Cartwright, G. E. and M. M. Wintrobe. The question of copper deficiency in man. *Amer. J. Clin. Nutr.* 15:94-110 (1964).

Caspary, W. F. and R. K. Crane. Active transport of *myo*-inositol and its relation to the sugar transport system in hamster small intestine. *Biochim. Biophys. Acta* 203:308-316 (1970).

Castle, W. B. Gastric intrinsic factor and vitamin B_{12} absorption. In *Handbook of Physiology*, Section 6, Vol. III, pp. 1529-1552, C. F. Code, Ed., American Physiological Society, Washington, D. C., 1968.

Cellier, K. M. and M. E. Hankin. Studies of nutrition in pregnancy. I. Some considerations in collecting dietary information. *Amer. J. Clin. Nutr.* 13:55-62 (1963).

Century, B. and M. K. Horwitt. Biological availability of various forms of vitamin E with respect to different indices of deficiency. *Fed. Proc.* 24:906-911 (1965).

Century, T. J., I. R. Fenichel, and S. B. Horowitz. The concentrations of water, sodium and potassium in the nucleus and cytoplasm of amphibian oocytes. *J. Cell Sci.* 7:5-13 (1970).

Cerecedo, L. R. Thiamine antagonists. *Amer. J. Clin. Nutr.* 3:273-281 (1955).

Chalmers, F., M. Clayton, L. Gates, R. Tucker, A. Wertz, C. Young, and W. Foster. The dietary record—how many and which days? *J. Amer. Diet. Ass.* 28:711-717 (1952).

Chanarin, I. and A. McLean. Origin of serum and urinary methyltetrahydrofolate in man. Some observations on the methylfolate block hypothesis in Addisonian pernicious anaemia. *Clin. Sci.* 32:57-67 (1967).

Chanarin, I. and J. Perry. Evidence for reduction and methylation of folate in the intestine during normal absorption. *Lancet* 2:776-778 (1969).

Chao, F. C. Dissociation of macromolecular ribonucleoprotein of yeast. *Arch. Biochem. Biophys.* 70:426-431 (1957).

Chapman, D. and R. B. Leslie. Structure and function of phospholipids in membranes. In *Membranes of Mitochondria and Chloroplasts*, pp. 91-126, E. Racker, Ed., Van Nostrand Reinhold Company, N. Y. (1970).

Charley, P. J., C. Stitt, E. Shore, and P. Saltman. Studies in the regulation of intestinal iron absorption. *J. Lab. Clin. Med.* 61:397-410 (1963).

Charlton, R. W., P. Jacobs, J. D. Torrance, and T. H. Bothwell. The role of the intestinal mucosa in iron absorption. *J. Clin. Invest.* 44:543-554 (1965).

Chase, H. P., W. F. B. Lindsley, Jr., and D. O'Brien. Undernutrition and cerebellar development. *Nature* 221:554-555 (1969).

Chase, L. R. and G. D. Aurbach. Renal adenyl cyclase: Anatomically separate sites for parathyroid hormone and vasopressin. *Science* 159:545-547 (1968).

Chase, L. R., S. A. Fedak, and G. D. Aurbach. Activation of skeletal adenyl cyclase by parathyroid hormone *in vitro*. *Endocrinology* 84:761-768 (1969).

Chatterjee, I. B. Biosynthesis of L-ascorbate in animals. In *Methods in Enzymology*, Vol. XVIII, Part A, pp. 28-34, D. B. McCormick and L. D. Wright, Eds., Academic Press, N. Y. (1970).

Chaudhuri, C. R. and I. B. Chatterjee. *L*-Ascorbic acid synthesis in birds: phylogenetic trend. *Science* 164:435-436 (1969).

Chaykin, G. Nicotinamide coenzymes. *Ann. Rev. Biochem.* 36:149-170 (1967).

Cheek, D. B. *Human Growth. Body Composition, Cell Growth, Energy, and Intelligence.* Lea and Febiger, Philadelphia (1968).

Cheek, D. B. Muscle cell growth in normal children. In *Human Growth*, D. B. Cheek, Ed., pp. 337-351, Lea and Febiger, Philadelphia (1968).

Cheek, D. B., J. A. Brasel, and J. E. Graystone. Muscle cell growth in rodents: sex differences and the role of hormones. In *Human Growth*, D. B. Cheek, Ed., pp. 306-325, Lea and Febiger, Philadelphia (1968).

Cheek, D. B. and D. E. Hill. Muscle and liver cell growth: role of hormones and nutritional factors. *Fed. Proc.* 29:1510-1515 (1970).

Chen, P. S. and H. B. Bosmann. Effect of vitamins D_2 and D_3 on serum calcium and phosphorous in rachitic chicks. *J. Nutr.* 83:133-139 (1964).

Cheung, W. J. Adenosine $3',5'$-monophosphate: On the mechanism of action. *Perspect. Biol. Med.* 15:221-235 (1972).

Chio, K. S. and A. L. Tappel. Inactivation of ribonuclease and other enzymes by peroxidizing lipids and by malonaldehyde. *Biochemistry* 8:2827-2832 (1969).

Chisolm, J. J., Lead poisoning. *Sci. Amer.* 224 (2):15-23 (1971).

Christakis, G., A. Miridjanian, L. Nath, H. S. Khurana, C. Cowell, M. Archer, O. Frank, H. Ziffer, H. Baker, and G. James. A nutritional epidemiologic investigation of 642 New York City children. *Amer. J. Clin. Nutr.* 21:107-126 (1968).

Christakis, G., S. H. Rinzler, M. Archer, G. Winslow, S. Jampel, J. Stephenson, G. Friedman, H. Fein, A. Kraus, and G. James. The anti-coronary club. A dietary approach to the prevention of coronary heart disease. A seven year report. *Amer. J. Public Health* 56:299-314 (1966).

Christakis, G., S. Sajecki, R. W. Hillman, E. Miller, S. Blumenthal, and M. Archer. Effect of a combined nutrition education and physical fitness program on the weight status of obese high school boys. *Fed. Proc.* 25:15-19 (1966).

Christensen, H. N. *Biological Transport.* W. A. Benjamin, N. Y. (1962).

Christensen, H. N. Amino acid transport and nutrition. *Fed. Proc.* 22:1110-1114 (1963).

Christian, J. E., L. W. Combs, and W. V. Kessler. Body composition: Relative *in vivo* determinations from potassium-40 measurements. *Science* 140:489-490 (1963).

Chvapil, M., J. N. Ryan, and C. F. Zukoski. The effect of zinc and other metals on the stability of lysosomes. *Proc. Soc. Exp. Biol. Med.* 140:642-646 (1972).

Cinnamon, A. D. and J. R. Beaton. Biochemical assessment of vitamin B_6 status in man. *Amer. J. Clin. Nutr.* 23:696-702 (1970).

Clark, B. and G. Hubscher. Glycerokinase in mucosa of the small intestine of the cat. *Nature* 195:599-600 (1962).

Clark, B. F. and K. A. Marcker. How proteins start. *Sci. Amer.* 218(1): 36-42 (1968).

Clark, C. T., H. Weissbach, and S. Udenfriend. 5-hydroxytryptophan decarboxylase: Preparation and properties. *J. Biol. Chem.* 210:139-148 (1954).

Clark, S. L. Jr. The ingestion of proteins and colloidal materials by columnar absorptive cells of the small intestine in suckling rats and mice. *J. Biophys. Biochem. Cytol.* 5:41-50 (1959).

Cleaver, J. E. Defective repair replication of DNA in xeroderma pigmentosum. *Nature* 218:652-656 (1968).

Clements, F. W. Naturally occurring goitrogens. *Brit. Med. Bull.* 16:133-137 (1960).

Clifton, G., S. R. Bryant, and C. G. Skinner. N'-(substituted) pantothenamides, antimetabolites of pantothenic acid. *Arch. Biochem. Biophys.* 137:523-528 (1970).

Cohen, A. C. Pyridoxine in the prevention and treatment of convulsions and neurotoxicity due to cycloserine. *Ann. N. Y. Acad. Sci.* 166:346-349 (1969).

Cohen, N., A. Gelb, and H. Sobotka. Intestinal absorption of folic acid *in vitro. Clin. Res.* 12:206A (1964).

Cohlan, S. Q. Excessive intake of vitamin A as a cause of congenital anomalies in the rat. *Science* 117:535-536 (1953).

Cohn, Z. A. and B. Benson. The *in vitro* differentiation of mononuclear phagocytes. II. The influence of serum on granule formation, hydrolase production, and pinocytosis. *J. Exper. Med.* 121:835-848 (1965).

Cohn, Z. A. and M. E. Fedorko. The formation and fate of lysosomes. In *Lysosomes in Biology and Pathology,* Vol. I, pp. 43-63, J. T. Dingle and H. B. Fell, Eds., *Frontiers of Biology,* Vol. 14A, Wiley-Interscience, N. Y. (1969).

Collins, G. H. and W. K. Converse. Cerebellar degeneration in thiamine-deficient rats. *Amer. J. Pathol.* 58:219-233 (1970).

Collip, J. B., L. I. Pugsley, H. Selye, and D. L. Thomson. Observations concerning the mechanism of parathyroid hormone action. *Brit. J. Exp. Path.* 15:335-336 (1934).

Comar, C. L., R. H. Wasserman, and M. M. Nold. Strontium-calcium discrimination factors in the rat. *Proc. Soc. Exp. Biol. Med.* 92:859-863 (1956).

Committee on Maternal Nutrition. Maternal nutrition and the course of pregnancy. National Research Council, National Academy of Sciences, Washington, D.C., 241 pp. (1970).

Committee on Maternal Nutrition. Nutritional supplementation and the outcome of pregnancy. National Research Council, National Academy of Sciences, Washington, D.C., 153 pp. (1973).

Committee on Nutritional Misinformation, Food and Nutrition Board. Supplementation of human diets with vitamin E. *Nutr. Rev.* 31:327-328 (1973).

Conn, E. E. and P. K. Stumpf. *Outlines of Biochemistry,* 3rd ed., p. 71, Wiley, N. Y. (1972).

Connor, W. E., D. T. Witiak, D. B. Stone, and M. L. Armstrong. Cholesterol balance and fecal neutral steroid and bile acid excretion in normal men fed dietary fats of different fatty acid composition. *J. Clin. Invest.* 48:1363-1375 (1969).

Conover, T. E. and M. Bárány. The absence of a myosin-like protein in liver mitochondria. *Biochem. Biophys. Acta* 127:235-238 (1966).

Conrad, M. E. and W. H. Crosby. The natural history of iron deficiency induced by phlebotomy. *Blood* 20:173-185 (1962).

Conrad, M. E. and W. H. Crosby. Intestinal mucosal mechanisms controlling iron absorption. *Blood* 22:406-415 (1963).

Conrad, M. E., L. R. Weintraub, and W. H. Crosby. The role of the intestine in iron kinetics. *J. Clin. Invest.* 43:963-974 (1964).

Consolazio, C. F. and H. L. Johnson. Measurement of energy cost in humans. *Fed. Proc.* 30:1444-1453 (1971).

Consolazio, C. F., R. E. Johnson, and E. Marek. *Metabolic Methods. Clinical procedure in the study of metabolic functions.* C. V. Mosby Co., St. Louis (1951).

Consolazio, C. F., L. O. Matoush, R. A. Nelson, R. S. Harding, and J. E. Canham. Excretions of sodium, potassium, magnesium and iron in human sweat and the relation of each to balance requirements. *J. Nutr.* 79:407-415 (1963b).

Consolazio, C. F., R. A. Nelson, L. O. Matoush, R. S. Harding, and J. E. Canham. Nitrogen excretion in sweat and its relation to nitrogen balance requirements. *J. Nutr.* 79:399-406 (1963a).

Consolazio, C. F., R. Shapiro, J. E. Masterson, and P. S. L. McKinzie. Energy requirements of men in extreme heat. *J. Nutr.* 73:126-134 (1961).

Contractor, S. D. and B. Shane. 4-pyridoxic acid-5'-phosphate: metabolite of pyridoxol in the rat. *Biochem. Biophys. Res. Commun.* 39:1175-1181 (1970).

Contrera, J. F. and A. S. Gordon. The renal erythropoietic factor. I. Studies on its purification and properties. *Ann. N. Y. Acad. Sci.* 149:114-119 (1968).

Cook, J. D., M. Layrisse, C. Martinez-Torres, R. Walker, E. Monsen, and C. A. Finch. Food iron absorption measured by an extrinsic tag. *J. Clin. Invest.* 51:805-815 (1972).

Coombs, R. R. A. and H. B. Fell. Lysosomes in tissue damage mediated by allergic reactions. In *Lysosomes in Biology and Pathology*, Vol. 2, pp. 3-18, J. T. Dingle and H. B. Fell, Eds., *Frontiers of Biology*, Vol. 14A, Wiley-Interscience, N. Y. (1969).

Coons, C. M. Iron retention by women during pregnancy. *J. Biol. Chem.* 97:215-226 (1932).

Cooper, B. A., G. S. D. Cantlie, and L. Brunton. The case for folic acid supplements during pregnancy. *Amer. J. Clin. Nutr.* 23:848-854 (1970).

Cooper, C. W., W. H. Schwesinger, A. M. Mahgoub, and D. A. Ontjes. Thyrocalcitonin: Stimulation of secretion by pentagastrin. *Science* 172:1238-1240 (1971).

Cooper, J. R. The role of ascorbic acid in the oxidation of tryptophan to 5-hydroxy-tryptophan. *Ann. N. Y. Acad. Sci.* 92:208-211 (1961).

Cooper, J. R. and H. L. Pincus. The role of thiamine in nerve conduction. In *Thiamine Deficiency: Biochemical Lesions and Their Clinical Significance*, pp. 112-121. Ciba Foundation Study Group No. 28. G. E. W. Wolstenholme and M. O'Connor, Eds., Little, Brown and Co., Boston (1967).

Cooperman, J. Microbiological assay of folic acid activity in serum and whole blood. In *Methods in Enzymology*, Vol. XVIII, Part B, D. B. McCormick and L. D. Wright, Eds., Academic Press, N. Y. (1971).

Copenhaver, J. S. and W. B. Bell. The production of bovine hyperkeratosis (X disease) with an experimentally made pellet feed. *Vet. Med.* 49:96-101 (1954).

Copp, D. H. Parathyroids and homeostasis of blood calcium. In *Bone as a Tissue*, pp. 289-299, K. Rodahl, J. T. Nicholson, and E. M. Brown, Jr. Eds., McGraw-Hill Book Company, Inc., N. Y. (1960).

Copp, D. H., E. C. Cameron, B. A. Cheney, A. G. F. Davidson, and E. G. Henze. Evidence for calcitonin—A new hormone from the parathyroid that lowers blood calcium. *Endocrinology* 70:638-649 (1962).

Copping, A. M. Inhibitors of pantothenic acid. In *Antivitamins,* J. C. Somogyi, Ed., *Bibl. Nutritio et Dieta,* Vol. 8, pp. 169-177, S. Karger, Basel (Switzerland), 1966.

Cordano, A., J. M. Baertl, and G. G. Graham. Copper deficiency in infancy. *Pediat.* 34:324-336 (1964).

Cori, C. F. The fate of sugar in the animal body. I. The rate of absorption of hexoses and pentoses from the intestinal tract. *J. Biol. Chem.* 66:691-715 (1925).

Cori, C. F. Mammalian carbohydrate metabolism. *Physiol. Revs.* 11:143-275 (1931).

Cori, C. F. and B. Illingworth. The prosthetic group of phosphorylase. *Proc. Nat. Acad. Sci.* 43:547-552 (1957).

Corradino, R. A. Embryonic chick intestine in organ culture: Response to vitamin D_3 and its metabolites. *Science* 179:402-405 (1973).

Costa, E. Turnover rate of neuronal monoamines: Pharmacological implications. *Excerpta Med. Intern. Congress Series.* No. 180:11-35 (1968).

Cotzias, G. C. Manganese in health and disease. *Physiol. Rev.* 38:503-532 (1958).

Coulston, A. and L. Lutwak. Dietary calcium deficiency and human periodontal disease. *Fed. Proc.* 31:721 (1972).

Coward, D. G., M. B. Sawyer, and R. G. Whitehead. Microtechniques for the automated analysis of serum total protein and albumin, urinary urea, creatinine, and hydroxyproline for nutrition surveys in developing countries. *Amer. J. Clin. Nutr.* 24:940-946 (1971).

Cox, E. V. and A. M. White. Methylmalonic acid excretion: an index of vitamin-B_{12} deficiency. *Lancet* II:853-856 (1962).

Cramer, C. F. Quantitative studies on the absorption and excretion of calcium for Thiry-Velle intestinal loops in the dog. In *The Transfer of Calcium and Strontium Across Biologic Membranes,* pp. 75-84, R. H. Wasserman, Ed., Academic Press, N. Y. (1963).

Crandon, J. H., C. C. Lund, and D. B. Dill. Experimental human scurvy. *New Eng. J. Med.* 223:353-369 (1940).

Crane, R. K. Intestinal absorption of sugars. *Physiol. Rev.* 40:789-825 (1960).

Crane, R. K. Na^+-dependent transport in the intestine and other animal tissues. *Fed. Proc.* 24:1000-1006 (1965).

Crane, R. K. Absorption of sugars. In *Handbook of Physiology,* Section 6: Alimentary Canal, Vol. III, pp. 1323-1351, C. F. Code, Ed., American Physiological Society, Washington, D. C., (1968).

Crane, R. K. Intestinal absorption of glucose. In *Intestinal Absorption,* Biomembranes, Vol. 4B, pp. 541-553, D. H. Smyth, Ed., Plenum Press, London (1974).

Crane, R. K. and P. Mandelstam. The active transport of sugars by various preparations of hamster intestine. *Biochim. Biophys. Acta* 45:460-476 (1960).

Cravioto, J., E. R. DeLicardie, and H. G. Birch. Nutrition, growth and neurointegrative development: An experimental and ecologic study. *Pediat.* 38:319-372 (1966).

Cravioto, J. and B. Robles. Evolution of adaptive and motor behavior during rehabilitation from kwashiorkor. *Amer. J. Orthopsychiatry* 35:449-464 (1965).

Cresta, M. New method of assessing food consumption by age-groups on the basis of overall family data. *Nutrition Newsletter* 8:37-49 (1970).

Crichton, R. Studies on the structure of ferritin and apoferritin from horse spleen. I. Tryptic digestion of ferritin and apoferritin. *Biochim. Biophys. Acta* 194:34-42 (1969).

Crick, F. H. C. On the genetic code. *Science* 139:461-464 (1963).

Crick, F. H. C. The genetic code—yesterday, today, and tomorrow. *Cold Spring Harbor Symp. Quant. Biol.* 31:3-9 (1966a).

Crick, F. H. C. Codon-anticodon paring: The wobble hypothesis. *J. Molec. Biol.* 19:548-555 (1966b).

Crick, F. Central dogma of molecular biology. *Nature* 227:561-563 (1970).

Crick, F. H. C., L. Barnett, S. Brenner, and R. J. Watts-Tobin. General nature of the genetic code for proteins. *Nature* 192:1227-1230 (1961).

Crokaert, R. Du dosage chimique de l'acide pantothénique. *Bull. soc. chim. biol.* 31:903-907 (1949).

Crosby, W. H. Regulation of iron metabolism. In *Regulation of Hematopoiesis*, Vol. 1, *Red Cell Production*, pp. 519-537, A. S. Gordon, Eds., Appleton-Century-Crofts, N.Y. 1970.

Csáky, T. Z. Significance of sodium ions in active intestinal transport of nonelectrolytes. *Amer. J. Physiol.* 201:999-1001 (1961).

Csáky, T. Z. A possible link between active transport of electrolytes and nonelectrolytes. *Fed. Proc.* 22:3-7 (1963).

Csallany, A. S., H. H. Draper, and S. N. Shah. Conversion of a d-a-tocopherol-C^{14} to tocopheryl-p-quinone *in vivo. Arch. Biochem. Biophys.* 98:142-145 (1962).

Csallany, A. S. and H. H. Draper. Dimerization of a-tocopherol *in vivo. Arch. Biochem. Biophys.* 100:335-337 (1963).

Cuatrecasas, P. Insulin-receptor interactions in adipose tissue cells: Direct measurement and properties. *Proc. Natl. Acad. Sci.* 68:1264-1268 (1971a).

Cuatrecasas, P. Properties of the insulin receptor of isolated fat cell membranes. *J. Biol. Chem.* 246:7265-7274 (1971b).

Cuatrecasas, P. Insulin receptor of liver and fat cell membranes. *Fed. Proc.* 32:1838-1846 (1973).

Cuatrecasas, P. and G. P. E. Tell. Insulin-like activity of concanavalin A and wheat germ agglutinin—Direct interactions with insulin receptors. *Proc. Natl. Acad. Sci.* 70:485-489 (1973).

Culley, W. J. and E. T. Mertz. Effect of restricted food intake on growth and composition of preweanling rat brain. *Proc. Soc. Exp. Biol. Med.* 118:233-235 (1965).

Curran, P. F. and A. K. Solomon. Ion and water fluxes in the ileum of rats. *J. Gen. Physiol.* 41:143-168 (1957).

Curran, P. F. and A. K. Solomon. Sodium, chloride and water transport by isolated rat ileum *in vitro. Fed. Proc.* 17:31 (1958).

Cuthbertson, W. F. J., J. Gregory, P. O'Sullivan, and H. F. Pegler. The anti-vitamin B_{12} activity of some compounds related to cobalamin. *Biochem. J.* 62:15P (1956).

Daems, W. Th., E. Wisse, and P. Brederoo. Electron microscopy of the vacuolar apparatus. In *Lysosomes in Biology and Pathology*, Vol. I, pp. 64-112, J. T. Dingle and H. B. Fell, Eds., *Frontiers of Biology*, Vol. 14A, Wiley-Interscience, N.Y. (1969).

Daft, F. S., E. G. McDaniel, L. G. Herman, M. K. Romine, and J. R. Hegner. Role of coprophagy in utilization of B vitamins synthesized by intestinal bacteria. *Fed. Proc.* 22:129-133 (1963).

Dagley, S. and D. E. Nicholson. *An Introduction to Metabolic Pathways*, Wiley, N.Y. (1970).

Dahlqvist, A. The intestinal disaccharidases and disaccharide intolerance. (Editorial) *Gastroenterology* 43:694-696 (1962).

Dahlqvist, A. Localization of the small-intestinal disaccharidases. *Amer. J. Clin. Nutr.* 20:81-88 (1967).

Dahlqvist, A. and B. Borgstrom. Digestion and absorption of disaccharides in man. *Biochem. J.* 81:411-418 (1961).

Dahlström, A. and J. Häggendal. Studies on the transport and life-span of amine storage granules in a peripheral adrenergic neuron system. *Acta Physiol. Scand.* 67:278-288 (1966).

Dairman, W., J. G. Christenson, and S. Udenfriend. Changes in tyrosine hydroxylase and dopa decarboxylase induced by pharmacological agents. *Pharmacol. Rev.* 24:269-289 (1972).

Dakshinamurti, K. and S. P. Mistry. Tissue and intracellular distribution of biotin-$C^{14}OOH$ in rats and chicks. *J. Biol. Chem.* 238:294-296 (1963).

Dalderup, C. B. M. Vitamins, Chapter XXVI. In *Side Effects of Drugs*, Vol. VI, L. Meyler and A. Herxheimer, Eds., Excerpta Medica Foundation, Amsterdam (1967).

Dalton, A. J. Golgi apparatus and secretion granules. In *The Cell*, Vol. II, pp. 603-619, J. Brachet and A. E. Mirsky, Eds., Academic Press, N.Y. (1961).

Dam, H. Vitamin K. *Vitamins Hormones* 6:27-53 (1948).

Dam, H. Interrelations between vitamin E and polyunsaturated fatty acids in animals. *Vitamins Hormones* 20:527-540 (1962).

Dam, H. and H. Granados. Peroxidation of body fat in vitamin E deficiency. *Acta Physiol. Scand.* 10:162-171 (1945).

Dam, H., F. Schønheyder, and E. Tage-Hansen. CLV. Studies on the mode of action of vitamin K, *Biochem. J.* 30:1075-1079 (1936).

Danielli, J. F. and H. Davson. A contribution to the theory of permeability of thin films. *J. Cell Comp. Physiol.* 5:495-508 (1935).

Darby, W. J., R. O. Cannon, and M. M. Kaser. The biochemical assessment of nutritional status during pregnancy. *Obstet. Gynec. Survey* 3:704-715 (1948).

Darlington, W. A. and J. H. Quastel. Absorption of sugars from isolated surviving intestine. *Arch. Biochem. Biophys.* 43:194-207 (1953).

Daum, K., W. W. Tuttle, and M. Wilson. Thiamine requirements and their implications. *J. Amer. Diet. Ass.* 25:398-404 (1949).

Dauwalder, M., W. G. Whaley, and J. E. Kephart. Functional aspects of the Golgi apparatus. *Sub-Cell. Biochem.* 1:225-275 (1972).

Davenport, E. Calculating the nutritive value of diets. *ARS Pub.* 62-10-1, U. S. Department of Agriculture (1964), 45 pp.

Davenport, H. W. *Physiology of the Digestive Tract*, 3rd ed., Year Book Medical Publishers, Inc., Chicago, 1971.

Davenport, H. W. Why the stomach does not digest itself. *Sci. Amer.* 226(1):86-94 (1972).

David, J. S. K., P. Malathi, and J. Ganguly. Role of the intestinal brush border in the absorption of cholesterol in rats. *Biochem. J.* 98:662-668 (1966).

Davidson, M. B. Effect of obesity on insulin sensitivity of human adipose tissue. *Diabetes* 21:6-12 (1972).

Davis, J. O. The renin-angiotensin system in the control of aldosterone secretion. In *Kidney Hormones*, J. W. Fisher, Ed., pp. 173-205, Academic Press, N. Y. (1971).

Davison, A. N. and J. Dobbing. Phospholipid metabolism in nervous tissue. 2. Metabolic stability. *Biochem. J.* 75:565-570 (1960).

Davison, A. N., R. S. Morgan, M. Wajda, and G. P. Wright. Metabolism of myelin lipids: Incorporation of [$3-^{14}C$] serine in brain lipids of the developing rabbit and their persistence in the central nervous system. *J. Neurochem.* 4:360-365 (1959).

Davison, P. F. Protein of nervous tissue: specificity, turnover, and function. In *The Neurosciences*, pp. 267-270, G. C. Quarton, T. Melnechuk, and F. O. Schmitt, Eds., Rockefeller University Press, N. Y. (1967).

Dawber, T. R., G. Pearson, P. Anderson, G. V. Mann, W. B. Kannel, D. Shurtleff, and P. McNamara. Dietary assessment in the epidemiologic study of coronary heart disease: The Framingham Study. II. Reliability of measurement. *Amer. J. Clin. Nutr.* 11:226-234 (1962).

Dawkins, M. J. R. and D. Hull. The production of heat by fat. *Sci. Amer.* 213 (2): 62-67 (1965).

Dawkins, M. J. R. and J. W. Scopes. Non-shivering thermogenesis and brown adipose tissue in the human newborn infant. *Nature* 206:201-202 (1965).

Dawson, E. B., R. R. Clark, and W. J. McGanity. Plasma vitamins and trace metal changes during teen-age pregnancy. *Amer. J. Obstet. Gynec.* 104:953-958 (1969).

Dawson, R. B., S. Rafal, and L. R. Weintraub. Absorption of hemoglobin iron: the role of xanthine oxidase in the intestinal heme-splitting reaction. *Blood* 35:94-103 (1970).

Daxenbichler, M. E., C. H. VanEtten, F. S. Brown, and Q. Jones. Oxazolidinethiones and volatile isothiocyanates in enzyme-treated seed meals from 65 species of cruciferae. *J. Agri. Food Chem.* 12:127-130 (1964).

De Duve, C. The lysosome concept. In *Ciba Foundation Symposium on Lysosomes*, pp. 1-31, A.V.S. de Reuck and M.P. Cameron, Eds., Little, Brown and Company, Boston (1963a).

De Duve, C. The Lysosome. *Sci. Amer.* 208(5): 64-72 (1963).

De Duve, C. From cytases to lysosomes. *Fed. Proc.* 23:1045-1049 (1964).

De Duve, C. The lysosome in retrospect. In *Lysosomes in Biology and Pathology*, Vol. 1, pp. 3-40, J. T. Dingle and H. B. Fell, Eds., *Frontiers of Biology*, Vol. 14A, Wiley-Interscience, N. Y. (1969a).

De Duve, C. Evolution of the peroxisome. *Ann. N. Y. Acad. Sci.* 168:369-381 (1969b).

De Duve, C. and P. Baudhuin. Peroxisomes (microbodies and related particles). *Physiol. Rev.* 46:323-357 (1966).

De Duve, C. and R. Wattiaux. *Functions of lysosomes.* Ann. Rev. Physiol. 28:435-492 (1966).

De Duve, C., R. Wattiaux, and M. Wibo. Effects of fat-soluble compounds on lysosomes *in vitro. Biochem. Pharmacol.* 9:97-116 (1962).

De Gubareff, N. and W. R. Platt. Influence of sodium flouride on healing of experimental fractures in rats, squirrel monkeys, and dogs. *Arch. Environ. Health.* 19:22-31 (1969).

DeLuca, H. F. 25-Hydroxycholecalciferol, the probable metabolically active form of vitamin D. *Amer. J. Clin. Nutr.* 22:412-424 (1969).

DeLuca, H. F. The role of vitamin D and its relationship to parathyroid hormone and calcitonin. *Recent Progr. Hormone Res.* 27:479-516 (1971).

DeLuca, H. F. The kidney as an endocrine organ for the production of 1,25-dihyroxyvitamin D_3, a calcium-mobilizing hormone. *New Eng. J. Med.* 289:359-365 (1973).

DeLuca, H. F. and J. W. Blunt. Vitamin D. In *Methods in Enzymology*, Vol. XVIII, Part C, pp. 709-733, D. B. McCormick and L. D. Wright, Eds. Academic Press, N. Y. (1971).

DeLuca, H. F., G. W. Engstrom, and H. Rasmussen. The action of vitamin D and parathyroid hormone *in vitro* on calcium uptake and release by kidney mitochondria. *Proc. Natl. Acad. Sci.* 48:1604-1609 (1962).

DeLuca, L., N. Maestri, F. Bonanni, and D. Nelson. Maintenance of epithelial cell differentiation: the mode of action of vitamin A. *Cancer* 30:1326-1331 (1972).

DeLuise, M., T. J. Martin, P. B. Greenberg, and V. Michelangeli. Metabolism of porcine, human and salmon calcitonin in the rat. *J. Endocr.* 53:475-482 (1972).

Demopoulos, H. B. The basis of free radical pathology. *Fed. Proc.* 32:1859-1861 (1973).

Dempsey, G. P., S. Bullivant, and W. B. Watkins. Endothelial cell membranes: polarity of particles as seen by freeze-fracturing. *Science* 179:190-192 (1973).

Dencker, L. and H. Tjalve. Distribution of vitamin D_3. Evidence of accumulation in renal proximal tubuli and thyroid parafollicular cells. *Experientia* 29:719-722 (1973).

Department of Health, Education, and Welfare. *Skinfold Thickness of Children 6-11 years, United States.* Vital and Health Statistics Series 11, No. 120, DHEW Publication No. (HSM) 73-1602, U. S. Govt. Printing Office, Washington, D. C. (1973a).

Department of Health, Education, and Welfare. *Height and Weight of Youths 12-17 Years, United States.* Vital and Health Statistics Series 11, No. 124, DHEW Publication No. (HSM) 73-1606, Superintendent of Documents, Washington, D. C. (1973b).

Department of Health and Social Security. Recommended intakes of nutrients for the United Kingdom. Her Majesty's Stationery Office, London, (1969) 43 pp.

Deren, J. J. Development of intestinal structure and function. In *Handbook of Physiology*, Section 6: *Alimentary Canal*, Vol. III, pp. 1099-1123, C. F. Code, Ed., American Physiological Society, Washington, D. C. (1968).

DeRobertis, E. Ultrastructure and cytochemistry of the synaptic region. *Science* 156:907-914 (1967).

DeRobertis, E. Molecular biology of synaptic receptors. *Science* 171:963-971 (1971).

DeRobertis, E. and H. S. Bennett. Submicroscopic vesicular component in the synapse. *Fed. Proc.* 13:35A (1954).

DeRobertis, E. and C. M. Franchi. The submicroscopic organization of axon material isolated from myelin nerve fibers. *J. Exper. Med.* 98:269-276 (1953).

DeRobertis, E. and H. Franco Ruffo. Submicroscopic organization of the mitochondrial body and other cytoplasmic structures of insect testis. *Exper. Cell Res.* 12:66-79 (1957).

DeRobertis, E. D. P., W. W. Nowinski, and F. A. Saez. *Cell Biology*, 5th Ed., W. B. Saunders Company, Philadelphia (1970), p. 53.

Deshmukh, D. S. and J. Ganguly. Demonstration of oxidation and reduction of retinal in rat intestine. *Indian J. Biochem.* 4:18-21 (1967).

Deshmukh, D. S., P. Malathi, K. Subba Rao, and J. Ganguly. Absorption of retinoic acid (vitamin A acid) in rats. *Indian J. Biochem.* 1:164-166 (1964).

Deshmukh, D. S., S. K. Murthy, S. Mahadevan, and J. Ganguly. Studies on metabolism of vitamin A: Absorption of retinal (vitamin A aldehyde) in rats. *Biochem. J.* 96:377-382 (1965).

DeVries, W. H., W. M. Grovier, J. S. Evans, J. D. Gregory, G. D. Novelli, M. Soodak, and F. Lipmann. Purification of coenzyme A from fermentation sources and its further partial identification. *J. Amer. Chem. Soc.* 72:4838 (1950).

Diamond, J. M. Tight and leaky junctions of epithelia: A perspective on kisses in the dark. *Fed. Proc.* 33: 2220-2224 (1974).

Dickerman, H., B. G. Redfield, J. Bieri, and H. Weissbach. The role of vitamin B_{12} in methionine biosynthesis in avian liver. *J. Biol. Chem.* 239:2545-2552 (1964).

Dickerson, R. E. X-ray studies of protein mechanisms. *Ann. Rev. Biochem.* 41:815-842 (1972).

Dietrich, L. S. Regulation of nicotinamide metabolism. *Amer. J. Clin. Nutr.* 24:800-804 (1971).

Dietrich, L. S., L. Martinez, and L. Franklin. Role of the liver in systemic pyridine nucleotide metabolism. *Naturwissenschaften* 55:231-232 (1968).

Dingle, J. T. Vacuoles, vesicles and lysosomes. *Brit. Med. Bull.* 24:141-145 (1968).

Dingle, J. T. Action of vitamin A on the stability of lysosomes *in vivo* and *in vitro*. In *Ciba Foundation Symposium on Lysosomes*, pp. 384-398, A. V. S. deReuck and M. P. Cameron, Eds., Little, Brown and Company, Boston (1963).

Dingle, J. T. and J. A. Lucy. Vitamin A, carotenoids and cell function. *Biol. Rev. Cambridge Phil. Soc.* 40:422-461 (1965).

Dinning, J. S. and P. L. Day. Vitamin E deficiency in the monkey. I. Muscular dystrophy, hematologic changes, and the excretion of urinary nitrogenous constitutents. *J. Exper. Med.* 105:395-402 (1957).

Dintzis, H. M. Assembly of the peptide chains of hemoglobin. *Proc. Natl. Acad. Sci.* 47:247-261 (1961).

Dirks, J. H., J. R. Clapp, and R. W. Berliner. The protein concentration in the proximal tubule of the dog. *J. Clin. Invest.* 43:916-921 (1964).

Dixit, B. N. and J. P. Buckley. Circadian changes in brain 5-hydroxytryptamine and plasma corticosterone in the rat. *Life Sci.* 6:755-758 (1967).

Dobbing, J. The influence of early nutrition on the development and myelination of the brain. *Proc. Roy. Soc.* (Series B) 159:503-509 (1964).

Dobbing, J. The developing brain: a plea for more critical interspecies extrapolation. *Nutr. Rep. Internat.* 7:401-406 (1973).

Dobbing, J. and J. Sands. Timing of neuroblast multiplication in developing human brain. *Nature* 226:639-640 (1970).

Dobzhansky, T. *Heredity and the Nature of Man,* Harcourt, Brace and World, Inc., N. Y. (1964).

Dodds, M. L. Sex as a factor in blood levels of ascorbic acid. *J. Amer. Diet. Ass.* 54:32-33 (1969).

Dodds, M. L., E. L. Price, and F. L. MacLeod. A study of the relation and adjustment of blood plasma level and urinary excretion of ascorbic acid to intake. *J. Nutr.* 40:255-263 (1950).

Dodge, F. A., Jr., and R. Rahaminoff. Cooperative action of calcium ions in transmitter release at the neuromuscular junction. *J. Physiol.* 193:419-432 (1967).

Donabedian, R. K. and A. Karmen. Fatty acid transport and incorporation into human erythrocytes *in vitro. J. Clin. Invest.* 46:1017-1027 (1967).

Donaldson, R. M., Jr., I. L. Mackenzie, and J. S. Trier. Intrinsic factor-mediated attachment of vitamin B_{12} to brush border and microvillous membranes of hamster intestine. *J. Clin. Invest.* 46:1215-1228 (1967).

Dounce, A. L. Nuclear gels and chromosomal structure. *Amer. Sci.* 59:74-83 (1971).

Dounce, A. L. and C. A. Hilgartner. A study of DNA nucleoprotein gels and the residual protein of isolated cell nuclei. *Exper. Cell Res.* 36:228-241 (1964).

Dowdle, E. B., D. Schachter, and H. Schenker. Active transport of Fe^{59} by everted segments of rat duodenum. *Amer. J. Physiol.* 198:609-613 (1960).

Dowling, J. E. and G. Wald. The biological function of vitamin A acid. *Proc. Nat. Acad. Sci.,* 46:587-608 (1960).

Downs, E. F. Nutritional dwarfing. A syndrome of early protein-calorie malnutrition. *Amer. J. Clin. Nutr.* 15:275-281 (1964).

Drapanas, T., J. S. Williams, J. C. McDonald, W. Heyden, T. Bow, and R. P. Spencer. Role of the ileum in the absorption of vitamin B_{12} and intrinsic factor (NF). *J.A.M.A.* 184:337-341 (1963).

Draper, H. H., J. G. Bergan, M. Chiu, A. S. Csallany, and A. V. Boaro. A further study of the specificity of the vitamin E requirement for reproduction. *J. Nutr.* 84:395-400 (1964).

Draper, H. H., A. S. Csallany, and M. Chiu. Isolation of a trimer of *a*-tocopherol from mammalian liver. *Lipids* 2:47-54 (1967).

Draper, H. H. and A. S. Csallany. Metabolism and function of vitamin E. *Fed. Proc.* 28:1690-1695 (1969).

Draper, H. H. and A. S. Csallany. Metabolism of Vitamin E. In *The Fat-Soluble Vitamins,* pp. 347-353, H. F. DeLuca and J. W. Suttie, Eds., The University of Wisconsin Press, Madison (1970).

Dreyer, W. J., D. S. Papermaster, and H. Kuhn. On the absence of ubiquitous structural protein subunits in biological membranes. *Ann. N. Y. Acad. Sci.* 195:61-74 (1972).

Dreyfus, P. M. Thiamine deficiency and the central nervous system, a review of pathophysiological concepts. *J. Vitaminol.* 15:335-336 (1969).

Droz, B. and C. P. Leblond. Migration of proteins along the axons of the sciatic nerve. *Science* 137:1047-1048 (1962).

Droz, B. and C. P. Leblond. Axonal migration of proteins in the central nervous system and peripheral nerves as shown by radioautography. *J. Comp. Neurol.* 121:325-346 (1963).

Drujan, B. D. Determination of vitamin A. In *Methods in Enzymology,* Vol. XVIII, Part C., pp. 565-573, D. B. McCormick and L. D. Wright, Eds., Academic Press, N. Y. (1971).

Drummond, J. C. The nomenclature of the so-called accessory food factors. *Biochem. J.* 14:660 (1920).

Drysdale, J. W. and H. N. Munro. Small-scale isolation of ferritin for the assay of the incorporation of ^{14}C-labelled amino acids. *Biochem. J.* 95:851-858 (1965).

Drysdale, J. W. and H. N. Munro. Regulation of synthesis and turnover of ferritin in rat liver. *J. Biol. Chem.* 241:3630-3637 (1966).

Drysdale, J. W., E. Olafsdottir, and H. N. Munro. Effect of ribonucleic acid depletion on ferritin induction in rat liver. *J. Biol. Chem.* 243:552-555 (1968).

Dubach, R. V., C. V. Moore, and S. Callender. Studies in iron transportation and metabolism. IX. Excretion of iron as measured by the isotope technique. *J. Lab. Clin. Med.* 45:599-615 (1955).

Dubé, R. B., E. C. Johnson, H. H. Yü, and C. A. Storwick, with technical assistance of S. Kosko and S. McFarland. Thiamine metabolism of women on controlled diets. II. Daily blood thiamine values. *J. Nutr.* 48:307-316 (1952).

Dubois, D. and E. F. Dubois. Clinical Calorimetry. A formula to estimate the approximate surface area if height and weight be known. *Arch. Inter. Med.* 17:863-871 (1916).

Duello, T. J. and J. T. Matschiner. Characterization of vitamin K from human liver. *J. Nutr.* 102:331-336 (1972).

Dugdale, A. E. An age-independent anthropometric index of nutritional status. *Amer. J. Clin. Nutr.* 24:174-180 (1971).

Dunagin, P. E., Jr., E. H. Meadows, Jr., and J. A. Olson. Retinoyl-beta-glucuronic acid: A major metabolite of vitamin A in rat bile. *Science* 148:86-87 (1965).

Dunagin, P. E., Jr., R. D. Zachman, and J. A. Olson. The identification of metabolites of retinol and retinoic acid in rat bile. *Biochim. Biophys. Acta* 124:71-85 (1966).

Dunn, M. S., E. A. Murphy, and L. B. Rockland. Optimal growth of the rat. *Physiol. Rev.* 27:72-94 (1947).

Dupont, J. and M. M. Mathias. Bio-oxidation of linoleic acid via methyl-malonyl-CoA. *Lipids* 4:478-483 (1969).

Dyer, R. F. Morphological features of brown adipose cell maturation *in vivo* and *in vitro*. *Amer. J. Anat.* 123:255-282 (1968).

Dziewiatkowski, D. D. Vitamin A and endochondral ossification in the rat as indicated by the use of sulphur-35 and phosphorus-32. *J. Exp. Med.* 100:11-24 (1954).

Eagles, J. A., M. G. Whiting, and R. E. Olson. Dietary appraisal. Problems in processing dietary data. *Amer. J. Clin. Nutr.* 19:1-9 (1966).

Eanes, E. D., J. D. Termine, and A. S. Posner. Amorphous calcium phosphate in skeletal tissues. *Clin. Orthopaedics Related Res.* 53:223-235 (1967).

Ebachi, S. and F. Lipmann. Adenosine triphosphate-linked concentration of calcium ions in a particulate fraction of rabbit muscle. *J. Cell Biol.* 14:389-400 (1962).

Ebel, J. G., A. N. Taylor, and R. H. Wasserman. Vitamin D-induced calcium-binding protein of intestinal mucosa. *Amer. J. Clin. Nutr.* 22:431-436, (1969).

Eccles, J. C. The Synapse. *Sci. Amer.* 212(1):56-66 (1965).

Eck, R. V. Genetic code: Emergence of a symmetrical pattern. *Science* 140:477-480 (1963).

Edelman, I. S., H. B. Haley, P. R. Schloerb, D. B. Sheldon, B. J. Friis-Hansen, G. Stoll, and F. D. Moore. Further observations on total body water. I. Normal values throughout the life span. *Surg. Gynec. Obstet.* 95:1-12 (1952).

Edholm, O. G., J. G. Fletcher, E. M. Widdowson, and R. A. McCance. The energy expenditure and food intake of individual men. *Brit. J. Nutr.* 9: 286-300 (1955).

Edstrom, J. E. and W. Beermann. The base composition of nucleic acids in chromosomes, puffs, nucleoli, and cytoplasm of *Chirononus* salivary gland cells. *J. Cell Biol.* 14:371-379 (1962).

Edwards, O. M., R. I. S. Bayliss, and S. Millen. Urinary creatinine excretion as an index of the completeness of 24-hour urine collections. *Lancet* 2:1165-1166 (1969).

von Ehrenstein, G. Transfer RNA and amino acid activation. In *Aspects of Protein Biosynthesis,* Part A, pp. 139-214, C. B. Anfinsen, Jr., Ed., Academic Press, N. Y. (1970).

Ehret, C. F. and E. L. Powers. Macronuclear and nucleolar development in *paramecium bursaria. Exper. Cell Res.* 9:241-259 (1955).

Eichholz, A. and R. K. Crane. Studies on the organization of the brush border in intestinal epithelial cells. I. Tris disruption of isolated hamster brush borders and density gradient separation of fractions. *J. Cell Biol.* 26:687-691 (1965).

El-Gorab, M. and B. A. Underwood. Solubilization of β-carotene and retinol into aqueous solutions of mixed micelles. *Biochim. Biophys. Acta* 306:58-66 (1973).

Elias, H. Three-dimensional structure identified from single sections. *Science* 174:993-1000 (1971).

Ellenbogen, L. and D. R. Highley. Intrinsic factor. *Vitamins Hormones* 21:1-49 (1963).

Ellis, F. R., S. Holesh, and J. W. Ellis. Incidence of osteoporosis in vegetarians and omnivores. *Amer. J. Clin. Nutr.* 25:555-558 (1972).

Elsom, K. O'S., J. G. Reinhold, J. T. L. Nicholson, and C. Chornock. Studies of the B vitamins in the human subject. V. The normal requirement for thiamine; some factors influencing its utilization and excretion. *Amer. J. Med. Sci.* 203:569-577 (1942).

Elson, D. Preparation and proterties of a ribonucleoprotein isolated from *Escherichia coli. Biochim. Biophys. Acta* 36:362-371 (1959).

Elson, D. A ribonucleic acid particle released from ribosomes by salt. *Biochim. Biophys. Acta* 53:232-234 (1961).

Elvehjem, C. A., R. J. Madden, S. M. Strong, and D. W. Woolley. The isolation and identification of the anti-black tongue factor. *J. Biol. Chem.* 123:137-149 (1938).

Elwood, P. C., D. Newton, J. D. Eakins, and D. A. Brown. Absorption of iron from bread. *Amer. J. Clin. Nutr.* 21:1162-1169 (1968).

Emerick, R. J., M. Zile, and H. F. DeLuca. Formation of retinoic acid from retinol in the rat. *Biochem. J.* 102:606-611 (1967).

Emerson, G. A., E. Wurtz, and O. H. Johnson. The antiriboflavin effect of galactoflavin. *J. Biol. Chem.* 160:165-167 (1945).

Emmett, A. D. and G. O. Luros. Water-Soluble Vitamines. *J. Biol. Chem.* 43:265-280 (1920).

Enesco, M. and C. P. Leblond. Increase in cell number as a factor in the growth of the organs and tissues of the young male rat. *J. Embryol. Exp. Morph.* 10:530-562 (1962).

Enright, L. V., V. Cole, and F. A. Hitchcock. Basal metabolism and iodine excretion during pregnancy. *Amer. J. Physiol.* 113:221-228 (1935).

Ensinck, J. W. and R. H. Williams. Hormonal and nonhormonal factors modifying man's response to insulin. In *Handbook of Physiology,* Section 7, Vol. I, R. O. Greep and E. B. Astwood, Eds., pp. 665-684, American Physiological Society, Washington, D. C., (1972).

Epstein, A. N., J. T. Fitzsimons, and B. J. Simons. Drinking caused by the intracranial injection of angiotensin in the rat. *J. Physiol.* 200:98-100P (1969).

Ericsson, J. L. E. Mechanism of cellular autophagy. In *Lysosomes in Biology and Pathology,* Vol. 2, pp. 345-394, J. T. Dingle and H. B. Fell, Eds., *Frontiers of Biology,* Vol. 14A, Wiley-Interscience, N. Y. (1969).

Ericsson, J. L. E. and B. F. Trump. Electron microscopic studies of the epithelium of the proximal tubule of the rat kidney. III. Microbodies, multivesicular bodies, and the Golgi apparatus. *Lab. Invest.* 15:1610-1633 (1966).

Ericsson, J. L. E., B. F. Trump, and J. Weibel. Electron microscopic studies of the proximal tubule of the rat kidney. II. Cytosegresomes and cytosomes: Their relationship to each other and to the lysosome concept. *Lab. Invest.* 14:1341-1365 (1965).

Ernster, L. and B. Kuylenstierna. Outer membrane of mitochondria. In *Membranes of Mitochondria and Chloroplasts*, pp. 172-212, E. Racker, Ed., Van Nostrand Reinhold Company, N. Y. (1970).

Erslev, A. J. Humoral regulation of red cell production. *Blood* 8:349-357 (1953).

Ertel, R., N. Brot, B. Redfield, J. E. Allende, and H. Weissbach. Binding of guanosine 5'-triphosphate by soluble factors required for polypeptide synthesis. *Proc. Natl. Acad. Sci.* 59:861-868 (1968).

Essner, E. and A. Novikoff. Cytological studies on two functional hepatomas. Interrelations of endoplasmic reticulum, Golgi apparatus, and lysosomes. *J. Cell Biol.* 15:289-312 (1962).

von Euler, U. S. Zur Kenntnis der pharmakologischen Wirkungen von Nativsekreten und Extrackten mannlicher accessorischer Geschlechtsdrüsen. *Arch. Exp. Path. Pharmak.* 175:75-84 (1934).

von Euler, U. S. A depressor substance in the vesicular gland. *J. Physiol.* (London) 84:21p-22p (1935).

von Euler, U. S. Distribution and metabolism of catechol hormones in tissues and axones. *Rec. Progr. Hormone Res.* 14:483-512 (1958).

von Euler, U. S. Adrenergic neurotransmitter functions. *Science* 173:202-206 (1971).

Evans, H. M. The pioneer history of vitamin E. *Vitamins Hormones* 20:379-387 (1963).

Everson, G. J. and R. E. Shrader. Abnormal glucose tolerance in manganese-deficient guinea pigs. *J. Nutr.* 94:89-94 (1968).

Exton, J. H. Gluconeogenesis. *Metabolism* 21:945-990 (1972).

Exton, J. H., S. B. Lewis, R. J. Ho, G. A. Robinson, and C. R. Park. The role of cyclic AMP in the interaction of glucagon and insulin in the control of liver metabolism. *Ann. N. Y. Acad. Sci.* 185:85-100 (1971).

Falkner, F. An air displacement method of measuring body volume in babies: a preliminary communication. *Ann. N. Y. Acad. Sci.* 110:75-79 (1963).

Fambrough, D. M., D. B. Drachman, and S. Satyamurti. Neuromuscular junction in myasthenia gravis: decreased acetylcholine receptors. *Science* 182:293-295 (1973).

Farquhar, M. G. Lysosome function in regulating secretion: disposal of secretory granules in cells of the anterior pituitary gland. In *Lysosomes in Biology and Pathology*, Vol. 2, pp. 462-482, J. T. Dingle and H. B. Fell, Eds., *Frontiers of Biology*, Vol. 14A, Wiley-Interscience, N. Y. (1969).

Farquhar, M. G. and G. E. Palade. Junctional complexes in various epithelia. *J. Cell Biol.* 17:375-412 (1963).

Farquhar, M. G. and G. E. Palade. Cell junctions in amphibian skin. *J. Cell Biol.* 26:263-291 (1965).

Fasella, P. Pyridoxal phosphate. *Ann. Rev. Biochem.* 36:185-210 (1967).

Fatt, P. and B. Katz. Spontaneous subthreshold activity of motor nerve endings. *J. Physiol.* 117:109-128 (1952).

Favarger, P. Relative importance of different tissues in the synthesis of fatty acids. In *Handbook of Physiology*, Sec. 5, *Adipose Tissue*, pp. 19-23, A. E. Renold and G. F. Cahill, Eds., American Physiological Society, Washington, D. C. (1965).

Fawcett, D. W. Physiologically significant specializations of the cell surface. *Circulation* 26:1105-1125 (1962).

Fawcett, D. W. *The Cell. Its Organelles and Inclusions.* W. B. Saunders Company, Philadelphia (1966).

Fawcett, D. W., J. A. Long, and A. L. Jones. The ultrastructure of endocrine glands. *Rec. Progr. Hormone Res.* 25:315-368 (1969).

Fedorko, M. E. and J. G. Hirsch. Cytoplasmic granule formation in myelocytes. *J. Cell Biol.* 29:307-316 (1966).

Fekete, S. The significance of mucopolysaccharides in the pathogenesis of toxaemias of pregnancy. *Acta Med. Acad. Sci.* Hung. 5:293 (1954). Cited in Hytten and Leitch, 1971.

Feldherr, C. M. Structure and function of the nuclear envelope: nucleo-cytoplasmic exchanges. *Adv. Cytopharmacol.* 1:89-98 (1971).

Feldherr, C. M. Structure and function of the nuclear evelope. *Adv. Cell. Molec. Biol.* 2:273-307 (1972).

Feldman, S. L. and R. J. Cousins. Influence of cadmium on the metabolism of 25-hydroxy-cholecalciferol in chicks. *Nutr. Rep. Internl.* 8:251-260 (1973).

Felig, P., T. Pozefsky, E. Marliss, and G. F. Cahill, Jr. Alanine: Key role in gluconeogenesis. *Science* 167:1003-1004 (1970).

Felig, P. and J. Wahren. Protein turnover and amino acid metabolism in the regulation of gluconeogenesis. *Fed. Proc.* 33:1092-1097 (1974).

Fell, H. B. The effect of vitamin A on the breakdown and synthesis of intercellular material in skeletal tissue in organ culture. *Proc. Nutr. Soc.* 24:166-170 (1965).

Fell, H. B. The direct action of vitamin A on skeletal tissue *in vitro*. In *The Fat-Soluble Vitamins,* pp. 187-202, H. F. DeLuca and J. W. Suttie, Eds., The University of Wisconsin Press, Madison (1970).

Ferguson, J. H. Blood coagulation, thrombosis, and hemorrhagic disorders. *Ann. Rev. Physiol.* 8:231-262 (1946).

Fernández-Moran, H. Sheath and axon structures in the internode portion of vertebrate myelinated nerve fibers. An electron microscope study of rat and frog sciatic nerves. *Exper. Cell Res.* 1:309-340 (1950).

Fernández-Moran, H. The submicroscopic organization of vertebrate nerve fibers. An electron microscope study of myelinated and unmyelinated nerve fibers. *Exper. Cell Res.* 3:282-359 (1952).

Fernández-Moran, H. Cell-membrane ultrastructure. *Circulation* 26:1039-1065 (1962).

Fernández-Moran, H. Membrane ultrastructure in nerve cells. In *The Neurosciences,* pp. 281-304, G. C. Quarton, T. Melnechuk, and F. O. Schmitt, Eds., Rockefeller University Press, New York (1967).

Fernstrom, J. D. and R. J. Wurtman. Nutrition and the brain. *Sci. Amer.* 230(2):84-91 (1974).

Ferro-Luzzi, G. Rapid evaluation of nutritional level. *Amer. J. Clin. Nutr.* 19:247-254 (1966).

Fidge, N. H. and D. S. Goodman. The enzymatic reduction of retinal to retinol in rat intestine. *J. Biol. Chem.* 243:4372-4379 (1968).

Fidge, N. H., T. Shiratori, J. Ganguly, and D. S. Goodman. Pathways of absorption of retinal and retinoic acid in the rat. *J. Lipid Res.* 9:103-109 (1968).

Field, J., H. S. Belding, and A. W. Martin. An analysis of the relation between basal metabolism and summated tissue respiration in the rat. *J. Cell Comp. Physiol.* 14:143-157 (1939).

Finch, C. A. Body iron exchange in man. *J. Clin. Invest.* 38:392-396 (1959).

Finch, C. A. Ferrokinetics and hemoglobin synthesis in man. *Vitamins Hormones* 26:515-523 (1968).

Fish, I. and M. Winick. Cellular growth in various regions of the developing rat brain. *Pediat. Res.* 3:407-412 (1969).

Fishbein, W. N. and S. P. Bessman. γ-Hydroxybutyrate in mammalian brain. *J. Biol. Chem.* 239:357-361 (1964).

Fisher, H., M. K. Brush, and P. Griminger. Reassessment of amino acid requirements of young women on low nitrogen diets. II. Leucine, methionine and valine. *Amer. J. Clin.*

984 BIBLIOGRAPHY

Nutr. 24:1216-1223 (1971).

Fisher, H., M. K. Brush, P. Griminger, and E. R. Sostman. Amino acid balance and nitrogen retention in man as related to prior protein nutrition. *J. Nutr.* 87:306-310 (1965).

Fisher, J. W. Introduction to Conference on Erythropoietin. *Ann. N. Y. Acad. Sci.* 149:9-11 (1968).

Fishman, M. A., P. Madyastha, and A. L. Prensky. The effects of undernutrition on the development of myelin in the rat central nervous system. *Lipids* 6:458-465 (1971).

Fishman, M. A., A. L. Prensky, M. E. Tumbleson, and B. Daftari. Relative resistance of the later phase of myelination to severe undernutrition in miniature swine. *Amer. J. Clin. Nutr.* 25:7-10 (1972).

Fitch, C. D. Experimental anemia in primates due to vitamin E deficiency. *Vitamins Hormones* 26:501-514 (1968).

Fitzsimons, J. T. The role of a renal thirst factor in drinking induced by extracellular stimuli. *J. Physiol.* 201:349-368 (1969).

Fitzsimons, J. T. and B. J. Simons. The effect on drinking in the rat of intravenous infusion of angiotensin, given alone or in combination with other thirst stimuli. *J. Physiol.* 203:45-57 (1969).

Fleischer, S., G. Rouser, B. Fleischer, A. Casu, and G. Kritchevsky. Lipid composition of mitochondria from bovine heart, liver, and kidney. *J. Lipid Res.* 8:170-180 (1967).

Fleshler, B. and R. A. Nelson. Sodium dependency of L-alanine absorption in canine Thiry-Vella loops. *Gut* 11:240-244 (1970).

Flickinger, C. J. The development of Golgi complexes and their dependence upon the nucleus in *Amebae. J. Cell Biol.* 43:250-262 (1969).

Florendo, N. T. Ribosome substructure in intact mouse liver cells. *J. Cell Biol.* 41:335-339 (1969).

Flores, M. Dietary studies for assessment of the nutritional status of populations in non-modernized societies. *Amer. J. Clin. Nutr.* 11:344-355 (1962).

Folin, O. A theory of protein metabolism. *Amer. J. Physiol.* 13:117-138 (1905).

Foltz, E. E., C. J. Barborka, and A. C. Ivy. The level of vitamin B-complex in the diet at which detectable symptoms of deficiency occur in man. *Gastroenterology* 2:323-344 (1944).

Fomon, S. J., R. L. Jensen, and G. M. Owen. Determination of body volume of infants by a method of helium displacement. *Ann. N. Y. Acad. Sci.* 110:80-90 (1963).

Foman, S. J., M. K. Younoszai, and L. N. Thomas. Influence of vitamin D on linear growth of normal full-term infants. *J. Nutr.* 88:345-350 (1966).

Food and Agriculture Organization of the United Nations, *Handbook of Human Nutritional Requirements.* FAO, Rome, 66 pp. (1974).

Food and Agriculture Organization of the United Nations, Second Committee on Calorie Requirements, *Calorie Requirements,* FAO Nutrition Studies 15 (1957).

Food and Agriculture Organization of the United Nations. Program of Food Consumption Surveys. FAO, Rome, 70 pp. (1964).

Food and Agriculture Organization/World Health Organization. *Calcium requirements.* Tech. Rep. WHO No. Tech. Rep. Ser. 230, Geneva (1962).

Food and Agriculture Organization/World Health Organization. *Requirements of vitamin A, thiamine, riboflavine and niacin.* Tech. Rep. Ser. No. 362 (1967).

Food and Agriculture Organization/World Health Organization. *Requirements of ascorbic acid, vitamin D, vitamin B$_{12}$, folate and iron.* Report of a Joint FAO/WHO Expert Committee, WHO Tech. Rep. Ser. No. 452, WHO, Geneva. 75 pp. (1970).

Food and Agriculture Organization/World Health Organization. *Energy and protein requirements.* WHO Tech. Rep. Ser. No. 522, Geneva (1973).

Food and Nutrition Board. National Research Council. *Recommended Dietary Allowances.*

Natl. Acad. Sci. Circular No. 115 (1943); 122 (1945); 129 (1948); 302 (1958); 1146 (1964); 1694 (1968).

Food and Nutrition Board. *Zinc in human nutrition.* National Research Council, Nat. Acad. Sci., Washington, D.C., 50 pp. (1970).

Food and Nutrition Board, NAS-NRC, and Council on Foods and Nutrition, AMA. Diet and coronary heart disease. *Nutr. Rev.* 30:223-225 (1972).

Food and Nutrition Board, National Research Council. *Recommended Dietary Allowances,* 8th ed., Natl. Acad. Sci., Washington, D. C. (1974).

Forbes, G. B. Another source of error in the metabolic balance method. *Nutr. Rev.* 31:297-300 (1973).

Forbes, G. B. Growth of the lean body mass in man. *Growth* 36:325-338 (1972).

Forbes, G. B., J. Gallup, and J. B. Hursh. Estimation of total body fat from potassium-40 content. *Science* 133:101-102 (1961).

Forbes, G. B. and J. B. Hursh. Age and sex trends in lean body mass calculated from K^{40} measurements: With a note on the theoretical basis for the procedure. *Ann. N. Y. Acad. Sci.* 110:255-263 (1963).

Forbes, R. M. Nutritional interactions of zinc and calcium. *Fed. Proc.* 19:643-647 (1960).

Forbes, R. M., A. R. Cooper, and H. H. Mitchell. The composition of the adult human body as determined by chemical analysis. *J. Biol. Chem.* 203:359-366 (1953).

Forbes, R. M., H. H. Mitchell, and R. A. Cooper. Further studies on the gross composition and mineral elements of the adult human body. *J. Biol. Chem.* 223:969-975 (1956).

Fordtran, J. S. and F. J. Ingelfinger. Absorption of water, electrolytes, and sugars from the human gut. In *Handbook of Physiology,* Section 6: *Alimentary Canal,* Vol. III, pp. 1457-1490, C. F. Code, Ed., American Physiological Society, Washington, D.C. (1968).

Fore, H. and R. A. Morton. Manganese in rabbit tissues. *Biochem. J.* 51:600-603 (1952).

Forsgren, L. Studies on the intestinal absorption of labelled fat-soluble vitamins (A, D, E, and K) via the thoracic-duct lymph in the absence of bile in man. *Acta Chir. Scand. Suppl.* 399, 3-29 (1969).

Forster, J. Versuche uber die Bedeutung der Aschebestandtheile in der Nahrung. *Z. Biol.* 9:297-380 (1873).

Foster, G. V., I. MacIntyre, and A. G. E. Pearse. Calcitonin production and the mito-chondrion-rich cells of the dog thyroid. *Nature* 203: 1029-1030 (1964).

Fourman, P. and P. Royer. *Calcium Metabolism and the Bone.* 2nd Ed., F. A. Davis Company, Philadelphia (1968).

Fox, H. C. and D. S. Miller. Acknee Toxin: a riboflavin antimetabolite? *Nature* 186:561-562 (1960).

Foy, H. and A. Kondi. Comparison between erythroid aplasia in marasmus and kwashiorkor and the experimentally induced erythroid aplasia in baboons in riboflavin deficiency. *Vitamins Hormones* 26:653-681 (1968).

Fraenkel-Conrat, J. and H. Fraenkel-Conrat. Metabolic fate of biotin and of avidin-biotin complex upon parenteral administration. *Biochim. Biophys. Acta* 8:66-70 (1952).

Francois, P. J. Food consumption surveys - study on a general formula for the estimation of per caput, household and group consumption. *Nutrition Newsletter* 8:10-26 (1970).

Franke, W. W. Isolated nuclear membranes. *J. Cell Biol.* 31:619-623 (1966).

Franke, W. W. On the universality of nuclear pore complex structure. *Z. Zellforsch. Mikrosk. Anat.* 105:405-429 (1970).

Franke, W. W., cited in Feldherr, C. M. Structure and function of the nuclear envelope: nucleocytoplasmic exchanges. *Adv. Cytopharmacol.* 1:89-98 (1971).

Franke, W. W., B. Deumling, B. Ermen, E. D. Jarasch, and H. Kleinig. Nuclear membranes from mammalian liver. I. Isolation procedure and general characteristics. *J. Cell. Biol.* 46:379-395 (1970).

Franke, W. W. and U. Scheer. The ultrastructure of the nuclear envelope of amphibian oocytes: a reinvestigation. I. The mature oocyte. *J. Ultrastruct. Res.* 30:288-316 (1970a).

Franke, W. W. and U. Scheer. The ultrastructure of the nuclear envelope of amphibian oocytes: A reinvestigation. II. The immature oocyte and dynamic aspects. *J. Ultrastruct. Res.* 30:317-327 (1970b).

Frankel, S. and S. Yasumura. Change in the thyroidal content of thyrocalcitonin produced by vitamin D in rats. *Endocrinology* 88:267-270 (1971).

Frankova, S. and R. H. Barnes. Influence of malnutrition in early life on exploratory behavior of rats. *J. Nutr.* 96:477-484 (1968a).

Frankova, S. and R. H. Barnes. Effect of malnutrition in early life on avoidance conditioning and behavior of adult rats. *J. Nutr.* 96:485-493 (1968b).

Fransson, L. Å. Structure and metabolism of the proteoglycans of dermatan sulfate. In *Chemistry and Molecular Biology of the Intracellular Matrix.* E. A. Balazs, Ed., Academic Press, N. Y. (1970).

Fraser, D., B. S. L. Kidd, S. W. Kooh, and L. Paunier. A new look at infantile hypercalcemia. *Pediat. Clin. N. Amer.* 13:503-525 (1966).

Fraser, D. R. and E. Kodicek. Investigations on vitamin D esters synthesized in rats. Detection and identification. *Biochem. J.* 106:485-490 (1968a).

Fraser, D. R. and E. Kodicek. Investigations on vitamin D esters synthesized in rats. Turnover and sites of synthesis. *Biochem. J.* 106:491-496 (1968b).

Fraser, D. R. and E. Kodicek. Enzyme studies on the esterification of vitamin D in rat tissues. *Biochem. J.* 109:457-467 (1968c).

Fraser, D. R. and E. Kodicek. Unique biosynthesis by kidney of a biologically active vitamin D metabolite. *Nature* 228:764-766 (1970).

Fraser, D. R. and E. Kodicek. Regulation of 25-hydroxycholecalciferol-1-hydroxylase activity in kidney by parathyroid hormone. *Nature* 241:163-166 (1973).

Frazer, A. C. Fat absorption and metabolism. *Analyst* 63:308-314 (1938).

Frenchman, R. and F. A. Johnston. Relation of menstrual losses to iron requirement. *J. Amer. Diet. Ass.* 25:217-220 (1949).

Frieden, E. Ceruloplasmin, a link between copper and iron metabolism. *Nutr. Rev.* 28:87-91 (1970).

Frieden, E. The ferrous to ferric cycles in iron metabolism. *Nutr. Rev.* 31:41-44 (1973).

Friedland, N. "Normal" lactose tolerance test. *Arch. Intern. Med.* 116:886-888 (1965).

Friedmann, T. Prenatal diagnosis of genetic disease. *Sci. Amer.* 225(5):34-42 (1971).

Friedrich, von, W. Antagonisten des vitamins B_{12}. *Bibl. Nutritio et Dieta* 8:178-225 (1966).

Friend, B. Nutrients in United States food supply. A review of trends, 1909-1913 to 1965. *Amer. J. Clin. Nutr.* 20:907-914 (1967).

Friis-Hansen, B. Hydrometry of growth and aging. In *Human Body Composition*, pp. 191-209, J. Brozek, Ed., Pergamon Press, Oxford (1965).

Friis-Hansen, B. Body water compartments in children: changes during growth and related changes in body composition. *Pediat.* 28: 169-181 (1961).

Friis-Hansen, B. Body composition during growth. *In vivo* measurements and biochemical data correlated to differential anatomical growth. *Pediat.* 47:264-274 (1971).

Fujimoto, D. and N. Tamiya. Incorporation of ^{18}O from air into hydroxyproline by chick embryo. *Biochem. J.* 84:333-335 (1962).

Fuller, R. W. Control of epinephrine synthesis and secretion. *Fed. Proc.* 32:1772-1781 (1973).

Fuller, W. and A. Hodgson. Conformation of the anticodon loop in tRNA. *Nature* 215:817-821 (1967).

Funk, C. The etiology of the deficiency diseases. *J. State Med.* 20:341-368 (1912).

Gad, P. and S. L. Clark, Jr. Involution and regeneration of the thymus in mice, induced by bacterial endotoxin and studied by quantitative histology and electron microscopy. *Amer. J. Anat.* 122:573-585 (1968).

Gall, J. G. Octagonal nuclear pores. *J. Cell Biol.* 32:391-399 (1967).

Gallo-Torres, H. E. Obligatory role of bile for the intestinal absorption of vitamin E. *Lipids* 5:379-384 (1970a).

Gallo-Torres, H. E. Intestinal absorption and lymphatic transport of d,1-3,4-^{3}H$_2$-α-tocopheryl nicotinate in the rat. *Int. Z. Vitaminforsch.* 40:505-514 (1970b).

Galton, D. J. *The Human Adipose Cell: A Model for Errors in Metabolic Regulation.* Appleton-Century-Crofts, N. Y. (1971).

Gamow, G. Possible relation between deoxyribonucleic acid and protein structures. *Nature* 173:318 (1954).

Ganguly, J. Absorption of vitamin A. *Amer. J. Clin. Nutr.* 22:923-933 (1969).

Garabedian, M., M. F. Holick, H. F. DeLuca and I. T. Boyle. Control of 25-hydroxy-cholecalciferol metabolism by parathyroid glands. *Proc. Natl. Acad. Sci.* 69:1673-1676 (1972).

Garby, L. and W. D. Noyes. Studies on hemoglobin metabolism: II. Pathways of hemoglobin iron metabolism in normal man. *J. Clin. Invest.* 38:1484-1486 (1959).

Garn, S. M. Comparison of pinch-caliper and X-ray measurements of skin plus subcutaneous fat. *Science* 124:178-179 (1956).

Garn, S. M. Selection of body sites for fat measurement. *Science* 125:550-551 (1957).

Garn, S. M. The evolutionary and genetic control of variability in man. *Ann. N. Y. Acad. Sci.* 134:602-615 (1966).

Garn, S. M., G. R. Greaney, and R. W. Young. Fat thickness and growth progress during infancy. In *Body Measurements and Human Nutrition*, pp. 122-140, J. Brozek, Ed., Wayne University Press, Detroit (1956).

Garn, S. M., C. C. Rohmann, and B. Wagner. Bone loss as a general phenomenon in man. *Fed. Proc.* 26:1729-1736 (1967).

Garn, S. M., N. N. Rosen, and M. B. McCann. Relative values of different fat folds in a nutritional survey. *Amer. J. Clin. Nutr.* 24:1380-1381 (1971).

Garren, L. D., G. N. Gill, and G. M. Walton. The isolation of a receptor for adenosine 3',5'-cyclic monophosphate (cAMP) from the adrenal cortex: The role of the receptor in the mechanism of action of cAMP. *Ann. N. Y. Acad. Sci.* 185:210-226 (1971).

Garrod, A. E. The incidence of alkaptonuria: A study of chemical individuality. *Lancet* ii:1616-1620 (1902).

Gaster, D., E. Havivi, and K. Guggenheim. Interrelations of calcium, fluorine and vitamin D in bone metabolism. *Brit. J. Nutr.* 21: 413-418 (1967).

Gay, C. V. and W. J. Mueller. Carbonic anhydrase and osteoclasts: Localization by labeled inhibitor autoradiography. *Science* 183:432-434 (1974).

Gedalia, I. and I. Zipkin. *The Role of Fluoride in Bone Structure.* Warren H. Green, Inc., St. Louis (1973).

Geffen, L. B. and G. V. Livett. Synaptic vesicles in sympathetic neurons. *Physiol. Rev.* 51:98-157 (1971).

Geren, B. B. and F. O. Schmitt. Electron microscope studies of the Schwann cell and its constituents with particular reference to their relation to the axon. In *8th Congress of Cell Biology*, Leiden, pp. 251-260, Wiley-Interscience, N. Y. (1954).

Gerson, C. D. and N. Cohen. The absorption of folic acid in man: Recent progress. *Mt. Sinai J. Med.* 39:343-351 (1972).

Gerstl, B., M. G. Tavaststjerna, R. B. Hayman, J. K. Smith, and L. F. Eng. Lipid studies of white matter and thalamus of human brains. *J. Neurochem.* 10:889-902 (1963).

Gholson, R. K. The pyridine nucleotide cycle. *Nature* 212:933-935 (1966).

Gibor, A. and S. Granick. Plastids and mitochondria: Inheritable systems. *Science* 145:

890-897 (1964).

Giese, A. C. *Cell Physiology*, 4th ed., W. B. Saunders, Philadelphia (1973).

Gilbert, W. and B. Muller-Hill. Isolation of the *lac* repressor. *Proc. Natl. Acad. Sci.* 56:1891-1898 (1966).

Gillman, T., M. Hathorn, and P. A. S. Canham. Experimental dietary siderosis. *Amer. J. Path.* 35:349-368 (1959).

Ginsburg, V. and H. G. Hers. On the conversion of fructose to glucose by guinea pig intestine. *Biochim. Biophys. Acta* 38:427-434 (1960).

Glaser, M., H. Simpkins, S. J. Singer, M. Sheetz, and S. I. Chan. On the interactions of lipids and proteins in the red blood cell membrane. *Proc. Natl. Acad. Sci.* 65:721-728 (1970).

Glaser, M. and S. J. Singer. Circular dichroism and the conformations of membrane proteins. Studies with red blood cell membranes. *Biochemistry* 10:1780-1787 (1971).

Glass, G. B. J. Gastric intrinsic factor and its function in metabolism of vitamin B_{12}. *Physiol. Rev.* 43:529-849 (1963).

Glass, G. B. J. *Gastric Intrinsic Factor and Other Vitamin B_{12} Binders.* Biochemistry, Physiology, Pathology and Relations to Vitamin B_{12} Metabolism. Georg Thieme Publishers, Stuttgart (1974).

Glomset, J. A. The mechanism of the plasma cholesterol esterification reaction: Plasma fatty acid transferase. *Biochim. Biophys. Acta* 65:128-135 (1962).

Gloor, U., J. Wursch, H. Mayer, O. Isler, and O. Wiss. Stoffwechsel-end-produkte von phyllochinon, menachinon-4, ubichinon-9 and hexahydroplastochinon-4 (phytylplastochinon). *Helv. Chim. Acta* 49:2582-2589 (1966).

Gnaedinger, R. H., E. P. Reineke, A. M. Pearson, W. D. Van Huss, J. A. Wessel, and H. J. Montoye. Determination of body density by air displacement, helium dilution and underwater weighing. *Ann. N. Y. Acad. Sci.* 110:96-108 (1963).

Go, V. L. W. and W. H. J. Summerskill. Digestion, maldigestion, and the gastrointestinal hormones. *Amer. J. Clin. Nutr.* 24:160-167 (1971).

Goldberg, A. L. Mechanisms of growth and atrophy of skeletal muscle. In *Muscle Biology*, Vol. 1, 89-118, R. G. Cassens, Ed., Marcel Dekker, Inc. New York (1972).

Goldberger, J. The transmissibility of pellagra. Public Health Reports 31:3159-3173 (1916).

Goldberger, J. and G. A. Wheeler. Experimental pellagra in the human subject brought about by a restricted diet. Public Health Reports 30:3336-3339 (1915).

Goldberger, J. and G. A. Wheeler. Experimental black tongue of dogs and its relation to pellagra. *Public Health Reports* 43:172-217 (1928).

Goldblatt, M. W. A depressor substance in seminal fluid. *J. Soc. Chem. Ind.* (London) 52:1056-1057 (1933).

Goldblatt, M. W. Properties of human seminal plasma. *J. Physiol.* (London) 84:208-218 (1935).

Goldman, R. F., B. Bullen, and C. Seltzer. Changes in specific gravity and body fat in overweight female adolescents as a result of weight reduction. *Ann. N. Y. Acad. Sci.* 110:913-917 (1963).

Goldrick, R. B., B. C. E. Ashley, and M. L. Lloyd. Effects of prolonged incubation and cell concentration on lipogenesis from glucose in isolated human omental fat cells. *J. Lipid Res.* 10:253-259 (1969).

Goldsmith, G. A. Experimental niacin deficiency. *J. Amer. Diet. Ass.* 32:312-316 (1956).

Goldsmith, G. A. *Nutritional Diagnosis.* C. C. Thomas, Springfield, Ill. (1959).

Goldsmith, G. A., O. N. Miller, and W. G. Unglaub. Efficiency of tryptophan as a niacin precursor in man. *J. Nutr.* 73:172-176 (1961).

Goldsmith, G. A., H. P. Sarett, U. D. Register, and J. Gibbens. Studies of niacin requirement in man. I. Experimental pellagra in subjects on corn diets low in niacin and tryptophan. *J. Clin. Invest.* 31:533-542 (1952).

Goldstein, L. Nucleocytoplasmic relationship. In *Cytology and Cell Physiology*, 3rd ed., pp. 559-635, G. H. Bourne, Ed., Academic Press, N. Y. (1964).

Goldwasser, E., L. O. Jacobson, W. Fried, and L. Pizak. Mechanism of the erythropoietic effect of cobalt. *Science* 125:1085-1086 (1957).

Goldwasser, E. and C. K. H. Kung. Properties of purified erythropoietin-E. Fed. Proc. 30:1128A (1971).

Gontzea, I. and P. Sutzescu. *Natural Antinutritive Substances in Foodstuffs and Forages*. S. Karger, Basel (Switzerland), (1968).

Gonzales, F. and M. J. Karnovsky. Electron microscopy of osteoclasts in healing fractures of rat bone. *J. Biophys. Biochem. Cytol.* 9:299-316 (1961).

Goodenough, U. W. and R. P. Levine. The genetic activity of mitochondria and chloroplasts. *Sci. Amer.* 223(5):22-29 (1970).

Goodman, DeW. S. Preparation of human serum albumin free of long-chain fatty acids. *Science* 125:1296-1297 (1957).

Goodman, DeW. S. Biosynthesis of vitamin A from β-carotene. *Amer. J. Clin. Nutr.* 22:963-965 (1969a).

Goodman, DeW. S. Retinol transport in human plasma. *Amer. J. Clin. Nutr.* 22:911-912 (1969b).

Goodman, DeW. S. Retinol transport in human plasma. In *The Fat-Soluble Vitamins*, pp. 203-212, H. F. DeLuca and J. W. Suttie, Eds., The University of Wisconsin Press, Madison (1970).

Goodman, DeW. S., R. Blomstrand, B. Werner, H. S. Huang, and T. Shiratori. The intestinal absorption and metabolism of vitamin A and β-carotene in man. *J. Clin. Invest.* 45:1615-1623 (1966).

Goodman, DeW. S. and H. S. Huang. Biosynthesis of vitamin A with rat intestinal enzymes. *Science* 149:879-880 (1965).

Goodman, DeW. S., H. S. Huang, M. Kanai, and T. Shiratori. The enzymatic conversion of all-*trans*-β-carotene into retinal. *J. Biol. Chem.* 242:3543-3554 (1967).

Goodman, DeW. S. and R. B. Leslie. Fluorescence studies of human plasma retinol-binding protein and of the retinol-binding protein-prealbumin complex. *Biochim. Biophys. Acta* 260:670-678 (1972).

Goodman, DeW. S. and R. P. Noble. Turnover of plasma cholesterol in man. *J. Clin. Invest.* 47:231-241 (1968).

Goodridge, A. G. and E. G. Ball. Lipogenesis in the pigeon: *in vitro* studies. *Amer. J. Physiol.* 211:803-808 (1966).

Gopalan, C., P. S. Venkatachalam, and B. Bhavani. Studies of vitamin A deficiency in children. *Amer. J. Clin. Nutr.* 8:833-840 (1960).

Gordon, E. E., K. Kowalski, and M. Fritts. Muscle proteins and DNA in rat quadriceps during growth. *Amer. J. Physiol.* 210:1033-1040 (1966).

Gorter, E. and F. Grendel. On bimolecular layers of lipoids on the chromocytes of the blood. *J. Exp. Med.* 41:439-443 (1925).

Gottlieb, A. A., A. Kaplan, and S. Udenfriend. Further evidence for the accumulation of a hydroxyproline-deficient, collangenase-degradable protein during collagen biosynthesis *in vitro*. *J. Biol. Chem.* 241:1551-1555 (1966).

Graham, R. C. and M. J. Karnovsky. The early stages of absorption of injected horseradish peroxidase in the proximal tubules of mouse kidney: ultrastructural cytochemistry by a new technique. *J. Histochem. Cytochem.* 14:291-302 (1966).

Granick, S. Iron metabolism and hemochromatosis. *Bull. N. Y. Acad. Med.* 25:403-428 (1949).

Granick, S. Iron metabolism. *Bull. N. Y. Acad. Med.* 30:81-105 (1954).

Gräsbeck, R., K. Simons, and I. Sinkkonen. Isolation of intrinsic factors from human gastric juice. *Acta. Chem. Scand.* 19:1777-1778 (1965).

Gräsbeck, R., K. Simons, and I. Sinkkonen. Isolation of intrinsic factor and its probable degradation product, as their vitamin B_{12} complexes, from human gastric juice. *Biochim. Biophys. Acta* 127:47-58 (1966).

Gray, R., I. Boyle, and H. F. DeLuca. Vitamin D metabolism: The role of kidney tissue. *Science* 172:1232-1234 (1972).

Gray, T. K. and P. L. Munson. Thyrocalcitonin. Evidence for physiological function. *Science* 166:512-513 (1969).

Graystone, J. E. and D. B. Cheek. The effects of reduced caloric intake and increased insulin-induced caloric intake on the cell growth of muscle, liver and cerebrum and on the skeletal collagen in the postweanling rat. *Pediat. Res.* 3:66-76 (1969).

Greaves, J. D. and L. A. Schmidt. Relation of bile to absorption of vitamin E in the rat. *Proc. Soc. Exp. Biol. Med.* 37:40-42 (1937).

Green, C. The transport of sterol across the mucosa. In *Biochemical Problems of Lipids*, pp. 144-148, A. C. Frazer, Ed., Elsevier, Amsterdam (1963).

Green, D. E. The mitochondrion. *Sci. Amer.* 210(1):63-74 (1964).

Green, D. E. Membrane proteins: A perspective. *Ann. N. Y. Acad. Sci.* 195:150-172 (1972).

Green, D. E. and Y. Hatefi. The mitochondrion and biochemical machines. *Science* 133:13-19 (1961).

Green, D. E., W. F. Loomis, and V. H. Auerbach. Studies on the cyclophorase system. I. The complete oxidation of pyruvic acid to carbon dioxide and water. *J. Biol. Chem.* 172:389-403 (1948).

Green, D. E. and D. H. MacLennan. Structure and function of the mitochondrial cristael membrane. *Bioscience* 19:213-222 (1969).

Green, D. E. and J. F. Perdue. Correlation of mitochondrial structure and function. *Ann. N. Y. Acad. Sci.* 137:667-684 (1966).

Green, D. E. and A. Tzagloff. Role of lipids in the structure and function of biological membranes. *J. Lipid Res.* 7:587-602 (1966).

Green, D. E. and J. H. Young. Energy transduction in membrane systems. *Amer. Sci.* 59:92-100 (1971).

Green, J. Antagonists of vitamin A. *Bibl. Nutritio et Dieta* 8:33-43 (1966).

Green, J. Antagonists of vitamin K. *Vitamins Hormones* 24:619-632 (1966).

Green, J. Vitamin E and the biological antioxidant theory. *Ann. N. Y. Acad. Sci.* 203:29-44 (1972).

Green, J. and J. Bunyan. Vitamin E and the biological antioxidant theory. *Nutr. Abstr. Rev.* 39:321-343 (1969).

Green, N. M. Evidence for a genetic relationship between avidins and lysozymes. *Nature* 217:254-256 (1968).

Green, N. M. Spectrophotometric determination of avidin and biotin. In *Methods in Enzymology*, Vol. XVIII, Part A, pp. 418-424, D. B. McCormick and L. D. Wright, Eds., Academic Press, N. Y. (1970).

Green, R., W. E. Carlson, and C. A. Evans. The inactivation of vitamin B_1 in diets containing whole fish. *J. Nutr.* 23:165-174 (1942).

Green, R., R. W. Charlton, H. Seftel, T. H. Bothwell, F. Mayet, E. B. Adams, C. A. Finch, and M. Layrisse. Body iron excretion in man: a collaborative study. *Amer. J. Med.* 45:336-353 (1968).

Greenberg, D. M. Studies in mineral metabolism with the aid of artificial radioactive isotopes. VIII. Tracer experiments with radioactive calcium and strontium on the mechanism of vitamin D action in rachitic rats. *J. Biol. Chem.* 157:99-104 (1945).

Greenberger, N. J., S. P. Balcerzak, and G. A. Ackerman. Iron uptake by isolated intestinal brush borders: Changes induced by alterations in iron stores. *J. Lab. Clin. Med.* 73:711-721 (1969).

Greenberger, N. J. and T. G. Skillman. Medium-chain triglycerides. Physiologic considerations and clinical implications. *New Eng. J. Med.* 280:1045-1058 (1969).

Greengard, P. and J. W. Kebabian. Role of cyclic AMP in synaptic transmission in the mammalian peripheral nervous system. *Fed. Proc.* 33: 1059-1067 (1974).

Greer, M. A. and Y. Grimm. Changes in thyroid secretion produced by inhibition of iodotyrosine deoxidase. *Endocrinology* 83:405-410 (1968).

Griffith, W. H. and J. F. Nyc. Choline X. Effects of deficiency. In *The Vitamins*, Vol. III, pp. 81-123, W. H. Sebrell and R. S. Harris, Eds., Academic Press, N. Y. (1971).

Griffith, W. H. and N. J. Wade. Choline metabolism. I. The occurrence and prevention of hemorrhagic degeneration in young rats on a low choline diet. *J. Biol. Chem.* 131:567-577 (1939).

Griminger, P. Biological activity of the various vitamin K forms. *Vitamins Hormones* 24:605-618 (1966).

Grobstein, C. Differentiation of vertebrate cells. In *The Cell*, Vol. I, pp. 437-496, J. Brachet and A. E. Mirsky, Eds., Academic Press, N. Y. (1959).

Grobstein, C. Cytodifferentiation and its controls. *Science* 143:643-650 (1964).

Gross, S. and D. K. Melhorn. Vitamin E, red cell lipids and red cell stability in prematurity. *Ann. N. Y. Acad. Sci.* 203:141-162 (1972).

Grossman, M. I. The spectrum of gastrointestinal hormone action. In 16th Nobel Symposium Frontiers of *Gastrointestinal Hormone Research*, S. Andersson, Ed., Almqvist and Wiksell, Stockholm (1970).

Grove, S. N., C. E. Bracker, and D. J. Morré. Cytomembrane differentiation in the endoplasmic reticulum-Golgi apparatus-vesicle complex. *Science* 161:171-173 (1968).

Grundfest, H. Synaptic and ephaptic transmission. In The *Neurosciences*, pp. 353-372, G. C. Quarton, T. Melnechuk, and F. O. Schmitt, Eds., Rockefeller University Press, New York (1967).

Grundy, S. M. and E. H. Ahrens, Jr. The effects of unsaturated dietary fats on absorption, excretion, synthesis, and distribution of cholesterol in man. *J. Clin. Invest.* 49:1135-1152 (1970).

Grundy, S., E. H. Ahrens, and J. Davignon. The interaction of cholesterol absorption and cholesterol synthesis in man. *J. Lipid Res.* 10:304-315 (1969).

Guarnieri, M. and R. M. Johnson. The essential fatty acids. *Advances Lipid Res.* 8:115-174 (1970).

Gubler, C. J. Enzyme studies in thiamine deficiency. *Internat. Zeitschr. Vitaminforschung.* 38:287-303 (1968).

Gubler, C. J. Thiamine and heart function. *J. Vitaminol.* 15:346-348 (1969).

Guha, A. and O. A. Roels. The influence of α-tocopherol on arylsulfatases A and B in the liver of vitamin A-deficient rats. *Biochim. Biophys. Acta* 111:364-374 (1965).

Gunsalus, I. C. The chemistry and function of the pyruvate oxidation factor (lipoic acid). *J. Cell. Comp. Physiol.* 41:113-136 (1953).

Gurney, J. M. and D. B. Jelliffe. Arm anthropometry in nutritional assessment: nomogram for rapid calculation of muscle circumference and cross-sectional muscle and fat areas. *Amer. J. Clin. Nutr.* 26:912-915 (1973).

Gurr, M. I. and A. T. James. *Lipid Biochemistry: An Introduction.* Cornell University Press, Ithaca, N. Y. (1971).

Guthrie, H. A. Severe undernutrition in early infancy and behavior in rehabilitated female rats. *Physiol. Behav.* 3: 619-623 (1968).

Guthrie, H. A. and M. L. Brown. Effect of severe undernutrition in early growth, brain size and composition in adult rats. *J. Nutr.* 94:419-426 (1968).

Guttmann, St., J. Pless, R. L. Huguenin, Ed. Sandrin, H. Bossert, and K. Zehnder. Synthesis of a highly potent hypocalcaemic dotriacontapeptide, having the properties of salmon calcitonin. In *Calcitonin: Proceedings of the Second International Symposium*, pp. 74-79, Springer-Verlag, New York (1970).

György, P. Vitamin B_2 and the pellagra-like dermatitis in rats. *Nature* 133:498-499 (1934).

György, P. Crystalline vitamin B_6. *J. Amer. Chem. Soc.* 60:983-984 (1938).

György, P. The curative factor (Vitamin H) for egg white injury, with particular reference to its presence in different foodstuffs and in yeast. *J. Biol. Chem.* 131:733-744 (1939).

György, P., Ed., *Vitamin Methods*, Vol. I., Academic Press, N. Y. (1950).

György, P. Early experiences with riboflavin—A retrospect. *Nutr. Rev.* 12:97-100 (1954).

György, P. Symposium on vitamin E and metabolism. *Vitamins Hormones* 20:599-601 (1962).

György, P. Developments leading to the metabolic role of vitamin B_6. *Amer. J. Clin. Nutr.* 24:1250-1256 (1971).

Habener, J. F., F. R. Singer, L. J. Deftos, and J. T. Potts, Jr. Immunological stability of calcitonin in plasma. *Endocrinology* 90:952-960 (1972).

Hackenbrock, C. R. Ultrastructural bases for metabolically linked mechanical activity in mitochondria. I. Reversible ultrastructural changes with change in metabolic steady state in isolated liver mitochondria. *J. Cell Biol.* 30:269-297 (1966).

Hackenbrock, C. R. Ultrastructural bases for metabolically linked mechanical activity in mitochondria. II. Electron transport-linked ultrastructural transformations in mitochondria. *J. Cell Biol.* 37:345-369 (1968).

Haessler, H. A. and K. J. Isselbacher. The metabolism of glycerol by the intestinal mucosa. *Biochim. Biophys. Acta* 73:427-436 (1963).

Hahn, P. E., W. F. Bale, E. O. Laurence, and G. H. Whipple. Radioactive iron and its metabolism in anemia. Its absorption, transportation and utilization. *J. Exp. Med.* 69:739-753 (1939).

Hahn, P. F., W. F. Bale, J. F. Ross, W. M. Balfour, and G. H. Whipple. Radioactive iron absorption by gastrointestinal tract. *J. Exp. Med.* 78:169-188 (1943).

Hahn, P. F., E. L. Carothers, W. J. Darby, M. Martin, C. W. Sheppard, R. O. Cannon, A. S. Beam, P. M. Densen, J. C. Peterson, and G. S. McClellan. Iron metabolism in human pregnancy as studied with radioactive isotopes. *Amer. J. Obst. Gynec.* 61:477-486 (1951).

Haley, F. L. and G. S. Samuelsen. Vitamin A and the detoxification of monobromobenzene. *J. Lab. Clin. Med.* 28:1079-1082 (1943).

Hallberg, L., A. M. Högdahl, L. Nilsson, and G. Rybo. Menstrual blood loss—a population study. Variation at different ages and attempts to define normality. *Acta Obstet. Gynec. Scand.* 45:320-351 (1966).

Hallberg, L. and L. Sölvell. Determination of the absorption rate of iron in man. *Acta Med. Scand.* (Suppl 358), 168:3-17 (1960a).

Hallberg, L. and L. Sölvell. Absorption of a single dose of iron in man. *Acta Med. Scand.* (Suppl. 358), 168:19-42 (1960b).

Hallberg, L. and L. Sölvell. Iron absorption during constant intragastric infusion of iron in man. *Acta Med. Scand.* (Suppl. 358), 168:43-69 (1960c).

Ham, A. W. *Histology*, 7th ed., J. B. Lippincott Company, Philadelphia, (1974).

Hambidge, K. M. Chromium nutrition in man. *Amer. J. Clin. Nutr.* 27:505-514 (1974).

Hambidge, K. M., C. Hambidge, M. Jacobs, and J. D. Baum. Low levels of zinc in hair, anorexia, poor growth, and hypogeusia in children. *Pediat. Res.* 6:868-874 (1972).

Hamerman, D. Views on the pathogenesis of rheumatoid arthritis. *Med. Clin. North Amer.* 52:593-605 (1968).

Hamilton, J. W. and R. D. Dallam. Isolation of vitamin K from animal tissue. *Arch. Biochem. Biophys.* 123:514-530 (1968).

Hanawalt, P. C. Repair of genetic material in living cells. *Endeavor XXXI* (113):83-87 (1972).

Hancock, R. Conservation of histones in chromatin during growth and mitosis *in vitro. J. Molec. Biol.* 40:457-466 (1969).

Hancox, N. M. and B. Boothroyd. Motion picture and electron microscope studies on the embryonic avian osteoclast. *J. Biophys. and Biochem. Cytol.* 11:651-661 (1961).

Hancox, N. M. and B. Boothroyd. Structure-function relationship in the osteoclast. In *Mechanisms of Hard Tissue Destruction,* pp. 497-514, R. F. Sognnaes, Ed., AAAS, Washington (1963).

Handler, P. Nutritional diseases. Conference on beriberi, endemic goiter, and hypovitaminosis A. *Fed. Proc.* 17:Part II 31-35 (1958).

Hankins, G. J., T. J. Eccles, Jr., B. C. Judlin, and M. C. Moore. Data processing of dietary survey data. *J. Amer. Diet. Ass.* 46:387-394 (1965).

Hansen, L. G. and W. J. Warwick. A fluorometric micromethod for serum vitamins A and E. *Clin. Chem.* 39:538-541 (1969).

Hanson, J. and J. Lowy. The structure of F-actin and of actin filaments isolated from muscle. *J. Molec. Biol.* 6:46-60 (1963).

Hardesty, B., W. Culp, and W. L. McKeehan. The sequence of reactions leading to the synthesis of a peptide bond on reticulocyte ribosomes. *Cold Spring Harbor Symp. Quant. Biol.* 34:331-345 (1969).

Hardinge, M. G., J. B. Swarner, and H. Crooks. Carbohydrates in foods. *J. Amer. Diet. Ass.* 46:197-204 (1965).

Hardman, J. G., G. A. Robison, and E. W. Sutherland. Cyclic nucleotides. *Ann. Rev. Physiol.* 33:311-336 (1971).

Harlan, W. R., Jr., P. S. Winesett, and A. J. Wasserman. Tissue lipoprotein lipase in normal individuals and in individuals with exogenous hypertriglyceridemia and the relationship of this enzyme to assimilation of fat. *J. Clin. Invest.* 46:239-247 (1967).

Haro, E. N., M. Brin, and W. W. Faloon. Fasting in obesity. Thiamine depletion as measured by erythrocyte transketolase changes. *Arch. Internal Med.* 117:175-181 (1966).

Harper, A. E. Remarks on the joule. *J. Amer. Diet. Ass.* 57:416-418 (1971).

Harper, A. E. Recommended dietary allowances: are they what we think they are? *J. Amer. Diet. Ass.* 64:151-156 (1974).

Harris, F., R. Hoffenberg, and E. Black. Calcium kinetics in Vitamin D deficiency rickets. II. Intestinal handling of calcium. *Metabolism* 14:1112-1121 (1965).

Harris, P. L. Bioassay of vitamin A compounds. *Vitamins Hormones* 18:341-370 (1960).

Harris, R. S. Reliability of nutrient analyses and food tables. *Amer. J. Clin. Nutr.* 11:377-381 (1962).

Harris, S. A. and K. Folkers. Synthesis of vitamin B_6. *J. Amer. Chem. Soc.* 61:1245-1247 (1939).

Harris, S. A., D. E. Wolf, R. Mozingo, G. E. Arth, R. C. Anderson, N. R. Easton, and K. Folkers. Biotin. V. Synthesis of dl-biotin, dl-allobiotin and dl-epi-allobiotin. *J. Amer. Chem. Soc.* 67:2096-2100 (1945).

Harrison, H. C., H. E. Harrison, and E. A. Park. Vitamin D and citrate metabolism: Effect of vitamin D in rats fed diets adequate in both calcium and phosphorus. *Amer. J. Physiol.* 192:432-436 (1958).

Harrison, H. E. and H. C. Harrison. Vitamin D and permeability of intestinal mucosa to calcium. *Amer. J. Physiol.* 208:370-374 (1965).

Harrison, H. E. and H. C. Harrison. Dibutyryl cyclic AMP, vitamin D and intestinal permeability to calcium. *Endocrinology* 86:756-760 (1970a).

Harrison, H. E. and H. C. Harrison. Role of vitamin D, parathyroid hormone, and cortisol in intestinal transport of calcium and phosphate. In *The Fat-Soluble Vitamins*, pp. 39-54, H. F. DeLuca and J. W. Suttie, Eds., The University of Wisconsin Press, Madison (1970b).

Harrison, H. E. and H. C. Harrison. Calcium. In *Intestinal Absorption*, Biomembranes, Vol. 4B, pp. 793-846, D. H. Smyth, Ed., Plenum Press, London (1974).

Hart, E. B., H. Steenbock, J. Waddell, and C. A. Elvehjem. Iron in nutrition. VII. Copper as a supplement to iron for hemoglobin building in the rat. *J. Biol. Chem.* 77:797-812 (1928).

Hasselbach, W. and L. G. Elfvin. Structural and chemical asymmetry of the calcium-transporting membranes of the sarcotubular system as revealed by electron microscopy. *J. Ultrastruct. Res.* 17:598-622 (1967).

Hathaway, M. L. and J. E. Strom. A comparison of thiamine synthesis and excretion in human subjects on synthetic and natural diets. *J. Nutr.* 32:1-8 (1946).

Haussler, M. R. Vitamin D: Mode of action and biomedical applications. *Nutr. Rev.* 32:257-266 (1974).

Haussler, M. R., D. W. Boyce, E. T. Littledike, and H. Rasmussen. A rapidly acting metabolite of vitamin D_3. *Proc. Nat. Acad. Sci.* 68:177-181 (1971).

Hayaishi, O. and Y. Shizuta. Binding of pyridoxal phosphate to apoenzymes as studied by optical rotatory dispersion and circular dichroism. *Vitamins Hormones* 28:245-264 (1970).

Hayward, J. S. and E. G. Ball. Quantitative aspects of brown adipose tissue thermogenesis during arousal from hibernation. *Biol. Bull.* 131: 94-103 (1966).

Hegsted, D. M. The estimation of relative nutrient intake and nutritional status by biochemical methods: Minerals. *Amer. J. Clin. Nutr.* 11:477-483 (1962).

Hegsted, D. M. Mineral intake and bone loss. *Fed. Proc.* 26:1747-1754 (1967).

Hegsted, D. M. and Y. Chang. Protein utilization in growing rats at different levels of intake. *J. Nutr.* 87:19-25 (1965a).

Hegsted, D. M. and Y. Chang. Protein utilization in growing rats. I. Relative growth index as a bioassay procedure. *J. Nutr.* 85:159-168 (1965b).

Hegsted, D. M., I. Moscoso, and C. C. Collazos. A study of the minimum calcium requirements of adult men. *J. Nutr.* 46:181-201 (1952).

Heinz, E. and P. M. Walsh. Exchange diffusion, transport, and intracellular level of amino acids in Ehrlich carcinoma cells. *J. Biol. Chem.* 233:1488-1493 (1958).

Helbock, H. J. and P. Saltman. The transport of iron by rat intestine. *Biochim. Biophys. Acta* 135:979-990 (1967).

Heller, J. Structure of visual pigments. II. Binding of retinal and conformational changes on light exposure in bovine visual pigment$_{500}$. *Biochemistry* 7:2914-2920 (1968).

Hellman, L. and J. J. Burns. Metabolism of L-ascorbic acid-1-C^{14} in man. *J. Biol. Chem.* 230:923-930 (1958).

Helminen, H. J. and J. L. E. Ericsson. Studies on mammary gland involution. II. Ultrastructural evidence for auto- and heterophagocytosis. *J. Ultrastruct. Res.* 25:214-227 (1968).

Henkin, R. H., P. J. Schecter, R. Hoye, and C. F. T. Mattern. Idiopathic hypogeusia with dysgeusia, hyposmia, and dysosmia. *J. Amer. Med. Assoc.* 217:434-440 (1971).

Henkin, R. I. Newer aspects of copper and zinc metabolism. In *Newer Trace Elements in Nutrition*, pp. 255-312, W. Mertz and W. E. Cornatzer, Eds., Marcel Dekker, Inc., New York (1971).

Herbert, V. Studies of the mechanism of the effect of hog intrinsic factor concentrate on the uptake of vitamin B_{12} by rat liver slices. *J. Clin. Invest.* 37:646-650 (1958).

Herbert, V. Mechanism of intrinsic factor action in everted sacs of rat small intestine. *J. Clin. Invest.* 38:102-109 (1959).

Herbert, V. Biochemical and hematologic lesions in folic acid deficiency. *Amer. J. Clin. Nutr.* 20:562-568 (1967).

Herbert, V. Folic acid deficiency in man. *Vitamins Hormones* 26:525-536 (1968).

Herbert, V. Nutritional requirements for vitamin B_{12} and folic acid. *Amer. J. Clin. Nutr.* 21:743-752 (1968).

Herbert, V. and W. B. Castle. Intrinsic factor. *New Eng. J. Med.* 270:1181-1185 (1964).

Herbert, V., C. W. Gottlieb, K. S. Lau, M. Fisher, N. R. Gevirtz, and L. R. Wasserman. The coated charcoal assay of unsaturated iron-binding capacity. *J. Lab. Clin. Med.* 67:855-862 (1966).

Herbert, V. and S. S. Shapiro. The site of absorption of folic acid in the rat *in vitro*. *Fed. Proc.* 21:250 (1962).

Herbert, V., R. R. Streiff, and L. W. Sullivan. Notes on vitamin B_{12} absorption; auto-immunity and childhood pernicious anemia; relation of intrinsic factor to blood group substance. *Medicine* 43:679-687 (1964).

Herbert, V., R. R. Streiff, L. W. Sullivan, and P. L. McGeer. Deranged purine metabolism manifested by aminoimidazole carboxamide excretion in megaloblastic anemias, hemolytic anemia and liver disease. *Lancet* 2:45-46 (1964).

Herbert, V. and R. Zalusky. Interrelations of vitamin B_{12} and folic acid metabolism: folic acid clearance studies. *J. Clin. Invest.* 41:1263-1276 (1962).

Herman, R. H. Mannose metabolism. *Amer. J. Clin. Nutr.* 24:488-498 (1971).

Hers, H. G. α-Glucosidase deficiency in generalized glycogen-storage disease (Pompe's Disease). *Biochem. J.* 86:11-16 (1963).

Hers, H. G. and T. Kusaka. Le metabolisme du fructose-1-phosphate dans le foie. *Biochim. Biophys. Acta* 11:427-437 (1953).

Hers, H. G. and F. Van Hoof. Genetic abnormalities of lysosomes. In *Lysosomes in Biology and Pathology*, Vol. 2, pp. 19-40, J. T. Dingle and H. B. Fell, Eds., *Frontiers of Biology*, Vol. 14A, Wiley-Interscience, N. Y. (1969).

Hersh, T. and D. A. Siddiqui. Magnesium and the pancreas. *Amer. J. Clin. Nutr.* 26:362-366 (1973).

Hertzig, E., H. G. Birch, S. A. Richardson, and J. Tizard. Intellectual levels of school children severely malnourished during the first two years of life. *Pediat.* 49:814-824 (1972).

Hess, A. F., M. Weinstock, and F. D. Helman. The antirachitic value of irradiated phytosterol and cholesterol. *J. Biol. Chem.* 63:305-308 (1925).

Hess, G. P. and J. A. Rupley. Structure and function of proteins. *Ann. Rev. Biochem.* 40:1013-1044 (1971).

Hicks, S. J., J. W. Drysdale, and H. N. Munro. Preferential synthesis of ferritin and albumin by different populations of liver polysomes. *Science* 164:584-585 (1969).

Highley, D. R., M. C. Davies, and L. Ellenbogen. Hog intrinsic factor. Some physico-chemical properties of vitamin B_{12}-binding fractions from hog pylorus. *J. Biol. Chem.* 242:1010-1015 (1967).

Hill, C. H. and G. Matrone. Chemical parameters in the study of *in vivo* and *in vitro* interactions of transition elements. *Fed. Proc.* 29:1474-1481 (1970).

Hill, H. A. O., J. M. Pratt, and R. J. P. Williams. Identification and investigation of cobalamins and cobamide coenzymes by nuclear magnetic resonance and electron paramagnetic resonance spectroscopy. In *Methods in Enzymology*, Vol. XVIII, Part C, pp. 5-31, D. B. McCormick and L. D. Wright, Eds., Academic Press, New York (1971).

Hillman, R. S. Mechanisms underlying abnormal erythropoiesis. In *Regulation of Hemato-poiesis*, Vol. I, pp. 579-609, A. S. Gordon, Ed. Appleton-Century-Crofts, N. Y. (1970).

Hillman, R. W. Tocopherol excess in man. Creatinuria associated with prolonged ingestion. *Amer. J. Clin. Nutr.* 5:597-600 (1957).

Hills, O. W., E. Liebert, D. L. Steinberg, and M. K. Horwitt. Clinical aspects of dietary depletion of riboflavine. *A. M. A. Arch. Inter. Med.* 87:682-693 (1951).

Hilz, H. and F. Lipmann. The enzymatic activation of sulfate. *Proc. Nat. Acad. Sci.* 41:880-890 (1935).

Hinman, J. W. Prostaglandins. *Ann. Rev. Biochem.* 41:161-178 (1972).

Hirano, S., P. Hoffman and K. Meyer. The structure of keratosulfate of bovine cornea. *J. Org. Chem.* 26:5064-5069 (1961).

Hirsch, J. and J. L. Knittle. Cellularity of obese and non-obese human adipose tissue. *Fed. Proc.* 29:1516-1521 (1970).

Hirsch, J., J. L. Knittle, and L. B. Salans. Cell lipid content and cell number in obese and non-obese human adipose tissue. *J. Clin. Invest.* 45:1023A (1966).

Hirsch, P. F., G. F. Gauthier, and P. L. Munson. Thyroid hypocalcemic principle and recurrent laryngeal nerve injury as factors affecting the response to parathyroidectomy in rats. *Endocrinology* 73:244-252 (1963).

Hirschmann, P. N. and G. Nichols, Jr. The isolation and partial characterization of calcium phosphate-containing granules from bone cells. *Fed. Proc.* 29:801A (1970).

Hittleman, K. J., O. Lindberg, and B. Cannon. Oxidative phosphorylation and compartmentation of fatty acid metabolism in brown fat mitochondria. *Europ. J. Biochem.* 11:183-192 (1969).

Ho, S. J., R. J. Ho, and H. C. Meng. Comparison of heparin-released and epinephrine-sensitive lipases in rat adipose tissue. *Amer. J. Physiol.* 212:284-290 (1967).

Hoagland, M. B. An enzymatic mechanism for amino acid activation in animal tissues. *Biochim. Biophys. Acta* 16:288-289 (1955).

Hoagland, M. B., E. B. Keller, and P. C. Zamecnik. Enzymatic carboxyl activation of amino acids. *J. Biol. Chem.* 218:345-358 (1956).

Hoagland, M. B. and P. C. Zamecnik. Intermediate reactions in protein biosynthesis. *Fed. Proc.* 16:197A (1957).

Hodges, R. E., J. Hood, J. E. Canham, H. E. Sauberlich, and E. M. Baker. Clinical manifestations of ascorbic acid deficiency in man. *Amer. J. Clin. Nutr.* 24:432-443 (1971).

Hodges, R. E. and H. Kolder. Experimental vitamin A deficiency in human volunteers. In Summary of Proceedings, Workshop on Biochemical and Clinical Criteria for Determining Human Vitamin A Nutriture. pp. 10-16, J. G. Bieri, Chmn., National Academy of Sciences, Washington, D.C. (1971).

Hodgkin, D. C., J. Kamper, J. Lindsey, M. MacKay, J. Pickworth, J. H. Robertson, C. B. Shoemaker, J. G. White, R. J. Prosen, and K. N. Trueblood. The structure of vitamin B_{12}. I. An outline of the crystallographic investigation of vitamin B_{12}. *Proc. Roy. Soc. London Ser. A* 242:228-263 (1957).

Hodgkin, D. C., J. Pickworth, J. H. Robertson, K. N. Trueblood, R. J. Prosen, and J. G. White. The crystal structure of the hexacarboxylic acid derived from B_{12} and the molecular structure of the vitamin. *Nature* 176:325-328 (1955).

Hoedemaker, P. J., J. Abels, J. J. Wachters, A. Arends, and H. O. Nieweg. Investigations about the site of production of Castle's gastric intrinsic factor. *Lab. Invest.* 13:1394-1399 (1964).

Hoffman, H. and G. W. Grigg. An electron microscopic study of mitochondria formation. *Exper. Cell Res.* 15:118-131 (1958).

Hofmann, A. and B. Borgstrom. Physico-chemical state of lipids in intestinal content during their digestion and absorption. *Fed. Proc.* 21:43-50 (1962).

Hoffmann, A. and B. Borgstrom. Hydrolysis of long-chain monoglycerides in micellar solution by pancreatic lipase. *Biochem. Biophys. Acta* 70:317-331 (1963).

Hogenkamp, H. P. C. Enzymatic reactions involving corrinoids. *Ann. Rev. Biochem.* 37:225-248 (1968).

Hohman, W. and H. Schraer. The intracellular distribution of calcium in the mucosa of the avian shell gland. *J. Cell Biol.* 30:317-331 (1966).

Hohman, W. and H. Schraer. Low temperature ultramicroincineration of thin-sectioned tissue. *J. Cell Biol.* 55:328-354 (1972).

Hokin, L. E. Dynamic aspects of phospholipids during protein secretion. *Internat. Rev. Cytol.* 23:187-208 (1968).

Holick, M. F., M. Garabedian, and H. F. DeLuca. 1,25-Dihydroxycholecalciferol: Metabolite of vitamin D_3 active on bone in anephric rats. *Science* 176:1146-1147 (1972).

Holick, M. F., A. Kleiner-Bosaller, H. K. Schnoes, P. M. Kasten, I. T. Boyle, and H. F. DeLuca. 1,24,25-Trihydroxyvitamin D_3. A metabolite of vitamin D_3 effective on intestine. *J. Biol. Chem.* 248:6691-6696 (1973).

Holick, M. F., H. K. Schnoes, H. F. DeLuca, R. W. Gray, I. T. Boyle and T. Suda. Isolation and identification of 24,25-dihydroxycholecalciferol: a metabolite of vitamin D_3 made in the kidney. *Biochemistry* 11:4251-4255 (1972).

Holick, M. F., H. K. Schnoes, H. F. DeLuca, T. Suda, and R. J. Cousins. Isolation and identification of 1,25-dihydroxycholecalciferol. A metabolite of vitamin D active in intestine. *Biochemistry* 10:2799-2804 (1971).

Hollenberg, C. H. Effect of nutrition on activity and release of lipase from rat adipose tissue. *Amer. J. Physiol.* 197:667-670 (1959).

Hollenberg, C. H. Adipose tissue lipases. II. In *Handbook of Physiology*, sec. 5, pp. 301-307, A. E. Renold and G. F. Cahill, Eds., American Physiological Society, Washington, D. C. (1965).

Hollenberg, C. H. Distribution of radioactive glycerol and fatty acids among adipose tissue triglycerides after administration of glucose-U-^{14}C. *J. Lipid Res.* 8:328-334 (1967).

Hollett, C. R. and J. V. Auditore. Localization and characterization of a lipase in rat adipose tissue. *Arch. Biochem. Biophys.* 121:423-430, (1967).

Holley, R. W., J. Apgar, G. A. Everett, J. T. Madison, M. Marquisee, S. H. Merrill, J. R. Penswick, and A. Zamir. Structure of a ribonucleic acid. *Science* 147:1462-1465 (1965).

Holman, C. A., E. B. Mawer, and D. J. Smith. Tissue distribution of cholecalciferol (vitamin D_3) in the rat. *Biochem. J.* 120:29P (1970).

Holmberg, C. G. and C. B. Laurell. Studies on the capacity of the serum to bind iron. A contribution to our knowledge of the regulation of serum iron. *Acta Physiol. Scand.* 10:307-319 (1945).

Holmes, E. G. An appraisal of the evidence upon which recently recommended protein allowances have been based. *World Rev. Nutr. Diet.* 5:237-274 (1965).

Holoubek, V. and T. Crocker. DNA-associated acidic proteins. *Biochim. Biophys Acta* 157:352-361 (1969).

Holst, A. and T. Frolich. Experimental studies relating to ship-beriberi and scurvy. 2. On the etiology of scurvy. *J. Hyg.* 7:634-671 (1907).

Holt, J. H. and D. Miller. The localization of phosphomonoesterase and aminopeptidase in brush borders isolated from intestinal epithelial cells. *Biochim. Biophys. Acta* 58:239-243 (1962).

Holt, L. E., Jr., P. György, E. L. Pratt, S. E. Snyderman, and W. M. Wallace. *Protein and Amino Acid Requirements in Early Life.* N. Y. University Press, N. Y. (1960).

Holter, H. Pinocytosis. In *Biological Structure and Function*, Vol. I, pp. 157-168, T. W. Goodwin and O. Lindberg, Eds., Academic Press, London (1961).

Holtzman, E. Golgi apparatus, GERL, and lysosomes in secretion and protein uptake by adrenal medulla cells. *J. Cell Biol.* 35:58A (1967).

Holzel, A., V. Schwarz, and K. W. Sutcliffe. Defective lactose absorption causing malnutrition in infancy. *Lancet* 1:1126-1128 (1959).

Hooper, C. E. S. Cell turnover in epithelial populations. *J. Histochem. Cytochem.* 4:531-540 (1956).

Hopkins, F. G. Feeding experiments illustrating the importance of accessory factors in normal dietaries. *J. Physiol.* 44:425-460 (1912).

Hopkins, L. L., Jr., and A. S. Majaj. Selenium in human nutrition. In *Symposium on Selenium in Biomedicine*, O. H. Muth, Ed., Avi Pub. Co., Westport, Conn. (1967).

Horowitz, S. B. and I. R. Fenichel. Analysis of sodium transport in the amphibian oocyte by extractive and radioautographic techniques. *J. Cell Biol.* 47:120-131 (1970).

Horton, E. W. Hypothesis on physiological roles of prostaglandins. *Physiol. Rev.* 49:122-161 (1969).

Horton, J. E., L. G. Raisz, H. A. Simmons, J. J. Oppenheim, and S. E. Mergenhagen. Bone resorbing activity in supernatant fluid from cultured human peripheral blood leukocytes. *Science* 177:793-795 (1972).

Horwitt, M. K. Vitamin E and lipid metabolism in man. *Amer. J. Clin. Nutr.* 8:451-461 (1960).

Horwitt, M. K. Interrelations between vitamin E and polyunsaturated fatty acids in adult men. *Vitamins Hormones.* 20:541-558 (1962).

Horwitt, M. K. Nutritional requirements of man, with special reference to riboflavin. *Amer. J. Clin. Nutr.* 18:458-466 (1966).

Horwitt, M. K., B. Century, and A. A. Zeman. Erythrocyte survival time and reticulocyte levels after tocopherol depletion in man. *Amer. J. Clin. Nutr.* 12:99-106 (1963).

Horwitt, M. K., C. C. Harvey, G. D. Duncan, and W. C. Wilson. Effects of limited tocopherol intake in man with relationships to erythrocyte hemolysis and lipid oxidations. *Amer. J. Clin. Nutr.* 4:408-419 (1956).

Horwitt, M. K., C. C. Harvey, O. W. Hills, and E. Liebert. Correlation of urinary excretion of ribovlavin with dietary intake and symptoms of ariboflavinosis. *J. Nutr.* 41:247-264 (1950).

Horwitt, M. K., C. C. Harvey, W. S. Rothwell, J. L. Cutler, and D. Haffron. Tryptophan-niacin relationships in man. *J. Nutr.* 60: Suppl. 1:1-43 (1956a).

Horwitt, M. K. and O. Kreisler. The determination of early thiamine-deficient states by estimation of blood lactic and pyruvic acids after glucose administration. *J. Nutr.* 37:411-427 (1949).

Horwitt, M. K., E. Liebert, O. Kreisler, and P. Wittman. Investigations of human require-ments for B-complex vitamins. National Research Council Bull. 116, National Academy of Sciences, Washington, D. C. 106 pp. (1948).

Hougie, C., E. M. Barrow, and J. B. Graham. Stuart clotting defect. I. Segregation of an hereditary hemorrhagic state from the heterogeneous group heretofore called "stable factor" (SPCA, proconvertin, factor VII) deficiency. *J. Clin. Invest.* 36:485-496 (1957).

Hryniuk, W. M. and J. R. Bertino. Growth rate and cell kill. *Ann. N. Y. Acad. Sci.* 186:330-342 (1971).

Hsia, D. Y-Y. The diagnosis of carrier of disease-producing genes. *Ann. N. Y. Acad. Sci.* 134:946-964 (1966).

Hsueh, A. M., M. Simonson, M. J. Kellum, and B. F. Chow. Perinatal undernutrition and the metabolic and behavioral development of the offspring. *Nutr. Rep. Internat.* 7:437-446 (1973).

Huang, R. C. and J. Bonner. Histone, a suppressor of chromosomal RNA synthesis. *Proc. Nat. Acad. Sci.* 48:1216-1222 (1962).

Huang, S. S. and T. M. Bayless. Milk and lactose intolerance in healthy Orientals. *Science* 160:83-84 (1968).

Hubbard, J. I. and S. Kwanbunbumpen. Evidence for the vesicle hypothesis. *J. Physiol.* 194:407-420 (1968).

Huehns, E. R., N. Dance, G. H. Beaven, F. Hecht, and A. G. Motulsky. Human embryonic hemoglobins. *Cold Spr. Harb. Symp. Quant. Biol.* 29:327-331 (1964).

Huldshinsky, K. Heilung von rachitis durch künstliche höhensonne. *Deut. Med. Wochschr.* 45:712-713 (1919).

Hull, D. The structure and function of brown adipose tissue. *Brit. Med. Bull.* 22:92-96 (1966).

Hull, D. and M. M. Segall. The contribution of brown adipose tissue to heat production in the new-born rabbit. *J. Physiol.* 181:449-457 (1965a).

Hull, D. and M. M. Segall. Sympathetic nervous control of brown adipose tissue and heat production in the new-born rabbit. *J. Physiol.* 181:458-467 (1965b).

Hull, D. and M. M. Segall. Distinction of brown from white adipose tissue. *Nature* 212:469-472 (1966).

Hullar, T. L. Potential antimetabolites of pyridoxal phosphate. *Ann. N. Y. Acad. Sci.* 166:191-198 (1969).

Hume, E. M. and H. A. Krebs, compilers. *Vitamin A requirement of human adults. An experimental study of vitamin A deprivation in man.* Medical Res. Council, Great Britain, Special Report Series No. 264, London (1949).

Hunt, E. E. and E. Giles. Allometric growth of body composition in man and other mammals. *Human Biol.* 30:253-273 (1956).

Hunt, E. E., Jr. and F. P. Heald. Physique, body composition, and sexual maturation in adolescent boys. *Ann. N. Y. Acad. Sci.* 110:532-544 (1963).

Hunt, J. A. and V. M. Ingram. A terminal peptide sequence of human haemoglobin? *Nature* 184:640-641 (1959).

Hunt, R. D., F. G. Garcia, and D. M. Hegsted. A comparison of vitamin D_2 and D_3 in new world primates. I. Production and regression of osteodystrophia fibrosa. *Lab. Animal Care* 17:222-234 (1967).

Hurley, L. S. and G. J. Everson. Delayed development of righting reflexes in offspring of manganese-deficient rats. *Proc. Soc. Exp. Biol. Med.* 102:360-362 (1959).

Hutton, J. J., A. L. Tappel, and S. Udenfriend. Cofactor and substrate requirements of collagen proline hydroxylase. *Arch. Biochem. Biophys.* 118:231-240 (1967).

Huxley, H. E. Electron microscope studies of natural and synthetic protein filaments from striated muscle. *J. Molec. Biol.* 7:281-308 (1963).

Huxley, H. E. The mechanism of muscular contraction. *Science* 164:1356-1366 (1969).

Hyden, H. RNA in brain cells. In *The Neurosciences*, pp. 248-266, G. C. Quarton, T. Melnechuk, and F. O. Schmitt, Eds., Rockefeller University Press, N. Y. (1967).

Hytten, F. E. and I. Leitch. *The Physiology of Human Pregnancy*, 2nd. ed. Blackwell Scientific Publications, Oxford (1971).

Hytten, F. E., A. M. Thomson, and N. Taggart. Total body water in normal pregnancy. *J. Obstet. Gynaec. Brit. Commonw.* 73:553-561 (1966).

Hyun, S. A., G. V. Vahouny, and C. R. Treadwell. Effect of α-ethylcaproic acid on cholesterol esterification and absorption. *Arch. Biochem. Biophys.* 104:139-145 (1964).

ICNND. *Manual for Nutrition Surveys*, 2nd Ed., U. S. Govt. Printing Office, Washington, D.C., (1963).

Illiano, G. and P. Cuatrecasas. Modulation of adenylate cyclase in liver and fat cell membranes by insulin. *Science* 175:906-908 (1972).

Imai, S. and K. Takeda. Actions of calcium and certain multivalent cations on potassium contracture of guinea pig's taenia coli. *J. Physiol.* 190:155-169 (1967).

Imami, R. H., S. Reiser, and P. A. Christiansen. Effects of vitamin E and essential fatty acid deficiencies on the intestinal transport of L-valine and α-methyl-D-glucoside in the rat. *J. Nutr.* 100:101-109 (1970).

Ingenbleek, Y., M. De Visscher, and Ph. De Nayer. Measurement of prealbumin as index of protein-calorie malnutrition. *Lancet* 2:106-109 (1972).

Ingram, V. M. Gene mutations in human haemoglobins: The chemical difference between normal and sickle cell haemoglobin. *Nature* 180:326-328 (1957).

Irving, J. T. *Calcium Metabolism.* Wiley, N. Y. (1957).

Irwin, M. I. and D. M. Hegsted. A conspectus of research on protein requirements of man. *J. Nutr.* 101:385-430 (1971).

Isselbacher, K. J. Metabolism and transport of lipid by intestinal mucosa. *Fed. Proc.* 24:16-22 (1965).

Ito, S. Structure and function of the glycocalyx. *Fed. Proc.* 28:12-25 (1969).

IUPAC-IUB Commission on Biochemical Nomenclature. Tentative Rules. *J. Biol. Chem.* 241:2987-2994 (1966).

IUPAC-IUB Commission on Biochemical Nomenclature. Rules for the nomenclature of lipids. *European J. Biochem.* 2:127-131 (1967).

Iversen, L. L. *The Uptake and Storage of Noradrenaline in Sympathetic Nerves.* Cambridge University Press, London, 1967.

Iwasaki, K., S. Sabol, A. J. Wahba, and S. Ochoa. Translation of the genetic message. VII. Role of initiation factors in formation of the chain initiation complex with *Escherichia coli* ribosomes. *Arch. Biochem. Biophys.* 125:542-547 (1968).

Jacob, F. and J. Monod. Genetic regulatory mechanisms in the synthesis of proteins. *J. Molec. Biol.* 3:318-356 (1961).

Jacob, M. I. Fatty acid synthesis in cell-free preparations of human adipose tissue. *Biochim. Biophys. Acta* 70:231-241 (1963).

Jacobs, F. A. Bidirectional flux of amino acids across the intestinal mucosa. *Fed. Proc.* 24:946-952 (1965).

Jacobson, L. O., E. Goldwasser, W. Fried, and L. Pizak. Role of the kidney in erythropoiesis. *Nature* 179:633-634 (1957).

Jacobson, W. and I. A. B. Cathie. The inactivation of folic acid antagonists by normal and leukaemic cells. *Biochem. Pharmacol.* 5:130-142 (1960).

Jaim-Etcheverry, G. and L. M. Zieher. Ultrastructural aspects of neurotransmitter storage in adrenergic nerves. *Adv. Cytopharmacol.* 1:343-361 (1971).

James, W. P. T. and A. M. Hay. Albumin metabolism: effect of the nutritional state and the dietary protein intake. *J. Clin. Invest.* 47:1958-1972 (1968).

Jamieson, J. D. Role of the Golgi complex in the intracellular transport of secretory proteins. *Adv. Cytopharmacol.* 1:183-190 (1971).

Jamieson, J. D. and G. E. Palade. Intracellular transport of newly synthesized proteins in the exocrine process. *J. Cell Biol.* 27:47A (1965).

Jamieson, J. D. and G. E. Palade. Role of the Golgi complex in the intracellular transport of secretory proteins. *Proc. Natl. Acad. Sci.* 55:424-431 (1966).

Jamieson, J. D. and G. E. Palade. Intracellular transport of secretory proteins in the **pancreatic** exocrine cell. I. Role of the peripheral elements of the Golgi complex. *J. Cell Biol.* 34:577-596 (1967a).

Jamieson, J. D. and G. E. Palade. Intracellular transport of secretory proteins in the pancreatic exocrine cell. II. Transport to condensing vacuoles and zymogen granules. *J. Cell Biol.* 34:597-615 (1967b).

Jansen, G. R., C. F. Hutchison, and M. E. Zanetti. Studies on lipogenesis *in vivo. Biochem. J.* 99:323-332 (1966a).

Jansen, G. R., M. E. Zanetti, and C. F. Hutchison. Studies on lipogenesis *in vivo. Biochem. J.* 102:864-869 (1966b).

Jeanloz, R. W. Mucopolysaccharides of higher animals. *The Carbohydrates,* Vol. IIB, pp.

589-625, W. Pigman, D. Horton, and A. Herp, Eds., Academic Press, N. Y. (1970).

Jeans, P. C. and G. Stearns. Effect of vitamin D on linear growth in infancy; effect of intakes above 1,800 U.S.P. units daily. *J. Pediat.* 13:730-740 (1938).

Jelliffe, D. B. Field anthropometry independent of precise age. *J. Pediat.* 75:334-335 (1969).

Jelliffe, D. B. and E. F. P. Jelliffe. Age-independent anthropometry. *Amer. J. Clin. Nutr.* 24:1377-1379 (1971).

Jewell, P. A. and E. B. Verney. An experimental attempt to determine the site of the neurohypophyseal osmoreceptors in the dog. *Phil. Trans. Roy. Soc.* (London) B 240:197-324 (1957).

Joel, C. D. The physiological role of brown adipose tissue. In *Handbook of Physiology*, Section 5, *Adipose Tissue*, A. E. Renold and G. F. Cahill, Eds., pp. 59-85, American Physiological Society, Washington, D. C. (1965).

Johansson, S., S. Lindstedt, U. Register, and L. Wadström. Studies on the metabolism of labeled pyridoxine in man. *Amer. J. Clin. Nutr.* 18:185-196 (1966).

Johns, D. G. and D. M. Valerino. Metabolism of folate antagonists. *Ann. N. Y. Acad. Sci.* 186:378-386 (1971).

Johnson, H. V., C. Boyd, J. Martinovic, G. Valkovich, and B. C. Johnson. A new blood protein which increases with vitamin K deficiency. *Arch. Biochem. Biophys.* 148:431-442 (1972).

Johnson, H. V., J. Martinovic, and B. C. Johnson. Vitamin K and the biosynthesis of the glycoprotein in prothrombin. *Biochem. Biophys. Res. Commun.* 43:1040-1048 (1971).

Johnson, N. E., E. N. Alcantara, and H. Linkswiler. Effect of level of protein intake on urinary and fecal calcium and calcium retention of young adult males. *J. Nutr.* 100:1425-1430 (1970).

Johnson, P. and W. F. R. Pover. Intestinal absorption of α-tocopherol. *Life Sci.* 4:115-117 (1962).

Johnston, J. M. Recent developments in the mechanism of fat absorption. In *Advances in Lipid Research*, Vol. 1, pp. 105-131, R. Paoletti and D. Kritchevsky, Eds., Academic Press, N. Y. (1963).

Johnston, J. M. Mechanism of fat absorption. In *Handbook of Physiology*, Section 6: *Alimentary Canal*, Vol. III, pp. 1353-1375, C. F. Code, Ed., American Physiological Society, Washington, D. C. (1968).

Johnston, P. V., K. C. Kopaczyk, and F. A. Kummerow. Effect of pyridoxine deficiency on fatty acid composition of carcass and brain lipids in the rat. *J. Nutr.* 74:96-102 (1961).

Johnston, P. V. and B. I. Roots. *Nerve Membranes.* A Study of the Biological and Chemical Aspects of Neuron-Glia Relationships. Pergamon Press, Oxford (1972).

Jones, D., J. Scholler, and K. Folkers. The vitamin activity of coenzyme Q_7 in reproduction in the rat. *Internat. J. Vit. Nutr. Res.* 41:215-220 (1971).

Jones, S. F. and S. Kwanbunbumpen. On the role of synaptic vesicles in transmitter release. *Life Sci.* 7:1251-1255 (1968).

Jorgensen, C. R., N. R. Landau, and T. H. Wilson. A common pathway for sugar transport in hamster intestine. *Amer. J. Physiol.* 200:111-116 (1961).

Jost, J-P. and H. V. Rickenberg. Cyclic AMP. *Ann. Rev. Biochem.* 40:741-774 (1971).

Juneja, H. S., N. R. Moudgal, and J. Ganguly. Studies on vitamin A. The effect of hormones on gestation in retinoate-fed female rats. *Biochem. J.* 111:97-105 (1969).

Juneja, H. S., S. K. Murthy, and J. Ganguly. Effect of retinoic acid on the reproductive performances of male and female rats. *Indian J. Exptl. Biol.* 2:153-154 (1964).

Jungas, R. L. Role of cyclic-3',5'-AMP in the response of adipose tissue to insulin. *Proc. Nat. Acad. Sci.* 56:757-763 (1966).

Jurkowitz, B. Determination of vitamin A acid in human plasma after oral administration. *Arch. Biochem. Biophys.* 98:337-341 (1962).

Jusko, W. J. and G. Levy. Absorption, metabolsim and excretion of riboflavin-5'-phosphate in man. *J. Pharm. Sci.* 56:58-62 (1967).

Jusko, W. J., G. Levy, and S. J. Yaffe. Effect of age on intestinal absorption of riboflavin in humans. *J. Pharm. Sci.* 59:487-490 (1970).

Kagan, A., T. R. Dawber, W. B. Kannel, and N. Revotskie. The Framingham Study: A Prospective Study of Coronary Heart Disease. *Fed. Proc.* 21:52-57 (1962).

Kagan, B. M., V. Stanincova, N. S. Felix, J. Hodgman, and D. Kalman. Body composition of premature infants: relation to nutrition. *Amer. J. Clin. Nutr.* 25:1153-1164 (1972).

Kagawa, Y. and N. Shimazono. Catabolism of L-ascorbate in animal tissues. In *Methods in Enzymology*, Vol. XVIII, Part A, pp. 46-50, D. B. McCormick, and L. D. Wright, Eds., Academic Press, N. Y. (1970).

Kahn, S. B., S. Fein, S. Rigberg, and I. Brodsky. Correlation of folate metabolism and socioeconomic status in pregnancy and in patients taking oral contraceptives. *Amer. J. Obstet. Gynec.* 108:931-935 (1970).

Kanai, M., A. Raz, and D. W. Goodman. Retinol-binding protein: The transport protein for vitamin A in human plasma. *J. Clin. Invest.* 47:2025-2044 (1968).

Kaplan, B. H. The control of heme synthesis. In *Regulation of Hematopoiesis*, Vol. I., pp. 677-700, A. S. Gordon, Ed., Appleton-Century-Crofts, N. Y. (1970).

Kaplowitz, P. B., R. D. Platz, and L. J. Kleinsmith. Nuclear phosphoproteins. III. Increase in phosphorylation during histone-phosphoprotein interaction. *Biochim. Biophys. Acta* 229:739-748 (1971).

Karlson, P. *Introduction to Modern Biochemistry.* 3rd ed., Academic Press, N. Y. (1968).

Karmen, A., I. McCaffrey, and R. L. Bowman. A flow-through method for scintillation counting of carbon-14 and tritium in gas-liquid chromatographic effluents. *J. Lipid Res.* 3:372-377 (1962).

Karmen, A., M. Whyte, and DeW. S. Goodman. Fatty acid esterification and chylomicron formation during fat absorption. I. Triglycerides and cholesterol esters. *J. Lipid Res.* 4:312-321 (1963).

Karrer, P., R. Morf, and K. Schöpp. Zur Kenntnis des Vitamins-A aus Fischtranen. *Helv. Chim. Acta* 14:1036-1040 (1931).

Karrer, P., K. Schöpp, and F. Benz. Synthesen von Flavinen IV. *Helv. Chim. Acta* 18:426-429 (1935).

Karvonen, M. J. Modification of the diet in primary prevention trials. *Proc. Nutr. Soc.* 31:355-362 (1972).

Kasper, C. B. Biochemical distinctions between the nuclear and microsomal membranes from rat hepatocytes. *J. Biol. Chem.* 246:577-581 (1971).

Katz, J., S. Rosenfeld, and A. L. Sellers. Albumin metabolism in amino-nucleoside nephrotic rats. *J. Lab. Clin. Med.* 62:910-934 (1963).

Katz, J., A. L. Sellers, and G. Bonorris. Effect of nephrectomy on plasma albumin catabolism in experimental nephrosis. *J. Lab. Clin. Med.* 63:680-693 (1964).

Katz, J. H. Transferrin and its functions in the regulation of iron metabolism. In *Regulation of Hematopoiesis*, Vol. 1, *Red Cell Production*, pp. 539-577, A. S. Gordon, Ed., Appleton-Century-Crofts, N. Y. (1970).

Katz, R., G. W. Cooper, A. S. Gordon, and E. D. Zanjani. Studies on the site of production of erythropoietin. *Ann. N. Y. Acad. Sci.* 149:120-127 (1968).

Kaufman, S. Coenzymes and hydroxylases: ascorbate and dopamine-β-hydroxylase; tetrahydropteridines and phenylalanine and tyrosine hydroxylases. *Pharmacol. Rev.* 18:61-69 (1966).

Kayden, H. J. and L. Bjornson. The dynamics of vitamin E transport in the human erythrocyte. *Ann. N. Y. Acad. Sci.* 203:127-140 (1972).

Keenan, T. W. and D. J. Morré. Phospholipid class and fatty acid composition of Golgi apparatus isolated from rat liver and comparison with other cell fractions. *Biochemistry* 9:19-25 (1970).

Keighley, G. and P. H. Lowy. Chemistry and purification of erythropoietin. In *Kidney Hormones*, pp. 269-293, J. W. Fisher, Ed., Academic Press, London (1971).

Kelley, L. and M. A. Ohlson. Experimental variables in predicting protein minima for rats. *J. Nutr.* 52:325-335 (1954).

Kelly, R. B., M. R. Atkinson, J. A. Huberman, and A. Kornberg. Excision of thymine dimers and other mismatched sequences by DNA polymerase of *Escherichia coli*. *Nature* 224:495-501 (1969).

Kelsay, J., A. Baysal, and H. Linkswiler. Effect of vitamin B_6 depletion on the pyridoxal, pyridoxamine and pyridoxine content of the blood and urine of men. *J. Nutr.* 94:490-494 (1968).

Kendrew, J. C., R. E. Dickerson, B. E. Strandberg, R. G. Hart, D. R. Davies, D. C. Phillips, and V. C. Shore. Structure of Myoglobin. A three-dimensional fourier synthesis at 2 Å resolution. *Nature* 185:422-427 (1960).

Kendrew, J. C., H. C. Watson, B. E. Strandberg, R. E. Dickerson, D. C. Phillips, and V. C. Shore. A partial determination by X-ray methods, and its correlation with chemical data. *Nature* 190:666-670 (1961).

Kennedy, E. P. and A. L. Lehninger. Oxidation of fatty acids and tricarboxylic acid cycle intermediates by isolated rat liver mitochondria. *J. Biol. Chem.* 179:957-972 (1949).

Kenny, A. D. and C. G. Dacke. Parathyroid hormone and calcium metabolism. *World Rev. Nutr. Dietet.* 20:231-298 (1975).

Keresztesy, J. C. and J. R. Stevens. Crystalline vitamin B_6. *Proc. Soc. Exp. Biol. Med.* 38:64-65 (1938).

Kerkut, G. A. and B. York. *The Electrogenic Sodium Pump.* Scientichnica, Ltd., Bristol (1971).

Keys, A. Diet and the epidemiology of coronary heart disease. *J.A.M.A.* 164:1912-1919 (1957).

Keys, A. and J. Brozek. Body fat in adult man. *Physiol. Rev.* 33:245-325 (1953).

Keys, A., J. Brozek, A. Henschel, O. Mickelsen, and H. L. Taylor. *The Biology of Human Starvation*, Vols. I and II., University of Minnesota Press, Minneapolis (1950).

Keys, A., A. F. Henschel, O. Mickelsen, and J. Brozek. The performance of normal young men on controlled thiamine intakes. *J. Nutr.* 26:399-415 (1943).

Keys, A., A. Henschel, H. L. Taylor, O. Mickelsen, and J. Brozek. Experimental studies on man with restricted intake of the B vitamins. *Amer. J. Physiol.* 144:5-42 (1945).

Khokhar, S. A. and R. L. Pike. Aldosterone producing capacity of adrenal glands of sodium-restricted pregnant rats. *J. Nutr.* 103:1126-1130 (1973).

Khoo, J. C., A. A. Aquino, and D. Steinberg. The mechanism of activation of hormone-sensitive lipase in human adipose tissue. *J. Clin. Invest.* 53:1124-1131 (1974).

Kies, C. Comparative value of various sources of nonspecific nitrogen for the human. *J. Agric. Food Chem.* 22:190-193 (1974).

Kimberg, D. V., D. Schachter, and H. Schenker. Active transport of calcium by intestine: Effects of dietary calcium. *Amer. J. Physiol.* 200:1256-1262 (1961).

King, J. C., D. H. Calloway, and S. Margen. Nitrogen retention, total body ^{40}K and weight gain in teenage pregnant girls. *J. Nutr.* 103:772-785 (1973).

Kingsbury, K. J., S. Paul, A. Crossley, and D. M. Morgan. Fatty acid composition of human depot fat. *Biochem. J.* 78:541-550 (1961).

Kinney, J. M., J. Lister, and F. D. Moore. Relationship of energy expenditure to total exchangeable potassium. *Ann. N. Y. Acad. Sci.* 110:711-722 (1963).

Kinney, T. D., D. M. Hegsted, and C. A. Finch. The influence of diet on iron absorption. I. The pathology of iron excess. *J. Exp. Med.* 90:137-145 (1949).

Kinsman, R. A. and J. Hood. Some behavioral effects of ascorbic acid deficiency. *Amer. J. Clin. Nutr.* 24:444-454 (1971).

Kint, J. A., G. Dacremont, D. Carton, E. Orye, and C. Hooft. Mucopolysaccharidoses: Secondarily induced abnormal distribution of lysosomal isoenzymes. *Science* 181:352-354 (1973).

Kirschner, D. A. and D. L. D. Caspar. Comparative diffraction studies on myelin membranes. *Ann. N. Y. Acad. Sci.* 195:309-320 (1972).

Kirshner, N., C. Halloway, W. J. Smith, and A. G. Kirshner. Uptake and storage of catecholamines. In *Mechanisms of Release of Biogenic Amines*, pp. 109-123, U. S. von Euler, S. Rosell, and B. Unvas, Eds., Pergamon Press, Oxford (1966).

Kiyasu, J. Y. and I. C. Chaikoff. On the manner of transport of absorbed fructose. *J. Biol. Chem.* 224:935-939 (1957).

Klavins, J. V., T. D. Kinney, and N. Kaufman. The influence of dietary protein on iron absorption. *Brit. J. Exp. Path.* 43:172-180 (1962).

Kleiber, M. Body size and metabolic rate. *Physiol. Rev.* 27:511-541 (1947).

Kleiber, M. *The Fire of Life: An Introduction to Animal Energetics.* Wiley, N. Y. (1961).

Kleiber, M. Joules vs. calories in nutrition. *J. Nutr.* 102:309-312 (1972).

Klein, R. L. and B. A. Afzelius. Nuclear membrane hydrolysis of adenosine triphosphate. *Nature* 212:609 (1966).

Kleiner, I. S. and J. M. Orten. *Biochemistry*, 7th Ed., C. V. Mosby Co., St. Louis (1966).

Kleiner-Boessaler, A. and H. F. DeLuca. Formation of retinoic acid from retinol in the kidney. *Arch. Biochem. Biophys.* 142:371-377 (1971).

Kleinig, H. Nuclear membranes from mammalian liver. II. Lipid composition. *J. Cell Biol.* 46:396-402 (1970).

Kleinsmith, L. J. and V. G. Allfrey. Nuclear phosphoproteins. I. Isolation and characterization of a phosphoprotein fraction from calf thymus nuclei. *Biochim. Biophys. Acta* 175:123-135 (1969).

Klevay, L. M. Hair as a biopsy material. I. Assessment of zinc nutriture. *Amer. J. Clin. Nutr.* 23:284-289 (1970a).

Klevay, L. M. Hair as a biopsy material. I. Assessment of copper nutriture. *Amer. J. Clin. Nutr.* 23:1194-1202 (1970b).

Klingenberg, M. On the density of the occupation of the mitochondrial membrane by respiratory components. In *Mitochondrial Structure and Compartmentation*, pp. 124-161, E. Quagliariello, S. Papa, E. C. Slater, and J. M. Tager, Eds., Adriatica Editrice, Bari (1967).

Klotz, I. M. and D. W. Darnall. Protein subunits: a table (second edition). *Science* 166:126-127 (1969).

Klotz, I. M., N. R. Langerman, and D. W. Darnall. Quaternary structure of proteins. *Ann. Rev. Biochem.* 39:25-62 (1970).

Knappe, J. Mechanism of biotin action. *Ann. Rev. Biochem.* 39:757-776 (1970).

Knittle, J. and J. Hirsch. Infantile nutrition as a determinant of adult adipose tissue metabolism and cellularity. *Clin. Res.* 15:323A (1967).

Knittle, J. L. and J. Hirsch. Effect of chain length on rates of uptake of free fatty acids during *in vitro* incubations of rat adipose tissue. *J. Lipid Res.* 6:565-571 (1965).

Knittle, J. L. and J. Hirsch. Effect of early nutrition on the development of rat epididymal fat pads: cellularity and metabolism. *J. Clin. Invest.* 47:2091-2098 (1968).

Kodicek, E. The metabolism of vitamin D. *Proc. 4th Internatl. Congr. Biochem.* XI:198-208 (1960).

Kodicek, E. Antivitamins of nicotinic acid and of biotin. In *Antivitamins*, Bibliotheca Nutritio et Dieta, p. 8, J. C. Somogyi, Ed., S. Karger, Basel (1966).

Kodicek, E. The story of vitamin D from vitamin to hormone. *Lancet* 1:325-329 (1974).

Koe, B. K. and A. Weissman. *p*-Chlorophenylalanine; a specific depletor of brain serotonin. *J. Pharmacol. Exper. Thera.* 154:499-516 (1966).

Koenig, H. Lysosomes in the nervous system. In *Lysosomes in Biology and Pathology*, Vol. 2, pp. 111-162, J. T. Dingle and H. B. Fell, Eds., *Frontiers of Biology*, Vol. 14A, Wiley-Interscience, N. Y. (1969).

Koenig, H. and A. Jibril. Acidic glycolipids and the role of ionic bonds in the structure-linked latency of lysosomal hydrolases. *Biochim. Biophys. Acta* 65:543-545 (1962).

Kofler, M., P. F. Sommer, H. R. Bolliger, B. Schmidli, and M. Vecchi. Physiochemical properties and assay of the tocopherols. *Vitamins Hormones* 20:407-439 (1962).

Kögl, F., J. de Gier, I. Mulder, and L. M. Van Deenen. Metabolism and functions of phosphatides. Specific fatty acid composition of the red blood cell membranes. *Biochim. Biophys. Acta* 43:95-103 (1960).

Kögl, F. and B. Tönnis. Über das Bios-Problem. Darstellung von Krystallisiertem Biotin aus Eigelb. *Z. Physiol. Chem.* 242:43-73 (1936).

Koketsu, K. and S. Miyamoto. Release of $_{45}$Ca from frog nerves. *Nature* 189:402-403 (1961).

Kolata, G. B. Cyclic GMP: Cellular regulator agent? *Science* 182:149-151 (1973).

Koller, F., A. Loeliger, and F. Duckert. Experiments on a new clotting factor (Factor VII). *Acta Haematol.* 6:1-18 (1951).

Kopin, I. J. The adrenergic synapse. In *The Neurosciences*, pp. 427-432, G. C. Quarton, T. Melnechuk, and F. O. Schmitt, Eds., Rockefeller University Press, N. Y. (1967).

Kopin, I. J. Biochemical aspects of storage and release of biogenic amines from sympathetic nerves. In *Mechanisms of Release of Biogenic Amines*, U. S. von Euler, S. Rossel, and B. Uvnas, Eds., p. 229, Pergamon Press, N. Y. (1966).

Kopple, J. D. and M. E. Swendseid. Evidence for a dietary histidine requirement in normal man. *Fed. Proc.* 33:671A (1973).

Korn, E. D. Structure of biological membranes. *Science* 153:1491-1498 (1966).

Korn, E. D. Current concepts of membrane structure and function. *Fed. Proc.* 28:6-11 (1969).

Kornberg, A. Biologic synthesis of deoxyribonucleic acid. *Science* 131:1503-1508 (1960).

Kornberg, A. Active center of DNA polymerase. *Science* 163:1410-1418 (1969).

Koschara, W. von. Isolierung eines gelben Farbstoffs (Uropterin) aus Menschenharn. *Z. Physiol. Chem.* 240:127-151 (1936).

Kozio, J. Fluorometric analyses of riboflavin and its coenzymes. In *Methods in Enzymology*, Vol. XVIII, Part B, pp. 253-285, D. B. McCormick and L. D. Wright, Eds., Academic Press, N. Y. (1970).

Krampitz, L. O. Catalytic functions of thiamin diphosphate. *Ann. Rev. Biochem.* 38:213-240 (1969).

Krantz, S. B. and E. Goldwasser. On the mechanism of erythropoietin-induced differentiation. II. The effect on RNA synthesis. *Biochim. Biophys. Acta* 103:325-332 (1965).

Kravitz, E. A. Acetylcholine, γ-aminobutyric acid, and glutamic acid: Physiological and chemical studies related to their roles as neurotransmitter agents. In The *Neurosciences*, pp. 433-444, G. C. Quarton, T. Melnechuk, and F. O. Schmitt, Eds., Rockefeller University Press, N. Y. (1967).

Krebs, H. A. The metabolic fate of amino acids. In *Mammalian Protein Metabolism*, Vol. I, pp. 125-176, H. N. Munro and J. B. Allison, Eds., Academic Press, N. Y. (1964).

Krebs, H. A. and K. Henseleit. Untersuchungen über die Harnstoffbildung im Tierkörper. *Z. Physiol. Chem.* 210:33-66 (1932).

Krehl, W. A., L. J. Tepley, and C. A. Elvehjem. Corn as an etiological factor in the production of nicotinic acid deficiency in the rat. *Science* 101:283 (1945a).

Krehl, W. A., L. J. Tepley, P. S. Sarma, and C. A. Elvejhem. Growth retarding effect of corn in nicotinic acid low rations and its counteraction by tryptophan. *Science* 101:489-490 (1945b).

Kretchmer, N. Lactose and lactase. *Sci. Amer.* 227(4):70-78 (1972).

Kretchmer, N., O. Ransome-Kuti, R. Hurwitz, C. Dungy, and W. Alakija. Intestinal absorption of lactose in Nigerian ethnic groups. *Lancet* 2:392-395 (1971).

Krishnamurthy, S., J. G. Bieri, and E. L. Andrews. Metabolism and biological activity of vitamin A acid in the chick. *J. Nutr.* 79:503-510 (1963).

Krishnamurthy, S., S. Mahadevan, and J. Ganguly. Association of vitamin A ester and vitamin A alcohol with proteins in rat liver. *J. Biol. Chem.* 233:32-36 (1958).

Krishnarao, G. V. G. and H. H. Draper. Influence of dietary phosphate on bone resportion in senescent mice. *J. Nutr.* 102:1143-1145 (1972).

Kromphardt, H., H. Grobecker, K. Ring, and E. Heinz. Uber den Einfluss von Alkali-Ionen auf den Glycintransport in Ehrlich-Ascites-Tumorzellen. *Biochim. Biophys. Acta* 74:549-551 (1963).

Krook, L., J. P. Whalen, G. V. Lesser and L. Lutwak. Human periodontal disease and osteoporosis. *Cornell Vet.* 62:371-391 (1972).

Kruse, H. D., E. R. Orent, and E. V. McCollum. Studies on magnesium deficient animals. I. Symptomatology resulting from magnesium deprivation. *J. Biol. Chem.* 96:519-539 (1932).

Kuhn, I. N., M. Layrisse, M. Roche, C. Martinez, and R. B. Walker. Observations on the mechanism of iron absorption. *Amer. J. Clin. Nutr.* 21:1184-1188 (1968).

Kuhn, R., K. Reinemund, F. Weygand, and R. Ströbele. Über die Synthese des Lactoflavins (Vitamin B_2). *Chem. Ber.* 68:1765-1774 (1935).

Kuman, A., H. Yamamura, and Y. Nishizuka. Mode of action of adenosine $3',5'$-cyclic phosphate on protein kinase from rat liver. *Biochem. Biophys. Res. Commun.* 41:1290-1297 (1970).

Kummerow, F. A. Possible role of vitamin E in unsaturated fatty acid metabolism. *Fed. Proc.* 23:1053-1058 (1964).

Kupiecki, F. P. and J. R. Weeks. Prolonged intravenous infusion of prostaglandin E_1 (PGE_1) on lipid metabolism in the rat. *Fed. Proc.* 25:719A (1966).

Kuratowska, Z. The renal mechanism of the formation and inactivation of erythropoietin. *Ann. N. Y. Acad. Sci.* 149:128-134 (1968).

Kuratowska, Z., B. Lewartowski, and B. Lipinski. Chemical and biological properties of an erythropoietin generating substance obtained from perfusates of isolated anoxic kidneys. *J. Lab. Clin. Med.* 64:226-237 (1964).

Kurzrok, R. and C. C. Lieb. Biochemical studies of human semen. II. The action of semen on the human uterus. *Proc. Soc. Exp. Biol. Med.* 28:268-272 (1930).

Lachman, E. Osteoporosis: the potentialities and limitations of its roentgenologic diagnosis. *Amer. J. Roentgenol. Radium Therapy Nuclear Med.* 74:712-715 (1955).

Lack, C. H. Lysosomes in relation to arthritis. In *Lysosomes in Biology and Pathology*, Vol. 1, pp. 493-508, J. T. Dingle and H. B. Fell, Eds., *Frontiers of Biology*, Vol. 14A, Wiley-Interscience, N.Y. (1969).

La Du, B. N. and V. G. Zannoni. The role of ascorbic acid in tyrosine metabolism. *Ann. N. Y. Acad. Sci.* 92:175-191 (1961).

Lafontaine, J. G. and C. Allard. A light and electron microscope study of the morphological changes induced in rat liver cells by the azo dye 2-Me-DAB. *J. Cell Biol.* 22:143-172 (1964).

Laitinen, H. A. Analytical methods for trace metals: an overview. *Ann. N. Y. Acad. Sci.* 199:173-181 (1972).

Laki, K. Size and shape of the myosin molecule. In *Contractile Proteins and Muscle,* pp. 179-217, K. Laki, Ed., Marcel Dekker, Inc., N. Y. (1971a).

Laki, K. Actin. In *Contractile Proteins and Muscle,* pp. 97-133, K. Laki, Ed., Marcel Dekker, Inc., N. Y. (1971b).

Laki, K. Tropomyosin A. In *Contractile Proteins and Muscle,* pp. 273-288, K. Laki, Ed., Marcel Dekker, Inc., N. Y. (1971c).

Lambooy, J. P. Riboflavin antagonists. *Amer. J. Clin. Nutr.* 3:282-290 (1955).

Lamola, A. A. and T. Yamane. Zinc protoporphyrin in the erythrocytes of patients with lead intoxication and iron deficiency anemia. *Science* 186:936-938 (1974).

Lan, T. H. and R. R. Sealock. The metabolism *in vitro* of tyrosine by liver and kidney tissues of normal and vitamin C-deficient guinea pigs. *J. Biol. Chem.* 155:483-492 (1944).

Lane, M. and C. P. Alfrey, Jr. The anemia of human riboflavin deficiency. *Blood* 25:432-442 (1970).

Lane, M. D. and F. Lynen. The biochemical function of biotin. VI. Chemical structure of the carboxylated active site of propionyl carboxylase. *Proc. Natl. Acad. Sci.* 49:379-385 (1963).

Langan, T. A. Cyclic AMP and histone phosphorylation. *Ann. N. Y. Acad. Sci.* 185:166-180 (1971).

Langer, B. W., Jr. and P. György. Biotin. VIII. Active compounds and antagonists. In *The Vitamins,* Vol. II, pp. 294-322, W. H. Sebrell, Jr. and R. S. Harris, Eds., Academic Press, N. Y. (1968).

Langworthy, C. F. The value of experiments on the metabolism of matter and energy. *Exp. Sta. Rec.* 9:1003-1019 (1897-1898).

Lardy, H. A. and S. M. Ferguson. Oxidative phosphorylation in mitochondria. *Ann. Rev. Biochem.* 38:991-1034 (1969).

Lát, J., A. Pavlik, and B. Jakoubek. Interrelations between individual differences in excitability levels, habituation-rates and in the incorporation of ^{14}C-leucine into brain and nonbrain proteins in rats. *Physiol. Behav.* 11:131-137 (1973).

Lát, Josef. Self-selection of dietary components. In *Handbook of Physiology,* Section 6, *Alimentary Canal,* Vol. I, pp. 367-386, C. F. Code, Ed., American Physiological Society, Washington, D.C. (1967).

Latta, H., A. B. Maunsbach, and L. Osvaldo. The fine structure of renal tubules in cortex and medulla. In *Ultrastructure of the Kidney,* pp. 1-65, A. J. Dalton and F. Haguenau, Eds., Academic Press, N. Y. (1967).

Laurell, C. B. Studies on the transportation and metabolism of iron in the body. *Acta Physiol. Scand.* (Suppl. 46) 14:1-129 (1947).

Lawrence, C. W., F. D. Crain, F. J. Lotspeich, and R. F. Krause. Absorption, transport, and storage of retinyl-15-^{14}C palmitate-9, 10-^{3}H in the rat. *J. Lipid Res.* 7:226-229 (1966).

Lawson, D. E. M., D. R. Fraser, E. Kodicek, H. R. Morris, and D. H. Williams. Identification of 1,25-dihydroxycholecalciferol, a new kidney hormone controlling calcium metabolism. *Nature* 230:228-230 (1971).

Layrisse, M., C. Martinez-Torres, and M. Roche. Effect of interaction of various foods on iron absorption. *Amer. J. Clin. Nutr.* 21:1175-1183 (1968).

Leach, E. H. and J. P. F. Lloyd. Citrol poisoning. *Proc. Nutr. Soc.* 15:xv-xvi (1956).

Leach, R. M., Jr. Role of manganese in the synthesis of mucopolysaccharides. *Fed. Proc.* 26:118-120 (1967).

Leach, R. M., Jr. Role of manganese in mucopolysaccharide metabolism. *Fed. Proc.* 30:991-994 (1971).

Leach, R. M., Jr. and A-M. Muenster. Studies on the role of manganese in bone formation. I. Effect upon the mucopolysaccharide content of chick bone. *J. Nutr.* 78:51-56 (1962).

Leach, R. M., Jr., A-M. Muenster, and E. Wien. Studies on the role of manganese in bone formation. II. Effect upon chondroitin sulfate synthesis in chick epiphyseal cartilage. *Arch. Biochem. Biophys.* 133:22-28 (1969).

Leblond, C. P. and B. Messier. Renewal of chief cells and goblet cells in the small intestine as shown by radioautography after injection of thymidine-H^3 into mice. *Anat. Rec.* 132:247-259 (1958).

Lederberg, J. A view of genetics. *Science* 131:269-276 (1960).

Lee, H. M., N. E. McCall, L. D. Wright, and D. B. McCormick. Urinary excretion of biotin and metabolites in the rat. *Proc. Soc. Exp. Biol. Med.* 142:642-644 (1973).

Lee, H. M., L. D. Wright, and D. B. McCormick. Metabolism of carbonyl-labeled ^{14}C-biotin in the rat. *J. Nutr.* 102:1453-1464 (1972).

Lee, Y. C., R. K. Gholson, and N. Raica. Isolation and identification of two new nicotinamide metabolites. *J. Biol. Chem.* 244:3277-3282 (1969).

Leevy, C. M. and H. Baker. Vitamins and alcoholism. *Amer. J. Clin. Nutr.* 21:1325-1328 (1968).

Lehman, I. R. DNA ligase: Structure, mechanism, and function. *Science* 186:790-797 (1974).

Lehninger, A. L. Water uptake and extrusion by mitochondria in relation to oxidative phosphorylation, *Physiol. Rev.* 42:467-517 (1962).

Lehninger, A. L. *The Mitochondrion.* W. A. Benjamin, Inc., N. Y. (1964).

Lehninger, A. L. The transfer of energy within cells. In *Ideas in Modern Biology*, Chap. 5, J. A. Moore, Ed., The Natural History Press, Garden City, N. Y. (1965a).

Lehninger, A. L. *Bioenergetics.* W. A. Benjamin, Inc., N. Y. (1965b).

Lehninger, A. L. Cell organelles: The mitochondrion. In *The Neurosciences*, pp. 91-100, G. C. Quarton, T. Melnechuk, and F. O. Schmitt, Eds., Rockefeller University Press, N. Y. (1967).

Lehninger, A. L. Acid-base changes in mitochondria and medium during energy-dependent and energy-independent binding of Ca^{++}. *Ann. N. Y. Acad. Sci.* 147:816-823 (1969).

Lehninger, A. L. *Biochemistry.* Worth Publishers, Inc., N. Y. (1970).

Lehninger, A. L. Mitochondria and calcium ion transport. *Biochem. J.* 119:129-138 (1970).

Lehninger, A. L. The molecular organization of mitochondrial membranes. *Adv. Cytopharmacol.* 1:199-208 (1971a).

Lehninger, A. L. A soluble, heat-labile, high-affinity Ca^{2+}-binding factor extracted from rat liver mitochondria. *Biochem. Biophys. Res. Commun.* 42:312-318 (1971b).

Lehninger, A. L. and E. Carafoli. The reaction of Ca^{++} with the mitochondrial membrane: a comparative study on mitochondria from different sources. *Fed. Proc.* 28:664A (1969).

Leichsenring, J. M. and E. D. Wilson. Food composition table for short method of dietary analysis (2nd revision). *J. Amer. Diet. Ass.* 27:386-389 (1951).

Leitch, I. The evolution of dietary standards. *Nutr. Abstr. Rev.* 11:509-521 (1942).

Leitch, I. Changing concepts in the nutritional physiology of human pregnancy. *Proc. Nutr. Soc.* 16:38-45 (1957).

Leitch, I. and F. C. Aitkin. Estimation of calcium requirement: re-examination. *Nutr. Abstr. Rev.* 29:393-411 (1959).

Lema, I. and H. H. Sandstead. Zinc deficiency, effect on collagen and glycoprotein synthesis and bone mineralization. *Fed. Proc.* 29:297A (1970).

Lenard, J. and S. J. Singer. Protein conformation in cell membrane preparations as studied by optical rotary dispersion and circular dichroism. *Proc. Nat. Acad. Sci.* 56:1828-1835 (1966).

Lengemann, F. W., R. H. Wasserman, and C. L. Comar. Studies on the enhancement of radiocalcium and radiostrontium absorption by lactose in the rat. *J. Nutr.* 68:443-456 (1959).

Lenhert, P. G. and D. C. Hodgkin. Structure of the 5,6-dimethylbenzimidazolylcobamide coenzyme. *Nature* 192:937-938 (1961).

Lentz, T. L. *Cell Fine Structure. An Atlas of Drawings of Whole-Cell Structure.* W. B. Saunders Company, Philadelphia (1971).

Lepkovsky, S. Crystalline factor I. *Science* 87:169-170 (1938).

Letarte, J. and A. E. Renold. Ionic effects on glucose transport and metabolism by isolated mouse fat cells incubated with or without insulin. III. Effects of replacement of Na^+. *Biochim. Biophys. Acta* 183:366-374 (1969).

Lev, M. and A. W. Milford. Water-soluble factors with vitamin K activity from pig liver and from *fusiformis nigrescens. Nature* 210:1120-1122 (1966).

Leveille, G. A. Modified thiochrome procedure for the determination of urinary thiamin. *Amer. J. Clin. Nutr.* 25:273-274 (1972).

Levenson, S. M. and B. Tennant. Some metabolic and nutritional studies with germfree animals. *Fed. Proc.* 22:109-119 (1963).

Leventhal, B. and F. Stohlman, Jr. Regulation of erythropoiesis. XVII. Determinants of red cell size in iron deficiency states. *Ped.* 37:62-67 (1966).

Lever, J. D. Cytological studies on the hypophysectomized rat adrenal cortex: the alterations of its fine structure following ACTH administration and on lowering the Na/K ratio. *Endocrinol.* 58:163-180 (1956a).

Lever, J. D. Physiologically induced changes in adrenocortical mitochondria. *J. Biophys. Biochem Cytol.* 2: No. 4 Suppl., 313-317 (1956b).

Leverton, R. M. Amino acid requirements of young adults. In *Protein and Amino Acid Nutrition,* A. A. Albanese, ed., Academic Press, N. Y. (1959).

Leverton, R. M. and A. G. Marsh. The iron metabolism and requirement of young women. *J. Nutr.* 23:229-238 (1942).

Levi, A. S., S. Geller, D. M. Root, and G. Wolf. The effect of vitamin A and other dietary constituents on the activity of adenosine triphosphate sulphurylase. *Biochem. J.* 109:69-74 (1968).

Levi, A. S. and G. Wolf. Purification and properties of the enzyme ATP-sulfurylase and its relation to vitamin A. *Biochim. Biophys. Acta* 178:262-282 (1969).

Levin, E. Y., B. Levenberg, and S. Kaufman. The enzymatic conversion of 3,4-dihydroxy-phenylethylamine to norepinephrine. *J. Biol. Chem.* 235:2080-2086 (1960).

Levine, R. A. Cyclic AMP in digestive physiology. *Amer. J. Clin. Nutr.* 26:876-881 (1973).

Levitsky, D. A. and R. H. Barnes. Effect of early malnutrition on the reaction of adult rats to aversive stimuli. *Nature* 225:468-469 (1970).

Levitsky, D. A. and R. H. Barnes. Nutritional and environmental interactions in the behavioral development of the rat: long term effects. *Science* 176:68-71 (1972).

Levitt, M. Detailed molecular model for transfer ribonucleic acid. *Nature* 224:759-763 (1969).

Levy, G. and W. J. Jusko. Factors affecting the absorption of riboflavin in man. *J. Pharm. Sci.* 55:285-289 (1966).

Levy, M. and M.-T. Sauner. Specificité de composition en phospholipides et en cholesterol des membranes mitochondriales. *Chem. Phys. Lipids.* 2:291-295 (1968).

Liang, C. C. Tissue breakdown and glyoxylic acid formation. *Biochem. J.* 83:101-106 (1963).

Lieberman, A., L. S. Freedman, and M. Goldstein. Serum dopamine-β-hydroxylase activity in patients with Huntington's chorea and Parkinson's disease. *Lancet* 1:153-154 (1972).

Lightner, D. A., A. Moscowitz, Z. J. Petryka, S. Jones, M. Weimer, E. Davis, N. A. Beach, and C. J. Watson. Mass spectrometry and ferric chloride oxidation applied to urobilinoid structures. *Arch. Biochem.* 131:566-576 (1969).

Lind, James. *Treatise of the Scurvy,* printed by Sands, Murray and Cochran, for A. Kincaid and A. Donaldson, pp. 456, Edinburgh (1753).

Linder, M. C. and H. N. Munro. Metabolic and chemical features of ferritins, a series of iron-inducible tissue proteins. *Amer. J. Path.* 72:263-282 (1973).

Lindley, D. C. and T. J. Cunha. Nutritional significance of inositol and biotin for the pig. *J. Nutr.* 32:47-59 (1946).

Lindquist, B. Effect of vitamin D on the metabolism of radiocalcium in rachitic rats. *Acta. Paediat.* 41:Suppl. 86, 1-82 (1952).

Linkswiler, H. M., C. L. Joyce, and C. R. Anand. Calcium retention of young adult males as affected by level of protein and of calcium intake. *Trans. N. Y. Acad. Sci.* (Series II) 36:333-340 (1974).

Lipkin, M. Cell proliferation in the gastrointestinal tract of man. *Fed. Proc.* 24:10-15 (1965).

Lipmann, F. Polypeptide chain elongation in protein synthesis. *Science* 164:1024-1031 (1969).

Lipmann, F. and N. O. Kaplan. A common factor in the enzymatic acetylation of sulfanilamide and of choline. *J. Biol. Chem.* 162:743-744 (1946).

Lipschitz, D. A., T. H. Bothwell, H. C. Seftel, A. A. Wapnick, and R. W. Charlton. The role of ascorbic acid in the metabolism of storage iron. *Brit. J. Haematol.* 20:155-163 (1971).

Littaru, G. P., L. Ho, and K. Folkers. Deficiency of coenzyme Q_{10} in human heart disease. *Internat. J. Vit. Nutr. Res.* 42:291-305 (1972).

Liu, S. H., H. I. Chu, H. C. Hsu, H. C. Chao, and S. H. Cheu. Calcium and phosphorus metabolism in osteomalacia. XI. The pathogenetic role of pregnancy and relative importance of calcium and vitamin D supply. *J. Clin. Invest.* 20:255-271 (1940).

Livingston, D. M. and E. C. W. Wacker. Trace metal methods for nutritional studies. *Amer. J. Clin. Nutr.* 24:1082-1085 (1971).

Lloyd, J. B. and F. Beck. Teratogenesis. In *Lysosomes in Biology and Pathology,* Vol. 1, pp. 433-449, J. T. Dingle and H. B. Fell, Eds., *Frontiers of Biology,* 14A, Wiley-Interscience, N. Y. (1969).

Locke, F. Towards the ideal artificial circulating fluid for the isolated frog's heart. *J. Physiol.* (London) 18:332-333 (1895).

Loewenstein, W. R. Intercellular communication. *Sci. Amer.* 222 (5):78-86 (1970).

Loewenstein, W. R. Membrane junctions in growth and differentiation. *Fed. Proc.* 32:60-64 (1973).

Loewenstein, W. R. and Y. Kanno. Studies on an epithelial (gland) cell junction. I. Modifications of surface membrane permeability. *J. Cell Biol.* 22:565-586 (1964).

Loewenstein, W. R. and Y. Kanno. Intercellular communication and tissue growth. I. Cancerous growth. *J. Cell Biol.* 33:225-234 (1967).

Loewenstein, W. R., S. J. Socolar, S. Higashino, Y. Kanno, and N. Davidson. Intercellular communication: Renal, urinary bladder, sensory, and salivary gland cells. *Science* 149:295-298 (1965).

Loewi, Otto. An autobiographic sketch. *Perspect. Biol. Med.* 4:3-25 (1960).

Lohmann, K. and P. Schuster. Untersuchungen iiber die cocarboxylase. *Biochem. Z.* 294:188-214 (1937).

Losito, R., C. A. Owen, Jr., and E. V. Flock. Metabolism of $[^{14}C]$ menadione. *Biochemistry* 6:62-68 (1967).

Losowsky, M. S., J. Kelleher, B. E. Walker, T. Davies, and C. L. Smith. Intake and absorption of tocopherol. *Ann. N. Y. Acad. Sci.* 203:212-222 (1972).

Lotspeich, W. D. and A. H. Wheeler. Insulin, anaerobiosis, and phlorizin in entry of D-galactose into skeletal muscle. *Amer. J. Physiol.* 202:1065-1069 (1962).

Loughlin, R. E., H. L. Elford, and J. M. Buchanan. Enzymatic synthesis of the methyl group of methionine. VII. Isolation of a cobalamin-containing transmethylase (5-methyl-tetrahydrofolate-homocysteine) from mammalian liver. *J. Biol. Chem.* 239:2888-2895 (1964).

Lovenberg, W., H. Weissbach, and S. Udenfriend. Aromatic L-amino acid decarboxylase. *J. Biol. Chem.* 237:89-93 (1962).

Lowenstein, J. M. Is insulin involved in regulating the rate of fatty acid synthesis? In *Handbook of Physiology*, Section 7: *Endocrinology*, Vol. I, pp. 415-424, R. O. Greep and E. B. Astwood, Eds., American Physiological Society, Washington, D. C. (1972).

Lowenthal, J. and J. A. MacFarlane. Use of a competitive vitamin K antagonist, 2-chloro-3-phytyl-1, 4-naphthoquinone, for the study of the mechanism of action of vitamin K and coumarin anticoagulants. *J. Pharmacol. Exp. Ther.* 157:672-680 (1967).

Lowey, H., S. Slayter, A. G. Weeds, and H. Baker. Substructure of the myosin molecule. I. Subfragments of myosin by enzymic degradation. *J. Molec. Biol.* 42:1-29 (1969).

Lowry, O. H. Biochemical evidence of nutritional status. *Physiol. Rev.* 32:431-448 (1952).

Lowry, O. H. and O. A. Bessey. Microchemical methods for nutritional studies. *Fed. Proc.* 4:268-271 (1945).

Lowy, P. H. Preparation and chemistry of erythropoietin. In *Regulation of Hematopoiesis*, Vol. I, pp. 395-412, A. S. Gordon, Ed., Appleton-Century-Crofts, N. Y. (1970).

Luck, D. J. L. Genesis of mitochondria in *Neurospora crassa. Proc. Nat. Acad. Sci.* 49:233-240 (1963a)

Luck, D. J. L. Formation of mitochondria in *Neurospora crassa. J. Cell Biol.* 16:483-499 (1963b).

Luck, D. J. L. and E. Reich. DNA in mitochondria of *Neurospora crassa. Proc. Nat. Acad. Sci.* 52:931-938 (1964).

Lucy, J. A. Ultrastructure of membranes: Micellar organization. *Brit. Med. Bull.* 24:127-129 (1968).

Lucy, J. A. Functional and structural aspects of biological membranes: A suggested structural role for vitamin E in the control of membrane permeability and stability. *Ann. N. Y. Acad. Sci.* 203:4-11 (1972).

Lucy, J. A. and F. U. Lichti. Reactions of vitamin A with acceptors of electrons. Interactions with iodine and the formation of iodine. *Biochem. J.* 112:231-241 (1969).

Lunin, N. Ueber die Bedeutung der anorganischen Salze fur die Ernahrung des Thieres (Inaugural-Dissertation, Dorpat, 1880), cited in McCollum, *History of Nutrition*, p. 204.

Lusk, G. *The Elements of the Science of Nutrition*, 4th ed., W. B. Saunders Company, Philadelphia (1928).

Lusk, G. The specific dynamic action. (Editorial Review) *J. Nutr.* 3:519-530 (1931).

Luzzati, V., H. Mustacchi, and A. Skoulios. The structure of the liquid-crystal phases of some soap + water systems. *Farad. Soc. Disc.* 25:43-50 (1958).

Lyttleton, J. W. Nucleoproteins of white clover. *Biochem. J.* 74:82-90 (1960).

Lyttleton, J. W. Isolation of ribosomes from spinach chloroplasts. *Exper. Cell Res.* 26:312-317 (1962).

Macara, I. G., T. G. Hoy, and P. M. Harrison. Formation of ferritin from apoferritin. Kinetics and mechanism of iron uptake. *Biochem. J.* 126:151-162 (1972).

Machado, E. A., E. A. Porta, W. S. Hartroft, and F. Hamilton. Studies on dietary hepatic necrosis. II. Ultrastructural and enzymatic alterations of the hepatocytic plasma membrane. *Lab. Invest.* 24:13-20 (1971).

MacIntosh, F. C. Formation, storage and release of acetylcholine at nerve endings. *Canad. J. Biochem. Physiol.* 37:343-356 (1959).

MacIntyre, I. Human calcitonin: Practical and theoretical consequences. In *Calcitonin, Proceedings of the Second International Symposium*, pp. 1-13, Springer-Verlag, N. Y. (1970).

Mackenzie, I. L. and R. M. Donaldson. Vitamin B_{12} absorption and the intestinal cell surface. *Fed. Proc.* 28:41-45 (1969).

Mackenzie, I. L., R. M. Donaldson, Jr., W. L. Kopp and J. S. Trier. Antibodies to intestinal microvillous membranes. II. Inhibition of intrinsic factor-mediated attachment of vitamin B_{12} to hamster brush border. *J. Exp. Med.* 128:375-386 (1968).

Mackrell, D. J. and J. E. Sokal. Antagonism between the effects of insulin and glucagon on the isolated liver. *Diabetes* 18:724-732 (1969).

MacMahon, M. T. and G. Neale. The absorption of α-tocopherol in control subjects and in patients with intestinal malabsorption. *Clin. Sci.* 38:197-210 (1970).

MacMahon, M. T., G. Neale and G. R. Thompson. Lymphatic and portal venous transport of α-tocopherol and cholesterol. *Europ. J. Clin. Invest.* 1:288-294 (1971).

MacMahon, M. T. and G. R. Thompson. Comparison of the absorption of a polar lipid, oleic acid, and a non-polar lipid, α-tocopherol from mixed micellar solutions and emulsions. *Europ. J. Clin. Invest.* 1:161-166 (1970).

Madden, S. C. and G. Whipple. Plasma proteins: their source, production and utilization. *Physiol. Rev.* 20:194-217 (1940).

Magendie, F. On the nutritive value of substances which contain no nitrogen. *Ann. de Chim. et de Phys.* 3:66 (1816).

Mahadevan, S. and J. Ganguly. Further studies on the absorption of vitamin A. *Biochem. J.* 81:53-58 (1961).

Mahadevan, S., P. Seshadri Sastry and J. Ganguly. Studies on the metabolism of vitamin A: 3. The mode of absorption of vitamin A esters in the living rat. *Biochem. J.* 88:531-533 (1963a).

Mahadevan, S., P. Seshadri Sastry and J. Ganguly. Studies on metabolism of vitamin A. 4. Studies on the mode of absorption of vitamin A by rat intestine *in vitro. Biochem. J.* 88:534-539 (1963b).

Maitra, U. and J. Hurwitz. The role of DNA in RNA synthesis. IX. Nucleoside triphosphate termini in RNA polymerase products. *Proc. Natl. Acad. Sci.* 54:815-822 (1965).

Majaj, A. S. Vitamin E-responsive macrocytic anemia in protein-calorie malnutrition. *Amer. J. Clin. Nutr.* 18:362-368 (1966).

Majaj, A. S., J. S. Dinning, S. A. Azzam, and W. J. Darby. Vitamin E responsive megaloblastic anemia in infants with protein-calorie malnutrition. *Amer. J. Clin. Nutr.* 12:374-379 (1963).

Majaj, A. S. and K. Folkers. Hematological activity of coenzyme Q in an anemia of human malnutrition. *Intern. Z. Vitaminforsch.* 38:182-195 (1968).

Mallette, L. E., J. H. Exton, and C. R. Park. Effects of glucagon on amino acid transport and utilization in the perfused rat liver. *J. Biol. Chem.* 244:5724-5728 (1969).

Malina, R. M., Quantification of fat, muscle and bone in man. *Clin. Orthoped. Rel. Res.* 65:9-38 (1969).

Malm, O. J. On phosphates and phosphoric acid as dietary factors in the calcium balance of man. *Scand. J. Clin. Lab. Invest.* 5:75-84 (1953).

Malm, O. J. Calcium requirements and adaptation in adult men. *Scand. J. Clin. Invest. Supp.* 36, 10:1-289 (1958).

Manganiello, V. C., F. Murad and M. Vaughan. Effects of lipolytic and antilipolytic agents on cyclic $3',5'$-adenosine monophosphate in fat cells. *J. Biol. Chem.* 246:2195-2202 (1971)

Manis, J. and D. Schachter. Fe^{59}-amino acid complexes: Are they intermediates in Fe^{59} absorption across intestinal mucosa? *Proc. Soc. Exp. Biol. Med.* 119:1185-1187 (1965).

Manis, J. F. and D. Schachter. Active transport of iron by intestine: effects of oral iron and pregnancy. *Amer. J. Physiol.* 203:81-86 (1962).

Manis, J. G. and D. Schachter. Active transport of iron by intestine: mucosal iron pools. *Amer. J. Physiol.* 207:893-900 (1964).

Mann, G. V., G. Pearson, T. Gordon and T. R. Dawber. Diet and cardiovascular disease in the Framingham study. I. Measurement of dietary intake. *Amer. J. Clin. Nutr.* 11:200-225 (1962).

March, B. E., E. Wong, L. Seier, J. Sim, and J. Biely. Hypervitaminosis E in the chick. *J. Nutr.* 103:371-377 (1973).

Marchesi, V. T., R. L. Jackson, J. P. Segrest and I. Kahane. Molecular features of the major glycoprotein of the human erythrocyte membrane. *Fed. Proc.* 32:1833-1837 (1973).

Marchis-Mouren, G., L. Pasero and P. Desnuelle. Further studies on amylase biosynthesis by pancreas of rats fed on a starch-rich or casein-rich diet. *Biochem. Biophys. Res. Commun.* 13:262-266 (1963).

Margaria, R. The sources of muscular energy. *Sci. Amer.* 226(3):84-91 (1972).

Margen, S., J. Y. Chu, N. A. Kaufmann, and D. H. Calloway. Studies in calcium metabolism. I. The calciuretic effect of dietary protein. *Amer. J. Clin. Nutr.* 27:584-589 (1974).

Markscheid, L. and E. Shafrir. Incorporation of lipoprotein-borne triglycerides by adipose tissue *in vitro. J. Lipid Res.* 6:247-257 (1965).

Marr, J. W. Individual dietary surveys: purposes and methods. *World Rev. Nutr. Dietet.* 13:105-164 (1971).

Marshall, F. N. Lipoprotein lipase activity in normal human adipose tissue and its absence in human lipomas. *Experientia* 21:130-131 (1965).

Marshall, M. W., V. A. Knox, D. L. Trout, A. M. A. Durand, and D. A. Benton. Biotin status and lipid metabolism in young inbred rats. *Nutr. Rep. Internat.* 5:201-212 (1972).

Marshall, R. D. Glycoproteins. *Ann. Rev. Biochem.* 41:673-702 (1972).

Marshall, R. D. and A. Neuberger. Aspects of the structure and metabolism of glycoproteins. *Adv. Carbohydrate Chem. Biochem.* 40:407-478 (1970).

Marston, H. R. and S. H. Allen. Factors affecting formiminoglutamic acid excretion in vitamin B_{12} deficiency. *Biochem. J.* 116:681-688 (1970).

Martin, H. E., J. Mehl, and M. Wertman. Clinical studies of magnesium metabolism. *Med. Clin. N. Am.* 36:1157-1171 (1952).

Maruyama, K. Regulatory proteins. In *Contractile Proteins and Muscle*, pp. 289-313, K. Laki, Ed., Marcel Dekker, Inc., N. Y. (1971).

Marx, S. J., C. J. Woodard, and G. D. Aurbach. Calcitonin receptors of kidney and bone. *Science* 178:999-1001 (1972).

Mason, M., J. Ford, and H. L. C. Wu. Effects of steroid and nonsteriod metabolites on enzyme conformation and pyridoxal phosphate binding. *Ann. N. Y. Acad. Sci.* 166:170-183 (1969).

Matschiner, J. T. and W. V. Taggart. Bioassay of vitamin K by intracardial injection in deficient adult male rats. *J. Nutr.* 94:57-59 (1968).

Matthews, D. M. Absorption of water-soluble vitamins. In *Intestinal Absorption*, Biomembranes, Vol. 4B, pp. 847-915, D. H. Smyth, Ed., Plenum Press, London (1974).

Matthews, J. L., J. H. Martin, H. W. Sampson, A. S. Kunin, and J. H. Roan. Mitochondrial granules in the normal and rachitic rat epiphysis. *Calcif. Tissue Res.* 5:91-99 (1970).

Matthews, R. G., R. Hubbard, P. K. Brown, and G. Wald. Tautomeric forms of metarhodopsin. *J. Gen. Physiol.* 47:215-240 (1964).

Maugh, T. H., II. Vitamin B_{12}: after 25 years, the first synthesis. *Science* 179:266-267 (1973).

Maunsbach, A. B. Observations on the ultrastructure and acid phosphatase activity of the cytoplasmic bodies in rat kidney proximal tubule cells. *J. Ultrastruct. Res.* 16:197-238 (1966a).

1014 BIBLIOGRAPHY

Maunsbach, A. B. Albumin absorption by renal proximal tubule cells. *Nature* 212:546-547 (1966b).

Maunsbach, A. B. Functions of lysosomes in kidney cells. In *Lysosomes in Biology and Pathology*, Vol. I, pp. 115-154, J. T. Dingle and H. B. Fell, Eds., Frontiers of Biology, Vol. 14A, Wiley-Interscience, N. Y. (1969).

Mawer, E. B., G. A. Lumb, K. Schaefer, and S. W. Stanbury. The metabolism of isotopically labelled vitamin D_3 in man: the influence of the state of vitamin D nutrition. *Clin. Sci.* 40:39-53 (1971).

Mawer, E. B. and K. Schaefer. Distribution of vitamin D_3 metabolites in human serum and tissues. *Biochem. J.* 114:75P (1969).

Mayer, J. Food composition tables. Basis, uses and limitations. *Postgrad. Med.* 28:295-307 (1960).

Mayer, J., P. Roy, and K. P. Mitra. Relation between caloric intake, body weight and physical work. Studies in an industrial male population in West Bengal. *Amer. J. Clin. Nutr.* 4:169-175 (1956).

Mayerle, J. A. and R. J. Havel. Nutritional effects on blood flow in adipose tissue of unanesthetized rats. *Amer. J. Physiol.* 217:1694-1698 (1969).

Mayerson, H. S. The lymphatic system. *Sci. Amer.* 208(6):80-90 (1963).

Maynard, L. Evalaution of dietary survey methods. *Fed. Proc.* 9:598-601 (1950).

Mazur, A. Role of ascorbic acid in the incorporation of plasma iron into ferritin. *Ann. N. Y. Acad. Sci.* 92:223-229 (1961).

Mazur, A. and A. Carleton. Relation of ferritin iron to heme synthesis in marrow and reticulocytes. *J. Biol. Chem.* 238:1817-1824 (1963).

McCall, J. T., N. P. Goldstein, and L. H. Smith. Implications of trace metals in human diseases. *Fed. Proc.* 30:1011-1015 (1971).

McCammon, R. W. The concept of normality. *Ann. N. Y. Acad. Sci.* 134:559-562 (1966).

McCance, R. A. The composition of the body: Its maintenance and regulation. *Nutr. Abstr. Rev.* 42:1269-1279 (1972).

McCance, R. A. and E. M. Widdowson. Absorption and excretion of iron. *Lancet* ii:680-684 (1937).

McCance, R. A. and E. M. Widdowson. Composition of the body. *Brit. Med. Bull.* 7:297-306 (1951).

McCance, R. A. and E. M. Widdowson. Nutrition and growth. *Proc. Roy. Soc. B* 156:326-337 (1962).

McCance, R. A. and E. M. Widdowson, Eds., *Calorie Deficiencies and Protein Deficiencies.* Little, Brown and Co., Boston (1968).

McCance, R. A. and E. M. Widdowson. Review lecture. The determinants of growth and form. *Proc. Roy. Soc. B* 185: 1-17 (1974).

McCandless, D. W., C. Hanson, K. V. Speeg, Jr., and S. Schenker. Cardiac metabolism in thiamin deficiency in rats. *J. Nutr.* 100:991-1002 (1970).

McCartney, C. P., R. E. Pottinger, and J. P. Harrod. Alterations in body composition during pregnancy. *Amer. J. Obstet. Gynec.* 77:1038-1053 (1959).

McCay, P. B., P. M. Pfeifer, and W. H. Stipe. Vitamin E protection of membrane lipids during electron transport functions. *Ann. N. Y. Acad. Sci.* 203:62-73 (1972).

McClure, F. J. Wheat cereal diets, rat caries, lysine and minerals. *J. Nutr.* 65:619-631 (1958).

McClure, F. J. Cariostatic effect of phosphates. *Science* 144:1337-1338 (1964).

McClure, F. J. *Water Fluoridation.* U. S. Department of Health, Education, and Welfare, National Institutes of Health, National Institute of Dental Research, Bethesda, Md. (1970).

McCollum, E. V. *A History of Nutrition.* Houghton-Mifflin, Boston (1957).

McCollum, E. V. and M. Davis. The necessity of certain lipids in the diet during growth.

J. Biol. Chem. 15:167-175 (1913).

McCollum, E. V., N. Simmonds, J. E. Becker, and P. G. Shipley. Studies on experimental rickets. XXIII. The production of rickets in the rat by diets consisting of essentially purified food substances. *J. Biol. Chem.* 54:249-252 (1922).

McCormick, D. B. and J. A. Roth. Specificity, stereochemistry, and mechanism of the color reaction between p-dimethylaminodinnamaldehyde and biotin analogs. *Anal. Biochem.* 34:226-236 (1970).

McCormick, D. B. and L. D. Wright, Eds., *Methods in Enzymology*, Vol. XVIII, Part A, Academic Press, N. Y. (1970).

McCormick, D. B. and L. D. Wright, Eds., *Methods in Enzymology*, Vol. XVIII, Part B, Academic Press, N. Y. (1971a).

McCormick, D. B. and L. D. Wright, Eds., *Methods in Enzymology*, Vol. XVIII, Part C, Academic Press, N. Y. (1971b).

McCoy, E. E. and C. Colombini. Interconversions of vitamin B_6 in mammalian tissue. *Agric. Food Chem.* 20:494-498 (1972).

McCoy, K. E. M. and P. H. Weswig. Some selenium responses in the rat not related to vitamin E. *J. Nutr.* 98:383-389 (1969).

McCoy, R. H., C. E. Meyer, and W. C. Rose. Feeding experiments with mixtures of highly purified amino acids. VIII. Isolation and identification of a new essential amino acid. *J. Biol. Chem.* 112:283-302 (1935-36).

McCulloch, E. A. Control of hematopoiesis at the cellular level. In *Regulation of Hematopoiesis*, Vol. I, pp. 133-159, A. S. Gordon, Ed., Appleton-Century-Crofts, N.Y. (1970).

McKanna, J. A. Membrane recycling: vesiculation of the amoeba contractile vacuole at systole. *Science* 179:88-90 (1973).

McKay, H., M. B. Patton, M. S. Pittman, G. Stearns, and N. Edelblute. The effect of vitamin D on calcium retentions. *J. Nutr.* 26:153-159 (1943).

McKhann, G. M., R. W. Albers, L. Sokoloff, O. Mickelsen, and D. B. Tower. The quantitative significance of the gamma-aminobutyric acid pathway in cerebral oxidative metabolism. In *Inhibition in the Nervous System and Gamma-aminobutyric Acid*, pp. 169-181, E. Roberts, et al., Eds., Pergamon Press, N. Y. (1960).

McKibbin, J. M. Glycolipids. In *The Carbohydrates*, Vol. IIB, pp. 711-738, W. Pigman, D. Horton, and A. Herp, Eds., Academic Press, N. Y. (1970).

McLaughlan, J. M. Relationship between protein quality and plasma amino acid levels. *Fed. Proc.* 22:1122-1125 (1963).

McLaughlan, J. M. and W. I. Illman. Use of free amino acid levels for estimating amino acid requirements of the growing rat. *J. Nutr.* 93:21-24 (1967).

McLean, F. C. and A. M. Budy. Chemistry and physiology of the parathyroid hormone. *Vitamins Hormones* 19:165-187 (1961).

McLean, F. C. and M. R. Urist. *Bone. Fundamentals of the Physiology of Skeletal Tissue*, 3rd Ed., University of Chicago Press, Chicago, 1968.

Melancon, M. J., Jr., H. Morii, and H. F. DeLuca. Physiologic effects of vitamin D, parathyroid hormone and calcitonin. In *The Fat-Soluble Vitamins*, pp. 111-123, H. F. DeLuca and J. W. Suttie, Eds., The University of Wisconsin Press, Madison (1970).

Melikian, V., A. Paton, R. J. Leeming, and H. Partman-Graham. Site of reduction and methylation of folic acid in man. *Lancet* 2:955-957 (1971).

Mellanby, E. An experimental investigation on rickets. *Lancet* 1:407-412 (1919).

Mellanby, E. *A Story of Nutritional Research: The Effect of Some Dietary Factors on Bones and the Nervous System.* Williams and Wilkins, Baltimore (1950).

Mendelson, J. H., M. Ogata, and N. K. Mello. Effects of alcohol ingestion and withdrawal on magnesium states of alcoholics: clinical and experimental findings. *Ann. N. Y. Acad. Sci.* 162:918-933 (1969).

Meneely, G. R., R. M. Heyssel, C. O. T. Ball, R. L. Weiland, A. R. Lorimer, C. Constantinides, and E. U. Meneely. Analysis of factors affecting body composition determined from potassium content in 915 normal subjects. *Ann. N. Y. Acad. Sci.* 110:271-281 (1963).

Meneghello, J. and H. Neimeyer. Liver steatosis in undernourished Chilean children. III. Evaluation of choline treatment with repeated liver biopsies. *Amer. J. Dis. Child.* 80:905-910 (1950).

Merriam, R. W. Nuclear envelope structure during cell division in *Chaetopterus* eggs. *Exp. Cell Res.* 22:93-107 (1961).

Merrill, A. L., C. F. Adams, and L. J. Fincher. Procedures for calculating nutritive values of home-prepared foods. *ARS 62-13,* U. S. Department of Agriculture, 35 pp. (1966).

Mertz, W. Chromium occurrence and function in biological systems. *Physiol. Rev.* 49:163-239 (1969).

Mertz, W. Some aspects of nutritional trace element research. *Fed. Proc.* 29:1482-1488 (1970).

Mertz, W. and W. E. Cornatzer, Eds., *Newer Trace Elements in Nutrition,* Marcel Dekker, Inc., N. Y. (1971).

Mertz, W. and E. E. Roginski. Chromium metabolism: The glucose tolerance factor. In *Newer Trace Elements in Nutrition,* pp. 123-153, W. Mertz and W. E. Cornatzer, Eds., Marcel Dekker, Inc., N. Y. (1971).

Meselson, M. and I. W. Stahl. Replication of DNA in E. coli. *Proc. Nat. Acad. Sci.* 44:671-676 (1958).

Messer, H. H., W. D. Armstrong and L. Singer. Fertility impairment in mice on a low fluoride diet. *Science* 177:893-894 (1972).

Metcalf, D. and M. A. S. Moore. *Haemopoietic Cells,* North-Holland Publishing Co., Amsterdam (1971).

Meunier, P., R. Ferrando, J. Jouanneteau, and G. Thomas. Influence de la vitamine A sur la détoxication du benzoate de sodium par l'organisme du rat. *Compt. Rend.* 228: 1254-1256 (1949).

Meyer, F. L., M. L. Brown, and M. L. Hathaway. Nutritive value of school lunches as determined by chemical analyses. *J. Amer. Diet. Ass.* 27:841-846 (1951).

Meyer, F. L., M. L. Brown, H. J. Wright, and M. L. Hathaway. A standardized diet for metabolic studies: Its development and application. *Technical Bulletin No. 1126,* U.S. Department of Agriculture, Washington, D. C. (1955).

Meyer, K., E. Davidson, A. Linker, and P. Hoffman. The acid mucopolysaccharides of connective tissue. *Biochim. Biophys. Acta* 21:506-518 (1956).

Mickelsen, O., W. O. Caster, and A. Keys. A statistical evaluation of the thiamine and pyramin excretion of normal young men on controlled intakes of thiamine. *J. Biol. Chem.* 168:415-431 (1947).

Miettinen, M., O. Turpeinin, M. J. Karvonen, R. Elosuo, and E. Paavilainen. Effect of cholesterol-lowering diet on mortality from coronary heart disease and other causes. A twelve-year clinical trial in men and women. *Lancet* 2:835-838 (1972).

Milhorat, A. T. Inositol. XI. Deficiency effects in human beings. In *The Vitamins,* Vol. III, pp. 398-405, W. H. Sebrell, Jr. and R. S. Harris, Eds., Academic Press, N. Y. (1971).

Miller, D. and R. K. Crane. The digestive function of the epithelium of the small intestine. I. An intracellular locus of disaccharide and sugar phosphate ester hydrolysis. *Biochim. Biophys. Acta* 52:281-293 (1961a).

Miller, D. and R. K. Crane. The digestive function of the epithelium of the small intestine. II. Localization of disaccharide hydrolysis in isolated brush border portion of intestinal epithelial cells. *Biochim. Biophys. Acta* 52:293-298 (1961b).

Miller, D. S. and A. E. Bender. The determination of the net utilization of protein by a shortened method. *Brit. J. Nutr.* 9:382-388 (1955).

Miller, E. J. Biochemical studies on the structure of chick bone collagen. *Fed. Proc.* 28:1839-1845 (1969).

Miller, E. J. and V. J. Matukas. Biosynthesis of collagen. The biochemist's view. *Fed. Proc.* 33:1197-1204 (1974).

Miller, F. and G. E. Palade. Lytic activities in renal protein absorption droplets. An electron microscopical cytochemical study. *J. Cell Biol.* 23:519-552 (1964).

Miller, L. I. and W. F. Bale. Synthesis of all plasma protein fractions except gamma globulins by the liver. *J. Exp. Med.* 99:125-132 (1954).

Miller, O. L., Jr. The visualization of genes in action. *Sci. Amer.* 228(3):34-43 (1973).

Miller, R. F. and R. W. Engel. Interrelationships of copper, molybdenum and sulfate sulfur in nutrition. *Fed. Proc.* 19:666-671 (1960).

Miller, W. J., J. D. Morton, W. J. Pitts, and G. M. Clifton. Effect of zinc deficiency and restricted feeding on wound healing in the bovine. *Proc. Soc. Exp. Biol. Med.* 118:427-430 (1965).

Milne, M. D. Genetic disorders of intestinal amino acid transport. In *Handbook of Physiology,* Section 6: *Alimentary Canal,* Vol. III, pp. 1309-1321, C. F. Code, Ed., American Physiological Society, Washington, D.C. (1968).

Milne, M. D. Hereditary disorders of intestinal transport. In *Intestinal Absorption.* Biomembranes, Vol. 4B, pp. 961-1013, D. H. Smyth, Ed., Plenum Press, London (1974).

Milne, M. D., A. Asatoor, and L. W. Loughridge. Hartnup disease and cystinuria. *Lancet* 1:51-52 (1961).

Minot, G. R. and W. P. Murphy. Treatment of pernicious anemia by a special diet. *J.A.M.A.* 87:470-476 (1926).

Mirand, E. A., T. C. Prentice, and W. R. Slaunwhite. Current studies on the role of erythropoietin on erythropoiesis. *Ann. N. Y. Acad. Sci.* 77:677-702 (1959).

Mirsky, A. E. and H. Ris. The desoxyribonucleic acid content of animal cells and its evolutionary significance. *J. Gen. Physiol.* 34:451-462 (1951).

Mistry, S. P. and K. Dakshinamurti. Biochemistry of biotin. *Vitamins Hormones* 22:1-56 (1964).

Mitchell, H. H. A method of determining the biological value of protein. *J. Biol. Chem.* 58:873-922 (1923).

Mitchell, H. H. Adult growth in man and its nutrient requirements. *Arch. Biochem.* 21:335-342 (1949).

Mitchell, H. H. *Comparative Nutrition of Man and Domestic Animals.* Academic Press, N. Y. (1962).

Mitchell, H. H. and E. G. Curzon. The dietary requirement of calcium and its significance. Actualitiés Scientifiques et Industrielles No. 771 Nutrition XVIII, Paris, Hermann (1939).

Mitchell, H. H. and M. Edman. Nutritional significance of the dermal losses of nutrients in man, particularly of nitrogen and minerals. *Amer. J. Clin. Nutr.* 10:163-172 (1962).

Mitchell, H. H., T. S. Hamilton, F. R. Steggerda, and H. W. Bean. The chemical composition of the adult human body and its bearing on the biochemistry of growth. *J. Biol. Chem.* 158:625-637 (1945).

Mitchell, H. K., E. E. Snell, and R. J. Williams. The concentration of "folic acid." *J. Amer. Chem. Soc.* 63:2284 (1941).

Mitchell, J. R., D. E. Becker, A. H. Jensen, B. G. Harmon, and H. W. Norton. Determination of amino acid needs of the young pig by nitrogen balance and plasma free amino acids. *J. Anim. Sci.* 27:1327-1331 (1968).

1018   BIBLIOGRAPHY

Mittelman, R., A. Chausmer, J. Bellavia, and S. Wallach. Thyrocalcitonin activity in hypercalcemia produced by calcium salts, parathyroid hormone and vitamin D. *Endocrinology* 81:599-604 (1967).

Mo, A., P. S. Peckos, and C. B. Glatkly. Computers in a dietary study. *J. Amer. Diet. Ass.* 59:111-115 (1971).

Molinoff, P. B., W. S. Brimijoin, R. M. Weinshilboum, and J. Axelrod. Neurally mediated increase in dopamine-β-hydroxylase activity. *Proc. Natl. Acad. Sci.* 66:453-458 (1970).

Mollenhauer, H. H. An intercisternal structure in the Golgi apparatus. *J. Cell Biol.* 24:504-511 (1965).

Mollenhauer, H. H. and D. J. Morré. Golgi apparatus and plant secretion. *Ann. Rev. Plant Physiol.* 17:27-46 (1966).

Monckeberg, F., S. Tisler, S. Toro, V. Guttas, and L. Vega. Malnutrition and mental development. *Amer. J. Clin. Nutr.* 25:766-772 (1972).

Monod, J., J. Wyman, and J.-P. Changeux. On the nature of allosteric transitions: A plausible model. *J. Molec. Biol.* 12:88-118 (1965).

Montgomery, R. Glycoproteins. In *The Carbohydrates*, Vol. IIB, pp. 627-709, W. Pigman, D. Horton, and A. Herp, Eds., Academic Press, N. Y. (1970).

Mookerjea, S. Action of choline in lipoprotein metabolism. *Fed. Proc.* 30:143-150 (1971).

Moore, C. V. and R. Dubach. Observations on the absorption of iron from foods tagged with radioiron. *Trans. Assoc. Am. Physicians.* 64:245-256 (1951).

Moore, C. V., R. Dubach, V. Minnich, and H. K. Roberts. Absorption of ferrous and ferric radioactive iron by human subjects and by dogs. *J. Clin. Invest.* 23:755-767 (1944).

Moore, F. D. and C. M. Boyden. Body cell mass and limits of hydration of the fat-free body: their relation to estimated skeletal weight. *Ann. N. Y. Acad. Sci.* 110:62-71 (1963).

Moore, F. D., K. H. Olesen, J. D. McMurrey, H. V. Parker, M. R. Ball, and C. M. Boyden. *The Body Cell Mass and Its Supporting Environment.* W. B. Saunders Company, Philadelphia (1963).

Moore, H. W. and K. Folkers. Vitamin B_{12}. VIII. Active compounds and antagonists. In *The Vitamins*, Vol. II, pp. 181-184, W. H. Sebrell, Jr. and R. S. Harris, Eds., Academic Press, N. Y. (1968).

Moore, M. A. S. and D. Metcalf. Ontogeny of the haemopoietic system: yolk sac origin of *in vivo* and *in vitro* colony forming cells in the developing mouse embryo. *Brit. J. Haematol.* 18:279-296 (1970).

Moore, T. Vitamin A and carotene. *Biochem. J.* 24:692-702 (1930).

Moore, T. *Vitamin A.* Elsevier Publishing Co., Princeton, N. J. (1957).

Morgan, E. H., E. R. Huehns, and C. A. Finch. Iron reflux from reticulocytes and bone marrow cells *in vitro*. *Amer. J. Physiol.* 210:579-585 (1966).

Morgan, F. J., R. E. Canfield, and D. S. Goodman. The partial structure of human plasma prealbumin and retinol-binding protein. *Biochim. Biophys. Acta* 236:798-801 (1971).

Morgan, H. E. and J. R. Neely. Insulin and membrane transport. In *Handbook of Physiology*, Section 7: *Endocrinology*, Vol. I, pp. 323-331, R. O. Greep and E. B. Astwood, Eds., American Physiological Society, Washington, D. C. (1972).

Mori, S. Primary changes in eyes of rats that result from deficiency of fat-soluble A. *J.A.M.A.* 79:197-200 (1922).

Morii, H. and H. F. DeLuca. Relationship between vitamin D deficiency, thyrocalcitonin, and parathyroid hormone. *Amer. J. Physiol.* 213:358-362 (1967).

Morley, C. G. D. Humoral regulation of liver regeneration and tissue growth. *Perspect. Biol. Med.* 17:411-428 (1974).

Morley, C. G. D. and H. S. Kingdon. The regulation of cell growth. 1. Identification and partial characterization of a DNA synthesis stimulating factor from the serum of partially hepatectomized rats. *Biochim. Biophys. Acta* 308:260-275 (1973).

Morré, D. J., W. W. Franke, B. Deumling, S. E. Nyquist, and L. Ovtracht. Golgi apparatus function in membrane flow and differentiation: Origin of plasma membrane from endoplasmic reticulum. In *Biomembranes*, Vol. 2, pp. 95-104, L. A. Manson, Ed., Plenum Press, N. Y. (1971a).

Morré, D. J., R. L. Hamilton, H. H. Mollenhauer, R. W. Mahley, W. P. Cunningham, R. D. Cheetham, and V. S. LeQuire. Isolation of a Golgi apparatus-rich fraction from rat liver. I. Method and morphology. *J. Cell Biol.* 44:484-490 (1970).

Morré, D. J., T. W. Keenan, and H. H. Mollenhauer. Golgi apparatus function in membrane transformations and product compartmentalization: Studies with cell fractions from rat liver. *Adv. Cytopharmacol.* 1:157-182 (1971b).

Morré, D. J., H. H. Mollenhauer, and C. E. Bracker. Origin and continuity of Golgi apparatus. In *Origin and Continuity of Cell Organelles*, Vol. 2, pp. 82-126, J. Reinert and H. Ursprung, Eds., Springer-Verlag, N. Y. (1971b).

Morrice, G., Jr., W. H. Havener, and F. Kapetansky. Vitamin A intoxication as a cause of pseudotumor cerebri. *J.A.M.A.* 173:1802-1805 (1960).

Morris, E. R. and B. L. O'Dell. Relationship of excess calcium and phosphorous to magnesium requirement and toxicity in guinea pigs. *J. Nutr.* 81:175-181 (1963).

Morris, M. D. and I. L. Chaikoff. The origin of cholesterol in liver, small intestine, adrenal gland, and testis of the rat: dietary versus endogenous contributions. *J. Biol. Chem.* 234:1095-1097 (1959).

Morrison, A. B. and J. A. Campbell. Vitamin absorption studies. I. Factors influencing the excretion of oral test doses of thiamine and riboflavin by human subjects. *J. Nutr.* 72:435-440 (1960).

Morse, B. S. and F. Stohlman, Jr. Regulation of erythropoiesis. XVIII. The effect of vincristine and erythropoietin on bone marrow. *J. Clin. Invest.* 45:1241-1250 (1966).

Moses, M. J. The nucleus and chromosomes: a cytological perspective. In *Cytology and Cell Physiology*, 3rd Ed., pp. 424-558, G. H. Bourne, Ed., Academic Press, N. Y. (1964).

Moulton, C. R. Age and chemical development in mammals. *J. Biol. Chem.* 57:79-97 (1923).

Mrsovosky, N. and U. Rowlatt. Changes in the microstructure of brown fat at birth in the human infant. *Biol. Neonat.* 13:230-252 (1968).

Mudd, S. H. Pyridoxine-responsive genetic disease. *Fed. Proc.* 30:970-976 (1971).

Mueller, J. F. Vitamin B_6 in fat metabolism. *Vitamins Hormones* 22:787-796 (1964).

Mueller, J. F. and R. W. Vilter. Pyridoxine deficiency in human beings induced with desoxypyridoxine. *J. Clin. Invest.* 29:193-201 (1950).

Mueller, W. J., R. L. Brubaker, C. V. Gay, and J. N. Boelkins. Mechanisms of bone resorption in laying hens. *Fed. Proc.* 32:1951-1954 (1973).

Muenter, M. D., H. O. Perry, and J. Ludwig. Chronic vitamin A intoxication in adults. Hepatic, neurologic and dermatologic complications. *Amer. J. Med.* 50:129-136 (1971).

Mulder, G. J. Ueber die Proteinverbindungen des Pflanzenreiches. *J. Prakt. Chem.* 16:129 (1839); 44:503-505 (1848).

Muller, S. A., A. S. Posner, and H. E. Firschein. Effect of vitamin D deficiency on the crystal chemistry of bone mineral. *Proc. Soc. Exp. Biol. Med.* 121:844-846 (1966).

Munro, H. M. and J. W. Drysdale. Role of iron in the regulation of ferritin metabolism. *Fed. Proc.* 29:1469-1473 (1970).

Munson, P. L. and T. K. Gray. Function of thyrocalcitonin in normal physiology. *Fed. Proc.* 29:1206-1208 (1970).

Murakami, U. and Y. Kameyama. Malformations of the mouse fetus caused by hypervitaminosis A of the mother during pregnancy. *Arch. Environ. Health.* 10:732-741 (1965).

von Muralt, A. The role of thiamine in neurophysiology. *Ann. N. Y. Acad. Sci.* 98:499-507 (1962).

Murray, J. M. and A. Weber. The cooperative action of muscle proteins. *Sci. Amer.* 230(2):58-71 (1974).

Murty, H. S., P. I. Caasai, S. K. Brooks, and P. P. Nair. Biosynthesis of heme in the vitamin E-deficient rat. *J. Biol. Chem.* 245:5498-5504 (1970).

Muto, Y., J. E. Smith, P. O. Milch, and D. S. Goodman. Regulation of retinol-binding protein metabolism by vitamin A status in the rat. *J. Biol. Chem.* 247:2542-2550 (1972).

Myant, N. B. Developmental aspects of lipid metabolism. In *The Biochemistry of Development*, P. Benson, Ed., Clinics in Developmental Medicine No. 37, J. B. Lippincott Co. (1971).

Myhre, E. Iron uptake and hemoglobin synthesis by human erythroid cell *in vitro. Scand. J. Clin. Lab. Invest.* 16:212-221 (1964).

Nagatsu, T., M. Levitt, S. Udenfriend. Tyrosine hydroxylase: The initial step in norepinephrine biosynthesis. *J. Biol. Chem.* 239:2910-2917 (1964).

Nair, P. P. Vitamin E and metabolic regulation. *Ann. N. Y. Acad. Sci.* 203:53-61 (1972).

Nair, P. P., H. S. Murty, P. I. Caasi, S. K. Brooks, and J. Quartner. Vitamin E. Regulation of biosynthesis of porphyrins and heme. *J. Agr. Food Chem.* 20:476-480 (1972).

Naismith, D. J. The role of body fat accumulated during pregnancy in lactation in the rat. *Proc. Nutr. Soc.* 30:93A (1971).

Najjar, V. A. and L. E. Holt. The biosynthesis of thiamine in man and its implication in human nutrition. *J.A.M.A.* 123:683-684 (1943).

Nakagawa, I., T. Takahashi, T. Suzuki, and K. Kobayashi. Amino acid requirements of children: nitrogen balance at the minimal level of essential amino acids. *J. Nutr.* 83:115-118 (1964).

Nandi, M. A. and E. S. Parham. Milk drinking by the lactose intolerant. *J. Amer. Diet. Ass.* 61:258-261 (1972).

Naora, H., H. Naora, M. Izawa, V. G. Allfrey, and A. E. Mirsky. Some observations on differences in composition between the nucleus and cytoplasm of the frog oocyte. *Proc. Natl. Acad. Sci.* 48:853-859 (1962).

Napolitano, L. The fine structure of adipose tissues. In *Handbook of Physiology*, Section 5, *Adipose Tissue*, A. E. Renold and G. F. Cahill, Jr., Eds., pp. 109-123, American Physiological Society, Washington, D. C. (1965).

Nass, M. M. K. Mitochondrial DNA. I. Intramitochondrial distribution and structural relations of single- and double-length circular DNA. *J. Molec. Biol.* 42:521-528 (1969).

Nasset, E. S. Role of the digestive system in protein metabolism. *Fed. Proc.* 24:953-958 (1965).

Nasset, E. S. and J. S. Ju. Mixture of endogenous and exogenous protein in the alimentary tract. *J. Nutr.* 74:461-465 (1961).

National Research Council. Nutrition Surveys: their techniques and value. Nat. Res. Council Bulletin No. 117, Nat. Acad. Sciences, 144 pp. Washington, D.C., (May, 1949).

Naughton, M. A. and H. M. Dintzis. Sequential biosynthesis of the peptide chains of hemoglobin. *Proc. Natl. Acad. Sci.* 48:1822-1830 (1962).

Neal, R. A. Isolation and identification of thiamine catabolites in mammalian urine; isolation and identification of some products of bacterial catabolism of thiamine. In *Methods in Enzymology*, XVIII, Part A, pp. 133-140, D. B. McCormick and A. D. Wright, Eds., Academic Press, New York (1970).

Neal, R. A. and W. N. Pearson. Studies of thiamine metabolism in the rat. I. Metabolic products found in urine. *J. Nutr.* 83:343-350 (1964).

Neame, K. D. and G. Wiseman. The transamination of glutamic and aspartic acids during absorption by the small intestine of the dog *in vivo. J. Physiol.* 135:442-450 (1957).

Neame, K. D. and G. Wiseman. The alanine and oxo acid concentrations in mesenteric blood during the absorption of L-glutamic acid by the small intestine of the dog, cat and rabbit *in vivo. J. Physiol.* 140:148-155 (1958).

Necheles, T. F. and L. M. Snyder. Malabsorption of folate polyglutamates associated with oral contraceptive therapy. *New Eng. J. Med.* 282:858-859 (1970).

Neher, R., B. Riniker, R. Maier, P. G. H. Byfield, T. V. Gudmundsson, and I. MacIntyre. Human calcitonin. *Nature* 200:984-986 (1968).

Neilands, J. B. and F. M. Strong. The enzymatic liberation of pantothenic acid. *Arch. Biochem.* 19:287-291 (1948).

Neilson, S. L., V. Bitsch, O. A. Larsen, H. A. Lassen, and F. Quaade. Blood flow through human adipose tissue during lipolysis. *Scand. J. Clin. Lab. Invest.* 22:124-130 (1968).

Neims, A. H. and L. Hellerman. Flavoenzyme catalysis. *Ann. Rev. Biochem.* 39:867-888 (1970).

Nelson, W. E. *Textbook of Pediatrics.* W. B. Saunders Company, Philadelphia (1946).

Nestel, P. J., W. Austin, and D. Foxman. Lipoprotein lipase content and triglyceride-fatty acid uptake in adipose tissue of rats of differing body weights. *J. Lipid Res.* 10:383-387 (1969).

Neuman, W. F. The *milieu interieur* of bone: Claude Bernard revisited. *Fed. Proc.* 28:1846-1850 (1969).

Neuman, W. F. and M. W. Neuman. *The Chemical Dynamics of Bone Mineral,* University of Chicago Press, Chicago (1958).

Neupert, W., G. D. Ludwig, and A. Pfaller. Structure and biogenesis of outer and inner mitochondrial membranes of *Neurospora crassa.* In *Biochemistry and Biophysics of Mitochondrial Membranes,* pp. 559-576, G. F. Azzone, E. Carafoli, A. L. Lehninger, E. Quagliariello, and N. Silliprandi, Eds., Academic Press, New York (1972).

Neurath, H. Protein-digesting enzymes. *Sci. Amer.* 211 (6):68-79 (1964).

Neutra, M. and C. P. Leblond. Synthesis of the carbohydrate of mucus in the Golgi complex as shown by electron microscope radioautography of goblet cells from rats injected with glucose-H^3. *J. Cell Biol.* 30:119-136 (1966).

Neutra, M. and C. P. Leblond. The Golgi apparatus. *Sci. Amer.* 220(2):100-107 (1969).

Newburgh, L. H., M. W. Johnston, and M. Falcon-Lesses. Measurement of total water exchange. *J. Clin. Invest.* 8:161-196 (1930).

Newcomer, A. D. and D. B. McGill. Lactose tolerance test in adults with normal lactase activity. *Gastroenterol.* 50:340-346 (1966).

Newman, R. W. Skinfold measurements in young American males. In *Body Measurements and Human Nutrition,* pp. 44-54, J. Brozek, Ed., Wayne University Press (1956).

Newton-John, H. F. and D. B. Morgan. Osteoporosis: disease or senescence? *Lancet* 1:232-233 (1968).

Niall, H., H. Keutman, R. Sauer, M. Hogan, B. Dawson, G. D. Aurbach, and J. T. Potts, Jr. The amino acid sequence of bovine parathyroid hormone. I. Hoppe-Seyler's *Z. Physiol. Chem.* 351:1586-1588 (1970).

Nicolaysen, R. Studies upon the mode of action of vitamin D. III. The influence of vitamin D on the absorption of calcium and phosphorus in the rat. *Biochem. J.* 31:122-129 (1937).

Nicholson, F. T. L. and F. W. Chornock. Intubation studies of the human intestine. XXII: An improved technique for the study of absorption; its application to ascorbic acid. *J. Clin. Invest.* 21:505-509 (1942).

Nielsen, F. H. and H. H. Sandstead. Are nickel, vanadium, silicon, fluorine, and tin essential for man? A review. *Amer. J. Clin. Nutr.* 27:515-520 (1974).

Nielson, F. H. and Z. Z. Ziporin. Effect of zinc deficiency on the uptake of $^{35}SO_4^-$ by the epiphyseal plate and primary spongiosa of the chick. *Fed. Proc.* 28:762A (1969).

Nikiforuk, G. and R. M. Grainger. Fluorine. In *Nutrition, A Comprehensive Treatise*, Vol. 1, pp. 417-461, G. H. Beaton and E. W. McHenry, Eds., Academic Press, N. Y. (1964).

Nir, I., I. Bruckental, I. Ascarelli, and A. Bondi. Effect of dietary protein level on *in vivo* and *in vitro* vitamin A esterase activity in the chick. *Brit. J. Nutr.* 21:565-581 (1967).

Nirenberg, M. The flow of information from gene to protein. In *Aspects of Protein Biosynthesis*, Part A, pp. 215-246, C. B. Anfinsen, Jr., Ed., Academic Press, N. Y. (1970).

Nirenberg, M. W. The Genetic Code: II. *Sci. Amer.* 208(3):80-94 (1963).

Nirenberg, M. W. and J. H. Matthaei. The dependence of cell-free protein synthesis in E. coli upon naturally-occurring or synthetic polyribonucleotides. *Proc. Nat. Acad. Sci.* 47:1588-1602 (1961).

Nirenberg, M. W., J. H. Matthaei, and O. W. Jones. An intermediate in the biosynthesis of polyphenylalanine directed by synthetic template RNA. *Proc. Natl. Acad. Sci.* 48:104-109 (1962).

Nishizawa, Y. and F. Matsuzaki. The antagonistic action of homopantothenic acid against pantothenic acid. *J. Vitaminol.* 15:8-25 (1969).

Nishizuka, Y. and O. Hayaishi. Studies on the biosynthesis of nicotinamide adenine dinucleotide. I. Enzymic synthesis of niacin ribonucleotides from 3-hydroxyanthranilic acid in mammalian tissues. *J. Biol. Chem.* 238:3369-3377 (1963).

Nishizuka, Y. and F. Lipmann. Comparison of guanosine triphosphate split and polypeptide synthesis with a purified *E. coli* system. *Proc. Natl. Acad. Sci.* 55:212-219 (1966).

Noell, W. K. and R. Albrecht. Vitamin A deficiency effect on retina: dependence on light. *Science* 172:72-79 (1971).

Noguchi, T., A. H. Cantor, and M. L. Scott. Mode of action of selenium and vitamin E in prevention of exudative diathesis in chicks. *J. Nutr.* 103:1502-1511 (1973).

Nomura, M. Ribosomes. *Sci. Amer.* 221(4):28-35 (1969).

Nomura, M. Bacterial ribosome. *Bact. Rev.* 34:228-277 (1970).

Nordin, B. E. C. Pathogenesis of osteoporosis. *Lancet.* 1:1011-1015 (1961).

Nordin, B. E. C. Calcium balance and calcium requirements in spinal osteoporosis. *Amer. J. Clin. Nutr.* 10:384-390 (1962).

Nordin, B. E. C., D. A. Smith, J. Shimmons, and C. Oxby. The effect of dietary calcium on the absorption and retention of radiostrontium. *Clin. Sci.* 32:39-48 (1967).

Nordin, E. C. and M. Peacock. The role of the kidney in serum calcium homeostasis. In *Calcitonin: Proceedings of the Second International Symposium*, pp. 472-482, Springer-Verlag, N. Y. (1970).

Norman, A. W. Actinomycin D and the response to vitamin D. *Science* 149:184-186 (1965).

Norman, A. W. and H. F. DeLuca. The preparation of H^3-vitamins D_2 and D_3 and their localization in the rat. *Biochemistry* 2:1160-1168 (1963).

Norman, A. W., M. R. Haussler, T. H. Adams, J. F. Myrtle, P. Roberts, and K. A. Hibberd. Basic studies on the mechanism of action of vitamin D. *Amer. J. Clin. Nutr.* 22:396-411 (1969).

Norman, A. W., J. F. Myrtle, R. J. Midgett, H. G. Nowicki, V. Williams, and G. Popjak. 1,25-Dihydroxycholecalciferol: Identification of the proposed active form of vitamin D_3 in the intestine. *Science* 173:51-54 (1971).

Norris, A. H., T. Lundy, and N. W. Shock. Trends in selected indices of body composition in men between the ages 30 and 80 years. *Ann. N. Y. Acad. Sci.* 110:623-639 (1963).

Norris, T. Dietary surveys. Their technique and interpretation. FAO Nutritional Studies No. 4, Washington, D. C. (1949).

North, R. The localization by electron microscopy of acid phosphatase activity in guinea pig macrophages. *J. Ultrastruct. Res.* 16:96-108, (1966).

Northcote, D. H. The Golgi apparatus. *Endeavor* 30:26-33 (1971).

Novikoff, A. B. Mitochondria (Chondriosomes). In *The Cell*, Vol. II, pp. 299-421, J. Brachet and A. E. Mirsky, Eds., Academic Press, N. Y. (1961a).

Novikoff, A. B. Lysosomes and related particles. In *The Cell*, Vol. II, pp. 423-488, J. Brachet and A. E. Mirsky, Eds., Academic Press, N. Y. (1961b).

Novikoff, A. B. Lysosomes in the physiology and pathology of cells: contributions of staining methods. In *Ciba Foundation Symposium on Lysosomes*, pp. 36-73, A. V. S. deReuck and M. P. Cameron, Eds., Little, Brown and Company, Boston (1963).

Novikoff, A. B., H. Beaufay, and C. DeDuve. Electron microscopy of lysosome-rich fractions from rat liver. *J. Biophys. Biochem. Cytol.* 2 (suppl):179-184 (1956).

Novikoff, A. B., E. Essner, S. Goldfischer, and M. Heus. Nucleosidephosphatase activities of cytomembranes. In *The Interpretation of Ultrastructure*, Vol. I, pp. 149-192, R. J. C. Harris, Ed., Academic Press, N. Y. (1962).

Novikoff, A. B., E. Essner, and N. Quintana. Golgi apparatus and lysosomes. *Fed. Proc.* 23:1010-1022 (1964).

Noyes, W. D., T. H. Bothwell, and C. A. Finch. The role of the reticuloendothelial cell in iron metabolism. *Brit. J. Haemat.* 6:43-55 (1960).

Noyes, W. D., F. Hosain, and C. A. Finch. Incorporation of radio iron into marrow heme. *J. Lab. Clin. Med.* 64:574-580 (1964).

Nyberg, W. The influence of Diphyllobothrium latum on the vitamin B_{12} intrinsic factor complex. II. *In vitro* studies. *Acta Med. Scand.* 167:189-192 (1960).

Nyquist, S. E., F. L. Crane, and D. J. Morré. Vitamin A: Concentration in the rat liver Golgi apparatus. *Science* 173:939-941 (1971).

O'Brien, J. S. A molecular defect of myelination. *Biophys. Res. Commun.* 15:484-490 (1964).

O'Brien, J. S. Stability of the myelin membrane. *Science* 147:1099-1107 (1965).

Ochs, S. Energy metabolism and supply of $\sim$P to the fast axoplasmic transport mechanism in nerve. *Fed. Proc.* 33:1049-1058 (1974).

Ockner, R. K., F. B. Hughes, and K. J. Isselbacher. Very low density lipoproteins in intestinal lymph: Role in triglyceride and cholesterol transport during fat absorption. *J. Clin. Invest.* 48:2367-2373 (1969).

Ockner, R. K., J. A. Manning, R. B. Poppenhausen, and W. K. L. Ho. A binding protein for fatty acids in cytosol of intestinal mucosa, liver, myocardium, and other tissues. *Science* 177:56-58 (1972).

Ohnishi, T. and T. Ohnishi. Extraction of a contractile protein from liver mitochondria. *J. Biochem.* (Tokyo) 51:380-381 (1962a).

Ohnishi, T. and T. Ohnishi. Extraction of actin- and myosin-like proteins from liver mitochondria. *J. Biochem.* (Tokyo) 52:230-231 (1962b).

Okazaki, R., T. Okazaki, K. Sakabe, K. Sugimoto, and A. Sugino. Mechanism of DNA chain growth. I. Possible discontinuity and unusual secondary structure of newly synthesized chains. *Proc. Nat. Acad. Sci.* 59:598-605 (1968).

Okey, R. and M. M. Lyman. Dietary fat and cholesterol metabolism. I. Comparative effects of coconut and cotton seed oil at three levels of intake. *J. Nutr.* 61:523-533 (1957).

Oldham, H., M. V. Davis, and L. J. Roberts. Thiamine excretions and blood levels of young women on diets containing varying levels of the B-vitamins with some observations on niacin and pantothenic acid. *J. Nutr.* 32:163-180 (1946).

Oldham, H. and B. B. Sheft. Effect of caloric intake on nitrogen utilization during pregnancy. *J. Amer. Diet. Ass.* 27:847-854 (1951).

Oldham, H. G. Thiamine requirements of women. *Ann. N. Y. Acad. Sci.* 98:542-549 (1962).

Olesen, K. H. Body composition in normal adults. In *Human Body Composition, Approaches and Applications*, J. Brozek, Ed., Pergamon Press, Oxford (1965).

Oliverio, V. T. and D. S. Zaharko. Tissue distribution of folate antagonists. *Ann. N. Y. Acad. Sci.* 186:387-399 (1971).

Olliver, M. Ascorbic Acid. IV. Estimation. In *The Vitamins*, Vol. I, pp. 338-385, W. H.

Sebrell, Jr. and R. S. Harris, Eds., Academic Press, N. Y. (1967).

Olson, E. B. and H. F. DeLuca. 25-Hydroxycholecalciferol: Direct effect on calcium transport. *Science* 165:405-407 (1969).

Olson, J. A. Metabolism and function of vitamin A. *Fed. Proc.* 28:1670-1677 (1969).

Olson, J. A. The alpha and the omega of vitamin A metabolism. *Amer. J. Clin. Nutr.* 22:953-962 (1969a).

Olson, J. A. Metabolism and function of vitamin A. *Fed. Proc.* 28:1670-1677 (1969b).

Olson, J. A. and O. Hayaishi. The enzymatic cleavage of β-carotene into vitamin A by soluble enzymes of rat liver and intestine. *Proc. Nat. Acad. Sci.* 54:1364-1370 (1965).

Olson, J. A. and M. R. Lakshmanan. Enzymatic transformations of vitamin A, with particular emphasis on carotenoid cleavage. In *The Fat-Soluble Vitamins*, pp. 213-226, H. F. DeLuca and J. W. Suttie, Eds., University of Wisconsin Press, Madison (1970).

Olson, R. E. Vitamin K induced prothrombin formation: Antagonism by actinomycin D. *Science* 145:926-928 (1964).

Olson, R. E. Studies of the *in vitro* biosynthesis of vitamin K-dependent clotting proteins. In *The Fat-Soluble Vitamins*, pp. 463-489, H. F. DeLuca and J. W. Suttie, Eds., University of Wisconsin Press, Madison (1970).

Olson, R. E. Vitamin E and its relation to heart disease. *Circulation* 48:179-184 (1973).

Omdahl, J. L. and H. F. DeLuca. Regulation of vitamin D metabolism and function. *Physiol. Rev.* 53:327-372 (1973).

Omdahl, J., M. F. Holick, T. Suda, Y. Tanaka, and H. F. DeLuca. Biological activity of 1,25-dihydroxycholecalciferol. *Biochemistry* 10:2935-2940 (1971).

O'Neal, R. M., O. C. Johnson, and A. E. Schaefer. Guidelines for classification and interpretation of group blood and urine data collected as part of the national nutrition survey. *Pediat. Res.* 4:103-106 (1970).

Onishi, T. Studies on the mechanism of decrease in the RNA content in liver cells of fasted rats. II. The mechanism of starvation-induced decrease in RNA polymerase activity in liver. *Biochim. Biophys. Acta* 217:384-393 (1970).

Oppenheimer, J. H., M. I. Surks, J. C. Smith, and R. Squef. Isolation and characterization of human thyroxine-binding prealbumin. *J. Biol. Chem.* 240:173-180 (1965).

Orci, L., M. Amherdt, F. Malaisse-Lagae, C. Rouiller, and A. E. Renold. Insulin release by emiocytosis: demonstration with freeze-etching technique. *Science* 179:82-84 (1973).

Orci, L., F. Malaisse-Lagae, M. Ravazzola, M. Amherdt, and A. E. Renold. Exocytosis-endocytosis coupling in the pancreatic beta cell. *Science* 181:561-562 (1973).

Orlic, D. Ultrastructural analysis of erythropoiesis. In *Regulation of Hematopoiesis*, Vol. I, pp. 271-296, A. S. Gordon, Ed., Appleton-Century-Crofts, N. Y. (1970).

Orlic, D., A. S. Gordon, and J. A. G. Rhodin. An ultrastructural study of erythropoietin-induced red cell formation in mouse spleen. *J. Ultrastruct. Res.* 13:516-542 (1965).

Orlic, D., A. S. Gordon, and J. A. G. Rhodin. Ultrastructural and autoradiographic studies of erythropoietin-induced red cell production. *Ann. N. Y. Acad. Sci.* 149:198-216 (1968).

Orloff, J. and J. Handler. The role of adenosine 3',5'-phosphate in the action of antidiuretic hormone. *Amer. J. Med.* 42:757-768 (1967).

Osaki, S., D. A. Johnson, and E. Frieden. The possible significance of the ferrous oxidase activity of ceruloplasmin in normal human serum. *J. Biol. Chem.* 241:2746-2751 (1966).

Osborne, T. B. *The Vegetable Proteins*. 2nd ed., Longmans, Green and Company, London (1924).

Osborne, T. B. and L. B. Mendel. Feeding experiments with isolated food-substances. Carnegie Institute of Washington, D. C., Publ. No. 156, Pts. I and II. (1911).

Osborne, T. B., L. B. Mendel, and E. L. Ferry. A method of expressing numerically the growth-promoting value of proteins. *J. Biol. Chem.* 37:223-229 (1919).

Oser, B. L., Ed., Hawk's Physiological Chemistry, 14th Ed., pp. 663-665, McGraw-Hill Co., N. Y. (1965).

Outhouse, J., H. Breiter, E. Rutherford, J. Dwight, R. Mills, and W. Armstrong. The calcium requirement of man. Balance studies on seven adults. *J. Nutr.* 21:565-575 (1941).

Owen, C. A., Jr. and J. L. Bollman. Serum and plasma antithrombin. *Proc. Soc. Exp. Biol. Med.* 67:367-369 (1948).

Pace, N. and E. N. Rathbun. Studies on body composition. III. The body water and chemically combined nitrogen content in relation to fat content. *J. Biol. Chem.* 158:685-691 (1945).

Padykula, H. A. Recent functional interpretations of intestinal morphology. *Fed. Proc.* 21:873-879 (1962).

Page, I. H. Serotonin and the Brain. In *The Structure and Function of Nervous Tissue*, Vol. III, pp. 289-307, G. H. Bourne, Ed., Academic Press, N. Y. (1969).

Page-Thomas, D. P. Lysosomal enzymes in experimental and rheumatoid arthritis. In *Lysosomes in Biology and Pathology*, Vol. 2, pp. 87-110, J. T. Dingle and H. B. Fell, Eds., *Frontiers of Biology*, 14A, North-Holland Publishing Company, Amsterdam (1969).

Palade, G. E. The fine structure of mitochondria. *Anat. Rec.* 114:427-451 (1952).

Palay, S. L. Principles of cellular organization in the nervous system. In *The Neurosciences*, pp. 24-31, G. C. Quarton, T. Melnechuk, and F. O. Schmitt, Eds., Rockefeller University Press, N. Y. (1967).

Palay, S. L. and L. J. Karlin. An electron microscopic study of the intestinal villus. 2. The pathway of fat absorption. *J. Biophys. Biochem. Cytol.* 5:373-384 (1959a).

Palay, S. L. and L. J. Karlin. An electron microscopic study of the intestinal villus. 1. The fasting animal. *J. Biophys. Biochem. Cytol.* 5:363-372 (1959b).

Pänkäläinen, M. and K. I. Kivirikko. Protocollagen proline hydroxylase: molecular weight, subunits and isoelectric point. *Biochim. Biophys. Acta* 221:559-565 (1970).

Pappenheimer, A. M. and M. Goettsch. A cerebellar disorder in chicks, apparently of nutritional origin. *J. Exptl. Med.* 53:11-16 (1931).

Pardee, A. B. Membrane transport proteins. *Science* 162:632-637 (1968).

Pařízková, J. Total body fat and skinfold thickness in children. *Metabolism* 10:794-807 (1961).

Pařízková, J. Impact of age, diet and exercise on man's body composition. *Ann. N. Y. Acad. Sci.* 110:661-674 (1963).

Pařízková, J. Physical activity and body composition. In *Human Body Composition, Approaches and Applications*, J. Brozek, Ed., Pergamon Press, Oxford (1965).

Pařízková, J. Obesity and physical activity. In *Nutritional Aspects of Physical Performance*, pp. 146-160, J. F. De Wijn and R. A. Binkhorst, Eds., Nutricia Ltd., Zoetermeer, The Netherlands (1972).

Pařízková, J. Body composition and exercise during growth and development. In *Physical Activity--Human Growth and Development*, pp. 97-124, G. L. Rarick, Ed., Academic Press, N. Y. (1973).

Parsons, B. J., D. H. Smyth, and C. B. Taylor. The action of phlorizin on the intestinal transfer of glucose and water *in vitro. J. Physiol.* 144:387-402 (1958).

Parsons, H. T., A. Williamson, and M. L. Johnson. The availability of vitamins from yeasts. I. The absorption of thiamine by human subjects from various types of bakers' yeast. *J. Nutr.* 29:373-381 (1945).

Parsons, H. T., J. G. Lease, and E. Kelly. Interrelationship between dietary egg white and requirement for protective factor in cure of nutritional disorder due to egg white. *Biochem. J.* 31:424-432 (1937).

Pascale, L. R., M. I. Grossman, H. S. Sloane, and T. Frankel. Correlations between thickness of skinfolds and body density in 88 soldiers. In *Body Measurements and Human Nutrition*, pp. 55-66, J. Brozek, Ed., Wayne University Press (1956).

Passmore, R. and J. V. G. A. Durnin. Human energy expenditures. *Physiol. Rev.* 35:801-840 (1955).

Passmore, R. and F. J. Ritchie. The specific dynamic action of food and the satiety mechanism. *Brit. J. Nutr.* 11:79-85 (1957).

Pastan, I. and R. L. Perlman. The role of the Lac promoter locus in the regulation of β-galactosidase synthesis by cyclic 3,5-adenosine monophosphate. *Proc. Nat. Acad. Sci.* 61:1336-1342 (1968).

Patriarca, P. and E. Carafoli. A study of the intracellular transport of calcium in rat heart. *J. Cell Physiol.* 72:29-38 (1968).

Patt, H. M. and H. Quastler. Radiation effects on cell renewal and related systems. *Physiol. Rev.* 43:357-396 (1963).

Patten, R. L. and C. H. Hollenberg. The mechanism of heparin stimulation of rat adipocyte lipoprotein lipase. *J. Lipid Res.* 10:374-382 (1967).

Patterson, E. I., M. H. Saltza, and E. L. R. Stokstad. The isolation and characterization of a pteridine required for the growth of *Crithidia fasciculata*. *J. Amer. Chem. Soc.* 78:5871-5873 (1956).

Patton, S. Milk. *Sci. Amer.* 221(1):58-68 (1969).

Pauling, L. Orthomolecular psychiatry. *Science* 160:265-271 (1968).

Pauling, L. *Vitamin C and the Common Cold.* W. H. Freeman and Company (1970).

Pauling, L., H. A. Itano, S. J. Singer, and I. C. Wells. Sickle cell anemia, a molecular disease. *Science* 110:543-548 (1949).

Payne, L. C. and C. L. Marsh. Absorption of gamma globulin by the small intestine. *Fed. Proc.* 21:909-912 (1962).

Pearson, W. N. Biochemical appraisal of the vitamin nutritional status in man. *J.A.M.A.* 180:49-55 (1962).

Pearson, W. N. Blood and urinary vitamin levels as potential indices of body stores. *Amer. J. Clin. Nutr.* 20:514-525 (1967).

Pekkarinen, M. Methodology in the collection of food consumption data. *World Rev. Nutr. Dietet.* 12:145-171 (1970).

Pennington, D., E. E. Snell, and R. J. Williams. An assay method for pantothenic acid. *J. Biol. Chem.* 135:213-222 (1940).

Penniston, J. T., R. A. Harris, J. Asai, and D. E. Green. The conformational basis of energy transformations in membrane systems. I. Conformational changes in mitochondria. *Proc. Nat. Acad. Sci.* 59:624-631 (1968).

Peraino, C. and A. E. Harper. Concentrations of free amino acids in blood plasma of rats force-fed L-glutamic acid, L-glutamine or L-alanine. *Arch. Biochem. Biophys.* 97:442-448 (1962).

Pereira, M. and D. Couri. Studies on the site of action of dicoumarol on prothrombin synthesis. *Biochim. Biophys. Acta* 237:348-355 (1971).

Pereira, S. M., A. Begum, T. Isaac, and M. E. Dumm. Vitamin A therapy in children with kwashiorkor. *Amer. J. Clin. Nutr.* 20:297-304 (1967).

Persson, B., P. Bjorntorp, and B. Hood. Lipoprotein lipase activity in human adipose tissue. I. Conditions for release and relationship to triglycerides in serum. *Metabolism* 15:730-741 (1966).

Persson, B., R. Tunell, and K. Ekengren. Chronic vitamin A intoxication during the first half year of life. *Acta Pediat. Scand.* 54:49-60 (1965).

Perutz, M. F. X-ray analysis of hemoglobin. *Science* 140:863-869 (1963).

Perutz, M. F. The hemoglobin molecule. *Sci. Amer.* 211(11):64-76 (1964).

Peterkofsky, B. and S. Udenfriend. Enzymatic hydroxylation of proline in microsomal polypeptides leading to formation of collagen. *Proc. Nat. Acad. Sci.* 53:335-342 (1965).

Petermann, M. L. How does a ribosome translate linear genetic information? *Sub-Cell Biochem.* 1:67-73 (1971).

Peters, A., S. L. Palay, and H. deF. Webster. *The Fine Structure of the Nervous System. The Cells and Their Processes*, Hoeber, N. Y. (1970).

Peters, A. and J. E. Vaughn. Microtubules and filaments in the axons and astrocytes of early post-natal rat optic nerves. *J. Cell Biol.* 32:113-119 (1967).

Peters, J. P., D. M. Kydd, and P. H. Lavietes. A note on the calculation of water exchange. *J. Clin. Invest.* 12:689-693 (1933).

Peters, R. A. The biochemical lesion in vitamin B_1 deficiency. Application of modern biochemical analysis in its diagnosis. *Lancet* 1:1161-1165 (1936).

Peters, R. A., K. H. Coward, H. A. Krebs, L. W. Mapson, L. G. Parson, B. S. Platt, J. C. Spence, and J. R. P. O'Brien (Accessory Food Factors Subcommittee of the British Medical Research Council) Vitamin C requirement of human adults. *Lancet* 1:853-860 (1948).

Peters, T. The biosynthesis of rat serum albumin. *J. Biol. Chem.* 237:1181-1185 (1962).

Petrack, B., F. Sheppy, and V. Fetzer. Studies on tyrosine hydroxylase from bovine adrenal medulla. *J. Biol. Chem.* 243:743-748 (1968).

Pettijohn, D. and P. Hanawalt. Evidence for repair-replication of ultra-violet damaged DNA in bacteria. *J. Molec. Biol.* 9:395-410 (1964).

Pfaff, E. and M. Klingenberg. Adenine nucleotide translocation of mitochondria. I. Specificity and control. *Europ. J. Biochem.* 6:66-79 (1968).

Pfiffner, J. J., D. G. Calkins, E. S. Bloom, and B. L. O'Dell. On the peptide nature of vitamin Bc conjugate from yeast. *J. Amer. Chem. Soc.* 68:1392 (1946).

Phelps, P. C., C. E. Rubin, and J. H. Luft. Electron microscopic techniques for studying absorption of fat in man with some observations on pinocytosis. *Gastroenterol.* 46:134-156 (1964).

Phillips, G. T., J. E. Nixon, J. A. Dorsey, P. H. W. Butterworth, C. J. Chesterton, and J. W. Porter. The mechanism of synthesis of fatty acids by the pigeon liver enzyme system. *Arch. Biochem. Biophys.* 138:380-391 (1970).

Piez, K. A. and H. Eagle. The free amino acid pool of cultured human cells. *J. Biol. Chem.* 231:533-545 (1958).

Pike, R. L., J. E. Miles, and J. M. Wardlaw. Juxtaglomerular degranulation and zona glomerulosa exhaustion in pregnant rats induced by low sodium intakes and reversed by sodium load. *Amer. J. Obstet. Gynec.* 95:604-614 (1966).

Pike, R. L. and H. A. Smiciklas. A reappraisal of sodium restriction during pregnancy. *Int. J. Gynecol. Obstet.* 10:1-8 (1972).

Pitkin, R. M., H. A. Kaminetsky, M. Newton, and J. A. Pritchard. Maternal nutrition. A selective review of clinical topics. *J. Obstet. Gynecol.* 40:773-785 (1972).

Pitts, R. F. *Physiology of the Kidney and Body Fluids*, 2nd Ed., Year Book Medical Publishers Inc., Chicago (1968).

Platt, B. S. and D. S. Miller. The net dietary-protein value (NDPV) of mixtures of foods—its definition, determination and application. *Proc. Nutr. Soc.* 18:vii-viii (1959).

Platt, B. S., D. S. Miller, and P. R. Payne. Protein value of human foods. In *Recent Advances in Human Nutrition*, p. 360, J. F. Brock, Ed. Churchhill, London (1961).

Playoust, M. R. and K. J. Isselbacher. Studies on the transport and metabolism of conjugated bile salts by intestinal mucosa. *J. Clin. Invest.* 43:467-476 (1964).

Plotkin, G. R. and K. J. Isselbacher. Secondary disaccharidase deficiency in adult celiac disease (non-tropical sprue) and other malabsorption states. *N. Engl. J. Med.* 271:1033-1037 (1964).

Plough, I. C. and E. B. Bridgforth. Relation of clinical and dietary findings in nutrition surveys. *Pub. Health Rpts.* 75:699-706 (1960).

Pohanka, D. G., H. Smiciklas-Wright, and R. L. Pike. Δ^5-3,β-Hydroxysteroid dehydrogenase activity in the adrenal cortex of the sodium-restricted pregnant rat. *Proc. Soc. Biol. Med.* 142:1092-1096 (1973).

1028   BIBLIOGRAPHY

Polimeni, P. I. and E. Page. Magnesium in heart muscle. *Circ. Res.* 33:367-374 (1973).

Polin, D., E. R. Wynosky, and C. C. Porter. Studies on the absorption of amprolium and thiamine in laying hens. *Poultry Sci.* 42:1057-1061 (1963).

Pollack, H., C. F. Consolazio, and G. J. Isaac. Metabolic demands as a factor in weight control. *J.A.M.A.* 167:216-219 (1958).

Pollack, S. and T. Campana. The relationship between mucosal iron and iron absorption in the guinea pig. *Scand. J. Haematol.* 7:208-211 (1970).

Pollack, S., J. N. George, R. C. Reba, R. M. Kaufman, and W. H. Crosby. The absorption of nonferrous metals in iron deficiency. *J. Clin. Invest.* 44:1470-1473 (1965).

Pollak, P. I. Thiamine. Encyclopedia of Chem. Technol. 20:173-193 (1969).

Pollock, H. Creatinine excretion as index for estimating urinary excretion of micronutrients or their metabolic end products. *Amer. J. Clin. Nutr.* 23:865-867 (1970).

Ponchon, G. and H. F. DeLuca. Metabolites of vitamin D_3 and their biologic activity. *J. Nutr.* 99:157-167 (1969).

Poole, B. Biogenesis and turnover of rat liver peroxisomes. *Ann. N. Y. Acad. Sci.* 168:229-243 (1969).

Popovtzer, M. M., J. B. Robinette, H. F. DeLuca and M. F. Holick. The acute effect of 25-hydroxycholecalciferol on renal handling of phosphorus. *J. Clin. Invest.* 53:913-921 (1974).

Pories, W. J., J. H. Henzel, C. C. Rob, and W. H. Strain. Acceleration of wound healing in man with zinc sulfate given by mouth. *Lancet* 1:121-124 (1967).

Porter, K. R. The ground substance: observations from electron microscopy. In *The Cell*, Vol. II, pp. 621-675, J. Brachet and A. E. Mirsky, Eds., Academic Press, N. Y. (1961).

Porter, K. R. Independence of fat absorption and pinocytosis. *Fed. Proc.* 28:35-40 (1969).

Porter, K. R., A. Claude, and E. F. Fullam. A study of tissue culture cells by electron microscopy. Methods and preliminary observations. *J. Exp. Med.* 81:233-246 (1945).

Posner, A. S. Relationship between diet and bone mineral ultrastructure. *Fed. Proc.* 26:1717-1722 (1967).

Posner, A. S. Crystal chemistry of bone mineral. *Physiol. Rev.* 49:760-792 (1969).

Posner, A. S. Bone mineral on the molecular level. *Fed. Proc.* 32:1933-1937 (1973).

Potter, L. T. Storage of norepinephrine in sympathetic nerves. *Pharmacol. Rev.* 18:439-451 (1966).

Potts, J. T. Jr. Polypeptide hormones and calcium metabolism. *Ann. Intern. Med.* 70:1243-1265 (1969).

Potts, J. T., Jr. Recent advances in thyrocalcitonin research. *Fed. Proc.* 29:1200-1205 (1970).

Potts, J. T., Jr., H. T. Keutmann, H. D. Niall and G. W. Tregear. The chemistry of parathyroid hormone and the calcitonins. *Vitamins Hormones* 29:41-93 (1971).

Potts, J. T., Jr., H. D. Niall, H. T. Keutmann, H. B. Brewer, and L. J. Deftos. The amino acid sequence of porcine thyrocalcitonin. *Proc. Nat. Acad. Sci.* 59:1321-1328 (1968).

Potts, J. T., Jr., H. D. Niall, H. T. Keutmann, L. J. Deftos, and J. A. Parsons. Calcitonin: Recent chemical and immunological studies. In *Calcitonin: Proceedings of the Second International Symposium*, pp. 56-73 Springer-Verlag, N. Y. (1970).

Prasad, A. D., A. R. Schulert, A. Miale, Z. Farid, and H. H. Sandstead. Zinc and iron deficiencies in male subjects with dwarfism and hypogonadism but without ancylostomiasis, schistosomiasis or severe anemia. *Amer. J. Clin. Nutr.* 12:437-444 (1963).

Primosigh, J. V. and E. D. Thomas. Studies on the partition of iron in bone marrow cells. *J. Clin. Invest.* 47:1473-1482 (1968).

Prockop, D. J. Role of iron in the synthesis of collagen in connective tissue. *Fed. Proc.* 30:984-990 (1971).

Prockop, D. J. and K. Juva. Synthesis of hydroxyproline *in vitro* by the hydroxylation of proline in a precursor of collagen. *Proc. Nat. Acad. Sci.* 53:661-668 (1965).

Prockop, D. J., A. Kaplan, and S. Udenfriend. Cofactor requirements of the O-demethylating liver microsomal enzyme system. *Arch. Biochem. Biophys.* 101:494-503 (1963).

Prockop, D. J. Intracellular biosynthesis of collagen and interactions of protocollagen proline hydroxylase with large polypeptides. In *The Chemistry and Molecular Biology of the Intracellular Matrix*, Vol. I, pp. 335-370, E. A. Balazs, Ed., Academic Press, London (1970).

Protein Advisory Group. *Milk Intolerance—Nutritional Implications*, Report on the PAG *ad hoc* working group meeting, United Nations System, Document 1.27/9 (1972).

Prusiner, S. B., B. Cannon, T. M. Ching, and O. Lindberg. Oxidative metabolism in cells isolated from brown adipose tissue. 2. Catecholamine regulated respiratory control. *Europ. J. Biochem.* 7:51-57 (1968).

Pryor, W. A. Free radical reactions and their importance in biochemical systems. *Fed. Proc.* 32:1862-1869 (1973).

Ptashne, M. Isolation of the γ phage repressor. *Proc. Nat. Acad. Sci.* 57:306-313 (1967).

Purdy, R. H., K. A. Woeber, M. T. Holloway, and S. H. Ingbar. Preparation of crystalline thyroxine-binding prealbumin from human plasma. *Biochemistry* 4:1888-1895 (1965).

Puszkin, S. and S. Berl. Actin-like properties of colchicine binding protein isolated from brain. *Nature* 225:558-559 (1970).

Puszkin, S., S. Berl, E. Puszkin, and D. D. Clarke. Actomyosin-like protein isolated from mammalian brain. *Science* 161:170-171 (1968).

Quaife, M. L. and P. L. Harris. Chemical assay of foods for vitamin E content. *Anal. Chem.* 20:1221-1224 (1948).

Quick, A. J. *Hemorrhagic Diseases.* Lea and Febiger, Philadelphia (1957).

Rabinowtiz, J. C. and E. E. Snell. The vitamin B_6 group. XIV. Distribution of pyridoxal, pyridoxamine and pyridoxine in some natural products. *J. Biol. Chem.* 176:1157-1167 (1948).

Racker, E. Resolution and reconstruction of the inner mitochondrial membrane. *Fed. Proc.* 26:1335-1340 (1967).

Racker, E. The membrane of the mitochondrion. *Sci. Amer.* 218(2):32-39 (1968).

Racker, E. Function and structure of the inner membrane of mitochondria and chloroplasts. In *Membranes of Mitochondria and Chloroplasts*, pp. 127-171, E. Racker, Ed., Van Nostrand Reinhold Company, N. Y. (1970).

Radouco-Thomas, S. Cellular and molecular aspects of transmitter release: Calcium/monoamine dynamics. *Adv. Cytopharmacol.* 1:457-475 (1971).

Raff, R. A. and H. R. Mahler. The nonsymbiotic origin of mitochondria. *Science* 177:575-582 (1972).

Raica, N., Jr. and H. E. Sauberlich. Blood cell transaminase activity in human vitamin B_6 deficiency. *Amer. J. Clin. Nutr.* 15:67-72 (1964).

Raisz, L. G. and C. L. Trummel. Role of vitamin D in bone metabolism. In *The Fat-Soluble Vitamins*, pp. 93-99, H. F. DeLuca and J. W. Suttie, Eds., The University of Wisconsin Press, Madison (1970).

Rambourg, A., W. Hernandez, and C. P. Leblond. Detection of complex carbohydrates in the Golgi apparatus of rat cells. *J. Cell Biol.* 40:395-414 (1969).

Rambourg, A. and C. P. Leblond. Electron microscopic observations of the carbohydrate rich cell coat present at the surface of cells in the rat. *J. Cell Biol.* 32:27-53 (1967).

Ramwell, P. and J. E. Shaw. Eds. Prostaglandins. *Ann. N. Y. Acad. Sci.* 180:5-568 (1971).

Rasmussen, H., J. Feinblatt, N. Nagata, and M. Pechet. Effect of ions upon bone cell function. *Fed. Proc.* 29:1190-1197 (1970).

Rasmussen, H. and N. Nagata. Renal gluconeogenesis: Effects of parathyroid hormone and dibutyryl 3′,5′-AMP. *Biochim. Biophys. Acta* 215:17-28 (1970).

Rasmussen, H., M. Wong, D. Bikle, and D. B. P. Goodman. Hormonal control of the renal conversion of 25-hydroxycholecalciferol to 1,25-dihydroxycholecalciferol. *J. Clin. Invest.* 51:2502-2504 (1972).

Rathbun, E. N. and N. Pace. Studies on body composition. I. The determination of total body fat by means of the body specific gravity. *J. Biol. Chem.* 158:667-676 (1945).

Raven, P. H. A multiple origin for plastids and mitochondria. *Science* 169:641-646 (1970).

Raychaudhuri, C. and I. D. Desai. Ceroid pigment formation and irreversible sterility in vitamin E deficiency. *Science* 173:1028-1029 (1971).

Reba, R. C., F. C. Leitnaker, and K. T. Woodward. In *Human Growth*, D. B. Cheek, Ed., pp. 674-681, Lea and Febiger, Philadelphia (1968).

Reddy, S. K., M. S. Reynolds, and J. M. Price. The determination of 4-pyridoxic acid in human urine. *J. Biol. Chem.* 233:691-696 (1958).

Regnault, H. W. and J. Reiset. Recherches chimiques sur la respiration des animaux des diverses classes. *Ann. Chim Phys.* (Ser. 3) 26:299-519 (1849).

Reh, E. Manual on household food consumption surveys. FAO Nutritional Studies No. 18, Rome, 96 pp. (1962).

Reid, B. L., A. A. Kurnick, R. L. Svacha, and J. R. Couch. The effect of molybdenum on chick and poult growth. *Proc. Soc. Exp. Biol. Med.* 93:245-248 (1956).

Reid, E. W. Intestinal absorption of solutions. *J. Physiol.* 28:241-256 (1902).

Reiser, S. and P. A. Christiansen. Intestinal transport of amino acids studied with *L*-valine. *Amer. J. Physiol.* 208:914-921 (1965).

Reissmann, K. R. Studies on the mechanism of erythropoietic stimulation in parabiotic rats during hypoxia. *Blood* 5:372-380 (1950).

Reizenstein, P. G. Excretion of non-labeled vitamin B_{12} in man. *Acta Med. Scand.* 165:313-320 (1959).

Rendi, R. On the occurrence of intramitochondrial RNA particles. *Exp. Cell Res.* 17:585-587 (1959).

Renold, A. E. A brief and fragmentary introduction to some aspects of adipose tissue metabolism with emphasis on glucose uptake. *Ann. N. Y. Acad. Sci.* 131:7-12 (1965).

Reutter, F. W., R. Siebenmann, and M. Pajarola. Fluoride in osteoporosis. In *Fluoride in Medicine*, pp. 143-152, T. L. Vischer, Ed., Hans Huber, Berne (1970).

Revel, J.-P. and S. Ito. The surface components of cells. in *The Specificity of Cell Surfaces*, pp. 211-234, B. D. Davis and L. Warren, Eds., Prentice-Hall, Inc., Englewood Cliffs, N. J. (1967).

Revel, M., M. Herzberg, A. Becarevic, and F. Gros. Role of a protein factor in the functional binding of ribosomes to natural messenger RNA. *J. Molec. Biol.* 33:231-249 (1968).

Reynafarje, B. and A. L. Lehninger. High affinity and low affinity binding of Ca^{++} by rat liver mitochondria. *J. Biol. Chem.* 244:584-593 (1969).

Rhead, W. J. and G. N. Schrauzer. Risks of long-term ascorbic acid overdosage. *Nutr. Rev.* 29:262-263 (1971).

Rhoads, R. E. and S. Udenfriend. Decarboxylation of α-ketoglutarate coupled to collagen proline hydroxylase. *Proc. Nat. Acad. Sci.* 60:1473-1478 (1968).

Rich, C. Discussion. *Fed. Proc.* 29:1188-1189 (1970).

Rich, C. and J. Ensinck. Effect of sodium fluoride on calcium metabolism of human beings. *Nature* 191:184-185 (1961).

Richardson, T. and A. L. Tappel. Swelling of fish mitochondria. *J. Cell Biol.* 13:43-53 (1962).

Richardson, T., A. L. Tappel, and E. R. Gruger, Jr. Essential fatty acids in mitochondria. *Arch. Biochem. Biophys.* 94:1-6 (1961).

Richardson, T., A. L. Tappel, L. M. Smith, and C. R. Houle. Polyunsaturated fatty acids in mitochondria. *J. Lipid Res.* 3:344-350 (1962).

Rickes, E. L., N. G. Brink, F. R. Koniuszy, T. R. Wood, and K. Folkers. Crystalline vitamin B_{12}. *Science* 107:396-397 (1948).

Riemann, W., C. Muir, and H. C. Macgregor. Sodium and potassium in oocytes of *Triturus cristatus*. *J. Cell Sci.* 4:299-304 (1969).

Rikkers, H. and H. F. DeLuca. An *in vivo* study of the carrier proteins of ^3H-vitamins D_3 and D_4 in rat serum. *Amer. J. Physiol.* 213:380-386 (1967).

Riklis, E. and J. H. Quastel. Effects of cations on sugar absorption by isolated surviving guinea pig intestine. *Canad. J. Biochem. Physiol.* 36:347-362 (1958).

Riley, C. A., G. Cohen, and M. Lieberman. Ethane evolution: a new index of lipid peroxidation. *Science* 183:208-210 (1974).

Rindi, G., L. de Giuseppe, and G. Sciorelli. Thiamine monophosphate, a normal constituent of rat plasma. *J. Nutr.* 94:447-454 (1968).

Rindi, G., G. Ferrari, U. Ventura, and A. Trotta. Action of amprolium on the thiamine content of rat tissues. *J. Nutr.* 89:197-202 (1966).

Rindi, G., U. Ventura, L. De Guiseppe, and G. Sciorelli. The phosphorylation of thiamine in the intestinal wall during absorption *in vitro*. *Experientia* 22:473-474 (1966).

Ringer, S. Further observations regarding the antagonism between calcium salts and sodium, potassium and ammonium salts. *J. Physiol.* 18:425-429 (1895).

Ritchie, A. K. and A. M. Goldberg. Vesicular and synaptoplasmic synthesis of acetylcholine. *Science* 173:489-490 (1970).

Ritchie, J. H., M. B. Fish, V. M. McMasters, and M. Grossman. Edema and hemolytic anemia in premature infants: a vitamin E deficiency syndrome. *New Eng. J. Med.* 279:1185-1190 (1968).

Ritchey, S. J. Metabolic patterns in preadolescent children. XV. Ascorbic acid intake, urinary excretion and serum concentration. *Amer. J. Clin. Nutr.* 17:57-114 (1965).

Rivers, J. M., E. D. Huang, and M. L. Dodds. Human metabolism of L-ascorbic and erythorbic acid. *J. Nutr.* 81:163-168 (1963).

Rivlin, R. S. Regulation of flavoprotein enzymes in hypothyroidism and in riboflavin deficiency. *Adv. Enzym. Regulat.* 8:239-250 (1970a).

Rivlin, R. S. Riboflavin metabolism. *New Eng. J. Med.* 283:463-472 (1970b).

Robbins, J. and J. E. Rall. Proteins associated with the thyroid hormones. *Physiol. Rev.* 40:415-489 (1960).

Robbins, R. C., L. M. Morrison, and C. F. Simpton. Effect of chondroitin sulfate A and flavonoids on hypervitaminosis D in rats. *Proc. Soc. Exp. Biol. Med.* 131:719-722 (1969).

Roberts, A. B. and H. F. DeLuca. Pathways of retinol and retinoic acid metabolism in the rat. *Biochem. J.* 102:600-610 (1967).

Roberts, L. J. The beginnings of the recommended dietary allowances. *J. Amer. Diet. Ass.* 34:903-908 (1958).

Robertson, E. G. The natural history of oedema during pregnancy. *J. Obstet. Gynaec. Brit. Commonw.* 78:520-529 (1971).

Robertson, J. D. The ultrastructure of cell membranes and their derivatives. *Biochem. Soc. Sympos.* 16:3-43 (1959).

Robertson, J. D. The molecular structure and contact relationships of cell membranes. *Progr. Biophys. Biophys. Chem.* 10:343-418 (1960).

Robertson, W. B. and J. Hewitt. Augmentation of collagen synthesis by ascorbic acid *in vitro*. *Biochim. Biophys. Acta* 49:404-406 (1961).

Robinson, F. A. *The Vitamin Co-factors of Enzyme Systems.* pp. 638-666, Pergamon Press, N. Y. (1966).

Robinson, J. and E. A. Newsholme. Glycerolkinase activities in rat heart and adipose tissue. *Biochem. J.* 104:2C-4C (1967).

Robinson, J. R. Body Fluid Dynamics. In *Mineral Metabolism*, Vol. 1, Part A, Chapter 7, C. L. Comar and F. Bronner, Eds., Academic Press, N. Y. (1960).

Robison, G. A., R. W. Butcher, and E. W. Sutherland. Cyclic AMP. *Ann. Rev. Biochem.* 37:149-174 (1968).

Robison, G. A., R. W. Butcher, and E. W. Sutherland. *Cyclic AMP.* Academic Press, N. Y. (1971).

Robison, G. A. and E. W. Sutherland. Cyclic AMP and the function of eukaryotic cells:

an introduction. *Ann. N. Y. Acad. Sci.* 185:5-9 (1971).

Rodbell, M. The problem of identifying the glucagon receptor. *Fed. Proc.* 32:1854-1858 (1973).

Rodgers, G. M., W. J. George, and J. W. Fisher. Increased kidney cyclic AMP levels and erythropoietin production following cobalt administration. *Proc. Soc. Exp. Biol. Med.* 140:977-981 (1972).

Rodriguez, M. E. and M. I. Irwin. A conspectus of research on vitamin A requirements in man. *J. Nutr.* 102:909-968 (1972).

Roe, D. A. Nutrient toxicity with excessive intake. I. Vitamins. *N. Y. State J. Med.* 66:869-873 (1966).

Roe, J. H. Appraisal of methods for the determination of *L*-ascorbic acid. *Ann. N. Y. Acad. Sci.* 92:277-283 (1961).

Roe, J. H. and C. A. Kuether. The determination of ascorbic acid in whole blood and urine through the 2,4-dinitrophenylhydrazine derivation of dehydroascorbic acid. *J. Biol. Chem.* 147:399-407 (1943).

Roe, J. H., M. B. Mills, M. J. Oesterling, and C. M. Damron. The determination of diketo-l-gulonic acid, dehydro-l-ascorbic acid and l-ascorbic acid in the same tissue extract by the 2,4-dinitrophenylhydrazine method. *J. Biol. Chem.* 174:201-208 (1948).

Roels, O. A. The influence of vitamins A and E on lysosomes. In *Lysosomes in Biology and Pathology*, Vol. 1, pp. 254-275, J. T. Dingle and H. B. Fell, Eds., *Frontiers of Biology*, 14A, Wiley-Interscience, N. Y. (1969).

Roels, O. A., S. Djaeni, M. R. Trout, T. G. Lauw, A. Heath, S. H. Poey, M. S. Tarwotjo, and B. Suhadi. The effect of protein and fat supplements on vitamin A-deficient Indonesian children. *Amer. J . Clin. Nutr.* 12:380-387 (1963).

Roels, O. A., M. E. Trout, and R. Dujaquier. Carotene balances on boys in Ruanda where vitamin A deficiency is prevalent. *J. Nutr.* 65:115-127 (1958).

Roels, O. A., M. Trout, and A. Guha. Vitamin A deficiency and acid hydrolases: β-glycerophosphate phosphatase in rat liver. *Biochem. J.* 93:23c-25c (1964).

Roels, O. A., M. Trout, and A. Guha. The effect of vitamin A deficiency and dietary α-tocopherol on the stability of rat-liver lysosomes. *Biochem. J.* 97:353-359 (1965).

Rogers, E. F. Thiamine antagonists. In *Methods in Enzymology*, Vol. XVIII, Part A, pp. 245-258, D. B. McCormick and L. D. Wright, Eds., Academic Press, N. Y. (1970).

Rogers, T. A., J. A. Setliff, and J. C. Klopping. The caloric cost and fluid and electrolyte balance in simulated subarctic survival situations. Arctic Aeromedical Laboratory Tech. Doc. Report 13-16 (December, 1963).

Rogers, W. E., Jr. Reexamination of enzyme activities thought to show evidence of a coenzyme role for vitamin A. *Amer. J. Clin. Nutr.* 22:1003-1013 (1969).

Rogers, W. E., Jr. and J. G. Bieri. Adrenal Δ^5-3β-hydroxysteroid dehydrogenase as related to vitamin A. *J. Biol. Chem.* 243:3404-3408 (1968).

Roncari, D. A. K. and C. H. Hollenberg. Esterification of free fatty acids by subcellular preparations of rat adipose tissue. *Biochim. Biophys. Acta* 137:446-463 (1967).

Rose, C. S. and P. György. Specificity of hemolytic reaction in vitamin E-deficient erythrocytes. *Amer. J. Physiol.* 168:414-420 (1952).

Rose, W. C. Introductory essay. In *An Experimental Inquiry Into Principles of Nutrition and the Digestive Process*, J. R. Young, 1803. University of Illinois Press, Urbana, Ill. (1959).

Rose, W. C., R. L. Wixon, H. B. Lockhart, and G. F. Lambert. The amino acid requirements of man. XV. The valine requirement; summary and final observations. *J. Biol. Chem.* 217:987-995 (1955).

Rosell, S., I. J. Kopin, and J. Axelrod. Fate of H³-noradrenaline in skeletal muscle before and following sympathetic stimulation. *Amer. J. Physiol.* 205:317-321 (1963).

Rosenberg, I. H., R. R. Streiff, H. A. Godwin, and W. B. Castle. Absorption of polyglutamic folate: participation of deconjugating enzymes of the intestinal mucosa. *New Eng. J. Med.* 280:985-988 (1969).

Rosenstreich, S. J., C. Rich, and W. Volwiler. Deposition in and release of vitamin D_3 from body fat: evidence for a storage site in the rat. *J. Clin. Invest.* 50:679-687 (1971).

Rosenthal, H. L. Vitamin B_{12}. IV. Estimation in foods and food supplements. In *The Vitamins*, Vol. II, pp. 139-144, W. H. Sebrell, Jr. and R. S. Harris, Eds., Academic Press, N. Y. (1968).

Rosenthal, H. L. and J. B. Allison. Some effects of caloric intake on nitrogen balance in dogs. *J. Nutr.* 44:423-431 (1951).

Ross, R. Wound healing. *Sci. Amer.* 220(6):40-50 (1969).

Rothenberg, S. P. Identification of a macromolecular factor in the ileum which binds intrinsic factor and immunologic identification of intrinsic factor in ileal extracts. *J. Clin. Invest.* 47:913-923 (1968).

Rothschild, M. A., M. Oratz, J. Mongelli, L. Fishman, and S. S. Schreiber. Amino acid regulation of albumin synthesis. *J. Nutr.* 98:395-403 (1969).

Rotruck, J. T., A. L. Pope, H. E. Ganther, and W. G. Hoekstra. Prevention of oxidative damage to rat erythrocytes by dietary selenium. *J. Nutr.* 102:689-696 (1972).

Rotruck, J. T., A. L. Pope, H. E. Ganther, A. B. Swanson, D. G. Hafeman and W. G. Hoekstra. Selenium: biochemical role as a component of glutathione peroxidase. *Science* 179:588-590 (1973).

Roubal, W. T. and A. L. Tappel. Polymerization of proteins induced by free-radical lipid peroxidation. *Arch. Biochem. Biophys.* 113:150-155 (1966).

Rubin, C. E. Electron microscopic studies of triglyceride absorption in man. *Gastroenterol.* 50:65-77 (1966).

Rubin, W. The epithelial "membrane" of the small intestine. *Amer. J. Clin. Nutr.* 24:45-64 (1971).

Rubner, M. *Die Gesetze des Energieverbrauchs bei der Ernahrung.* Leipzig and Vienna, Deuticke (1902).

Rude, S., R. E. Coggeshall, and L. S. Van Orden. Chemical and ultrastructural identification of 5-hydroxytryptamine in an identified neuron. *J. Cell Biol.* 41:832-854 (1969).

Rupp, W. D. and P. Howard-Flanders. Discontinuities in the DNA synthesized in an excision-defective strain of *Escherichia coli* following ultraviolet irradiation. *J. Molec. Biol.* 31:291-304 (1968).

Rupp, W. D., C. E. Wilde, III, D. L. Reno, and P. Howard-Flanders. Exchanges between DNA strands in ultraviolet-irradiated *Escherichia coli. J. Molec. Biol.* 61:25-44 (1971).

Sabatini, D. D., G. Blobel, Y. Nonomura, and M. R. Adelman. Ribosome-membrane inter-action: structural aspects and functional implications. *Adv. Cytopharmacol.* 1:119-129 (1971).

Sabatini, D. D., Y. Tashiro, and G. E. Palade. On the attachment of ribosomes to microsomal membranes. *J. Molec. Biol.* 19:503-524 (1966).

Said, A. K. and D. M. Hegsted. Evaluation of dietary protein quality in adult rats. *J. Nutr.* 99:474-480 (1969).

Salans, L. B., C. A. Bray, S. W. Cushman, E. Danforth, Jr., J. A. Glennon, E. S. Horton, and E. A. H. Sims. Glucose metabolism and the response to insulin by human adipose tissue in spontaneous and experimental obesity. Effects of dietary composition and adipose cell size. *J. Clin. Invest.* 53:848-856 (1974).

Salans, L. B., E. S. Horton, and E. A. H. Sims. Experimental obesity in man: Cellular character of the adipose tissue. *J. Clin. Invest.* 50:1005-1011 (1971).

Salans, L. B., J. L. Knittle, and J. Hirsch. The role of adipose cell size and adipose tissue insulin sensitivity in the carbohydrate intolerance of human obesity. *J. Clin. Invest.* 47:153-165 (1968).

Sampson, H. W., J. L. Matthews, J. H. Martin, and A. S. Kunin. An electron microscopic localization of calcium in the small intestine of normal, rachitic and vitamin D-treated rats. *Calcified Tissue Res.* 5:305-316 (1970).

Sandell, E. B. *Colorimetric Determination of Traces of Metals.* Wiley-Interscience, N. Y. (1959).

Sandiford, I. and T. Wheeler. The basal metabolism before, during, and after pregnancy. *J. Biol. Chem.* 62:329-352 (1924).

Sandstead, H. H., R. F. Burk, G. H. Booth, and W. J. Darby. Current concepts on trace minerals. Clinical considerations. *Med. Clin. North Amer.* 54:1509-1531 (1970).

Sandstead, H. H., V. C. Lanier, G. H. Shepard, and D. D. Gillespie. Zinc and wound healing. *Amer. J. Clin. Nutr.* 23:514-519 (1970).

Sandstead, H. H., A. S. Prasad, A. R. Schulert, Z. Farid, A. Miale, Jr., S. Bassily, and W. J. Darby. Human zinc deficiency, endocrine manifestations and response to treatment. *Amer. J. Clin. Nutr.* 20:422-442 (1967).

Sarett, H. P. The metabolism of pantothenic acid and its lactone moiety in man. *J. Biol. Chem.* 159:321-325 (1945).

Sargent, D. W. An evaluation of basal metabolic data for children and youth in the United States. Home Economics Research Report No. 14, U.S.D.A., Washington, D.C., (1961).

Sargent, D. W. An evaluation of basal metabolic data for infants in the United States. Home Economics Research Report No. 18, U.S.D.A., Washington, D.C., (1962).

Sargent, F., II and K. P. Weinman. Physiological individuality. *Ann. N. Y. Acad. Sci.* 134:696-720 (1966).

Sato, Y. A possible role of pyridoxine in lipid metabolism. *Nagoya J. Med. Sci.* 33:105-130 (1970).

Sauberlich, H. E. Biochemical alterations in thiamine deficiency—their interpretation. *Amer. J. Clin. Nutr.* 20:528-542 (1967).

Sauberlich, H. E. Vitamin B_6 group: VIII. Active compounds and antagonists. In *The Vitamins,* Vol. II, pp. 33-44, W. H. Sebrell and R. S. Harris, Eds., Academic Press, N. Y. (1968).

Sauberlich, H. E., J. E. Canham, E. M. Baker, N. Raica, Jr., and Y. F. Herman. Human vitamin B_6 nutriture. *J. Scientific and Ind. Res.* 29:S28-37 (1970).

Sauberlich, H. E., J. E. Canham, E. M. Baker, N. Raica, Jr., and Y. F. Herman. Biochemical assessment of the nutritional status of vitamin B_6 in the human. *Amer. J. Clin. Nutr.* 25:629-642 (1972a).

Sauberlich, H. E., R. P. Dowdy, and J. H. Skala. Laboratory tests for the assessment of nutritional status. In *Critical Reviews in Clinical Laboratory Sciences,* Vol. 4, Issue 3, CRS Press, Cleveland (1973).

Sauberlich, H. E., J. H. Judd, G. E. Nicholalds, H. P. Broquist, and W. J. Darby. Application of the erythrocyte glutathione reductase assay in evaluating riboflavin nutritional status in a high school student population. *Amer. J. Clin. Nutr.* 25:756-762 (1972).

Scanu, A. M. and C. Wisdom. Serum lipoproteins: structure and function. *Ann. Rev. Biochem.* 41:703-730 (1972).

Schachter, D. Calcium transport, vitamin D, and the molecular basis of active transport. In *The Fat-Soluble Vitamins,* pp. 55-65, H. F. DeLuca and J. W. Suttie, Eds., The University of Wisconsin Press, Madison (1970).

Schachter, D., E. B. Dowdle, and H. Schanker. Active transport of calcium by the small intestine of the rat. *Amer. J. Physiol.* 198:263-268 (1960).

Schachter, D., J. D. Finkelstein, and S. Kowarski. Metabolism of vitamin D. I. Preparation of radioactive vitamin D and its absorption in the rat. *J. Clin. Invest.* 43:787-796 (1964).

Schachter, D., D. V. Kimberg, and S. Schenker. Active transport of calcium by intestine: Action and bioassay of vitamin D. *Amer. J. Physiol.* 200:1263-1271 (1961).

Schachter, D., S. Kowarski, J. D. Finkelstein, and R.-I. W. Ma. Tissue concentration differences during active transport of calcium by intestine. *Amer. J. Physiol.* 211:1131-1136 (1966).

Schachter, D., S. Kowarski, and P. Reid. Molecular basis for vitamin D action in the small intestine. *J. Clin. Invest.* 46:1113-1114A (1967).

Schachter, D., S. Kowarski, and P. Reid. Active transport of calcium by intestine: studies with a calcium activity electrode. In *A Symposium on Calcium and Cellular Function*, pp. 108-123, A. W. Cuthbert, Ed., Macmillan, London (1969).

Schachter, D. and S. M. Rosen. Active transport of Ca^{45} by the small intestine and its dependence on vitamin D. *Amer. J. Physiol.* 196:357-362 (1959).

Schade, S. G., R. J. Cohen, and M. E. Conrad. Effect of hydrochloric acid on iron absorption. *New Eng. J. Med.* 279:672-674 (1968).

Schatz, G. Biogenesis of mitochondria. In *Membranes of Mitochondria and Chloroplasts*, pp. 251-314, E. Racker, Ed., Van Nostrand Reinhold Company, New York (1970).

Scheib, D. Properties and role of acid hydrolases on the Mullerian ducts during sexual differentiation in the male chick embryo. In *Ciba Foundation Symposium on Lysosomes*, pp. 264-277, A. V. S. de Reuck and M. P. Cameron, Eds., Little, Brown and Company, Boston (1963).

Schekman, R., A. Weiner and A. Kornberg. Multienzyme systems of DNA replication. *Science* 186:987-993 (1974).

Schenk, R. K., D. Spiro, and J. Wiener. Cartilage resorption in the tibial epiphyseal plate of growing rats. *J. Cell Biol.* 34:275-291 (1967).

Schiff, D., L. Stern, and L. Leduc. Chemical thermogenesis in newborn infants: catecholamine excretion and the plasma non-esterified fatty acid response to cold exposure. *Pediat.* 37:577-582 (1966).

Schlaphoff, D. and F. A. Johnston. The iron requirement of six adolescent girls. *J. Nutr.* 39:67-82 (1949).

Schlenk, H. Odd numbered and new essential fatty acids. *Fed. Proc.* 31:1430-1435 (1972).

Schmidt, U., P. Grafer, K. Altland, and H. W. Goedde. Biochemistry and chemistry of lipoic acids. *Adv. Enzymol.* 32:423-469 (1969).

Schmitt, F. O., R. S. Bear, and G. L. Clark. X-ray diffraction studies on nerve. *Radiology* 25:131-151 (1935).

Schnaitman, C. Comparison of rat liver mitochondrial and microsomal membrane proteins. *Proc. Nat. Acad. Sci.* 63:412-419 (1969).

Schnaitman, C. and J. W. Greenawalt. Enzymatic properties of the inner and outer membranes of rat liver mitochondria. *J. Cell Biol.* 38:158-175 (1968).

Schneider, W. C. and V. R. Potter. Intracellular distribution of enzymes. IV. The distribution of oxalacetic oxidase activity in rat liver and rat kidney fractions. *J. Biol. Chem.* 177:893-903 (1948).

Schoenheimer, R. *The Dynamic State of Body Constituents*. Harvard University Press, Cambridge (1942).

Schoenheimer, R. and D. Rittenberg. Deuterium as an indicator in the study of intermediary metabolism. III. The role of the fat tissues. *J. Biol. Chem.* 111:175-181 (1935).

Scholler, J., T. M. Farley, and K. Folkers. Therapeutic activity of coenzyme Q for reproduction. *Intern. Z. Vitaminforsch.* 38:362-368 (1968).

Schraer, R., J. A. Elder, and H. Schraer. Aspects of mitochondrial function in calcium movement and calcification. *Fed. Proc.* 32:1938-1943 (1973).

Schroeder, H. A. Chromium deficiency in rats: a syndrome simulating diabetes mellitus with retarded growth. *J. Nutr.* 88:439-445 (1966).

Schroeder, H. A., J. J. Balassa, and F. H. Tipton. Abnormal trace metals in man: Chromium. *J. Chron. Dis.* 15:941-964 (1962).

Schulman, I. and C. H. Smith. Hemorrhagic disease in an infant due to deficiency of a previously undescribed clotting factor. *Blood* 7:794-807 (1952).

Schultz, J. and N. J. Smith. A quantitative study of the absorption of food iron in infants and children. *AMA J. Dis. Child.* 95:109-119 (1958).

Schultz, S. G. and P. F. Curran. Intestinal absorption of sodium chloride and water. In *Handbook of Physiology*, Section 6: *Alimentary Canal,* Vol. III, pp. 1245-1275, C. F. Code, Ed., American Physiological Society, Washington, D. C. (1968).

Schultz, S. G., R. E. Fuisz, and P. F. Curran. Amino acid and sugar transport in rabbit ileum. *J. Gen. Physiol.* 49:849-866 (1966).

Schultze, H. E. and J. F. Heremans. *Molecular Biology of Human Proteins*, Vol. 1. Elsevier Publishing Co., Amsterdam (1966).

Schumaker, V. N. and G. H. Adams. Circulating liproproteins. *Ann. Rev. Biochem.* 38:113-136 (1969).

Schwarz, K. Development and status of experimental work on Factor 3-selenium. *Fed. Proc.* 20:666-673 (1961).

Schwarz, K. and C. M. Foltz. Selenium as an integral part of factor 3 against dietary necrotic liver degeneration. *J. Amer. Chem. Soc.* 79:3292-3293 (1957).

Schwarz, K. and W. Mertz. Chromium III and the glucose tolerance factor. *Arch. Biochem. Biophys.* 85:292-295 (1959).

Schwarz, K. and D. B. Milne. Fluorine requirement for growth in the rat. *Bioinorganic Chem.* 1:331-338 (1972).

Schwarz, K., D. B. Milne, and E. Vinyand. Growth effects of tin compounds in rats maintained in a trace element controlled environment. *Biochem. Biophys. Res. Commun.* 40:22-29 (1970).

Scott, B. L. The occurrence of specific cytoplasmic granules in the osteoclast. *J. Ultrastruct. Res.* 19:417-431 (1967).

Scott, B. L. and D. C. Pease. Electron microscopy of the epiphyseal apparatus. *Anat. Rec.* 126:465-495 (1956).

Scott, D. Clinical biotin deficiency ("egg white injury"). *Acta Med. Scand.* 162:69-70 (1958).

Scott, M. L. Anti-oxidants, selenium and sulphur amino acids in the vitamin E nutrition of chicks. *Nutr. Abstr. Rev.* 32:1-8 (1962).

Scott, M. L. Studies on vitamin E and related factors in nutrition and metabolism. In *The Fat-Soluble Vitamins*, pp. 355-368, H. F. DeLuca and J. W. Suttie, Eds., The University of Wisconsin Press, Madison (1970).

Scott, M. L. The selenium dilemma. *J. Nutr.* 103:803-810 (1973).

Scott, P. J., L. P. Visentin, and J. M. Allen. The enzymatic characteristics of peroxisomes of amphibian and avian liver and kidney. *Ann. N. Y. Acad. Sci.* 168:244-264 (1969).

Scrimshaw, N. S. and M. Behar. World-wide occurrence of protein malnutrition. *Fed. Proc.* 18:82-87 (1959).

Scrimshaw, N. S., M. Behar, G. Arroyave, F. Viteri, and C. Tejada. Characteristics of kwashiorkor (sindrome pluricarencial de la infancia). *Fed. Proc.* 15:977-985 (1956).

Scrimshaw, N. S., V. R. Young, R. Schwartz, M. Piche, and J. B. Das. Minimum dietary essential amino acid-to-total nitrogen ratio for whole egg protein fed to young men. *J. Nutr.* 89:9-18 (1966).

Scriver, C. R. and J. H. Hutchinson. The vitamin B_6 deficiency syndrome in human infancy:

biochemical and clinical observations. *Pediat.* 31:240-250 (1963).

Scrutton, M. C., M. F. Utter, and A. S. Mildvan. Pyruvate carboxylase. VI. The presence of tightly bound manganese. *J. Biol. Chem.* 241:3480-3487 (1966).

Sealock, R. and H. E. Silberstein. The control of experimental alcaptonuria by means of vitamin C. *Science* 90:517 (1939).

Sedvall, G. and I. J. Kopin. Acceleration of norepinephrine synthesis in the rat submaxillary gland *in vivo* during sympathetic nerve stimulation. *Life Sci.* 6:45-51 (1967).

Seelig, M. S. Review: relationships of copper and molybdenum to iron metabolism. *Amer. J. Clin. Nutr.* 25:1022-1037 (1972).

Seelig, M. S. and H. A. Heggtveit. Magnesium interrelationships in ischemic heart disease: a review. *Amer. J. Clin. Nutr.* 27:59-79 (1974).

Segal, H. L. Enzymatic interconversion of active and inactive forms of enzymes. *Science* 180:25-32 (1973).

Seljelid, R. Endocytosis in thyroid follicle cells. IV. On the acid phosphatase activity in the thyroid follicle cells, with special reference to the quantitive aspects. *J. Ultrastruct. Res.* 18:237-256 (1967).

Seltzer, C. C., R. F. Goldman, and J. Mayer. Triceps skinfold as predictive measure of body density and body fat in obese adolescent girls. *Pediat.* 36:212-218 (1965).

Seltzer, C. C. and J. Mayer. Simple criterion of obesity. *Postgrad. Med.* 38:A101-A107 (1965).

Semenza, G., S. Auricchio, A. Rubino, A. Prader, and J. D. Welsh. Lack of some intestinal maltases in a human disease transmitted by a single genetic factor. *Biochim. Biophys. Acta* 105:386-389 (1965).

Setlow, R. B. and W. L. Carrier. The disappearance of thymine dimers from DNA: an error-correcting mechanism. *Proc. Nat. Acad. Sci.* 51:226-231 (1964).

Shah, D. V. and J. W. Suttie. Mechanism of action of vitamin K: Evidence for the conversion of a precursor protein to prothrombin in the rat. *Proc. Nat. Acad. Sci.* 68:1653-1657 (1971).

Shantz, E. M. Isolation of pure A_2. *Science* 108:417-419 (1948).

Shapiro, B., I. Chowers, and G. Rose. Fatty acid uptake and esterification in adipose tissue. *Biochim. Biophys. Acta* 23:115-120 (1957).

Shapiro, B., M. Staffer, and G. Rose. Pathways of triglyceride formation in adipose tissue. *Biochim. Biophys. Acta* 44:373-375 (1960).

Sharon, N. Glycoproteins. *Sci. Amer.* 230(5):78-86 (1974).

Shaw, J. H. and E. A. Sweeney. Nutrition in relation to dental medicine. In *Modern Nutrition in Health and Disease*, 5th Ed., pp. 733-769, R. S. Goodhart and M. E. Shils, Eds., Lea and Febiger, Philadelphia (1973).

Shearer, M. J. and P. Barkhan. Studies on the metabolites of phylloquinone (vitamin K_1) in the urine of man. *Biochim. Biophys. Acta* 297:300-312 (1973).

Sheehan, R. G. and R. P. Frenkel. The control of iron absorption by the gastrointestinal mucosal cell. *J. Clin. Invest.* 51:224-231 (1972).

Sheldon, W. Congenital pancreatic lipase deficiency. *Arch. Disease Childhood* 39:268-271 (1964).

Shelling, D. H. Calcium and phosphorus studies. III. The source of excess serum calcium in viosterol hypercalcemia. *J. Biol. Chem.* 96:229-243 (1932).

Sheppard, A. J. Gas chromatography of vitamin K_1. In *Methods in Enzymology*, Vol. XVIII, Part C, pp. 461-464, D. B. McCormick and L. D. Wright, Eds., Academic Press, N. Y., (1971).

Sheppard, A. J. and W. D. Hubbard. Gas chromatography of vitamins D_2 and D_3. In *Methods in Enzymology*, Vol. XVIII, Part C, pp. 733-746, D. B. McCormick and L. D. Wright, Eds., Academic Press, N. Y. (1971).

Sheppard, A. J., A. R. Prosser, and W. D. Hubbard. Gas chromatography of vitamin E. In

Methods in Enzymology, Vol. XVIII, Part C, pp. 356-365, D. B. McCormick and L. D. Wright, Eds., Academic Press, N.Y. (1971).

Sherman, H. C. Calcium requirement of maintenance in man. *J. Biol. Chem.* 44:21-27 (1920).

Sheving, L. E., W. H. Harrison, P. Gordon, and J. E. Pauly. Daily fluctuation (circadian and ultradian) in biogenic amines of the rat brain. *Amer. J. Physiol.* 214:166-173 (1968).

Shils, M. E. Experimental human magnesium depletion. I. Clinical observations and blood chemistry alterations. *Amer. J. Clin. Nutr.* 15:133-143 (1964).

Shishiba, Y., D. H. Solomon, and G. N. Beall. Comparison of early effects of thyrotropin and long-acting thyroid stimulation on thyroidal secretion. *Endocrinology* 80:957-961 (1967).

Shnitka, T. K. Pinocytotic labelling of liver-cell lysosomes with colloidal gold: Observations on the uptake of the marker, and its subsequent discharge into bile canaliculi. *Fed. Proc.* 24:556A (1965).

Shojania, A. M., G. Harnady, and G. H. Barnes. Oral contraceptives and serum-folate levels. *Lancet* 1:1376-1377 (1968).

Shorb, M. S. Activity of vitamin B_{12} for the growth of lactobacillus lactis. *Science* 107:397-398 (1948).

Shrago, E., J. A. Glennon, and E. S. Gordon. Enzyme studies in human liver and adipose tissue. *Nature* 212:1263 (1966).

Siekevitz, P. Protoplasm: endoplasmic reticulum and microsomes and their properties. *Ann. Rev. Physiol.* 25:15-40 (1963).

Siekevitz, P. and G. E. Palade. A cytochemical study on the pancreas of the guinea pig. III. *In vivo* incorporation of leucine-1-C^{14} into the proteins of cell fractions. *J. Biophys. Biochem. Cytol.* 4:557-566 (1958).

Siekevitz, P. and G. E. Palade. A cytochemical study on the pancreas of the guinea pig. V. *In vivo* incorporation of leucine-1-C^{14} into the chymotrypsinogen of various cell fractions. *J. Biophys. Biochem. Cytol.* 7:619-630 (1960).

Silber, R. H. and K. Unna. Studies on the urinary excretion of pantothenic acid. *J. Biol. Chem.* 142:623-628 (1942).

Silverman, M., F. Ebaugh, and R. C. Gardiner. The nature of labile citrovorum factor in human urine. *J. Biol. Chem.* 223:259-270 (1956).

Silverman, W. A., A. Zamelis, J. C. Sinclair, and F. J. Agate. Warm nape of the newborn. *Pediat.* 33:984-987 (1964).

Simon, E. J., A. Eisengart, L. Sundheim, and A. T. Milhorat. The metabolism of vitamin E. II. Purification and characterization of urinary metabolites of a-tocopherol. *J. Biol. Chem.* 221:807-817 (1956).

Simonson, E. The concept and definition of normality. *Ann. N. Y. Acad. Sci.* 134:541-558 (1966).

Simonson, M., J. K. Stephan, H. M. Hanson, and B. F. Chow. Open field studies in offspring of underfed mother rats. *J. Nutr.* 101:331-335 (1971).

Simoons, F. J. Primary adult lactose intolerance and the milking habit: A problem in biologic and cultural interrelations. II. A cultural historical hypothesis. *Amer. J. Dig. Dis.* 15:695-710 (1970).

Singer, J. E., M. Westphal, and K. Niswander. Relationship of weight gain during pregnancy to birth weight and infant growth and development in the first year of life. *Obstet. Gynec.* 31:417-423 (1968).

Singer, S. J. The molecular organization of biological membranes. In *Structure and Function of Biological Membranes*, pp. 145-222, L. I. Rothfield, Ed., Academic Press, N. Y. (1971).

Singer, S. J. A fluid lipid-globular protein mosaic model of membrane structure. *Ann. N. Y. Acad. Sci.* 195:16-23 (1972).

Singer, S. J. and G. L. Nicolson. The fluid mosaic model of the structure of cell membranes. *Science* 175:720-731 (1972).

Singleton, J. W. and L. Laster. Biliverdin reductase of guinea pig liver. *J. Biol. Chem.* 240:4780-4789 (1965).

Sinsheimer, R. L. Is the nucleic acid message in a two-symbol code? *J. Molec. Biol.* 1:218-220 (1959).

Siperstein, M. D. and M. J. Guest. Studies on the site of the feedback control of cholesterol synthesis. *J. Clin. Invest.* 39:642-652 (1960).

Siri, W. E. Fat, water and lean tissue studies. *Fed. Proc.* 12:133 (1953).

Siri, W. E. The gross composition of the body. *Adv. Biol. Med. Phys.* IV:239-280 (1956).

Sjostrand, F. S. *Biochemical Problems of Lipids*, Vol. 1, pp. 91-115, Elsevier, Amsterdam (1963).

Sjostrand, F. S. A comparison of plasma membrane, cytomembranes, and mitochondrial membranes with respect to ultrastructural features. *J. Ultrastruct. Res.* 9:561-580 (1963).

Sjostrand, F. S. The endoplasmic reticulum. In *Cytology and Cell Physiology*, 3rd Ed., pp. 311-375, G. H. Bourne, Ed., Academic Press, N. Y. (1964).

Sjostrand, F. S. Ultrastructure and function of cellular membranes. In *The Membranes*, pp. 151-210, A. J. Dalton and F. Haguenau, Eds., Academic Press, N. Y. (1968).

Skeggs, H. R. and L. D. Wright. The use of *Lactobacillus arabinosus* in the microbiological determination of pantothenic acid. *J. Biol. Chem.* 156:21-26 (1944).

Skou, J. C. Enzymatic basis for active transport of Na^+ and K^+ across cell membrane. *Physiol. Rev.* 45:596-617 (1965).

Slater, E. C., J. J. M. De Vijlder, and W. Boers. The binding of NAD^+ and NADH to glyceraldehydephosphate dehydrogenase. *Vitamins Hormones* 28:315-328 (1970).

Slater, T. F. Lysosomes and experimentally induced tissue injury. In *Lysosomes in Biology and Pathology*, Vol. I, pp. 469-492, J. T. Dingle and H. B. Fell, Eds., *Frontiers of Biology*, Vol. 14A, Wiley-Interscience, N. Y. (1969).

Slautterback, D. B. Mitochondria in cardiac muscle cells of the canary and some other birds. *J. Cell Biol.* 24:1-21 (1965).

Slover, H. T., J. Lehmann, and R. J. Valis. Vitamin E in foods: Determination of tocols and tocotrienols. *Amer. Oil Chem. Soc.* 46:417-420 (1968).

Smiciklas, H. A., R. L. Pike, and H. Schraer. Ultrastructure of adrenal glands in sodium-deficient pregnant rats. *J. Nutr.* 101:1045-1056 (1971a).

Smiciklas, H. A., D. G. Pohanka and R. L. Pike. Progressive histochemical and ultrastructural changes in the zona glomerulosa induced by sodium deficiency during pregnancy in the rat. *J. Nutr.* 101:1439-1444 (1971b).

Smith, A. D. and H. Winkler. Lysosomes and chromaffin granules in the adrenal medulla. In *Lysosomes in Biology and Pathology*, Vol. I, pp. 155-166, J. T. Dingle and H. B. Fell, Eds., *Frontiers of Biology*, Vol. 14A, Wiley-Interscience, N. Y. (1969).

Smith, B. M. and E. M. Malthus. Vitamin A content of human liver from autopsies in New Zealand. *Brit. J. Nutr.* 16:213-218 (1962).

Smith, D. H. Introduction. In *Transport Across the Intestine*, pp. 1-12, W. L. Burland and P. D. Samuel, Eds., Churchill Livingstone, Edinburgh (1972).

Smith, D. S. The structure of flight muscle sarcosomes in the blowfly *Calliphora Erythrocephala* (Diptera). *J. Cell Biol.* 19:115-138 (1963).

Smith, D. S., U. Jarlfors, and R. Beranek. The organization of synpatic axoplasm in the Lamprey (Petromyzon Marinus) central nervous system. *J. Cell Biol.* 46:199-219 (1970).

Smith, E. L. and L. F. J. Parker. Purification of anti-pernicious anemia factor. *Biochem. J.* 43:viii-ix (1948).

Smith, J. A., J. W. Drysdale, A Goldberg, and H. N. Munro. The effect of enteral and parenteral iron on ferritin synthesis in the intestinal mucosa of the rat. *Brit. J. Haematol.* 14:79-86 (1968).

Smith, M. D. and I. M. Pannacciulli. Absorption of inorganic iron from graded doses. Its significance in relation to iron absorption tests and the "mucosal block" theory. *Brit. J. Haematol.* 4:428-434 (1958).

Smith, R. and M. Dick. Total urinary hydroxyproline in osteomalacia and the effect upon it of treatment with vitamin D. *Clin. Sci.* 34:43-56 (1968).

Smith, R. E. Thermogenic activity of the hibernating gland in the cold-acclimated rat. *Physiologist* 4:113A (1961).

Smith, R. E. and M. G. Farquhar. Modulation in nucleoside diphosphatase activity of mammotrophic cells of the rat adenohypophysis during secretion. *J. Histochem. Cytochem.* 18:237-250 (1970).

Smith, R. E. and B. A. Horwitz. Brown fat and thermogenesis. *Physiol. Rev.* 49:330-425 (1969).

Smith, S. E. and E. J. Larson. Zinc toxicity in rats. Antagonistic effects of copper and liver. *J. Biol. Chem.* 163:29-38 (1946).

Smith, U., D. S. Smith, H. Winkler, and J. W. Ryan. Exocytosis in the adrenal medulla demonstrated by freeze-etching. *Science* 179:79-82 (1973).

Smuts, D. B. The relation between the basal metabolism and the endogenous nitrogen metabolism with particular reference to the maintenance requirement of protein. *J. Nutr.* 9:403-433 (1935)

Snell, E. E. The vitamin B_6 group. *J. Biol. Chem.* 157:491-505 (1945).

Snell, E. E. and F. M. Strong. A microbiological assay for riboflavin. *Ind. Eng. Chem. Anal. Ed.* 11:346-350 (1939).

Snell, E. E. and L. D. Wright. A microbiological method for the determination of nicotinic acid. *J. Biol. Chem.* 139:675-686 (1941).

Snyder, S. H., S. P. Banerjee, H. I. Yamamura, and D. Greenberg. Drugs, neurotransmitters, and schizophrenia. *Science* 184:1243-1253 (1974).

Snyder, S. H., A. B. Young, J. P. Bennett, and A. H. Mulder. Synaptic biochemistry of amino acids. *Fed. Proc.* 32:2039-2047 (1973).

Synderman, S. E., L. E. Holt, Jr., J. Dancis, E. Roitman, A. Boyer, and M. E. Balis. "Unessential" nitrogen: a limiting factor for human growth. *J. Nutr.* 78:57-72 (1962).

Sognnaes, R. F. Fluoride protection of bones and teeth. *Science* 150:989-993 (1965).

Solomon, A. K. Pores in the cell membrane. *Sci. Amer.* 203(12):146-156 (1960).

Sommer, P. and M. Kofler. Physicochemical properties and methods of analysis of phylloquinones, menaquinones, ubiquinones, plastoquinones, menadione, and related compounds. *Vitamins Hormones* 24:349-400 (1966).

Somogyi, J. C., Ed., *Antivitamins. Biblio. Nutritio et Dieta.* S. Karger, Basel, (1966).

Sottocasa, G. L., B. Kuylenstierna, and A. Bergstrand. Separation and some enzymatic properties of the outer and inner membranes of liver mitochondria. In *Methods in Enzymology*, Vol. X, pp. 448-463, R. Estabrook and M. Pullman, Eds., Academic Press, N. Y. (1967).

Sottocasa, G. L., G. Sandri, E. Panfill, and B. de Bernard. Glycoprotein in the mitochondrial compartments of rat liver. In *Biochemistry and Biophysics of Mitochondrial Membranes*, pp. 431-443, G. F. Azzone, E. Carafoli, A. L. Lehninger, E. Quagliariello, and N. Siliprandi, Eds., Academic Press, N. Y. (1972).

Sourkes, T. L. Dopa decarboxylase: Substrates, coenzyme, inhibitors. *Pharmacol. Rev.* 18:53-60 (1966).

Sourkes, T. L. Influence of specific nutrients on catecholamine synthesis and metabolism. *Pharmacol. Rev.* 24:349-359 (1972).

Spencer, H., J. Menczel, I. Lewin, and J. Samachson. Effect of high phosphorous intake on calcium and phosphorous metabolism in man. *J. Nutr.* 86:125-132 (1965).

Spencer, R. P., S. Purdy, R. Hoerdtke, T. M. Bow, and M. A. Markulis. Studies on intestinal absorption of L-ascorbic acid-C^{14}. *Gastroenterol.* 44:768-773 (1963).

Spencer, R. P. and N. Zamchek. The intestinal absorption of riboflavin by the rat and hamster. *Gastroenterol.* 40:794-797 (1961).

Spies, T. D., C. Cooper, and M. A. Blankenhorn. The use of nicotinic acid in the treatment of pellagra. *J.A.M.A.* 110:622-627 (1938).

Spirichev, W. B. and N. V. Blazheievich. Mechanism of toxicity of vitamin D. *Internat. Ztschr. Vitaminforsch.* 39:30-36 (1969).

Spirin, A. S. and L. P. Gavrilova. *The Ribosome.* Springer-Verlag, N. Y. (1969).

Sprecher, H. W. Regulation of polyunsaturated fatty acid biosynthesis in the rat. *Fed. Proc.* 31:1451-1457 (1972).

Squires, B. T. Differential staining of buccal epithelial smears as an indicator of poor nutritional status due to protein-calorie deficiency. *J. Pediat.* 66:891-897 (1965).

Stadtman, T. C. Vitamin B_{12}. *Science* 171:859-867 (1971).

Stadtman, T. C. Selenium biochemistry. *Science* 183:915-922 (1974).

Staudinger, H., K. Krisch, and S. Leonhäuser. Role of ascorbic acid in microsomal electron transport and the possible relationship to hydroxylation reactions. *Ann. N. Y. Acad. Sci.* 92:195-207 (1961).

Stanfield, J. P., M. S. R. Hutt, and R. Tunnicliffe. Intestinal biopsy in kwashiorkor. *Lancet* ii:519-523 (1965).

Starcher, B. C. Studies on the mechanism of copper absorption in the chick. *J. Nutr.* 97:321-326 (1969).

Stassen, F. L. H., G. J. Cardinale, and S. Udenfriend. Activation of prolyl hydroxylase in L-929 fibroblasts by ascorbic acid. *Proc. Nat. Acad. Sci.* 70:1090-1093 (1973).

Steele, R. Reflections on pools. *Fed. Proc.* 23:671-679 (1964).

Steenbock, H. The induction of growth promoting and calcifying properties in a ration by exposure to light. *Science* 60:224-225 (1924).

Stefanik, P. A. and M. F. Trulson. Determining the frequency intakes of foods in large group studies. *Amer. J. Clin. Nutr.* 11:335-343 (1962).

Steggerda, F. R. and H. H. Mitchell. Variability in the calcium metabolism and calcium requirement of adult human subjects. *J. Nutr.* 31:407-422 (1946).

Stein, G. S. and R. Baserga. Cytoplasmic synthesis of acidic chromosomal proteins. *Biochem. Biophys. Res. Commun.* 44:218-223 (1971).

Stein, G. S., T. C. Spelsberg, and L. J. Kleinsmith. Nonhistone chromosomal proteins and gene regulation. *Science* 183:817-824 (1974).

Stein, O. and Y. Stein. Lecithin synthesis, intracellular transport and secretion in rat liver. IV. A radioautographic and biochemical study of choline-deficient rats injected with choline-^{3}H. *J. Cell Biol.* 40:461-483 (1969).

Stein, W. D., Y. Eilam, and W. R. Lieb. Active transport of cations across biological membranes. *Ann. N. Y. Acad. Sci.* 227:328-336 (1974).

Steinberg, D., M. Vaughan, and S. Margolis. Studies of triglyceride biosynthesis in homogenates of adipose tissue. *J. Biol. Chem.* 236:1631-1637 (1961).

Steinkamp, R., R. Dubach, and C. V. Moore. Studies in iron transportation and metabolism. VIII. Absorption of radioiron from iron-enriched bread. *Arch. Internatl. Med.* 95:181-193 (1955).

Stephens, R. E. Reassociation of microtubule protein. *J. Molec. Biol.* 33:517-519 (1968).

Stephenson, L. S. and M. C. Latham. Lactose intolerance and milk consumption: the relation of tolerance to symptoms. *Amer. J. Clin. Nutr.* 27:296-303 (1974).

Stetten, M. R. Some aspects of the metabolism of hydroxyproline studied with the aid of isotopic nitrogen. *J. Biol. Chem.* 181:31-37 (1949).

Stetten, M. R. and R. Schoenheimer. The metabolism of l(-)-proline studied with the aid of deuterium and isotopic nitrogen. *J. Biol. Chem.* 153:113-132 (1944).

Stevenson, N. R. and M. K. Brush. Existence and characteristics of Na^+-dependent active transport of ascorbic acid in guinea pig. *Amer. J. Clin. Nutr.* 22:318-326 (1969).

Steyn-Parvé, E. P. The mode of action of some thiamine analogues with antivitamin activity. In *Thiamine Deficiency: Biochemical Lesions and Their Clinical Significance*, pp. 26-42. Ciba Foundation Study Group No. 28, G. E. W. Wolstenholme and M. O'Connor, Eds., Little, Brown and Company, Boston (1967).

Stiebeling, H. K. *Food budget for nutrition and production programs.* U.S.D.A. Misc. Pub. 183 (1933).

Stiller, E. T., S. A. Harris, J. Finkelstein, J. C. Keresztesy, and K. Folkers. Pantothenic acid. VIII. The total synthesis of pure pantothenic acid. *J. Amer. Chem. Soc.* 62:1785 (1940).

Stoeckenius, W. Some observations on negatively stained mitochondria. *J. Cell Biol.* 17:443-454 (1963).

Stoeckenius, W. Morphological observations on mitochondria and related structures. *Ann. N. Y. Acad. Sci.* 137:641-642 (1966).

Stoeckenius, W. Electron microscopy of mitochondrial and model membranes. In *Membranes of Mitochondria and Chloroplasts*, pp. 53-90, E. Racker, Ed., Van Nostrand Reinhold Company, N. Y. (1970).

Stoffel, W. and H.-G. Schiefer. Biosynthesis and composition of phosphatides in outer and inner mitochondrial membranes. *Hoppe-Seyler's Zeitschrift fur Physiol. Chemie* 349:1017-1026 (1968).

Stohlman, F., Jr. Humoral regulation of erythropoiesis: XIV. A model for abnormal erythropoiesis in thalassemia. *Ann. N. Y. Acad. Sci.* 119:578-585 (1964).

Stohlman, F., Jr. Kinetics of erythropoiesis. In *Regulation of Hematopoiesis*, Vol. I, pp. 317-326, A. S. Gordon, Ed., Appleton-Century-Crofts, N. Y. (1970a).

Stohlman, F., Jr. Regulation of red cell production. In *Formation and Destruction of Blood Cells*, pp. 65-84, T. J. Greenwalt and G. A. Jamieson, Eds., J. B. Lippincott Company, Philadelphia (1970b).

Stohlman, F., Jr. Erythropoietin and erythroid cell kinetics. In *Kidney Hormones*, pp. 331-341, J. W. Fisher, Ed., Academic Press, London, 1971.

Stohlman, F., Jr., S. Ebbe, B. Morse, D. Howard, and J. Donovan. Regulation of erythropoiesis. XX. Kinetics of red cell production. *Ann. N. Y. Acad. Sci.* 149:156-172 (1968).

Stohlman, F., Jr., D. Howard, and A. Beland. Humoral regulation of erythropoiesis. XII. Effect of erythropoietin and iron on cell size in iron deficiency anemia. *Proc. Soc. Exp. Biol. Med.* 113:986-988 (1963).

Stone, N. and A. Meister. Function of ascorbic acid in the conversion of proline to collagen hydroxyproline. *Nature* 194:555-557 (1962).

Storvick, C. A. and J. M. Peters. Methods for the determination of vitamin B_6 in biological materials. *Vitamins Hormones* 22:833-854 (1964).

Straus, W. Lysosomes, phagosomes and related particles. In *Enzyme Cytology*, pp. 239-319, D. B. Roodyn, Ed., Academic Press, N. Y. (1967).

Strauss, E. W. Absorption of fat from solutions of mixed bile salt micelles by hamster intestine *in vitro. J. Cell Biol.* 23:90A (1964).

Strauss, E. W. Electron microscopic study of intestinal fat absorption *in vitro* from mixed micelles containing linolenic acid, monolein, and bile salt. *J. Lipid Res.* 7:307-323 (1966).

Strauss, E. W. Morphological aspects of triglyceride absorption. In *Handbook of Physiology*, Section 6: *Alimentary Canal*, Vol. III, pp. 1377-1406, C. F. Code, Ed., American Physiological Society, Washington, D. C. (1968).

Strauss, E. W. and S. Ito. Autoradiographic and biochemical study of linolenic acid-C^{14} absorption by hamster intestine from mixed micelles *in vitro*. *J. Cell Biol.* 27:101A (1965).

Streffer, C. and D. H. Williamson. The effect of calcium ions on the leakage of protein and enzymes from rat-liver slices. *Biochem. J.* 95:552-560 (1965).

Streiff, R. R. Folate deficiency and oral contraceptives. *J.A.M.A.* 214:105-108 (1970).

Stryer, L. Implications of x-ray crystallographic studies of protein structure. *Ann. Rev. Biochem.* 37:25-50 (1968).

Subba Rao, K., S. Seshadri, and P. Ganguly. Studies on metabolism of vitamin A. II. Enzymic synthesis and hydrolysis of phenolic sulphates in vitamin A-deficient rats. *Biochem. J.* 87:312-317 (1963).

Subba Row, Y., A. B. Hastings, and M. Elkin. Chemistry of anti-pernicious anemia substances of liver. *Vitamins Hormones* 3:237-296 (1948).

Suda, T., H. F. DeLuca, H. Schnoes, and J. W. Blunt. 25-Hydroxyergocalciferol: a biologically active metabolite of vitamin D_2. *Biochem. Biophys. Res. Commun.* 35:182-185 (1969).

Suda, T., H. F. DeLuca, H. K. Schnoes, Y. Tanaka, and M. F. Holick. 25,26-Dihydroxy-cholecalciferol, a metabolite of vitamin D_3 with intestinal calcium transport activity. *Biochemistry* 9:4776-4780 (1970).

Sueoka, N. Correlation between base composition of deoxyribonucleic acid and amino acid composition of protein. *Proc. Nat. Acad. Sci.* 47:1141-1149 (1961a).

Sueoka, N. Compositional correlation between deoxyribonucleic acid and protein. *Cold Spring Harbor Symp. Quant. Biol.* 26:35-43 (1961b).

Svirbely, J. L. and A. Szent-Györgyi. The chemical nature of vitamin C. *Biochem. J.* 26:865-870 (1932).

Sulakhe, P. V. and N. S. Dhalla. Excitation-contraction coupling in heart. X. Further studies on the energy-linked calcium transport by sub-cellular particles in the failing heart of myopathic hamster. *Biochem. Med.* 8:18-27 (1973).

Sund, H. *The Pyridine Nucleotide Coenzymes.* Interscience, New York, 1968.

Sutherland, E. W. Studies on the mechanism of hormone action. *Science* 177:401-408 (1972).

Sutherland, E. W., I. Øye, and R. W. Butcher. Action of epinephrine and the role of the adenyl cyclase system in hormone action. *Rec. Progr. Hormone Res.* 21:623-646 (1965).

Sutherland, E. W. and G. A. Robison. The role of cyclic AMP in the control of carbohydrate metabolism. *Diabetes* 18:797-819 (1969).

Swell, L., E. C. Trout, Jr., H. Field, Jr., and C. R. Treadwell. Absorption of H^3-β2sitosterol in the lymph fistula rat. *Proc. Soc. Exp. Biol. Med.* 100:140-142 (1959a).

Swell, L., E. C. Trout, Jr., H. Field, Jr., and C. R. Treadwell. Intestinal absorption of C^{14} phytosterols. *J. Biol. Chem.* 234:2286-2289 (1959b).

Swendseid, M. E., W. H. Griffith, and S. G. Tuttle. The effect of low protein diet on the ratio of essential to nonessential amino acids in blood plasma. *Metabolism* 12:96-97 (1963).

Swendseid, M. E., I. Williams, and M. S. Dunn. Amino acid requirements of young women based on nitrogen balance data. I. The sulfur-containing amino acids. *J. Nutr.* 58:495-505 (1956a).

Swendseid, M. E., I. Williams, and M. S. Dunn. Amino acid requirements of young women based on nitrogen balance data. II. Studies on isoleucine and on minimum amounts of the eight amino acids fed simultaneously. *J. Nutr.* 58:507-517 (1956b).

Swift, H. and Z. Hruban. Focal degradation as a biological process. *Fed. Proc.* 23:1026-1037 (1964).

Swift, R. W. and C. E. French. *Energy Metabolism and Nutrition.* Scarecrow Press, Washington, D. C. (1954).

Sydenstricker, V. P. The history of pellagra, its recognition as a disorder of nutrition and its conquest. *Amer. J. Clin. Nutr.* 6:409-414 (1958).

Sydenstricker, V. P., S. A. Singal, A. P. Briggs, N. M. de Vaughn, and H. Isbell. Preliminary observations on "egg white injury" in man and its cure with a biotin concentrate. *Science* 95:176-177 (1942).

Szent-Györgyi, A. Observations on the function of peroxidase systems and the chemistry of the adrenal cortex. *Biochem. J.* 22:1387-1409 (1928).

Szent-Györgyi, A. *Chemistry of Muscular Contraction,* Academic Press, N.Y. (1947).

Szent-Györgyi, A. *Bioenergetics,* Academic Press, N. Y. (1957).

Szent-Györgyi, A. Muscle research. *Science* 128:600-702 (1958).

Szentkiralyi, E. M. and A. Oplatka. On the formation and stability of the enzymically active complexes of heavy meromyosin with actin. *J. Molec. Biol.* 43:551-566 (1969).

Taggart, N. R., R. M. Holliday, W. Z. Billewicz, F. E. Hytten, and A. M. Thomson. Changes in skinfolds during pregnancy. *Brit. J. Nutr.* 21:439-451 (1967).

Taggart, W. V. and J. T. Matschiner. Metabolism of menadione-6,7-^{3}H in the rat. *Biochemistry* 8:1141-1146 (1969).

Takagi, M. and K. Ogata. Direct evidence for albumin biosynthesis by membrane bound polysomes in rat liver. *Biochem. Biophys. Res. Commun.* 33:55-60 (1968).

Takaki, K. Health of the Japanese Navy. *Lancet* ii:86 (1887).

Tanaka, Y. and H. F. DeLuca. The control of 25-hydroxyvitamin D metabolism by inorganic phosphate. *Arch. Biochem. Biophys.* 154:566-574 (1973).

Tanaka, Y., H. Frank, and H. F. DeLuca. Biological activity of 1,25-dihydroxy-vitamin D_3 in the rat. *Endocrinology* 92:417-422 (1973).

Tandler, C. J. and J. L. Sirlin. Some observations on the nuclear pool of ribonucleic acid phosphorus. *Biochim. Biophys. Acta* 55:228-230 (1962).

Tao, M. Mechanism of activation of a rabbit reticulocyte protein kinase by adenosine 3',5'-cyclic monophosphate. *Ann. N. Y. Acad. Sci.* 185:227-231 (1971).

Tappel, A. L. Vitamin E as the biological lipid antioxidant. *Vitamins Hormones* 20:493-510 (1962).

Tappel, A. L. Lysosomal enzymes and other components. In *Lysosomes in Biology and Pathology,* Vol. 2, pp. 207-244, J. T. Dingle and H. B. Fell, Eds., *Frontiers of Biology,* Vol. 14A, Wiley-Interscience, N. Y. (1969).

Tappel, A. L. Reactions of vitamin E, ubiquinol, and selenoamino acids, and protection of oxidant-labile enzymes. In *The Fat-Soluble Vitamins,* pp. 369-374, H. F. DeLuca and J. W. Suttie, Eds., The University of Wisconsin Press, Madison (1970).

Tappel, A. L. Vitamin E and free radical peroxidation of lipids. *Ann. N. Y. Acad. Sci.* 203:12-28 (1972).

Tappel, A. L. Lipid peroxidation damage to cell components. *Fed. Proc.* 32:1870-1874 (1973).

Tappel, A. L., P. L. Sawant, and S. Shibko. Lysosomes: distribution in animals, hydrolytic capacity and other properties. In *Ciba Foundation Symposium on Lysosomes,* pp. 78-108, A. V. S. DeReuck and M. P. Cameron, Eds., Little, Brown and Company, Boston (1963).

Tappel, A. L. and H. Zalkin. Inhibition of lipide peroxidation in mitochondria by vitamin E. *Arch. Biochem. Biophys.* 80:333-336 (1959).

Targan, S. R., S. Merrill, and A. D. Schwabe. Fractionation and quantification of β-carotene and vitamin A derivatives in human serum. *Clin. Chem.* 15:479-486 (1969).

Tashiro, Y. and P. Siekevitz. Ultracentrifugal studies on the dissociation of hepatic ribosomes *J. Molec. Biol.* 11:149-165 (1965).

Taussig, H. B. Possible injury to the cardiovascular system from vitamin D. *Ann. Internal Med.* 65:1195-1200 (1966).

Taylor, A. C. and P. Weiss. Demonstration of axonal flow by the movement of tritium-labeled protein in mature optic nerve fibers. *Proc. Nat. Acad. Sci.* 54:1521-1527 (1965).

Taylor, A. N. and R. H. Wasserman. Correlations between the vitamin D-induced calcium binding protein and intestinal absorption of calcium. *Fed. Proc.* 28:1834-1838 (1969).

Taylor, A. N. and R. H. Wasserman. Immunofluorescent localization of vitamin D-dependent calcium-binding protein. *J. Histochem. Cytochem.* 18:107-115 (1970).

Temin, H. M. RNA-directed DNA synthesis. *Sci. Amer.* 226(1):24-33 (1972).

Teng, C-S and T. H. Hamilton. Role of chromatin in estrogen action in the uterus. II. Hormone-induced synthesis of nonhistone acidic proteins which restore histone-inhibited DNA-dependent RNA synthesis. *Proc. Nat. Acad. Sci.* 63:465-472 (1969).

Tepperman, J. *Metabolic and Endocrine Physiology*, 3rd ed., Year Book Medical Publishers Incorporated (1973).

Terroine, E. F. and R. Bonnet. Le mechanism de l'action dynamique specifique. *Ann. Physiol.* 2:488-598 (1926).

Thach, R. E., K. F. Dewey, J. C. Brown, and P. Doty. Formylmethionine codon AUG as an initiator of polypeptide synthesis. *Science* 153:416-418 (1966).

Thedering, F. Pernicious anemia and its variants. *Vitamins Hormones* 26:539-546 (1968).

Theorell, H. Reindarstellung (Kristallisation) des gelben atmungsfermentes un die reversible Spaltung desselben. *Biochem. Z.* 272:155-156 (1934).

Thomas, C. D. The precursors of hypertension and coronary artery disease: insights from studies of biological variation. *Ann. N. Y. Acad. Sci.* 134:1028-1040 (1966).

Thomas, L., R. T. McCluskey, J. L. Potter, and G. Weissmann. Comparison of the effects of papain and vitamin A on cartilage. *J. Exper. Med.* 111:705-718 (1960).

Thompson, G. R., B. Lewis, and C. C. Booth. The absorption of ^{3}H-labelled vitamin D_3 in control subjects and in patients with intestinal malabsorption. *J. Clin. Invest.* 45:94-102 (1966a).

Thompson, G. R., B. Lewis, and C. C. Booth, Vitamin D absorption after partial gastrectomy. *Lancet* 1:457-458 (1966b).

Thompson, G. R., B. Lewis, G. Neale, and C. C. Booth. Mechanisms of vitamin D deficiency in patients with lesions of the gastrointestinal tract. *Quart. J. Med.* 34:486-487 (1965).

Thompson, J. N., J. McC. Howell, and G. A. J. Pitt. Vitamin A and reproduction in rats. *Proc. Roy. Soc.* B159:510-535 (1964).

Thompson, J. N. and M. L. Scott. Impaired lipid and vitamin E absorption related to atrophy of the pancreas in selenium-deficient chicks. *J. Nutr.* 100:797-809 (1970).

Thompson, R. H. S. The function of a vitamin: the legacy of this concept to biochemistry. *Biochem. Pharmacol.* 20:513-517 (1971).

Thomson, A. D., H. Baker, and C. M. Leevy. Pattern of ^{35}S-thiamine hydrochloride absorption in the malnourished alcoholic patient. *J. Lab. Clin. Med.* 76:34-45 (1970).

Thomson, A. D., O. Frank, H. Baker, and C. M. Leevy. Thiamine propyl disulfide: absorption and utilization. *Ann. Int. Med.* 74:529-534 (1971).

Thomson, A. D. and C. M. Leevy. Observations on the mechanism of thiamine hydrochloride absorption in man. *Clin. Sci.* 43:153-163 (1972).

Thomson, A. M. Diet in pregnancy. 1. Dietary survey technique and the nutritive value of diets taken by primigravidae. *Brit. J. Nutr.* 12:446-461 (1958).

Thomson, A. M. Diet in pregnancy. 2. Assessment of the nutritive value of diets, especially in relation to differences between social classes. *Brit. J. Nutr.* 13:190-204 (1959a).

Thomson, A. M. Diet in pregnancy. 3. Diet in relation to the course and outcome of pregnancy. *Brit. J. Nutr.* 13:509-525 (1959b).

Thomson, A. M., F. E. Hytten, and W. Z. Billewicz. The energy cost of human lactation. *Brit. J. Nutr.* 24:565-572 (1970).

Tillotson, J. A. and E. M. Baker. An enzymatic measurement of the riboflavin status in man. *Amer. J. Clin. Nutr.* 25:425-431 (1972).

Tillotson, J. A., H. E. Sauberlich, E. M. Baker, and J. E. Canham. Use of carbon-14 labeled vitamins in human nutrition studies: pyridoxine. *Proc. VIIth Int. Cong. Nutr.* (Hamburg) 5:554-557 (1968).

Timiras, P. S. *Developmental Physiology and Aging.* The Macmillan Co., N. Y. (1972).

Tissieres, A. and J. D. Watson. Ribonucleoprotein particles from *Escherichia coli. Nature* 182:778-780 (1958).

Todhunter, E. N. Development of knowledge in nutrition. I. Animal experiments. II. Human experiments. *J. Amer. Diet. Ass.* 41:328-334; 335-340 (1962).

Toepfer, E. W. and J. Lehmann. Procedure for chromatographic separation and microbiological assay of pyridoxine, pyridoxal and pyridoxamine in food extracts. *J. Ass. Offic. Agr. Chem.* 44:426-430 (1961).

Toepfer, E. W. and M. M. Polansky. Recent developments in the analysis for vitamin B_6 in foods. *Vitamins Hormones* 22:825-832 (1964).

Tontisirin, K., V. R. Young, W. M. Rand, and N. W. Scrimshaw. Plasma threonine response curve and threonine requirements of young men and elderly women. *J. Nutr.* 104:495-505 (1974).

Topham, R. W. and E. Frieden. Identification and purification of a non-ceruloplasmin ferroxidase of human serum. *J. Biol. Chem.* 245:6698-6705 (1970).

Toscani, F. Comparison of analyzed with calculated diets. *Food Research.* 13:187-192 (1948).

Toskes, P. P. and J. Deren. The role of the pancreas in vitamin B_{12} absorption: Studies of vitamin B_{12} absorption in partially pancreatectomized rats. *J. Clin. Invest.* 51:216-223 (1972).

Toskes, P. P., J. Hansell, J. Cerda, and J. Deren. Vitamin B_{12} malabsorption in chronic pancreatic insufficiency. *New Eng. J. Med.* 284:627-632 (1971).

Tower, D. B., S. A. Luse, and H. Grundfest. *Properties of Membranes.* Springer Publishing Co., Inc., N. Y. (1962).

Trams, E. G., L. E. Giuffrida, and A. Karmen. Gas chromatographic analysis of long-chain fatty acids in gangliosides. *Nature* 193:680-681 (1962).

Tranzer, J. P., H. Thoenen, R. L. Snipes, and J. G. Richards. Recent developments on the ultrastructural aspect of adrenergic nerve endings in various experimental conditions. In *Mechanisms of Synaptic Transmission*, K. Akert and P. G. Waser, Eds., *Progress in Brain Res.* 31:33-46 (1969).

Travis, S., M. M. Mathias, and J. Dupont. Effect of biotin deficiency on the catabolism of linoleate in the rat. *J. Nutr.* 102:767-771 (1972).

Treadwell, C. R., L. Swell, and G. V. Vahouny. Factors in sterol absorption. *Fed. Proc.* 21:903-908 (1962).

Treadwell, C. R. and G. V. Vahouny. Cholesterol absorption. In *Handbook of Physiology*, Section 6: *Alimentary Canal*, Vol. III, pp. 1407-1438, C. F. Code, Ed., American Physiological Society, Washington, D. C. (1968).

Treble, D. H. and E. G. Ball. The occurrence of glycerolkinase in rat brown adipose tissue. *Fed. Proc.* 22:357A (1963).

Tria, E. and A. M. Scanu. *Structural and Functional Aspects of Lipoproteins in Living*

Systems. Academic Press, N. Y. (1969).

Triner, L., G. G. Nahas, Y. Vulliemoz, N. I. A. Overweg, M. Verosky, D. V. Habif, and S. H. Ngai. Cyclic AMP and smooth muscle function. *Ann. N. Y. Acad. Sci.* 185:458-476 (1971).

Trowell, H. C., T. Moore, and I. M. Sharman. Vitamin E and carotenoids in the blood plasma in kwashiorkor. *Ann. N. Y. Acad. Sci.* 57:734-736 (1954).

Trulson, M. F. and M. B. McCann. Comparison of dietary survey methods. *J. Amer. Diet. Ass.* 35:672-676 (1959).

Ts'o, P. O. P., J. Bonner, and J. Vinograd. Structure and properties of microsomal nucleoprotein particles from pea seedlings. *Biochim. Biophys. Acta* 30:570-582 (1958).

Tubbs, P. K. and P. B. Garland. Membranes and fatty acid metabolism. *Brit. Med. Bull.* 24:158-164 (1968).

Tullis, I. G., V. Lawson, and R. Williams. The digital computer in calculating dietary data. *J. Amer. Diet. Ass.* 46:384-386 (1965).

Turnbull, A., F. Cleton, and C. A. Finch. Iron absorption. IV. The absorption of hemoglobin iron. *J. Clin. Invest.* 41:1897-1907 (1967).

Turner, J. B. and D. E. Hughes. The absorption of some B-group vitamins by surviving rat intestine preparations. *Quart. J. Exptl. Physiol.* 47:107-123 (1962).

Udenfriend, S. Tyrosine hydroxylase. Pharmacol. Rev. 18:43-51 (1966).

Ugolev, A. M. Membrane (contact) digestion. *Physiol. Rev.* 45:555-595 (1965).

Ullrich, J., Y. M. Ostrovsky, J. Eyzaguirre, and H. Holzer. Thiamine pyrophosphate-catalyzed enzymatic decarboxylation of *a*-oxo acids. *Vitamins Hormones* 28:365-398 (1970).

Umbreit, W. W. Vitamin B_6 antagonists. *Amer. J. Clin. Nutr.* 3:291-297 (1955).

Umbreit, W. W. and I. C. Gunsalus. The function of pyridoxine derivatives: arginine and glutamic acid decarboxylases. *J. Biol. Chem.* 159:333-341 (1945).

Underwood, B. A. The determination of vitamin A and some aspects of its distribution, mobilization and transport in health and disease. *World Rev. Nutr. Dietet.* 19:123-172 (1974).

Underwood, B. A., H. Siegel, R. C. Weisell, and M. Dolinski. Liver stores of vitamin A in a normal population dying suddenly or rapidly from unnatural causes in New York City. *Amer. J. Clin. Nutr.* 23:1037-1042 (1970).

Underwood, E. J. *Trace Elements in Human and Animal Nutrition,* 3rd ed., Academic Press, N. Y. (1971).

Unglaub, W. G. and G. A. Goldsmith. Evaluation of vitamin adequacy; urinary excretion tests. In *Methods for Evaluation of Nutritional Adequacy and Status - Symposium,* pp. 69-81, Advisory Board on Quartermaster Research and Development, Committee on Foods, Natl. Acad. of Sci. Nat. Res. Council, Washington, D. C. (1954).

Uri, N. Physico-chemical aspects of autoxidation. In *Autoxidation and Antioxidants,* Vol. I, pp. 55-106, W. O. Lundberg, Ed., Wiley-Interscience (1961).

U. S. Department of Health, Education, and Welfare. *Ten-state nutrition survey 1968-1970. III. Clinical anthropometry dental.* DHEW Publication No. 72-8131, Washington, D. C. (n.d.).

U. S. Department of Health, Education, and Welfare. *Ten-state nutrition survey 1968-1970. V. Dietary.* DHEW Publication No. (HSM) 72-8133, Washington, D. C. (n.d.).

U. S. Department of Health, Education, and Welfare. *Screening children for nutritional status.* U. S. Government Printing Office, Washington, D. C. (1971).

U. S. Pharmacopeial Convention, Inc. *The Pharmacopeia of the U. S. A.,* XVI. Mack Publishing Co., Easton, Pa. (1960).

Vaes, G. Studies on bone enzymes. The activation and release of latent acid hydrolases and catalase in bone tissue homogenates. *Biochem. J.* 97:393-402 (1965).

Vaes, G. On the mechanisms of bone resorption. The action of parathyroid hormone on the excretion and synthesis of lysosomal enzymes and on the extracellular release of acid by bone cells. *J. Cell Biol.* 39:676-697 (1968).

Vaes, G. Lysosomes and the cellular physiology of bone resorption. In *Lysosomes in Biology and Pathology*, Vol. I, pp. 217-253, J. T. Dingle and H. B. Fell, Eds., *Frontiers of Biology*, Vol. 14A, Wiley-Interscience, N. Y. (1969).

Vaes, G. and P. Jacques. Studies on bone enzymes. The assay of acid hydrolases and other enzymes in bone tissue. *Biochem. J.* 97:380-386 (1965).

Vallee, B. L., W. E. C. Wacker, A. F. Bartholomay, and F. L. Hoch. Zinc metabolism in hepatic dysfunction. II. Correlation of metabolic patterns with biochemical findings. *New Eng. J. Med.* 257:1055-1065 (1957).

Van Bruggen, E. F. J., P. Borst, G. F. C. M. Ruttenberg, M. Gruber, and A. M. Kroon. Circular mitochondrial DNA. *Biochim. Biophys. Acta* 119:437-439 (1966).

Van Campen, D. Regulation of iron absorption. *Fed. Proc.* 33:100-105 (1974).

Van Campen, D. R. Effects of zinc, cadmium, silver and mercury on the absorption and distribution of copper-64 in rats. *J. Nutr.* 88:125-130 (1966).

Vandenheuvel, F. A. Study of biological structure at the molecular level with stereomodel projections. I. The lipids in the myelin sheath of nerve. *J. Amer. Oil Chem. Soc.* 40:455-471 (1963).

Vanderkooi, G. Molecular architecture of biological membranes. *Ann. N. Y. Acad. Sci.* 195:6-15 (1972).

Vanderkooi, G. and D. E. Green. Biological membrane structure. I. The protein crystal model for membranes. *Proc. Nat. Acad. Sci.* 66:615-621 (1970).

Van Dorp, D. A. The biosynthesis of prostaglandins. *Mem. Soc. Endocrinol.* 14:39-47 (1966).

Van Dorp, D. A., R. K. Beerthuis, D. H. Nugsteren, and H. Vonkeman. The biosynthesis of prostaglandins. *Biochim. Biophys. Acta* 90:204-207 (1964).

van Leersum, E. C. The discovery of vitamines. *Science* 64:357-358 (1926).

Vasington, F. D. and J. V. Murphy. Ca^{++} uptake by rat kidney mitochondria and its dependence on respiration and phosphorylation. *J. Biol. Chem.* 237:2670-2677 (1962).

Vaughan, M. Lipid metabolism. I. Introductory remarks. *Pharmacol. Rev.* 18:215-216 (1966).

Vaughan, M. The mechanism of the lipolytic action of catecholamines. *Ann. N. Y. Acad. Sci.* 139:841-848 (1967).

Vaughan, M., J. E. Berger, and D. Steinberg. Hormone-sensitive lipase and monoglyceride lipase activities in adipose tissue. *J. Biol. Chem.* 239:401-409 (1964).

Vaughan, M., D. Steinberg, and R. Pittman. On the interpretation of studies measuring uptake and esterification of [I-^{14}C] palmitic acid by rat adipose tissue *in vitro. Biochim. Biophys. Acta* 84:154-166 (1964).

Ventura, U. and G. Rindi. Transport of thiamine by the small intestine *in vitro. Experientia* 21:645-646 (1965).

Verney, E. B. The antidiuretic hormone and the factors which determine its release. *Proc. Roy. Soc. B* 135:25-106 (1947).

Verzar, F. and E. J. McDougall. *Absorption from the Intestine.* London, Longmans Green (1936).

Vidaver, G. A. Mucate inhibition of glycine entry into pigeon red cells. *Biochemistry* 3:799-803 (1964a).

Vidaver, G. A. Glycine transport by hemolyzed and restored pigeon red cells. *Biochemistry* 3:795-799 (1964b).

Vidaver, G. A. Some tests of the hypothesis that the sodium-ion gradient furnishes the energy for glycine-active transport by pigeon cells. *Biochemistry* 3:803-808 (1964c).

Villar-Palasi, J. Larner, and L. C. Shen. Glycogen metabolism and the mechanism of action of cyclic AMP. *Ann. N. Y. Acad. Sci.* 185:74-84 (1971).

Vitale, J. J. and D. M. Hegsted. Effects of dietary methionine and vitamin B_{12} deficiency on folate metabolism. *Brit. J. Haematol.* 17:467-475 (1969).

Viveros, O. H., L. Arqueros, and N. Kirshner. Release of catecholamines and dopamine-β-oxidase from the adrenal medulla. *Life Sci.* 7:609-619 (1968).

Vivier, E. Observations ultrastructurales sur l'enveloppe nucléaire et ses "pores" chez des sporozoaires. *J. Microscopie* 6:371-390 (1967).

Voit, C. Physiologie des allgemeinen stoffwechsels und der ernährung. In *Handbuch der Physiologie*, Vol. 6, Part 1, L. Hermann, Ed. (1881).

Vos, J., I. Molenaar, M. Searle-vanLeeuwen, and F. A. Hommes. Mitochondrial and microsomal membranes from livers of vitamin D-deficient ducklings. *Ann. N. Y. Acad. Sci.* 203:74-80 (1972).

Wachman, A. and D. S. Bernstein. Diet and osteoporosis. *Lancet* 1:958-959 (1968).

Wachstein, M. Evidence for a relative vitamin B_6 deficiency in pregnancy and some disease states. *Vitamins Hormones* 22:705-721 (1964).

Wacker, W. E. C. Nucleic acids and metals. III. Changes in nucleic acid, protein, and metal content as a consequence of zinc deficiency in *Euglena gracilus. Biochemistry* 1:859-865 (1962).

Wacker, W. E. C. and A. F. Parisi. Magnesium metabolism. *New Eng. J. Med.* 278:658-663; 712-717; 772-776 (1968).

Wada, H., T. Morisue, Y. Nichimura, Y. Morino, Y. Sakamoto, and K. Ichihara. Enzymatic studies on pyridoxine metabolism. *Proc. Jap. Acad.* 35:299-304 (1959).

Waddell, J. The provitamin D of cholesterol. I. The antirachitic efficacy of irradiated cholesterol. *J. Biol. Chem.* 105:711-739 (1934).

Waelsch, H., W. M. Sperry, and V. A. Stoyanoff. A study of the synthesis and deposition of lipids in brain and other tissues with deuterium as an indicator. *J. Biol. Chem.* 135:291-296 (1940a).

Waelsch, H., W. M. Sperry, and V. A. Stoyanoff. Lipid metabolism in brain during myelination. *J. Biol. Chem.* 135:297-302 (1940b).

Waelsch, H., W. M. Sperry, and V. A. Stoyanoff. The influence of growth and myelination on the deposition and metabolism of lipids in the brain. *J. Biol. Chem.* 140:885-897 (1941).

Wagner, R. P. Genetics and phenogenetics of mitochondria. *Science* 163:1026-1031 (1969).

Waite, L. C. Carbonic anhydrase inhibitors, parathyroid hormone and calcium metabolism. *Endocrinology* 91:1160-1165 (1972).

Wakil, S. J. A malonic acid derivative as an intermediate in fatty acid synthesis. *J. Amer. Chem. Soc.* 80:6465 (1958).

Wald, G. Vitamin A in the retina. *Nature* 132:316-317 (1933).

Wald, G. The biochemistry of vision. *Ann. Rev. Biochem.* 22:497-526 (1953).

Walker, A. R. P. Does low intake of calcium retard growth or conduce to stuntedness? *Amer. J. Clin. Nutr.* 2:265-271 (1954).

Walker, A. R. P. and U. B. Arvidsson. Studies on human bone from South African Bantu subjects. I. Chemical composition of ribs from subjects habituated to diet low in calcium. *Metabolism* 3:385-391 (1954).

Walker, R. M. and H. M. Linkswiler. Calcium retention in the adult human male as affected by protein intake. *J. Nutr.* 102:1297-1302 (1972).

Wall, R. Overlapping genetic codes. *Nature* 193:1268-1270 (1962).

Wallace, W. M. Nitrogen content of the body and its relation to retention and loss of nitrogen. *Fed. Proc.* 18:1125-1136 (1959).

Wang, M. M., K. H. Fisher, and M. L. Dodds. Comparative metabolic response to erythorbic acid and ascorbic acid by the human. *J. Nutr.* 77:443-447 (1962).

Warburg, O. and W. Christian. Über ein neues Oxydationsferment und sein Absorptionspektrum. *Biochem. Z.* 254:438-458 (1932).

Warburg, O. and W. Christian. Co-Fermentproblem. *Biochem. Z.* 275:112-113; 464 (1935).

Wasserman, R. H. The vitamin D-dependent calcium-binding protein. In *The Fat-Soluble Vitamins*, pp. 21-37, H. F. DeLuca and J. W. Suttie, Eds., The University of Wisconsin Press, Madison (1970).

Wasserman, R. H. and R. A. Corradino. Metabolic role of vitamins A and D. *Ann. Rev. Biochem.* 40:501-532 (1971).

Wasserman, R. H., R. A. Corradino, and A. N. Taylor. Vitamin D-dependent calcium-binding protein. Purification and some properties. *J. Biol. Chem.* 243:3978-3986 (1968a).

Wasserman, R. H. and A. N. Taylor. Vitamin D_3-induced calcium-binding protein in chick intestinal mucosa. *Science* 152:791-793 (1966).

Wasserman, R. H. and A. N. Taylor. Vitamin D-dependent calcium-binding protein. Response to some physiological and nutritional variables. *J. Biol. Chem.* 243:3987-3993 (1968).

Wasserman, R. H. and A. N. Taylor. Metabolic roles of fat-soluble vitamins D, E, and K. *Ann. Rev. Biochem.* 41:179-202 (1972).

Waterlow, J. C. Protein nutrition and enzyme changes in man. *Fed. Proc.* 18:19-31 (1959).

Waterlow, J. C. and G. A. O. Alleyne. Protein malnutrition in children: advances in knowledge in the last ten years. *Adv. Protein Chem.* 25:117-242 (1971).

Waterlow, J. C. and T. Weisz. The fat, protein and nucleic acid content of the liver in malnourished human infants. *J. Clin. Invest.* 35:346-354 (1956).

Watson, C. J. Gold from dross: The first century of the urobilinoids. *Ann. Int. Med.* 70:839-851 (1969).

Watson, J. D. *Molecular Biology of the Gene*, 2nd. ed., W. A. Benjamin, Inc., N. Y. (1970).

Watson, J. D. and F. H. C. Crick. Molecular structure of nucleic acids: A structure for deoxypentose nucleic acids. *Nature* 171:737-738 (1953).

Watt, B. L. and A. L. Merrill. *Composition of foods - raw, processed, prepared.* Agriculture Handbook No. 8, Agricultural Research Service, U. S. Dept. of Agric. (Revised 1963).

Waugh, W. A. and C. G. King. Isolation and identification of vitamin C. *J. Biol. Chem.* 97:325-331 (1932).

Weber, A. and J. M. Murray. Molecular control mechanisms in muscle contraction. *Physiol. Rev.* 53:612-673 (1973).

Weber, F. and O. Wiss. Über den Stoffwechsel des Vitamins E in der Ratte. *Helv. Physiol. Pharmacol. Acta* 21:131-141 (1963).

Weber, R. Behaviour and properties of acid hydrolases in regressing tails of tadpoles during spontaneous and induced metamorphosis *in vitro*. In *Ciba Foundation Symposium on Lysosomes*, pp. 282-300, A. V. S. De Reuck and M. P. Cameron, Eds., Little, Brown and Company, Boston (1963).

Weibel, E. R., W. Stäubli, R. Gnägi, and F. A. Hess. Correlated morphometric and biochemical studies on the liver cell. I. Morphometric model, stereologic methods and normal morphometric data for rat liver. *J. Cell Biol.* 42:68-91 (1969).

Weiner, N. and A. Alousi. Influence of nerve stimulation on rate of synthesis of norepinephrine. *Fed. Proc.* 25:259A (1967).

Weiner, N., G. Cloutier, R. Bjur, and R. I. Pfeffer. Modification of norepinephrine synthesis in intact tissue by drugs and during short-term adrenergic nerve stimulation. *Pharmacol. Rev.* 24:203-221 (1972).

Weinstock, I. M. and A. A. Iodice. Acid hydrolase activity in muscular dystrophy and denervation atrophy. In *Lysosomes in Biology and Pathology*, Vol. 1, pp. 450-468, J. T. Dingle and H. B. Fell, Eds., *Frontiers of Biology*, Vol. 14A, Wiley-Interscience, N. Y. (1969).

Weinstock, M. and C. P. Leblond. Formation of collagen. *Fed. Proc.* 33:1205-1218 (1974).

Weintraub, L. R., M. E. Conrad, and W. H. Crosby. Absorption of hemoglobin by the rat. *Proc. Soc. Exp. Biol. Med.* 120:840-842 (1965).

Weintraub, L. R., M. B. Weinstein, H.-J. Huser, and S. Rafal. Absorption of hemoglobin iron: The role of a heme-splitting substance in the intestinal mucosa. *J. Clin. Invest.* 47:531-539 (1968).

Weiss, P. and H. B. Hiscoe. Experiments on the mechanism of nerve growth. *J. Exp. Zool.* 107:315-395 (1948).

Weissbach, H. and R. T. Taylor. Metabolic role of vitamin B_{12}. *Vitamins Hormones* 26:395-412 (1968).

Weissbach, H. and R. T. Taylor. Roles of vitamin B_{12} and folic acid in methionine synthesis. *Vitamins Hormones* 28:415-440 (1970).

Weissbach, H., J. Toohey and H. A. Barker. Isolation and properties of vitamin B_{12} coenzymes containing benzimidazole or dimethylbenzimidazole. *Proc. Nat. Acad. Sci.* 45:521-525 (1959).

Weissmann, G. Lysosomal mechanisms of tissue injury in arthritis. *New Eng. J. Med.* 286:141-147 (1972).

Weissmann, G. and L. Thomas. Studies on lysosomes. II. The effect of cortisone on the release of acid hydrolases from storage granule fraction of rabbit liver induced by an excess of vitamin A. *J. Clin. Invest.* 42:661-669 (1963).

Welham, W. C. and A. R. Behnke. The specific gravity of healthy men. *J.A.M.A.* 118:498-501 (1942).

Wellner, D. Flavoproteins. *Ann. Rev. Biochem.* 36:669-690 (1967).

Wellner, V. P., J. I. Santos, and A. Meister. Carbamyl phosphate synthetase. A biotin enzyme. *Biochemistry* 7:2848-2857 (1968).

Wells, I. C. Hemorrhagic kidney degeneration in choline deficiency. *Fed. Proc.* 30:151-154 (1971).

Wessel, J. A., A. Ufer, W. D. Van Huss, and D. Cederquist. Age trends of various components of body composition and functional characteristics in women aged 20-69 years. *Ann. N. Y. Acad. Sci.* 110:608-622 (1963).

West, D. W. and E. C. Owen. The urinary excretion of metabolites of riboflavine by man. *Brit. J. Nutr.* 23:889-898 (1969).

West, D. W. and E. C. Owen. Reduction of 7,8-dimethyl-10-(formylmethyl)isoalloxazine by an enzyme in liver. *Brit. J. Nutr.* 29:43-50 (1973).

West, R. Activity of vitamin B_{12} in Addisonian pernicious anemia. *Science* 107:398 (1948).

Westmoreland, N. Connective tissue alterations in zinc deficiency. *Fed. Proc.* 30:1001-1010 (1971).

Wetzel, B. K., S. S. Spicer, and S. H. Wollman. Changes in fine structure and acid phosphatase localization in rat thyroid cells following thyrotropin administration. *J. Cell Biol.* 25:593-618 (1965).

Whaley, W. G. Proposals concerning replication of the Golgi apparatus. In *Probleme der Biologischen Reduplication*, pp. 340-371, P. Sitte Ed., Spring, Berlin-Heidelberg-N. Y. (1966).

Whaley, W. G. The Golgi apparatus. In *The Biological Basis of Medicine*, Vol. 1, pp. 179-208, E. E. Bittar and N. Bittar, Eds., Academic Press, N. Y. (1968).

Whaley, W. G., M. Dauwalder, and J. E. Kephart. Assembly, continuity, and exchanges in certain cytoplasmic membrane systems. In *Origin and Continuity of Cell Organelles*, Vol. 2, pp. 1-45, J. Reinert and H. Ursprung, Eds., Springer-Verlag, N. Y. (1971).

Whaley, W. G., M. Dauwalder, and J. E. Kephart. Golgi apparatus: Influence on cell surfaces. *Science* 175:596-599 (1972).

Wheby, M. S. and L. G. Jones. Role of transferrin in iron absorption. *J. Clin. Invest.* 42:1007-1015 (1963).

Whedon, G. D. Effects of high calcium intakes on bones, blood and soft tissue: relationship of calcium intake to balance in osteoporosis. *Fed. Proc.* 18:1112-1118 (1959).

Wheeldon, L. W. and A. L. Lehninger. Energy-linked synthesis and decay of membrane proteins in isolated rat liver mitochondria. *Biochemistry* 5:3533-3545 (1966).

White, L. W. and B. R. Landau. Sugar transport and fructose metabolism in human intestine *in vitro*. *J. Clin. Invest.* 44:1200-1213 (1965).

Whitehead, R. G. Hydroxyproline creatinine ratio as an index of nutritional status and rate of growth. *Lancet* 2:567-570 (1965).

Whitehead, R. G. and R. F. A. Dean. Serum amino acids in kwashiorkor. I. Relationship to clinical condition. *Amer. J. Clin. Nutr.* 14:313-319 (1964).

Whiting, M. G. and R. M. Leverton. Reliability of dietary appraisal: Comparisons between laboratory analysis and calculation from tables of food values. *Amer. J. Pub. Health.* 50:815-823 (1960).

Whittaker, V. P. and M. N. Sheridan. The morphology and acetylcholine content of isolated cerebral cortical synaptic vesicles. *J. Neurochem.* 12:363-372 (1965).

Whittam, R. The molecular mechanisms of active transport. In *The Neurosciences*, pp. 313-325, G. C. Quarton, T. Melnechuk, and F. O. Schmitt, Eds., Rockefeller Institute, N. Y. (1967).

Wicks, W. D. Regulation of hepatic enzyme synthesis by cyclic AMP. *Ann. N. Y. Acad. Sci.* 185:152-165 (1971).

Wicks, W. D., C. A. Barnett, and J. B. McKibbin. Interaction between hormones and cyclic AMP in regulating specific hepatic enzyme synthesis. *Fed. Proc.* 33:1105-1111 (1974).

Widdowson, E. M. Nutritional individuality. *Proc. Nutr. Soc.* 21:121-128 (1962).

Widdowson, E. M. Early nutrition and later development. In *Diet and Bodily Constitution*, G. E. W. Wolstenholme, Ed., Little, Brown and Co., Boston (1964).

Widdowson, E. M. Chemical analysis of the body. In *Human Body Composition*, Josef Brozek, Ed., Pergamon Press, Oxford (1965).

Widdowson, E. M. Harmony of growth. *Lancet* 1:901-905 (1970).

Widdowson, E. M. and J. W. T. Dickerson. Chemical composition of the body. In *Mineral Metabolism*, Vol. II, Part A, pp. 1-247, C. L. Comar and F. Bronner, Eds., Academic Press, N. Y. (1964).

Widdowson, E. M., O. G. Edholm, and R. A. McCance. The food intake and energy expenditure of cadets in training. *Brit. J. Nutr.* 8:147-155 (1954).

Widdowson, E. M. and R. A. McCance. The composition of foods. Medical Research Council Special Report Series No. 297, H. M. Stationery Office, London (1960).

Widdowson, E. M. and R. A. McCance. The effect of finite periods of undernutrition at different ages on the composition and subsequent development of the rat. *Proc. Roy. Soc. B* 158:329-342 (1963).

Widdowson, E. M., R. A. McCance, and C. M. Spray. The chemical composition of the human body. *Clin. Sci.* 10:113-125 (1951).

Wiese, H. F., A. E. Hansen, and D. J. D. Adams. Essential fatty acids in infant nutrition. I. Linoleic acid requirement in terms of serum di, tri and tetraenoic acid levels. *J. Nutr.* 66:345-360 (1958).

Wildman, S. G., T. Hongladarom, and S. I. Honda. Chloroplasts and mitochondria in living plant cells. *Science* 138:434-435 (1962).

Wilhelmj, C. M., J. L. Bollman, and G. C. Mann. Studies on the physiology of the liver. XVII. The effect of the removal of the liver on the specific dynamic action of amino acids adminstered intravenously. *Amer. J. Physiol.* 87:497-509 (1928).

Willcock, E. G. and F. G. Gowland Hopkins. The importance of individual amino acids in metabolism. Observations of the effect of adding tryptophane to a dietary in which zein is the sole nitrogenous constituent. *J. Physiol.* 35:88-102 (1906-7).

Williams, C. D. A nutritional disease of childhood associated with a maize diet. *Arch. Dis. Childhood* 8:423-433 (1933).

Williams, G. A., E. Bowser, W. J. Henderson, and F. Uzgiries. Effects of vitamin D and cortisone on intestinal absorption of calcium in the rat. *Proc. Soc. Exp. Biol. Med.* 106:664-666 (1961).

Williams, M. A. and G. E. Scheier. Effect of methyl arachidonate supplementation on the fatty acid composition of livers of pyridoxine-deficient rats. *J. Nutr.* 74:9-15 (1961).

Williams, R. J. *Biochemical Individuality: The Basis for the Genotrophic Concept.* Wiley, N. Y. (1956).

Williams, R. J., J. H. Truesdail, H. H. Weinstock, E. Rohrmann, C. M. Lyman, and C. H. McBurney. Pantothenic acid. II. Its concentration and purification from liver. *J. Amer. Chem. Soc.* 60:2719-2723 (1938).

Williams, R. R. *Toward the Conquest of Beriberi.* Harvard University Press, Cambridge, Mass., (1961).

Williams, R. R. and J. K. Cline. Synthesis of vitamin B_1. *J. Amer. Chem. Soc.* 58:1504-1505 (1936).

Williams, R. R., H. L. Mason, B. F. Smith, and R. M. Wilder. Induced thiamine deficiency and the thiamine requirement of man. *Arch. Int. Med.* 69:721-738 (1942).

Wills, L. The nature of the hemopoietic factor in Marmite. *Lancet* 224:1283-1286 (1933).

Wills, V. G. and J. C. Waterlow. The death rate in the age group 1-4 years as an index of malnutrition. *J. Trop. Pediat.* 3:167 (1958).

Wilmanns, W. Effects of amethopterin treatment on thymidylate synthesis in human leucocytes and bone marrow cells. *Ann. N. Y. Acad. Sci.* 186:365-371 (1971).

Wilson, C. S., A. E. Schaefer, W. J. Darby, E. B. Bridgeforth, W. N. Pearson, G. F. Combs, E. C. Letherwood, Jr., J. C. Greene, L. J. Teply, I. C. Plough, W. J. McGanity, D. B. Hand, Z. I. Kertesz, and C. W. Woodruff. A review of methods used in nutrition surveys conducted by the interdepartmental committee on nutrition for national defense (ICNND). *Amer. J. Clin. Nutr.* 15:29-44 (1964).

Wilson, D. E. Prostaglandins and the gastrointestinal tract. *Prostaglandins* 1:281-293 (1972).

Wilson, R. P. Absence of ascorbic acid synthesis in channel catfish, *Ictalurus punctatus* and blue catfish, *Ictalurus frucatus. Comp. Biochem. Physiol.* 46B:635-638 (1973).

Wilson, T. H. *Intestinal Absorption.* W. B. Saunders Company, Philadelphia (1962).

Wilson, T. H. Intestinal absorption of vitamin B_{12}. *Physiologist* 6:11-26 (1963).

Wilson, T. H. Intrinsic factor and B_{12} absorption—a problem in cell physiology. *Nutr. Rev.* 23:33-35 (1965).

Wilson, T. H. and B. R. Landau. Specificity of sugar transport by the intestine of the hamster. *Amer. J. Physiol.* 198:99-102 (1960).

Wilson, T. H. and D. W. Wilson. Studies *in vitro* of digestion and absorption of pyrimidine nucleotides by the intestine. *J. Biol. Chem.* 233:1544-1547 (1958).

Wilson, T. H. and G. Wiseman. The use of sacs of everted small intestine for the study of the transference of substances from the mucosal to the serosal surface. *J. Physiol.* 123:116-125 (1954).

Winegrad, S. Intracellular calcium movements of frog skeletal muscle during recovery from tetanus. *J. Gen. Physiol.* 51:65-83 (1968).

Wingo, W. J. and J. Awapara. Decarboxylation of *L*-glutamic acid by brain. *J. Biol. Chem.* 187:267-271 (1950).

Winick, M. Cellular growth of the placenta as an indication of abnormal fetal growth. In *Diagnosis and Treatment of Fetal Disorders*, pp. 83-101, Proc. Internatl. Symp. on Diagnosis and Treatment of Disorders Affecting the Intrauterine Patient, K. Adamson, Ed., Springer-Verlag, N. Y. (1968).

Winick, M. Nutrition and nerve cell growth. *Fed. Proc.* 29:1510-1515 (1970).

Winick, M., J. A. Brasel, and P. Rosso. Nutrition and cell growth. In *Nutrition and Development*, Vol. 1, pp. 49-97, M. Winick, Ed., Wiley, N. Y. (1972).

Winick, M., A. Coscia, and A. Noble. Cellular growth in human placenta. I. Normal placental growth. *Pediat.* 39:248-251 (1967).

Winick, M. and A. Noble. Quantitative changes in DNA, RNA, and protein during prenatal and postnatal growth in the rat. *Develop. Biol.* 12:451-466 (1965).

Winick, M. and A. Noble. Cellular response in rats during malnutrition at various ages. *J. Nutr.* 89:300-306 (1966).

Winick, M. and P. Rosso. The effect of severe early malnutrition on cellular growth of human brain. *Pediat. Res.* 3:181-184 (1969).

Winkler, H., A. D. Smith, F. DuBois, and H. van den Bosch. The positional specificity of lysosomal phospholipase A activities. *Biochem. J.* 105:38C-40C (1967).

Winkler, H. H. Localization of the atractyloside-sensitive nucleotide binding sites in rat liver mitochondria. *Biochim. Biophys. Acta* 189:152-161 (1969).

Winkler, H. H., F. L. Bygrave, and A. L. Lehninger. Characterization of the atractyloside-sensitive adenine nucleotide transport system in rat liver mitochondria. *J. Biol. Chem.* 243:20-28 (1968).

Winkler, H. H. and A. L. Lehninger. The atractyloside-sensitive nucleotide binding site in a membrane preparation from rat liver mitochondria. *J. Biol. Chem.* 243:3000-3008 (1968).

Wischnitzer, S. The nuclear envelope: its ultrastructure and functional significance. *Endeavor* 33:137-142 (1974).

Wiseman, G. Absorption of protein digestion products. In *Intestinal Absorption*, Biomembranes, Vol. 4A, pp. 363-481, D. H. Smyth, Ed., Plenum Press, London (1974).

Wiseman, G. Active transport of amino acids by sacs of everted small intestine of the golden hamster (*Mesocricetus auratus*). *J. Physiol.* 133:626-630 (1956).

Wisniewski, H., M. L. Shelanski, and R. D. Terry. Effects of mitotic spindle inhibitors on neurotubules and neurofilaments in anterior horn cells. *J. Cell Biol.* 38:224-229 (1968).

Wiss, O. and H. Gloor. Absorption, distribution, storage, and metabolites of vitamins K and related quinones. *Vitamins Hormones* 24:575-586 (1966).

Witten, P. W. and R. T. Holman. Polyethenoid fatty acid metabolism. VI. Effect of pyridoxine on essential fatty acid conversions. *Arch. Biochem. Biophys.* 41:266-273 (1952).

Woese, C. R. *The Genetic Code. The Molecular Basis for Genetic Expression*. Harper and Row, N. Y. (1967).

Wolf, G. and L. DeLuca. Recent studies on some metabolic functions of vitamin A. In *The Fat-Soluble Vitamins*, pp. 257-265, H. F. DeLuca and J. W. Suttie, Eds., The University of Wisconsin Press, Madison (1970).

Wolf, S. *The Stomach*. Oxford University Press, N. Y. (1965).

Wollman, S. H. Secretion of thyroid hormones. In *Lysosomes in Biology and Pathology*, Vol. 2, pp. 483-512, J. T. Dingle and H. B. Fell, Eds., *Frontiers of Biology*, Vol. 14A, Wiley-Interscience, N. Y. (1969).

Woodrow, I. L. and J. M. de Man. Distribution of *trans*-unsaturated fatty acids in milk fat. *Biochim. Biophys. Acta* 152:472-478 (1968).

Woodward, R. B. Recent advances in the chemistry of natural products. *Pure Appl. Chem.* 17:519-547 (1968).

Woodward, R. B. Recent advances in the chemistry of natural products. *Pure Appl. Chem.* 25:283-304 (1971).

Woolley, D. W. Identification of the mouse antialopecia factor. *J. Biol. Chem.* 139:29-34 (1941).

Woolley, D. W. Some new aspects of the relationship of chemical structure to biological activity. *Science* 100:579-583 (1944a).

Woolley, D. W. Production of a scurvy-like condition of guinea pigs with glucoascorbic acid, and its prevention with ascorbic acid. *Fed. Proc.* 3:97A (1944b).

Woolley, D. W. Production of nicotinic acid deficiency with 3-acetyl-pyridine the ketone analogue of nicotinic acid. *J. Biol. Chem.* 157:445-459 (1945).

Woolley, D. W. *Metabolic Inhibitors.* Academic Press, N. Y. (1963).

Woolley, D. W. and L. O. Krampitz. Production of a scurvy-like condition by feeding of a compound structurally related to ascorbic acid. *J. Exp. Med.* 78:333-339 (1943).

World Health Organization. Expert Committee on medical assessment of nutritional status. WHO Technical Report Series No. 258 (1963).

Worthington, C. R. X-ray studies on nerve and photoreceptors. *Ann. N. Y. Acad. Sci.* 195:293-308 (1972).

Wostmann, B. S., P. L. Knight, L. L. Keeley, and D. F. Kan. Metabolism and function of thiamine and naphthoquinones in germfree and conventional rats. *Fed. Proc.* 22:120-124 (1963).

Wright, L. D., E. L. Cresson, and C. A. Driscoll. Biotin derivatives in human urine. *Proc. Soc. Exp. Biol. Med.* 91:248-252 (1956).

Wuest, H. M. and D. Perlman. Vitamin B_{12}. III. Industrial preparation and preparation. In *The Vitamins,* Vol. II, pp. 139-144, W. H. Sebrell, Jr. and R. S. Harris, Eds., Academic Press, N. Y. (1968).

Wurzberger, R. J. and J. M. Musacchia. Subcellular distribution and aggregation of bovine adrenal tyrosine hydroxylase. *J. Pharmacol. Exp. Ther.* 177:155-167 (1971).

Yagi, K., T. Nagatsu, I. Nagatsu-Ishibashi, and A. Ohashi. Migration of C^{14}-labelled riboflavin into rat-tissues. *J. Biochem.* (Tokyo) 59:313-315 (1966).

Yamamoto, T. On the thickness of the unit membrane. *J. Cell Biol.* 17:413-421 (1963).

Yang, C. S. and D. B. McCormick. Degradation and excretion of riboflavin in the rat. *J. Nutr.* 93:445-453 (1967).

Yanofsky, C. Gene structure and protein structure. *Harvey Lect.* 61:145-168 (1967).

Yĉas, M. *The Biological Code,* Frontiers of Biology, Vol. 12, North-Holland Publishing Company, Amsterdam (1969).

Young, C. M. A comparison of dietary study methods. 2. Dietary history vs. seven-day record vs. 24-hr. recall. *J. Amer. Diet. Ass.* 28:218-221 (1952a).

Young, C. M., J. Blondin, R. Tensuan, and J. H. Fryer. Body composition studies of "older" women thirty to seventy years of age. *Ann. N. Y. Acad. Sci.* 110:589-607 (1963a).

Young, C. M., F. W. Chalmers, H. N. Church, M. M. Clayton, R. E. Tucker, A. W. Wertz, and W. D. Foster. A comparison of dietary study methods. I. Dietary history vs. seven-day-record. *J. Amer. Diet. Ass.* 28:124-128 (1952).

Young, C. M., M. E. K. Martin, R. Tensuan, and J. Blondin. Predicting specific gravity and body fatness in young women. *J. Amer. Diet. Ass.* 40:102-107 (1962).

Young, C. M., S. S. Scanlan, H. S. Im, and L. Lutwak. Effect on body composition and other parameters in obese young men of carbohydrate level of reduction diet. *Amer. J. Clin. Nutr.* 24:290-296 (1971).

Young, C. M., R. S. Tensuan, F. Sault, and F. Holmes. Estimating body fat of normal young women. *J. Amer. Diet. Ass.* 42:409-413 (1963b).

Young, E. G. Dietary standards. In *Nutrition, An Advanced Treatise*, Vol. II, G. H. Beaton and E. W. McHenry, Eds., Academic Press, N. Y. (1964).

Young, H. B. Body composition, culture, and sex: Two comments. In *Human Body Composition, Approaches and Applications*, J. Brozek, Ed., Pergamon Press, Oxford (1965).

Young, J. R. *An Experimental Inquiry into Principles of Nutrition and the Digestive Process, 1803*. University of Illinois Press, Urbana (1959).

Young, V. R., M. A. Hussein, E. Murray, and N. S. Scrimshaw. Plasma tryptophan response curve and its relation to tryptophan requirements in young adult men. *J. Nutr.* 101:45-60 (1971).

Young, V. R. and N. S. Scrimshaw. Endogenous nitrogen metabolism and plasma free amino acids in young adults given a "protein-free" diet. *Brit. J. Nutr.* 22:9-20 (1968).

Young, V. R., K. Tontisirin, L. Ozalp, F. Lakshmanan, and N. S. Scrimshaw. Plasma amino acid response curve and amino acid requirements in young men: Valine and lysine. *J. Nutr.* 102:1159-1169 (1972).

Yunghans, W. N., T. W. Keenan, and D. J. Morré. Isolation of a Golgi apparatus-rich fraction from rat liver. III. Lipid and protein composition. *Exp. Mol. Path.* 12:36-45 (1970).

Zachman, R. D., P. E. Dunagin, Jr., and J. A. Olson. Formation and enterohepatic circulation of metabolites of retinol and retinoic acid in bile duct-cannulated rats. *J. Lipid Res.* 7:3-9 (1966).

Zaklama, M. S., M. K. Gabr, S. El Maraghy, and V. N. Patwardhan. Liver vitamin A in protein-calorie malnutrition. *Amer. J. Clin. Nutr.* 25:412-418 (1972).

Zakrzewski, S. F. Mechanism of reduction of folate and dihydrofolate. In *Biochemical Aspects of Antimetabolites and of Drug Hydroxylation*, Fed. Eur. Biochem. Soc. Vol. 16, pp. 49-64, D. Shugar, Ed., Academic Press, N. Y. (1969).

Zalkin, H. and A. L. Tappel. Studies of the mechanism of vitamin E action. IV. Lipide peroxidation in the vitamin E-deficient rabbit. *Arch. Biochem. Biophys.* 88:113-117 (1960).

Zamenhof, S., E. Van Marthens, and L. Grauel. DNA (cell number) and protein in neonatal rat brain: alteration by timing of maternal dietary protein restriction. *J. Nutr.* 101:1265-1270 (1971).

Zile, M., R. J. Emerick, and H. F. DeLuca. Identification of 13-cis retinoic acid in tissue extracts and its biological activity in rats. *Biochim. Biophys. Acta* 141:639-641 (1967).

Zilversmit, D. B. Formation and transport of chylomicrons. *Fed. Proc.* 26:1599-1605 (1967).

Ziporin, Z. Z., W. T. Nunes, R. C. Powell, P. P. Waring, and H. E. Sauberlich. Excretion of thiamine and its metabolites in the urine of young adult males receiving restricted intakes of the vitamin. *J. Nutr.* 85:287-296 (1965).

Zull, J. E., E. Czarnowska-Misztal and H. F. DeLuca. Actomycin D inhibition of vitamin D action. *Science* 149:182-184 (1965).

Zuntz, N. Ueber den Stoffverbrauch des Hundes bei Muskelarbeit. Pfluger's Archiv f. d. ges. Physiol. 68:191-211 (1897). Cited in Benedict, F. G. and E. P. Cathcart, *Muscular Work, A Metabolic Study with Special Reference to the Efficiency of the Human Body as a Machine*, p. 33. Carnegie Institute of Washington, Washington, D. C. (1913).

Zurier, R. B., R. G. Campbell, S. A. Hashim, and T. Van Itallie. Enrichment of depot fat with odd and even numbered medium-chain fatty acids. *Amer. J. Physiol.* 212:291-294 (1967).

Zweifach, B. W. *Functional Behavior of the Microcirculation*. Charles C. Thomas, Springfield (1961).

index

Absorption, 230-297
  amino acids, 238-244
  ascorbic acid, 252-254
  calcium, 277-284
  carbohydrates, 235-238
  cholesterol, 249-251
  electrolytes, 276-277
  fat, 244-249
  folacin, 255-256
  iron, 284-296
  minerals, 277-296
  myo-inositol, 261-262
  nucleic acids, 251-252
  pyridoxine, 255
  riboflavin, 254
  sites in small intestine, 233
  vitamin A, 262-271
  vitamin B_{12}, 256-261
  vitamin D, 271-274
  vitamin E, 274-275
  vitamin K, 275-276
  water, 276-277
Accessory food factors, vitamins, 15
Acetoacetate, 53
Acetoacetyl CoA, and ketone body
    formation, 576-578
Acetyl amino sugars, structure, 24
Acetylcholine, 183
  in nerve function, 698-700
Acetyl CoA, 86, 114
  in fatty acid synthesis, 466-467
  in tricarboxylic acid cycle, 515-518
Acetyl CoA carboxylase, 131
β-*N*-Acetylglucosaminidase, 535
  in lysosomal membrane, 537
3-Acetyl pyridine, 105
4-Acetyl pyridine, 105
Aconitase, 193
Actin, 647, 655-656
Active acetate, 114
Activity, energy costs of, 837-839
  as defined by FAO/WHO, 921
Actomyosin, 656-657
Acyl glycerols, 41-42
Adenine, 72, 75-76, 78-79
  structure, 73
Adenosine diphosphate, *see* ADP
Adenosine monophosphate, *see* AMP
Adenosine phosphates, *see* ATP; ADP;
    and AMP
Adenosine triphosphate, *see* ATP
Adenyl cyclase, 74
Adenylic acid, 72
Adenosine-3', 5'-monophosphate, *see* AMP
Adenosine triphosphate, *see* ATP
ADP, 21

Adipose cells, 709-726
  brown adipose cells, 709, 720-725
    see also Fat cells, brown
  white adipose cells, 709, 710-720
    see also Fat cells, white
Adult growth, 856
Alanine, cycle, 576-577
  formula, 50
β-Alanine, 113
Albumin(s), 59
  guidelines for interpretation of serum
    levels, 951
  synthesis in protein-calorie malnutrition,
    582
Alcohol dehydrogenase, 97, 206
Alcoholic withdrawal and magnesium, 187
Alcoholism, thiamin absorption in, 253
Aldehyde oxidase, 197
  and molybdenum, 202
Aldosterone and sodium metabolism, 188
Amethopterin (Metrotrexate, MTX), 121
Alkaline phosphatase, 228
Alopecia, 177
Amine oxidation, 108
Amino acid(s), 49-53
  absorption, 238-244
  basic structure, 52
  bidirectional flux across intestinal mucosa,
    240
  carrier system in absorption, 241
  classification, 52
  deficiency, 61
  functions, 53
  glucogenic, 53, 519
  intestinal transport system, 242
  ketogenic, 53, 519
  oxidation in mitochondria, 519-523
  oxidative pathways, 520
  pool, 239
  preferential catabolism in heart, 665
  purified, 17
  relative absorption rates, 243
  requirements, and plasma amino acid
    levels, 862-863
    of adults, 860
    of infants, 859
    of young women, 861
  score, 863-864
  sodium, role in transport of, 243
Aminoacyl synthetase, 447

Aminoethanol, 43
6-Aminonicotinamide, 105
7-Aminonicotinamide, 105
Amino acid oxidases, 93
2-Amino-3-carboxymuconate semialdehyde,
  101
Aminoimidazole carboxamide (AIC), 102
Aminopterin, 121
Aminopeptidase(s), 224-225, 228
Amino sugars, structure, 24
Ammonia, in urea synthesis, 584
  toxicity and nitrogen excretion, 331
AMP, 21, 74-75
Amniotic fluid, weight gain during
  gestation, 785-787
Amprolium, 89
Amylase(s), 217, 226-227
Anemia, and vitamin E, 167
  iron-deficiency, 194
  megaloblastic, 120, 127
  pernicious, 128
  vitamin B_6-responsive, 110
Angiotensin, in sodium and water balance,
  329-330
Animal feeding experiments, early studies,
  15
Anisotropic bands in muscle, 647
Annulus, 394-395
Anthropometry, 761-765
  age-independent measurements, 761
  in normal and obese children, 809
Anticodon and wobble hypothesis, 443
Antidiuretic hormone (ADH), 327
Antimetabolites, definition, 82
Antioxidants and vitamin E deficiency, 164
Appetite, and energy expenditure, 850
Arabinose, 20
Arachidic acid, formula, 32
Arachidonic acid, 33-34
Arginase, 197
Arginine, in creatine synthesis, 583
  formula, 51
  in urea synthesis, 584
Arthritis, rheumatoid, 561
Ascorbic acid, 134-139
  absorption, 252
  active transport and Na^+, 252
  in collagen synthesis, 619
  and the common cold, 138
  antagonists, 139

assay, 136
biochemical function, 136-138
blood levels, and dietary intake, 885-888
    use in nutrition surveys, 948
chemistry, 135
deficiency, and behavior, 880
    and bone metabolism, 644
    dietary intake and clinical evidences
        of, 878
    symptoms of, 83
excretion, 138
FAO standards, 929
guidelines for interpretation of serum
        levels, 951
in iron absorption, 293
load test, 890
metabolites, 138-139
Recommended Dietary Allowance, 900,
        907-908
structure, 135
Aspartic acid, formula, 51
    in urea synthesis, 584
Astrocytes, 669
ATP, 21, 74
ATPase, 186
Avidin, 129, 134
Axon, 670, 672-677

Balance studies, 7, 819-822
Basal metabolism and body surface area,
        827-831
    definition, 827
    effect, of age, 831
        of fever, 834
        of hyperthyrodism, 834
        of sleep, 848
        of sex, 832-833
        of weight, 832-833
    factors affecting, 831-834
    and nutritional state, 834
    and race, 833
Basic Four, 898
Behavior, and early malnutrition, 754-756
Behenic acid, formula, 32
Beriberi, 14, 15
Betaine and choline deficiency, 175
Bile acids, 47
    in lipid absorption, 245
    synthesis in hepatocytes, 592
Bile pigment, formation of, 592-593

Bile salts and gastric ulceration, 222
    in absorption of carotenoids and vitamin
        A, 267
    in activation of pancreatic hydrolase, 263
    and lipid digestion, 221
Bimolecular leaflet, 358
Biochemical individuality, 309
Biocytin, 131
Biological value (BV), 865
Biopterin, 121
Biotin, 129-134
    antagonists, 134
    assay, 130
    biochemical function, 130-133
    chemistry, 129-130
    deficiency, 133
    estimated needs, 915
    excretion, 133
    metabolites, 133-134
    structure, 130
Biotin sulfone, 134
Bisnorbiotin, 133
Blood, increase during gestation, 787
Blood coagulation, calcium, role of, 183
    vitamin K, role of, 171
Blood-group substances, 67
Body cell mass, 760
    definition, 771
    gross composition of, 773
Body composition, 757-813
    of adult, 795
    and age, 779-780
    and body density, 765-769
    calculation by simultaneous multiple
        isotope dilution, 769
        from body potassium, 771
    changes during the life cycle, 777-804
    chemical analysis of, 759-761
    and exercise, 810-813
    fat-free basis, 777
    in fetal development, 782-785
    of infant, 794
    of lactating female, 790
    of newborn, 781, 794
    in obesity, 806-810
    in pregnancy, 787-790
    of premature infant, 784
    of preschool child, 795
    [40] potassium analysis of, 774
    ratios and derivations of body

components, 770
and skinfold thickness, 762-765
and weight change, 804-810
Body fat, and age, 802-803
calculation from body water, 765-771
percent of body weight, 770
and sex, 802-803
see also Adipose cell
Body fluid compartments, 316
Body heat loss, 841
and energy expenditure, 824
Body size, and energy requirements for
activity, 837
Body solids, percent of body weight, 770
Body surface area, and basal metabolism,
827-831
calculation of, 829-831
Body volume, calculation of, 763-765
measurement, by air displacement, 769
by helium displacement method, 768
Body water, and age, 796-799
and calculation of body fat, 765
determination of, 769
in pregnancy, 789
and sex, 803-804
Body weight, and composition, 804-810
Bone, calcification, 623
cells, 616-645
composition of, 617-619
effect of, parathyroid hormone on, 631-
636
thyrocalcitonin on, 638-639
vitamin D on, 639-643
fluid compartments of, 624
formation and calcium balance, 628
growth of, 625-629
Haversian system, 627
loss of, 629-630
maturation of, 623
mineral deposition in, 623-625
resorption of, 556-559, 625
and lysosomal enzymes, 626-627
surface area of, 624
Boron, content of fat-free tissue in adults,
760
Brain, cellular growth pattern, 740-742
effects of malnutrition, 751-752
Buccal smears, use in nutrition surveys, 948
Butyric acid, 34
formula, 32

Cadmium, antagonism to copper absorption,
296
and synthesis of $1, 25(OH)_2 D_3$, 641
Calciferol-25-hydroxylase, 158
Calcitonin, 528, 636
and vitamin D toxicity, 160
see also Thyrocalcitonin
Calcium, 182-184
absorption, 277-284
effect of, dietary calcium, 278
lactose, 278
vitamin D, 279-284
and parathyroid hormone (PTH), 283-284
and protein intake, 870
role of NaCl, 282
adaptation to intake, 869
balance data, 869
balance and bone formation, 628
in blood, 182-631
body content, 182, 795
in cell nucleus, 401
determination of requirements, 868
FAO standards, 926-927
fat-free tissue content, 760
functions, 182-183
in human fetus, 784
and ^{90} strontium, 183-184
maintenance of blood levels, 631, 633-
635
ratio to phosphorus, 184
Recommended Dietary Allowance, 900,
905-906
release of neurotransmitters, role in, 689-
691
retention and protein intake, 869-871
role in muscle contraction, 661-662
and IF-B_{12} complex, 258
transport in mitochondria, 527-529
turnover in bone, 634-635
Calcium-binding protein (CaBP), 279
Calcium cation pump, 281
Caloric equivalents in calorimetric studies,
845
Caloric value of foodstuffs, 9, 850-854
Calorigenic effect of food, 834-837
and energy requirement for synthesis of
ATP, 836-837
Calorimetry, 839-847
development of, 5, 10-11
direct, 843

indirect, 843-847
principles of, 823-825
Capric acid, formula, 32
Caprylic acid, formula, 32
Caproic acid, formula, 32
Carbamyl phosphate, 132
  in urea synthesis, 584
Carbohydrate(s), 19-30
  absorption, 235-238
  classification, 19
  definition, 19
  digestion, 216-221
  disaccharides, 19, 23-25
  estimated needs, 914
  heteropolysaccharides, 26
  hexoses, 22-24
  homopolysaccharides, 26
  lactose, 20
  monosaccharides, 19, 20-22
  monosaccharide derivatives, 23-24
  mucopolysaccharides, 27-30
  oligosaccharides, 19, 23-25
  pentoses, 21-22
  polysaccharides, 19, 26-27
  starch, 19
  sucrose, 19-20
Carbohydrate metabolism index, 891
Carbonates, in iron absorption, 293
Carbonic anhydrase, 60, 197, 206
  bone resorption, role in, 627
Carboxypeptidases, 224, 227
Carotene, blood levels, use in nutrition
    surveys, 948
  guidelines for interpretation of plasma
    levels, 951
  serum levels and nutritional status, 888
Carotene cleavage enzyme, 263
β-carotene, absorption, 263
  cleavage to vitamin A, 143, 262
β-carotene-15-15' dioxygenase, 263
  see also Carotene cleavage enzyme
Carotenoids, absorption and dietary fat,
    268
  vitamin A activity, 144-145
Casein, digestion, 223
Catecholamines, 74
  in nerve function, 692-698
  storage, 695-696
  synthesis, 693-694
Celiac disease and digestive

  enzyme deficiency, 218
Cell(s), autophagy of, 559-560
  coat, 27, 368
  communication, 384
  determination of number and size, 734
  differentiation, 566
  ependymal in central nervous system, 669
  growth, 729-758
    fetal, 738
    phases of, 735-738
    placental, 738-739
  hyperplasia, 399
  hypertrophy, 399
  inclusions, 350
  junctions, 369
  number and fetal growth, 738
  organelle(s), turnover of, 559-560
  Schwann, 669
  structure, 348-350
  web, 425
Cellulose, 26
Cephalins, 43
Ceramides, 68-69
Cerebrosides, 68
Ceroid pigmentation, 166
Ceruloplasmin, 67, 196-197, 297
  iron metabolism, role in, 193-194
Chastek paralysis, 90
Chemical maturity, definition, 778
  and physiological development at birth,
    778
Chemical score, 863
  see also Amino acid score
Chloride, body content, 795
  fat-free tissue, content, 760
  functions, 190
  distribution in body, 189
Chloride shift, 189-190
Cholecalciferol, 154
  structure, 155
  see also Vitamin D
Cholecystokinin, 215-216, 228
Cholecystokinin-pancreozymin, 216, 224,
    227
Cholesterol, absorption, 249-251
  and absorption of fatty acids, 249
  degradation, 587-592
  endogenous, 249
  exogenous, 249
  factors influencing hepatic synthesis in

the rat, 590
in lymph, 250
in miscelles, 222
in myelin sheath, 679
serum, and coronary artery disease, 48
and unsaturated fats, 590-591
structure, 46
synthesis, 46, 587-592
Cholesterol esterase, 221, 227, 249
Choline, 43, 174-176
deficiency, 174-175
estimated needs, 915
structure, 174
Choline acetylase, 698
Chondroitin, 29
Chondroitin A and vitamin A toxicity, 160
Chondroitin sulfates, 29
Chromium, 207
absorption, 297
Chromosomal puffs, 420
Chromosomes, 398
Chromatin, 395, 398-400
Chromoprotein(s), 60
Chylomicrons, 71, 247-248
Chyme, 217
Chymodenin, 224
Chymotripsin, 227
Chymotripsinogen, 224, 227
synthesis in response to diet, 217
Cisternae, 472
Cis-trans isomerism, 37
Citral, 153
Citric acid, energy yield, 853
Citric acid cycle, 514
see also Tricarboxylic acid cycle
Citrovorum factor, 116, 118
Citrulline, 52
Clearing factor, see Lipoprotein lipase
Cobalt, 122-123
estimated needs, 914
fat-free tissue content, 760
functions, 197
Codons, 436
and the Adaptor Hypothesis, 440
Coenzyme, definition, 81
Coenzyme A, 113-114
Coenzyme I, see NAD
Coenzyme II, see NADP
Collagen, 29, 60, 67, 197
in bone formation, 617

cross-linking in bone, 621-622
synthesis, 619-622
and ascorbic acid, 136
and iron, 194
Collagenase, 227
Copper, 196-198
absorption, 296
body content, 196, 795
body depletion, 198
deficiency, in animals, 196-197
estimated needs, 914
fat-free tissue content, 760
functions, 197
in blood, 196, 297
serum level and disease states, 198
Coprophagy, 300
Cori Cycle, 461
Coronary artery disease, 48
Corticosterone, 47
Cortisone, 47
Corrinoids, 122
Creatine synthesis in hepatocytes, 582-583
Creatine kinase in muscle contraction, 663
Creatine phosphate in muscle contraction, 662
Creatinine, excretion, as predictor of muscle mass, 773-774
use in nutrition surveys, 948
guidelines for interpretation of urinary levels, 952
reabsorption, by kidney, 332
Cristae and cellular respiratory activity, 494
Crypts of Lieberkuhn, 232
Cyanocobalamin, see vitamin B_{12}
Cyclic AMP, 74-75
blood glucose regulation, role in, 574
calcium absorption, role in, 284
catabolite repression, role in, 453-456
epinephrine action, role in, 325
fat hydrolysis, role in, 717-720
functions, 75
glucose transport in adipose cell, role in, 715
glycogenesis, role in, 453
glycogenolysis, role in, 453
insulin action in adipose cells, role in, 714-717
repression of protein synthesis, role in, 453-456
structure, 75

Cyclopentanoperhydrophenanthrene nucleus, 46
Cycloserine, 111
Cystathionase, 110
Cystathionine synthetase, 110
Cystathionuria, 110
Cysteine, 53
  formula, 50
  oxidation-reduction reactions, role in, 191
Cystine, formula, 50
  oxidation-reduction actions, role in, 191
Cystinuria, and absorption of amino acids, 241
Cytidylic acid, 72
Cytochromes, 60
  in mitochondrial membrane, 502
Cytochrome oxidase, 197
Cytoplasmic matrix, 350, 424-427
  composition, 426
  structure, 425-426
Cytosine, 72-73, 75-76, 78-79

Deamination, 108
  oxidative, 521
  and urea synthesis, 583-584
Decarboxylation, 108
7-Dehydrocholesterol, 47
Dehydroascorbic acid, 135
Dehydroretinol (Vitamin A$_2$), 142
Dendrites, 670
Dental caries, and fluoride, 203
  and phosphates, 185
  and phytates, 177
Deoxycorticosterone, 47
2-Deoxy-D-ribose, 21
4-Deoxypyridoxine, 111
Deoxyribonuclease, 227
Deoxyribonucleic acid, see DNA
Deoxyribose, 21, 75, 79
Dermatan sulfate, 29
Desamino-NAD, 102
Desmosome(s), 369-370, 372, 385, 425
Desulfhydration, 108
Desthiobiotin, 134
Desthioisobiotin, 134
Development, periods in human, 732-733
  stages, 730-734
Dextrin, digestion, 226
Dextrose, 20
  see Glucose

Diacyl glycerol, 41
Dicoumarol, 173
Dictyosome, 473
Dietary standards, 895-932
  British, 913, 918-920
  Canadian, 913, 916-917
  FAO/WHO standards, 920-931
  history, 896-897
  Recommended Dietary Allowances, 899-913
  uses of, 897-898
Dietary surveys, 937-942
  calculation and interpretation of nutrient intake, 942-947
  comparison of analysed and calculated intake, 943-946
  guide to interpretation of nutrient intake, 944-945
  household food consumption, 937-939
  individual food consumption, 939-942
    24-hour recall, 940
    food record, 940
    weighed intake, 940
    diet history, 941
  physiological consumption, 939
Diethyl riboflavin, 95
Differential ultracentrifugation, 343-344
Diffusion, exchange, 374, 377-378
  facilitated, 374, 376
  simple, 374-375
Digestion, 215-230
  early studies, 9-10
  in mouth, 216, 226
  neural-hormonal relationships, 229
  in small intestine, 227-228
  source and action of enzymes, 226-227
  in stomach, 226
Diglycerides, see Diacyl glycerols
Dihydroxyacetone, 20
Dihydroxyacetone phosphate, 457
1,25-Dihydroxycholecalciferol, 157-158
  and bone resorption, 640
  regulation of synthesis, 157
  site of hydroxylation, 274
24,25-Dihydroxycholecalciferol, 158
25,26-Dihydroxycholecalciferol, 158
Diiodotyrosine, 199
Diketogulonic acid, 135-136
Dipeptidase(s), 225, 228
Disaccharides, 23-25

Disaccharidases, 228
  activity in villus cells, 217
  deficiency and carbohydrate digestion,
    218
Disease(s), demyelinating, 670
  Niemann-Pick, 679
  storage, 560
DNA, 21, 75-79
  fetal organ content, 738-739
  in mitochondria, 526
  organ content during growth, 735-736
  replication, 77, 403-408
  structure, 76
  transcription of, 411-421
DNA polymerase, 404
Dopamine in nerve function, 692-698
Dopamine-β-hydroxylase, 694
Down's syndrome, 695
DPNH-cytochrome reductase, 193

Edema, physiological adjustment in
    pregnancy, 790
Egg-white injury, 129
Elaidic acid, 37
Elastase, 227
Elastin, 60, 197, 617
Electrolyte(s), absorption, 276
  conservation, 327
Electron transport, 521-524
  and ascorbic acid, 137
  particles in mitochondria, 496
Eluate factor, 112
Embden-Meyerhof glycolytic pathway, 456-
    461
Emiocytosis, 383-384
Endocytosis, 382
Endopeptidases, 224, 227
Endoplasmic reticulum, 349, 424, 427-470
  angular or smooth, 428
  composition, 432-433
  fatty acid synthesis in, 466-467
  functions, 433-470
  glycogenesis in, 465-467
  glycolysis in, 456-461
  granular or rough, 428
  pentose phosphate shunt in, 461-465
  protein synthesis in, 434-456
  structure, 428-432
  unsaturated fatty acid synthesis in, 467-
    468

Energy, balance, 847-850
  costs for various activities, 837-839
  dietary standards for pregnant and non-
    pregnant women, 931
  effect of body weight and activity (FAO),
    922
  expenditure, components of, 824
    estimation, 848
  FAO standards, 921-923
  heat equivalent of work, 825
  Recommended Dietary Allowances, 900,
    902-904
  requirement, and activity, 837
    and calorigenic effect of food, 834
    estimation, 822-850
    factors contributing to, 826
    and heat production, 823
  value of foods, 9, 850-854
Enzyme(s), activity and vitamin require-
    ments, 891-893
  and alterations in diet, 217
  induction of, 451
  in lysosomal membrane, 534-535
  pancreatic, 217
  proteolytic, 224
  regulatory, 452
  repression, 451
Enterocrinin, 228
Enterogastrone, 215
  and gastric emptying time, 221
Epinephrine, 53, 74, 553
  in nerve function, 692-698
Ergocalciferol, structure, 155
  see also Vitamin D
Erythrocyte hemolysis test and vitamin E
    deficiency, 893
Erythrocytes, 595-615
  degradation of, 613-614
  and globin synthesis, 611-613
  and hemoglobin synthesis, 606-613
  iron incorporation in, 608-609
  maturation, 602
Erythrogenin, 598
  see also Renal erythropoietic factor (REF)
Erythropoietin, 67, 597-602
  composition of, 597
  mechanism of action, 599-602
  source of, 597
Erythropoiesis-stimulating factor, 597
  see also Erythropoietin

Erythrose, 20
Erythrulose, 20
Essential amino acids, 50-51
  identification, 16
  minimum requirements of adults, 860
  see also Amino acids
Essential fatty acids, 34-38, see also Fatty
    acids
  deficiency, 35
  discovery, 17
Estrogens, 47
Ethanolamine, 43-44
Ethoxyquin, 166
Exercise and body composition, 810-813
  energy source of, 663
Exocytosis in lysosomes, 547
Exopeptidases, 224, 227
Extracellular fluid, 316, 769
  compartmentalization, 317-319
  weight gain during gestation, 787

Fabry's disease, 69
Factorial method for estimation of nutrient
    requirements, 855-856
Factor 3, 204
Factor U, 116
FAD, structure, 93
  and dietary intake of riboflavin, 892
Fat, adult body content, 759
  consumption patterns, 48
  estimated needs, 914
Fat cell, brown, distribution in embryo, 721
  function, 722-725
  role of cAMP in metabolism of, 724-725
  structure, 720-722
Fat cell, white, calculation of cell number,
    710
  glucose transport into, 714-717
  fatty acid synthesis in, 717
  fatty acid transport into, 713-714
  lipogenesis, role of liver, 712-713
  lipolysis in, 717-720
  structure, 710-711
  triacyl glycerol synthesis in, 717-719
Fat-free body, 760, 771
  limits of hydration, 772
Fat-free solids, percent of body weight, 770
Fat-soluble vitamins, 140-173
  absorption, 262-276
  in micelles, 222

Fatty acids, 31-38
  in diet, 34
  energy yield of oxidation, 525
  free, as energy source for heart, 665
  isomers, 37
  medium chain, 222
  in myelin sheath, 679
  odd-numbered, occurrence, 34
  oxidation in mitochondria, 510-512
  saturated, naturally occurring, 32
  synthesis, 466-467
    in mammals, 469
  transport into adipose cell, 713-714
  transport, 720
  unsaturated, naturally occurring, 33
Fatty acid binding protein (FABP), 246
Fecal excretion, 299
Ferritin, 60, 193, 284
  iron binding, 287
  iron status and incorporation into
    mucosal cells, 289
  regulation of protein turnover in, 287
Ferroxidases, 197
  and iron metabolism, 193-194
Fetuin, 67
Fetus, composition of weight gain, 785
  developmental status and body com-
    position, 782-785
  growth, 782
  weight gain during gestation, 787
Fibrin, 67
Fibrinogen, 67, 171
Filtrate factor, 112
Flavin adenine dinucleotide, see FAD
Flavin mononucleotide, see FMN
Flavoproteins, 60
  in mitochondrial membrane, 502
Fluid mosaic, 360
Fluoride, 203-204
  effects of excess, 203
  estimated needs, 914
  in prevention of, bone loss, 630
    dental caries, 203
FMN, sturcture, 92
Folacin, 115-122
  absorption, 255
  antagonists, 121
  assay, 117
  biochemical function, 117
  and cell division, 602

chemistry, 116-117
and choline deficiency, 175
coenzymes, 117-119
deficiency symptoms, 83, 120
dietary intake and clinical evidences of
    deficiency, 879
excretion, 120
FAO standards, 929
guidelines for interpretation of blood
    levels, 951
metabolites, 120-121
minimum requirement, 880
and oral contraceptives, 120, 256
Recommended Dietary Allowance, 900,
    909
rate of absorption and length of side chain,
    255
structure, 116
Folic acid, site of methylation, 256
structure, 116
    see also Folacin
Folic acid reductase, 117
Folinic acid, 118
Food account, in dietary surveys, 937
Food and Nutrition Board, 899-900
Food composition, 11
Food composition tables, limitation in
    evaluating dietary intakes, 943
Food list, in dietary surveys, 938
Food plans, 898
Food record, in dietary surveys, 938
Formiminoglutamate (FIGLU), 120
N-formyl-L-kynurenine, 100
Formylmethylflavine, 94
N^5-Formyl THFA, 118-120
N^{10}-Formyl THFA, 118-119
Free radicals and vitamin E, 167-168
Fructose, 20
rate of absorption, 236
structure, 22
Fructose-6-phospahte, 457
Fructokinase, 236
Fumarate, 53

Galactoflavin, 95
Galactogens, 26
Galactose, 20
structure, 22
D-Galactosamine, 28
Gamma aminobutyric acid, 700

synthesis, 701
Gamma globulin, 67
absorption, 240
Gangliosides, 68
Gastric lipase, 221
Gastrin, 215-216, 223
Gaucher's disease, 69
Gelatinase, 223
Gene(s) activity, induction of, 415
regulatory, 412
Genetic code, 435
Genome, 398
Glial cells, 669
Gibbs-Donnan Equilibrium, 319
Globin synthesis, 611-613
Globulin(s), 59
Glucagon, 74
and regulation of blood glucose level, 574
Glucoascorbic acid, 139
Gluconeogenesis, in hepatocytes, 575-576,
    578
D-Glucosamine, 28
Glucose, 20
absorption and Na^+ requirement, 237
energy yield of oxidation, 524-525
homeostasis, 575
metabolic pathways, 456
regulation of blood level, 572-575
structure, 22
tolerance test and chromium, 207
Glucose-6-phosphatase, 237
Glucose-6-phosphate, 23, 457
α-Glucosidase, in lysosomal membrane, 535,
    537
Glutamic acid, 51, 53
Glutamic decarboxylase, 110
Glutamic-oxaloacetic transaminase, and
    vitamin B_6 intake, 892
Glutamic-pyruvate transaminase, and vitamin
    B_6 intake, 892
Glutathione, 53, 136
Glutathione peroxidase, 197, 205
Glutathione reductase in assessment of
    riboflavin status, 892
Glyceraldehyde, 20
Glyceraldehyde-3-phosphate, 457
Glyceraldehyde-3-phosphate dehydrogenase,
    97
Glyceric acid-1,3-diphosphate, 457
Glycerides, see Acyl glycerols

Glycerokinase, 246, 720
Glycerol, release from adipose cell, 720
  structure, 41
Glycerol ester hydrolase, 221
Glycerol phosphate, formation of, 716
Glycerolphosphate dehydrogenase, 97
Glycerophosphate, 246
  formation for glycerol and ATP, 247
Glycine, 53
  in creatine synthesis, 583
  structure, 50
Glycine oxidase, 93
Glycoaminoglycans, see Mucopoly-
    saccharides
Glycocalyx, see Cell coat
Glycogen, 26-27
  digestion, 226
  structure, 27
Glycogenesis, 465-467
Glycolipids, 31, 67, 69
Glycolysis, 456-461
  in muscle contraction, 662
Glyconic acids, structure, 24
Glycoprotein(s), 60, 62
  classification, 64
  composition, 65
  distribution, 67
  function, 67
  in mitochondria, 499
Goiter, 200
Goitrin, 200
Goitrogens, 200
Golgi apparatus, 350, 471-489
  and cell secretions, 480
  function(s), 477-488
  hormone synthesis in, 486-487
  lysosome formation, role in, 484
  membrane flow, role in, 477-479
  milk synthesis in, 487-488
  origin, 475-477
  phospholipid synthesis in, 485
  secretory cycle in, 482
  sturcture, 472-477
Guanine, 72, 75-76, 78-79
  structure, 73
Guanylic acid, 72
Ground substance, 424
  composition in bone, 622-623
  see also Cytoplasmic matrix
Growth and cell protein content, 736-737

comparison of species, 731
definition, 730
and DNA organ content, 735-737
effect of malnutrition in early life, 744-
    753
in assessment of nutritional status, 952-955
Growth hormone, and muscle cell size, 753

Haversian system in bone, 627
Heart disease and fat consumption
        patterns, 48
Heat of combustion, 851-852
Heat production, 6
  calculation from, oxygen consumption,
      847
    respiratory quotient, 845-847
  and surface area, 9
Hematocrit, guidelines for interpretation of
      blood levels, 950
Hematopoiesis, schematic model, 600
Heme, synthesis, 607
Hemicelluloses, 26
Hemoglobin(s), 60, 194
  blood levels, use in nutrition surveys, 948
  composition, 606
  digestion and absorption of iron from, 291
  embryonic, 611-612
  guidelines for interpretation of blood
      levels, 950
  mutant, 437
  sickle cell, 437
  synthesis and erythropoietin, 599
    and iron deficiency, 600
Hemosiderin, 60, 193, 284
Heparin, 28, 30
  in mast cells, 713
Hepatocrinin, 228
Hepatocyte(s), 570-593
  bile pigment formation in, 592-593
  cholesterol synthesis in, 587-592
  creatine synthesis in, 582-583
  and degradation of cholesterol, 587-592
  gluconeogenesis in, 575-576
  and ketone body formation, 577-578
  phosphatidic acid synthesis in, 586
  plasma lipids synthesis in, 585-587
  plasma lipoproteins synthesis in, 587
  plasma proteins synthesis in, 581-583
  and regulation of blood glucose level, 572-
      575

structure, 349, 571-572
triacyl glycerols synthesis in, 586-587
urea synthesis in, 583-585
Heterophagosomes, 44
 see also Lysosomes, secondary
Heteropolysaccharides, 26
Hexose monophosphate shunt, 461
 see also Pentose phosphate shunt
Hexoses, 22-24
Hexuronic acid, 135
Hiberative gland, 721
 see also Fat cell, brown
Histamine, 74
 in mast cells, 713
Histidine, structure, 51
 evidence for essentiality, 860
Histone(s), 60
 in cell nucleus, 414, 422
Homeostasis, 303
Homocystinuria, 110
Homogentisic acid, 137
Homopantothenic acid, 115
Homopolysaccharides, 26
Hormones, adrenocorticosteroids, 47
 gastrointestinal, 215-216, 225
 synthesis, 486-487
Hyaluronic acid, 28
Hydrochloric acid, in stomach, 226
3-Hydroxyanthranilate, 101
Hydroxyapatite, 182, 623
25-Hydroxycholecalciferol, 156, 158
 and bone resorption, 640
 vitamin D, transport form, 273
Hydroxycobalamin, 123
Hydroxyethylflavine, 93
3-Hydroxy-L-kynurenine, 100
Hydroxylation reactions
 and ascorbic acid, 137
 and iron, 194-195
Hydroxylysine, in collagen synthesis, 619
p-Hydroxyphenylpyruvic acid oxidase, 137
Hydroxyproline, 136
 formula, 51
 in collagen synthesis, 619
Hydroxyproline/creatinine index, use in
  nutrition surveys, 948
5-hydroxytryptamine, see Serotonin
Hypertension, 695
Hypervitaminosis A, effect on bone, 644
Hypervitaminosis D, 159-160, 643

Hypogeusia, 206
Hypoxanthine, 72
 structure, 73
H zone, in muscle, 647

Iduronic acid, 28-29
4-Imidazolidone-2-caproic acid, 134
Inosinic acid, 72
Inositides, 44
Myo-inositol, 44, 176-178
 absorption, 261-262
 biochemical function, 177
 deficiency, 177
 structure, 176
Insulin, action in obesity, 715
 and cAMP activity in adipose cells, 714-
  717
 effect on, muscle cell size, 753
  serotonin release, 705
 glucose transport into adipose cell, role in,
  714-717
 and regulation of blood glucose level, 572-
  575
Integrating motor pneumotachograph, 842
Intercalated disks, 653
Interstitial fluid, 316
Intracellular fluid, 316, 769
 percent of body weight, 770
Intrinsic factor (IF), 226
 binding of vitamin B_{12}, 257
 Ca^{2+} and vitamin B_{12} binding, 258
 chemistry, 256
 mechanism of action, 259
 secretion, 257
 and vitamin B_{12} absorption, 256-261
Iron, 192-195
 absorption, 284-296
  estimated in relation to dietary animal
   protein, 927
  factors affecting, 292
  from hemoglobin, 291
  radioisotope studies, 873
  regulation of, 285
 body content, 192, 795
 deficiency, 194
 and erythrocyte formation, 608-609
 forms in diet, 291
 functions, 194
 FAO standards, 928
 fat-free tissue content, 760

fortification of foods, 292
guidelines for interpretation of serum
  levels, 950
interconversion of ferrous and ferric iron,
  193
intestinal transport, regulation of, 286
losses in menses, 872
metabolism, 194
Recommended Dietary Allowance, 900,
  906-907
requirements, determination of, 871-873
  in pregnancy, 872
in serum, 192
storage, 193
  and ascorbic acid, 138
Iron-binding capacity, 193, 295
Inulin, 26
Iodine, 198-201
  body content, 198
  deficiency, 200
  function, 197, 199
  Recommended Dietary Allowance, 900,
    907
  and simple goiter, 200
  in thyroxine, 198
Iodopsin, 146
Isoleucine, 53
  formula, 50
Isomaltase, deficiency, 221
Isoniazid, structure, 111
Isotope dilution techniques, in calculation
  of body composition, 769-776
Isotropic bands, in muscle, 647
Isoxanthopterin, 121

Keratan sulfate, 28, 30
Keratin(s), 60
α-Ketoglutarate, 53, 86
Ketone bodies, 22
  as energy source for heart, 665
  formation in liver, 577-578
  oxidation, 579
Ketonemia, 580
Ketonuria, 580
Ketosis, 580
Kilocalorie, definition, 508
  in calorimetric studies, 823
Kilojoule, definition, 508
Krebs cycle, 514
  see also Tricarboxylic acid cycle

Kwashiorkor, 61
  clinical and biochemical lesions, 62
  and mucosal cell proliferation, 233
  see also Protein-calorie malnutrition
Kynureninase, 109-110
L-Kynurenine, 100

Lactase, 228
  activity and disaccharide intake, 218
  synthesis and milk intake, 219
Lactate, as energy source for heart, 665
Lactation, and body composition, 790
Lacteal(s), 234
Lactic dehydrogenase, 97, 460
Lactobacillus casei factor, 116
Lactogenesis, 487
Lactose in diet, 20
  intolerance, 218-221
    and genetic selection, 220
    and milk intake, 219-220
  structure, 25
  tolerance test, 220
Lauric acid, 34
  formula, 32
LDH, 460
  see also Lactic dehydrogenase
Lean body mass, 760, 771
  and age, 799-801
  definition, 765
  in pregnancy, 788
Lean body weight, calculation from body
  potassium, 776
Lecithins, 43, 174
Lecithinase, 222, 228
Leucine, 53
  formula, 50
Levulose, 20
  see also Fructose
Lignoceric acid, formula, 32
Linoleic acid, conversion to arachidonic
  acid, 36-37
  formula, 33
  significance, 34
Linolenic acid, 34, 36
  formula, 33
Lipase, 222, 227
Lipid(s), 31-48
  absorption, 244-252
  acyl glycerols, 41-43
  classification, 31

digestion, 221-223
fatty acids, 32-38
lipoproteins, 69-71
sphingolipids, 45-46
sphingomyelines, 45-46
phospholipids, 42-45
polyunsaturated fatty acids, 34-37
Lipid-globular protein mosaic, 360-361
Lipid peroxidation, 166-168
of plasma membrane, 364-368
and vitamin E, 367
Lipoic acid, 177-178
biochemical function, 178
in pyruvate oxidation, 512-514
structure, 177
Lipolysis, in adipose cell, 717-720
Lipolytic theory, 244
Lipoprotein lipase and adipose cell
metabolism, 713
and heparin, 30
in plasma, 183
Lipoproteins, 31, 60
classification, 70-71
composition of human serum, 70
synthesis in, intestinal mucosa, 248
Golgi apparatus, 485-486
Lipositols, 44
Lipoyl-L-lysine, 178
Lipoyl dehydrogenase, 93
Liver, 570
role in fatty acid synthesis, 712-713
see also Hepatocyte(s)
Load tests, 890
Luteinizing hormone, 74
Lysine, formula, 51
Lysosome(s), 350, 533-563
and bone resorption, 555-557
discharge of digestion products, 546
enzymes in, 535
structure-linked latency of, 538
exocytosis or defecation in, 547-548
formation, role of Golgi apparatus, 484
function of, 547-560
and hormone secretion, 551-555
identification, 533-535
and kidney function, 549-550
membrane and lysosomal function, 537-539
membrane stabilizers and labilizers, 540-542

effect of vitamin A, 540-541
effect of vitamin E, 541-542
effect of selenium, 542
organ content, 534
origin, 542-547
primary, 542-544
secondary, 544-545
storage granules, 543
structure, 535-537

Macula adherens, 369
Macrophage(s), 291, 550-551
Magnesium, 185-187
body content, 185, 795
in carboxylase system, 86
in cell nucleus, 401
deficiency, 186-187
functions, 186
fat-free tissue content, 760
Recommended Dietary Allowance, 900, 907
in serum, 185
Malic acid, energy yield, 853
Malnutrition, and behavior, 753-756
and cell growth, 746-753
effect on, brain growth, 751-752
muscle growth, 752-753
organ weight and DNA content, 747-749
placental growth, 750-751
and growth retardation, 744-753
and mental development, 753-756
Malonyl CoA, in fatty acid synthesis, 466-467
Manganese, 201-202
absorption, 297
biochemical role, 201
body content, 201
in carboxylase system, 86
deficiency, 201-202
estimated needs, 915
functions, 197
in mucopolysaccharide synthesis, 623
toxicity, 202
Maltase, 228
activity, 218
deficiency, 221
Maltose, 217
structure, 25
Mammary gland, weight gain during gestation, 787

Mannosans, 26

Mannose, 20

  structure, 22

Marasmus, clinical and biochemical lesions, 62

  see also Protein-calorie malnutrition

Mast cells, role in lipoprotein lipase action, 713

Matrix binding theory of lysosomes, 538-539

Mature hydration, definition of, 799

Medium chain fatty acids, absorption, 248

  see also Fatty acids, medium chain

Membrane, cell, see Plasma membrane

Membrane pores, 368

Membrane(s), selective permeability, 373-374

Menadione, structure, 169

Menaquinone, 169, 173

  structure, 170

Mental development, interaction of nutrition and environment, 755

  and malnutrition, 753-756

β-Mercaptoethylamine, 113

Metabolic antagonists, see Antimetabolites

Metabolism, resting, 8

Metachromatic leucodystrophy, 69

Metalloprotein(s), 60

Methemoglobin, 194

Metabolic body size, 830

Metabolic pools, definition, 310

Metabolism, basal, see Basal metabolism

  resting, see Resting metabolism

Methionine, formula, 50

  and choline deficiency, 175

4-Methoxypyridoxine, 111

β-Methyl crotonyl CoA carboxylase, 131

Methyl glyoxal, 87

Methylmalonyl-CoA, 125-127

  conversion to succinyl CoA, 127

Methylmalonyl-oxalacetic transcarboxylase, 132

N^1-Methylnicotinamide, 104-105

  excretion, use in nutrition surveys, 948

  structure, 105

N^1-Methylnicotinamide 2-pyridone, 104

N^1-Methylnicotinamide 6-pyridone, structure, 105

ω-Methyl pantothenic acid, 115

N^5-Methyl THFA, 127

$N^{5,10}$-Methylene THFA, 118-119

$N^{5,10}$-Methenyl THFA, 118-119

Methyl transferase, 125

Metrotrexate (MTX), see Amethopterin

Microbodies, 562-563

Microscopy, electron, 340

  freeze-etch electron, 340

  interference, 341

  phase contrast, 341

  scanning electron, 340

Milk, synthesis in Golgi apparatus, 487-488

Minerals, absorption, 277-297

  essential, 181

  deposition in bone, 623-625

  requirements, recognition of, 13-14

Minimum requirement, 876

  definition, 817

Mitochondria, 350, 490-531

  amino acid oxidation in, 519-523

  calcium transport in, 527-529

  cholesterol in, 502

  compartments, 503-504

  composition, 498-503

  contraction, 504-506

  DNA in, 392

  enzymes in, 500-502

  function, 506-529

  glycoprotein content, 499

  lipid content, 499

  location in cells, 492

  membrane shuttle systems, 518

  number in cells, 492

  origin, 529-530

  oxidation of fatty acids in, 509-512

  oxidation of pyruvic acid in, 512-515

  oxidative phosphorylation in, 523-525

  phospholipid composition of, 502

  protein synthesis in, 525-527

  swelling of, 505

  structure, 492-498

  tricarboxylic acid cycle in, 515-519

Molybdenum, 93, 202-203

  biochemical role, 202

  body content, 202

  estimated needs, 915

  functions, 197

  species difference in requirement, 202

  toxicity, 203

Monoacyl glycerol, structure, 41

Monoamine oxidase, 702
Monobromobenzene, 153
Monoglyceride, *see* Monoacyl glycerol
Monoglyceride lipase, 228
Monoiodotyrosine structure, 199
Monosaccharides, 20-22
  absorption, 235
  classification, 20
  definition, 20
Monosaccharide(s) derivatives, 23-24
Mortality rate of preschool children, index
    of malnutrition, 937
Mottled enamel and fluoride, 203
Mucopolysaccharide(s), 27-30, 67
  in bone formation, 617
  synthesis in bone, 622-623
    and vitamin A, 148-149
Mucoprotein(s), 60
Mucosal Block Theory, 285
Mucosal structure, and malabsorption
    syndromes, 233
Muscle mass, calculation from K_e and
    creatinine excretion, 773
Multiple sclerosis, 679
Muscle, cardiac, composition and structure
    cell growth in, 742-744
  cell number and age, 742
  cell size and sex differences, 743
  cells, 647-666
  contraction, 658-665, 825
    role of calcium, 661-662
    source of energy, 662-664
  effect of malnutrition, 752-753
  fatigue of, 663
  preferential amino acid catabolism in, 665
  skeletal, composition and structure, 653
  structure of, 647-658
Mutations, 405-408
  and repair synthesis, 408-411
Myasthenia gravis, 700
Myelin sheath, 670-671
  composition, 679
  formation of, 677-678
  lipid composition of, 679
Myofilaments, 647
Myoglobin, 192
Myosin, 647, 654-655
  composition, 654
  structure of, 655
Myristic acid, 34

formula, 32

NAD, *see* Nicotinamide adenine dinucleo-
  tide
NADP, *see* Nicotinamide adenine dinucleo-
  tide phosphate
Nerve cells, *see* Neuron(s)
Nerve impulse, conduction of, 683-692
Net dietary protein calories percent
    (NDpCal%), 866-867
Net protein utilization (NPU), 865
Neurin, 691
Neuroblastoma, 695
Neuroglia, 669
Neurofilaments, 675
Neuron(s), 669-707
  function of, 680-692
  membrane potential, 681-683
  organelles in, 673
  structure, 672-680
  synaptic transmission in, 689-692
Neuroplasm, 673
Neurostenin, 690-691
Neurotransmitters, 687, 692-706
Neurotubules, 675
Neutral fats, 31
Niacin, 95-106
  biochemical function, 97-104
  chemistry, 96-97
  coenzymes, 97-99
  deficiency symptoms, 83
  dietary intake and clinical evidences of
    deficiency, 878
  excretion, 104
  metabolites, 104-105
    urinary excretion and niacin intake, 883-
    884
  milligram equivalents, 103
  in pyruvate oxidation, 512-514
  Recommended Dietary Allowance, 900,
    909
  structure, 97
  synthesis from tryptophan, 99-103
Niacinogen, 105
Nickel, 207-208
Nicotinamide, 95
  structure, 97
  see also Niacin
Nicotinamide nucleotides, turnover,
  104

Nicotinamide adenine dinucleotide, 21, 97-99
  structure, 98
Nicotinamide adenine dinucleotide phosphate, 21, 97-99
  structure, 99
Nicotinate ribonucleotide, 102
Nicotinic acid, 53, 95
  structure, 97
  see also Niacin
Nicotinic acid mononucleotide, 99
Nicotinuric acid, structure, 105
Niemann-Pick disease, 45, 679
Night blindness, 146
Nissl bodies, 674
Nitritocobalamin, 123
Nitrogen, body content, 795
  endogenous losses, 855
  excretion, 331-332
  fat-free tissue content, 760
  maintenance requirement, 855
  metabolic fecal losses, 855
  nonessential, significance of, 861-862
Nitrogen balance, and body protein reserves, 857
  and determination of requirements, 856
  and energy intake, 858
  and essential amino acid intake, 858-860
  in growing animals, 737
  limitations of, 856-857
  and physiological state, 857
  in pregnancy, 788
  and total nitrogen intake, 858-860
Nitrogen balance index, 865
Nitrogen equilibrium, 16
Nodes of Ranvier, 671
Nonessential amino acid nitrogen, and nitrogen requirement, 861-862
Nonshivering thermogenesis, role of brown fat, 723-725
Norepinephrine, 137, 183, 553
  and cAMP, 325
  metabolism of, 697
  in nerve function, 692-698
  role in oxidation of brown fat, 723
  synthesis, 693
Normality, concept of, 305
Nuclear envelope, 393, 430-432
  see also Nucleus, membrane
Nuclear matrix, 400-402

Nuclear pores, 394
Nucleic acid(s), 71-79
  absorption, 251
Nucleolus, 349, 395-398
  components of, 398
Nucleoprotein(s), 60
Nucleosidase, 228
Nucleosides, 72
Nucleotidase, 228
Nucleotide(s), 71-75
Nucleus, 348, 391-422
  calcium in, 401
  determination of number and weight of, 734
  and formation of RNA, 412
  function, 402-422
  location in cell, 393
  magnesium in, 401
  membrane of, 393-395
  and oxidative phosphorylation, 401
  potassium in, 401
  RNA content, 412
  size and cell function, 393
  structure, 393-402
  weight, calculation of, 399
Nutrient exchange, 319-326
  and fluid movement, 320-326
  and ion distribution, 319
Nutrient intake, calculation of, 942-946
Nutrient metabolism, outline of, 819
Nutrient requirements, 816-932
  definition of, 817
  methodology for determination of, 817-819
  variability in, 309
Nutrients, renal conservation of, 330
  stores in the human body, 314
Nutrition, definition of, 1
Nutritional status, biochemical evaluation, 819, 947-949
  clinical evaluation, 819, 945-955
  information needed for assessment, 936
Nutrition surveys, 933-956
  clinical signs related to nutrition (WHO), 953-954
  correlation of dietary, biochemical, and clinical data, 955
  guide for interpretation of nutrient intake, 944-945
  guidelines for interpretation

of blood and urine data, 950-952

Obesity, adipose cell number and size in, 710
  body composition in, 806-810
  insulin response in, 715
Oleic acid, 36-37
  formula, 33
Oligodendrocytes, 669
Oligosaccharides, 23-25
Operon, 413
  programmed derepression of, 414
Operon-regulator gene hypothesis, 414
Opsin, 146
Ornithine, formula, 52
  in urea synthesis, 584
Osmoreceptors, 327
Osteoblasts, 617
Osteoclast-activating factor, 630
Osteoclasts, 555
Osteocytes, 617
Osteogenic cells, 617
Osteomalacia, 645
Osteon, 627
  see also Haversian system
Osteoporosis, and dietary calcium to phosphorus ratio, 185
  and fluoride intake, 630
Ovalbumin, 67
Oxaloacetate, 53
  in tricarboxylic acid cycle, 515-518
Oxidative decarboxylation, 86
Oxidative phosphorylation, 509, 521-524
  energy yield of, 523-525
Oxygen debt after exercise, 663-664
Oxythiamin, 89
  and thiamin absorption, 253

Palmitic acid, formula, 32
Palmitoleic acid, 36
  formula, 33
Pancreas, exocrine secretion, 227
  digestive enzymes, 224
Pancreatic hydrolase, 263
Pancreatic lipase, 183
Pancreozymin, 215-216
Panthenol, 115
Pantotheine, 114
Pantothenic acid, 112-115
  antagonists, 115

assay, 113
  biochemical function, 113-114
  chemistry, 113
  estimated needs, 915
  excretion, 115
  in pyruvate oxidation, 512-514
  metabolites, 115
  structure, 113
Pantoic acid, 113
Pantothenamides, 115
Paracasein, 223
Parakeratosis, 206
Parathyroid hormone, and calcium absorption, 283-284
  and cAMP, 74
  cAMP and calcium absorption, 284
  effect on bone, 631-636
  interrelationship with thyrocalcitonin and vitamin D, 642
  and plasma free calcium concentration, 528
  structure of, 632
  and vitamin D, 158
Particulate theory, 244
Pellagra, 95-96
  and maize diets, 105-106
Pentosans, 26
Pentose phosphate shunt, 86, 461-465
Pentoses, 21-22
Peptide linkages, 49
  formation of, 448
Peptidyl transferase factors, 446
Pepsinogens, conversion to pepsin, 223
Perikaryon, 670, 672-677
Periodontal disease and dietary calcium to phosphorus ratio, 185
Peroxisomes, see Microbodies
Phagocytes, 550-551
Phagocytosis, 382-383
Phenylalanine, 53
  formula, 50
Phlogiston theory of combustion, 4
Phosphatidic acids, 31
  structure, 42
  synthesis, 586
Phosphatidyl choline, 43
  energy requirement for synthesis, 824
Phosphatidyl ethanolamine, 43
Phosphatidyl inositol, 44
Phosphatidyl serine, 43

Phosphogluconate pathway, 461
  see also Pentose phosphate shunt
Phospholipase A, 183, 227
Phospholipids, 31, 42-45
  classification, 43
Phosphoprotein(s), 60
Phosphorus, 184-185
  in blood, 184
  body content, 184, 795
  deficiency in animals, 184
  fat-free tissue content, 760
  functions, 184
  in cell nucleolus, 401-402
  Recommended Dietary Allowance, 900,
    905-906
Phosphorylase kinase, 183
Phylloquinone, 169, 173
  structure, 170
Physical activity, and body composition,
    810-813
Phytates, and calcium absorption, 177
  and iron absorption, 293
Phytosterols, absorption, 250
Pinocytosis, 382-383
  and gamma globulin absorption in the
    newborn, 240
  in lysosomes, 547
Placenta, cellular growth pattern, 738
  composition of, 785
  effects of malnutrition, 750-751
  weight gain in, 785
Plasma, as transport medium, 304-305
Plasma amino acids and amino acid
    requirements, 862
Plasma constituents, 306-307
  constancy of, 315
  renal control of, 326
Plasma lipid, synthesis of, 585-587
Plasma lipoprotein(s), synthesis of, 587
Plasmalogens, 31, 44
Plasma membrane, 348, 352-390
  function, 386
  integrity, 364
  models, 360
  role of, 353-354
  structure, 354-371
Plasma pH, regulation of, 332
Plasma protein(s), synthesis, 581-583
PLP, *see* Pyridoxal phosphate
Polypeptide(s) digestion, 224

synthesis, 446-456
Polysaccharides, 26-27, 216
Polyunsaturated fatty acids, biosynthesis,
    35-36
  ratio to saturated acids (PUFA:UFA), 48
  and vitamin E deficiency, 164
Pools, metabolic, 310
Potassium, body content, 190, 795
    and age, 801
    and body weight, 775-778
    in pregnancy, 788
    and sex, 801
  concentration in cell water, 771
  content of human fetus, 784
  depletion, 190-191
  estimated needs, 914
  fat-free body content, 760
  functions, 190
  isotope (^{40}K) in calculation of body fat,
    774-776
  in neuron function, 681-683, 685
  in serum, 190
  therapy, 191
  total exchangeable, 771-773
Pregnancy, and basal heat production, 833
  and changes in body composition, 787-
    790
  metabolic alterations in, 791
  nutritional requirements of, 790
  physiological adaptations in, 791
  recommended allowances, 792
  sodium intake in, 791
  weight gain in, 785-786
Pregnenolone, 47
Premature infant, effect of diet on body
    composition, 784-785
Procarboxypeptidase, 224, 227
Proerythroblast, and erythrocyte formation,
    602
Progesterone, 47
Proinsulin, structure, 55
Proline, structure, 51
  hydroxylation of, 136
Propionyl-CoA carboxylase, 132
Prostaglandins, 38-40, 74
Prosthetic group, definition, 81
Protein(s), 49-62
  as source of nitrogen, 16
  calculation of cell content, 734
  cellular turnover, 450

classification, 59-61
conformation, 58
contractile, 656
chromosomal, 400
deficiency, 61
determination of requirement, 854-863
dietary standards for pregnant and
    nonpregnant women, 931
endogenous and digestive secretions, 238
digestion, 223-234
extrinsic in plasma membrane, 361
fibrous, 56
FAO standards, 922-926
functions, 53
globular, 56
intake and calcium retention, 868-871
intrinsic in plasma membrane, 361
isomerism, 49
maintenance requirement, 854-855
organ content during growth, 735-736
Recommended Dietary Allowance, 900,
    904-905
repressor, 412
reserves, 311
serum, use in nutrition surveys, 948
    guidelines for interpretation of levels in,
    951
structure, 49, 54-59
    hydrogen bonding, 56
    pleated sheet, 57
    secondary bonding, 56
    tertiary structure, 57
    quaternary structure, 59
synthesis, 434-456
    in mitochondria, 525-527
    in ribosomes, 443-456
    regulation of, 450-451 ·
    repression of, 451-456
    time factor in, 439
Protein-calorie malnutrition, 61
    and albumin synthesis, 582
    and brain cell number and size, 752
    and digestive enzyme deficiency, 218
    and mucosal cell proliferation, 233
    techniques for assessing, 948
Protein efficiency ratio (PER), 864-865
Protein quality, methods of evaluation,
    863-868
Protein X and vitamin K, 172
Proteolipid(s), 60

Prothrombin, 67, 170
    biosynthesis and vitamin K, 172
Protoporphyrin, 194
    synthesis, 606
Provitamin A, 142
Pteroylglutamic acid, see Folacin
Purines, 71-72
    biosynthesis and THFA, 118
    structure, 73
Pyridine nucleotide cycle, 104
Pyridine-3-sulphonamide, 105
Pyridoxal, 111
    and amino acid absorption, 244
    structure, 106
    see also Vitamin B$_6$
Pyridoxal kinase, 111
Pyridoxal phosphate, 107
    structure, 108
Pyridoxamine, 111
    structure, 107
    see also Vitamin B$_6$
Pyridoxamine phosphate, 111
Pyridoxic acid, 107, 111
    structure, 110
Pyridoxine, 111
    absorption, 255
    deficiency symptoms, 83
    structure, 106
    see also Vitamin B$_6$
Pyrimidines, 71-72
    biosynthesis and THFA, 118
    structure, 73
Pyrithiamine, 89
    and thiamin absorption, 253
Pyrophosphatase, inorganic, 186
Pyruvate carboxylase, 132, 201
Pyruvate dehydrogenase and thiamin
    deficiency, 87
Pyruvate phosphokinase, 186
Pyruvic acid, 53, 86
    oxidation in mitochondria, 512-515
        energy yield via the TCA cycle, 524

Quinolinate ribonucleotide, 102
Quinolinic acid, 99, 101

Radioautography, 341
Raffinose, 26
Receptor membranes, 386
Recommended Dietary Allowances, 899-913

Releasing factor and vitamin B_{12}
     absorption, 260
Renal erythropoeitic factor, 598
Renin-angiotensin system, 329
Rennin, 223
Repressor-corepressor complex, 452
Repressor-inducer complex, 414
Residual body, in lysosomes, 545
Reticulocytes and erythrocyte formation,
     602, 604
Respiratory exchange, 8
Respiratory quotient, 7, 844-845
   and calculation of heat production, 845-
     847
Resting metabolism, definition of, 825
Retinaldehyde, 141-142, 146
   absorption, 264
   formation from carotene cleavage, 262
   see also Vitamin A
Retinoic acid, 141-142, 146
   absorption, 264
   metabolic pathways, 151
   see also Vitamin A
Retinol, 141-150
   transport, 264
   see also Vitamin A
Retinol-binding protein (RBP), 264-265
Retinol equivalent, calculation from pro-
     vitamin A, 911
Retinyl acetate, metabolic pathways, 151
Retinyl esters, 142
   in food, 263
Retinyl ester hydrolase, 263
Retinyl-β-glucuronide, 150
Retinyl ester hydrolase, 227
Rhodopsin, 141, 146-147
Ribitol, 21
Riboflavin, 90-95
   absorption, 254
   antagonists, 95
   assay, 91-92
   biochemical functions, 92-94
   chemistry, 91
   correlation of dietary intake and
     deficiency symptoms, 882
   coenzymes, 92
   deficiency symptoms, 83
   dietary intake and clinical evidences of
     deficiency, 878
   and plasma levels, 885

excretion, 94
   use in nutrition surveys, 948
   guidelines for interpretation of urinary
     levels, 952
   metabolites, 94-95
   in pyruvate oxidation, 512-514
   Recommended Dietary Allowance, 900,
     908-909
   structure, 91
   urinary excretion and deficiency
     symptoms, 882-883
Ribonuclease, 227
Ribose, 20-21, 79
Ribosomes, 349
   protein synthesis, role in, 443-446
Ribulose, 20
RNA, 21, 75, 79
   amount in nucleus, 412
   and chromosome puffs, 420-421
   calculation of cell content, 734
   classes of, 420
   messenger, 79, 420
     and polysomes, 445
     and protein synthesis, 446-451
     in mitochondria, 527
     synthesis, induction of by structural
       genes, 414
   ribosomal, 79, 420
     and protein synthesis, 446-451
     precursor in nucleus, 398
   synthesis, 416-421
   structure, 78-79
   transfer, 420, 440
     and the adaptor hypothesis, 440
     and protein synthesis, 446-451
     structure, 442
RNA-amino acid code, 436
RNA-directed DNA polymerase, 421
RNA/DNA ratio in rat organs, 738
RNA polymerase, 416-417

Saltatory conduction, 683, 685-686
Saturated fatty acids, melting point, 41
   naturally occurring, 32
Sarcomere, 647
Sarcoplasm, 647
Sarcoplasmic reticulum, 649
Schwann cells, 669
Scurvy, 14-15, 134
   and bone metabolism, 644

Secretion, 215-216, 227
Secretory cycle, in Golgi apparatus, 482
Sedoheptulose, 20
Sedoheptulose-7-phosphate, 463
Selenium, 204-205
 biochemical role, 205
 essentiality, 205
 estimated needs, 915
 functions, 197
 toxicity, 205
 and vitamin E metabolism, 204
 and vitamin E in lysosomal membrane
  stabilization, 542-543
 and vitamin E deficiency, 164
Serine, 43
 formula, 50
Serotonin, 53, 74, 183
 biosynthesis of, 703
 catabolism, 704
 diurnal fluctuations in plasma and brain
  concentrations, 702
 effect of, diet on brain concentration,
  705-706
  insulin on release of, 705
 in nerve function, 701-706
Sialic acid, 63
Sialidase, in lysosomal membrane, 535, 537
Silicon, 207-208
Skinfold thickness, 762-765
 and age, 795-796
 correlation with body density, 798
 correlation with X-ray measurements, 764
 in obese children, 808
 sex differences in, 795-796
 standardization of measurements, 763-764
Slope-ratio assay for determination of
  protein quality, 867
Small intestine, epithelial cell structure, 230
 mucosal structure, 230
 rate of cell renewal, 232
Sodium, 187-189
 balance and role of angiotensin, 330
 body content, 188, 795
 in bone, 188
 content of human fetus, 784
 depletion, 188
 dietary intake, 187
 estimated needs, 914
 fat-free tissue content, 760
 in neuron function, 681-683, 685

 in serum, 188
 metabolic regulation, 188
 requirement, 187
  in pregnancy, 189
Sodium benzoate and vitamin A, 153
Sodium pump, 237, 379-380
 in neuron function, 685
Sorbose, 20
Specific dynamic action (SDA) of food,
  see Calorigenic effect of food
Specific dynamic effect of food, 6-7
 see also Calorigenic effect of food
Specific gravity, and determination of body
  fat, 765
 calculation of, body fat, 768
  body water, 768
 conversion to body fat, 767
 prediction from skinfold thickness, 768
4-Sphingenine, 45, 68-69
Sphingolipids, 45-46
 in myelin sheat, 679
Sphingomyelins, 31, 45-46
Sphingomyelinase, 45
Sphingosine, 68
 see also 4-Sphingenine
Starch, in diet, 19
 digestion, 226
Starvation, and RNA synthesis, 412
Stearic acid, formula, 32
Steatorrhea, 222
Stenin, 691
Sterols, 46-48
Steroids, 46-48
[90]Strontium and calcium, 183-184
Stem cells, in bone, 617
 and cell differentiation, 567
 pluripotential, 595
Substrate level phosphorylations, 457, 460
Succinic dehydrogenase, 93, 193
Succinate, 53
Succinyl CoA, 86
 reaction with malonyl CoA, 127
Sucrase, 228
 activity and disaccharide intake, 218
 deficiency, 221
Sucrose, in diet, 19-20
 structure, 25
Sugar alcohols, structure, 24
Sulfur, 191-192
 in bile acids, 192

in mucopolysaccharides, 192
in oxidation-reduction reactions, 191
Sulfur amino acids and vitamin E deficiency, 164
Syncytium, 393
Synapse, 671, 686-687
Synaptic transmission, 683, 686-692
Synaptic vesicles, 687

Taurine, 53
Telolysosomes, in lysosomal development, 544-545
Ten State Nutrition Survey, 946
Testosterone, 47
Tetrahydrofolic acid (THFA), 117
Tetranorbiotin, 134
Thiamin, 84-90
   absorption, 252-253
      in alcoholics, 253
   antagonists, 89
   assay, 85
   biochemical function, 85-88
   coenzymes, 86
   chemistry, 85
   deficiency, 83, 87
      and transketolase test, 891-892
   dietary intake and clinical evidences of deficiency, 878
   and urinary excretion, 883
   and plasma levels, 885
   excretion, 88
      use in nutrition surveys, 948
   guidelines for interpretation of urinary levels, 951
   metabolites, 88-90
   in pyruvate oxidation, 512-514
   Recommended Dietary Allowance, 900, 908
   structure, 85
Thiaminase, 89-90
Thiamin hydrochloride, 85
Thiamin monophosphate, 86
Thiamin pyrophosphate (TPP) structure, 86
Thiamin triphosphate, 86
Thirst regulation, 329
Threonine, 17
   formula, 50
Threose, 20
Thrombin, 171
Thymidylic acid, 72

Thymine, 72, 75-76, 79
   structure, 73
Thyrocalcitonin, 74, 636-639
   amino acid sequence of, 637
   interrelationships with parathyroid hormone and vitamin D, 642
   structure, 636
Thyroglobulin, 67, 198
   and thyroxine binding, 551
Thyroid-stimulating hormone, 199
Thyroxine, 53, 197
   binding with prealbumin, 265
   in biosynthesis of FMN and FAD, 93-94
   function, 199
   secretion of, 551-553
   structure, 199
Tin, 207-208
Tissue culture, 344
α-Tocopherol, structure, 161
Tocopherols, 161
   see also Vitamin E
α-Tocopherol-p-quinone, 168
α-Tocopheronic acid, 168
Totipotent germ cells and cell differentiation, 567
Toxopyrimidine, 111
Trace elements, 181, 195-208
   functions, 197
Transamination, 519-521
   vitamin B_6, role in, 108
Transcorrin, 261
Transcription, reverse, 421
Transferrin, 60, 67, 192
   chemistry of, 295
   guidelines for interpretation of serum levels, 950
   in human plasma, 295
   and iron transport, 285
   site of synthesis, 295
Transfer vesicles, 474
Transketolase, 86
   activity and thiamin deficiency, 87
   in pentose phosphate shunt, 463-464
Transport, 303-307, 374
   active, 377-382
      and ATP, 379
      and Na$^+$, 379
   in amino acid absorption, 241
   sodium-dependent system, 238
   structural requirements of sugars, 235

of amino acids, 382
bulk, 382
of cations, 381
coupled, 382
of glucose, 382
noncoupled, 382
passive, 374-377
Triacyl glycerols, 41-43
end products of digestion, 222
hydrolysis in adipose cell, 718-720
in mucosal cell, 246
structure, 41
synthesis of, 586-587, 717-719
in mucosal cell, 248
Tributyrase, 221
Tricarboxylic acid cycle, 514-519
Triceps fatfold measurements, 795-796
Triglycerides, see Triacyl glycerols
1,24,25-Trihydroxycholecalciferol, 158
Triiodothyronine, 551-553
structure, 199
Tromexan, 173
Tropomyosin, 657
Troponin, 658
Tryptophan, 17, 53, 100, 137
conversion, to NAD, 103
to niacin, 99-103
formula, 51
metabolism and vitamin B_6 deficiency,
109
and serotonin synthesis, 702-703
Trypsin, 227
Trypsinogen, 224, 227
T-system in muscle, 649
Tubulin, 675
Tyrosine, 53
formula, 50
Tyrosinase, 197
Tyrosine hydroxylase, 694

Ubiquinone, 178-179
biochemical function, 179
in clinical medicine, 179
deficiency, 179
structure, 178
Ultracentrifugation, 343
Ultramicroincineration, low temperature,
341
Unit membrane, development of concept,
355-360

Unsaturated fatty acids, and vitamin B_6,
109
interconversions, 35
naturally occurring, 33
synthesis of, 467-470
Unsaturated iron binding capacity (UIBC),
295
Uracil, 72, 78-79
structure, 73
Urea nitrogen/creatinine ratio, use in
nutrition surveys, 948
Urea, synthesis in hepatocytes, 583-585
Uridine diphosphate glucose, 465
Uridylic acid, 72
Urinary excretion, in assessing vitamin
requirements, 881-885
Uronic acids, structure, 24
Ureylenecyclohexylvaleric acid, 134
Uterus, weight gain during gestation, 787

Valine, formula, 50
intestinal transport, 241
Vanadium, 207-208
Vasopressin, 74
Wills factor, 115
Vitamin H, 129
Vitamin M, 115
Vitamin A, 15, 141-153
absorption, 262-271
and protein deficiency, 269-271
and vitamin E nutriture, 268-269
antagonists, 153
biochemical function, 145-150
blood levels, and deficiency symptoms,
889
use in nutrition surveys, 948
chemistry, 142-145
deficiency, 83, 148-150
effect on bone, 644
dietary intake and blood levels, 888
and clinical evidence of deficiency, 879
FAO standards, 929
guidelines for interpretation of plasma
levels, 951
interrelationship between various forms,
147
lysosomal membrane labilization, role in,
540-541
metabolites, 150-151
nutritional status and release

of retinol-binding protein from liver, 265-267
physiological functions, 145-146
plasma levels in protein-calorie malnutrition, 269-271
provitamins, 142
Recommended Dietary Allowance, 900, 911-912
requirement to cure deficiency symptoms, 880-881
structure, 141
toxicity, 152-153
visual cycle, role in, 147
Vitamin A$_2$, 142
Vitamin B$_6$, 106-112
antagonists, 111
assay, 107
biochemical function, 107-110
chemistry, 107
coenzymes, 107
deficiency, 106, 178
dietary intake and clinical deficiency, 878
and excretion of 4-pyridoxic acid, 883
and urinary excretion, 884
and essential fatty acid metabolism, 109
excretion, 110
and genetic diseases, 109-110
and marijuana, 112
metabolites, 110-111
and oral contraceptives, 112
Recommended Dietary Allowance, 900, 909-910
Vitamin B$_{12}$, 122-129
absorption, 226, 256-261
antagonists, 129
assay, 124-125
biochemical function, 125-128
and cell division, 602
chemical synthesis, elucidation of, 124
chemistry, 122-123
and choline deficiency, 175
cobalt in, 197
coenzymes, 125-126
deficiency, 83, 127
dietary intake and clinical deficiency, 879
excretion, 129
FAO standards, 929
and folacin metabolism, 118, 127-128
forms of the vitamin, 123
metabolites, 128-129

minimum requirement, 880
Recommended Dietary Allowance, 900, 910-911
ribonucleotide synthesis, role in, 128
structure, 123
Vitamin D, 154-160, 528
absorption, 271-274
and bile salts, 272
active form, 156
assay, 155
biochemical function, 155-158
and calcium absorption, 156
and calcium mobilization from bone, 156
chemistry, 154-155
distribution in tissues, 158
deficiency and bone maturation, 623
effect on, bone, 639-643
collagen metabolism, 641
collagen synthesis, 622
FAO standards, 929
interrelationships with parathyroid hormone and thyrocalcitonin, 642
and intestinal transport of phosphate, 282
metabolites, 158-159
and parathyroid hormone, 158
Recommended Dietary Allowance, 900, 912
toxicity, 159-160, 643
transport in blood, 273
Vitamin D$_2$, structure, 155
Vitamin D$_3$, structure, 155
Vitamines, 15
Vitamin E, 160-169
absorption, 274-275
bile, role in, 274
assay, 161-163
biochemical function, 163-167
chemistry, 161
in chylomicra, 274
deficiency, 164, 166
and anemia, 607
and collagen cross-linking, 622
and muscular dystrophy, 560-562
and unsaturation of mitochondrial membrane fatty acids, 499
dietary intake and blood levels, 889
and clinical deficiency, 879
and erythrocyte hemolysis, 893
and intestinal transport of valine, 241
lysosomal membrane, role in

stabilization of, 541-542
metabolites, 168
naturally occurring forms, 162
and polyunsaturated fatty acids, 166
Recommended Dietary Allowance, 900, 912
and selenium in lysosomal membrane stabilization, 542
toxicity, 168-169
Vitamin K, 169-173
absorption, 275-276
antagonists, 173
assay, 170
biochemical function, 170-173
chemistry, 169-170
estimated needs, 915
intestinal synthesis, 275, 300-301
metabolite, 172-173
naturally occurring forms, 169
structures, 169-170
Vitamin(s), accessory food factors, 15
blood levels in assessing requirements, 885-889
following a test dose of vitamin, 889
clinical evaluation of deficiency, 877-881
deficiency symptoms in man, 83
enzyme activity in assessing requirements, 891-893
intestinal synthesis, 300-301
methods for assessing requirements, 874-894
sequence in development of deficiency, 875
techniques to evaluate response to diet, 875
tissue saturation of, 876
urinary excretion and nutritional status, 881-885
following a test dose, 889-890
Vitamin theory, development of, 14

Warfarin, 171
Water, 208-210
absorption, 276
balance, 209, 327-330
and role of angiotensin, 330
body content, 209, 759, 795
body distribution, 328
conservation, 327
endogenous secretion, 276
estimated needs, 914
extracellular, 769
fat-free tissue content, 760
functions, 209
effects of body depletion, 209-210
gastrointestinal circulation, 276
in regulation of body temperature, 209
intracellular, 769
metabolic, 208
of oxidation, 208
Water-soluble vitamins, 80-139
absorption, 252-262
Waxes, 31
Weighed intake, 938
Wilson's disease, 198
Wobble hypothesis, 443

Xanthine oxidase, 93, 193, 197
and molybdenum, 202
Xanthurenic acid, excretion in vitamin B_6 deficiency, 892
Xanthurenic aciduria, 110
Xanthopterin, 121
X-disease (bovine hyperkeratosis), 153
Xerophthalmia, 141
X-ray diffraction, 343
Xylose, 20-21
Xylulose, 20

Zinc, 206-207
antagonism to copper absorption, 296
biochemical role, 206
body content, 206, 795
deficiency, 206
fat-free tissue content, 760
functions, 197
metabolism in disease states, 207
and mucopolysaccharide synthesis, 623
in plasma, 297
Recommended Dietary Allowance, 900, 907
Z line in muscle, 647
Zona adherens, 369, 385
Zona occludens, 369
Zymogen granules, 473-474
Zymogens, 224